ACE® MEDICAL EXERCISE SPECIALIST MANUAL

THE DEFINITIVE RESOURCE FOR HEALTH AND EXERCISE PROFESSIONALS WORKING WITH SPECIAL POPULATIONS

AMERICAN COUNCIL ON EXERCISE®

EDITORS
JAMES S. SKINNER, PH.D., FACSM
CEDRIC X. BRYANT, PH.D., FACSM
SABRENA JO, M.S.
DANIEL J. GREEN

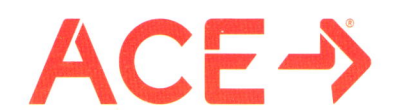

Library of Congress Catalog Card Number: 2015932186

ISBN 9781890720865

Copyright © 2021, 2015 American Council on Exercise (ACE)

Printed in the United States of America

All rights reserved. Except for use in a review, the reproduction or utilization of this work in any form or by any electronic, mechanical, or other means, now known or hereafter invented, including xerography, photocopying, and recording, and in any information retrieval system, is forbidden without the written permission of the American Council on Exercise.

ACE, ACE IFT, ACE Integrated Fitness Training, and American Council on Exercise are registered trademarks of the American Council on Exercise. Other product names used herein are for identification purpose only and may be trademarks of their respective companies.

C D E F

Distributed by:
American Council on Exercise
4851 Paramount Drive
San Diego, CA 92123
(858) 576-6500
(858) 576-6564 FAX
ACEfitness.org

Project Editor: Daniel J. Green

Technical Editors: James S. Skinner, Ph.D., FACSM, Cedric X. Bryant, Ph.D., FACSM, & Sabrena Jo, M.S.

Creative Direction: Ian Jensen

Art Direction & Cover Design: Karen McGuire

Internal Reviewers: Chris Gagliardi, B.S., & Belinda Thompson, B.S.

Production: Nancy Garcia

Photography: Dennis Covey, Rob Andrew, & Matt Gossman

Anatomical Illustrations: James Staunton

Index: Kathi Unger

Exercise models: Beth Baxter, Dana Cobb, Kris Fukuda, Tamra Herb, Aliya Lawson, Monika Lucs, Michael Marsh, Anthony Padilla, Jenn Samore, Jay Simon, Danielle Vojta, Renee West, & Richard Zuniga

Acknowledgments:
Thanks to the entire American Council on Exercise staff for their support and guidance through the process of creating this manual.

A special thanks to Rehab United for allowing us to photograph on location at their Sorrento Valley facility.

NOTICE

The fitness industry is ever-changing. As new research and clinical experience broaden our knowledge, changes in programming and standards are required. The authors and the publisher of this work have checked with sources believed to be reliable in their efforts to provide information that is complete and generally in accord with the standards accepted at the time of publication. However, in view of the possibility of human error or changes in industry standards, neither the authors nor the publisher nor any other party who has been involved in the preparation or publication of this work warrants that the information contained herein is in every respect accurate or complete, and they are not responsible for any errors or omissions or the results obtained from the use of such information. Readers are encouraged to confirm the information contained herein with other sources.

DISCLAIMER

Moving forward, ACE will use "they" and "their" in place of "he/she" and "his/her." This change eliminates gender biases associated with these pronouns and is more inclusive of all individuals across the gender spectrum. Note that all ACE content moving forward will reflect this update, and previous content will be updated as needed. It is ACE's goal to share our mission to Get People Moving with all people, regardless of race, gender, sexual orientation, physical or intellectual abilities, religious beliefs, ethnic background, or socioeconomic status.

MISSION

Get People Moving.

P21-007

TABLE OF CONTENTS

FOREWORD vii
INTRODUCTION ix
STUDYING FOR THE ACE MEDICAL EXERCISE SPECIALIST EXAM xi

PART I: INTRODUCTION
CHAPTER 1 Role and Scope of Practice for the Certified Medical Exercise Specialist   *Kelly Spivey* 2
CHAPTER 2 Applying the ACE Integrated Fitness Training® Model in the Medical Exercise Setting   *Todd Galati* .. 20
CHAPTER 3 Working With Clients With Health Challenges   *Nancey Trevanian Tsai* 56

PART II: LEADERSHIP AND IMPLEMENTATION
CHAPTER 4 Behavioral Change   *Tracie Rogers* 94
CHAPTER 5 Communication Strategies   *Barbara A. Brehm* 118
CHAPTER 6 Professional Relationships and Business Strategies   *Lisa Coors* 142

PART III: MAJOR CARDIOVASCULAR AND PULMONARY DISEASES AND DISORDERS
CHAPTER 7 Coronary Heart Disease   *Ralph La Forge* 168
CHAPTER 8 Blood Lipid Disorders   *Ralph La Forge* 208
CHAPTER 9 Hypertension   *W. Larry Kenney & Lacy M. Alexander* 244
CHAPTER 10 Pulmonary Disease: Asthma and Chronic Obstructive Pulmonary Disease   *Natalie Digate Muth* 276

PART IV: METABOLIC DISEASES AND DISORDERS
CHAPTER 11 Overweight and Obesity   *Len Kravitz* 314
CHAPTER 12 The Metabolic Syndrome   *Barry A. Franklin, Wendy M. Miller, & Peter A. McCullough* 344
CHAPTER 13 Diabetes Mellitus   *Larry S. Verity* 362

PART V: MUSCULOSKELETAL DISORDERS
CHAPTER 14 Posture and Movement   *Fabio Comana & Chris McGrath* 404
CHAPTER 15 Balance and Gait   *Michol Dalcourt & Fabio Comana* 478
CHAPTER 16 Arthritis   *John G. Aronen & Kent A. Lorenz* 526
CHAPTER 17 Osteoporosis and Osteopenia   *Kara A. Witzke* 556
CHAPTER 18 Musculoskeletal Injuries of the Lower Extremity   *Scott Cheatham* 586
CHAPTER 19 Musculoskeletal Injuries of the Upper Extremity   *Michael Levinson* 632
CHAPTER 20 Low back Pain   *Jennifer Solomon* 660

PART VI: PERINATAL CONSIDERATIONS
CHAPTER 21 Prenatal and Postpartum Exercise   *Sabrena Jo* 684

APPENDIX A ACE Code of Ethics 728
APPENDIX B Exam Content Outline 734
APPENDIX C Nutrition for Health and Fitness   *Natalie Digate Muth* 744

GLOSSARY 784
INDEX 816

FOREWORD

THE BENEFITS OF PHYSICAL ACTIVITY AND PROPER NUTRITION—AND THE negative consequences of a sedentary lifestyle and poor eating habits—are widely accepted and supported by research. While many fitness texts, including *The Exercise Professional's Guide to Personal Training*, focus on working with clients who are "apparently healthy," the benefits of activity and nutrition extend to individuals at risk for, and living with, many common diseases and disorders.

ACE developed the Medical Exercise Specialist certification to enable exercise professionals to collaborate with the healthcare community to support their clients' health and fitness goals. Whether your career objective is to work with youth in order to combat the epidemic of childhood obesity, to empower older clients to take control of their health and wellness as they navigate one or more chronic conditions, or anything in between, this manual will enable you to home in on the specific clients you want to serve and then do so from a strong foundation of evidence-based practice.

The sad truth is that healthcare in America is still focused on disease treatment rather than disease prevention, and therefore has not yet made the paradigm shift needed to modify personal behaviors in a way that affects overall health and well-being. It is becoming increasingly clear that qualified fitness professionals, particularly the CMES, are an essential element of the healthcare continuum and are perfectly positioned to serve in the quest not only for disease management, but disease prevention as well. Inactivity, obesity, and poor nutrition are the foundational elements of many disease states, including many of those covered in this manual, and are all elements that a CMES can directly impact through behavior modification and lifestyle change.

The mission of this manual is twofold: to serve (1) as your core study material while preparing for the ACE Medical Exercise Specialist Certification exam and (2) as a trusted resource throughout your career. Make good use of this textbook and everything else ACE has to offer and you will be well on your way to a promising and rewarding career in fitness and/or allied health. I wish you the best as you pursue your passion, expand your knowledge base, and work to better serve your at-risk clients.

SCOTT GOUDESEUNE
CHIEF EXECUTIVE OFFICER

INTRODUCTION

THE AMERICAN COUNCIL ON EXERCISE IS PROUD TO INTRODUCE THE
ACE Medical Exercise Specialist Manual and its associated certification program. As stated in Chapter 1 of this text, the ACE Medical Exercise Specialist certification was developed to enable fitness professionals to collaborate with the healthcare community to support their clients' health and fitness goals.

The launch of this program is perfectly timed to take advantage of the opportunities offered by the U.S. Affordable Care Act (ACA), landmark legislation with a primary focus on preventive care. Health and preventive services are now a national priority and the ACE Certified Medical Exercise Specialist (CMES) should play an integral role in promoting healthy behaviors.

PART I: INTRODUCTION begins by explaining the role and scope of practice for the CMES, including the CMES's role in the healthcare continuum and the standards of care. Chapter 2 discusses how to apply the ACE Integrated Fitness Training® (ACE IFT®) Model, the centerpiece of *The Exercise Professional's Guide to Personal Training*, in the medical exercise setting. The ACE IFT Model is featured in the case studies associated with each disease or disorder covered in the manual. This section of the text closes with a chapter on working with clients with health challenges, including the psychological impact of health challenges and the impact of various lifestyle choices on a client's physiological capacity. This chapter also features a 10-step decision-making approach to exercise programming for special populations that can serve as a guide for working with any client.

PART II: LEADERSHIP AND IMPLEMENTATION includes three chapters covering elements of working with special-population and at-risk clients that are universal, regardless of a client's individual challenges. Chapter 4 discusses the determinants of health behavior and models of behavior change. Strategies to help clients make positive behavior changes are also offered. The next chapter provides application-based communication strategies that the CMES can implement to better understand and motivate clients. The final chapter in this section teaches readers how to most effectively communicate with allied healthcare professionals in order to best serve their clients and build a strong professional network. Also included in this chapter are the CMES's professional responsibilities and a business-planning guide.

PART III: MAJOR CARDIOVASCULAR AND PULMONARY DISEASES AND DISORDERS
consists of four chapters covering coronary heart disease, blood lipid disorders, hypertension, and asthma and chronic obstructive pulmonary disease. It is in this section of the manual that readers are introduced to chapter elements that appear throughout the text, including the following:

- Condition overview
- Diagnostic testing and criteria
- Treatment options
- Nutritional considerations
- Exercise training recommendations
- Exercise guidelines summaries
- Case studies

This consistent chapter outline provides not only the background information the CMES needs to understand a particular disease or disorder, but also the practical tools they need to safely and effectively work with affected clients.

PART IV: METABOLIC DISEASES AND DISORDERS includes chapters on overweight and obesity, the metabolic syndrome, and diabetes mellitus using the same chapter outline described above.

PART V: MUSCULOSKELETAL DISORDERS consists of seven chapters. Chapter 14 covers posture and movement and features instruction on how to conduct a postural assessment as well as movement screens and flexibility and muscle-length testing. This chapters also features exercise examples for stability and mobility and practical approaches for designing and implementing restorative exercise programs. Chapter 15 explains how to assess a client's balance and gait and offers exercises designed to improve gait. Myofascial slings, and exercises designed to strengthen each, are also discussed. Chapters 16 and 17 discuss arthritis and osteoporosis/osteopenia, respectively, using the chapter outline listed above, and include sample exercises tailored to the needs of each population. Chapters 18, 19, and 20 cover lower-extremity injuries, upper-extremity injuries, and low-back pain, providing the CMES with an introduction to the most common types and causes of injury, along with exercise guidelines associated with each.

PART VI: PERINATAL CONSIDERATIONS consists of a single chapter that covers prenatal and postpartum exercise, including physiological changes and biomechanical considerations associated with pregnancy, as well as exercise techniques for pregnant women.

The following features are included throughout the manual in an effort to create a more interactive, application-based reading experience:

- *Expand Your Knowledge:* This feature highlights key research or new insights of which a CMES should be aware, sometimes showing how an old concept was revised with new information or how conflicting evidence sometimes exists.
- *Apply What You Know:* These textboxes feature real-world examples to illustrate specific concepts. Essentially, "this is what you've learned, and this is how it's used in the actual work setting."
- *Think It Through:* This feature asks thought-provoking questions that force the reader to pause and really chew on the concepts being learned.
- *Do the Math:* This feature provides an application-based perspective to math calculations, giving the reader the context for how the numbers are used in the real world, and why they matter.

The goal of this manual is to enable the ACE Certified Medical Exercise Specialist to become an integral and respected member of a client's healthcare team and join in the overall effort to help the client reach their optimal health and fitness level. We wish you good luck in your efforts and sincerely hope that this manual serves you well as you prepare for the certification exam and remains a trusted resource throughout your career.

JAMES S. SKINNER, PH.D., FACSM
TECHNICAL EDITOR

CEDRIC X. BRYANT, PH.D., FACSM
CHIEF SCIENCE OFFICER

SABRENA JO, M.S.
DIRECTOR OF SCIENCE AND RESEARCH

DANIEL J. GREEN
SENIOR PROJECT MANAGER AND EDITOR FOR PUBLICATIONS AND CONTENT DEVELOPMENT

STUDYING FOR THE ACE MEDICAL EXERCISE SPECIALIST EXAM

TO HELP YOU ON YOUR JOURNEY TO BECOMING AN ACE CERTIFIED MEDICAL EXERCISE SPECIALIST (CMES), WE HAVE PUT TOGETHER A COMPREHENSIVE SET OF RESOURCES YOU CAN USE WHILE YOU STUDY.

In addition to this manual, you'll also utilize the *ACE Medical Exercise Specialist Manual Study Companion*, which contains multiple-choice questions for each corresponding chapter of the *ACE Medical Exercise Specialist Manual*, as well as a summary review of each chapter to help you focus your studies.

FOR MANUAL AND ACE UNIVERSITY

If you purchased ACE University, you will use our online programs to guide you through your studies.

ACE University will transform your study process into a digital experience designed to help ACE Medical Exercise Specialist Certification candidates get the ultimate study experience. With interactive lessons that include the electronic *ACE Medical Exercise Specialist Manual Study Companion*, assigned reading, case studies, lesson quizzes, exam review modules, and two practice tests, it will help you learn like you would in a classroom. See below for tips on optimizing your use of the electronic study companion.

If you are utilizing ACE University, log in to your My ACE account at www.ACEfitness.org/myace to begin.

FOR MANUAL AND ELECTRONIC STUDY COMPANION ONLY

If you are using the manual and electronic study companion, take the following steps to best prepare for the exam:

- **STEP 1:** Read Chapters 1–6 of this book, *ACE Medical Exercise Specialist Manual*. These chapters cover multiple facets of becoming an ACE Certified Medical Exercise Specialist—from the role of the CMES in the health and fitness industry to basic communication and behavioral change techniques. Also included in these chapters is information on how to apply the ACE Integrated Fitness Training® (ACE IFT®) Model in the medical exercise setting. The ACE IFT Model is revisited in each of the case studies presented in later chapters.

  After reading each chapter, complete the corresponding quiz questions in Chapters 1–6 of the *ACE Medical Exercise Specialist Manual Study Companion*.

  Also, review Appendices A and B in this manual, which cover the ACE Code of Ethics and the Exam Content Outline, as well as pages 745 to 747, where you will find the ACE Position Statement on Nutrition Scope of Practice for Exercise Professionals. Appendix C presents the principles of nutrition for the CMES. If nutrition is a new area of study for you, take the time to study Appendix C at this point, as more advanced nutrition concepts are presented in subsequent chapters of the *ACE Medical Exercise Specialist Manual*.

- **STEP 2:** Read Chapters 7–13 of this book. This material covers the major cardiovascular and pulmonary diseases and disorders, as well as metabolic diseases and disorders, that a CMES is likely to encounter while working with clients.

  After reading each chapter, complete the corresponding quiz questions in Chapters 7–13 of the *ACE Medical Exercise Specialist Manual Study Companion*.

- **STEP 3:** Read Chapters 14–21 of this book, which cover musculoskeletal disorders and perinatal considerations. The seven chapters that make up the musculoskeletal disorders section cover everything from posture and gait, to arthritis and osteoporosis, to common injuries, including low-back pain.

After reading each chapter, complete the corresponding quiz questions for Chapters 14–21 of the *ACE Medical Exercise Specialist Manual Study Companion.* At this point, we also recommend that you register for the ACE Certified Medical Exercise Specialist Certification Exam by visiting www.ACEfitness.org. Setting a date will give you a clear goal to work toward while you study.

IMPORTANT TIPS

- To register for your exam, do not forget that you must be at least 18 years old and hold a current certificate in cardiopulmonary resuscitation (CPR) and, if living in North America, proper use of an automated external defibrillator (AED). The course must include a live skills check. Online courses are not accepted. As you begin your studies, start looking into local providers and register for a course. You must also submit supporting documentation for each of the following:
  - ✓ A bachelor's degree in exercise science or a related field
  - ✓ 500 hours of work experience designing and implementing exercise programs for apparently healthy individuals and/or high-risk individuals, as documented by a qualified professional
- As you make your way through your study materials, be sure to keep an eye out for the boldface terms in the chapters, which are defined in the glossary.
- As a general rule, ACE recommends that candidates invest 80 to 100 hours of study time over a three- to four-month period to adequately prepare for the ACE Medical Exercise Specialist Certification Exam.
- For additional tips and resources, visit ACE Answers to review commonly asked study questions, video demonstrations and lectures, exam prep blogs, connect with ACE study coaches and certified professionals on Facebook, and to participate in live study webinars (www.ACEfitness.org/fitness-certifications/ace-answers).

PART I
INTRODUCTION

CHAPTER 1
ROLE AND SCOPE OF PRACTICE FOR THE CERTIFIED MEDICAL EXERCISE SPECIALIST

CHAPTER 2
APPLYING THE ACE INTEGRATED FITNESS TRAINING® MODEL IN THE MEDICAL EXERCISE SETTING

CHAPTER 3
WORKING WITH CLIENTS WITH HEALTH CHALLENGES

1 ROLE AND SCOPE OF PRACTICE FOR THE CERTIFIED MEDICAL EXERCISE SPECIALIST

IN THIS CHAPTER

THE HEALTHCARE CONTINUUM

THE ROLE OF THE CMES WITHIN ALLIED HEALTHCARE
PHYSICIAN-CRITICAL PATHWAY
WORKING WITHIN THE HEALTHCARE COMMUNITY

SCOPE OF PRACTICE

FOCUS ON DISEASE PREVENTION
PRIMARY PREVENTION
SECONDARY PREVENTION
TERTIARY PREVENTION

STANDARDS OF CARE
COMPONENTS OF PROGRAM DESIGN
SAFETY CONCERNS RELATED TO PROGRAM IMPLEMENTATION
THE 10-STEP DECISION-MAKING APPROACH TO EXERCISE PROGRAMMING FOR SPECIAL POPULATIONS
RISK MANAGEMENT
LIFELONG LEARNING
CONSULTATIONS/PRIVACY ISSUES

SUMMARY

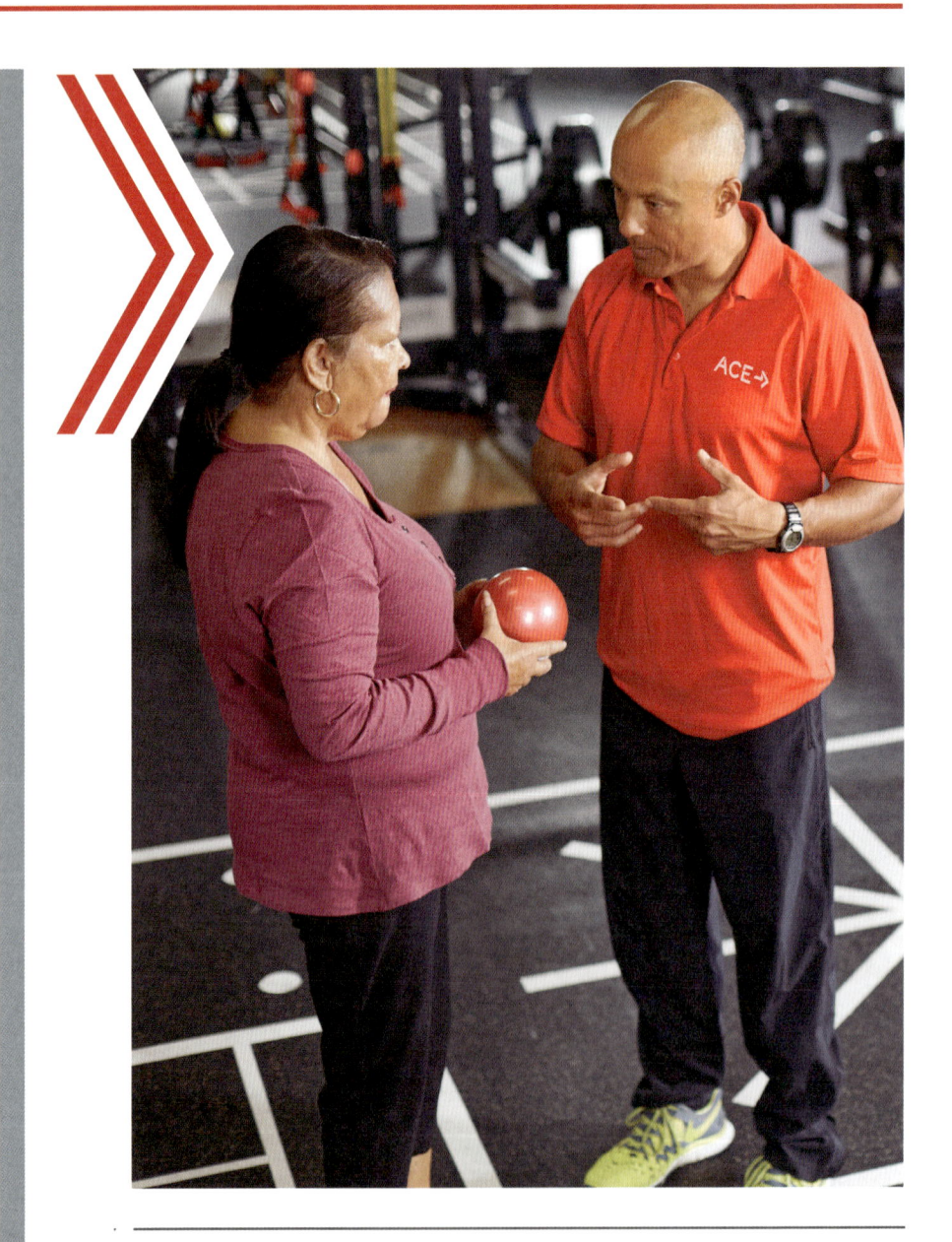

ABOUT THE AUTHOR
Kelly Spivey, N.D., has a doctorate in Natural Health and a master's degree in Fitness Management. She has an extensive career in the health and fitness arena, ranging from cardiopulmonary rehabilitation manager to owner/operator of three medically based fitness centers. Dr. Spivey is a Territory Manager for Freemotion Fitness, works with the University of Tampa in the Health Science & Human Performance Department, and serves as a subject matter expert for ACE.

By Kelly Spivey

THE ACE® MEDICAL EXERCISE SPECIALIST certification was developed to enable exercise professionals to collaborate with the healthcare community to support their clients' health and fitness goals. In the past, the primary role of an advanced trainer was to bridge the gap between the clinical setting and the traditional fitness center. That role is now changing. Due to the current state of the healthcare system, the majority of healthcare dollars are spent in treating disease and dysfunction.

The United States spends more on healthcare than any other nation in the world, largely due to the resources given to treat well-established diseases and dysfunctions, as opposed to preventing the diseased state. Analysts predict that a continued increase in chronic disease and dysfunction will cost the U.S. healthcare system an estimated 4.2 trillion dollars annually by the year 2023 (Bodenheimer, Chen, & Bennett, 2009). Despite the logic associated with disease-prevention practices, the current healthcare system has not made the paradigm shift necessary to modify personal behaviors that affect overall health and well-being. As a result of this void, the role of the ACE Certified Medical Exercise Specialist (CMES) has evolved into one of health promotion and disease prevention, using a variety of lifestyle interventions (e.g., exercise, nutrition, and stress management) and behavior-modification techniques.

The U.S. Affordable Care Act (ACA) is considered landmark legislation with a primary focus on preventive care. One of the programs associated with the ACA is the Prevention and Public Health Fund, which financially supports programs focused on prevention, improved health outcomes, public health, and the enhancement of healthcare quality, with new resources available for programs such as chronic disease self-management, screening and counseling, smoking cessation, and **diabetes** prevention. State and local community involvement is also important to the success of health and preventive services, and the CMES should play an integral role in promoting healthy behaviors.

A CMES has the knowledge, training, and experience to work with clients who currently have, or are at risk for developing, one or more health conditions. The CMES must develop a keen understanding of each client's current disease state and then design a safe, effective, and enjoyable program that will enable the client to resume optimal function. The CMES does not act as an independent entity, but as a viable part of the healthcare community.

The CMES can position themself as an integral component of the healthcare continuum, working with allied health professionals in facilitating lifestyle-modification and disease-prevention strategies. Furthermore, the CMES can offer programs that support the existing services provided by licensed healthcare professionals (e.g., supervised exercise to promote weight loss for a client currently working with a certified diabetes educator). There is also a need in the healthcare industry to provide a continuation of care for those who have not reached maximal rehabilitation potential. The many components of a balanced health and fitness program are best facilitated by a certified health and exercise professional, like the CMES.

LEARNING OBJECTIVES:

» Explain the ACE Certified Medical Exercise Specialist's place and role within the healthcare continuum.

» Describe the ACE Certified Medical Exercise Specialist's scope of practice, including examples of actions that are outside and within this defined scope.

» List and briefly explain the three tiers of disease prevention.

» Explain the standards of care for the ACE Certified Medical Exercise Specialist and how they apply to program design, risk management, continuing education, and client privacy issues.

The populations served by the CMES include, but are not limited to:
- Those who are at risk for chronic disease or dysfunction, based on lifestyle or family history
- Those who have borderline health conditions that may be reversed and/or managed with a progressive health and fitness program
- Those with newly diagnosed cardiovascular, metabolic, or orthopedic conditions and who are in need of professional health and fitness guidance
- Those with chronic cardiovascular, metabolic, or orthopedic conditions and in need of continued health and fitness guidance
- Post-rehabilitation patients following discharge from an outpatient rehabilitation program
- Those with certain psychological disorders that may benefit from a program of regular exercise

The benefits of exercise are well established, but the majority of healthcare providers have no formal education or practical experience in exercise program design and implementation. An individual may be advised to "begin a regular exercise program," but is unlikely to receive much direction from their healthcare provider. Clearly, the proper application of exercise is a key to a successful health and fitness program. Because of their knowledge and experience in exercise science, a CMES can be positioned as a tremendous asset in the healthcare continuum, filling the gap between advice and application. The CMES can also be a tremendous asset when it comes to facilitating motivation and compliance.

A client may be referred by a physician or rehabilitation specialist, or seek out a CMES on their own. To establish a working relationship with other allied healthcare professionals and develop the most appropriate treatment plan, the CMES should seek communication with the client's primary healthcare provider and develop strong ties with members of the healthcare team. This book defines an acceptable **scope of practice** for the CMES, offers guidelines for developing safe and effective health and fitness programs for special populations, and provides useful strategies that allow the CMES to position themselves as a vital member of the healthcare team.

THE HEALTHCARE CONTINUUM

The CMES has a unique place within the healthcare continuum. Any given client may have one or more physicians, depending on the disease or dysfunction. They may have worked with a rehabilitation specialist, such as a physical therapist or cardiac rehabilitation nurse, or be under the care of a **registered dietitian (RD)** or psychiatrist. The role of the CMES is to work in conjunction with the current healthcare team to establish the most effective health and fitness plan. This healthcare team takes direction from the client's personal physician. In essence, the physician acts as a "gatekeeper" (Figure 1-1). Therefore, ongoing communication is vital to the success of the team and ultimately the client.

When working with special populations, it is expected that the CMES will have the following knowledge and skills as they relate to the populations being served:
- Knowledge of basic disease **pathophysiology**
- Knowledge of the physician-critical pathway (see Figure 1-2, page 7) as it relates to treatment of disease and dysfunction, and skill in establishing themselves as an integral part of this pathway
- Knowledge of common medications used in the treatment of diseases and dysfunctions, along with the side effects, and skill in applying this information to exercise design and programming

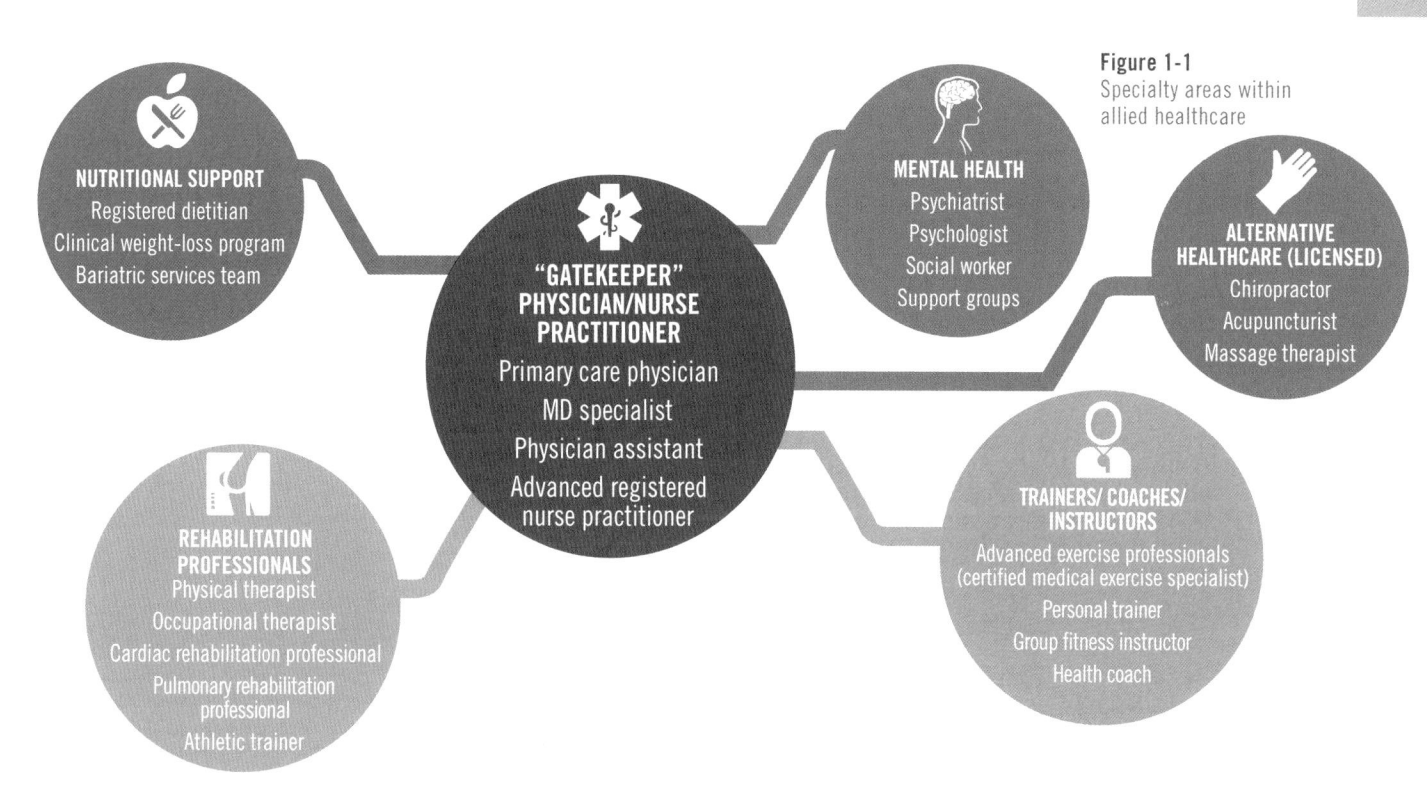

Role and Scope of Practice for the Certified Medical Exercise Specialist — CHAPTER 1

Figure 1-1
Specialty areas within allied healthcare

NUTRITIONAL SUPPORT
Registered dietitian
Clinical weight-loss program
Bariatric services team

"GATEKEEPER" PHYSICIAN/NURSE PRACTITIONER
Primary care physician
MD specialist
Physician assistant
Advanced registered nurse practitioner

MENTAL HEALTH
Psychiatrist
Psychologist
Social worker
Support groups

ALTERNATIVE HEALTHCARE (LICENSED)
Chiropractor
Acupuncturist
Massage therapist

REHABILITATION PROFESSIONALS
Physical therapist
Occupational therapist
Cardiac rehabilitation professional
Pulmonary rehabilitation professional
Athletic trainer

TRAINERS/ COACHES/ INSTRUCTORS
Advanced exercise professionals (certified medical exercise specialist)
Personal trainer
Group fitness instructor
Health coach

- Knowledge of common diagnostic tests and skill in designing exercise programs based on the results and/or physician-recommended parameters
- Knowledge and skill in performing an appropriate fitness assessment, including the selection of appropriate methods, measures, endpoints, and special considerations as they relate to the client's disease state and medications, as well as any environmental conditions
- Knowledge of expected exercise progression, from hospital to rehabilitation to mainstream fitness settings and skill in developing a safe, effective, and enjoyable program based on these parameters: frequency, intensity, time, and type of exercise, as well as appropriate goals and the customary time needed to achieve predetermined and realistic goals
- Knowledge of exercise contraindications as they relate to a variety of accepted values (e.g., blood pressure and blood **glucose**)
- Knowledge and skill in modifying exercise programs to accommodate clients facing health challenges
- Knowledge of current dietary guidelines and skill in educating clients on making appropriate food choices based on solid scientific evidence and sound nutritional practices
- Knowledge of psychological implications related to disease and disability and an ability to empathize with clients who are struggling with their personal health challenges
- Knowledge of recognizable signs and symptoms of improperly managed stress and skill in developing effective coping strategies to eliminate or manage daily stressors
- Knowledge of signs or symptoms that require medical interventions beyond the capability of the CMES
- Knowledge of, and ability to perform, first aid and **cardiopulmonary resuscitation (CPR)**, and use an **automated external defibrillator (AED)** when necessary
- Knowledge of appropriate communication tools and skill in interviewing and communicating effectively with the client and/or healthcare team
- Detailed knowledge of appropriate health and fitness goals (e.g., blood glucose level, joint functioning and **range of motion,** and appropriate **body composition**) and the knowledge and skills to help clients progress toward them

EXPAND YOUR KNOWLEDGE

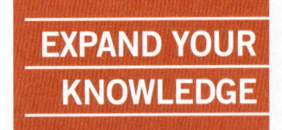

USING THE EXAM CONTENT OUTLINE AS A STUDY TOOL

The ACE Medical Exercise Specialist Exam Content Outline is a valuable tool for candidates preparing for the ACE Medical Exercise Specialist Certification Exam. It is the result of an in-depth job analysis conducted with a panel of subject matter experts that was then validated via an industry-wide survey. The final ACE Medical Exercise Specialist exam content outline, presented as Appendix B of this manual, is the blueprint used in assembling each ACE Medical Exercise Specialist exam.

Candidates are encouraged to refer to this exam content outline as they prepare for the ACE Medical Exercise Specialist exam, as it details the key concepts and competencies assessed by the exam. It does not provide the exact questions on an ACE exam; however, it does provide the four main content "Domains" assessed by the exam and the percentage of questions that come from each Domain.

Each Domain is comprised of several "Tasks" that are essential for a medical exercise professional to perform competently in order to meet the required level of competence to earn the ACE Medical Exercise Specialist Certification. The percentages listed with each Domain represent the criticality of the tasks in the Domain, and the frequency with which a CMES will perform them.

The following steps should help you use the exam content outline in preparing for the ACE Medical Exercise Specialist exam:

- Review the exam content Domains and their associated percentages. This will help you determine the relative weight of each Domain on the total examination
- Review and understand each Task Statement. Each question on the ACE Medical Exercise Specialist exam maps to one of the Task Statements, as these have been identified as the critical tasks a well-qualified CMES must perform consistently to provide safe and effective exercise programming to help clients prevent and manage disease, avoid injuries, improve overall wellness and function throughout all phases of medical interventions, and return to desired activities following rehabilitation.
- Review the Knowledge and Skill Statements associated with each Task. These describe the knowledge and skills in which a health and exercise professional must be competent to perform the essential tasks of a CMES.
- Refer back to the Exam Content Outline as you study to ensure that you have learned the knowledge and skills necessary to perform the essential Tasks of a well-qualified CMES.
- Refer back to the Exam Content Outline after completing the online practice tests to review the concepts and competencies covered in any Domains that have been identified as areas of focus as you continue your studies.

THE ROLE OF THE CMES WITHIN ALLIED HEALTHCARE

Physician-critical Pathway

It is important for a CMES working within the healthcare system to understand the role of the exercise professional as it relates to the other members of the healthcare team. In many cases, the client has a primary care physician who is responsible for their general medical care. If the client is exhibiting signs or symptoms of disease or is at risk for developing a particular disease or dysfunction, the doctor will perform a number of diagnostic tests to confirm or deny this suspicion. Once the disease or dysfunction is confirmed, the treatment options will be considered. If the doctor feels that the patient requires medical intervention outside their scope of care, the doctor will likely make a referral. This referral might be to a specialized physician (e.g., cardiologist or orthopedist) or to an RD, a mental health specialist, a rehabilitation professional, or a CMES. The referring physician is kept abreast of the patient's progress via regularly written or electronic reports. The primary physician will also make decisions on appropriate follow-up (e.g., subsequent office visits or further diagnostic tests). The physician-critical pathway is a decision-making tool to help the physician with the patient's case management (Figure 1-2).

Figure 1-2
Physician-critical pathway

PATIENT PRESENTS WITH ONE OR MORE OF THE FOLLOWING:
- Signs/symptoms
- Abnormal screening results
- Multiple risk factors
- Positive family history

DETERMINATION OF APPROPRIATE DIAGNOSTIC TESTS:
- Blood work
- Non-invasive tests (e.g., magnetic resonance imaging, x-ray, or exercise stress test)
- Invasive tests (e.g., heart catheter, or exploratory knee arthroscopy)

DETERMINATION OF TREATMENT OPTIONS:
- Medication
- Surgery
- Rehabilitation
- Behavior modification

POTENTIAL REFERRALS/CONSULTS:
- Physician (e.g., cardiologist, orthopedist, or endocrinologist)
- Non-physician (e.g., registered dietitian, physical therapist, occupational therapist, certified diabetes educator, personal trainer, health coach, or certified medical exercise specialist)

FOLLOW-UP

THINK IT THROUGH

Considering that a client will likely spend more time with a CMES than their primary healthcare provider, what steps will you take to ensure that the health information and exercise guidelines you pass along to a client are appropriate for their health limitations?

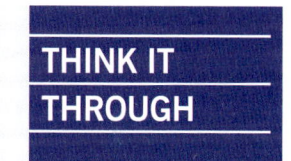

On average, a personal physician spends approximately 11 minutes with a patient (Gottschalk & Flocke, 2005); an RD may meet with a patient or client for a one-hour block of time and perhaps one follow-up visit; and a physical therapist or cardiac rehabilitation nurse may see the patient on a regular basis, but often juggles multiple patients at once. The CMES is one of the few healthcare professionals who have the opportunity to spend a considerable amount of one-on-one time with a client, which allows for a great deal of information sharing. The CMES is likely to know the client on a more personal level and discover detailed information about their daily lifestyle habits and behaviors. More importantly, regular appointments give the CMES an opportunity to share copious amounts of health information and facilitate the behavior-change process, allowing for permanent adoption of new behaviors. Other allied healthcare professionals will share information and initiate the path to wellness, but the CMES will help hold the client accountable and provide regular feedback, enabling the client to reach their maximal potential.

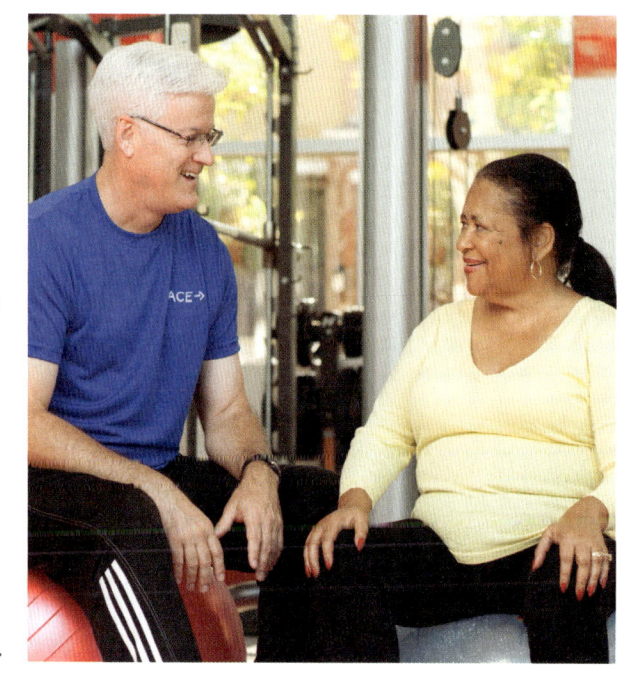

Working Within the Healthcare Community

Members of the healthcare community will not always appreciate the value of having a CMES on their team. Fortunately, exercise continues to gain recognition and endorsement from the healthcare community as an integral preventive and post-rehabilitative tool. Challenges for the CMES to be viewed as an integral part of the healthcare team may include the following:
- *The CMES must demonstrate their value to the healthcare team.* The CMES will have the benefit of regular meetings with the client, which aids in exercise compliance and

enhanced behavior modification. The physician will have peace of mind knowing that their patient will be continuously supervised and referred back to the appropriate healthcare practitioner if complications arise.
- *The CMES must not exceed their professional boundaries or go outside the scope of practice.* Providing a specific exercise plan will give the healthcare professional a clearer understanding of the exercise program components.
- *The CMES must communicate on a regular basis with either the referring physician or the healthcare team.* An accepted reporting structure includes the following: pre-exercise assessment report; monthly progress reports using a summary of daily **SOAP notes**; post-exercise program summary of progress; and written and/or verbal communication on complications or emergency situations.

Referral sources are certainly not limited to physicians. A CMES can also market themself to nurse practitioners, physician assistants, RDs, certified diabetes educators, physical or occupational therapists, cardiac rehabilitation providers, massage therapists, prenatal educators, chiropractors, social workers, clinical psychologists, support groups, weight-loss clinics, and personal trainers.

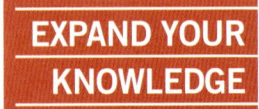

EXPAND YOUR KNOWLEDGE

PHYSICIANS INCREASINGLY PRESCRIBE EXERCISE

Physicians and other healthcare professionals can be influential sources of health information. Specifically, exercise counseling by primary care physicians has been shown to be moderately effective at increasing patients' participation in physical activity (Sanchez et al., 2015; Orrow et al., 2012).

A 2012 report from the Centers for Disease Control and Prevention (CDC) suggests that over the past decade, the medical community has increased its efforts to recommend participation in exercise and other physical activity (Barnes & Schoenborn, 2012). The key findings of the report include:
- In 2010, one in three adults who had seen a physician or other health professional had been advised to begin or continue to engage in exercise or physical activity.
- Between 2000 and 2010, the percentage of adults receiving exercise advice increased by about 10%.
- Receiving exercise recommendations occurred more frequently for adults with chronic diseases (e.g., **hypertension,** cardiovascular disease, cancer, and diabetes).
- Adults with overweight or **obesity** were often given exercise advice, and had the largest percentage point increases over the same period in being advised to exercise.

Although the prevalence of receiving advice from physicians to become or continue to be physically active remains well below one-half of U.S. adults and varies substantially across population subgroups (Barnes & Schoenborn, 2012), exercise professionals can seize the opportunity to connect with those healthcare providers who regularly recommend exercise to their patients. See Chapter 6 for information on networking with the healthcare community.

SCOPE OF PRACTICE

To maintain support from the healthcare community, it is paramount that the CMES stays within their professional scope of practice (Figure 1-3). The CMES *must* preclude themself from activities that are limited to licensed healthcare professionals. For example, a CMES may have seen dozens of clients with **sciatica.** Therefore, they are familiar with the symptoms related to sciatica and know the appropriate treatment plan. However, a CMES must not diagnose any disease, dysfunction, or condition. It would be appropriate to report significant signs or symptoms to the healthcare team, but not to label a specific condition. Additionally, a CMES cannot prescribe specific meal plans or give specific recommendations on supplements or trendy diet plans (see Appendix C for more information on nutrition-related scope of practice issues). A CMES cannot provide massage therapy unless they are licensed to do so.

ACE CERTIFIED MEDICAL EXERCISE SPECIALIST SCOPE OF PRACTICE

The ACE Certified Medical Exercise Specialist is an integral member of the healthcare team who has met all the requirements of the American Council on Exercise to develop and deliver specific and complementary clinical exercise programs independently and in collaboration with other healthcare providers. The CMES has expertise in conducting assessments and designing comprehensive health and fitness programs to help clients prevent and manage disease, avoid injuries, improve overall wellness and function throughout all phases of medical interventions, and return to desired activities following rehabilitation. The CMES applies the principles of exercise science, health coaching, nutrition, psychology, corrective exercise, and pathophysiology to develop health and fitness programs for special-population clients with clinical issues (e.g., cardiovascular, pulmonary, metabolic, and musculoskeletal) in order to facilitate lasting behavioral change and improve client function, health, fitness, and well-being. ACE Certified Medical Exercise Specialists have a scope of practice that includes:

- Conducting health-history interviews to identify risk factors or known diagnoses of cardiovascular, pulmonary, metabolic, musculoskeletal, and other diseases, disorders, injuries, and ailments that require specialized considerations for exercise participation and the need for healthcare referrals
- Evaluating health, fitness, and lifestyle information to assess an individual's readiness for physical activity, facilitate program design, optimize adherence, identify at-risk clients, and make appropriate referrals
- Assessing posture (static and dynamic), balance (static and dynamic), kinetic-chain stability and mobility, functional movement patterns, coordination, and gait (walking and running)
- Identifying and conducting appropriate assessments to determine cardiorespiratory fitness, muscular endurance, muscular strength, and flexibility
- Guiding clients through realistic goal setting based on their expectations and limitations, assessment data, and recommendations from healthcare professionals
- Designing and delivering preventive programs for at risk clients in order to help them improve health, fitness, and function while mitigating the risk of diseases, disorders, ailments, and injuries
- Developing and implementing programs for clients in all stages of medical intervention in order to complement treatment and improve function, health, and fitness
- Applying coaching strategies to develop rapport and facilitate lasting health-behavior changes
- Educating clients on specific health behaviors and self-monitoring tools in order to enhance program adherence, safety, and success
- Instructing clients on safe and effective exercise techniques using appropriate communication, coaching, and cueing strategies in order to optimize program outcomes and build self-efficacy
- Maintaining confidential, detailed client records according to the Health Insurance Portability and Accountability Act (HIPAA), electronic medical records, and other guidelines to track progress, make appropriate adjustments, and communicate (as necessary) with other healthcare professionals
- Recognizing and responding to acute medical conditions and injuries

Figure 1-3
ACE Certified Medical Exercise Specialist Scope of Practice

Visit www.ACEfitness.org/CMESresources to download a free PDF of the ACE Certified Medical Exercise Specialist Scope of Practice, as well as other forms and tools that you can use throughout your career as a CMES.

Also, they cannot make recommendations that contradict those of the client's healthcare provider. Table 1-1 lists some examples of practices that fall outside, or within, the CMES scope of practice.

The CMES should never go against the recommendations of the healthcare team. They may recommend certain progressions to the referring physician, based on subjective and objective assessments, but it is essential that no changes be instituted without prior written approval from the licensed healthcare professional.

Each jurisdiction has specific laws and parameters of professional responsibility within any given field. It is the responsibility of the CMES to know the laws in their geographical area and conform to the professional scope of practice and the laws of the state, province, or country.

TABLE 1-1

EXAMPLES OF ACTIONS THAT FALL OUTSIDE, AND WITHIN, THE ACE CERTIFIED MEDICAL EXERCISE SPECIALIST SCOPE OF PRACTICE

Outside the Scope of Practice	Within the Appropriate Scope of Practice
Diagnosing or labeling an unknown condition	Referring to the appropriate healthcare practitioner for diagnostic tests or additional screening; reporting notable signs or symptoms
Designing a specific meal plan with daily menus and exact portion sizes	Designing a daily eating plan based on the MyPlate Food Guidance System (www.myplate.gov)
Recommending a diet consisting of mostly protein for weight loss and/or muscle gain	Recommending carbohydrate, protein, and fat intake based on the Dietary Reference Intakes (DRI) and scientific parameters
Recommending specific supplements and dosages	Referring to a licensed healthcare practitioner for specific guidelines on supplement usage, dosage, and contraindications
Performing hands-on therapeutic massage	Recommending/demonstrating the use of neuromuscular devices (e.g., foam rollers) to release muscle tension
Recommending the use of over-the-counter medications for a post-exercise muscle strain	Discussing the appropriate first-aid techniques for dealing with an acute injury
Adding the use of the rowing machine to emphasize cross-training, even though the referring physician stated "treadmill only"	Contacting the referring healthcare provider (with the client's written permission) to discuss equipment alternatives and appropriate exercise progressions

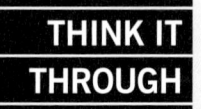

THINK IT THROUGH

How would you handle a situation in which a client specifically asks you to make a recommendation that you know is outside your scope of practice? For example, consider a scenario in which a client asks which medication you find more effective for post-workout soreness, ibuprofen or acetaminophen. Draft a standard response you can use in these situations.

FOCUS ON DISEASE PREVENTION

Many clients served by a CMES may be concerned with one or more health challenges. Their entry into supervised health and fitness programs may be motivated by a number of factors:
- Financial (e.g., trying to lower their blood pressure so their health/life insurance premiums are not negatively affected)
- Quality of life (e.g., trying to restore normal function so they can return to leisure activities like golfing or tennis)
- Morbidity/mortality (e.g., trying to control their diabetes so they do not suffer from complications like **neuropathy** or vision disturbances; or starting an exercise program following a gastric bypass procedure to make a serious health change)
- Psychological (e.g., trying to get off medications to regain a sense of health and control)

These clients are not looking for guidance to fit into their "skinny jeans." Rather, they are looking for guidance in quality-of-life issues and disease prevention.

Primary Prevention

The U.S. Preventive Services Task Force defines primary prevention measures as "those provided to individuals to prevent the onset of a targeted condition" (U.S. Preventive Services Task Force, 2012; U.S. Preventive Services Task Force, 1996). Primary prevention measures include activities that help avoid a particular disease or dysfunction. Examples include immunization against disease and health education programs promoting the benefits of exercise. Primary prevention is typically considered the most cost-effective form of healthcare because it helps reduce the costs and burdens associated with disease and dysfunction.

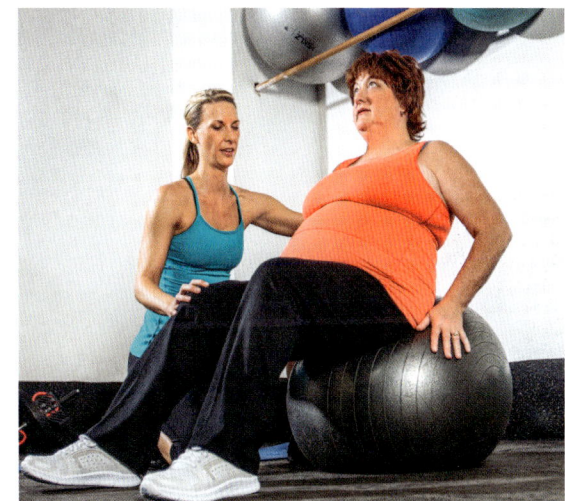

Secondary Prevention

Secondary prevention means to "identify and treat asymptomatic persons who have already developed risk factors or preclinical disease but in whom the condition is not clinically apparent" (U.S. Preventive Services Task Force, 2012; U.S. Preventive Services Task Force, 1996). The healthcare community focuses on screening for and detecting common asymptomatic diseases that, if left untreated, pose a significant risk for negative outcome. With early detection, the natural course of a disease or dysfunction can often be slowed down or even reversed. This can maximize well-being and minimize suffering.

An example of secondary prevention is a physician determining that their patient has developed stage 1 hypertension. The physician will implement an appropriate treatment program aimed at reducing the blood pressure values. This plan may include medications, smoking cessation, weight loss, and a supervised exercise program.

Tertiary Prevention

Tertiary prevention focuses on the care of established disease, with attempts made to minimize the negative effects of disease, restore optimal function, and prevent disease-related complications. Since the disease is established, primary and secondary prevention activities may have been unsuccessful or simply ignored. Most likely, involvement in these primary and secondary activities would have minimized the impact of the disease. It is not likely that the CMES will work with clients until their disease/dysfunction and associated health risks are deemed manageable or under control. The physician may recommend clinically based therapy programs prior to referral to a CMES. The healthcare team needs to keep the individual's primary, secondary, and tertiary prevention needs in mind when prioritizing and guiding care.

Some clients may be trying to prevent disease, while others may be trying to keep their current diseases or dysfunctions at bay, or even reverse the disease process. Some may even be trying to prevent future events from occurring. Whatever the client's motive, the primary task of a CMES is to work with the healthcare team to design and implement a comprehensive program aimed at preventing disease and optimizing health outcomes.

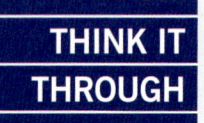

> **THINK IT THROUGH**
>
> Just like a physician focuses on different forms of treatment based on the type of prevention, a CMES must take into account the appropriate applications of exercise training for clients working on primary, secondary, or tertiary prevention. How will you approach designing and implementing fitness programs for clients who fall into the various phases of prevention as they relate to type 2 diabetes?

> **EXPAND YOUR KNOWLEDGE**
>
> ### CHEMOPROPHYLAXIS
>
> **Chemoprophylaxis** involves the use of drugs, nutritional supplements, or other natural substances to prevent future disease. For example, a client may take it upon themself to take a daily aspirin prophylactically to prevent heart disease. Because aspirin is a drug with potentially serious side effects, the client should consult with their personal healthcare provider to discuss the risks and benefits of daily aspirin use.
>
> This example brings up another important point. If a client informs the CMES of self-prescribing supplements in megadoses, the CMES should recommend that the client consult with their doctor or personal pharmacist. Many Americans turn to supplements and herbal remedies because they tend to be less expensive than prescription medications, are often easier to obtain, and the side effects, in many cases, may be negligible when compared to prescription medication. There is a widening gap between the consumer demand and the professional expertise on herbs, vitamins, minerals, and the like. Sales of vitamin, mineral, and herbal supplements exceed 30 million dollars annually (*Nutrition Business Journal*, 2012). In the United States, 40 to 50% of men and women 50 years of age or older regularly use multivitamin/mineral supplements (Karmangar & Emadi, 2012). With so much information available on the Internet, many people will self-treat their conditions using potentially harmful combinations of prescription drugs, over-the-counter medications, and supplements, which may cause serious side effects.
>
> A CMES is likely to encounter clients who use over-the-counter medications and/or supplements to prevent disease or dysfunction or to self-medicate. A client may even substitute an herbal supplement for medication prescribed by their personal physician. None of these practices should be condoned and the CMES should recommend that clients consult with a licensed healthcare professional who specializes in the field of supplementation.
>
> As people age, they are more likely to be prescribed more than one kind of prescription medication, and many seniors take three or more. This increases the risk for drug interactions, mix-ups, and the potential for side effects. In addition, the effects of aging cause older adults' bodies to process and respond to medicines differently than those of younger people. Age-related changes in the liver, kidneys, **central nervous system,** and heart are among the contributing factors causing elderly people to be more vulnerable to overdose and side effects.
>
> Note that a drug is defined as a substance other than food that is intended to affect the structure or function of the body. This definition includes prescription medications, supplements (e.g., vitamins, minerals, and herbs), over-the-counter medications (e.g., aspirin, acetaminophen, and ibuprofen), and regularly used chemicals (e.g., caffeine, alcohol, and nicotine). All drugs have the potential for side effects and negative interaction with other drugs.
>
> A single herbal supplement or over-the-counter medication may pose minimal health risks, but the risks and side effects can increase exponentially when certain combinations of drugs are taken on a daily basis. Consider the following examples of harmful drug combinations.

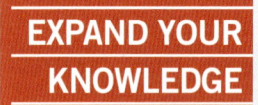

A client is taking the following substances, all of which have blood-thinning properties that can cause excessive bleeding:
- Prescription Motrin for chronic knee pain
- Self-prescribed aspirin for heart-disease prevention
- Self-prescribed vitamin E as an antioxidant
- Self-prescribed ginkgo biloba as a memory booster

Another example involves a client who is taking the following substances, all of which have stimulant properties and can cause anything from jitteriness to heart palpitations—or worse, cardiac arrest:
- Self-prescribed diet pills containing Siberian ginseng
- Self-prescribed guarana for energy enhancement
- Daily consumption of caffeinated beverages or energy drinks
- Self-administered over-the-counter allergy medication
- Cigarette smoking or use of smokeless tobacco

STANDARDS OF CARE

The CMES should be familiar with health risks associated with a client's specific disease or dysfunction. Before challenging a client's cardiovascular or musculoskeletal system, a number of safety concerns must be considered and contraindications for exercise testing and programming must be known. Subsequent chapters provide detailed information on risks and contraindications related to exercise programming, progression, and appropriate modifications for each specific disease or dysfunction.

Components of Program Design

The CMES is responsible for designing and implementing a progressive health and fitness program. The client should be well-advised of the exercise plan, including short- and long-term goals. To enhance the health and well-being of a client, a comprehensive program should include most, if not all, of the following components:

- Cardiorespiratory endurance
- Muscular endurance
- Body composition
- Posture
- Stress management
- Daily physical-activity plan
- Muscular strength
- Flexibility
- Balance
- Breathing techniques
- Nutrition
- Scheduled rest and recovery time

The CMES should know how to safely and effectively improve the essential components of physical fitness: cardiorespiratory endurance, muscular strength and endurance, posture, flexibility, balance, and body composition. The remaining components are just as important, but likely will be included as a supplement to the essential fitness components. As an advanced health and exercise professional, the CMES should also know how to make appropriate programming adjustments for specific health conditions, ranging from rotator cuff impingement to obesity. Application of these key elements as they relate to program design and implementation for specific diseases and dysfunctions is discussed in detail in subsequent chapters.

A thorough understanding of the client's condition will enable the CMES to design a safe and effective fitness program. Though each program will vary depending on the specific goals, objectives, and limitations of the client, the basic framework for exercise progression is based on the FITT principle: frequency, intensity, time, and type of exercise.

F: 3–5 days per week (daily for some clients)

I: 60–90% of predicted **maximal heart rate (MHR); first ventilatory threshold (VT1)** training

T: 20–60 minutes of continuous or accumulated activity

T: Specific modes of exercise to improve muscular strength and endurance, cardiorespiratory endurance, flexibility, and body composition

When determining the appropriate plan for exercise progression, the CMES must assess the objective data (e.g., heart rate and blood pressure, treadmill speeds, and sets and repetitions), as well as the subjective data (e.g., **rating of perceived exertion,** leg pain, difficulty in breathing, and excess fatigue). The client-reported information may be more valuable when determining the appropriate modifications in the fitness plan.

One program component that is often overlooked is the home-exercise program. The time spent with a client may total only two to three hours per week. To optimize health and wellness, it is important to establish a fitness plan for the remaining time away from the live training sessions. Might the client benefit from a yoga class or a post-rehabilitation support group? Would a weekly aquatic exercise class be an appropriate supplement to a land-based training program? The CMES will do well to consider a variety of options when designing a comprehensive health and wellness program. The CMES may consider using a software program that can be utilized to program and track activity during off days.

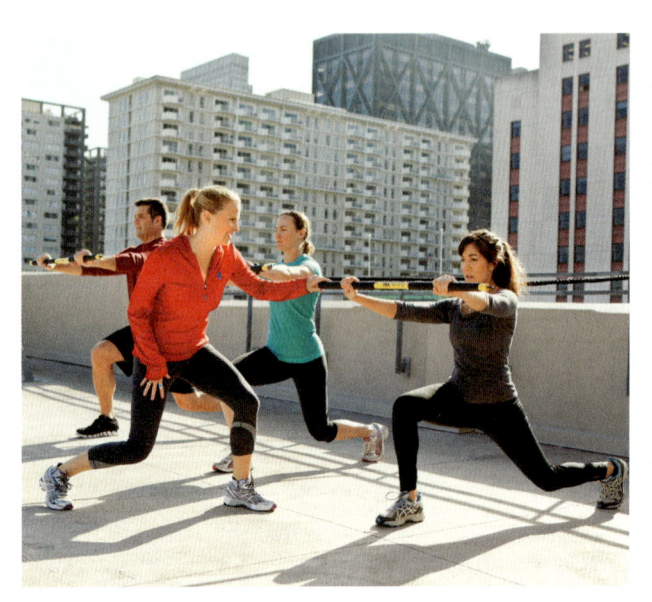

The fact that the CMES meets with the client on a regular basis creates a favorable position within the healthcare continuum for optimizing behavioral change and disease management. Using information-gathering techniques, the CMES will be able to modify the client's program and enable the successful completion of the agreed-upon goals and objectives. If a problem arises, the CMES can discuss their concerns with the referring physician before symptoms deteriorate. The CMES can help coach the client through the inevitable struggles associated with behavioral modification and provide the necessary tools and support to facilitate positive change. This responsibility starts with the initial evaluation and continues with each session.

Safety Concerns Related to Program Implementation

It is the responsibility of the CMES to ensure the safety of their clients. Prior to each exercise session, it is necessary to conduct a brief pre-exercise assessment. When appropriate, vital signs should be checked and recorded. The client should be asked about any recent symptoms and any problems related to the exercise program itself. The CMES should also make observations on the client's current condition. This information should be documented in the client's chart. Based on the client's subjective and objective data, the exercise program may need to be modified from the intended plan.

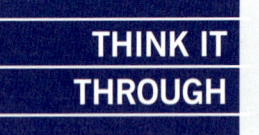

THINK IT THROUGH

As a CMES, it may be necessary to provide a "reality check" to a client who has unrealistic expectations. Obstacles that may prove to be a challenge are genetics, pre-existing conditions, timeframe, and the risk/benefit ratio associated with a certain program. What type of advice would you provide in the following instances?
- A client who has extreme weight-loss goals (i.e., lose 40 pounds within the next month)
- A client with significant knee degeneration who wants to return to triathlon training

While you do not want to discourage exercise participation, it is extremely important to develop realistic goals and objectives. What alternatives might you suggest that would continue to challenge each client while maintaining their overall health and safety?

The 10-step Decision-making Approach to Exercise Programming for Special Populations

This manual provides detailed information for designing safe and effective health and fitness programs for addressing the most common diseases and dysfunctions encountered by health and exercise professionals. It is the responsibility of the CMES to apply this information to individual clients. Most chapters provide one or more case studies, but it is simply impossible to cover every situation that may arise when working with special populations. The "10-Step Decision-making Approach to Exercise Programming for Special Populations," which is detailed in Chapter 3, is a model of reasoning to guide the CMES through the critical decision-making steps of client risk assessment, goal-setting, and exercise design and implementation.

Risk Management

The CMES must be familiar with the common exercise-induced risks associated with each client's disease or dysfunction. **Risk management** involves being proactive about potential threats to the health and safety of clients, staff, and visitors. There are numerous industry-accepted standards (the minimal performance expectations each facility must meet) and guidelines (recommendations to help each facility achieve higher than minimal expectations) for staffing, programming, equipment, facility layout, and emergency preparedness.

The CMES may be working within a facility, from a home studio, or entering a client's home. Each location poses its own risk-management challenges. A written policy will help make certain that all variables have been assessed and addressed, ultimately ensuring the safety and security of the clients. This policy should include sections on risk management and emergency planning, pre-activity screening, client orientation, education, supervision, staff qualifications, facility design, fitness equipment, and operational practices.

The CMES may need guidance on federal laws, including the Occupational Safety and Health Administration (OSHA) Blood-borne Pathogen Standard, employment laws, and the Federal Privacy Act. It is important to evaluate state laws and industry standards as they relate to AED availability and CPR certification. Ultimately, being proactive helps exercise professionals protect their clients as well as their own business interests.

Lifelong Learning

The field of health education and disease prevention is constantly changing and evolving. As a responsible CMES, it is important to stay abreast of the current research associated with health and fitness, especially as it relates to disease prevention. Knowing where to go for valid health and fitness information is paramount. There are abundant educational sources filled with medical quackery, which makes it challenging to differentiate between what is valid and what is hype. It is important to stay with well-established organizations and industry-accepted publications when searching for information. The information written in consumer magazines should be scrutinized for its content and integrity. Is the author trying to sell something? Is the study sample size appropriate? Are research findings statistically significant? Who conducted the study? For example, consider the biased findings of a pharmaceutical company's self-funded study of its own supplement. Has the same study been replicated by independent companies with the same or similar results?

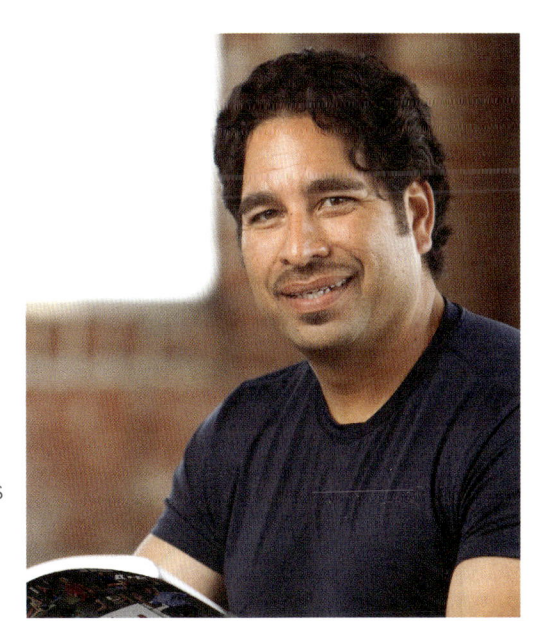

The CMES should take much care in deciding which reference materials and Internet sources to integrate into their collection of educational resources. There is a comprehensive list of references and suggested readings provided at the end of each chapter in this manual.

Additionally, it is recommended that every CMES have the following personal references for quick and easy access to pertinent medical information:
- *Physician's Desk Reference* (PDR) and Medline Plus (www.medlineplus.gov), among other comprehensive guides to prescription drugs
- PDR or other comprehensive guides to supplements
- Medical terminology reference (e.g., *Tabor's Cyclopedic Medical Dictionary*)
- Reputable reference guide to integrative medicine (*The American Pharmaceutical Association Practical Guide to Natural Medicines*)
- Reputable disease-specific medical textbooks, journal subscriptions, or Internet sites

When a client brings their list of medications and supplements, the CMES should consider the significant side effects of these drugs, especially as they relate to exercise program design and implementation. If a client brings the written results from their **magnetic resonance imaging (MRI),** there may be some medical terminology in the report that is unfamiliar. It is important to understand test results, as they can have an impact on the development of the exercise plan. The CMES is also likely to encounter a client who is trying one or more alternative medical practices.

The CMES should develop and implement a comprehensive exercise and lifestyle-modification plan, and most importantly, include an educational component. Unfortunately, many exercise professionals want their clients to become dependent on their presence. This may temporarily help the CMES's bottom line, but they are doing the client a disservice. One of the roles of the CMES is to educate clients and help them establish reasonable expectations and develop their own lifelong health and fitness plan.

Consultations/Privacy Issues

During the training sessions, information can be shared with the client to enhance their personal knowledge base. The client will likely have many questions about their disease or dysfunction, especially if they are newly diagnosed with a disease. Due to the vast amount of information that is available on disease prevention and management, there may be a need for further educational support from other health and exercise professionals. The CMES should develop a strong network of licensed healthcare professionals who can be consulted with specific questions that may be outside the CMES's area of expertise. Refer to Table 1-2 for a partial listing of licensed professionals.

As part of the CMES's professional responsibility, all client information should remain confidential when consulting with another professional. Pertinent information can be shared, but names and recognizable traits must remain anonymous. If the consulting healthcare professional recommends a referral to a licensed professional, it may be necessary to terminate the training program until the client has received professional help and is referred back to the CMES.

An essential aspect of the standard of care is knowing one's limitations. The depth of essential knowledge outlined in the performance domains included in the Exam Content Outline (see Appendix B) ranges from basic to advanced. When working with a client with health challenges, it is essential that the CMES has more than a familiarity with the disease or dysfunction. Before venturing into unfamiliar territory, it is best to refer the client to another CMES who

TABLE 1-2

POSSIBLE NETWORK OF LICENSED PROFESSIONALS

- M.D./D.O.: General practitioner or internist
- M.D. specialist: Cardiologist, orthopedist, neurologist
- Clinical psychologist or psychiatrist
- Chiropractor
- Physical therapist
- Occupational therapist
- Cardiac rehabilitation specialist
- Registered dietitian
- Pharmacist
- Massage therapist

specializes in the specific condition in question. Trial and error is not an option when dealing with special populations, or any client for that matter.

That said, a CMES need not limit themselves to well-known populations. Another important characteristic of the CMES is the ability to acquire additional knowledge and training and learn how to safely and effectively apply this knowledge to any future clientele. Experience can be acquired from continuing education courses or through working in conjunction with another exercise professional who has the sought-after experience. Most hospitals have volunteer opportunities that enable further applied training with the target population. A few likely places to volunteer would be in the outpatient physical therapy department or in a cardiac or pulmonary rehabilitation center.

SUMMARY

The current healthcare system spends the majority of its resources treating chronic illness and disease. Resources would be much better spent educating the general population and implementing programs to prevent disease and dysfunction. The ACE Certified CMES is in a perfect position to facilitate this paradigm shift, as well as playing a supporting role as a member of the healthcare team in the management of chronic conditions.

It is the responsibility of the CMES to stay within their scope of practice; educate both the healthcare community as well as the general public on the benefits of supervised, progressive fitness programs; and advocate high standards of professionalism within the field.

There are very few professions that have the opportunity to significantly impact the health and well-being of the clientele they serve. With the necessary knowledge and skills to focus on disease prevention and management, plus the dedication to make a difference in the lives of others, a CMES can and should become an integral part of the healthcare continuum.

REFERENCES

Barnes, P.M. & Schoenborn, C.A. (2012). *Trends in Adults Receiving a Recommendation for Exercise or Other Physical Activity from a Physician or Other Health Professional.* National Center for Health Statistics Data Brief, No. 86. Hyattsville, Md.: National Center for Health Statistics.

Bodenheimer, T., Chen, E., & Bennett H.D. (2009). Confronting the growing burden of chronic disease: Can the U.S. health care workforce do the job? *Health Affairs (Millwood),* 28, 1, 64–74

Gottschalk, A. & Flocke, S. (2005). Time spent in face-to-face patient care and work outside the examination room. *Annals of Family Medicine,* 3, 6, 488–493.

Karmangar, F. & Emadi, A. (2012). Vitamin and mineral supplements: Do we really need them? *International Journal of Preventive Medicine,* 3, 3, 221–226.

Nutrition Business Journal (2012). *NBJ's Supplement Business Report.* New York: Penton Media.

Orrow, G. et al. (2012). Effectiveness of physical activity promotion based in primary care: Systemic review and meta-analysis of randomised controlled trials. *BMJ,* 3, 344, e1389.

Sanchez, A. et al. (2015). Effectiveness of physical activity promotion interventions in primary care: A review of reviews. *Preventive Medicine,* 7, 76 Suppl, S56–S67.

U.S. Preventive Services Task Force (2012). *The Guide to Clinical Preventive Services.* Rockville, Md.: Agency for Healthcare Research and Quality (www.ahrq.gov)

U.S. Preventive Services Task Force (1996). *The Guide to Clinical Preventive Services.* Rockville, Md.: Agency for Healthcare Research and Quality (www.ahrq.gov).

SUGGESTED READING

American College of Sports Medicine (2019). *ACSM's Health/Fitness Facility Standards and Guidelines* (5th ed.). Champaign, Ill.: Human Kinetics.

American College of Sports Medicine (2022). *ACSM's Guidelines for Exercise Testing and Prescription* (11th ed.). Philadelphia: Wolters Kluwer.

American College of Sports Medicine (2016). *ACSM's Exercise Management for Persons with Chronic Disease and Disabilities* (4th ed.). Champaign, Ill.: Human Kinetics.

American College of Sports Medicine (1998). AHA/ACSM joint statement: Recommendations for cardiovascular screening, staffing, and emergency policies at health/fitness facilities. *Medicine & Science in Sports & Exercise*, 30, 6, 7–8.

American Council on Exercise (2020). *The Exercise Professional's Guide to Personal Training.* San Diego: American Council on Exercise.

American Council on Exercise (2019). *The Professional's Guide to Health and Wellness Coaching.* San Diego: American Council on Exercise.

Barnes, P.M. & Schoenborn, C.A. (2012). *Trends in Adults Receiving a Recommendation for Exercise or Other Physical Activity from a Physician or Other Health Professional.* National Center for Health Statistics data brief, No. 86. Hyattsville, MD: National Center for Health Statistics.

Koh, H.K. & Sebelius, K.G. (2010). Promoting prevention through the Affordable Care Act. *New England Journal of Medicine,* 363, 1296–1299.

Medline Plus Reference on Drugs and Supplements (A service of the National Library of Medicine and National Institutes of Health) www.medlineplus.gov.

Tabor's Cyclopedic Medical Dictionary (23rd ed.) (2017). Philadelphia: F.A. Davis Co.

2 APPLYING THE ACE INTEGRATED FITNESS TRAINING® MODEL IN THE MEDICAL EXERCISE SETTING

IN THIS CHAPTER

FUNCTION–HEALTH–FITNESS–PERFORMANCE CONTINUUM

ACE IFT MODEL OVERVIEW
A CLIENT-CENTERED APPROACH
CARDIORESPIRATORY TRAINING
MUSCULAR TRAINING

SUMMARY

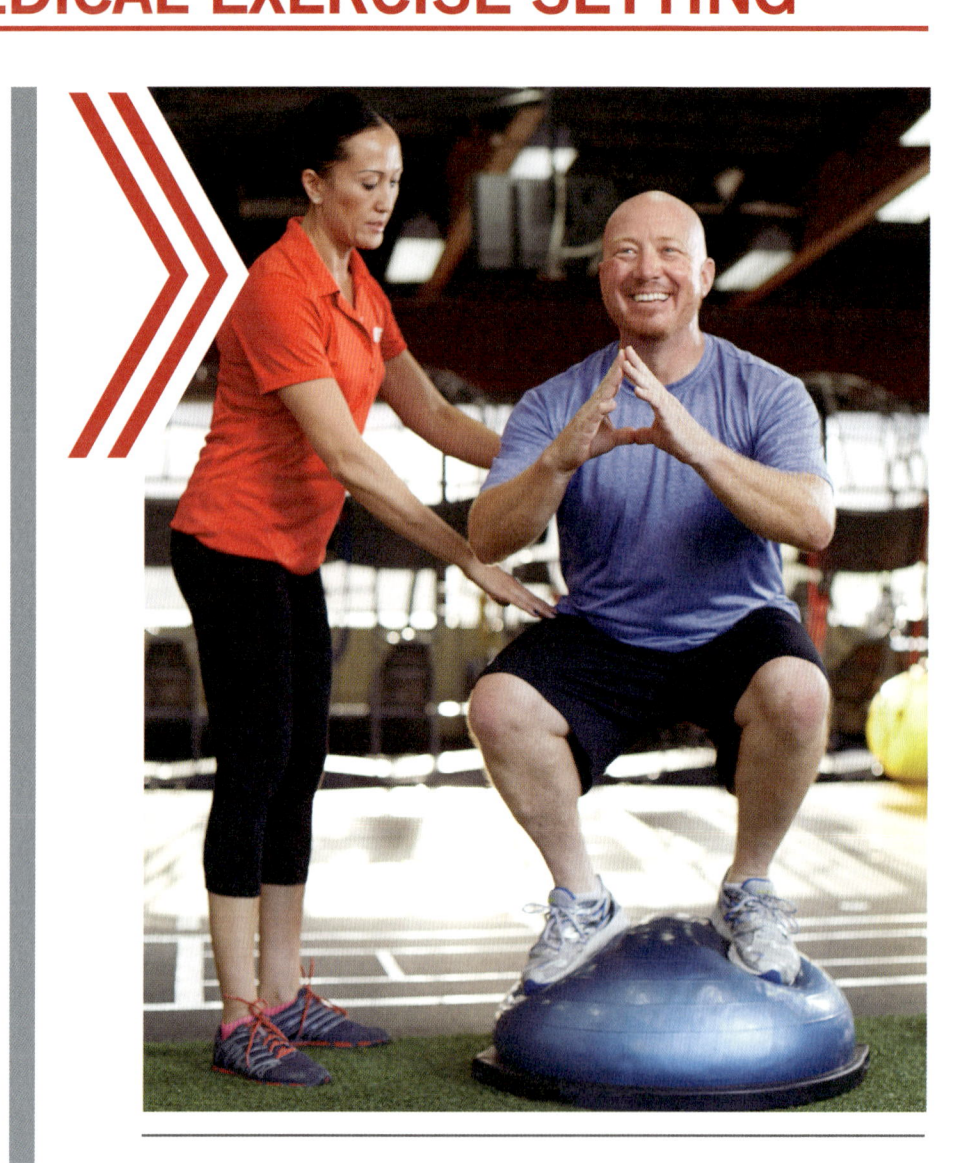

ABOUT THE AUTHOR

Todd Galati, M.A., is the Senior Director of Standards and Practice Advancement for the American Council on Exercise. He holds a bachelor's degree in athletic training, a master's degree in kinesiology, and four ACE certifications (Certified Medical Exercise Specialist, Personal Trainer, Health Coach, and Group Fitness Instructor). Prior to joining ACE, Galati was a program director with the University of California, San Diego School of Medicine, where he researched the effectiveness of youth fitness programs in reducing risk for cardiovascular disease, obesity, and type 2 diabetes. Galati's experience includes teaching biomechanics, applied kinesiology, and anatomy classes at California State University, San Marcos and San Diego State University, working as a research physiologist with the U.S. Navy, personal training in medical fitness facilities, and coaching endurance athletes.

By Todd Galati, M.A., CMES

DURING THE PAST SEVERAL DECADES, THE ROLE of the exercise professional in healthcare has seen slow, steady growth. Recently, a new light has been shined on the importance of regular exercise as part of a comprehensive medical plan. Driven by evidence that exercise plays a critical role in improving function, fitness, and health in clients who have health conditions such as **obesity, hypertension, dyslipidemia, diabetes,** and **osteoarthritis,** fitness has become recognized as a key component of the healthcare solution for an aging and increasingly inactive population. All of this has created an increased need for well-qualified medical exercise professionals to provide exercise programs for clients with special needs.

The ACE Certified Medical Exercise Specialist (CMES) is an integral member of the healthcare team, serving as the medical exercise practitioner developing and delivering specific and complementary programming in collaboration with other healthcare providers. The CMES has expertise in conducting assessments and designing comprehensive health and fitness programs to help clients prevent and manage disease, avoid injuries, improve overall wellness and function, and return to desired activities following rehabilitation. The CMES applies the principles of exercise science, health coaching, nutrition, psychology, and pathophysiology to develop health and fitness programs for clients with clinical issues (e.g., cardiovascular, pulmonary, metabolic, and musculoskeletal).

A CMES must be prepared to work with clients who have one or more health conditions that require specialized exercise programming. Often, when clients have more than one special need, the secondary health issue is related to the client's primary medical condition. The National Heart, Lung, and Blood Institute (NHLBI) has reported some well-recognized associations between obesity and risk factors for **cardiovascular disease (CVD).** In individuals who had **type 2 diabetes mellitus (T2DM),** hypertension, or dyslipidemia, the percentage of those subjects who also had **overweight** or obesity was 82%, 85%, and 84%, respectively (NHLBI, 1998). Evidence suggests that CVD, T2DM, and the **metabolic syndrome** are all linked to the proinflammatory state associated with abdominal obesity (Lee & Pratley, 2007; Wisse, 2004; Fasshauer & Paschke, 2003).

At the same time, advancements in health coaching and behavioral science have resulted in knowledge, skills, and abilities that the CMES can apply to help build client **self-efficacy** and fuel exercise program **adherence.** This has led to advances that have shifted the focus from more traditional training parameters to greater emphasis on contemporary training parameters, resulting in a client-centered approach to exercise programming to effectively address each client's needs and goals (Table 2-1).

Exercise professionals are well aware that the benefits of exercise include improved health, fitness, mood, weight management, stress management, and other health-related parameters. The *Physical Activity Guidelines for Americans* reinforce these positive benefits by acknowledging that regular exercise is a critical component of good health and that individuals can reduce their risk of developing **chronic disease** by staying physically active and participating in structured exercise on a regular basis (U.S. Department of Health & Human Services, 2018).

LEARNING OBJECTIVES:

» Define the function–health–fitness–performance continuum and how it applies to all clients, regardless of health limitations or fitness level.

» Explain the general recommendations for cardiorespiratory and muscular training exercise for healthy adults.

» Describe the ACE Integrated Fitness Training (ACE IFT) Model and its application to clients across the entire function–health–fitness–performance continuum.

» Specify how rapport and behavior-change strategies fit within the ACE IFT Model.

» Explain the phases of the two ACE IFT Model training components: Cardiorespiratory Training and Muscular Training.

TABLE 2-1
TRADITIONAL TRAINING PARAMETERS VERSUS CONTEMPORARY TRAINING PARAMETERS

Traditional Training Parameters	Contemporary Training Parameters	
Cardiorespiratory (aerobic) fitness Muscular endurance Muscular strength Flexibility	Health-behavior change Postural (kinetic chain) stability Kinetic chain mobility Movement efficiency Core conditioning Balance Cardiorespiratory (aerobic and anaerobic) fitness	Metabolic markers (ventilatory thresholds) Muscular endurance Muscular strength Flexibility Agility, coordination, and reaction time Speed and power

The second edition of the *Physical Activity Guidelines for Americans* expands on the previous edition by providing key guidelines for preschool-aged children, children and adolescents, adults, older adults, women during pregnancy and the postpartum period, adults with chronic health conditions, and adults with disabilities. The key guidelines suggest that adults should move more and sit less throughout the day. For substantial health benefits, adults should do at least 150 minutes a week of moderate-intensity cardiorespiratory physical activity, 75 minutes a week of vigorous-intensity aerobic physical activity, or an equivalent combination of the two (U.S. Department of Health & Human Services, 2018). In addition, adults should participate in muscle-strengthening activities of at least moderate intensity, involving all major muscle groups, on two or more days per week (U.S. Department of Health & Human Services, 2018). While the latest *Guidelines* endorse exercise as a means to achieving good health, they do not provide specific instructions for *how* to exercise.

The American College of Sports Medicine (ACSM, 2022) publishes general evidence-based recommendations for cardiorespiratory exercise [noted as aerobic (cardiovascular endurance) exercise in its publication] and muscular-training exercise (noted as resistance training it its publication). While these guidelines provide broad ranges for exercise frequency, intensity, time, and type (FITT), they do not provide specific instructions for *how* to exercise. In addition, there are exercise guidelines for many specific groups, including youth, older adults, women during pregnancy and the postpartum period, and people who have obesity, hypertension, **hyperlipidemia, osteoporosis,** and a variety of other chronic disease conditions and health considerations. These guidelines are based on medical and scientific research, are published by the governing body for each respective group, and provide specific exercise recommendations to help individuals engage in physical activity safely and effectively in order to improve their health and quality of life.

So, how does a CMES pull it all together? How does a novice or even an experienced CMES know what type of initial exercise program is appropriate for each client; if and when fitness assessments are beneficial; how to address foundational movement, balance, or postural issues; and how to progress or modify a program based on observed and reported feedback? To address these questions and more, the American Council on Exercise® (ACE) developed the ACE Integrated Fitness Training (ACE IFT®) Model to provide the CMES with a systematic and comprehensive approach to training that integrates exercise programming and progressions with a client-centered approach to facilitate health-behavior changes, while also improving posture, movement, **flexibility,** balance, core function, cardiorespiratory fitness, and **muscular fitness** (**muscular strength** and **muscular endurance**). To gain an understanding of the ACE IFT Model, it is helpful to first review the full continuum of human movement and fitness.

Applying the ACE Integrated Fitness Training Model® in the Medical Exercise Setting   CHAPTER 2

FUNCTION–HEALTH–FITNESS–PERFORMANCE CONTINUUM

The function–health–fitness–performance continuum is based on the premise that human movement and fitness can progress and regress along a spectrum that starts with developing or reestablishing basic functional movements and extends to performing highly advanced and specialized movements and physical work seen in athletics (Figure 2-1). Each individual is at a unique point on this continuum based upon factors that include health status and physical limitations; frequency, intensity, and types of physical activities; and any participation in, and goals for, athletic performance. Both lifecycle and lifestyle factors can influence where an individual currently falls on the continuum.

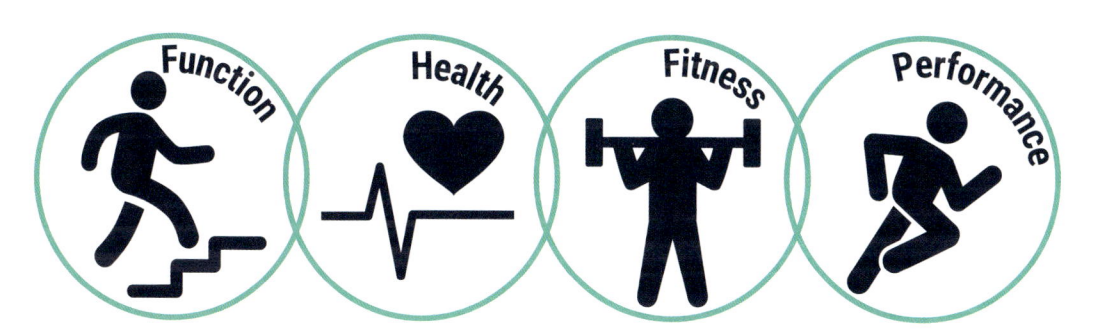

Figure 2-1
The function–health–fitness–performance continuum

Lifecycle factors include infant and child development, adolescent and pubescent growth spurts, adulthood, pregnancy, and aging. Early child development is focused primarily on gaining the strength, **stability,** and balance to perform basic human functional movements like holding one's head up, rolling over, sitting, crawling, standing, and eventually taking first steps. As children grow, their movements help them to build healthier bodies and develop the fitness to jump, climb, and run longer and faster. As adolescents and teens, human development includes considerable skeletal growth and muscular development. This developmental progression helps people progress from low-functioning infants to young adults who have good health, fitness, and even some performance-related skills and abilities. Unfortunately, far too often, lifestyle factors (e.g., smoking, excessive alcohol consumption, poor nutrition, and inadequate sleep and physical activity) disrupt natural human development, resulting in individuals regressing along the continuum to where they are less fit, are at risk for, or have, chronic disease and other health issues, and may even have impaired functional movement.

While the function–health–fitness–performance continuum is not a training method, the CMES can utilize this concept to understand that clients ebb and flow along this continuum based on the lifecycle and lifestyle factors that are impacting, positively or negatively, their opportunities for, and participation in, physical activity. The CMES can help clients progress along this continuum by meeting them where they are and providing personalized exercise programs and coaching based on each client's current health, fitness, and goals.

A CMES working with a client who has difficulties performing **activities of daily living (ADL)** should first establish goals aimed at helping the client improve basic functional movements. If a client has been insufficiently active for an extended period or is at risk for health issues, the CMES should provide the client with personalized programming that improves both health and functional movements. A CMES working with clients who have adequate functional movements and health can help them to improve fitness and, if appropriate, incorporate performance-related exercises.

CHAPTER 2
Applying the ACE Integrated Fitness Training® Model in the Medical Exercise Setting

ACE IFT MODEL OVERVIEW

Meeting each client's personalized needs can be a welcome challenge for an experienced CMES—and at the same time a potentially confusing and frustrating endeavor for a newly certified exercise professional. While the function–health–fitness–performance continuum provides a suggested sequence for training clients ranging from physically inactive to performance-oriented, it does not address the individual components of fitness and how they fit together.

The ACE IFT Model is a comprehensive system for exercise programming that pulls together the multifaceted training parameters required to be a successful exercise professional. It organizes the latest exercise science and health-behavior research into a systematic approach to designing, implementing, and modifying exercise programs based on the unique abilities, needs, and goals of each individual. Since its launch in 2010, the ACE IFT Model has evolved to incorporate new evidence-based practices in fitness assessments, exercise programming, and coaching skills. It has also evolved, based on user feedback, into a model that is just as robust in terms of science, content, and comprehensive programming, while being simplified in its presentation and terminology.

The ACE IFT Model has two training components:
- Cardiorespiratory Training
- Muscular Training

Each training component has three phases that are named to accurately reflect the training focus of each phase (Figure 2-2). The two training components of the ACE IFT Model are structured based on evidence-based exercise programming and progressions, along with associated fitness and functional assessments, that produce physiological adaptations to exercise that improve function,

Figure 2-2
ACE Integrated Fitness Training Model

ACE→ Integrated Fitness Training® Model

Cardiorespiratory Training
- PERFORMANCE
- FITNESS
- BASE

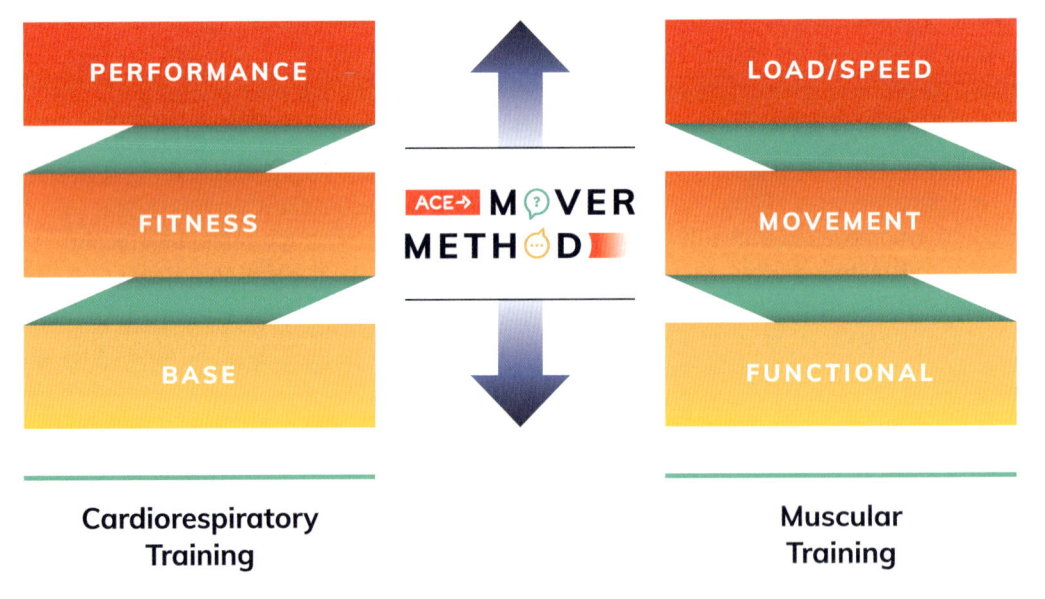

ACE→ MOVER METHOD

Muscular Training
- LOAD/SPEED
- MOVEMENT
- FUNCTIONAL

health, fitness, and performance. The training components are independent of each other, allowing for the integration of any Cardiorespiratory Training phase with any Muscular Training phase to meet the personalized health and fitness goals and capabilities of each client. This adaptable programming allows the ACE IFT Model to be used with everyone from previously physically inactive clients who have limited exercise experience to high-performance endurance athletes who have poor postural stability and seasoned weight lifters who have low cardiorespiratory fitness.

The ACE IFT Model also provides exercise professionals with tools and methods to help clients make fitness-related behavior changes that facilitate physical-activity participation and adherence to make lasting improvements in health and well-being.

RESTORING FUNCTION ORIGINALLY GAINED DURING HUMAN DEVELOPMENT

EXPAND YOUR KNOWLEDGE

Human development provides a framework for gaining a more comprehensive understanding of the ACE IFT Model's two principal training components: muscular training and cardiorespiratory training. The phases of these training components are designed to give health and exercise professionals the knowledge and skills to appropriately provide assessments, programs, and progressions that help clients move from where they currently are to where they want to be. To gain a better understanding of the phases of each training component, it is helpful to take a closer look at how people gain and lose functional movement and cardiorespiratory fitness in the first place.

The foundations of human movement include mobile joints, muscular function to initiate and control movements, and endurance for sustained efforts. Birth itself requires newborns to have highly mobile joints. This is facilitated by a developing skeleton that includes long bones with slightly pliable ends, irregular and flat bones that are in segments (e.g., the skull) with fibrous connections that will later become ossified, developing articular surfaces at the joints, and soft tissue that is highly elastic.

Following birth, human movements are small and repeated, driven by genetic coding aimed at gaining the strength and neuromuscular control required to stabilize the skeleton. Early achievements of infants include lifting and controlling the head while in prone and upright positions, reaching for and grasping objects, and pushing with the legs. These neuromuscular developments progress over the first 12 to 18 months of life to include rolling over, sitting up, getting into quadruped position (on all fours), crawling, standing, and eventually walking. Each new accomplishment builds on previous neuromuscular achievements. As walking progresses from initial steps to walking longer distances, the cardiorespiratory system and locomotive muscles develop endurance to sustain and advance this movement. Over time, movement patterns are combined and muscular strength increases to meet the demands of moving and controlling a body that is in a state of rapid growth. As development continues, muscular and cardiovascular endurance must be developed to support and enhance sustained movements. It is during these early stages of development that humans first gain the function that should sustain them throughout life as the foundation for performance of ADL and the platform upon which individuals build health and fitness.

Throughout childhood, muscular strength and endurance increase to meet the demands posed by the growing body and essential movements that include running, jumping, hopping, climbing, swinging, skipping, throwing, catching, and swimming. As children play, they develop the cardiorespiratory fitness to play longer and run faster. Human development is programmed to help highly mobile newborns gain the strength and stability necessary to progress to the movement patterns that are the foundation of Movement Training. Growth provides the early stimuli required to progressively increase the loads placed on the human body that are replicated by Load/Speed Training.

Cardiorespiratory fitness is first gained by infants performing continual movements of increasing duration that require additional oxygen and nutrients to be delivered to the working muscles. This load increases little by little in order to build the aerobic base required for sustained human movements at moderate intensity. As children's games increase in duration and intensity, they begin performing and progressing aerobic intervals that are the key stimuli required to build cardiorespiratory fitness.

The development that occurs as children meet the expanding movement and cardiorespiratory challenges that are categorized in both Fitness Training and Movement Training give youth the foundation for healthy and active lives. Unfortunately, somewhere between adolescence and adulthood many people lose what they were born to be: a mobile human with relatively effective functional movement and cardiorespiratory endurance. Physical inactivity and too many hours spent in seated positions are root causes, leading to lost joint mobility, decreased joint stability, postural issues, and poor movement patterns. This is exacerbated by reductions in cardiorespiratory fitness, making it more difficult to sustain the physical work required to perform jobs, keep up with children, and participate in activities that were previously achievable and enjoyable.

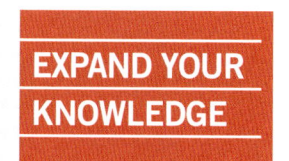

It is important to keep all of this in mind when working with clients, as most of them once possessed much of the stability, **mobility**, movement, and cardiorespiratory fitness that they now want and need to regain. For many clients, the initial goals will be to help them recover what has been lost so they can initiate and control movements (stability and mobility) with good posture and desired movement patterns, while also helping them gain the aerobic base and then aerobic efficiency required of their goal activities. The hurdles faced by each client will be unique, just as when the client gained these neuromuscular skills and cardiorespiratory fitness the first time. From there, movement, strength, and cardiorespiratory fitness can be progressed as the CMES helps the client make physical activity a regular part of their life.

Only clients who have competitive or performance-oriented goals will progress to advanced levels of programming in Performance and Load/Speed Training. This is similar for youth participating in organized physical activities of higher intensity and competitive sports. Over time, even people who have trained for years in Performance and Load/Speed Training may begin to regress to Fitness and Movement Training as they age and no longer train for competitive performance.

It is always important to look at clients in each training component of the ACE IFT Model, as injuries (e.g., low-back or orthopedic), illness (e.g., coronary artery disease or arthritis), or years of specialized training (e.g., running or bodybuilding) can lead to imbalances in one component that require training in an earlier phase than in the other. It is also critical to assess each client's current phases and readiness for change, as that is the starting point (where they are today) and helps define what is possible for them as they aim to reach both short- and long-term goals. It is always important to meet people where they are versus trying to move them to where the CMES believes they should go. This especially applies to people as they age, recover from injuries or medical treatments, have chronic health conditions, or live with illness, as they may no longer have interest in focusing on fitness. They may instead want to focus all training on improving their quality of life and function in ADL.

A key thing to remember is that cardiorespiratory fitness and functional movement are gained throughout the normal development process, and then are impaired or lost due to physical inactivity, injury, illness, and aging. Health and exercise professionals can apply the assessments, programming, and progressions in the ACE IFT Model to help clients regain fitness and function, and to achieve many physical and performance goals. Before jumping into physical programming, be sure to determine the client's readiness for change, provide motivation and encouragement, and build a program with achievable and meaningful small goals that can provide regular successes that build self-efficacy and drive adherence.

A Client-centered Approach

The greatest impact that a CMES can regularly have on the lives of their clients is to help them positively change health-related behaviors and establish positive relationships with exercise. For this reason, the client–CMES relationship is the foundation of the ACE IFT Model. It is built upon **rapport,** trust, and **empathy,** with the CMES serving as a "coach" to the client throughout their physical activity and health behavior-change journey. This approach starts with realizing that the "client" is the first person in the client–CMES relationship. Clients are paying the CMES for an important service: to guide them through a personalized journey to improve health and fitness and to reach their unique goals.

ACE→ MOVER METHOD

Introducing the ACE Mover Method™ Philosophy and ACE ABC Approach™

A key element of using the ACE IFT Model to empower clients to make behavioral changes to improve their health, fitness, and overall quality of life is the adoption of the ACE Mover Method, which is founded on the following tenets:
- Each professional interaction is client-centered, with a recognition that clients are the foremost experts on themselves.
- Powerful open-ended questions and active listening are utilized in every session with clients.
- Clients are genuinely viewed as resourceful and capable of change.

ACE → ABC APPROACH

Exercise professionals can easily apply the ACE Mover Method through the ACE ABC Approach:
- **A**sk open-ended questions
- **B**reak down barriers
- **C**ollaborate

Every client–CMES interaction offers an opportunity to utilize coaching skills to help build rapport while positioning the client as an active partner in their behavior-change journey. Asking questions leads to the identification of goals and options for breaking down barriers, which in turn leads to collaborating on next steps. The ACE Mover Method provides the foundational skills for communicating effectively with clients, but it is not the equivalent of a health coaching certification. The CMES should work in concert with other professionals, such as health coaches and **registered dietitians** and other allied health professionals, whenever appropriate, to take a team approach to improving their clients' health and wellness.

Step 1 of this process involves asking powerful questions to identify what the client hopes to accomplish by working with an exercise professional and what, if any, physical activities the client enjoys. Open-ended questions are the key to sparking this discussion.

Step 2 involves asking more questions to discover what potential barriers may get in the way of the client reaching their specific goals. Questions like "What do you need to *start* doing now to move closer to your goals?" and "What do you need to *stop* doing that will enable you to reach your goals?" can be very revealing.

Step 3 is all about collaboration as the client and exercise professional work together to set **SMART goals** and establish specific steps to take action toward those goals. Allowing the client to lead the discussion of how to monitor and measure progress empowers them to take ownership of their personal behavior-change journey.

Clients want to know that the CMES cares about them. This is similar to what individuals seek when hiring the services of other professionals who have an impact on their quality of life, and it is at the heart of a client-centered approach. From physicians to financial planners, people will continue to work with the same professional if they can see that the professional truly cares about them and their health, whether it be physical or financial. Clients should already have a belief that the CMES they hire has the knowledge, skills, and abilities to help them reach their goals. With rare exception, they do not care to hear *all* the science, training methods, and other health-related information that the CMES knows. Instead, they want to hear that their CMES is invested in them. A successful CMES keeps the conversation focused on the client. They have paid for the session, so it is their time.

Building rapport is a critical component of a client-centered approach, as this process promotes open communication, develops trust, and fosters the client's desire to participate in an exercise program. Rapport should be developed early through open communication and initial positive experiences with exercise, and then enhanced through behavioral strategies that help build long-term adherence.

A primary goal of every session should be to have the client wanting to return for the next session. Starting with the first session, the CMES should include exercise programming that provides an appropriate level of challenge for the client at that time. Exercises and intensities should provide an adequate yet achievable level of challenge, and progressions should be appropriately matched to the gains that the client has made since the last session.

Fitness assessments, once thought to be a mandatory starting point for any exercise program, are not actually necessary for many clients. This should not be confused with health screening, which should be conducted with each client to determine if they have any limitations for, or should receive medical clearance prior to, exercise participation. Before conducting a fitness assessment with a client, it is important to determine if the assessment is necessary to help the client reach their goals, and if the client is interested in completing the fitness assessment.

The ACE IFT Model provides the CMEs with the option to either conduct evidence-based fitness assessments or lead clients through early sessions that incorporate exercise programming that delivers appropriate movement and fitness challenges while also providing the CMES with valuable feedback about a client's current postural stability, joint mobility, functional movement, balance, cardiorespiratory fitness, and muscular fitness. Early training sessions that include exercises that provide "assessment" information can be the key to success for many clients by helping them to get moving right away. They also provide the CMES with useful information to help them modify each client's program during subsequent sessions to build on that success.

APPLY WHAT YOU KNOW

FACILITATING BEHAVIORAL CHANGE

Applying behavior-change strategies in the design and delivery of comprehensive exercise programs that help clients reach their unique fitness and wellness goals is a primary function performed by a successful CMES. Some of the key steps that facilitate fitness-related health-behavior change include:

- Implementing strategies for developing and enhancing rapport
- Identifying each client's readiness to change behavior and stage of behavior change
- Creating a caring, supportive climate in which a client's motivation can flourish
- Fostering exercise adherence by creating positive exercise experiences that build self-efficacy
- Determining the need for, and appropriate selection and timing of, assessments and reassessments
- Designing, leading, and modifying exercise programs based on each client's current health and fitness status, needs, and goals
- Fostering a sense of self-reliance to empower clients to take ownership of their lifestyle changes
- Utilizing appropriate strategies to help clients transition from one stage of behavior change to the next
- Implementing **relapse**-prevention strategies
- Helping clients transition from **extrinsic motivation** to **intrinsic motivation**
- Establishing realistic short- and long-term goals to prevent discouragement and/or burnout, providing multiple opportunities for success and promoting adherence
- Factoring a client's external stressors into total fatigue to avoid training plateaus and prevent **overtraining syndrome**
- Empowering clients by helping them increase self-efficacy and knowledge to train on their own
- Supporting clients in making physical activity a life-long habit

Cardiorespiratory Training

The *2018 Physical Activity Guidelines for Americans,* as well as guidelines from the World Health Organization (WHO), provide comprehensive evidence-based recommendations to reduce the risk of many adverse health outcomes (WHO, 2020; U.S. Department of Health & Human Services, 2018). Many of the recommendations are derived from the knowledge that most health benefits occur with at least 150 minutes a week of moderate-intensity cardiorespiratory activity and that the benefits of physical activity far outweigh the possibility of adverse outcomes. Specific guidelines for adults aged 18 to 64 include the following:

- Any amount of physical activity is more desirable when compared to none. Additionally, a concerted effort should be made to sit less throughout the day.
- Perform 150 to 300 minutes per week of moderate-intensity cardiorespiratory physical activity, or 75 to 150 minutes per week of vigorous-intensity cardiorespiratory physical activity, or a combination of both. Additional health benefits are obtained from performing greater amounts of activity than these quantities.
- Participate in muscle-strengthening activities involving all major muscle groups at least two days per week.

Applying the ACE Integrated Fitness Training Model® in the Medical Exercise Setting

With regard to cardiorespiratory programming, however, widely accepted guidelines for physical activity and basic fitness training are presented by ACSM and the American Heart Association (AHA). These guidelines frequently use the FITT acronym to discuss cardiorespiratory programming (ACSM, 2022; Haskell et al., 2007). Additionally, clients should always enjoy the exercise experience, as this influences the thoughts and emotions that can ultimately dictate participation and adherence rates. Frequency, intensity, and duration collectively represent the exercise volume, load, or magnitude of training that is likely to provoke the physiological adaptations to the training response. A **dose-response relationship** exists between volume and the health/fitness benefits achieved, implying that greater benefits are achieved with increased volumes.

The CMES generally progresses and patterns their clients' programs by manipulating these variables (i.e., frequency, intensity, time, and type) (Table 2-2). The rate of program progression depends on each client's individual health status, exercise tolerance, available time, and program goals. Improvement in cardiorespiratory fitness occurs most quickly from progressive increases in exercise intensity and fades when training intensity is reduced. Changes in fitness are more sensitive to changes in intensity than to changes in the frequency or duration of training.

TABLE 2-2
AEROBIC (CARDIOVASCULAR ENDURANCE) EXERCISE RECOMMENDATIONS

FITT	Recommendation
Frequency	• At least 3 days/week • For most adults, spreading the exercise sessions across 3–5 days/week may be the best most conducive strategy to reach the recommended amounts of physical activity.
Intensity	• Moderate (40–59% HRR) and/or vigorous (60–89% HRR) intensity is recommended for most adults.
Time	• Most adults should accumulate 30–60 minutes/day (≥150 minutes/week) of moderate-intensity exercise, 20–60 minutes/day (≥75 minutes/week) of vigorous-intensity exercise, or a combination of moderate- and vigorous-intensity exercise daily to attain the recommended targeted volumes of exercise.
Type	• Aerobic exercise performed in a continuous or intermittent manner that involves major muscle groups is recommended for most adults.

Note: HRR = Heart-rate reserve

Reprinted with permission from American College of Sports Medicine (2022). *ACSM's Guidelines for Exercise Testing and Prescription* (11th ed.). Philadelphia: Wolters Kluwer.

While programs following these guidelines have shown positive results for decades, they are subject to substantial errors in training intensities, as the training heart rates are calculated as percentages of predicted **maximal heart rates (MHR),** which have been shown to have standard deviations of approximately 12 beats per minute (bpm) using the long-standing equation of MHR = 220 – Age (Fox, Naughton, & Haskell, 1971), or closer to 7 bpm using newer formulas from Gellish et al. (2007) and Tanaka, Monahan, and Seals (2001).

Gellish et al.: Maximal heart rate = 206.9 – (0.67 x Age)
Tanaka, Monahan, and Seals: Maximal heart rate = 208 – (0.7 x Age)

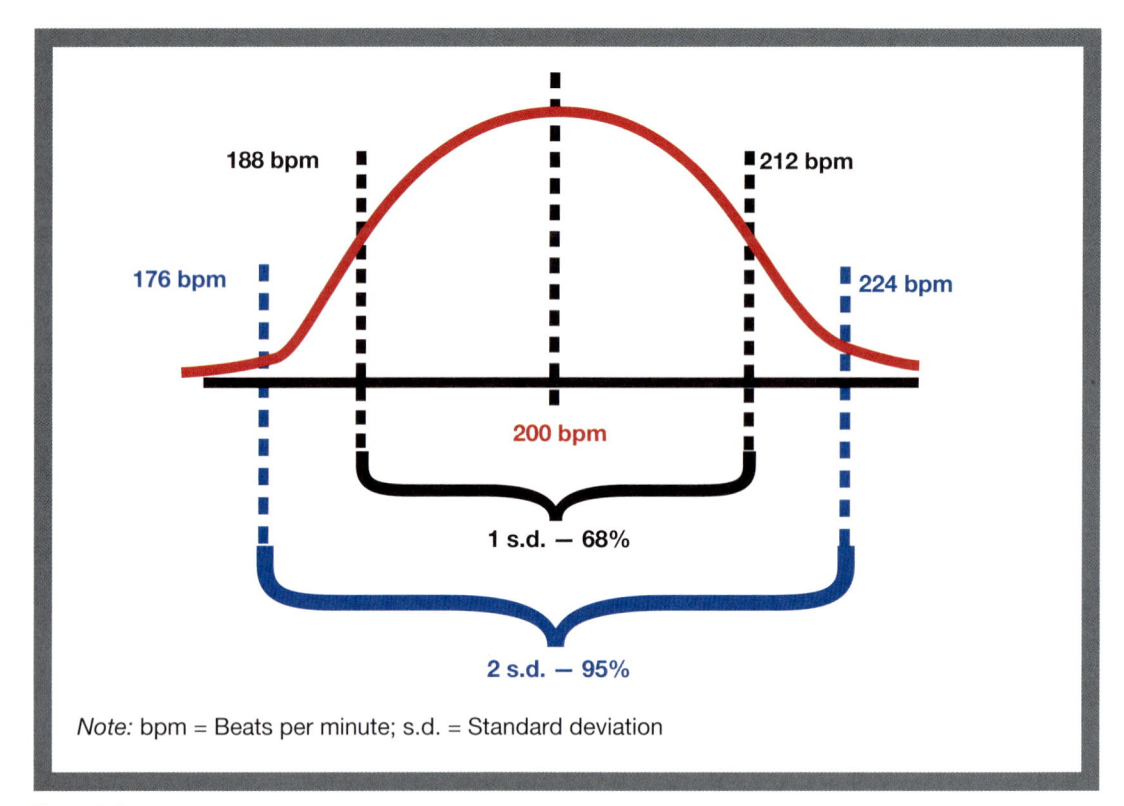

Figure 2-3
The standard deviation (i.e., 12 beats per minute) for the 220 – age maximal heart rate prediction equation for 20 year olds

In practical terms, this means that 95% of the population, represented by ±2 standard deviations from the estimate, has a true MHR that is ±14 bpm from the predicted MHR using the Gellish et al. or Tanaka, Monahan, and Seals equations, or ±24 bpm using the Fox, Naughton, and Haskell equation (Figure 2-3). This error in predicted MHR becomes amplified when this value is used to calculate **target heart rate (THR)** ranges for cardiorespiratory exercise as either a direct percentage of MHR or using the Karvonen formula, which uses MHR and **resting heart rate (RHR)** to first calculate **heart-rate reserve (HRR),** then calculate THR as a percentage of HRR.

KARVONEN FORMULA
Heart-rate reserve = Maximal heart rate – Resting heart rate
Target heart rate = (Heart-rate reserve x % intensity) + Resting heart rate

Approaches that use a relative percent of predicted MHR, HRR, or even predicted $\dot{V}O_2max$ or $\dot{V}O_2reserve$ ($\dot{V}O_2R$), are essentially flawed, as they do not take into account the individual metabolic responses to exercise. Instead, exercise programming can be tailored to each client's unique metabolic markers to improve health, fitness, and performance by identifying and using the client's **heart rate (HR)** at the **first ventilatory threshold (VT1)** and **second ventilatory threshold (VT2).** These metabolic markers are the recommended intensity markers around which exercise programs are designed in the different cardiorespiratory training phases of the ACE IFT Model. There are many different exercise intensity markers that can be used to delineate moderate- from vigorous-intensity exercise, or vigorous from very vigorous (anaerobic) exercise, and to develop programs using the cardiorespiratory phases of the ACE IFT Model; however, HR at VT1 and VT2, the **talk test,** and **rating of perceived exertion (RPE)** using the Borg 6 to 20 scale or the 0 to 10 category ratio scale are the recommended methods, as they are more accurate and enable unique programming for each client.

Applying the ACE Integrated Fitness Training Model® in the Medical Exercise Setting **CHAPTER 2**

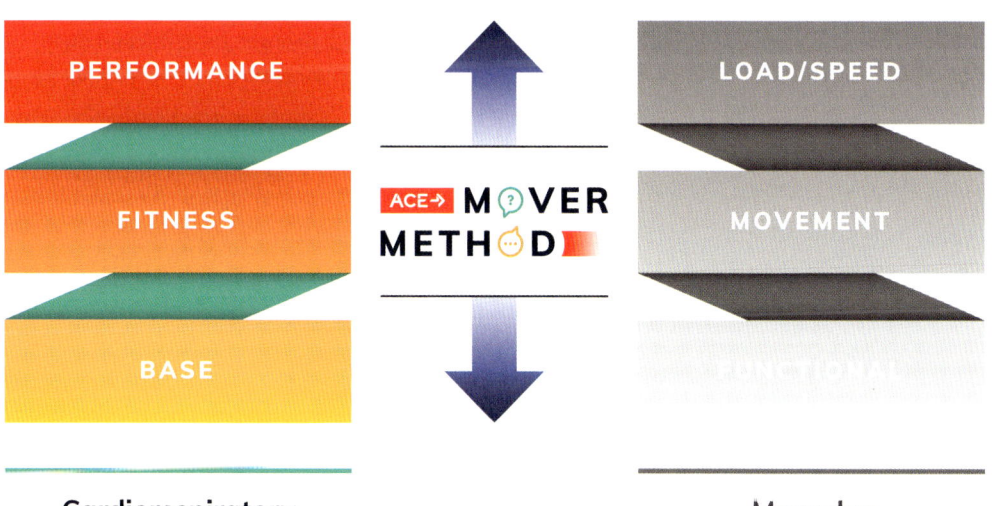

> **EXPAND YOUR KNOWLEDGE**
>
> **UNDERSTANDING THE NOMENCLATURE**
>
> Many texts use varied terminology related to the metabolic markers used to describe the physiological response to cardiorespiratory exercise. In this manual, VT1 and VT2 are used, but it is important that the CMES be able to recognize the other terms when reviewing the literature:
> - VT1 is also referred to as the **lactate threshold** and the anaerobic threshold
> - VT2 is also referred to as the respiratory compensation threshold and the **onset of blood lactate accumulation (OBLA)**
>
> Another potential source of confusion involves the term "anaerobic threshold," which has come to mean different things in various parts of the world based on the way it was used in early research on the topic. This is another reason ACE has chosen to utilize VT1 and VT2 throughout this manual.

The ACE IFT Model provides a systematic approach to cardiorespiratory training that can help move a client all the way from being physically inactive to training for a personal record in an event like a half marathon. While this will not be a training goal of most previously physically inactive individuals, having an organized system of training that can allow for long-term progression is empowering for the CMES because it provides them with strategies for training the entire spectrum of clientele—from the physically inactive person to the competitive athlete.

The Cardiorespiratory Training component of the ACE IFT Model is divided into three phases, each with a title that defines its training focus (Figure 2-4).

Figure 2-4
ACE IFT Model Cardiorespiratory Training phases

Clients are categorized into a given phase based on their current health, fitness levels, and goals. By utilizing the assessment and programming tools in each phase, the CMES can develop individualized cardiorespiratory programs for clients ranging from **sedentary** to endurance athletes. Programming in each phase will be based on the three-zone training model shown in Figure 2-5, using HR at VT1 and VT2 to develop individualized programs based on each client's metabolic responses to exercise. It is important to note that training principles in the ACE IFT Model's Cardiorespiratory Training phases can be implemented by a CMES using various exercise intensity markers, including ones based on predicted values such as %HRR or %MHR, but the exercise intensities will not be as accurate for individual clients as when they utilize measured HR at VT1 and VT2 (Table 2-3).

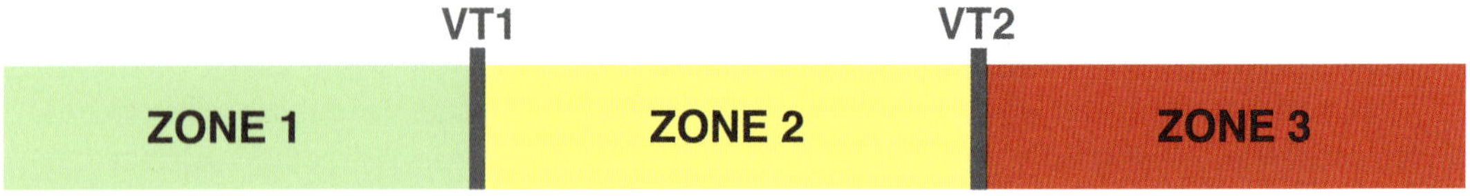

Figure 2-5
Three-zone intensity model

```
              VT1                    VT2
    ZONE 1    |       ZONE 2          |    ZONE 3
```

Note: VT1 = First ventilatory threshold; VT2 = Second ventilatory threshold

TABLE 2-3
THREE-ZONE INTENSITY MODEL USING VARIOUS INTENSITY MARKERS

Intensity Markers		Zone 1	Zone 2	Zone 3	Advantages/Limitations
Category terminology for exercise programming	Light	Moderate	Vigorous	Near maximal/ maximal	
Metabolic markers: VT1 and VT2* (HR relative to VT1 and VT2)*		Below VT1 (HR <VT1)	VT1 to just below VT2 (HR ≥VT1 to <VT2)	VT2 and above (HR ≥VT2)	• Based on measured VT1 and VT2 • Ideally, VT1 and VT2 are measured in a lab with a metabolic cart and blood lactate • Field assessments are relatively easy to administer, require minimal equipment, and provide accurate corresponding HRs at VT1 and VT2 • Programming with metabolic markers allows for personalized programming
Talk test*		Can talk comfortably Can talk but not sing	Not sure if talking is comfortable Cannot say more than a few words without pausing for a breath	Definitely cannot talk comfortably	• Based on actual changes in ventilation due to physiological adaptations to increasing exercise intensities • Very easy for practical measurement • No equipment required • Can easily be taught to clients • Allows for personalized programming
RPE (terminology)*	Very, very weak to light	"Moderate" to "somewhat hard/strong"	"Hard/strong" to "very hard"	"Very strong to very, very hard/strong to maximal"	• Good subjective intensity marker • Correlates well with talk test, metabolic markers, and measured %$\dot{V}O_2$max • Easy to teach to clients
RPE (0 to 10 scale)*	0.5 to 2	3 to 4	5 to 6	7 to 10	• Good subjective intensity marker • Correlates well with talk test, metabolic markers, and measured %$\dot{V}O_2$max • 0 to 10 scale is easy to teach to clients
RPE (6 to 20 scale)	9 to 11	12 to 13	14 to 17	≥18	• Good subjective intensity marker • Correlates well with talk test, metabolic markers, and measured %$\dot{V}O_2$max • 6 to 20 scale is not as easy to teach to clients as the 0 to 10 scale • *Note:* An RPE of 20 represents maximal effort and cannot be sustained as a training intensity.

TABLE 2-3
THREE-ZONE INTENSITY MODEL USING VARIOUS INTENSITY MARKERS

Intensity Markers		Zone 1	Zone 2	Zone 3	Advantages/Limitations
%$\dot{V}O_2R$	30 to 39%	40 to 59%	60 to 89%	≥90%	• Requires *measured* $\dot{V}O_2$max for most accurate programming • Impractical due to expensive equipment needed for assessment • Increased error with use of *predicted* $\dot{V}O_2$max or *predicted* MHR • Relative percentages for programming are population-based and not individually specific
%HRR	30 to 39%	40 to 59%	60 to 89%	≥90%	• Requires *measured* MHR and RHR for most accurate programming • Measured MHR is impractical for the vast majority of trainers and clients • Use of RHR increases individuality of programming vs. strict %MHR • Use of *predicted* MHR introduces potentially large error; the magnitude of the error is dependent on the specific equation used • Relative percentages for programming are population-based and not individually specific
%MHR	57 to 63%	64 to 76%	77 to 95%	≥96%	• Requires *measured* MHR for accuracy in programming • Measured MHR is impractical for the vast majority of trainers and clients • Use of *predicted* MHR introduces potentially large error; the magnitude of the error is dependent on the specific equation used • Does not include RHR, as is used in %HRR • Relative percentages for programming are population-based and not individually specific
METs	2 to 2.9	3 to 5.9	6 to 8.7	≥8.8	• Requires *measured* $\dot{V}O_2$max for most accurate programming • Can use in programming more easily than other intensity markers based off $\dot{V}O_2$max • Limited in programming by knowledge of METs for given activities and/or equipment that gives MET estimates • Relative MET ranges for programming are population-based and not individually specific (e.g., a 5-MET activity might initially be perceived as vigorous by a previously sedentary client)
%$\dot{V}O_2$max	37 to 45%	46 to 63%	64 to 90%	≥91%	• Refer to %$\dot{V}O_2R$ • Actual measurement is individualized and not based on a prediction

Note: VT1 = First ventilatory threshold; VT2 = Second ventilatory threshold; HR = Heart rate; RPE = Rating of perceived exertion; $\dot{V}O_2$max = Maximal oxygen uptake; $\dot{V}O_2R$ = Oxygen uptake reserve; HRR = Heart-rate reserve; MHR = Maximal heart rate; RHR = Resting heart rate; METs = Metabolic equivalents

*These are the preferred intensity markers to use with the three-zone model when designing, implementing, and progressing cardiorespiratory training programs using the ACE Integrated Fitness Training Model.

Base Training

Base Training is focused on developing an initial aerobic base in clients who have been insufficiently active. This should not be confused with the "aerobic-base training" that is performed by endurance athletes as the foundation of their offseason training. Instead, it is focused on getting people to move consistently to establish basic cardiorespiratory endurance to improve health, energy, mood, and caloric expenditure and to serve as a foundation for progressing to Fitness Training.

Any client who is not consistently performing moderate-intensity cardiorespiratory exercise for bouts of at least 20 minutes on at least three days per week should begin with Base Training. The initial cardiorespiratory exercise performed should be of an appropriate duration and intensity that the client can tolerate. The CMES can learn about their clients' current cardiorespiratory exercise participation during the investigation stage of the client–CMES relationship. No cardiorespiratory assessments are recommended during the Base Training phase, since many of the clients who start in this phase will be unfit and may have difficulty completing an assessment of this nature.

A client who has been physically inactive for an extended period might only be able to initially perform five minutes of continuous cardiorespiratory exercise at a moderate or low-to-moderate intensity. In a scenario of this nature, the CMES should give the client positive feedback for completing the five-minute exercise bout, remind the client that bouts of physical activity of any length are beneficial in reducing health risks, and document the total time completed. This would serve as the client's baseline cardiorespiratory fitness data and the starting point for Cardiorespiratory Training progressions to build an aerobic base.

Regardless of the initial duration, the goal for all clients in Base Training is to create early positive exercise experiences to help clients become regular exercisers while gradually increasing exercise duration and frequency until the client is performing cardiorespiratory exercise three to five days per week for a duration of 20 minutes or more. The easiest method for monitoring intensity with clients during Base Training is to use the talk test. If the client can perform the exercise and talk comfortably, they are likely below VT1. When exercising below VT1, clients should be exercising at a moderate intensity classified by an RPE of 3 to 4 (0 to 10 scale).

Fitness Training

Fitness Training is focused on enhancing the client's aerobic efficiency by progressing the program through increased duration of sessions, increased frequency of sessions when possible, and the integration of exercise performed at and above VT1 (see Table 2-4, page 39). The inclusion of cardiorespiratory exercise performed at and above VT1 allows the CMES to blend moderate-intensity exercise (below VT1) with moderate- to vigorous-intensity exercise (at or above VT1 to just below VT2; RPE = 5 to 6 on the 0 to 10 scale) in a client's program to create variety and facilitate physiological adaptations leading to greater cardiorespiratory fitness levels. Both new and existing clients who can consistently perform moderate-intensity physical activity for bouts of 20 minutes or more on at least three days per week can perform Fitness Training. As with Base Training, the initial Fitness Training program should be performed at an appropriate duration, intensity, and frequency for the client based on their current level of exercise participation.

The CMES can incorporate intervals into exercise programs for clients with Fitness Training goals to add variety to individual sessions and to introduce more intense training stimuli to elicit desired physiological adaptations to exercise. The CMES should keep in mind each client's current cardiorespiratory fitness level when selecting interval intensities and durations to ensure that the increased challenge is appropriate for the client. By providing clients with intervals that offer increased yet achievable challenges, the CMES can help their clients simultaneously increase fitness and self-efficacy.

Individual goals for Fitness Training will vary greatly among clients. Those looking to improve fitness and overall health can benefit from increased exercise frequency, duration, and the introduction of intervals. Clients with goals for longer endurance events, such as completing a 10K run or a half marathon, will need to include some exercise sessions of longer duration to reach the total exercise duration required to complete the event. The CMES can help each client work toward their unique goals by manipulating training variables and then adjusting them regularly based on the client's progress, recovery, challenges, and timeline. Many clients will spend years focused on various cardiorespiratory goals within Fitness Training, while those with endurance performance–oriented goals should be progressed to Performance Training.

The CMES will select and administer cardiorespiratory fitness assessments according to each client's needs and desires using information obtained during the preparticipation health screening. Cardiorespiratory fitness assessments are also determined by a number of other factors, including availability of equipment, client lifestyles, time allotment, and the CMES's level of comfort with the assessment procedures. Recommendations for the specific timing of cardiorespiratory fitness assessments should be aligned with client goals.

During the administration of any exercise assessment involving exertion (e.g., cardiorespiratory or muscular endurance and/or muscular strength assessment), the CMES must always be aware of identifiable signs or symptoms that merit immediate assessment termination and possible referral to a qualified healthcare professional (ACSM, 2022). These signs and symptoms include:

- Onset of angina, chest pain, or angina-like symptoms
- Significant drop (≥10 mmHg) in **systolic blood pressure (SBP)** despite an increase in exercise intensity or a decrease in SBP below the value obtained in the same position prior to assessment
- Excessive rise in BP: SBP reaches >250 mmHg and/or **diastolic blood pressure (DBP)** reaches >115 mmHg
- Shortness of breath, wheezing (does not include heavy breathing due to intense exercise), leg cramps, or claudication
- Signs of poor **perfusion:** lightheadedness, confusion, **ataxia,** pallor (pale skin), **cyanosis** (bluish coloration, especially around the mouth), nausea, or cold and clammy skin
- Failure of HR to increase with increased exercise intensity
- Noticeable change in heart rhythm by **palpation** or **auscultation**
- Subject requests to stop
- Physical or verbal manifestations of severe fatigue
- Failure of assessment equipment

Ventilatory threshold assessment is based on the physiological principle of ventilation. During submaximal exercise, ventilation increases linearly with O_2 uptake and CO_2 production. This occurs primarily through an increase in **tidal volume.** At higher or near-maximal intensities, the frequency of breathing becomes more pronounced and **minute ventilation ($\dot{V}_E$)** rises disproportionately to the increase in O_2 uptake (Figure 2-6).

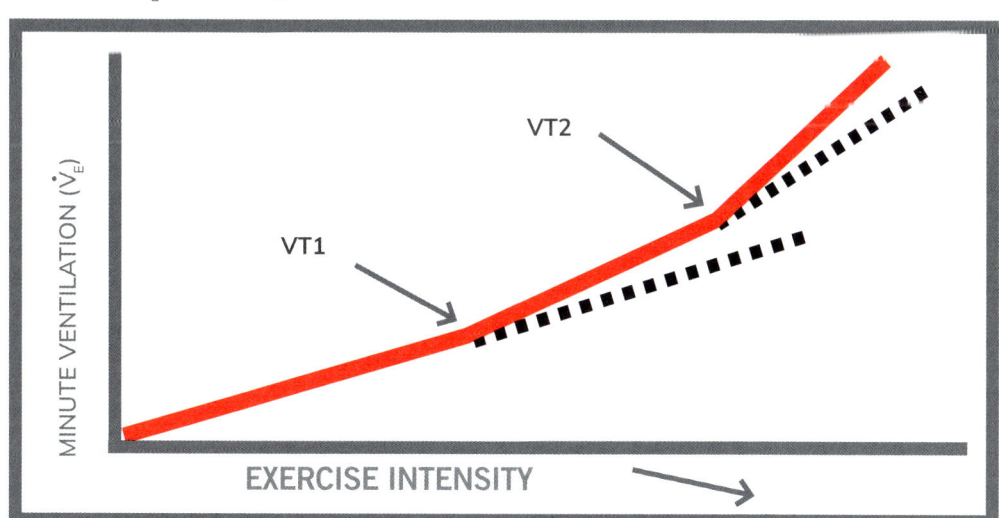

Figure 2-6
Ventilatory response to increasing exercise intensity

Note: VT1 = First ventilatory threshold; VT2 = Second ventilatory threshold

This disproportionate rise in breathing rate represents a state of ventilation that is no longer directly linked with O_2 demand at the cellular level and is generally termed the ventilatory threshold. The overcompensation in breathing frequency results from an increase in CO_2 production related to the **anaerobic glycolysis** that predominates during near-maximal-intensity exercise. During strenuous exercise, breathing frequency may increase from 12 to 15 breaths per minute at rest to 35 to 45 breaths per minute, while tidal volume increases from resting values of 0.4 to 1.0 L up to 3 L or greater (McArdle, Katch, & Katch, 2019).

As exercise intensity increases, ventilation increases in a somewhat linear manner, demonstrating deflection points at certain intensities associated with metabolic changes within the body. One point, called the "crossover" point, or VT1, represents a level of intensity at which blood lactate accumulates faster and must be offset by blood buffers, which are compounds that neutralize acidosis in the blood and muscle fibers. This metabolic change causes the person to alter breathing in an effort to blow off the extra CO_2 produced by the buffering of acid metabolites. The cardiorespiratory challenge to the body at this point lies primarily with inspiration and not with the expiration of additional amounts of CO_2 (associated with buffering lactate in the blood). The need for O_2 is met primarily through an increase in tidal volume and not respiratory rate. As exercise intensity continues to increase past the crossover point, ventilation rates begin to increase exponentially as O_2 demands outpace the O_2-delivery system and lactate begins to accumulate in the blood. Consequently, respiratory rates increase.

The second disproportionate increase in ventilation (VT2) occurs at the point where lactate is rapidly increasing with intensity and results in hyperventilation even relative to the extra CO_2 that is being produced. This second threshold represents the point at which blowing off the CO_2 is no longer adequate to buffer the increase in acidity that is occurring with progressively intense exercise.

In well-trained individuals, VT1 is approximately the highest intensity that can be sustained for one to two hours of exercise. In elite marathon runners, VT1 is very close to their competitive pace. The VT2 is the highest intensity that can be sustained for 30 to 60 minutes in well-trained individuals.

An important note for assessment purposes is that the exercise intensity associated with the ability to talk comfortably is highly related to VT1. As long as the exerciser can speak comfortably, they are almost always below VT1. The first point where it becomes more difficult to speak approximates the intensity of VT1, and the point at which speaking is definitely not comfortable approximates the intensity of VT2.

The majority of exercise professionals will not have access to metabolic analyzers for identifying VT1 and VT2 and will need valid field assessments to identify these markers. As such, the most useful and practical approaches for assessing cardiorespiratory fitness are presented here. This section reviews field assessments for measuring HR at VT1.

Contraindications

This type of assessment is not recommended for:
- Individuals with certain breathing problems [asthma or **chronic obstructive pulmonary disease (COPD)**]
- Individuals prone to panic/anxiety attacks, as the labored breathing may create discomfort or precipitate an attack
- Those recovering from a recent respiratory infection
- Individuals who are not fit enough to perform or benefit from the assessment

---

TALK TEST

Following up on suggestions from a generation ago, several groups have explored the value of the talk test as a method of monitoring (and controlling) exercise training intensity (Cannon et al.,

2004; Persinger et al., 2004; Recalde et al., 2002; Voelker et al., 2002; Porcari et al., 2001; Dehart et al., 2000). The usual experience with the talk test is that if two people are exercising and having a conversation, one of them will eventually turn to the other and say something like, "If we are going to keep talking, you are going to have to slow down." The talk test works on the premise that at about the intensity of VT1, the increase in ventilation is accomplished by an increase in breathing frequency. One of the requirements of comfortable speech is to be able to control breathing frequency. Thus, at the intensity of VT1, it is no longer possible to speak comfortably.

The simple talk test has been shown to work fairly well as an index of the exercise intensity at VT1. Options include asking clients to recite something familiar, such as reciting the alphabet or "A is for apple, B is for boy, etc.," then answer the question, "Can you speak comfortably?" If the answer is yes, the intensity is below the VT1. At the first response that is less than an unequivocal "yes," the intensity is probably right at that of the VT1, and if the answer is "no," the intensity is probably above VT1. When the client can no longer say more than a word or two between breaths, they are at or above VT2.

Another option is to compare the number to which an individual can count during the expiration phase of one breath during exercise against the number counted during the expiration phase at rest. Normally, when the number counted to during exercise drops to about 70% of the number that is possible at rest, the intensity is approximately equal to the VT1. For example, if an individual can count to 14 during the expiration phase at rest, 70%—the indicator of VT1—represents the exercise intensity at which they can no longer count past 10.

The talk test has several advantages as a method of programming and monitoring exercise compared to a given %$\dot{V}O_2$max or %MHR, since it is based off an individual's unique metabolic or ventilatory responses to exercise. Thus, for most people, training at intensities at which the answer to the question, "Can you speak comfortably?" becomes less than an unequivocal "yes" may represent the ideal training intensity marker. Therefore, the talk test is an appropriate marker to use for many individuals, especially for those seeking to lose weight or develop their cardiorespiratory efficiency. Training at or near this intensity (unique to the individual's own metabolism) increases the likelihood of a better exercise experience. Higher-intensity training for those individuals with performance goals can be regulated in terms of VT2.

SUBMAXIMAL TALK TEST FOR VT1

This test is best performed using HR **telemetry** (HR strap and watch) for continuous monitoring. To avoid missing VT1, the exercise increments need to be small, increasing **steady-state heart rate (HRss)** by approximately 5 bpm per stage. Consequently, this test will require some preparation to determine the appropriate increments that elicit a 5-bpm increase. Once the increments are determined, the time needed to reach HRss during a stage must also be determined (60 to 120 seconds per stage is usually adequate).

The end-point of the test is not a predetermined HR but is instead based on monitoring changes in breathing rate (technically metabolic changes) that are determined by the client's ability to recite a predetermined combination of phrases. *Note:* Reading, as opposed to reciting from memory, is not advised, as it compromises balance if testing is being performed on a treadmill.

The objectives of the test are to measure the HR response at VT1 by progressively increasing exercise intensity and achieving steady state at each stage, as well as to identify the HR where the ability to talk continuously becomes compromised. This point represents the intensity where the individual can continue to talk while breathing with minimal discomfort and reflects an associated increase in tidal volume that should not compromise breathing rate or the ability to talk. Progressing beyond this point where breathing rate increases significantly, making continuous talking difficult, is not necessary and will render the test inaccurate.

Equipment:
- Treadmill, cycle ergometer, elliptical trainer, or arm ergometer
- Stopwatch
- HR monitor with chest strap (optional)

- Predetermined text that the individual will recite (e.g., alphabet)

Pre-test procedure:
- As this test involves small, incremental increases in intensity specific to each individual, the testing stages need to be predetermined. The goal is to incrementally increase workload in small quantities to determine VT1. Large incremental increases may result in the individual passing through VT1, thereby invalidating the test:
  - ✓ Recommended workload increases are approximately 0.5 mph, 1% grade, or 10 to 20 watts.
  - ✓ The objective is to increase HRss at each stage by approximately 5 bpm.
  - ✓ Plan to complete this test within eight to 16 minutes to ensure that localized muscle fatigue from longer durations of exercise is not an influencing factor.
- Measure pre-exercise HR and BP (if necessary), both sitting and standing, and then record the values on the testing form.
- Describe the purpose of this graded exercise test, review the predetermined protocol and the passage to be recited, and allow the client the opportunity to address any questions or concerns. Each stage of the test lasts one to two minutes to achieve HRss at each workload.
- Allow the client to walk on the treadmill or use the ergometer to warm up and get used to the apparatus. If using a treadmill, they should avoid holding the handrails. If the client is too unstable without holding onto the rails, consider using another testing modality, as this will invalidate the test results.
- Take the client through a light warm-up (RPE of 2 to 3 on the 0 to 10 scale) for three to five minutes, maintaining an intensity comfortably below a moderate level.

Test protocol and administration:
- Once the client has warmed up, adjust the workload intensity so the client is working at a moderate-to-strong intensity level (RPE of 3 to 4 on the 0 to 10 scale).
- Toward the latter part of each stage (i.e., last 20 to 30 seconds), measure/record the HR and then ask the client to recite the predetermined passage. Upon completion of the recital, ask the client to identify whether they felt this task was easy or uncomfortable-to-challenging. *Note:* Conversations with questions and answers are not suggested, as the test needs to evaluate the challenge of talking continuously, not in brief bursts as in conversation. Also, reading as opposed to reciting from memory, is not advised, as it may compromise balance if testing is being performed on a treadmill.
  - ✓ The test concludes when the client reports that they can speak, but not entirely comfortably.
- If VT1 is not achieved, progress through the successive stages, repeating the protocol at each stage until VT1 is reached.
- Once the HR at VT1 is identified, progress to the cool-down phase (matching the warm-up intensity) for three to five minutes.
- This test should ideally be conducted on two separate occasions with the same exercise modality to determine an average VT1 HR.
  - ✓ HR varies between treadmills, bikes, etc., so it is important to conduct the tests with the exercise modality that the client uses most frequently.
  - ✓ The VT1 HR will also be noticeably higher if the test is conducted after weight training due to fatigue and increased metabolism. Therefore, clients should be tested before performing muscular-training exercises.

The HR at VT1 can be used as a target HR when determining exercise intensity. Those interested in sports conditioning and/or competition would benefit from training at higher intensities, while those interested in health and general fitness are well-served to stay at or slightly below this exercise intensity.

Performance Training

Individuals who progress to Performance Training will have goals that are focused on success in endurance sports and events. This may include achieving a personal record in a cycling, swimming, or rowing event, running a local marathon in a time that qualifies them for a national-level event, or finishing top-five at a state or national championship. In these examples, the training programs will progress beyond the parameters of fitness to focus on performance through increased speed, **power,** and endurance.

Performance Training requires adequate training volume to prepare clients to comfortably complete their events. This is only the first step, as clients focused on Performance Training will have goals that go far beyond simply finishing an event. To help them achieve higher-level performance goals, the CMES will want to continue building on the moderate- and vigorous-intensity exercise in their programs while integrating intervals that push clients up to and beyond VT2, where efforts are of very high intensity (RPE = 7 to 10 on the 0 to 10 scale) and short duration.

A CMES can help clients advance their endurance performance by designing programs that include periodized training plans with each day's training focused on specific variables such as distance, recovery, increased speed, or improved power. Periodized training plans allow the CMES to manipulate key training variables, including total training volume, as well as frequency and duration of intervals performed both between VT1 and just below VT2 and at or above VT2, to help each client reach their unique performance goals. As a client's total weekly training time increases, a greater percentage of their training time will typically be at moderate intensities to accommodate the increased training volume and to allow for recovery from higher-intensity interval-training sessions. Table 2-4 provides a summary of the three phases of Cardiorespiratory Training.

TABLE 2-4	
CARDIORESPIRATORY TRAINING	
Base Training	• Focus on moderate-intensity cardiorespiratory exercise (RPE = 3 to 4), while keeping an emphasis on enjoyment. • Keep intensities below the talk-test threshold (below VT1). • Increase duration and frequency of exercise bouts. • Progress to Fitness Training when the client can complete at least 20 minutes of cardiorespiratory exercise below the talk-test threshold at least three times per week.
Fitness Training	• Progress cardiorespiratory exercise duration and frequency based on the client's goals and available time. • Integrate vigorous-intensity (RPE = 5 to 6) cardiorespiratory exercise intervals with segments performed at intensities below, at, and above VT1 to just below VT2.
Performance Training	• Progress moderate- and vigorous-intensity cardiorespiratory exercise. • Program sufficient volume for the client to achieve goals. • Integrate near-maximal and maximal intensity (RPE = 7 to 10) intervals performed at and above VT2 to increase aerobic capacity, speed, and performance. • Periodized training plans can be used to incorporate adequate training time below VT1, from VT1 to just below VT2, and at or above VT2.

Note: RPE = Rating of perceived exertion (0 to 10 scale); VT1 = First ventilatory threshold; VT2 = Second ventilatory threshold

VT2 THRESHOLD ASSESSMENT

VT2 is equivalent to OBLA, or the point at which blood lactate accumulates at rates faster than the body can buffer and remove it (blood lactate >4 mmol/L). This marker represents an exponential increase in the concentration of blood lactate, indicating an exercise intensity that can no longer be sustained for long periods, and represents the highest sustainable level of exercise intensity, a strong marker of exercise performance. Continually measuring blood lactate is an accurate method to determine OBLA and the corresponding VT2. However, the cost of lactate analyzers and handling of biohazardous materials make it impractical for most exercise professionals. Consequently, field tests have been created to challenge an individual's ability to sustain high intensities of exercise for a predetermined duration to *estimate* VT2. This method of testing requires an individual to sustain the highest intensity possible during a single bout of steady-state exercise. This obviously mandates high levels of conditioning and experience in pacing. Consequently, VT2 testing is *only* recommended for well-conditioned individuals with fitness and performance goals.

Well-trained individuals can probably estimate their own HR response at VT2 during their training by identifying the highest intensity they can maintain for an extended duration. In cycling, coaches often select a 10-mile time trial or 60 minutes of sustained intensity, whereas in running, a 30-minute run is often used. Given that testing for 30 to 60 minutes is impractical in most fitness facilities, the CMES can opt to use shorter single-stage tests of highest sustainable intensity to estimate the HR response at VT2.

In general, the intensity that can be sustained for 15 to 20 minutes is higher than what could be sustained for 30 to 60 minutes in conditioned individuals. To predict the HR response at VT2 using a 15- to 20-minute test, the CMES can estimate that the corrected HR response would be equivalent to approximately 95% of the 15-to 20-minute HR average. For example, if an individual's average sustainable HR for a 20-minute bike test is 168 bpm, their HR at VT2 would be 160 bpm (168 bpm x 0.95).

This assessment is best performed using HR telemetry (HR strap and watch) for continuous monitoring. Individuals participating in this test need experience with the selected modality to effectively pace themselves at their maximal sustainable intensity for the duration of the bout. In addition, this test should only be performed by clients who are cleared for exercise and ready for Performance Training.

Pre-assessment procedure:
- Briefly explain the purpose of the assessment, review the predetermined protocol, and allow the client the opportunity to address any questions or concerns.
- Take the client through a light warm-up (2- to 3-out-of-10 effort) for three to five minutes, maintaining a heart rate below 120 bpm.

Assessment protocol and administration:
- Begin the assessment by increasing the intensity to the predetermined level.
  - ✓ Allow the individual to make changes to the exercise intensity as needed during the first few minutes of the bout. Remember, they need to be able to maintain the selected intensity for 20 minutes.
- During the last five minutes of exercise, record the heart rate at each minute interval.
- Use the average HR collected over the last five minutes to account for any **cardiovascular drift** associated with fatigue, thermoregulation, and changing blood volume.
- Multiply the average HR attained during the 15- to 20-minute high-intensity exercise bout by 0.95 to determine the VT2 estimate.

Muscular Training

The Muscular Training component of the ACE IFT Model provides a systematic approach to training that starts with helping clients to improve poor postural stability and **kinetic chain** mobility, and then incorporates programming and progressions to help people train for general fitness, strength, body building, and athletic performance. While many clients will not progress to training for athletic performance, using a training model that provides the CMES with the knowledge and tools to work with clients across a broad spectrum of movement skills and challenges is empowering.

The ACE IFT Model Muscular Training component is divided into three phases, each with a title that defines its training focus (Figure 2-7).

ACE → Integrated Fitness Training® Model

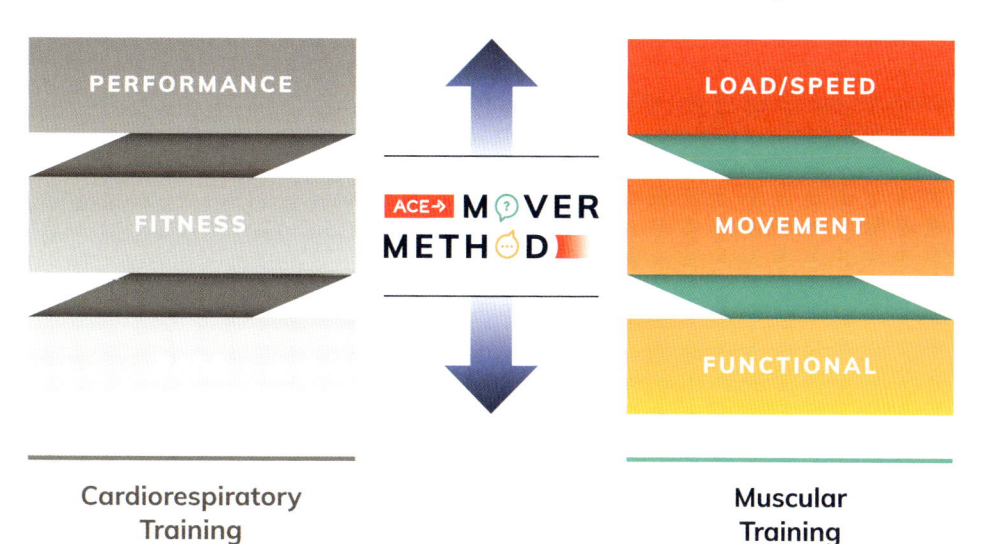

Figure 2-7
ACE IFT Model Muscular Training phases

Cardiorespiratory Training — PERFORMANCE / FITNESS

ACE → MOVER METHOD

Muscular Training — LOAD/SPEED / MOVEMENT / FUNCTIONAL

Functional Training

Functional Training focuses on the Muscular Training goals of establishing, or in many cases reestablishing, postural stability and kinetic chain mobility through the introduction of exercise programs that improve joint function through improved muscular endurance, flexibility, core function, **static balance,** and **dynamic balance.** This basic muscular function is typically gained as part of normal child development. Unfortunately, physical inactivity coupled with an increasingly technology-driven world has resulted in more adults having compromised posture, balance, and muscular function.

Exercise selection for Functional Training will focus on core and balance exercises that improve the strength and function of the muscles responsible for stabilizing the spine and **center of gravity (COG)** during static positions and dynamic movements. Exercises for Functional Training will initially use primarily body-weight resistance. As clients progress to Movement Training and Load/Speed Training, it is important to still include Functional Training exercises in their workouts. These can be included as part of either the warm-up or cool-down, or by incorporating progressions that increase the challenge of the Functional Training exercises by increasing the resistance or balance challenges.

Movement involves integrated action along the kinetic chain, where action at one segment affects successive segments within the chain. Joint mobility is the range of uninhibited movement around a joint or body segment. Joint stability is the ability to maintain or control joint movement or position. Both joint mobility and stability are attained by the interaction of all components surrounding the joints and the neuromuscular system. Joint mobility should not be attained by compromising joint stability. Some joints are designed to be more stable than mobile (e.g., foot, knee, lumbar spine, and scapulothoracic), while others are designed to be more mobile than stable (e.g., ankle, hip, thoracic spine, and glenohumeral). Figure 2-8 provides an illustration of the alternating pattern of stable and mobile joints along the kinetic chain, with joints labeled as favoring "stability" or "mobility."

GLENOHUMERAL = MOBILITY
SCAPULOTHORACIC = STABILITY
THORACIC SPINE = MOBILITY
LUMBAR SPINE = STABILITY
HIP = MOBILITY
KNEE = STABILITY
ANKLE = MOBILITY
FOOT = STABILITY

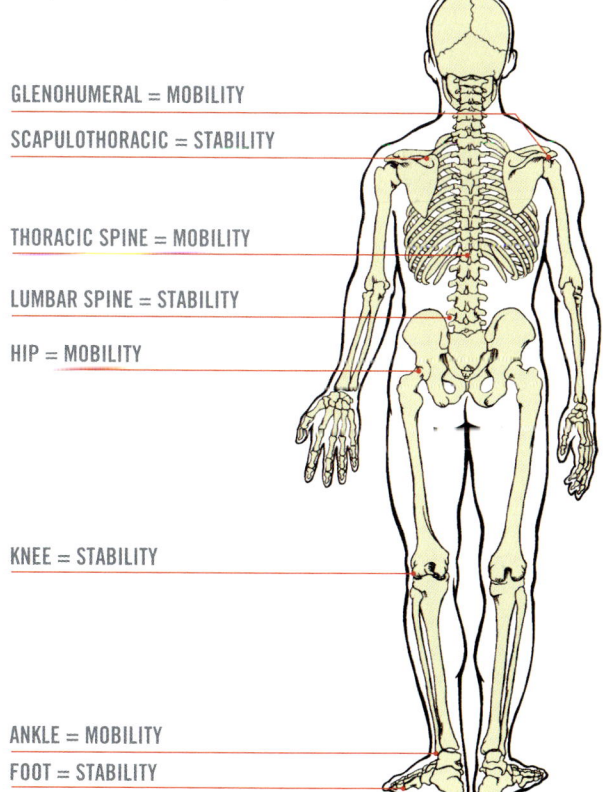

Figure 2-8
Mobility and stability of the kinetic chain

A static postural assessment is an excellent test for observing a client's joints and how they relate to each other, and for viewing how those joints maintain their positions against gravity in a relaxed, standing position. Individuals who exhibit good posture generally demonstrate an appropriate relationship between stability and mobility throughout the kinetic chain. On the other hand, individuals who exhibit poor posture typically lack the mobility required for normal joint movement, the stability to maintain good posture, or both.

Observing active movement is an effective method to determine the contribution that muscle imbalances and poor posture have on neural control, and also helps identify movement compensations (Whiting & Rugg, 2006; Sahrmann, 2002). If altered movement patterns are present, it is usually indicative of some form of adjusted neural action, commonly referred to as "faulty neural control," which normally manifests itself out of muscle tightness or an imbalance between muscles acting on the joint.

Compromised joint movement alters neuromuscular control and function, prompting additional postural misalignments and faulty loading at the joints that inevitably increases overload and the likelihood for injury and pain (Figure 2-9). It is therefore imperative that the CMES works to restore and maintain normal joint alignment, joint movement, muscle balance, and muscle function, all of which are critical for optimal health and longevity. Effective programming and attention to exercise technique will help the CMES achieve this goal.

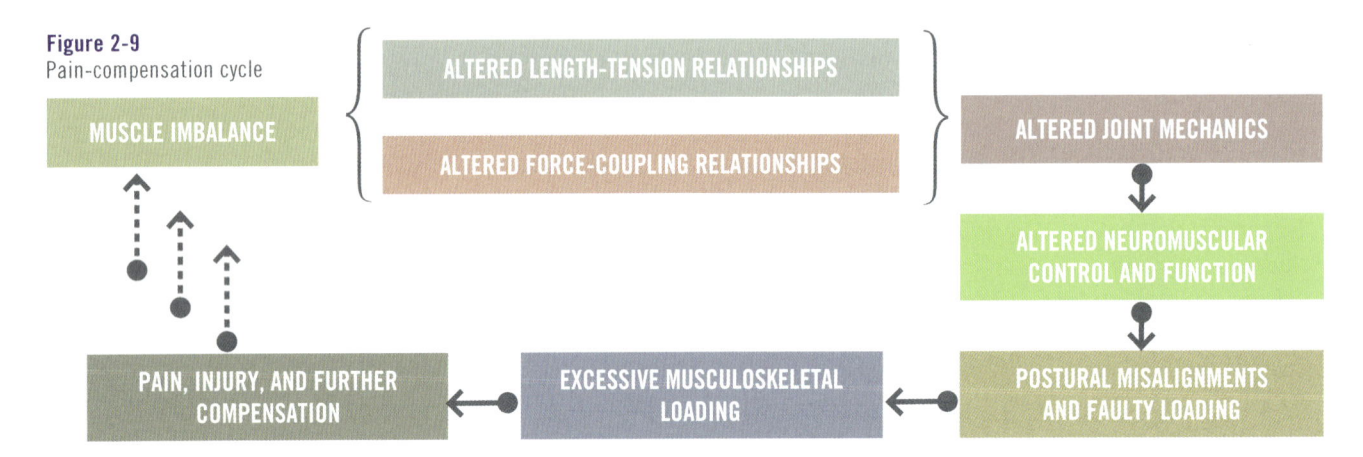

Figure 2-9
Pain-compensation cycle

MUSCLE IMBALANCE → ALTERED LENGTH-TENSION RELATIONSHIPS / ALTERED FORCE-COUPLING RELATIONSHIPS → ALTERED JOINT MECHANICS → ALTERED NEUROMUSCULAR CONTROL AND FUNCTION → POSTURAL MISALIGNMENTS AND FAULTY LOADING → EXCESSIVE MUSCULOSKELETAL LOADING → PAIN, INJURY, AND FURTHER COMPENSATION

A lack of mobility can be attributed to numerous factors, including reduced levels of physical activity, and increased actions that promote muscle imbalance (e.g., repetitive movements, habitually poor posture, side-dominance, poor exercise technique, and imbalanced strength training programs) (Kendall et al., 2005). This loss of mobility leads to compensations in movement and potential losses of stability at subsequent joints.

It is important to remember that while all joints demonstrate varying levels of stability and mobility, they tend to favor one over the other, depending on their function within the body (Cook & Jones, 2007a; Cook & Jones, 2007b). Individuals who have good balance between the more stable and more mobile joints along the kinetic chain will be better prepared to support controlled movements and will have decreased risk of musculoskeletal injuries. When joints designed to be more stable are lacking stability, they fail to provide an adequate base of support for the movements of the adjacent joints that favor mobility, placing the more mobile adjacent joints at greater risk for injury. An example of this is seen when instability in the scapulothoracic joint leads to rotator cuff or other shoulder injuries. The mechanism of injury stems from the unstable scapulothoracic joint failing to provide the stable foundation required for proper movements of the glenohumeral joint. From a mechanical perspective, this type of scenario can be analogous to climbing stairs versus climbing a rope ladder, or standing on a solid floor versus standing on a balance board.

Injuries can also occur when a more mobile joint is lacking adequate mobility, causing the adjacent, more stable joints to sacrifice stability for mobility to allow for full-body movements. A common example of this is seen when an individual loses hip mobility because of a sedentary lifestyle, injury, or repetitive motions that cause tightness in the muscles acting on the hip (e.g., hip flexors and hamstrings). The lower back is often the victim in this scenario, as it sacrifices stability to allow for more mobility to compensate for the lack of hip mobility, as is seen with exaggerated **lordosis** in individuals who have tight hip flexors.

Compromised joint stability and mobility is common following injury or surgery. Specific protocols for improving joint stability and mobility following medical or therapeutic treatment are provided with the training protocols for each injury or joint in Chapters 18 through 20. In all situations, the underlying goals are to first restore adequate mobility and stability to support proper movement during ADL. As the client progresses, mobility and stability can be enhanced to facilitate movements required to help the client meet their goals for desired activities and resultant improvements in health and fitness.

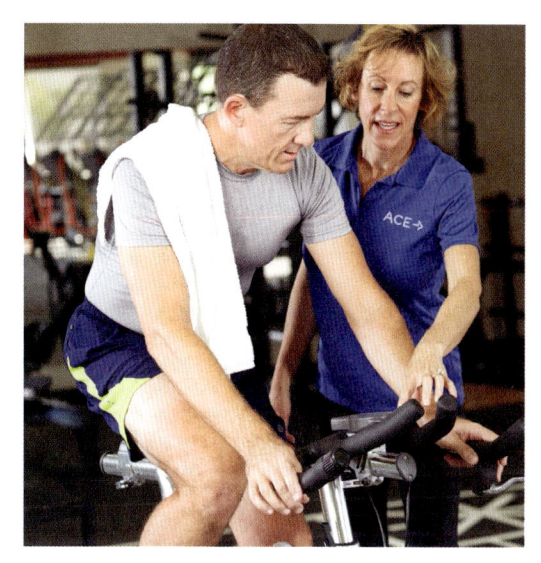

Individuals who have overweight or obesity may experience structural changes due to the increased loads on the skeleton that can result in low-back pain, decreased mobility, modified gait pattern, and changes in the relative energy expenditures for a given activity. In addition, osteoarthritis, particularly of the knee, is strongly associated with increases in **body mass index (BMI)**. While the association between obesity and low-back pain is unclear, researchers have reported a linear correlation between increasing BMI and low-back pain, especially in large population studies (Leboeuf-Yde, 2000; Toda et al., 2000; Han et al., 1997). There also appears to be a higher incidence of obesity-related low-back pain in women versus men (Shiri et al., 2010; Shiri, 2008).

There are many causes for compromised stability and mobility. Whether the root cause is physical inactivity, injury, or a chronic condition, the general focus of Functional Training is on the introduction of low-intensity exercise programs to improve muscle balance, muscular endurance, core function, flexibility, and static and dynamic balance to improve the client's posture. This facilitates proper joint mechanics throughout the kinetic chain. Figure 2-10 illustrates the importance of muscle balance and its contribution to movement efficiency, reinforcing the importance of conducting static postural assessments with clients during the onboarding process and during reassessments.

Figure 2-10
Movement efficiency pattern

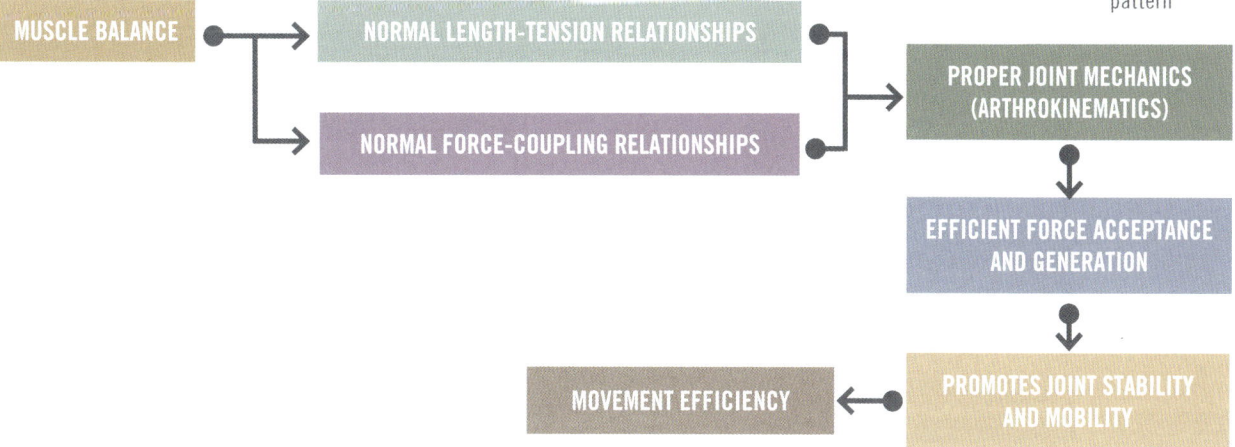

MUSCLE BALANCE → NORMAL LENGTH-TENSION RELATIONSHIPS / NORMAL FORCE-COUPLING RELATIONSHIPS → PROPER JOINT MECHANICS (ARTHROKINEMATICS) → EFFICIENT FORCE ACCEPTANCE AND GENERATION → PROMOTES JOINT STABILITY AND MOBILITY → MOVEMENT EFFICIENCY

Teaching a client how to find and hold a relatively neutral posture will create the foundation for the movement skills that will be introduced in the phases that follow. It is important to note that this neutral position will be unique for each client, so the focus should be on assisting each client to learn and practice this position. Exercise selection in this phase will focus on core and balance exercises that improve the strength and function of the muscles responsible for stabilizing the spine and COG during movement. Exercises will use primarily body weight or body-segment weight as resistance. No assessments of muscular strength or endurance are needed prior to designing and implementing exercise programs during this phase. Assessments that should be conducted early in this phase include basic assessments of:

- Posture
- Balance
- Movement
- **Range of motion (ROM)** of the ankle, hip, shoulder complex, and thoracic and lumbar spine

Exercise programs should be developed based on the results of these assessments to address each client's weaknesses and imbalances.

The principal goal of this phase of the training program will be to develop postural stability throughout the kinetic chain without compromising mobility at any point in the chain (Figure 2-11). Exercises should emphasize supported surfaces that offer stability against gravity (e.g., floor or backrests) and focus on restorative flexibility, **isometric** contractions, strengthening muscles first through limited ROM, static balance, core activation, spinal stabilization, and muscular endurance to promote stability. Exercise-programming tools and strategies for improving stability and mobility are presented throughout Chapters 14, 15, 18, 19, and 20, with specific regimens presented for different musculoskeletal injuries and conditions. Clients are ready to progress to Movement Training once they are able to hold stable neutral posture while standing and throughout multiple movements and exercises.

Figure 2-11
Programming components of the stability and mobility training phase

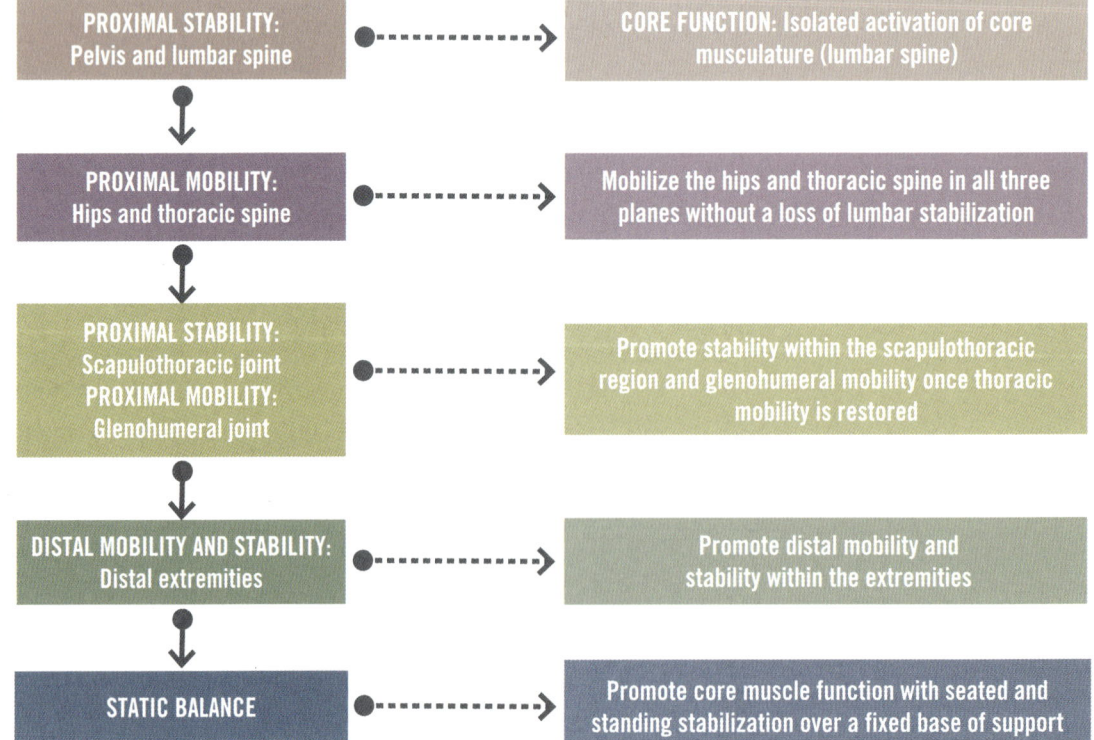

PROXIMAL STABILITY: Pelvis and lumbar spine	**CORE FUNCTION:** Isolated activation of core musculature (lumbar spine)
PROXIMAL MOBILITY: Hips and thoracic spine	Mobilize the hips and thoracic spine in all three planes without a loss of lumbar stabilization
PROXIMAL STABILITY: Scapulothoracic joint **PROXIMAL MOBILITY:** Glenohumeral joint	Promote stability within the scapulothoracic region and glenohumeral mobility once thoracic mobility is restored
DISTAL MOBILITY AND STABILITY: Distal extremities	Promote distal mobility and stability within the extremities
STATIC BALANCE	Promote core muscle function with seated and standing stabilization over a fixed base of support

UNDERSTANDING SELF–MYOFASCIAL RELEASE

Understanding the concept behind self–myofascial release requires an understanding of the fascial system itself. **Fascia** is a densely woven, specialized system of **connective tissue** that covers and unites all of the body's compartments. The result is a system where each part is connected to the other parts through this web of tissue. Essentially, the purpose of the fascia is to surround and support the bodily structures, which provides stability as well as a cohesive direction for the line of pull of muscle groups. For example, the fascia surrounding the quadriceps keeps this muscle group contained in the anterior compartment of the thigh (stability) and orients the muscle fibers in a vertical direction so that the line of pull is more effective at extending the knee. In a normal healthy state, fascia has a relaxed and wavy configuration. It has the ability to stretch and move without restriction. However, with physical trauma, scarring, or inflammation, fascia may lose its pliability.

Self–myofascial release is a technique that applies pressure to tight, restricted areas of fascia and underlying muscle in an attempt to relieve tension and improve flexibility. It is thought that applying direct sustained pressure to a tight area can inhibit the tension in a muscle. Tightness in soft tissue may be diminished through the application of pressure (e.g., self–myofascial release) followed by **static stretching.**

The practical application of myofascial release in the fitness setting is commonly done through the use of a foam roller, where the client controls their own intensity and duration of pressure. A common technique is to instruct clients to perform small, continuous, back-and-forth movements on a foam roller, covering an area of 2 to 6 inches (5 to 15 cm) over the tender region for 30 to 60 seconds (Figure 2-12). Because exerting pressure on an already tender area requires a certain level of pain tolerance, the intensity of the application of pressure determines the duration for which the client can withstand the discomfort. The CMES should always be cognizant of the pain tolerance for rolling of their clients. For some individuals, using a foam roller will simply feel too painful. In these cases, a softer foam roller or a soft, small ball can be used in place of the traditional, denser foam roller.

Evidence is lacking on the mechanisms and benefits of performing self–myofascial release, with some experts disparaging the use of the word "release" as an accurate depiction of what actually occurs. A CMES who encourages the use of this technique to improve flexibility with clients should make every effort to stay current with research as it becomes available in this area.

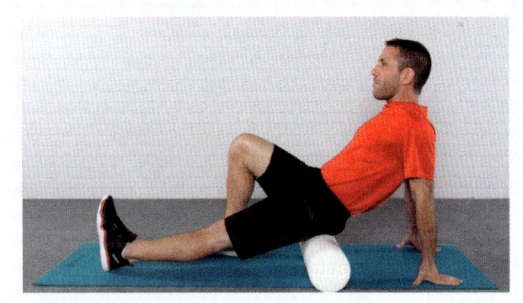

EXPAND YOUR KNOWLEDGE

a. Gluteals

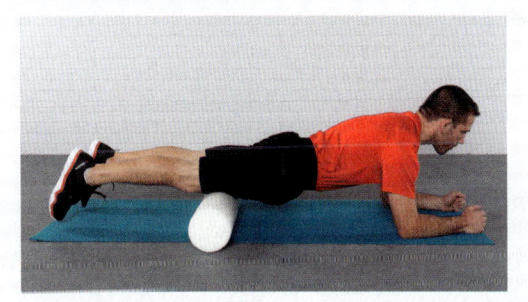

b. Quadriceps

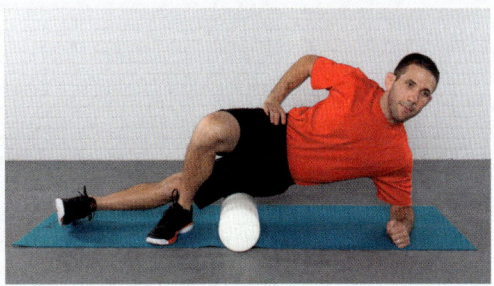

c. Iliotibial band

Figure 2-12
Self–myofascial release using a foam roller

Movement Training

The primary focus of Movement Training is on helping clients develop good movement patterns without compromising postural or joint stability. Movement Training focuses on the five primary movement patterns (Figure 2-13):

- *Bend-and-lift movements:* These movements are performed throughout the day as a person sits, stands, or squats down to lift an object off the floor.
- *Single-leg movements:* These movements involve single-leg balance and movement as performed during walking or going up and down stairs. In addition, lunging movements are performed when a person steps forward to reach down with one hand to pick up something small off the floor.
- *Pushing movements:* These upper-body movements occur in four primary directions: forward (e.g., when pushing open a door), overhead (e.g., lifting something to a high shelf), **lateral** (e.g., lifting one's torso when getting up from a side-lying position), and downward (e.g., pushing oneself up and out of the side of a swimming pool).

Figure 2-13
Five primary movement patterns

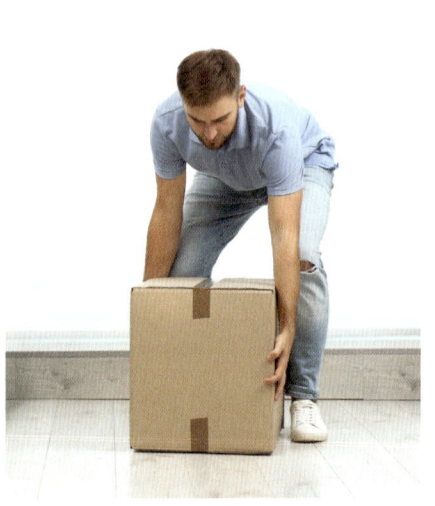

a. Bend-and-lift movement

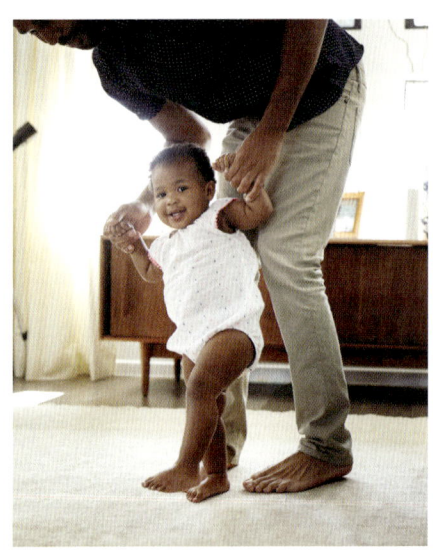

b. Single-leg movement

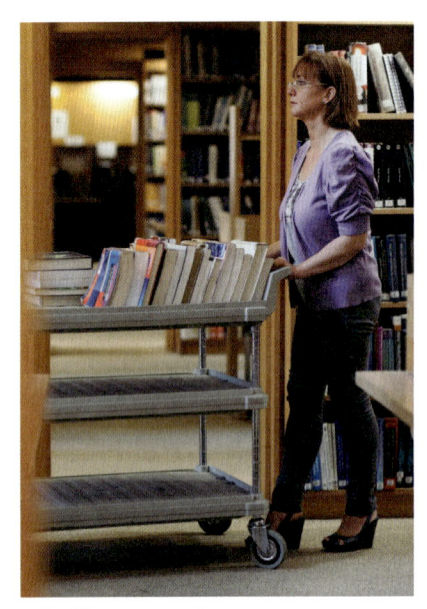

c. Pushing movement

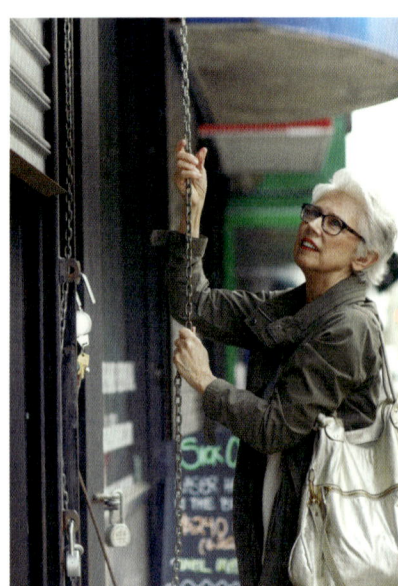

d. Pulling movement

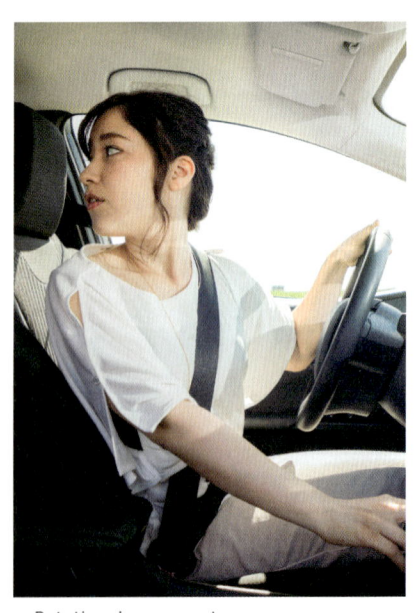

e. Rotational movement

- *Pulling movements:* These movements occur during exercises like a seated row or pull-up, or when pulling open a door.
- *Rotational movements:* These movements often occur in the torso as force transfers from the legs to the arms (e.g., throwing a ball) or during twisting movements like a dancer performing pirouettes or a golfer striking a ball.

Movement Training exercises should emphasize the proper sequencing of movements and control of the body's COG throughout the normal ROM being performed. The CMES should integrate Functional Training exercises into Movement Training programs to help clients maintain and improve postural stability and kinetic chain mobility, as they are essential for performing the five primary movement patterns well (see Table 2-6, page 49). One option for including Functional Training exercises is to add them to the warm-up to prepare the body for the more rigorous movements that follow. Body-weight exercises are often used initially during Movement Training, with external resistance introduced typically to build muscular endurance with an emphasis on controlled motion. The CMES should make sure that clients can perform the five primary movement patterns well before adding external loads to the movement patterns to decrease the risk of injury that can result from loading poorly executed movements.

Load/Speed Training

Traditional resistance-training programs for muscle **hypertrophy,** strength, or endurance all require external loads to facilitate increased muscular force production. Therefore, during load training, the variables of exercise program design are applied in a manner consistent with the standard FITT-VP model for increasing muscular hypertrophy, enhancing muscular endurance, or improving muscular strength (Table 2-5). Exercise selection is consistent with traditional resistance-training exercises and is dictated by the client's specific goals and needs. Resistance, or loading, can be applied through a number of different options, including selectorized equipment, plate-loaded cables and machines, barbells, dumbbells, kettlebells, medicine balls, elastic tubing, or even non-traditional strength-training equipment such as

TABLE 2-5
RESISTANCE TRAINING EXERCISE RECOMMENDATIONS

FITT	Recommendation
Frequency	• For novices, each major muscle group should be trained at least 2 days/week. • For experienced exercisers, frequency is secondary to training volume, thus individuals can choose a weekly frequency per muscle group based on personal preference.
Intensity	• For novices, 60–70% 1-RM, performed for 8–12 repetitions are recommended to improve muscular fitness. • For experienced exercisers, a wide range of intensities and repetitions are effective dependent on the specific muscular-fitness goals.
Type	• Multijoint exercises affecting more than one muscle group and targeting agonist and antagonist muscle groups are recommended for all adults. • Single-joint and core exercises may also be included in a resistance-training program, typically after performing multijoint exercise(s) for that particular muscle group. • A variety of exercise equipment and/or body weight can be used to perform these exercises.

Note: 1-RM = One-repetition maximum

Reprinted with permission from American College of Sports Medicine (2022). *ACSM's Guidelines for Exercise Testing and Prescription* (11th ed.). Philadelphia: Wolters Kluwer.

tires or water-filled containers. Regardless of the exercises selected or the type of loads used, the focus during this phase is on good exercise form and increasing muscular force and endurance.

The broad focus of Load/Speed Training is on applying external loads to movements that create a need for increased force production that results in muscular adaptations. Loads can be applied through resistance training, **high-intensity interval training (HIIT),** speed work, **plyometrics,** power lifting, and other sport-specific resistance (e.g., using swim training paddles or pedaling large gears while cycling uphill).

As with Movement Training, Load/Speed Training should integrate Functional Training exercises to help clients maintain and enhance postural stability and kinetic chain mobility to adequately support the increased workloads and force production (see Table 2-6, page 49). Load/Speed Training also integrates the five primary movements that are the focus of Movement Training, with the emphasis being on loading the movements through different planes of motion, angles, speeds, and combined movements [e.g., squat with dumbbells (Figure 2-14) and seated single-arm overhead press in the scapular plane (Figure 2-15)].

Clients can have a variety of individual goals that are reached through Load/Speed Training. Fitness-related goals for this type of training include muscular strength, muscular endurance, muscle hypertrophy, and positive changes in **body composition.** The

Figure 2-14
Squat with dumbbells

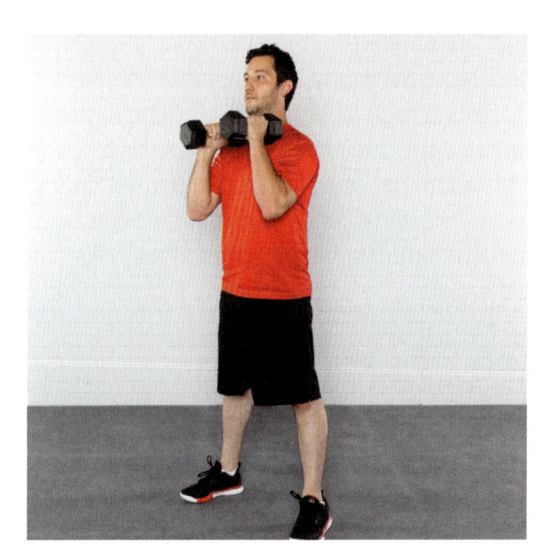

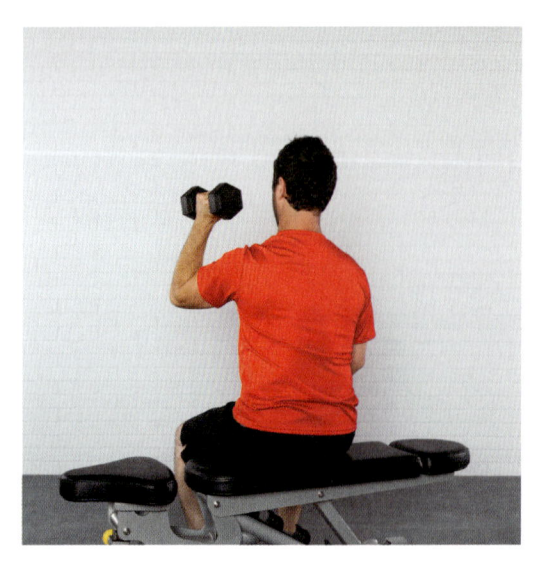

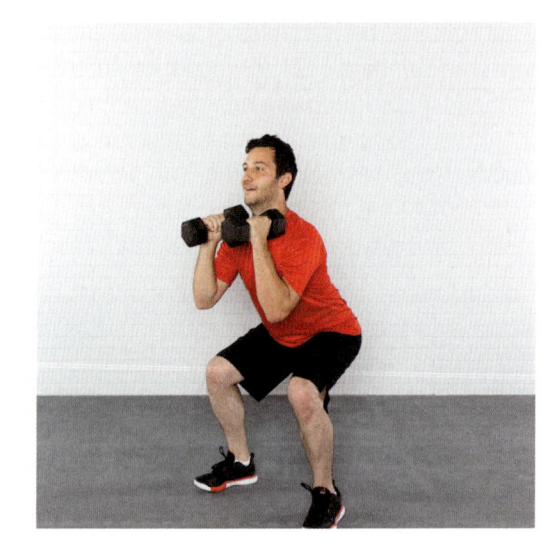

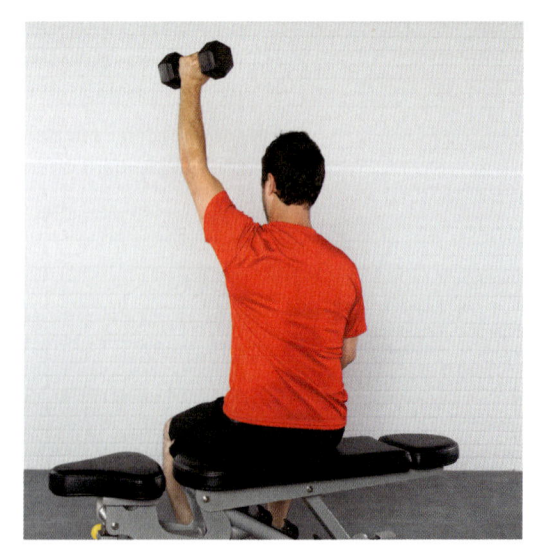

Figure 2-15
Seated single-arm overhead press in scapular plane

Applying the ACE Integrated Fitness Training Model® in the Medical Exercise Setting   CHAPTER 2

CMES can help clients reach their fitness-related Load/Speed Training goals by designing exercise programs for each client that incorporate appropriate muscular-training variables, including exercise selection and the frequency and intensity with which each exercise is performed. Clients who have athletic performance goals can benefit from training that builds speed, **agility, quickness,** and power. Before advancing to training for athletic performance goals, clients should consistently exhibit good postural stability, kinetic chain mobility, and movement patterns. They should also have a good foundation of muscular strength to produce and control the force generated during athletic performance–focused exercises and drills. Exercise selection for clients with athletic performance goals can include power lifting, plyometrics, speed work, and drills for agility, **coordination,** and quickness.

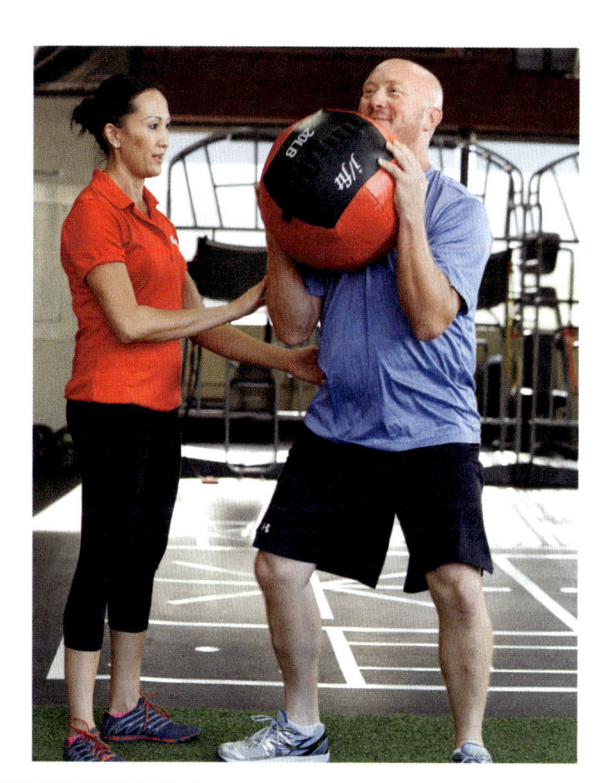

Table 2-6 provides a summary of the three phases of Muscular Training.

TABLE 2-6	
MUSCULAR TRAINING	
Functional Training	Focus on establishing/reestablishing postural stability and kinetic chain mobility.
	Exercise programs should improve muscular endurance, flexibility, core function, and static and dynamic balance.
	Progress exercise volume and challenge as function improves.
Movement Training	Focus on developing good movement patterns without compromising postural or joint stability.
	Programs should include exercises for all five primary movement patterns in varied planes of motion.
	Integrate Functional Training exercises to help clients maintain and improve postural stability and kinetic chain mobility.
Load/Speed Training	Focus on application of external loads to movements to create increased force production to meet desired goals.
	Integrate the five primary movement patterns through exercises that load them in different planes of motion and combinations.
	Integrate Functional Training exercises to enhance postural stability and kinetic chain mobility to support increased workloads.
	Programs should focus on adequate resistance-training loads to help clients reach muscular strength, endurance, and hypertrophy goals.
	Clients with goals for athletic performance will integrate exercises and drills to build speed, agility, quickness, and power.

ACE-sponsored Research

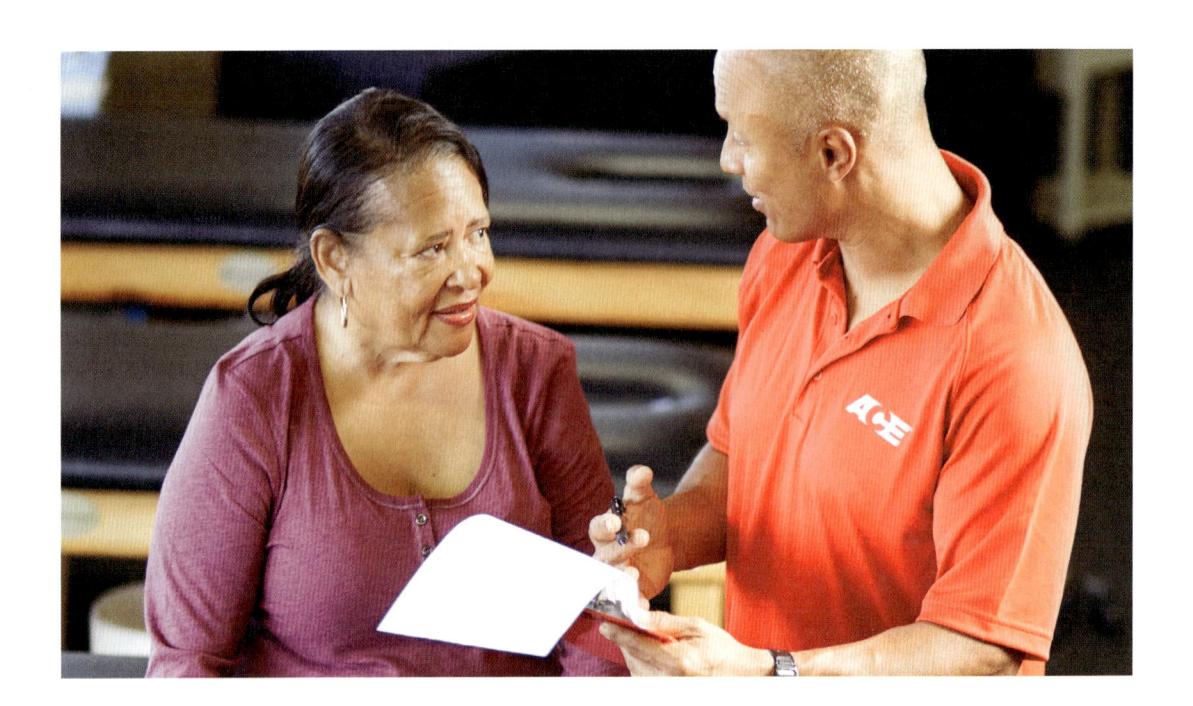

Effectiveness of the ACE Integrated Fitness Training Model

In a randomized trial, Dalleck and colleagues compared the effectiveness of two exercise training programs for improving cardiorespiratory fitness, muscular fitness, and cardiometabolic health (Dalleck et al., 2016). Participants were randomized into one of two training programs: (1) an ACE IFT Model personalized training program, and (2) a standardized training program designed according to American College of Sports Medicine guidelines (ACSM, 2014). Each training program was 13 weeks in length, with weeks 1 through 3 focused on cardiorespiratory training and weeks 4 through 13 including both cardiorespiratory training and muscular training.

The standardized training group performed cardiorespiratory exercise at an intensity based on a percentage of their HRR, progressing from 40 to 45% HRR in week 1 to 60 to 65% HRR in weeks 9 through 13. Each participant in the ACE IFT Model group received a personalized exercise program based on HR at their unique ventilatory thresholds (VT1 and VT2), with exercise intensity progressing from HR <VT1 in week 1 to HR >VT2 in weeks 9 through 13. Both groups performed cardiorespiratory exercise three days per week, starting with 25 minutes per session in week 1 and progressing to 50 minutes per session in weeks 9 through 13. The muscular training program for the standardized training group was comprised of two sets of 12 repetitions on a resistance-training machine circuit of traditional exercises performed three days per week. The ACE IFT Model group performed a muscular-training circuit comprised of two sets of 12 repetitions of multijoint/multiplanar exercises using free weights and machine modalities that allowed for free motion during exercise.

Baseline and follow-up assessment results revealed that when compared to the standardized training group, the ACE IFT Model personalized training group had significantly ($p<0.05$) greater beneficial changes in **body-fat percentage, fat-free mass, $\dot{V}O_2$max, SBP, DBP, right and left leg stork-stand performance, bench press at five-repetition maximum (5-RM), and leg press (5-RM)**. Additionally, 100% of individuals in the ACE IFT Model training group experienced positive improvements in $\dot{V}O_2$max (i.e., all individuals were responders), which was significantly ($p<0.05$) greater than the 64.3% of individuals in the standardized training group who showed positive improvements in $\dot{V}O_2$max (Figure 2-16).

Interestingly, the remaining 35.7% of individuals in the standardized training group experienced undesirable changes in $\dot{V}O_2$max and were categorized as non-responders to cardiorespiratory exercise training. The ACE IFT Model personalized training group also had significantly more individuals elicit favorable responses (i.e., responders) in cardiometabolic, anthropometric, muscular, and neuromotor outcome measurements when compared to the standardized training group (Table 2-7).

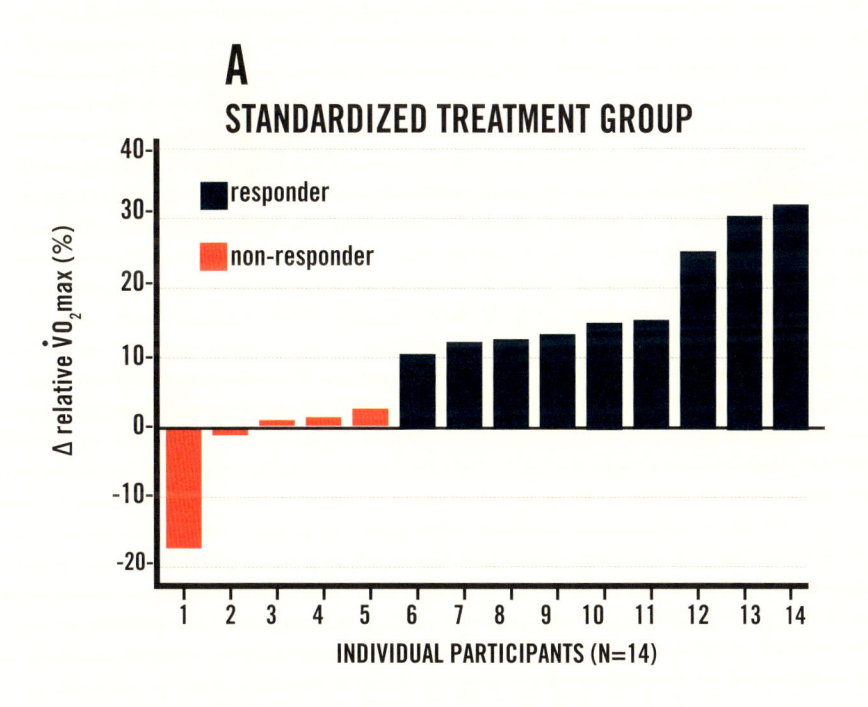

Figure 2-16
Individual variability in relative $\dot{V}O_2$max response (% change) to exercise training in the standardized (A) and ACE IFT Model (B) treatment groups

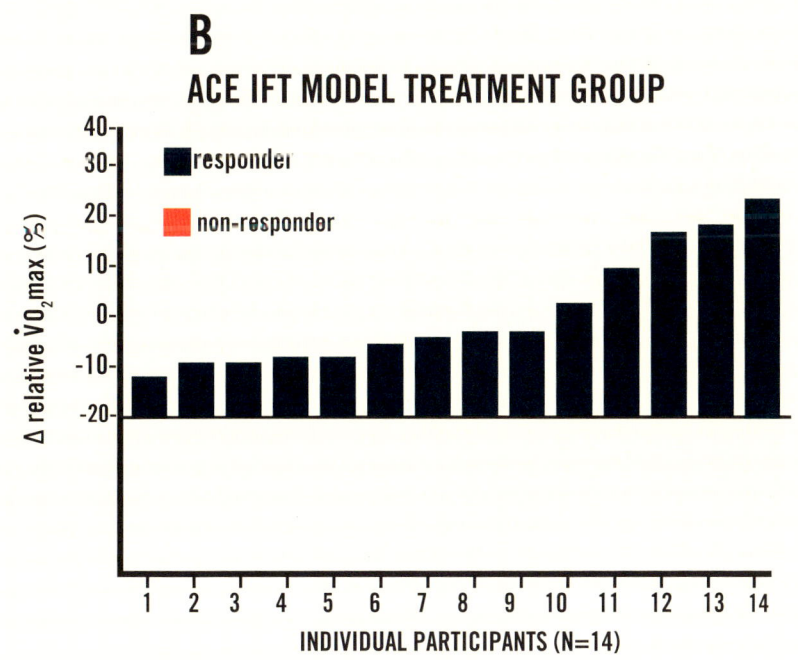

TABLE 2-7
CARDIOMETABOLIC, ANTHROPOMETRIC, AND MUSCULAR AND NEUROMOTOR EXERCISE RESPONDERS

	Responders in the "Standardized" Group (%)	Responders in the "ACE IFT Model" Group (%)
Cardiometabolic responders		
Systolic BP	42.9	100
HDL cholesterol	50.0	100
Triglycerides	85.7	85.7
Blood glucose	42.9	92.9
Anthropometric responders		
Waist circumference	78.6	92.9
Percent body fat	78.6	100
Muscular and neuromotor responders		
Right-leg stork stand	78.6	100
Left-leg stork stand	85.7	92.9
5-RM bench press	64.3	100
5-RM leg press	64.3	100

Note: BP = Blood pressure; HDL = High-density lipoprotein; 5-RM = 5-repetition maximum

Conclusions

- Personalized exercise programming using the ACE IFT Model elicited significantly greater improvements in $\dot{V}O_2$max, muscular fitness, and key cardiometabolic risk factors when compared to standardized exercise programming following 13 weeks of exercise training.
- The ACE IFT Model personalized training group had significantly increased training responsiveness compared to the standardized exercise training group, with 100% of the participants favorably responding to the training stimulus.
- Dalleck et al. (2016) concluded that "these novel findings are encouraging and underscore the importance of personalized exercise programming to enhance training efficacy and limit training unresponsiveness."

SUMMARY

The ACE IFT Model provides medical exercise professionals with a systematic approach to providing integrated assessment and programming solutions for clients across the entire function–health–fitness–performance continuum. Throughout this manual, the ACE IFT Model is applied through exercise programming solutions for the specific conditions covered. The phases of the ACE IFT Model provide appropriate levels of programming to improve function, health, basic fitness, advanced fitness, and performance, while the training components—Cardiorespiratory Training and Muscular Training—allow the CMES to provide comprehensive training solutions that are appropriate for each client's current health, fitness, and goals in each area of training. The central focus of creating positive experiences that promote self-efficacy and enhance program adherence is at the heart of what drives clients to have successful experiences with physical activity. There are many exercise programming tools that have been delivered through a variety of books, courses, and workshops, requiring exercise professionals to spend years learning new material and figuring out how to convert that knowledge into practical programs. The ACE IFT Model provides a comprehensive solution that synthesizes appropriate assessments, exercise programming, and health-coaching tools to help engage clients and empower them to make meaningful changes.

REFERENCES

American College of Sports Medicine (2022). *ACSM's Guidelines for Exercise Testing and Prescription* (11th ed.). Philadelphia: Wolters Kluwer.

American College of Sports Medicine (2014). *ACSM's Guidelines for Exercise Testing and Prescription* (9th ed.). Philadelphia: Lippincott Williams & Wilkins.

Cannon, C. et al. (2004). The talk test as a measure of exertional ischemia. *American Journal of Sports Medicine,* 6, 52–57.

Cook, G. & Jones, B. (2007a). *Secrets of the Shoulder.* www.functionalmovement.com

Cook, G. & Jones, B. (2007b). *Secrets of the Hip and Knee.* www.functionalmovement.com

Dalleck, L.C. et al. (2016). Does a personalized exercise prescription enhance training efficacy and limit training unresponsiveness? A randomized controlled trial. *Journal of Fitness Research,* 5, 3, 15–27.

Dehart, M. et al. (2000). Relationship between the talk test and ventilatory threshold. *Clinical Exercise Physiology,* 2, 34–38.

Fasshauer, M. & Paschke, R. (2003). Regulation of adipocytokines and insulin resistance. *Diabetologia,* 46, 1594–1603.

Fox III, S.M., Naughton, J.P., & Haskell, W.L. (1971). Physical activity and the prevention of coronary heart disease. *Annals of Clinical Research,* 3, 404–432.

Gellish, R.L. et al. (2007). Longitudinal modeling of the relationship between age and maximal heart rate. *Medicine & Science in Sports & Exercise,* 39, 5, 822–829.

Han, T.S. et al. (1997). The prevalence of low back pain and associations with body fatness, fat distribution and height. International Journal of Obesity & Related Metabolic Disorders, 21, 600–607.

Haskell, W.L. et al. (2007). Physical activity and public health: Updated recommendations of the American College of Sports Medicine and the American Heart Association. *Medicine & Science in Sports & Exercise,* 39, 1423–1434

Kendall, F.P. et al. (2005). *Muscles Testing and Function with Posture and Pain* (5th ed.). Baltimore, Md.: Lippincott Williams & Wilkins.

Leboeuf-Yde, C. (2000). Body weight and low back pain: A systematic literature review of 56 journal articles reporting on 65 epidemiologic studies. *Spine,* 25, 226–237.

Lee, Y.H. & Pratley, R.E. (2007). Abdominal obesity and cardiovascular disease risk: The emerging role of the adipocyte. *Journal of Cardiopulmonary Rehabilitation,* 27, 2–10.

McArdle, W., Katch, F., & Katch, V. (2019). *Exercise Physiology: Nutrition, Energy, and Human Performance* (8th ed.). Philadelphia: Lippincott, Williams & Wilkins.

National Heart, Lung and Blood Institute (1998). Obesity Education Initiative Expert Panel. *Clinical Guidelines on the Identification, Evaluation, and Treatment of Overweight and Obesity in Adults: The Evidence Report.* Bethesda, Md.: National Institutes of Health. NIH publication No. 98-4083.

Persinger, R. et al. (2004). Consistency of the talk test for exercise prescription. *Medicine & Science in Sports & Exercise,* 36, 1632–1636.

Porcari, J.P. et al. (2001). Prescribing exercise using the talk test. *Fitness Management,* 17, 9, 46–49.

Recalde, P.T. et al. (2002). The talk test as a simple marker of ventilatory threshold. *South African Journal of Sports Medicine,* 9, 5–8.

Sahrmann, S.A. (2002). *Diagnosis and Treatment of Movement Impairment Syndromes.* St. Louis, Mo.: Mosby.

Shiri, R. (2008). Obesity and the prevalence of low-back pain in young adults. *American Journal of Epidemiology,* 167, 1110–1119.

Shiri, R. et al. (2010). The association between obesity and low-back pain: A meta-analysis. *American Journal of Epidemiology,* 171, 135–154.

Tanaka, H., Monahan, K.D., & Seals, D.R. (2001). Age-predicted maximal heart revisited. *Journal of the American College of Cardiology,* 37, 153–156.

Toda, Y. et al. (2000). Lean body mass and body fat distribution in participants with chronic low back pain. *Archives of Internal Medicine,* 160, 3265–3269.

U.S. Department of Health & Human Services (2018). *Physical Activity Guidelines for Americans* (2nd ed.). www.health.gov/paguidelines/

Voelker, S.A. et al. (2002). Relationship between the talk test and ventilatory threshold in cardiac patients. *Clinical Exercise Physiology,* 4, 120–123.

Whiting W.C. & Rugg, S. (2006). *Dynatomy: Dynamic Human Anatomy.* Champaign, Ill.: Human Kinetics.

World Health Organization (2020). *WHO Guidelines on Physical Activity and Sedentary Behavior.* www.who.int/publications/i/item/9789240015128

Wisse, B.E. (2004). The inflammatory syndrome: The role of adipose tissue cytokines in metabolic disorders linked to obesity. *Journal of the American Society of Nephrology,* 15, 2792–2800.

SUGGESTED READING

American Council on Exercise (2020). *The Exercise Professional's Guide to Personal Training.* San Diego, Calif.: American Council on Exercise.

American Council on Exercise (2019). *The Professional's Guide to Health and Wellness Coaching.* San Diego, Calif.: American Council on Exercise.

U.S. Department of Health & Human Services (2018). *Physical Activity Guidelines for Americans* (2nd ed.). www.health.gov/paguidelines/

3 WORKING WITH CLIENTS WITH HEALTH CHALLENGES

IN THIS CHAPTER

PSYCHOLOGICAL IMPACT OF HEALTH CHALLENGES
IMPACT OF DISEASE
STRESS
IMPACT OF EXERCISE

LIFESTYLE CHOICES AND THEIR IMPACT ON PHYSIOLOGICAL CAPACITY
TOBACCO USE
FOOD CHOICES
INACTIVITY
ALCOHOL
CAFFEINE
PERFORMANCE-ENHANCING SUPPLEMENTS/DRUGS
SUGARY DRINKS
ILLICIT DRUGS
SUN EXPOSURE

THE 10-STEP DECISION-MAKING APPROACH TO EXERCISE PROGRAMMING FOR SPECIAL POPULATIONS
STEP 1: PERFORM A PRE-EXERCISE HEALTH-RISK ASSESSMENT
STEP 2: OBTAIN PHYSICIAN CLEARANCE
STEP 3: IDENTIFY EXERCISE BENEFITS AND GOALS
STEP 4: DETERMINE ACUTE EXERCISE RISKS
STEP 5: PREPARE FOR MEDICAL EMERGENCIES
STEP 6: OBTAIN INFORMED CONSENT
STEP 7: PLAN BASELINE FITNESS SCREENING AND TESTING
STEP 8: DESIGN THE EXERCISE PROGRAM
STEP 9: PLAN EXERCISE PROGRAM IMPLEMENTATION
STEP 10: DOUBLE-CHECK ESTABLISHED GUIDELINES

SUMMARY

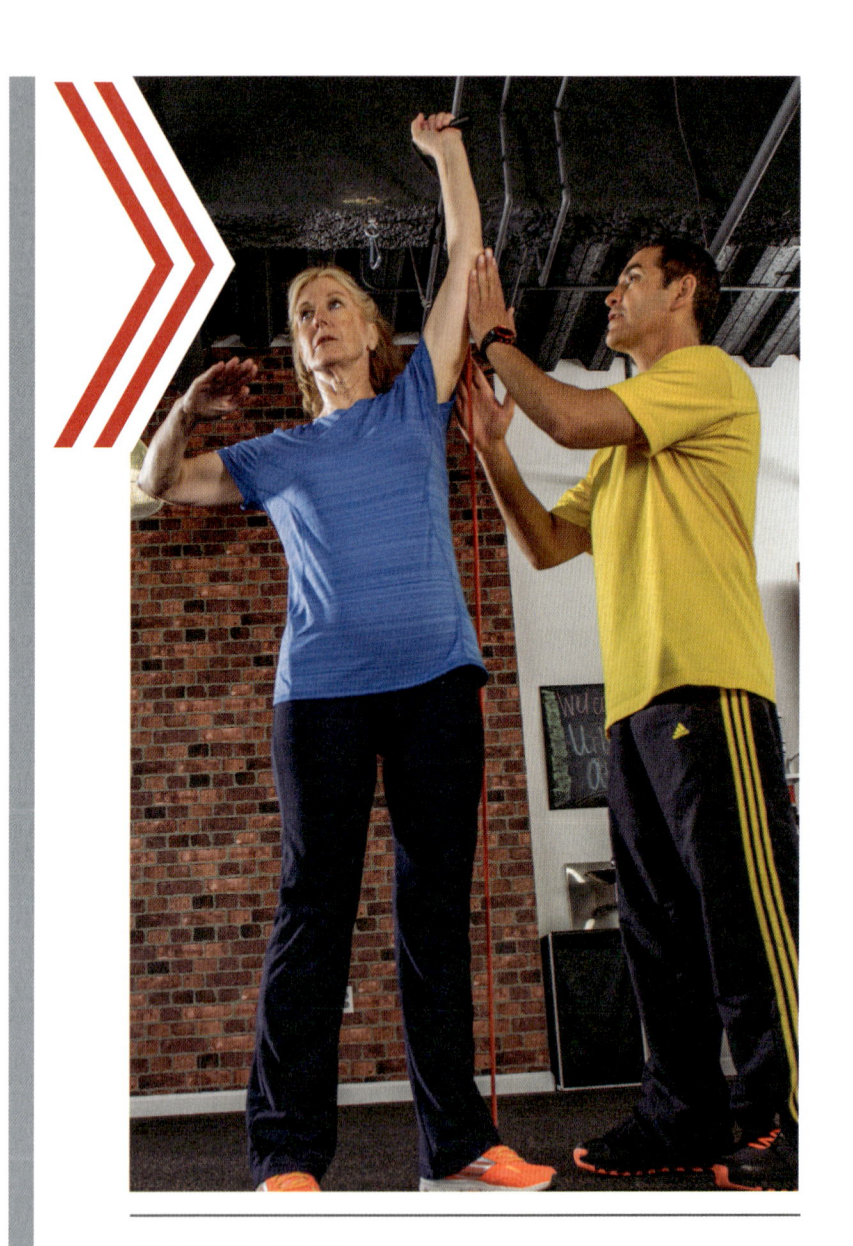

ABOUT THE AUTHOR
Nancey Trevanian Tsai, M.D., received her medical degree from Eastern Virginia Medical School in Norfolk, Va. She completed an internship in General Surgery at Swedish Medical Center in Seattle, commenced Orthopaedic Surgery training at Louisiana State University in New Orleans, and completed a Physical Medicine and Rehabilitation residency at Stanford University in Palo Alto, Calif., with a subspecialty in sports medicine. She is a diplomate of the American Board of Physical Medicine and Rehabilitation and is a clinical associate professor of neurosurgery at the Medical University of South Carolina in Charleston.

By Nancey Trevanian Tsai

WHILE HEALTH CHALLENGES ARE TYPICALLY viewed individually—in this text, readers will find chapters on **diabetes mellitus, coronary heart disease (CHD),** and **overweight** and **obesity,** for example—the truth is that many clients will present with multiple health challenges. These clients are some of the most difficult clients to manage. They are often taking numerous medications ("polypharmacy"), and it can be difficult to differentiate the symptoms associated with the diseases from the side effects of their medications.

Physical fatigue intermingles with **depression** and often both are escalated. Furthermore, people with multiple health challenges can place an emotional strain on those who work and live with them, be it their caregivers, physicians, or family members.

Regardless of whether a client has one or more diseases or disorders, the cost is significant. It can be hard for those who are otherwise healthy to imagine the burden imposed on those with chronic and/or multiple disease states. There is the physical burden of the disease itself, which alters function in daily activities, the financial burden of medical bills and medications, the time limitations due to medication dosing and/or side effects, and the emotional burden that comes with a loss of independence in one or more aspect(s) of daily living. Some diseases may have one name but impact multiple organ systems, such as diabetes. It is worth taking time to ask clients how their disease(s) and treatments have impacted their daily function.

One psychological aspect of having health challenges, especially more than one, is the social isolation the client may feel. Some of this is due to decreased mobility and **functional capacity.** Some of it can be due to the scheduling of medications and their anticipated side-effects, and some of it can be due to **body dysmorphism** and/or shame. Still others will perseverate on "if only" statements, such as "if only I quit smoking earlier," or "if only I stayed active." Unfortunately, social isolation can be depressing, lead to rumination, and commence a vicious cycle of negative self-talk. The ACE® Certified Medical Exercise Specialist (CMES) may have clients who lament that their calendar revolves around doctors' appointments rather than pleasurable activities. These are some of the most difficult clients to serve, as there is a complex social emotional pattern that has to be altered. Such clients may have difficulty "finding time" to exercise regularly, but really enjoy it once they attend. It is very important to help them verbalize the positive aspects of exercise on their disease and their overall sense of well-being at the end of each session as positive reinforcement. Remember, behind every great person is a large network of support; in fact, the greatness of the achievement is most frequently proportional to the size of the supporting team. The CMES should encourage clients to become part of a network, either through the facility or in their general community outside of the medical concerns. With time, the personal-training appointment will become a significant portion of their positive social activity. A CMES can be powerfully persuasive in a client's life, not only as a fitness instructor, but also as a coach and encourager. The key is to replace negative self-talk with positive affirmations and explore new social networks.

LEARNING OBJECTIVES:

» Explain the psychological impact of health challenges, as well as the importance of exercise on positively influencing those challenges.

» Briefly describe how lifestyle choices such as drug use, food choices, and physical inactivity can impact physiological capacity.

» Explain the 10-step decision-making approach to exercise programming for a CMES who works with special populations.

There are disease processes that are chronic, without definitive cure, and/or with devastating consequences. Some examples include cancer, HIV/AIDS, **rheumatoid arthritis,** and **multiple sclerosis.** The diagnosis often becomes a sentinel event, and life is seen as having a "before" and "after" this event. It becomes even more important to foster an environment in which these clients are not defined by their disease through sensitive and effective communication. This process involves acceptance of their feelings, empathy for their hardships, and respect for each of them as an individual. It is also important to maintain reasonable boundaries, especially in terms of time, so that the appointments do not degenerate into self-absorption and lose functional exercise as a focus.

> **EXPAND YOUR KNOWLEDGE**
>
> **MONETARY IMPACT OF MULTIPLE HEALTH CHALLENGES**
>
> According to the World Bank, the United States spent 17.9% of its gross domestic product on healthcare in 2011 (Fuchs, 2013). Relatively little of this is actual payment for interaction with physicians. An increasing amount is for prescription pharmaceuticals, "nutriceuticals," and functional assistance in the form of skilled nursing and/or devices. Money spent on preventive measures is comparatively little, despite its potential impact on sustained health. However, as co-pays for medications are increasing—up to $75 for some brand name prescriptions—the session with the CMES can seem like a relative bargain when considering the long-term beneficial effects of regular exercise. A person who exercises is less likely to require long-term care or other functional assistance during their lifetime. The benefits of exercise range from immediate to lifelong when maintained.

PSYCHOLOGICAL IMPACT OF HEALTH CHALLENGES

Impact of Disease

The diagnosis of a disease can impact a person's sense of self and wellness. For some, the diagnosis comes after a catastrophic event, such as a heart attack or a **stroke.** For others, it is an insidious process that may be noticed only by loved ones. The reactions to the diagnosis of a disease can be as diverse as abject denial to a clear lifestyle alteration, and is related to the person's coping mechanisms. Furthermore, there is a growing body of evidence that indicates a strong correlation between physical and emotional health. Stress affects wellness physically and emotionally. It is appropriate to ask how a client is coping with the disease and how it impacts their life. This is a helpful step in establishing **rapport** and may alter the way a program is designed and progressed. Some clients will experience a crisis and separate themselves from toxic life situations and/or experience a new appreciation for their friends and families. Others may feel helpless, even paralyzed and unable to move toward better choices and better lifestyle decisions. Health challenges bring attention to the need to change bad habits as the person's physiology and life circumstances change.

Although a disease is not necessarily a permanent state, a client can begin to identify themself by a diagnosis. For example, a client may say, "I am diabetic" rather than "I have diabetes." This disease-ridden identity is often one of the barriers that keep a client from seeing themself getting better. With more diagnoses often comes depression and chronic pain. Depression often leads to decreased immunity and a greater predisposition to seasonal illnesses. The CMES should have frank discussions about a client's disease by identifying the client's knowledge base of the disease, its signs and symptoms, the expectations of its progression or regression with a fitness program, and any concerns the client may have regarding how this disease impacts one's life. If a client is identified as having been traumatized by the sudden onset of the disease process, they may need a referral to a psychologist to develop appropriate coping skills. Some clients will use humor as a way to minimize their reaction to their diagnosis, and it is important to offer them a confidential forum to air their feelings. Others will have tremendous **anxiety** and need reassurance that their concerns are heard. It is important to separate the signs and symptoms of the disease from the client's sense of self. A focus on functional gains and separating the person from their diseases can dramatically impact a client's outlook in a positive way.

During the initial interview and throughout the program, it is important to ask how the client feels, preferably as an open-ended question. Depending upon the client's personality, a series of questions may be needed to follow up on the first response. It is helpful to have the client recall a functional gain, a limitation, and a moment when they felt good with the circumstances. This verbalization helps to reinforce a positive image of the fitness activity relative to the client's function and helps with program progression. It also extends rapport beyond superficial acquaintance. It is important to affirm clients' feelings, even if the CMES does not agree with their beliefs about their state of health. By allowing clients to openly talk about their feelings, the CMES offers a way to discharge the negative impact of the health challenge prior to the workout, allowing for more productivity during the exercise session.

There is a growing trend to employ multidisciplinary approaches to treating disease. Integral to this idea is teamwork involving the treating physician, patient/client, physical therapist, exercise professional, and psychologist. Once clearance has been obtained from the physician for an exercise program, the CMES has the option of recommending other team members. For some clients, a counselor—a psychologist, social worker, or therapist—may be a valuable team member to assist in functional restoration. This multidisciplinary approach has been demonstrated to be more effective than medication alone or the utilization of any one aspect individually (Schultz et al., 2007; Li et al., 2006; Lillefjell, Krokstad, & Espnes, 2006).

Stress

Dr. Hans Selye (1975) defined stress as "a nonspecific response of the body to any demand made upon it." Stress can be good and/or performance-enhancing ("eustress") or bad ("distress"), although most people typically associate stress with bad events. A stressor is a particularly difficult concept to define, because it is largely dependent on a person's coping mechanisms. What is stressful for one person may not be stressful at all for another. Furthermore, there are categories of stressors, including positive and negative, and high- and low-impact. The greatest stressors include those events that occur to those closest to the individual, such as the death of a spouse or close family member, a change in marital status, the birth of a child, or a change in employment. The suddenness of these events also changes the impact, depending upon the situation. Some clients will cope with the sudden, unexpected death of a loved one better than others. Others, for example, will have "grieved" for a parent with **Alzheimer's disease** long before they pass on. A common theme inherent in stress is the idea of being out of control in one or more situations. As such, the general concept behind coping with stress is to be able to control one's reaction to a stressor, even if one cannot control the context of the stress.

Stressors, or triggers, fall into two categories: external and internal. Examples of external stressors include the following:
- *Physical environment:* Noise, lights (bright, direct sunlight, fluorescent lights), temperature (hot or cold), space (confined or open)
- *Social interactions:* With those in a position of power; with rude or angry people
- *Occupational/organizational:* Rules (explicit and implicit), deadlines, power structure, and the expectations of those who are higher ranked
- *Life events:* Death of a spouse or close relative, new job, new child, or new home

Examples of internal stressors include the following:
- *Lifestyle choices:* Smoking, excessive alcohol or caffeine intake, poor sleep habits, or poor hygiene

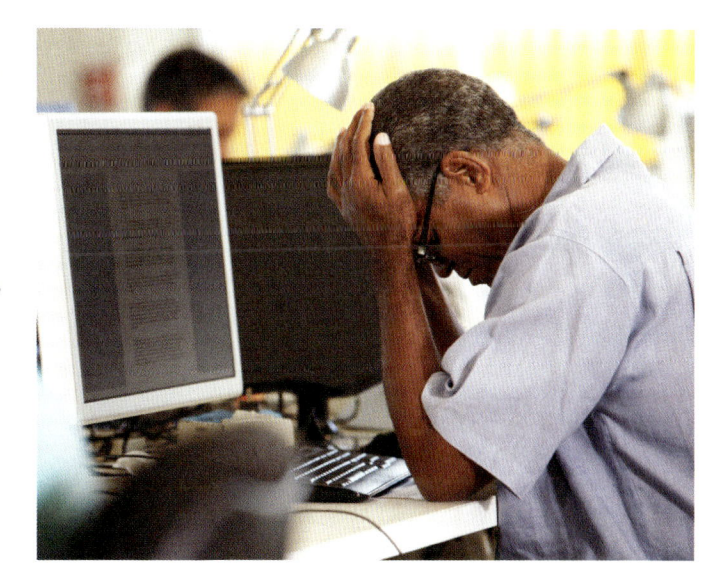

- *Negative self-image:* Excessive self-criticism, inherent pessimistic outlook, or unrealistic expectations
- *Inability to adapt:* Concrete thinking, taking criticism personally, or an unwillingness to change or compromise
- *Personality traits:* Type A personalities or perfectionism

In all cases, there are physiological consequences to stress. **Cortisol** levels are altered in individuals in high-stress environments. Immunity and resistance to disease are lowered during times of stress. Stress can lead to disease states and negatively impact pre-existing diseases by lowering the body's defense mechanisms. The stress reaction consists of a physiological response, including the outpouring of sympathetic **hormones** and alterations of **glucose** and fatty acids in the blood to provide energy. **Epinephrine,** also known as adrenaline, initiates the "fight-or-flight" response—increasing the **heart rate** and **blood pressure**; increasing mental alertness; and shunting blood flow to the brain, heart, and muscles in preparation for stress. Some people feel euphoric during this time and will continually seek situations that cause these physiological changes. However, others will feel different symptoms more commonly associated with stress, typically some combination of the following categories:

- *Physical:* Headache, chest pains, palpitations, nausea, trembling, and diffuse muscle and joint aches and/or stiffness
- *Mental:* Decreased attention, concentration, memory, confusion, and indecisiveness
- *Emotional:* Anxiety, depression, irritability, worry, anger, and frustration
- *Behavioral:* Tics and other nervous habits such as nail-biting, increased hand-to-mouth activity (eating, smoking, and drinking), and verbal and/or physical abuse of self or others

Although the triggers can be external or internal, the reaction to stress is almost entirely self-generated. As such, recognizing the stressor and one's reaction to it becomes the first step in coping with stress. If the stress load is overwhelming, it may be important to keep a journal of one's situations and feelings for a week to clearly identify the triggers and their effects. Understanding the stress reaction and altering one's behaviors and thinking are not necessarily easy tasks, because they involve a change in one's outlook on life and general perspective. The development of management and coping skills associated with stress is a multistep process that takes practice. The steps include avoiding stressful situations when possible (boundary creation), altering the situation if it is not avoidable, controlling reactions to stressors, and adaptation.

- *Avoiding stress:* Most people know what situations stress them positively or negatively. When dealing with an avoidable negative stressor, such as a person or a place, limiting interactions with that person or place will decrease the total stress load. People must learn to establish healthy boundaries and plan exit strategies ahead of time. Learning to say no is an important part of creating healthy boundaries and maintaining balance. In addition, planning and practicing certain phrases, such as, "I'm sorry to cut this short, but I have a lot to do today and want to get home at a reasonable time," is helpful to maintaining those boundaries. In some cases, it may be necessary to leave the job or relationship that is causing the significant burden in one's life.
- *Altering the context of the stress:* Most stressors are potentially manageable. There are many books and websites devoted to time- and money-management, which are major stressors in many people's lives. Balancing the schedule to reflect positive and negative stress activities is another important step to effective stress management. The CMES can teach clients to schedule in regular exercise, sit down to eat and be conscious of food choices, and plan rewards at regular intervals. These actions will help make negative stressors more manageable.
- *Controlling reactions to stressors:* Learning to separate one's feelings and reactions to a stressor is a skill that takes practice. For example, many people are easily angered or upset by criticism from a parent. However, if the emotional reaction is immediately assessed and depersonalized, the stress has less impact ("I'm not being criticized. They are just having a bad day."). It is also helpful to learn phrases, such as, "I can't talk about this right now. I'll get back to you later." It takes effort and practice to stop the immediate emotional reaction

that leads to the complex set of behaviors that ensue. However, being able to recognize those internal cues and separate from them will make it easier to practice new behaviors. It is important to remind clients that while a person cannot control the stressors, they can control the reaction to them.
- *Adaptation:* This step involves resiliency to challenges. Physical resiliency comes from a well-balanced diet, adequate sleep and relaxation, and regular exercise. Mental resiliency comes from the ability to look at each situation objectively and being able to identify opportunities when problems arise. Emotional resiliency is the ability to reject negative thinking and have a sense of humor when situations do not go as well as planned. This is the most creative of all the steps and also the most satisfying.

THINK IT THROUGH

Evaluate the fitness facility where you work for elements that might induce stress in clients with specific diseases or disabilities. Are the lights too bright in one area of the facility? Is the music too loud? Can clients performing mindful exercise in the group fitness room overhear loud conversations from elsewhere in the facility? Think of ways to minimize these potentially stressful situations.

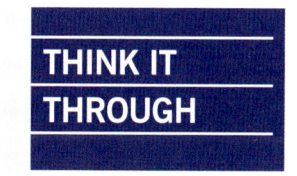

Impact of Exercise

The *2018 Physical Activity Guidelines for Americans* report states that physical activity supports normal growth and development; helps people function, feel, and sleep better; and reduces the risk of a wide span of chronic diseasess (U.S. Department of Health and Human Services, 2018). According to the World Health Organization (2010), physical fitness and exercise can reduce the risk of heart disease, **type 2 diabetes,** some cancers, **osteoarthritis, osteoporosis,** and obesity. On the other hand, a **sedentary** lifestyle prevents the body from utilizing its energy stores and regulating its metabolism effectively. Exercise is crucial to maintaining health, performance capacity, and overall quality of life.

Exercise also improves a person's psychological profile. There are many reasons for this, including the release of **neurotransmitters, endocrine** regulation, and improved sleep. Exercise also discharges the heightened arousal state that results from stress. Satisfaction can also come from the simple act of reaching a goal during each session. Nearly everyone will feel better physically and psychologically after a session of exercise that is appropriate to their level of fitness.

Physical activity stimulates the secretion of many "feel-good" hormones. The most obtuse example of this is the reported "runner's high," which is associated with the release of **endorphins** during a mid- to long-distance run. Other hormones released during exercise include **growth hormone, norepinephrine,** epinephrine, and **glucagon.** Glucagon is secreted to convert stored **glycogen** into glucose, which improves the efficiency of **insulin** for several hours after each session. Norepinephrine and epinephrine are released in the brain and throughout the body to elevate mood during and immediately after exercise. With regular exercise, the body seeks to continue staying active, sustaining a positive feedback loop.

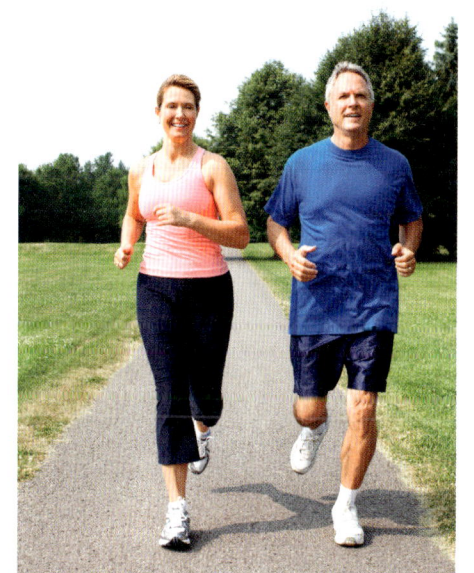

It has been demonstrated that regular exercise leads to improved sleep quality and duration, which also contributes to the release of nocturnal, reparative neurotransmitters, including growth hormone, **insulin-like growth factors,** and **melatonin.** Although a sleeping person seems inactive, radiography and neurophysiologic studies have demonstrated that some parts of the brain are more active during REM (rapid eye movement) sleep than when a person is performing mundane daily tasks (Dang-Vu et al., 2010). Sleep-deprivation experiments have demonstrated that pain tolerance is decreased with increased irritability when REM and deep sleep are denied for more than 36 hours in healthy and chronically ill subjects (Irwin et al., 2012; Azevedo et al., 2011). Chronic sleep deprivation (e.g., four hours of sleep over a five-day workweek) could have deleterious effects not only on daytime alertness but also on cognitive performance, even when subjects report not necessarily feeling sleepy (Philip et al., 2012). Although there are a number of sleep-induction medications available over-the-counter and by prescription, virtually all of them disrupt the normal sleep patterns. Most of these medications allow a person to fall or stay asleep, but do not allow them to achieve REM or deep sleep. So while a person may feel as if they have rested, the cellular repair mechanisms typically taking place during sleep have not occurred. Other clients have no problems falling or staying asleep, but have sleep disturbances, such as **sleep apnea** or nocturnal seizures that require monitoring and interventions with medical devices.

Because sleep is a restorative activity, those who do not sleep well will frequently have other health challenges. In their review of the literature on sleep and glucose metabolism, Cappuccio et al. (2010) found that decreased quantity and quality of sleep consistently and significantly predict the risk of the development of type 2 diabetes. Other studies have suggested that sleep deprivation may be linked to obesity, heart disease, and mental illnesses such as bipolar disorder [Perry, Patil, & Presley-Cantrell, 2013; Institute of Medicine (IOM), 2006]. Many studies suggest that sleep deprivation increases activity on the hypothalamic-pituitary-adrenal axis and suppresses growth hormones, which could lead to poor stress management and even obesity (Lucassen & Cizza, 2012; IOM, 2006). The great majority of clients will note improved sleep after regular exercise within several weeks of starting their program. They will also experience improved mental clarity and increased creativity with adequate restorative sleep, in addition to improved physical health.

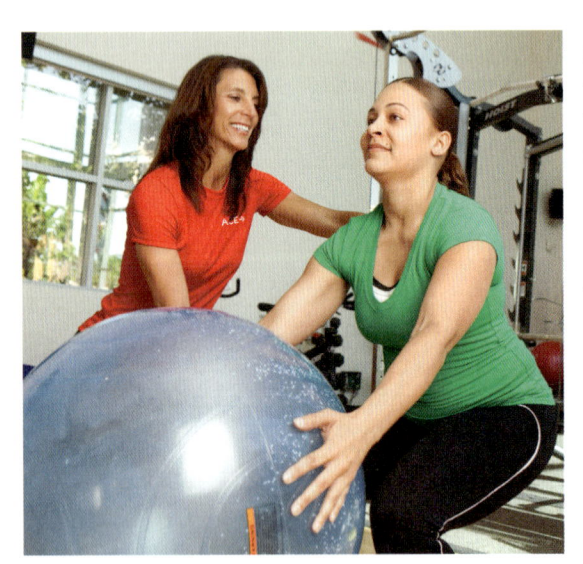

For some clients, the psychological effects of exercise go beyond the hormonal effects of each session. There is the sense of accomplishment in achieving small goals with each session and reaching intermediate goals at set intervals. Some clients may accomplish more during the day due to improved overall function. Some may even report that they "overdid it" and need to work on setting reasonable limits. The improved sleep resulting from a well-designed exercise program can improve pain thresholds and general life satisfaction. The CMES should spend a few minutes with clients to review their subjective feelings since their last session, as doing so may reinforce their perception of progress.

LIFESTYLE CHOICES AND THEIR IMPACT ON PHYSIOLOGICAL CAPACITY

Under normal circumstances, physiological capacity increases through childhood and early adulthood and begins to decline in mid- to late-adulthood. As a person ages, **aerobic power** can continue to improve at decreased rates, but performance declines. Although aerobic power increases in childhood and early adulthood with increases in blood and lung volumes, aerobic power declines by about 1% per year and **maximal heart rate** decreases by one beat per year after reaching maturity. Because muscle cells change in composition, shunting **fast-twitch muscle fibers** toward **intermediate-** and **slow-twitch muscle fibers,** performance of endurance activities tends to decline more slowly than performance of power-related activities. Strength exercise, although still important, typically produces less actual gains in the elderly than with young adults. However, as the rate of loss is similar between men and women regardless of baseline, it is important to optimize muscle mass and performance during early- and mid-adulthood in anticipation of the eventual decline in performance.

Clients with health challenges have altered physiology. For example, those with signs of **cardiovascular disease (CVD)** or with known CVD have a ceiling to their aerobic power because chest pain or poorer performance of the heart itself does not allow those with CVD to exercise at higher levels. A client who recently had hip surgery may continue to have range-of-motion limitations. Elderly persons may complain of instability and balance issues. In contrast, those who exercise regularly and/or have an active lifestyle typically have fewer functional limitations and less significant health concerns.

Working with a client who is known to have CVD requires both due diligence and sensitivity on the part of the CMES. Typically, a stress test will have been done to demonstrate the limits on heart rate and/or perceived intensity. However, as a client continues in their program, improvements may allow for incremental increases in duration and/or intensity. Documentation of the client's comments and complaints, as well as communication with the attending physician, will maximize functional exercise capacity while minimizing the risk of further complications and making the exercise safer. Other modifying factors include age, nutritional status, and other disease-associated risk factors.

While the heart is responsible for the mechanical aspects of pushing blood through the vascular channels, the lungs are crucial for the oxygen–carbon dioxide exchange. For younger clients—including youth—restrictive lung disease at the level of the **bronchioles** is often responsible for exercise-related **asthma.** With age, typically, the rate-limiting step is the air exchanged at the alveolar level, which is usually related to a prolonged history of smoking and/or industrial pollutant exposure. Both of these factors can lead to decreased oxygen flow to the skeletal muscles at rest and during exercise. At times, it may be challenging, even for the seasoned healthcare provider, to ascertain the basis of a person's exercise limitations. Unlike otherwise healthy clients who should be encouraged to work through perceived difficulty, those with cardiovascular and/or pulmonary disease may be signaling an active disease process. Ceasing exercise to monitor vitals or perhaps calling for more acute care may be indicated at times. For some, it may be worth pursuing a monitored environment for program development until underlying causes are addressed appropriately and definitively. Medical clearance and clarification of limitations should be obtained.

Sensory integration dysfunction is a growing concern across all ages as people become more sedentary. Injuries due to falls and accidents are increasing in even young children. Falling is a factor that has traditionally been associated with the aged, but is now seen in middle-age and even young adults whose lifestyle choices have impacted their neurological systems. Some of these choices included prolonged and/or excessive use of alcohol and use of certain illicit drugs (e.g., ecstasy). For others, it can be a side effect after years of using certain prescription medications. In children, increasingly sedentary lifestyles may have contributed to premature deterioration of **synapses** that coordinate body movement. Fortunately, there are training exercises that can improve **proprioception** and increase overall function.

Some complicated diseases have associated health risks that impact exercise programming. It is important for the CMES to understand that chronic progressive and/or relapsing-remitting illnesses can alter a client's ability to perform consistently. For example, a client with multiple sclerosis may demonstrate less strength and endurance when the weather is hot or if they do not remain well hydrated and overheats. The client may have an exacerbation with increased stress at home or work and be unable to return to the maintenance program for several weeks. While it is not within the realm of expertise of a CMES to know all of the manifestations of these systemic and other diseases, it behooves one to seek medical clearance and clarification of limitations if there are any concerns prior to program creation.

Tobacco Use

Smoking is likely one of the costliest lifestyle choices a person can make. In addition to the immediate cost of tobacco products, virtually every system in the body is adversely affected by smoking. Insurance costs—including health, auto, home, and life—are universally higher for smokers than non-smokers. Not commonly reported is the physical and mental anguish suffered by smokers as a result of their choice.

A cigarette contains thousands of chemicals that interact with the body, the most widely discussed of which is nicotine. Nicotine can be a highly addictive substance in some individuals, creating an artificial need for a substance that is not critical to sustaining life. There are also thermal effects of inhaling a burned substance. Over time, doing so changes the cell types of all the surfaces the inhaled smoke contacts along the oropharynx and respiratory tract, leading to cancerous growths in those who are genetically susceptible.

The mechanism, causal or correlative, between the use of tobacco and neck and/or back pain is still speculative. One theory is that vasospasm of the small vessels that supply the disks, joints, and small nerves that innervate the spine anatomy causes **transient ischemia** to those tissues with each dose of nicotine that has a cumulative effect over many pack years (Ditre et al., 2011). When those small vessels lose function or become inadequate to supply nutrients to relatively avascular tissue—such as the intervertebral disks—it accelerates the natural aging process of those tissues. A similar line of reasoning exists for a client with diabetes, who is also more likely to have neck and back pain due to the development of small vessel disease with prolonged **hyperglycemia.** Once the disk or joint capsule is dessicated, there is no remodeling process, as there might be in better vascularized tissue. The bony elements then produce osteophytic changes, which can lead to foraminal and central **stenosis,** both of which can contribute to impingement of nerve tissue, causing pain and weakness. Additionally, those who smoke increase both the carbon monoxide load and alveolar dead space, which is the area for air exchange in the lungs, leading to decreased oxygenation tension and saturation in the blood. Smoking also impedes bony fusion, the staple of neck and back surgery. It is well known that smokers who do not quit go on to form mal-unions and non-unions more frequently than those who do not smoke. What cannot be described clinically is the persistent pain that interrupts all activities of life, including sleep. Eventually, the pain centralizes and there is no respite, no position that makes it better, and no medication that offers complete relief.

With very rare exceptions (e.g., in a person diagnosed with paranoid schizophrenia, for whom the psychotic symptoms are known to be attenuated with smoking), there are no health benefits associated with the use of tobacco. For those who choose to quit, most organ systems will reach some level of normalization within one year. Some damage is irreversible, such as the increased alveolar dead space in **chronic obstructive pulmonary disease (COPD).** Smoking cessation will halt the progression of damage, but cannot reverse the changes. It is always advisable that clients find the motivation and surround themselves with those who will help them to stop smoking.

Food Choices

As mentioned earlier in this chapter, the majority of Americans have overweight or obesity. Although there are a few persons for whom a diagnosis of **hypothyroidism** accounts for a small amount of their weight disparity, it is clearly not the case that more than half of the American population has an endocrine dysfunction.

Carbohydrate consumption is a common research focus because of the tendency for many Americans to frequently eat the easily accessible and relatively inexpensive forms of carbohydrate that occur in refined foods. When consumed in their least processed form, whole grains are an excellent source of **fiber,** plant **proteins,** and **complex carbohydrates** that offers sustained energy. During the late 1980s and early 1990s, when **fat** was considered the root cause of overweight and obesity, many people found themselves continuing to gain weight and even developing diabetes due to overconsumption of highly refined, highly processed sugary snacks that were "fat-free." Examples of refining processes include the hulling of brown rice, which removes the bran (source of fiber) and the germ (source of protein) from the kernel, leaving only the **carbohydrate** and a minimum of protein inherent in the grain. Many "whole-wheat breads" are made from white flour with a small amount of whole-wheat flour in preparing the dough. A high-quality grain-based diet means choosing whole grain in its natural, unprocessed state.

Impaired insulin signaling and metabolism contributes to the development of the **metabolic syndrome (MetS),** a constellation of cardiovascular risk factors including abdominal obesity, impaired glucose control, **hypertension,** and **dyslipidemia** (Rask-Madsen & Kahn, 2012; Grundy et al., 2005). Thus, frequent consumption of highly processed or refined foods may be a significant contributor to the increased incidence of this disorder in developed nations. The mildly increased blood pressure, borderline **hypercholesterolemia,** and persistent hyperglycemia are all symptoms of insulin dysregulation. It is well known that exercise suppresses the release of insulin and improves the cellular uptake of glucose after a meal. Although pharmaceutical companies are developing new drugs to offset the symptoms of MetS, daily physical activity can play an important role in helping to normalize blood glucose levels and also increases the release of natural endorphins to improve mood.

Many people have found success with low-carbohydrate diets. However, they can be expensive and difficult to sustain over long periods of time. Although high-quality proteins should be consumed daily to maintain muscle mass, very few individuals need more than 10–35% of their total daily calories from protein to sustain optimal health. This amount is easily obtained by those who consume a normal diet. It is typically recommended that adults keep total fat between 20–35% of total caloric intake. In addition, less than 10% of calories should come from saturated fats (U.S. Department of Agriculture, 2020). Fat acts to insulate nerve tissue and internal organs. When not consumed in the diet, it can be converted from an excess of carbohydrate or protein products. However, while skeletal muscle preferentially uses fatty acids as fuel at rest, the brain and other tissues prefer glucose to produce **adenosine triphosphate (ATP).** Individuals following a carbohydrate-restrictive diet that induces **ketosis,** resulting in fatigue and mental sluggishness, can have difficulty maintaining an active lifestyle.

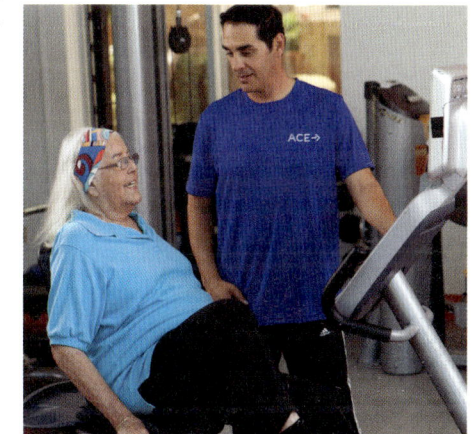

Inactivity

Using bedrest as the extreme example of inactivity, one can infer the relative effects of sedentary lifestyles. For every day a person is immobile, strength decreases by 1 to 1.5%; five weeks of total inactivity will cause a 50% loss of previous muscle strength, with a plateau reached at 25 to 40% of original strength. Simply performing one contraction a day at 50% of maximal strength is enough to prevent this decrease (Strax, Gonzalez, & Cuccurullo, 2004). Lack of gravity resistance causes **osteopenia** and **hypercalcemia.** It is well known that excess calcium in the blood can lead to diffuse abdominal discomfort, depression, pain syndromes, and kidney stones, and calcium is the last mineral to normalize after prolonged inactivity. Osteopenia leads to weakened bones and a higher fracture risk. Blood flow from the lower extremities is attenuated, potentially leading to the development of blood clots. Although it is unlikely that being a "couch potato" will lead to all of these pathologies, lesser manifestations can still be present to some level in a person who chooses to be sedentary.

There is growing evidence that prolonged sitting, standing, and other non-exercise activities may independently increase the risk of such lifestyle diseases as obesity, cancer, diabetes, impaired glucose uptake, and **insulin resistance.** Even when adults meet physical-activity guidelines, prolonged sitting can compromise one's metabolic health. Even short breaks of one to two minutes each hour can have positive effects. Therefore, clients should be encouraged to be more active and less inactive. Both are important.

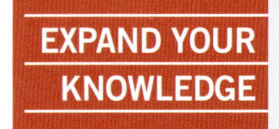

> **EXPAND YOUR KNOWLEDGE**
>
> **PHYSICAL ACTIVITY AFFECTS RISK FACTORS FOR CARDIOVASCULAR DISEASE**
>
> As mentioned earlier, MetS is a collection of cardiovascular risk factors comprised of abdominal obesity, impaired glucose control, hypertension, and dyslipidemia (Grundy et al., 2005). Each MetS component separately increases the risk for CVD and all-cause mortality, but the full syndrome is associated with an increase in risk that is greater than the risk of each individual risk factor. Therapeutic lifestyle changes, including exercise, are recommended as a first-line strategy in the treatment of cardiovascular risk factors. In a meta-analysis that reviewed exercise's effects on cardiovascular risk factors in patients with MetS, Pattyn and colleagues (2013) found that aerobic endurance training (e.g., between 40–60 minutes, 3–5 days per week, at moderate to high intensities for 8–52 weeks) favorably influenced waist circumference, **high-density lipoprotein (HDL)** levels, **systolic blood pressure (SBP)**, and **diastolic blood pressure (DBP)**. The researchers also found that regular endurance training positively affected other important cardiovascular risk factors, including **low-density lipoprotein (LDL)** levels, total cholesterol, and BMI.
>
> In addition to aerobic exercise, participation in regular resistance training has also been shown to yield positive effects on markers for MetS. In their review of the literature on resistance training in the treatment of MetS, Strasser, Siebert, and Schobersberger (2010) found that weight training has a clinically and statistically significant effect on risk factors such as obesity, **glycosylated hemoglobin (A1c)** levels, and SBP. The researchers concluded that resistance training should be recommended in the management of type 2 diabetes and metabolic disorders.
>
> The results of these research reviews are impressive, considering that only one form of treatment [i.e., exercise (either aerobic or resistance training)] was found to positively affect the variables related to MetS. These findings also suggest that both aerobic and resistance-training exercise should be included in a physical activity program to reduce the risk of MetS and subsequent CVD. See Chapter 12 for information on exercise programming for MetS.

Alcohol

It is unclear whether moderate alcohol consumption is better for health than teetotaling. There is no doubt that long-term, heavy usage of alcohol, or even occasional binging, leads to altered end-organ function with age. The effects are amplified when the alcohol usage is commenced at an early age.

The most commonly reported disease associated with heavy alcohol use is liver disease (Gao & Bataller, 2011). The liver is the first area of processing of most toxins, including alcohol. Some persons are unable to break down alcohol completely and have physiologic reactions, such as flushing and discomfort, and so they will avoid alcohol consumption altogether. Cells that process alcohol also process drugs such as acetaminophen (Tylenol). If the liver attempts to process more than 4 grams of acetaminophen (about 12 regular or eight extra-strength tablets) or some combination of alcohol and acetaminophen per day, acute liver failure can ensue, leading to increased mortality. More commonly, long-term usage leads to changes in the cytohistologic features, first as a **fatty liver,** then as a shrunken cirrhotic liver. Because the liver produces nearly all of the noncellular blood proteins, every tissue in the body becomes more fragile with long-term heavy alcohol consumption. Alcohol consumption also leads to decreased reaction time, decreased motor coordination, and impaired memory at the time of usage.

Caffeine

Caffeine is another substance that is prevalent in most diets. For many, a morning does not begin until after the first cup of coffee. Others choose sodas or energy drinks. Even some of the effects of chocolate can be attributed to the small amount of caffeine present. Caffeine is a xanthine compound, part of a group of **central nervous system (CNS)** stimulants that also includes nicotine. When consumed in moderation, caffeine can lead to moderate improvements in executive tasks and motor coordination. When consumed in excess, it can lead to nervousness, insomnia, and symptoms that parallel panic and/or heart attacks. It can be an addictive substance for susceptible persons, leading to symptoms of withdrawal if completely and suddenly removed. Numerous studies have shown that caffeine ingested prior to and during prolonged submaximal and high-intensity exercise can improve performance (Hodgson, Randell, & Jeukendrup, 2013). Because of caffeine's performance-enhancing qualities, many over-the-counter medications containing caffeine have been added to the "banned-substances" list for athletes.

Performance-enhancing Supplements/Drugs

The fine line between supplements and compounds designed to enhance performance continues to be blurred with the advent of genetic technology. A client may have goals that are admirable, but the means of achieving them may not necessarily be acceptable. Over-the-counter supplements designed to increase metabolism, build muscle mass, and/or burn fat are easily accessible. Claims made by manufacturers are not subject to the rigorous testing standards of the Food and Drug Administration (FDA). On the other hand, for the high-performance athlete for whom a few one-hundredths of a second can mean the difference between Olympic gold and obscurity, the risk of getting caught is often the basis for making the decision on whether to use supplements, rather than any ethical or health concerns. Unfortunately, this decision is not limited to high-profile athletes, but also affects high school athletes for whom performance can sometimes represent the pathway to a college scholarship or professional sports contract.

The United States Olympic Committee has a published list of banned substances, some of which are sport-specific (such as beta blockers for archery). Additional information can be obtained at the U.S. Anti-Doping Agency's website (www.usada.org).

Sugary Drinks

Sugary drinks are ubiquitous in American life. Soft drinks constitute a multibillion dollar industry that has replaced water for hydration in many people's lives. The refined sugar content in the larger soda sizes has been linked with the increase in the metabolic syndrome and type 2 diabetes. Currently, American adults ages 19 years and older consume an average of about 400 calories per day as beverages, with the highest intake coming from regular soda. In fact, sugar-sweetened beverages and sweetened coffees and teas are responsible for more than 40% of the added sugars the typical American consumes in a day (U.S. Department of Agriculture, 2020). Research into the consumption of high-calorie beverages, such as regular soda, suggests that it can contribute to childhood obesity, and limitation of sweetened beverages may help decrease obesity in children (Morgan, 2013).

There is also concern over soft-drink consumption, specifically of cola products, and its potential adverse effects on **bone mineral density (BMD).** In addition to displacing healthier beverages, colas contain caffeine and phosphoric acid, which may negatively affect bone. Although more research is needed, investigators in the Framingham Osteoporosis Study concluded that intake of cola, but not of other carbonated soft drinks, is associated with low BMD in women. Similar results were seen for diet cola and, although weaker, for decaffeinated cola (Tucker et al., 2006).

Illicit Drugs

Occasional use of recreational drugs in the United States is typically done by educated, higher-socioeconomic professionals. The most common drugs used include marijuana, cocaine, and amphetamine-based substances. Legality issues aside, there are physiological risks that can be harmful. Marijuana leads to decreased reaction time and poor executive function in the immediate phase, with gynecomastia (atypical breast tissue development in males) and microgonadism (smaller testicles) with long-term use. Cocaine and other CNS stimulants can lead to insomnia in the short-term, and have higher addiction potentials due to their dysphoria-inducing withdrawal symptoms. With long-term amphetamine abuse, irreversible mental states resembling schizophrenia, such as paranoia, poor pain tolerance, and lethargy, can ensue. Users of cocaine are at risk for hypertension and stroke, typically with bleeding into the brain (intracerebral hemorrhage), which has debilitating long-term effects. A CMES can reduce professional risk by refusing to work with clients who are known to be using illicit substances.

Sun Exposure

Ultraviolet rays activate vitamin-D precursors at the level of the skin. The amount of exposure this requires is much less than it takes to alter the melanin content of the skin. Most researchers and dermatologists would agree that there is no such thing as "a healthy tan." Contrary to popular belief, getting a "base tan" at a tanning booth does not protect from burns at the beach. According to the American Academy of Dermatology (AAD), the UVA and UVB exposure from a booth is more detrimental to skin health than typical sunburns. In fact, the AAD opposes indoor tanning and supports prohibiting the sale and use of commercial indoor tanning equipment (AAD, 2012). Prolonged sun exposure leads to premature aging and increased risk of skin cancers. It also leads to changes in the eye, including photokeratitis and cataract development. Some medications will make the skin more susceptible to burning. When the body is busy repairing its largest organ (the skin), the immune system is rendered more susceptible to viral illnesses and/or reactivations. As such, it is not infrequent that cold sores or herpes will flare up after excessive sun exposure. It is important that clients think of tanning as an inflammatory response to an environmental insult. When training clients outdoors, the CMES should strongly recommend that sunblock be applied before exposure and reapplied after water exposure or excessive sweating.

APPLY WHAT YOU KNOW

DEVELOP A PLAN FOR HAVING DIFFICULT CONVERSATIONS WITH CLIENTS

A CMES will sometimes find themself discussing lifestyle choices with clients, and must do so without offending or embarrassing them. Effectively discussing topics like drug use, alcohol consumption, and even physical inactivity and poor food choices can be very difficult for some clients and requires a high degree of rapport between the client and the CMES, who should try to develop a means of initiating these often difficult conversations with a combination of tact and authority.

Consider the following scenario, in which a client reveals a concern with excess alcohol consumption during a conversation about his struggles with diabetes and hypertension.

CMES: Can you tell me what you are doing now that you think is good for you and what you are doing that you think is not so good for you?

Client (C): When I avoid the junk food that is always around the house, or when I remember to take my medicine, that's certainly good for me. Let's see…bad things? I know I shouldn't be drinking as much as I do. I do enjoy a few beers with my buddies. But the truth is, it's always more than a few beers. But I honestly don't know if I have what it takes to make these big changes.

CMES: I understand. Making important changes isn't an easy thing to do. People try and then ultimately give up all the time. I'm ready to work with you to help you discover some important reasons you have for considering doing things to help yourself, and what those things could be. It sounds like you are thinking that it might be time for a change. I'm wondering that if you don't change, what do you think is the worst thing that might happen?

C: I'm worried that I'll become an alcoholic or that my hypertension and diabetes will do me in. My father died of his diabetes and my grandfather died when I was a young kid from being an alcoholic. And I'm so overweight that I don't know if I can ever lose all of this baggage.

CMES: Sounds like you see some pretty negative things happening in your life if you don't change, like what happened to your father and grandfather. That must be tough to think about, especially if you wonder if you can really do it. So, what's the best thing you could imagine happening to you that could result from making some changes?

C: Well, my wife and kids sure would like it, that's for sure. And I wouldn't always be worrying about dying. Every time I get drunk lately, I feel guilty. I know I have do something. But I just don't know how.

CMES: So what I hear you saying is you've been thinking a lot about making some changes in your activity level, and eating and drinking habits, and that you have some real rock-solid reasons to do so, but on the other hand you aren't sure you really have the ability or tools to make those changes. Many people report feeling like you do. They want to make changes in their lifestyle but find it difficult.

C: So I'm not the only one who is in this spot, huh? Well, that's good to know. I just don't know what to do from here.

CMES: No, you sure aren't alone. Why don't we discuss some ideas for getting started…

… Working With Clients With Health Challenges — CHAPTER 3

THE 10-STEP DECISION-MAKING APPROACH TO EXERCISE PROGRAMMING FOR SPECIAL POPULATIONS

The 10-step decision-making approach detailed here provides the CMES with a stepwise process of working with clients with chronic diseases that is based on the principles of exercise science and clinical medicine. This approach will also provide the CMES with a model for reasoning and thinking through (versus memorizing) the critical steps of exercise programming for clients with any of a variety of health conditions.

When working with any client, the CMES must understand the effects of exercise—both acute and long-term—as well as the disease or disability's pathophysiology and any associated medications. Armed with this knowledge, the CMES should then be able to determine the mechanisms by which the disease/disability alters the exercise response, as well as the exercise-related benefits (which are typically associated with long-term exercise adaptations) and risks (which are usually associated with acute exercise responses) for each individual. It is important to note that knowledge of the benefits and risks of exercise for each organ system will then direct all subsequent steps in the management of clients with chronic disease, disabilities, or special health conditions.

The 10 steps, some of which involve answering a series of questions for each client, are as follows:
- Step 1: Perform a pre-exercise health-risk assessment
- Step 2: Obtain physician clearance
- Step 3: Identify exercise benefits and goals
- Step 4: Determine acute exercise risks
- Step 5: Prepare for medical emergencies
- Step 6: Obtain informed consent
- Step 7: Plan baseline fitness screening and testing
- Step 8: Design the exercise program
- Step 9: Plan exercise program implementation
- Step 10: Double-check established guidelines

Step 1: Perform a Pre-exercise Health-risk Assessment

The purpose of this step is to maximize client safety by assisting in the detection of known and unknown conditions that may increase exercise-related risks. In addition, this step will assist in individualizing each client's exercise program and provide the CMES with some level of protection from potential liabilities. This is probably the most important of the 10 steps, as it "defines the problems" and acts as the foundation from which all subsequent decisions are made.

The American College of Sports Medicine (ACSM, 2022) preparticipation guidelines are designed to remove any unnecessary barriers to becoming more physically active. Risk-factor profiling or classification is not part of the exercise preparticipation health-screening process because supporting evidence is lacking for the presence of risk factors without underlying disease increasing the risk for activity-related cardiovascular events and screening must not become a barrier to participation. Further, the guidelines note that when an individual becomes more physically active, their risks decline. The new health-screening process is based on three factors that have been identified as important risk modulators of exercise-related cardiovascular events:
- The individual's current level of physical activity
- Diagnosed cardiovascular, metabolic, or renal disease and/or the presence of signs or symptoms of cardiovascular, metabolic, or renal disease
- The desired exercise intensity

This screening protocol makes general recommendations for medical clearance, leaving the specifics—such as the need for medical exams or exercise tests—up to the discretion of the healthcare provider.

The goal of this process is to identify individuals:
- Who should receive medical clearance before initiating an exercise program or increasing the frequency, intensity, and/or volume of their current program
- With clinically significant disease(s) who may benefit from participating in a medically supervised exercise program
- With medical conditions that may require exclusion from exercise programs until those conditions are resolved or better controlled

Figure 3-1 presents the preparticipation health-screening algorithm, while an exercise preparticipation checklist is presented in Figure 3-2. This algorithm shows that medical clearance is needed only under the following circumstances, with regular exercise defined as performing planned, structured physical activity for at least 30 minutes at moderate intensity on at least three days/week for at least the past three months:
- **For those who do not exercise regularly:** If a client has cardiovascular, metabolic, or renal disease, or signs or symptoms that suggest they do, then medical clearance is necessary.
- **For regular exercisers:** If a client has signs or symptoms suggestive of cardiovascular, metabolic, or renal disease, they should discontinue exercise and seek medical clearance. If a client has a known history of cardiovascular, metabolic, or renal disease and has a desire to progress to vigorous-intensity aerobic exercise, medical clearance is recommended.

While the identification of the signs and symptoms referenced in this algorithm may be within the **scope of practice** of most CMES, interpretation of those same signs and symptoms should be made only by qualified healthcare professionals within the context in which they appear (ACSM, 2022):
- Pain; discomfort (or other **angina** equivalent) in the chest, neck, jaw, arms, or other areas that may result from **myocardial ischemia**; or other recent onset pain of unknown origin
- Shortness of breath at rest or with mild exertion **(dyspnea)**
- **Orthopnea** (dyspnea in a reclined position) or **paroxysmal nocturnal dyspnea** (onset is usually two to five hours after the beginning of sleep)
- Dizziness, or **syncope,** most commonly caused by reduced perfusion to the brain
- Ankle **edema**
- **Palpitations** or **tachycardia**
- **Intermittent claudication** (pain sensations or cramping in the lower extremities during exercise that is associated with inadequate blood supply)
- Known heart murmur
- Unusual fatigue or shortness of breath with usual activities

Resistance Training

Current evidence is insufficient regarding cardiovascular complications during low-to-moderate intensity resistance training to warrant formal prescreening recommendations (ACSM, 2022). Limited data are available on the topic, but it appears that the risk of complications is low.

Self-guided Screening

Preparticipation health screening for individuals wanting to initiate an exercise program may be conducted using the **Physical Activity Readiness Questionnaire for Everyone (PAR-Q+)** form (Figure 3-3). This form is evidence-based and was developed with a goal of reducing unnecessary barriers to exercise. The PAR-Q+ can be used as either a self-guided screening tool or as an additional element of screening for use by personal trainers seeking additional client information.

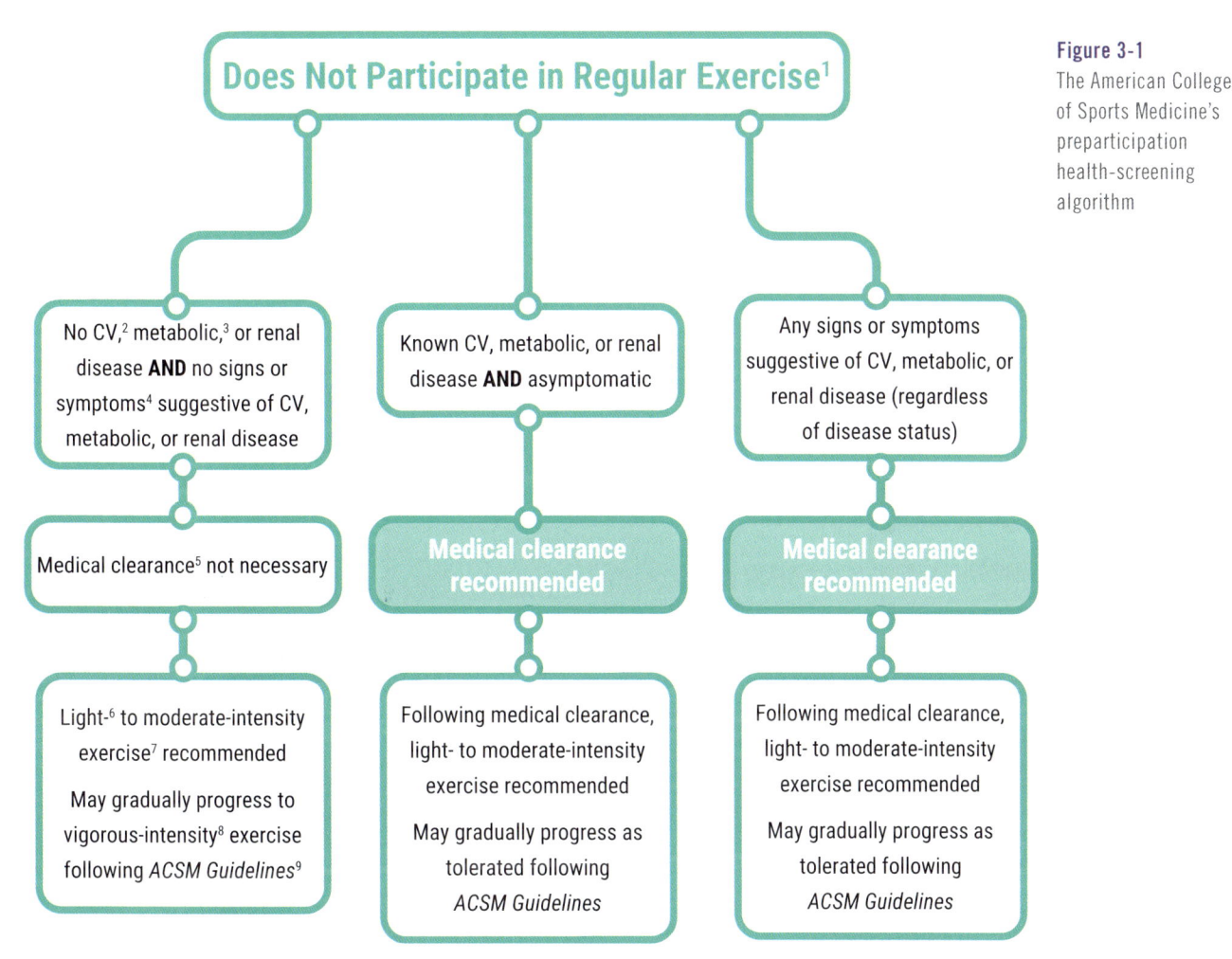

Working With Clients With Health Challenges   CHAPTER 3

Figure 3-1
The American College of Sports Medicine's preparticipation health-screening algorithm

Does Not Participate in Regular Exercise[1]

No CV,[2] metabolic,[3] or renal disease AND no signs or symptoms[4] suggestive of CV, metabolic, or renal disease
↓
Medical clearance[5] not necessary
↓
Light-[6] to moderate-intensity exercise[7] recommended

May gradually progress to vigorous-intensity[8] exercise following *ACSM Guidelines*[9]

Known CV, metabolic, or renal disease AND asymptomatic
↓
Medical clearance recommended
↓
Following medical clearance, light- to moderate-intensity exercise recommended

May gradually progress as tolerated following *ACSM Guidelines*

Any signs or symptoms suggestive of CV, metabolic, or renal disease (regardless of disease status)
↓
Medical clearance recommended
↓
Following medical clearance, light- to moderate-intensity exercise recommended

May gradually progress as tolerated following *ACSM Guidelines*

---

[1] **Exercise participation** Performing planned, structured physical activity for at least 30 minutes at moderate intensity on at least 3 days/week for at least the past 3 months

[2] **Cardiovascular disease** Cardiac, peripheral vascular, or cerebrovascular disease

[3] **Metabolic disease** Type 1 and 2 diabetes mellitus

[4] **Sign and symptoms** At rest or during activity. Includes pain, discomfort in the chest, neck, jaw, arms, or other areas that may result from ischemia; shortness of breath at rest or with mild exertion; dizziness or syncope; orthopnea or paroxysmal nocturnal dyspnea; ankle edema; palpitations or tachycardia; intermittent claudication; known heart murmur; unusual fatigue or shortness of breath with usual activities

[5] **Medical clearance** Approval from a healthcare professional to engage in exercise

[6] **Light intensity exercise** 30–39% HRR or $\dot{V}O_2R$, 2–2.9 METs, RPE 9–11, an intensity that causes slight increases in HR and breathing

[7] **Moderate-intensity exercise** 40–59% HRR or $\dot{V}O_2R$, 3–5.9 METs, RPE 12–13, an intensity that causes noticeable increases in HR and breathing

[8] **Vigorous-intensity exercise** ≥60% HRR or $\dot{V}O_2R$, ≥6 METs, RPE ≥14, an intensity that causes substantial increases in HR and breathing

[9] **ACSM Guidelines** *ACSM's Guidelines for Exercise Testing and Prescription,* 11th edition

Note: CV = Cardiovascular; HRR = Heart-rate reserve; $\dot{V}O_2R$ = Oxygen uptake reserve; METs = Metabolic equivalents; RPE = Rating of perceived exertion; HR = Heart rate; ACSM = American College of Sports Medicine

Reprinted with permission from American College of Sports Medicine (2022). *ACSM's Guidelines for Exercise Testing and Prescription* (11th ed.). Philadelphia: Wolters Kluwer.

Continued on the next page

Figure 3-1
The American College of Sports Medicine's preparticipation health-screening algorithm *(continued)*

```
                    Participates in Regular Exercise[1]
        ┌──────────────────────────┼──────────────────────────┐
        │                          │                          │
  No CV,[2] metabolic,[3]     Known CV, metabolic,      Any signs or symptoms
  or renal disease AND        or renal disease AND      suggestive of CV, metabolic,
  no signs or symptoms[4]     asymptomatic              or renal disease (regardless
  suggestive of CV,                                     of disease status)
  metabolic, or renal
  disease
        │                          │                          │
  Medical clearance[5]        Medical clearance for      Discontinue exercise and
  not necessary               moderate-intensity         seek medical clearance
                              exercise[7] not necessary
                              
                              Medical clearance (within
                              the past 12 months if no
                              change in signs/symptoms)
                              recommended before
                              engaging in vigorous-
                              intensity exercise[8]
        │                          │                          │
  Continue moderate- or       Continue with              May return to exercise
  vigorous-intensity          moderate-intensity         following medical clearance
  exercise                    exercise
                                                         Gradually progress as
  May gradually progress      Following medical          tolerated following
  following ACSM              clearance, may gradually   ACSM Guidelines
  Guidelines[9]               progress as tolerated
                              following ACSM Guidelines
```

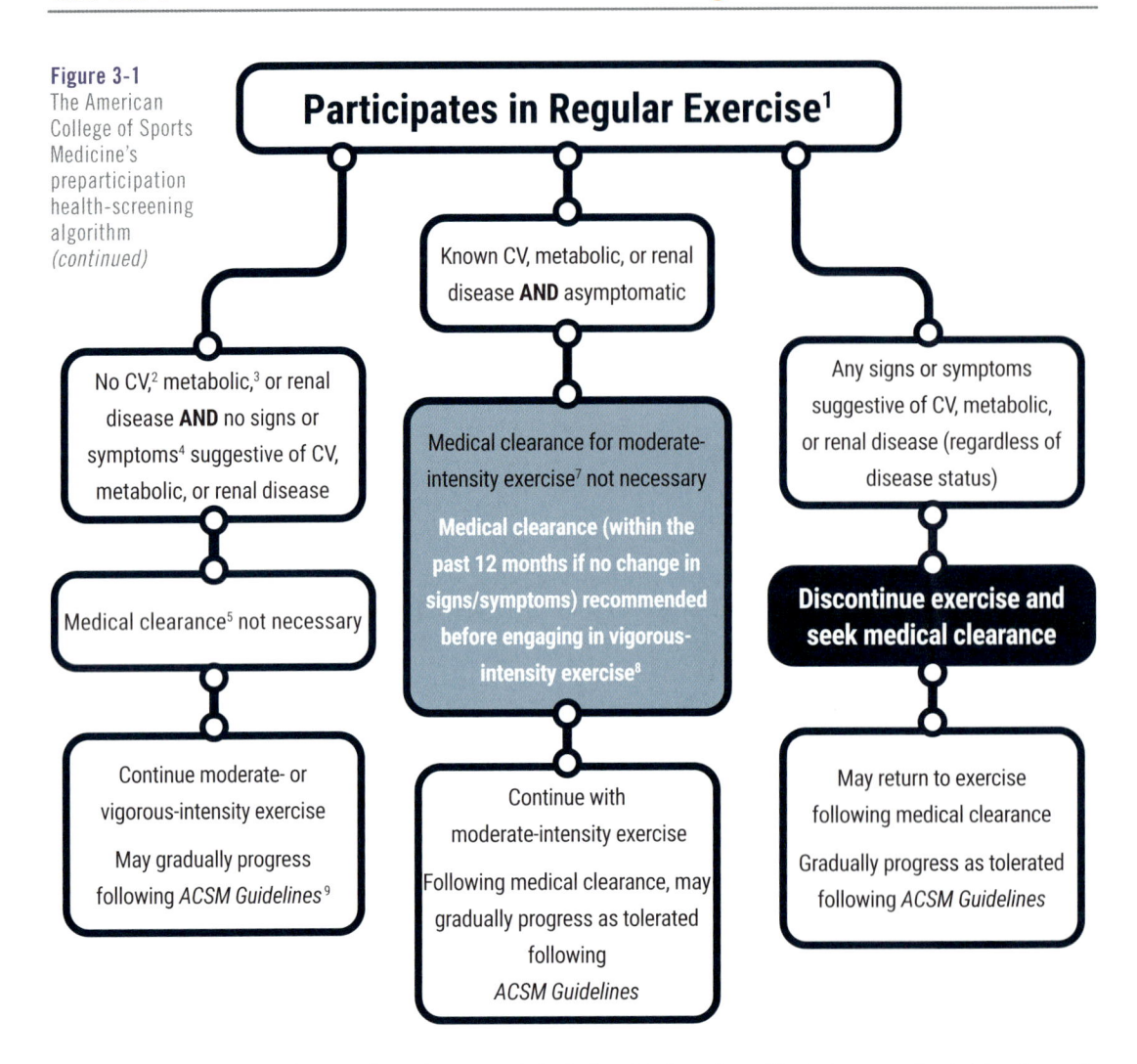

[1] **Exercise participation** Performing planned, structured physical activity for at least 30 minutes at moderate intensity on at least 3 days/week for at least the past 3 months

[2] **Cardiovascular disease** Cardiac, peripheral vascular, or cerebrovascular disease

[3] **Metabolic disease** Type 1 and 2 diabetes mellitus

[4] **Sign and symptoms** At rest or during activity. Includes pain, discomfort in the chest, neck, jaw, arms, or other areas that may result from ischemia; shortness of breath at rest or with mild exertion; dizziness or syncope; orthopnea or paroxysmal nocturnal dyspnea; ankle edema; palpitations or tachycardia; intermittent claudication; known heart murmur; unusual fatigue or shortness of breath with usual activities

[5] **Medical clearance** Approval from a healthcare professional to engage in exercise

[6] **Light-intensity exercise** 30–39% HRR or $\dot{V}O_2R$, 2–2.9 METs, RPE 9–11, an intensity that causes slight increases in HR and breathing

[7] **Moderate-intensity exercise** 40–59% HRR or $\dot{V}O_2R$, 3–5.9 METs, RPE 12–13, an intensity that causes noticeable increases in HR and breathing

[8] **Vigorous-intensity exercise** ≥60% HRR or $\dot{V}O_2R$, ≥6 METs, RPE ≥14, an intensity that causes substantial increases in HR and breathing

[9] **ACSM Guidelines** *ACSM's Guidelines for Exercise Testing and Prescription*, 11th edition

Note: CV = Cardiovascular; HRR = Heart-rate reserve; $\dot{V}O_2R$ = Oxygen uptake reserve; METs = Metabolic equivalents; RPE = Rating of perceived exertion; HR = Heart rate; ACSM = American College of Sports Medicine

Reprinted with permission from American College of Sports Medicine (2022). *ACSM's Guidelines for Exercise Testing and Prescription* (11th ed.). Philadelphia: Wolters Kluwer.

EXERCISE PREPARTICIPATION HEALTH-SCREENING QUESTIONNAIRE FOR EXERCISE PROFESSIONALS

Assess your client's health needs by marking all *true* statements.

Step 1

SYMPTOMS
Does your client experience:
☐ chest discomfort with exertion
☐ unreasonable breathlessness
☐ dizziness, fainting, blackouts
☐ ankle swelling
☐ unpleasant awareness of a forceful, rapid, or irregular heart rate
☐ burning or cramping sensations in your lower legs when walking short distances
☐ known heart murmur

If you **did** mark any of these statements under the symptoms, **STOP,** your client should seek medical clearance before engaging in or resuming exercise. Your client may need to use a facility with a **medically qualified staff**.

If you **did not** mark any symptoms, continue to steps 2 and 3.

Step 2

CURRENT ACTIVITY
Has your client performed planned, structured physical activity for at least 30 minutes at moderate intensity on at least 3 days per week for at least the past 3 months?

Yes ☐ No ☐

Continue to Step 3.

Step 3

MEDICAL CONDITIONS
Has your client had or does he or she currently have:
☐ a heart attack
☐ heart surgery, cardiac catheterization, or coronary angioplasty
☐ pacemaker/implantable cardiac defibrillator/rhythm disturbance
☐ heart valve disease
☐ heart failure
☐ heart transplantation
☐ congenital heart disease
☐ diabetes
☐ renal disease

Evaluating Steps 2 and 3:
- If you **did not mark any of the statements in Step 3,** medical clearance is not necessary.

- If you marked Step 2 **"yes"** and **marked any of the statements in Step 3,** your client may continue to exercise at light to moderate intensity without medical clearance. Medical clearance is recommended before engaging in vigorous exercise.

- If you marked Step 2 **"no"** and **marked any of the statements in Step 3,** medical clearance is recommended. Your client may need to use a facility with a **medically qualified staff.**

Figure 3-2
Exercise preparticipation health-screening questionnaire for exercise professionals

Reprinted with permission from American College of Sports Medicine (2022). *ACSM's Guidelines for Exercise Testing and Prescription* (11th ed.). Philadelphia: Wolters Kluwer.

CHAPTER 3　　　　　　　　　　　　　　　　　　　Working With Clients With Health Challenges

This important screening document is regularly updated and revised and there are different versions depending on the clientele with whom you are working. The PAR-Q+ and ePARmed-X+ (for clients who have had a positive response to the PAR-Q+ or have been referred to use this more comprehensive form by a healthcare professional) were created to reduce barriers for all individuals to become more physically active. These forms are publicly available at www.eparmedx.com.

Figure 3-3
The Physical Activity Readiness Questionnaire for Everyone

2021 PAR-Q+

The Physical Activity Readiness Questionnaire for Everyone

The health benefits of regular physical activity are clear; more people should engage in physical activity every day of the week. Participating in physical activity is very safe for MOST people. This questionnaire will tell you whether it is necessary for you to seek further advice from your doctor OR a qualified exercise professional before becoming more physically active.

GENERAL HEALTH QUESTIONS

Please read the 7 questions below carefully and answer each one honestly: check YES or NO.	YES	NO
1) Has your doctor ever said that you have a heart condition ☐ OR high blood pressure ☐ ?	☐	☐
2) Do you feel pain in your chest at rest, during your daily activities of living, OR when you do physical activity?	☐	☐
3) Do you lose balance because of dizziness OR have you lost consciousness in the last 12 months? Please answer NO if your dizziness was associated with over-breathing (including during vigorous exercise).	☐	☐
4) Have you ever been diagnosed with another chronic medical condition (other than heart disease or high blood pressure)? PLEASE LIST CONDITION(S) HERE: _____	☐	☐
5) Are you currently taking prescribed medications for a chronic medical condition? PLEASE LIST CONDITION(S) AND MEDICATIONS HERE: _____	☐	☐
6) Do you currently have (or have had within the past 12 months) a bone, joint, or soft tissue (muscle, ligament, or tendon) problem that could be made worse by becoming more physically active? Please answer NO if you had a problem in the past, but it **does not limit your current ability** to be physically active. PLEASE LIST CONDITION(S) HERE: _____	☐	☐
7) Has your doctor ever said that you should only do medically supervised physical activity?	☐	☐

✓ If you answered NO to all of the questions above, you are cleared for physical activity.
Please sign the PARTICIPANT DECLARATION. You do not need to complete Pages 2 and 3.

- ▶ Start becoming much more physically active – start slowly and build up gradually.
- ▶ Follow Global Physical Activity Guidelines for your age (https://www.who.int/publications/i/item/9789240015128).
- ▶ You may take part in a health and fitness appraisal.
- ▶ If you are over the age of 45 yr and NOT accustomed to regular vigorous to maximal effort exercise, consult a qualified exercise professional before engaging in this intensity of exercise.
- ▶ If you have any further questions, contact a qualified exercise professional.

PARTICIPANT DECLARATION
If you are less than the legal age required for consent or require the assent of a care provider, your parent, guardian or care provider must also sign this form.

I, the undersigned, have read, understood to my full satisfaction and completed this questionnaire. I acknowledge that this physical activity clearance is valid for a maximum of 12 months from the date it is completed and becomes invalid if my condition changes. I also acknowledge that the community/fitness center may retain a copy of this form for its records. In these instances, it will maintain the confidentiality of the same, complying with applicable law.

NAME _____ DATE _____
SIGNATURE _____ WITNESS _____
SIGNATURE OF PARENT/GUARDIAN/CARE PROVIDER _____

● If you answered YES to one or more of the questions above, COMPLETE PAGES 2 AND 3.

⚠ **Delay becoming more active if:**
- ✓ You have a temporary illness such as a cold or fever; it is best to wait until you feel better.
- ✓ You are pregnant - talk to your health care practitioner, your physician, a qualified exercise professional, and/or complete the ePARmed-X+ at www.eparmedx.com before becoming more physically active.
- ✓ Your health changes - answer the questions on Pages 2 and 3 of this document and/or talk to your doctor or a qualified exercise professional before continuing with any physical activity program.

Copyright © 2021 PAR-Q+ Collaboration 1 / 4
01-11-2020

Continued on the next page

2021 PAR-Q+

FOLLOW-UP QUESTIONS ABOUT YOUR MEDICAL CONDITION(S)

Figure 3-3
The Physical Activity Readiness Questionnaire for Everyone (continued)

1. Do you have Arthritis, Osteoporosis, or Back Problems?
If the above condition(s) is/are present, answer questions 1a-1c   If **NO** ☐ go to question 2

1a.	Do you have difficulty controlling your condition with medications or other physician-prescribed therapies? (Answer **NO** if you are not currently taking medications or other treatments)	YES ☐ NO ☐
1b.	Do you have joint problems causing pain, a recent fracture or fracture caused by osteoporosis or cancer, displaced vertebra (e.g., spondylolisthesis), and/or spondylolysis/pars defect (a crack in the bony ring on the back of the spinal column)?	YES ☐ NO ☐
1c.	Have you had steroid injections or taken steroid tablets regularly for more than 3 months?	YES ☐ NO ☐

2. Do you currently have Cancer of any kind?
If the above condition(s) is/are present, answer questions 2a-2b   If **NO** ☐ go to question 3

2a.	Does your cancer diagnosis include any of the following types: lung/bronchogenic, multiple myeloma (cancer of plasma cells), head, and/or neck?	YES ☐ NO ☐
2b.	Are you currently receiving cancer therapy (such as chemotheraphy or radiotherapy)?	YES ☐ NO ☐

3. Do you have a Heart or Cardiovascular Condition? This includes Coronary Artery Disease, Heart Failure, Diagnosed Abnormality of Heart Rhythm
If the above condition(s) is/are present, answer questions 3a-3d   If **NO** ☐ go to question 4

3a.	Do you have difficulty controlling your condition with medications or other physician-prescribed therapies? (Answer **NO** if you are not currently taking medications or other treatments)	YES ☐ NO ☐
3b.	Do you have an irregular heart beat that requires medical management? (e.g., atrial fibrillation, premature ventricular contraction)	YES ☐ NO ☐
3c.	Do you have chronic heart failure?	YES ☐ NO ☐
3d.	Do you have diagnosed coronary artery (cardiovascular) disease and have not participated in regular physical activity in the last 2 months?	YES ☐ NO ☐

4. Do you currently have High Blood Pressure?
If the above condition(s) is/are present, answer questions 4a-4b   If **NO** ☐ go to question 5

4a.	Do you have difficulty controlling your condition with medications or other physician-prescribed therapies? (Answer **NO** if you are not currently taking medications or other treatments)	YES ☐ NO ☐
4b.	Do you have a resting blood pressure equal to or greater than 160/90 mmHg with or without medication? (Answer **YES** if you do not know your resting blood pressure)	YES ☐ NO ☐

5. Do you have any Metabolic Conditions? This includes Type 1 Diabetes, Type 2 Diabetes, Pre-Diabetes
If the above condition(s) is/are present, answer questions 5a-5e   If **NO** ☐ go to question 6

5a.	Do you often have difficulty controlling your blood sugar levels with foods, medications, or other physician-prescribed therapies?	YES ☐ NO ☐
5b.	Do you often suffer from signs and symptoms of low blood sugar (hypoglycemia) following exercise and/or during activities of daily living? Signs of hypoglycemia may include shakiness, nervousness, unusual irritability, abnormal sweating, dizziness or light-headedness, mental confusion, difficulty speaking, weakness, or sleepiness.	YES ☐ NO ☐
5c.	Do you have any signs or symptoms of diabetes complications such as heart or vascular disease and/or complications affecting your eyes, kidneys, **OR** the sensation in your toes and feet?	YES ☐ NO ☐
5d.	Do you have other metabolic conditions (such as current pregnancy-related diabetes, chronic kidney disease, or liver problems)?	YES ☐ NO ☐
5e.	Are you planning to engage in what for you is unusually high (or vigorous) intensity exercise in the near future?	YES ☐ NO ☐

Figure 3-3
The Physical Activity Readiness Questionnaire for Everyone
(continued)

2021 PAR-Q+

6. Do you have any Mental Health Problems or Learning Difficulties? This includes Alzheimer's, Dementia, Depression, Anxiety Disorder, Eating Disorder, Psychotic Disorder, Intellectual Disability, Down Syndrome

If the above condition(s) is/are present, answer questions 6a-6b   If **NO** ☐ go to question 7

6a. Do you have difficulty controlling your condition with medications or other physician-prescribed therapies? (Answer **NO** if you are not currently taking medications or other treatments)   YES ☐ NO ☐

6b. Do you have Down Syndrome **AND** back problems affecting nerves or muscles?   YES ☐ NO ☐

7. Do you have a Respiratory Disease? *This includes Chronic Obstructive Pulmonary Disease, Asthma, Pulmonary High Blood Pressure*

If the above condition(s) is/are present, answer questions 7a-7d   If **NO** ☐ go to question 8

7a. Do you have difficulty controlling your condition with medications or other physician-prescribed therapies? (Answer **NO** if you are not currently taking medications or other treatments)   YES ☐ NO ☐

7b. Has your doctor ever said your blood oxygen level is low at rest or during exercise and/or that you require supplemental oxygen therapy?   YES ☐ NO ☐

7c. If asthmatic, do you currently have symptoms of chest tightness, wheezing, laboured breathing, consistent cough (more than 2 days/week), or have you used your rescue medication more than twice in the last week?   YES ☐ NO ☐

7d. Has your doctor ever said you have high blood pressure in the blood vessels of your lungs?   YES ☐ NO ☐

8. Do you have a Spinal Cord Injury? *This includes Tetraplegia and Paraplegia*

If the above condition(s) is/are present, answer questions 8a-8c   If **NO** ☐ go to question 9

8a. Do you have difficulty controlling your condition with medications or other physician-prescribed therapies? (Answer **NO** if you are not currently taking medications or other treatments)   YES ☐ NO ☐

8b. Do you commonly exhibit low resting blood pressure significant enough to cause dizziness, light-headedness, and/or fainting?   YES ☐ NO ☐

8c. Has your physician indicated that you exhibit sudden bouts of high blood pressure (known as Autonomic Dysreflexia)?   YES ☐ NO ☐

9. Have you had a Stroke? *This includes Transient Ischemic Attack (TIA) or Cerebrovascular Event*

If the above condition(s) is/are present, answer questions 9a-9c   If **NO** ☐ go to question 10

9a. Do you have difficulty controlling your condition with medications or other physician-prescribed therapies? (Answer **NO** if you are not currently taking medications or other treatments)   YES ☐ NO ☐

9b. Do you have any impairment in walking or mobility?   YES ☐ NO ☐

9c. Have you experienced a stroke or impairment in nerves or muscles in the past 6 months?   YES ☐ NO ☐

10. Do you have any other medical condition not listed above or do you have two or more medical conditions?

If you have other medical conditions, answer questions 10a-10c   If **NO** ☐ read the Page 4 recommendations

10a. Have you experienced a blackout, fainted, or lost consciousness as a result of a head injury within the last 12 months **OR** have you had a diagnosed concussion within the last 12 months?   YES ☐ NO ☐

10b. Do you have a medical condition that is not listed (such as epilepsy, neurological conditions, kidney problems)?   YES ☐ NO ☐

10c. Do you currently live with two or more medical conditions?   YES ☐ NO ☐

PLEASE LIST YOUR MEDICAL CONDITION(S) AND ANY RELATED MEDICATIONS HERE: _____

GO to Page 4 for recommendations about your current medical condition(s) and sign the PARTICIPANT DECLARATION.

Copyright © 2021 PAR-Q+ Collaboration   3/ 4
01-11-2020

Working With Clients With Health Challenges CHAPTER 3

2021 PAR-Q+

Figure 3-3
The Physical Activity Readiness Questionnaire for Everyone
(continued)

✅ **If you answered NO to all of the FOLLOW-UP questions (pgs. 2-3) about your medical condition, you are ready to become more physically active - sign the PARTICIPANT DECLARATION below:**

- It is advised that you consult a qualified exercise professional to help you develop a safe and effective physical activity plan to meet your health needs.
- You are encouraged to start slowly and build up gradually - 20 to 60 minutes of low to moderate intensity exercise, 3-5 days per week including aerobic and muscle strengthening exercises.
- As you progress, you should aim to accumulate 150 minutes or more of moderate intensity physical activity per week.
- If you are over the age of 45 yr and **NOT** accustomed to regular vigorous to maximal effort exercise, consult a qualified exercise professional before engaging in this intensity of exercise.

🛑 **If you answered YES to one or more of the follow-up questions** about your medical condition:
You should seek further information before becoming more physically active or engaging in a fitness appraisal. You should complete the specially designed online screening and exercise recommendations program - the **ePARmed-X+ at www.eparmedx.com** and/or visit a qualified exercise professional to work through the ePARmed-X+ and for further information.

⚠️ **Delay becoming more active if:**

- You have a temporary illness such as a cold or fever; it is best to wait until you feel better.
- You are pregnant - talk to your health care practitioner, your physician, a qualified exercise professional, and/or complete the ePARmed-X+ **at www.eparmedx.com** before becoming more physically active.
- Your health changes - talk to your doctor or qualified exercise professional before continuing with any physical activity program.

- You are encouraged to photocopy the PAR-Q+. You must use the entire questionnaire and NO changes are permitted.
- The authors, the PAR-Q+ Collaboration, partner organizations, and their agents assume no liability for persons who undertake physical activity and/or make use of the PAR-Q+ or ePARmed-X+. If in doubt after completing the questionnaire, consult your doctor prior to physical activity.

PARTICIPANT DECLARATION

- All persons who have completed the PAR-Q+ please read and sign the declaration below.
- If you are less than the legal age required for consent or require the assent of a care provider, your parent, guardian or care provider must also sign this form.

I, the undersigned, have read, understood to my full satisfaction and completed this questionnaire. I acknowledge that this physical activity clearance is valid for a maximum of 12 months from the date it is completed and becomes invalid if my condition changes. I also acknowledge that the community/fitness center may retain a copy of this form for records. In these instances, it will maintain the confidentiality of the same, complying with applicable law.

NAME _____ DATE _____

SIGNATURE _____ WITNESS _____

SIGNATURE OF PARENT/GUARDIAN/CARE PROVIDER _____

For more information, please contact
www.eparmedx.com
Email: eparmedx@gmail.com

Citation for PAR-Q+
Warburton DER, Jamnik VK, Bredin SSD, and Gledhill N on behalf of the PAR-Q+ Collaboration. The Physical Activity Readiness Questionnaire for Everyone (PAR-Q+) and Electronic Physical Activity Readiness Medical Examination (ePARmed-X+). Health & Fitness Journal of Canada 4(2):3-23, 2011.

The PAR-Q+ was created using the evidence-based AGREE process (1) by the PAR-Q+ Collaboration chaired by Dr. Darren E. R. Warburton with Dr. Norman Gledhill, Dr. Veronica Jamnik, and Dr. Donald C. McKenzie (2). Production of this document has been made possible through financial contributions from the Public Health Agency of Canada and the BC Ministry of Health Services. The views expressed herein do not necessarily represent the views of the Public Health Agency of Canada or the BC Ministry of Health Services.

Key References
1. Jamnik VK, Warburton DER, Makarski J, McKenzie DC, Shephard RJ, Stone J, and Gledhill N. Enhancing the effectiveness of clearance for physical activity participation; background and overall process. APNM 36(S1):S3-S13, 2011.
2. Warburton DER, Gledhill N, Jamnik VK, Bredin SSD, McKenzie DC, Stone J, Charlesworth S, and Shephard RJ. Evidence-based risk assessment and recommendations for physical activity clearance; Consensus Document. APNM 36(S1):S266-s298, 2011.
3. Chisholm DM, Collis ML, Kulak LL, Davenport W, and Gruber N. Physical activity readiness. British Columbia Medical Journal. 1975;17:375-378.
4. Thomas S, Reading J, and Shephard RJ. Revision of the Physical Activity Readiness Questionnaire (PAR-Q). Canadian Journal of Sport Science 1992;17:4 338-345.

Copyright © 2021 PAR-Q+ Collaboration 4/4
01-11-2020

Exercise professionals should be familiar with each of the signs and symptoms listed on page 70 and document them in a client's file if the client (1) has a history of any of these symptoms or (2) develops these signs or symptoms while under the CMES's supervision.

> It is imperative that the client's personal physician be made aware of any signs or symptoms suggestive of cardiovascular, metabolic, or renal disease that may have been discovered as a result of this prescreening session or during an ongoing exercise program.

Health-history Questionnaires

> It is recommended that a CMES consult a legal professional familiar with local and regional laws prior to utilizing the informed consent and agreement and release of liability forms.

Visit www.ACEfitness.org/CMESresources to download a free PDF of a health-history questionnaire and musculoskeletal health questionnaire, as well as other forms and tools that you can use throughout your career as a CMES.

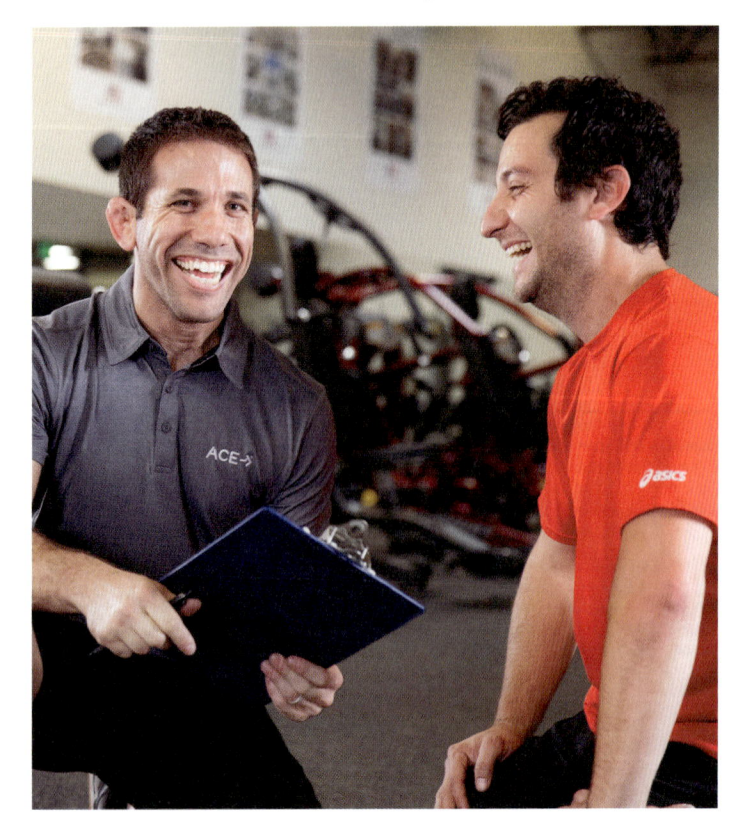

Once the client's risk for exercise has been assessed, the need for outside referral has been determined (yes or no), and the client is cleared for exercise, an appropriate health and fitness plan can then be developed. There are several important forms that the CMES should review, keep accessible, and utilize as needed with clients. These forms include the following:

Health-history questionnaire (Figure 3-4):
- This form collects more detailed medical and health information beyond the preparticipation health screening, including the following:
  - ✓ Past and present exercise and physical-activity information
  - ✓ Medications and supplements
  - ✓ Recent or current illnesses or injuries, including chronic or acute pain
  - ✓ Surgery and injury history
  - ✓ Family medical history
  - ✓ Lifestyle information (related to nutrition, stress, work, sleep, etc.)

Musculoskeletal health questionnaire (Figure 3-5):
- As many older adults will present with some type of joint or muscle pain, this form provides exercise professionals with a more detailed account of the client's musculoskeletal health.
- This questionnaire is excerpted from Dr. Nicholas DiNubile's book *FrameWork: Your 7-Step Program for Healthy Muscles, Bones, and Joints* (DiNubile & Patrick, 2005). Exercise professionals can use this book as a resource when working with clients to assess their musculoskeletal health.

Exercise history and attitude questionnaire (Figure 3-6):
- This form provides the CMES with a detailed background of the client's previous exercise history, including behavioral and adherence experience.
- This information is important when developing goals, designing programs incorporating the client's preferences and attitudes toward exercise, and implementing strategies for improving motivation and adherence.

HEALTH-HISTORY QUESTIONNAIRE

Name:_____ Phone (H):_____

Address:_____

City:_____ ZIP:_____

Emergency Contact:_____ Emergency Phone:_____

Personal Physician: _____

DOB:_____ Age:_____ Sex: ❑ M ❑ F Physician's Phone: _____

SECTION I. MEDICAL HISTORY

1. Mark any of the following for which you have been diagnosed or treated:

   ____ Kidney problem   ____ Heart problem   ____ Phlebitis   ____ Concussion
   ____ Mononucleosis   ____ Cirrhosis, liver   ____ Stroke   ____ Asthma

2. Mark any medications taken in the last 6 months:

   ____ Blood thinner   ____ Epilepsy medicine   ____ Nitroglycerin   ____ Cholesterol medicine
   ____ Diabetes medicine   ____ Heart rhythm medicine   ____ Insulin   ____ Other
   ____ Blood pressure medicine ____ Diuretic (water pill)   ____ Digitalis

3. List any surgeries you have had in the past (e.g., knee, heart, or back):

   _____
   _____
   _____

4. Have you ever had back problems, any problems with joints (knee, hip, shoulder, elbow, or neck), or been diagnosed with arthritis? _____ If yes, describe:

   _____
   _____
   _____

5. Do you have any other medical conditions or health problems that may affect your exercise plan or safety in any way? _____ If yes, describe:

   _____
   _____
   _____

SECTION II. CARDIOPULMONARY AND METABOLIC SYMPTOMS

YES	NO	
❑	❑	Do you ever get unusually short of breath with very light exertion?
❑	❑	Do you ever have pain, pressure, heaviness, or tightness in the chest area?
❑	❑	Do you regularly have unexplained pain in the abdomen, shoulder, or arm?
❑	❑	Do you ever have dizzy spells or episodes of fainting?
❑	❑	Do you ever feel "skips," palpitations, or runs of fast or slow heartbeats in your chest?
❑	❑	Has a physician ever told you that you have a heart murmur?
❑	❑	Do you regularly get lower-leg pain during walking that is relieved with rest?
❑	❑	Do you have any joints that often become swollen and painful? Where:_____

Figure 3-4
Health-history questionnaire

Continued on next page

Reprinted with permission from Bryant, C.X., Franklin, B.A., & Newton-Merrill, S. (2007). *ACE's Guide to Exercise Testing & Program Design* (2nd ed.). Monterey, Calif.: Healthy Learning.

SECTION III. CARDIOPULMONARY/METABOLIC DISEASE

❏ YES ❏ NO   Have you ever had a heart attack, bypass surgery, angioplasty, or been diagnosed with coronary artery disease or other heart disease? If yes, describe:

_____
_____
_____

❏ YES ❏ NO   Do you have emphysema, asthma, or any other chronic lung condition or disease?

_____
_____

❏ YES ❏ NO   Are you an insulin-dependent diabetic?

_____
_____

SECTION IV. CORONARY RISK FACTOR PROFILE

❏ YES ❏ NO   Have you had high blood pressure (≥140 mmHg systolic or ≥90 mmHg diastolic) on more than one occasion?

_____

Please list any medications you take for high blood pressure:

_____
_____

❏ YES ❏ NO   Have you ever been told that your blood cholesterol was high (200 mg/dL or higher)?
Cholesterol level_____

❏ YES ❏ NO   Do you currently smoke 10 or more cigarettes per day?
cigarettes/day_____   years smoked_____

❏ YES ❏ NO   Have you ever been told that you have high blood sugar or diabetes? If yes, describe:

_____
_____

❏ YES ❏ NO   Has anyone in your immediate family (parents and siblings) had any heart problems or coronary disease before age 55? If yes, describe:

_____
_____

❏ YES ❏ NO   Do you feel you are more than 20 lb (9 kg) overweight?
What do you feel is your realistic ideal weight? _____

SECTION V. FITNESS

Circle the average number of times per week you participate in planned moderate-to-strenuous exercise of at least 20 minutes duration (e.g., brisk walking, jogging, cycling, swimming, stair climbing, weightlifting, active sports such as tennis, or aerobic classes).

     0   1   2   3   4   5   6   7   8   9   10

❏ YES ❏ NO   Can you briskly walk 1 mile without fatigue?
❏ YES ❏ NO   Can you jog 2 miles continuously at a moderate pace without discomfort?
❏ YES ❏ NO   Can you do 20 push-ups?

Please list your body weight (circle the appropriate units):
Now:_____lb/kg   1 year ago:_____lb/kg   Age 21:_____lb/kg

Figure 3-4
Health-history questionnaire *(continued)*

Working With Clients With Health Challenges — CHAPTER 3

SECTION VI. LIFESTYLE AND BEHAVIORAL

1. Describe any aerobic exercise you have done in the past (what, when, how often, and for how long). _____
_____
_____

2. Describe any muscular strength/weight training you have done in the past (what, when, how often, and for how long)._____
_____
_____

3. List any major obstacles that you feel you will have to overcome to stick with your exercise plan long-term (e.g., what has stopped you in the past).
_____
_____
_____

4. Have you ever participated in aerobic or aerobic step classes? _____Yes _____No

5. Please list any recreational physical activities (e.g., tennis or golf) in which you regularly participate and how often.
_____
_____
_____

6. List any favorite activities you would like to include in your exercise plan. _____
_____
_____

7. List any activities that you definitely do not like and do not want to include._____
_____
_____
_____

8. Which do you prefer? _____ Group exercise _____ Exercising on your own

9. List the two most important goals or reasons why you want to exercise regularly. _____
_____
_____

10. Your occupation:_____

11. Do you spend more than 25% of work time doing the following (mark all that apply)?
_____Sitting at a desk _____Lifting/carrying loads _____Standing _____Driving _____Walking

12. Number of hours worked per week: _____Hours Any flexible hours? _____Yes _____No

13. Write in the best exercise times for you during a typical week.

	Mon.	Tues.	Wed.	Thurs.	Fri.	Sat.	Sun.
AM							
PM							

14. Where do you plan to exercise? _____Club _____Home _____Outside

    Other_____

15. If at home, list all available equipment.
_____
_____

Figure 3-4
Health-history questionnaire *(continued)*

MUSCULOSKELETAL HEALTH QUESTIONNAIRE

1. Have you had to see a doctor in the past three years for any bone, joint, or spine problems?
   - ❏ No
   - ❏ One or two visits, but no problems now
   - ❏ Do doctors give frequent-flyer miles?

2. Have you ever had an orthopedic injury severe enough to result in one of the following?
   - Kept you out of sports or exercise for a month?
   - Required crutches for two or more weeks?
   - Required surgery?
   - ❏ No   ❏ Yes (to any of the questions)

3. Have you ever dislocated or separated your shoulder?
   - ❏ No   ❏ Yes
   If yes, please explain._____

4. Do you have joint swelling?   ❏ No   ❏ Yes

5. Have you lost mobility (range of motion) in any joint? For example, can you fully straighten (extend) and fully bend (flex)? Compare right to left.
   - ❏ No
   - ❏ A little stiff at times, but motion is full
   - ❏ Motion is limited in one or two major joints or the spine

6. Do your knees creak or make noise when you are going up or down stairs?
   - ❏ No
   - ❏ Yes, but no discomfort or pain
   - ❏ Yes, and does cause discomfort and/or pain

7. Do you have trouble actually ascending or descending stairs?
   - ❏ No
   - ❏ Only after going up and down multiple times, especially while carrying heavier items
   - ❏ Yes

8. Do you have stiffness in any joints associated with any of the following conditions?
   - Upon awakening (i.e., until showering or moving for about 15–20 minutes)
   - After sitting still for more than 30 minutes
   - For no apparent reason
   - ❏ No
   - ❏ Only the day after a hard workout
   - ❏ Yes

9. Does high barometric pressure (i.e., damp, rainy weather) make your joints ache?
   - ❏ No
   - ❏ Rarely
   - ❏ Friends consult me instead of the weatherman

10. Have you ever had an episode of lower-back or neck pain or spasm?
    - ❏ No
    - ❏ Yes, it kept me off my feet for less than 24 hours
    - ❏ Yes, I miss work due to recurrent episodes

11. Do you have pain while lying on either shoulder at night in bed?
    - ❏ No
    - ❏ Rarely
    - ❏ Almost nightly; tossing and turning to get comfy

12. Do you have difficulty falling asleep at night or awaken during the night because of any joint or muscle discomfort?
    - ❏ No
    - ❏ Rarely or minor difficulty
    - ❏ Yes

13. Do you awaken at night with your hands or fingers "asleep"?
    - ❏ No
    - ❏ Rarely and I easily shake it off
    - ❏ My hands get more sleep than I do

Note: If a client answers "Yes" to any of the items, this may suggest a musculoskeletal issue that warrants further evaluation. Be sure to refer to an appropriate healthcare professional as needed.

Figure 3-5
Sample musculoskeletal health questionnaire

Reprinted with permission from *FrameWork* by Nicholas A. DiNubile, M.D., with William Patrick © 2005 by Nicholas A. DiNubile, M.D. Permission granted by Rodale, Inc., Emmaus, PA 18098.

EXERCISE HISTORY AND ATTITUDE QUESTIONNAIRE

Name _____ Date _____

General Instructions: Please fill out this form as completely as possible. If you have any questions, DO NOT GUESS; ask your trainer or coach for assistance.

1. Please rate your exercise level on a scale of 1 to 5 (5 indicating very strenuous) for each age range through your present age:

    15–20 _____ 21–30 _____ 31–40 _____ 41–50 _____ 51–60 _____ 61–70 _____ 70+ _____

2. Were you a high school and/or college athlete?

    ❏ Yes ❏ No   If yes, please specify _____

3. Do you have any negative feelings toward, or have you had any bad experience with, physical-activity programs?

    ❏ Yes ❏ No   If yes, please explain _____

4. Do you have any negative feelings toward, or have you had any bad experience with, fitness testing and evaluation?

    ❏ Yes ❏ No   If yes, please explain _____

5. Rate yourself on a scale of 1 to 5 (1 indicating the lowest value and 5 the highest).

    Circle the number that best applies.

Characterize your present athletic ability.	1	2	3	4	5
When you exercise, how important is competition?	1	2	3	4	5
Characterize your present cardiovascular capacity.	1	2	3	4	5
Characterize your present muscular capacity.	1	2	3	4	5
Characterize your present flexibility capacity.	1	2	3	4	5

6. Do you start exercise programs but then find yourself unable to stick with them?   ❏ Yes ❏ No

7. How much time are you willing to devote to an exercise program? _____ minutes/day _____ days/week

8. Are you currently involved in regular endurance (cardiovascular) exercise?

    ❏ Yes ❏ No   If yes, specify the type of exercise(s) _____

    _____ minutes/day _____ days/week

    Rate your perception of the exertion of your exercise program (check the box):
    ❏ Light   ❏ Fairly light   ❏ Somewhat hard   ❏ Hard

9. How long have you been exercising regularly? _____ months _____ years

10. What other exercise, sport, or recreational activities have you participated in?

    In the past 6 months? _____

    In the past 5 years? _____

11. Can you exercise during your work day?   ❏ Yes ❏ No

12. Would an exercise program interfere with your job?   ❏ Yes ❏ No

13. Would an exercise program benefit your job?   ❏ Yes ❏ No

Figure 3-6
Sample exercise history and attitude questionnaire

Continued on the next page

14. What types of exercise interest you?
    - ❏ Walking
    - ❏ Jogging
    - ❏ Swimming
    - ❏ Cycling
    - ❏ Aerobics
    - ❏ Strength training
    - ❏ Stationary biking
    - ❏ Rowing
    - ❏ Racquetball
    - ❏ Tennis
    - ❏ Other aerobic activity
    - ❏ Stretching

15. Rank your goals in undertaking exercise: What do you want exercise to do for you?
    Use the following scale to rate each goal separately.

	Not at all important				Somewhat important				Extremely important	
a. Improve cardiovascular fitness	1	2	3	4	5	6	7	8	9	10
b. Facilitate body-fat weight loss	1	2	3	4	5	6	7	8	9	10
c. Reshape or tone my body	1	2	3	4	5	6	7	8	9	10
d. Improve performance for a specific sport	1	2	3	4	5	6	7	8	9	10
e. Improve moods and ability to cope with stress	1	2	3	4	5	6	7	8	9	10
f. Improve flexibility	1	2	3	4	5	6	7	8	9	10
g. Increase strength	1	2	3	4	5	6	7	8	9	10
h. Increase energy level	1	2	3	4	5	6	7	8	9	10
i. Feel better	1	2	3	4	5	6	7	8	9	10
j. Increase enjoyment	1	2	3	4	5	6	7	8	9	10
k. Other	1	2	3	4	5	6	7	8	9	10

16. By how much would you like to change your current weight?

    (+) _____ lb   (−) _____ lb

Figure 3-6
Sample exercise history and attitude questionnaire *(continued)*

Visit www.ACEfitness.org/CMESresources to download a free PDF of an exercise history and attitude questionnaire, a medical release form, as well as other forms and tools that you can use throughout your career as a CMES.

Step 2: Obtain Physician Clearance

As a general rule, it is prudent, from both a medical and legal perspective, to obtain a medical clearance for all clients with an identified chronic disease, disability, or injury, even if a clearance is not explicitly recommended in any of the established guidelines (Figure 3-7). When in doubt, a CMES should be conservative with these higher-risk clients.

Step 3: Identify Exercise Benefits and Goals

- *What are the client's goals?* To identify the client's goals, the CMES should use interviews, surveys, and informal discussions.
- *What are the health team's goals?* Include questions on the medical clearance form and interview health team members if at all possible. Note that the medical team's goals will most likely be related to the health benefits gained from exercise.
- *What role does exercise play in the management of the disease/disability?* The CMES can apply an organ-systems model: Based on what is known about the normal long-term effects of exercise on each organ system, and what is known about how the disease affects each organ system, how might exercise affect the disease progression and/or the general health of the client?
- *Is there documented evidence of the benefits of exercise?* Perform medical/scientific literature reviews, refer to exercise science and sports medicine texts and journals, and review any established guidelines.

Step 4: Determine Acute Exercise Risks

- *What are the effects of exercise?* Apply the organ-systems model described in Step 3 to the client's primary disease, associated conditions, and medications.
- *Are there any absolute and/or relative contraindications to exercise?* Review the established guidelines for each of the client's conditions.
- *Has the physician identified any special limitations or contraindications?* It is essential that the CMES consults with the healthcare team to develop a safe and appropriate program.

Figure 3-7
Sample medical release form

SAMPLE MEDICAL RELEASE FORM

Date _____

Dear Doctor:

Your patient, _____, wishes to start a personalized training program.

However, your patient must first obtain a medical clearance prior to initiating exercise due to the following risk factors or conditions:
_____

The activity will involve the following:

(type, frequency, duration, and intensity of activities)

If your patient is taking medications that will affect their exercise capacity or heart-rate response to exercise, please indicate the manner of the effect (raises or lowers exercise capacity or heart-rate response):

Type of medication(s)_____

Effect(s) _____

Please identify any recommendations or restrictions that are appropriate for your patient in this exercise program:
_____
_____

Please identify any medications that could increase your patient's risk for problems while exercising:
_____
_____

Thank you.

Sincerely,

Fred Fitness
Personalized Gym, Address, Phone

_____ has my approval to begin an exercise program with the recommendations or restrictions stated above.

Signed_____Date_____Phone_____

Step 5: Prepare for Medical Emergencies

- *What are the potential exercise-related medical emergencies?* Completion of Step 4 will identify the most common potential emergencies.
- *How will a CMES recognize a medical emergency?* Learn the signs and symptoms of each of the identified emergencies. The CMES should take a basic first aid course and refer to first aid, medical, and sports medicine texts and manuals to learn more.
- *How should a CMES respond?* The CMES should develop and practice an emergency plan based on their qualifications. At minimum, the CMES must know standard **cardiopulmonary resuscitation (CPR)**, basic first aid, and how to use an **automated external defibrillator (AED).**

Step 6: Obtain Informed Consent

When a client signs an **informed consent** form, they are acknowledging having been specifically informed about the risks associated with activity. Clients should be informed of the potential risks associated with exercise identified in Step 4. These risks should be clearly documented on the informed consent form, which should be completed prior to the performance of any fitness screening tests. This form provides evidence of the disclosure of the purposes, procedures, risks, and benefits associated with the assessments.

A sample informed consent form is presented in Figure 3-8. It is important to note that this is not a liability waiver and therefore does not provide legal immunity.

Figure 3-8
Sample informed consent form

Note: This document has been prepared to serve as a guide to improve understanding. Exercise professionals should not assume that this form will provide adequate protection in the event of a lawsuit. Please see an attorney before creating, distributing, and collecting any agreements to participate, informed consent forms, or waivers.

No form should be adopted without independent review by a lawyer and such other experts as may be appropriate.

CIRCULATORY AND RESPIRATORY FITNESS TEST

Informed Consent for Exercise Testing of Apparently Healthy Adults
(without known heart disease)

Name_____

1. Purpose and Explanation of Test

I hereby consent to voluntarily engage in an exercise test to determine my circulatory and respiratory fitness. I also consent to the taking of samples of my exhaled air during exercise to properly measure my oxygen uptake. I also consent, if necessary, to have a small blood sample drawn by needle from my arm for blood chemistry analysis and to the performance of lung function and body fat (skinfold pinch) tests. It is my understanding that the information obtained will help me evaluate future physical activities and sports activities in which I may engage.

Before I undergo the test, I certify that I am in good health and have had a physical examination conducted by a licensed medical physician within the last _____ months. Further, I hereby represent and inform the facility that I have accurately completed the pre-test history interview presented to me by the facility staff and have provided correct responses to the questions as indicated on the history form or as supplied to the interviewer. It is my understanding that I will be interviewed by a physician or other person prior to my undergoing the test who will in the course of interviewing me determine if there are any reasons that would make it undesirable or unsafe for me to take the test. Consequently, I understand that it is important that I provide complete and accurate responses to the interviewer and recognize that my failure to do so could lead to possible unnecessary injury to myself during the test.

The test that I will undergo will be performed on a motor-driven treadmill or bicycle ergometer with the amount of effort gradually increasing. As I understand it, this increase in effort will continue until I feel and verbally report to the operator any symptoms such as fatigue, shortness of breath, or chest discomfort that may appear. It is my understanding and I have been clearly advised that it is my right to request that a test be stopped at any point if I feel unusual discomfort or fatigue. I have been advised that I should, immediately upon experiencing any such symptoms or if I so choose, inform the operator that I wish to stop the test at that or any other point. My wishes in this regard shall be absolutely carried out.

It is further my understanding that prior to beginning the test, I will be connected by electrodes and cables to an electrocardiographic recorder that will enable the facility personnel to monitor my cardiac (heart) activity. During the test itself, it is my understanding that a trained observer will monitor my responses continuously and take frequent readings of blood pressure, the electrocardiogram, and my expressed feelings of effort. I realize that a true determination of my exercise capacity depends on progressing the test to the point of fatigue.

Once the test has been completed, but before I am released from the test area, I will be given special instructions about showering and recognition of certain symptoms that may appear within the first 24 hours after the test. I agree to follow these instructions and promptly contact the facility personnel or medical providers if such symptoms develop.

2. Risks

It is my understanding and I have been informed that there exists the possibility of adverse changes during the actual test. I have been informed that these changes could include abnormal blood pressure, fainting, disorders of heart rhythm, stroke, and very rare instances of heart attack or even death. Every effort, I have been told, will be made to minimize these

Initial: _____

occurrences by preliminary examination and by precautions and observations taken during the test. I have also been informed that emergency equipment and personnel are readily available to deal with these unusual situations should they occur. I understand that there is a risk of injury, heart attack, stroke, or even death as a result of my performance of this test, but knowing those risks, it is my desire to proceed to take the test as herein indicated.

3. Benefits to Be Expected and Alternatives Available to the Exercise Testing Procedure

The results of this test may or may not benefit me. Potential benefits relate mainly to my personal motives for taking the test (e.g., knowing my exercise capacity in relation to the general population, understanding my fitness for certain sports and recreational activities, planning my physical conditioning program, or evaluating the effects of my recent physical habits). Although my fitness might also be evaluated by alternative means (e.g., a bench step test or an outdoor running test), such tests do not provide as accurate a fitness assessment as the treadmill or bike test, nor do those options allow equally effective monitoring of my responses.

4. Confidentiality and Use of Information

I have been informed that the information that is obtained from this exercise test will be treated as privileged and confidential and will consequently not be released or revealed to any person without my express written consent or as required by law. I do, however, agree to the use of any information for research or statistical purposes so long as same does not provide facts that could lead to the identification of my person. Any other information obtained, however, will be used only by the facility staff to evaluate my exercise status or needs.

5. Inquiries and Freedom of Consent

I have been given an opportunity to ask questions about the procedure. Generally, these requests, which have been noted by the testing staff, and their responses are as follows:

_____

_____

_____

I further understand that there are also other remote risks that may be associated with this procedure. Despite the fact that a complete accounting of all remote risks is not entirely possible, I am satisfied with the review of these risks, which was provided to me, and it is still my desire to proceed with the test.

I acknowledge that I have read this document in its entirety or that it has been read to me if I have been unable to read same.

I consent to the rendition of all services and procedures as explained herein by all facility personnel.

Date_____

_____
Client's Signature

_____
Witness' Signature

_____
Test Supervisor's Signature

Reprinted with permission from Herbert, D.L. & Herbert, W.G. (2002). *Legal Aspects of Preventive and Rehabilitative Exercise Programs* (4th ed.). Canton, Oh.: PRC Publishing. All rights reserved.

Figure 3-8
Sample informed consent form
(continued)

Step 7: Plan Baseline Fitness Screening and Testing

- *Is fitness testing safe?* Remember that fitness testing is exercise. The answers derived in Step 4 will provide guidance when determining whether fitness testing is safe for a specific client.
- *Is fitness testing necessary?* Refer to Steps 3 and 4 for guidance.
- *What should the CMES measure? Fitness variables? Health variables? Ability to perform **activities of daily living (ADL)?*** Include those measurements that allow for tracking of goals and expected benefits.

Step 8: Design the Exercise Program

- *What exercise program will most effectively maximize the benefits and minimize the risks?* Refer to Steps 3 and 4 for guidance when answering this question. Consider all components of a balanced exercise program (i.e., aerobic, muscle conditioning, flexibility, balance and gait, and warm-up and cool-down). Determine frequency, intensity, mode, and duration. For clients with advanced diseases and/or disabilities, focus on improving the ability to perform ADL. Remember that many individuals with chronic diseases and disabilities have sedentary lifestyles. In many cases, exercise capacity will be more limited by poor general conditioning than the disease or disability itself.

Step 9: Plan Exercise Program Implementation

To answer all of the questions in this step, refer back to Steps 3 and 4 for guidance, review established guidelines, and consult with members of the healthcare team as needed.

- *What should a CMES include in the pre-exercise session screen (prior to every exercise session)?* This should primarily be a safety screen. The CMES should communicate with the client prior to each exercise session to find out how they are feeling that day. Asking the client if they are experiencing any pain or exacerbation of symptoms, or if health status has changed since the last exercise appointment, can guide the CMES in creating the best program for each individual client.
- *What should a CMES monitor during each exercise session?* It is essential that the CMES monitors signs and symptoms of the client's specific medical problems (e.g., ratings of perceived dyspnea in a client with COPD; pre- and post-exercise blood pressure in a client with hypertension).
- *What program variables should a CMES monitor over time? Fitness variables? Health variables? Ability to perform ADL?* Measurements (preferably objective measurements) should be used to track goals and expected benefits. In addition, the CMES should monitor signs or symptoms of evolving medical problems (e.g., increased severity or frequency of disease symptoms or increased medication requirements).
- *How quickly should the CMES progress the client's program?* Consider all the components of a balanced exercise program (i.e., aerobic, muscle conditioning, flexibility, balance and gait, and warm-up and cool-down). Determine how to progress the frequency, intensity, mode, and duration of the program based on both the client's health limitations and their unique goals.
- *What are the indications for program modification or referral to a physician?* Review the established guidelines for each of the client's conditions (Step 2), including those found in the literature review process as well as the physician's limitations and recommendations (Step 3). The exercise program will need to be modified if the client reports the presence of acute pain related to exercise and/or increased fatigue. An exacerbation of symptoms related to the client's condition, novel symptoms, increased fatigue, and/or the presence of unexplained acute pain or chronic pain should alert the CMES for the need to refer the client to their healthcare provider.

Working With Clients With Health Challenges   CHAPTER 3

- *What type of follow-up should the CMES provide to the client's physician?* The CMES should offer to the client's physician any consultation notes, **SOAP notes,** and program notes related to the client. This will aid the physician in their own record-keeping process and will keep the lines of communication open between the CMES and the client's healthcare provider.

Step 10: Double-check Established Guidelines

Keeping up-to-date with established guidelines is important for both client safety and liability-related reasons. The CMES should refer to the chapters in this manual that relate to a client's conditions, in addition to ACSM guidelines and advice from medical specialty colleges such as the American College of Obstetricians and Gynecologists (ACOG) and the American College of Cardiology (ACC). Other medical and public educations groups, including the American Heart Association (AHA), American Cancer Society (ACS), American Diabetes Association (ADA), and Arthritis Foundation (AF) are excellent resources as well.

Most exercise research to date addresses the prevention of chronic diseases, while the role of exercise in the management of these diseases has not been as well studied. For most chronic diseases, there is insufficient scientific data for the development of specific exercise guidelines. The CMES must continually review the exercise medicine literature to stay informed of new research findings and practice guidelines.

SUMMARY

It is optimistic to state that society has moved from "taking medicine" to "receiving healthcare," and that exercise is less about aesthetics and more about fitness and health. While traditional healthcare professionals are helpful in the reactive phase of disease and disability, the CMES can be an effective partner in proactive maintenance and/or development of function. The CMES has the power to empower, and to create a positive vision that will help lead each client to a better quality of life.

The CMES can utilize the 10-step decision-making approach detailed in this chapter to guide their programming for all clients, regardless of what diseases or disabilities they are managing. It is essential that the CMES understands the purpose and proper use of the documents presented in this chapter, as they not only represent the appropriate standard of care for all clients, but also help protect health and exercise professionals from potential liability associated with injury.

REFERENCES

American Academy of Dermatology (2012). *Position Statement on Indoor Tanning* www.aad.org/forms/policies/uploads/ps/ps-indoor%20tanning.pdf

American College of Sports Medicine (2022). *ACSM's Guidelines for Exercise Testing and Prescription* (11th ed.). Philadelphia: Wolters Kluwer.

Azevedo, E. et al. (2011). The effects of total and REM sleep deprivation on laser-evoked potential threshold and pain perception. *Pain,* 152, 9, 2052–2058.

Bryant, C.X., Franklin, B.A., & Newton-Merrill, S. (2007). *ACE's Guide to Exercise Testing & Program Design* (2nd ed.). Monterey, Calif.: Healthy Learning.

Cappuccio, F.P. et al. (2010). Quantity and quality of sleep and incidence of type 2 diabetes: A systematic review and meta-analysis. *Diabetes Care,* 33, 414–420.

Dang-Vu, T.T. et al. (2010). Functional neuroimaging insights into the physiology of human sleep. *Sleep,* 33, 12, 1589–1603.

DiNubile, N.A. & Patrick, W. (2005). *FrameWork: Your 7-Step Program for Healthy Muscles, Bones, and Joints.* Emmaus, Pa.: Rodale Press.

Ditre, J.W. et al. (2011). Pain, nicotine, and smoking: Research findings and mechanistic considerations. *Psychological Bulletin,* 137, 6, 1065–1093. DOI: 10.1037/a0025544

Fuchs, V.R. (2013). The gross domestic product and health care spending. *New England Journal of Medicine,* 369, 107–109.

Gao, B. & Bataller, R. (2011). Alcoholic liver disease: Pathogenesis and new therapeutic targets. *Gastroenterology,* 141, 5, 1572–1585. DOI: 10.1053/j.gastro.2011.09.002

Grundy, S.M. et al. (2005). Diagnosis and management of the metabolic syndrome: An American Heart Association/ National Heart, Lung, and Blood Institute Scientific Statement. *Circulation,* 112, 17, 2735–2752.

Herbert, D.L. & Herbert, W.G. (2002). *Legal Aspects of Preventive and Rehabilitative Exercise Programs* (4th ed.). Canton, Oh.: PRC Publishing.

Hodgson, A.B., Randell, R.K., & Jeukendrup, A.E. (2013). The metabolic and performance effects of caffeine compared to coffee during endurance exercise. *PLoS One,* 8, 4, e59561. DOI: 10.1371/journal.pone.0059561

Institute of Medicine (2006). *Sleep Disorders and Sleep Deprivation: An Unmet Public Health Problem.* Washington, D.C.: The National Academy of Sciences.

Irwin, M.R. et al. (2012). Sleep loss exacerbates fatigue, depression, and pain in rheumatoid arthritis. *Sleep,* 35, 537–543.

Li, E.J.Q. et al. (2006). The effect of a "training on work readiness" program for workers with musculoskeletal injuries: A randomized control trial (RCT) study. *Journal of Occupational Rehabilitation,* 16, 4, 529–541.

Lillefjell, M., Krokstad, S., & Espnes, G.A. (2006). Factors predicting work ability following multidisciplinary rehabilitation for chronic musculoskeletal pain. *Journal of Occupational Rehabilitation,* 16, 4, 543–555.

Lucassen, E.A. & Cizza, G. (2012). The hypothalamic-pituitary-adrenal axis, obesity, and chronic stress exposure: Sleep and the HPA axis in obesity. *Current Obesity Reports,* 1, 4, 208–215.

Morgan, R.E. (2013). Does consumption of high-fructose corn syrup beverages cause obesity in children? *Pediatric Obesity,* 8, 4, 249–254.

Pattyn, N. et al. (2013). The effect of exercise on the cardiovascular risk factors constituting the metabolic syndrome: A meta-analysis of controlled trials. *Sports Medicine,* 43, 121–133.

Perry, G.S., Patil, S.P., Presley-Cantrell, L.R. (2013). Raising awareness of sleep as a healthy behavior. *Preventing Chronic Disease,* 10: E133. DOI: 10.5888/pcd10.130081 PMCID: PMC3741412

Philip, P. et al. (2012). Acute versus chronic sleep deprivation in middle-aged people: Differential impact on performance and sleepiness. *Sleep,* 35, 997–1002.

Rask-Madsen, C. & Kahn, C.R. (2012). Tissue-specific insulin signaling, metabolic syndrome and cardiovascular disease. *Arteriosclerosis, Thrombosis, and Vascular Biology,* 32, 9, 2052–2059. DOI: 10.1161/ATVBAHA.111.241919

Schultz, I.Z. et al. (2007). Models of return to work for musculoskeletal disorders. *Journal of Occupational Rehabilitation,* 17, 4, 782.

Selye, H. (1975). *Stress Without Distress.* New York: Signet.

Strasser, B., Siebert, U., & Schobersberger, W. (2010). Resistance training in the treatment of the metabolic syndrome: A systematic review and meta-analysis of the effect of resistance training on metabolic clustering in patients with abnormal glucose metabolism. *Sports Medicine,* 1, 40, 5, 397–415.

Strax, T.E., Gonzalez, P. & Cuccurullo, S. (2004). Effects of extended bed rest—Immobilization and inactivity. In: *Physical Medicine and Rehabilitation Board Review,* New York: Demos Medical Publishing.

Tucker, K.L. et al. (2006). Colas, but not other carbonated beverages, are associated with low bone mineral density in older women: The Framingham Osteoporosis Study. *American Journal of Clinical Nutrition,* 84, 4, 936–942.

U.S. Department of Agriculture (2020). *2020-2025 Dietary Guidelines for Americans.* www.dietaryguidelines.gov

U.S. Department of Health & Human Services (2018). *Physical Activity Guidelines for Americans* (2nd ed.). www.health.gov/paguidelines

World Health Organization (2010). *Global Recommendations on Physical Activity for Health.* Geneva: World Health Organization.

SUGGESTED READINGS

American Council on Exercise (2021). *Coaching Senior Fitness.* San Diego, Calif.: American Council on Exercise.

Malina, R. (1996). Tracking of physical activity and physical fitness across the lifespan. *Research Quarterly for Exercise and Sport,* 67, 3, 48–61.

McNamee, D. (1996). A change in lifestyle may prevent cancer. *Lancet,* 348, 1436.

Pattyn, N. et al. (2013). The effect of exercise on the cardiovascular risk factors constituting the metabolic syndrome: A meta-analysis of controlled trials. *Sports Medicine,* 43, 121–133.

Perry, G.S., Patil, S.P., & Presley-Cantrell, L.R. (2013). Raising awareness of sleep as a healthy behavior. *Preventing Chronic Disease,* 10: E133. DOI: 10.5888/pcd10.130081 PMCID: PMC3741412

Strasser, B., Siebert, U., & Schobersberger, W. (2010). Resistance training in the treatment of the metabolic syndrome: A systematic review and meta-analysis of the effect of resistance training on metabolic clustering in patients with abnormal glucose metabolism. *Sports Medicine,* 1, 40, 5, 397–415.

World Health Organization (2010). *Global Recommendations on Physical Activity for Health.* Geneva: World Health Organization.

ADDITIONAL RESOURCES

American Heart Association: www.heart.org

American Cancer Society: www.cancer.org

American Diabetes Association: www.diabetes.org

General medical information: www.WebMD.com; www.medscape.com

PART II
LEADERSHIP AND IMPLEMENTATION

CHAPTER 4
BEHAVIORAL CHANGE

CHAPTER 5
COMMUNICATION STRATEGIES

CHAPTER 6
PROFESSIONAL RELATIONSHIPS AND BUSINESS STRATEGIES

4 BEHAVIORAL CHANGE

IN THIS CHAPTER

DETERMINANTS OF HEALTH BEHAVIOR
OPERANT CONDITIONING
HABIT
SOCIAL AND INDIVIDUAL FACTORS

TRANSTHEORETICAL MODEL OF BEHAVIORAL CHANGE
STAGES OF CHANGE
PROCESSES OF CHANGE
SELF-EFFICACY
DECISIONAL BALANCE

HEALTH BELIEF MODEL
SELF-EFFICACY

STRATEGIES FOR BEHAVIORAL CHANGE
COMMUNICATION
AVOID MAKING ASSUMPTIONS
RELAPSE PREVENTION
EMPOWERING THE CLIENT
MANAGING HIGH-RISK SITUATIONS

ADHERENCE
BEHAVIORAL MODIFICATION
COGNITIVE BEHAVIORAL TECHNIQUES

SUMMARY

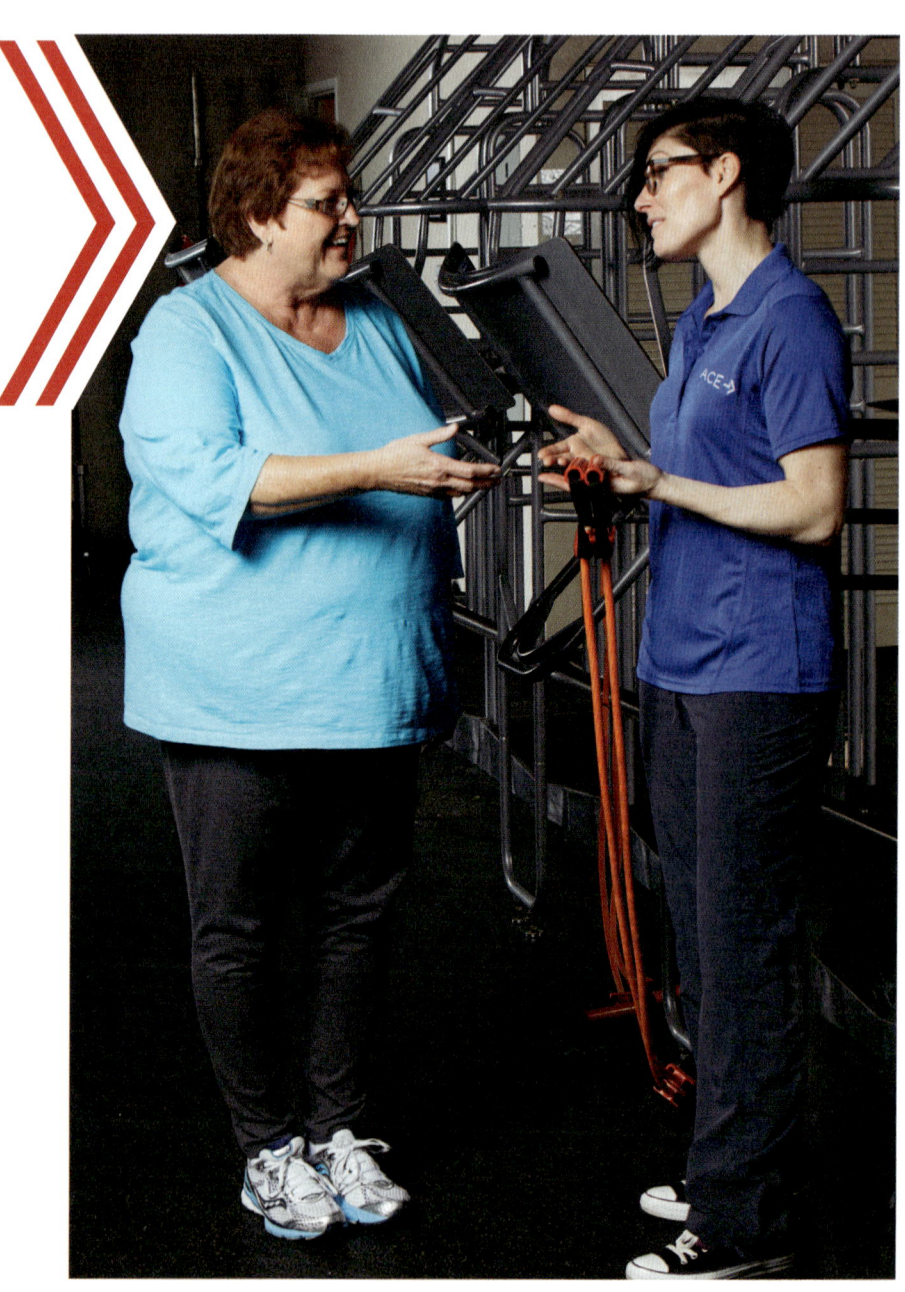

ABOUT THE AUTHOR
Tracie Rogers, Ph.D., is a sport and exercise psychology specialist and an assistant professor in the Human Movement program at the Arizona School of Health Sciences at A.T. Still University. Dr. Rogers teaches, speaks, and writes on psychological constructs related to behavioral change and physical-activity participation and adherence.

By Tracie Rogers

ACE® CERTIFIED MEDICAL EXERCISE SPECIALISTS (CMES) have a solid understanding of the physiological factors and outcomes related to exercise. Research consistently demonstrates the physical and mental benefits of regular exercise programs, and the CMES serves as an advocate to clients for engaging in regular activity programs. Despite the amount of knowledge and sound research available and the fact that the majority of the population knows that they should exercise more, only 20% of adults are engaging in enough activity to meet the recommended aerobic and muscle-strengthening guidelines (Centers for Disease Control and Prevention, 2013).

This demonstrates that knowledge about health benefits and disease prevention is not enough on its own to actually get people moving. Health psychology as a field addresses the complexity of behavioral change and identifies biological, psychological, and social factors that affect health and health behaviors (Engel, 1977). The CMES must have an understanding of these factors and how they influence exercise program adoption and **adherence** to be better able to serve their clientele.

A CMES is in a unique role to intervene when clients need help the most. Whether a client has health issues, is at risk for disease, is in need of a post-rehabilitative fitness program, or is recovering from a cardiovascular, pulmonary, metabolic, or musculoskeletal issue, the CMES is able to create programming specific to clients' needs in order to generate positive health and mobility outcomes. In this role, the CMES is able to not only help prevent additional future health problems, but to promote health, reduce risk, and improve quality of life. Encouraging, motivating, and teaching clients to engage in regular physical activity, choose healthy nutrition and eating habits, and properly manage emotional stress, among other lifestyle decisions, can help clients reduce disease risk and increase overall wellness.

DETERMINANTS OF HEALTH BEHAVIOR

If it was simple to understand why some people engage in healthy behaviors and others do not, and if this simple understanding led to a quick fix, a CMES and other health and exercise professionals would have no problem encouraging people to start and adhere to programs. This, unfortunately, is not the case. Instead, the attempt to understand the choices that people make with regard to health behaviors is often frustrating. The complexity of predicting health behaviors is further complicated with physical activity, as exercise is perceived to take more time and effort than other health behaviors (Turk, Rudy, & Salovey, 1984). However, despite the complicated task of successfully promoting activity adoption and maintenance, researchers do have some understanding of factors that influence exercise behavior. There are numerous predictors of health behaviors, including learning, social and individual factors, and motivations and emotions. The more the CMES understands about these principles, the better they will be able to help people successfully make changes.

LEARNING OBJECTIVES:

» Describe common theories on the determinants of health behavior including operant conditioning, habit formation, and social and individual factors.

» List and describe the five stages of change of the transtheoretical model of behavioral change and explain how these stages relate to client self-efficacy and decisional balance.

» Explain strategies for helping clients progress from one stage of change to the next to facilitate behavior-change goals.

» Help clients adhere to a behavior-change program through the use of effective communication, relapse prevention, and cognitive behavioral techniques.

Operant Conditioning

In any type of lifestyle-modification or post-rehabilitation exercise program, the primary goal of a CMES is to safely and effectively increase healthy behaviors in clients' lives in order to improve health, prevent future disease states, and regain physical capabilities. As with anything new, these health behaviors must be learned and perfected. Individuals' knowledge of health behaviors come from a variety of sources and each client will bring knowledge, both good and bad, that has been learned over time from other people and life experiences. A CMES will be most effective in successfully establishing new behaviors if they take the time to understand the history behind the development of clients' current behaviors and attitudes and the principles associated with learning new behaviors. One way that people learn behavior is through **operant conditioning,** a process by which behavior is influenced by its consequences. Operant conditioning studies the learning process by looking at the relationships between **antecedents,** behaviors, and consequences (Skinner, 1938). In other words, operant conditioning examines the variables that trigger exercise behavior (or lack thereof) and also the variables that follow exercise behavior (or lack thereof). This behavior chain (trigger–behavior–consequence) can then be used to help predict and teach future behaviors (Martin & Pear, 2010).

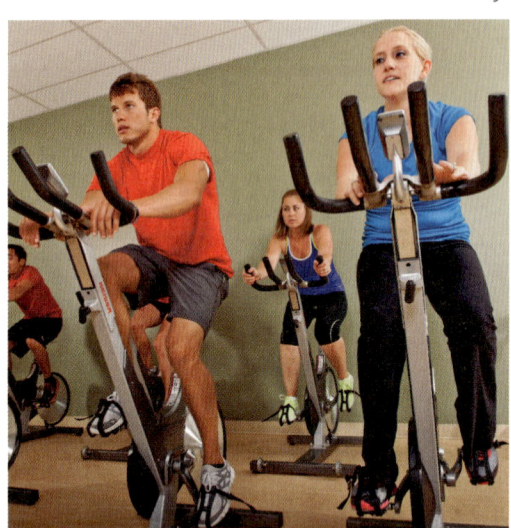

APPLY WHAT YOU KNOW

USING OPERANT CONDITIONING TO INCREASE HEALTHY BEHAVIOR

In an exercise program, the goal is to increase healthy behaviors in clients' lives. According to the principle of operant conditioning, behaviors are strengthened when they are reinforced. In the training context, using positive reinforcements means that positive or healthy behaviors have consequences that are going to increase the likelihood of the behavior happening again. At the most basic level with a new client, a positive behavior is simply showing up to the gym. If the success of this behavior (which can be a real victory for a new exerciser) is ignored by the CMES, the likelihood of it happening again will decrease. However, if the client is verbally rewarded for showing up and is further rewarded with a positive, pleasant, and supportive workout experience, then the behavior has been positively reinforced and the likelihood of it happening again has been increased. As exercise professionals, the opportunity to trigger lasting change is always present, and the basic principle of operant conditioning can serve as a good reminder of the influence a CMES has with each client they encounter.

Antecedents

An important part of the learning experience is developing awareness about the consequences of behaviors in different conditions. Antecedents, an important part of operant conditioning, are stimuli that precede or trigger a behavior and often signal the likely consequences of the behavior. Antecedents help guide behavior so that it will most likely lead to desired consequences. Furthermore, antecedents can be manipulated in the environment to maximize the likelihood of desirable behaviors and consequences. This type of influence on behavior is called **stimulus control** and can be a valuable tool in learning and achieving behavioral change. Because antecedents serve as influencers for behavior, it is important that the CMES learn triggers that lead to exercise and non-exercise outcomes for specific clients. A straightforward example of stimulus control is having exercise clothes ready for the exercise session. Whether it means have everything laid out on the floor ready for an early morning session or packed in a bag in the car for a stop on the way home from work, this type of trigger can help lead to the desired behavior of exercise.

Response Consequences

The most important component of operant conditioning is what happens after a behavior is executed. This is especially important because the CMES can manipulate consequences to shape behavior, as different consequences lead to different future behavioral outcomes. Consequences involve the presentation, nonoccurrence, or removal of a positive or negative stimulus. In operant conditioning, there are four categories of consequences.

- **Positive reinforcement** is the presentation of a positive stimulus and *increases* the likelihood that a behavior will reoccur in the future. As previously mentioned, an enjoyable exercise experience itself can be a powerful positive reinforcement for beginning exercisers.
- **Negative reinforcement** consists of the removal or avoidance of negative stimuli following a behavior. In other words, the removal of something negative that once followed a behavior makes a person more likely to perform the behavior again. For example, if a client associates physical activity with low-back pain (negative stimulus) from previous workouts, they are not likely to want to participate in physical activity in the future. However, if the CMES works together with the client to create an individualized exercise program beginning at an appropriate level of intensity, while also focusing on postural stability and kinetic-chain mobility, the low-back pain may be avoided (avoidance of the negative stimulus). This will increase the likelihood that the the client will adhere to the program.
- **Extinction** occurs when a positive stimulus that once followed a behavior is removed, and this *decreases* the likelihood of the behavior occurring again. Consider a client who receives positive feedback from their family whenever they prepare a healthy meal, but then start to hear complaints from their kids, who want to return to their old, unhealthier ways of eating. This change in response decreases the likelihood that they will cook healthy dinners in the future.
- **Punishment** consists of an aversive stimulus following an undesirable behavior and also *decreases* the likelihood of the behavior occurring again. If a tardy client was told that their appointment was cancelled due to their tardiness and that they must be on time for their workout sessions, they will likely not be late again. However, despite the fact that punishment is effective at decreasing an unwanted behavior, it also increases fear and decreases enjoyment, so it must be used sparingly and only when appropriate (never for poor performance, only for lack of effort). Despite being effective in decreasing the likelihood of an unwanted behavior, punishment also increases fear and decreases enjoyment, both of which should be avoided in an exercise setting. Therefore, there is rarely a place for punishment in the client–exercise professional relationship.

The CMES plays a direct role in the consequence portion of operant conditioning, and, as a result, should understand each type of consequence to ensure they provide appropriate **feedback** to client behaviors. Positive reinforcement should follow the things that clients are doing well, while the things that need improvement should not be ignored, but identified and corrected. Effective feedback and presentation of consequences is even more important at the start of a program when new habits and thought processes are being formed related to exercise participation. Communication, as always, is a crucial component of the learning process because clients need to be empowered with information about the goal behavior (exercise) and the desired behavioral consequences. Consistency of consequences will promote clarity, understanding, and proper execution, which will help put the goal-setting plan and other program components into action (Smith, 2010).

APPLY WHAT YOU KNOW

IMPLEMENTING OPERANT CONDITIONING

Your new client has been referred to you for an exercise program to help improve blood sugar regulation. After assessing the client's needs and resources, you have the client start a walking program for 30 minutes each day. The client chooses to walk around her neighborhood after she gets home from work. Based on daily check-ins with your client, you learn that she did great for the first two days, but got home a bit late on the third day and was hungry so she skipped her walk. This happened again on the fourth and fifth days. She is feeling discouraged and tells you that she is unable to stick to this program.

There are many ways you can address this situation. From an operant conditioning perspective, you should address the environmental triggers and consequences related to the behavior and then use appropriate tools to help generate success.

After talking with your client and evaluating the situation, you decide that it is not a great choice to wait until she gets home from work to engage in the exercise program. After a long day at work, there are too many potential distractions (e.g., food and need for relaxation) to create the opportunity for success. You recommend that she packs her exercise clothes and changes into them before she leaves work. Then you identify a park between her work and home that has great walking paths. You also help her choose a healthy snack to eat before her workout so that she is not starving for dinner. Remembering that she does not have to walk 30 minutes in one session, you can also suggest that she walk 15 minutes to a park or restaurant for lunch and then 15 minutes back to work. These simple stimulus-control modifications are easy for her to incorporate and will maximize her likelihood of program adoption.

Habit

As the CMES works to change negative health behaviors and promote positive health behaviors, it is important to remember that most daily behaviors are habits. Over time, behaviors become established in one's life and are executed without much thought or, more importantly, resistance. The CMES should be aware that many healthy and unhealthy behaviors are habitual and that most people are unable to just stop doing something unhealthy "cold turkey." However, just because something is a habit does not mean it is permanent. Habits can be changed and replaced, but doing so requires an active decision and effort to change (Duhigg, 2012). Common unhealthy behaviors are food choices, snacking, and extended periods of inactivity. It is much more effective if the CMES works with clients to identify habitual unhealthy behaviors in their lives and work to replace them with more productive, healthy behaviors. In order for this transition to occur, new antecedents and consequences must be implemented to instigate the change of habitual behaviors, and **social support** networks are important for this challenging task.

APPLY WHAT YOU KNOW

A STEP-BY-STEP APPROACH TO CHANGING HABITS

Helping clients to change health behavior habits does not need to be a complicated process. Instead, it should be taught in a simple step-by-step approach. The first step should be to work with the client to create cues for healthy behavior. These can be anything from laying out clothes and setting a calendar reminder to scheduling an appointment for activity with a friend. These tasks are basic, but simple cues can serve as effective triggers to initiate behavior. Another important step is to encourage clients to make healthy behaviors part of their routine. In other words, encourage repetitive behaviors on a daily basis. Routine behaviors, over time, will become the new normal for clients' daily activities. Finally, build in rewards for consistent execution of new behaviors. Rewards can come in the form of recognition of positive results and do not need to be external or material items, although in some situations that may be appropriate as well (i.e., a client rewarding themself with a pedicure or massage after a month of consistent behavior execution). The CMES should work with the client at the start of the program to identify meaningful and motivating rewards.

Social and Individual Factors

Social Support

When deciding to make a behavioral change and when adopting a new program, the perceived support that one feels is an important predictor of program success. In fact, social support from family and friends is an important predictor of physical-activity behavior and has been consistently related to activity in both cross-sectional and prospective research designs (Duncan & McAuley, 1993). Social support itself is a subjective construct that refers to perceived aid, assistance, help, or support received from others (Sarafino & Smith, 2014). It is an uphill battle for an individual to adopt and maintain a new exercise program if they do not feel supported at home or at work. A lack of support can be seen through clients' motivation, participation, confidence, and willingness to change. Social support is an interesting challenge for a CMES, because while it is impossible to directly create support in clients' home and personal lives, it is feasible to build support within the workout environment. The CMES should be aware of client situations in which a support network is needed and work to create that network within the program.

Personality Traits

All individuals have a set of general tendencies that make up their personalities. These traits account for individual differences between people and are difficult to define and measure in both practice and in research. Studies have shown that there are a few identifiable traits that have consistent relationships with exercise behavior. Self-motivation is defined as one's ability to set goals, monitor progress, and self-reinforce and it has been shown to have a positive relationship with physical-activity adherence (Dishman, 1982). Obviously, the more self-motivated an individual is, the easier it will be for the CMES to implement the program and engage the client. A self-motivated client is prepared to be accountable and to be an active participant in the program. The challenge is trying to build one's level of self-motivation. Research suggests that by building competence and autonomy, individuals' intrinsic motivation levels will increase (Deci & Ryan, 2002). This has also been demonstrated with patients diagnosed as being at high risk for **coronary artery disease (CAD).** Those who perceive their primary care providers as being autonomy-supportive are more self-motivated to live a healthier lifestyle (Williams et al., 2004). This demonstrates the importance of the CMES understanding the clients' needs and offering choices to create the perception of client control. Health and exercise professionals often take too much control over the program and simply present it to the client as a finished product. A good example of this is when the CMES lists a few reasons why exercise is beneficial. Instead of mentioning reasons that the CMES thinks are important, the list should be long and inclusive, allowing clients to select those that are important to them. It is much more effective to include the client in the process to build autonomy and confidence.

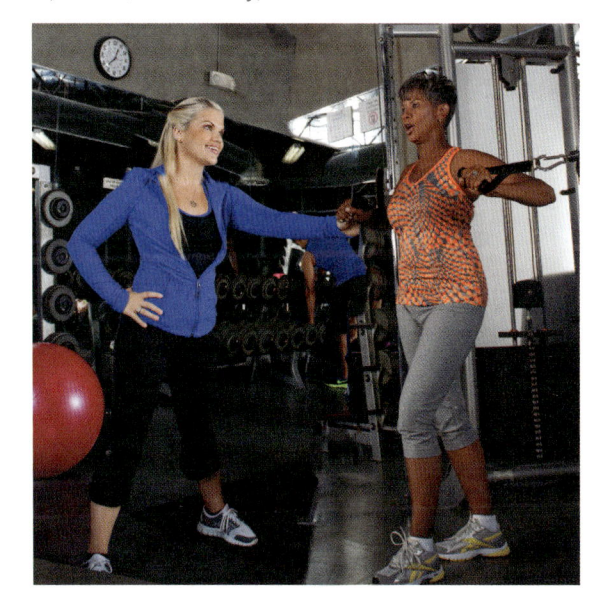

Another trait related to exercise behavior is conscientiousness. This personality profile, which represents one's tendency to be organized and dutiful and to have the ability to complete tasks, has been linked to higher fitness levels and healthy food selection (Bogg & Roberts, 2004). Additionally, research has shown that people with high levels of conscientiousness are more likely to stick with an exercise program in unstable situations compared to those who are less conscientious (Conner, Rodgers, & Murray, 2007). This means that when schedules change and obstacles arise, conscientious individuals are more likely to adhere to their programs. Furthermore, conscientious clients will be more aware of program expectations and will work on a regular basis to meet the demands of all aspects of program participation. Additionally, these clients will be more prepared to make changes in their lives to fully adopt the lifestyle modifications.

Cognitive Variables

All experienced health and exercise professionals know that people have a wide range of knowledge, attitudes, and beliefs about both the importance of, and processes involved with, adopting and maintaining an active lifestyle. A key variable in this context is health perception, which has been linked to adherence, such that those who perceive their health to be poor are unlikely to start or adhere to an activity program. Furthermore, if they do participate, it will likely be at an extremely low intensity and frequency (Dishman & Buckworth, 1997). This is particularly important for a CMES who is working with clients who are recovering from injury, who are ill, or who are at high risk for developing a disease. It is easy to believe that this population would be more motivated to participate for health improvement, but instead, a low health perception has the opposite effect, thus requiring additional support and work on the part of the CMES. This relationship can be further explained by **locus of control,** which is a belief in personal control over health outcomes. An internal locus of control means that one believes they can make a difference or change an outcome. This positive state is related to higher rates of exercise adherence (Kloek et al., 2006).

On the other hand, if an individual has poor health, they may simply perceive that nothing can be done to change it, which reflects an external locus of control. An external locus of control can lead to **learned helplessness**, a state in which an individual feels completely powerless to control things or make changes in their life. For example, learned helplessness is relevant to health-related problems and has been shown to be an important predictor of health outcomes in patients with **rheumatoid arthritis.** Specifically, learned helplessness significantly predicts disability, pain, and fatigue (Camacho et al., 2013). The good news for health and exercise professionals is that locus of control and learned helplessness are dynamic constructs that can be altered and, more importantly, improved. Locus of control is also associated with the concept of autonomy and self-motivation. This relationship makes sense, as the belief of having control is related to the desire to be in control and the motivation to make changes. It is important for a CMES to realize that when people make the decision to do something and have a sense of control over what they are doing, they are much more likely to stick with it and succeed. As previously mentioned, this is counterintuitive for some health and exercise professionals who believe they must control and dictate every aspect of the client's program.

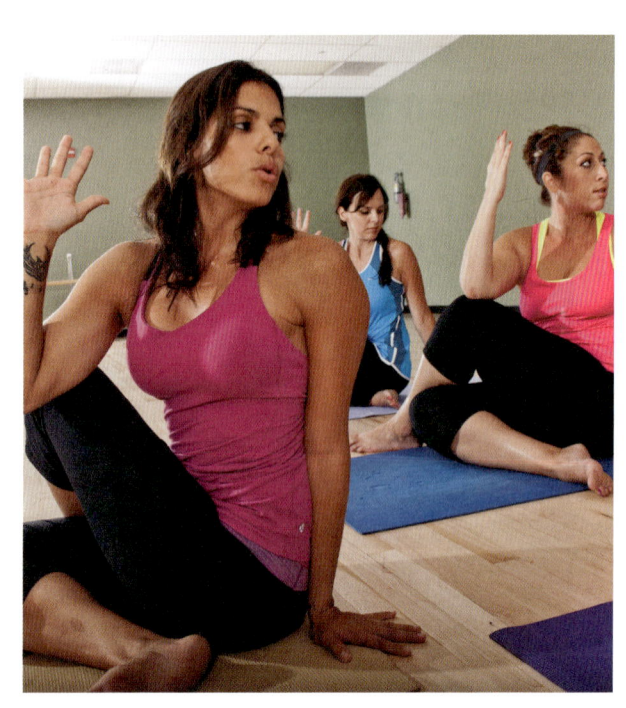

Another cognitive variable is perceived barriers, such as lack of time or energy, which are consistently related to low exercise-program adherence. The best way for a CMES to deal with perceived barriers is through communication and education. These perceptions cannot be discounted or dismissed as irrelevant, but instead people must learn to problem solve and make decisions and program modifications as needed. This should be a one-step-at-a-time approach to help people build the confidence and positive perceptions needed for success.

TRANSTHEORETICAL MODEL OF BEHAVIORAL CHANGE

For a CMES, each client will present unique challenges and circumstances that require customized programming to meet individual needs and health conditions and to promote program adherence. Changing behaviors and, more specifically, adopting healthy behaviors, is a complicated process, and as a result, several theoretical models have been developed

Behavioral Change   CHAPTER 4

to explain and predict the factors influencing health behavior and health-behavior change. It is not the role of a CMES to have a complete and thorough understanding of each model of behavioral change; however, it is important for a CMES to be able to identify principal components of the theories and how they may relate to program adoption and maintenance.

One important factor in behavioral change is the client's readiness to make a change. This individual readiness for change is the focus of a well-accepted theory examining health behaviors called the **transtheoretical model of behavioral change (TTM)** (Prochaska & DiClemente, 1984). The TTM is straightforward and directly applicable to many client situations. The model provides a comprehensive approach to working with clients who want and need to make healthier lifestyle choices. A CMES who develops the ability to apply the concepts of the TTM may be better equipped to help clients with health-related changes that have the potential for improved quality of life, improved health, and reduced risk of **morbidity** and **mortality.**

The components of the TTM that are commonly applied to an exercise context are stages of change and processes of change. Additionally, **decisional balance, self-efficacy,** and situational temptations to **relapse** can be important concepts for the CMES to consider when working with clients who are attempting healthy behavioral change. A common issue with the TTM is that practitioners only use the stages-of-change component of the model and ignore the other concepts. This is an ineffective use of the model, as the stage of change is simply the identification of where a person is in terms of readiness to change. Working through decisional balance with clients, promoting increased self-efficacy, and educating clients on how to avoid relapses can allow the CMES to make a difference and promote progression.

Stages of Change

The TTM consists of five stages of behavioral change. These stages help health and exercise professionals identify clients' readiness to change based on their behaviors and thoughts; this information is the first step in helping people adopt health behaviors (Table 4-1). People in the **precontemplation** stage are **sedentary** and not considering participation in an activity program. These people do not see activity as relevant in their lives and may even discount the importance or practicality of being physically active. This group may have such a lack of information that they may even be unaware that a sedentary lifestyle is a serious risk factor for chronic illness. This may be particularly true if an individual does not have **overweight** and has the perception that the primary outcome of exercise is weight loss. The main goal of the CMES is to encourage the client to start thinking about change and about how change is relevant in their life. Encouragement, personalizing healthy lifestyle information, expressing concern about specific symptoms, and asking the client what they see sees as advantages to change, are all appropriate techniques at this stage. Essentially, the CMES provides information and helps the client analyze personal risk. Media resources, referrals to other health professionals, and personalized handouts are examples of what the CMES can offer to clients at this stage. Validating the client's lack of readiness, ensuring the client understands the decision is entirely theirs, and encouraging exploration, not action, are additional key methods to help the client move to the **contemplation** stage. Not all people are ready to move out of this stage and some simply may not. In the precontemplation stage, the individual says, "I won't."

The second stage is contemplation. In the contemplation stage, people are still sedentary; however, they are starting to consider the importance of activity and have begun to identify the personal implications of being inactive. Nevertheless, they are still not prepared to commit to making a change. A CMES can encourage clients to review the pros and cons of healthy behavioral change by asking them to list benefits and obstacles to change. Also, by asking clients how they might overcome the barriers listed, the CMES can start a dialogue that presents exercise as a feasible solution. The goal of the CMES when working with clients in the contemplation stage is to get clients saying "maybe this is right for me."

TABLE 4-1
STAGES OF CHANGE

Stage	Traits	Goals	Strategies
Precontemplation	Unaware or under-aware of the problem, or believe that it cannot be solved (e.g., latent pain)	Increase awareness of the risks of inactivity, and of the benefits of activity Focus on addressing something relevant to them Have them start thinking about change	Validate lack of readiness to change and clarify that this decision is theirs Encourage reevaluation of current behavior and self-exploration, while not taking action Explain and personalize the inherent risks Utilize general sources, including media, Internet, and brochures to increase awareness
Contemplation	Aware of the problem and weighing the benefits versus risks of change Have little understanding of how to go about changing	Inform them of available options Provide cues to action and some basic structured direction	Validate lack of readiness to change and clarify that this decision is theirs Encourage evaluation of the pros and cons of making change Identify and promote new, positive outcome expectations and boost self-confidence Offer invitations to become more active (e.g., free trials)
Preparation	Seeking opportunities to participate in activity (combine intent and behavior with activity)	Structured, regular programming with frequent positive feedback and reinforcements on their progress	Verify that the individual has the underlying skills for behavioral change and encourage small steps toward building self-efficacy Identify and assist with problem-solving obstacles Help the client identify social support and establish goals
Action	Desire for opportunities to maintain activities Changing beliefs and attitudes High risk for lapses or returns to undesirable behavior	Establish exercise as a habit through motivation and adherence to the desired behavior	Behavior-modification strategies Focus on restructuring cues and social support toward building long-term change Increase awareness to inevitable lapses and bolster self-efficacy in coping with lapses Reiterate long-term benefits of adherence Require continual feedback on progress
Maintenance	Empowered, but desire a means to maintain adherence Good capability to deal with lapses	Maintain support systems Maintain interest and avoid boredom or burnout	Reevaluate strategies currently in effect Plan for contingencies with support systems, although this may no longer be needed Reinforce the need for a transition from external to internal rewards Plan for potential lapses Encourage program variety Remind the client that it takes less time and effort to maintain a higher level of fitness or health than it did to acquire it

Behavioral Change

CHAPTER 4

The third stage is the **preparation** stage. People in this stage are performing some amount of physical activity, as they are mentally and physically preparing to adopt an activity program. Exercise during the preparation stage may be a sporadic walk, or even a visit to the gym, but it is inconsistent and unfocused. People in the preparation stage have typically made the decision that they want to adopt and live an active lifestyle but they still need a great deal of information about how to actually do it. Therefore, this is the perfect opportunity for a CMES to start educating the client and creating a plan to introduce consistent healthy lifestyle behaviors. Clients in the preparation stage have said yes to change and it is the role of the CMES to turn that desire into achievable action. People in the preparation stage say, "I will."

The next stage is the **action** stage. The action stage consists of people engaging in regular physical activity for less than a six-month period. It is during this stage that the CMES is most needed and important. In addition to program design and implementation, the CMES should be helping clients set specific goals that track and monitor progress, providing encouragement and feedback, celebrating success, building social support, focusing on long-term benefits of participation, and offering support to overcome obstacles. Clients in the action stage should all have a clear goal-setting plan that utilizes **SMART goals** (see page 113). Although clients in this stage are engaging in exercise behavior, this participation is still new and the likelihood of dropout is high. This means that a CMES must be aware of even small disruptions to the schedule that could potentially alter participation, and education and communication must remain consistent. In the action stage, the person says, "I am now."

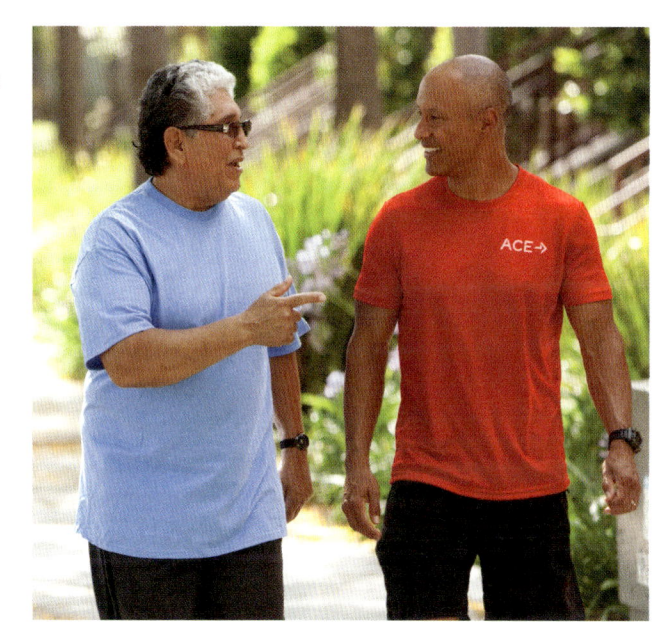

The final stage is the **maintenance** stage, which is marked by regular physical-activity participation for longer than six months. The primary focus at this point is relapse prevention. The CMES must continue to be aware that a client can slip backward at any time and should identify the risks of this for each client. Additionally, the CMES should help clients create the ability to provide internal feedback and develop internal rewards. Building client autonomy at this stage will increase the likelihood of continued adherence. In the maintenance stage, the person says, "I am."

Factors that influence a client to begin exercising are usually quite different from those associated with continuing to exercise. Many people begin because others (physician, family, or friends) think that it is a good thing, or they want to improve their appearance or health. The same people continue to exercise, however, because of themselves and how they perceive that the program helps them. For example, effective leadership makes the activities enjoyable and enables clients to feel better and see improvements (Skinner, 2005).

It is important to remember that behavioral change is a process, not a single event. Clients in all stages will encounter challenges in maintaining their new behaviors and can relapse, often all the way back to the precontemplation stage. Any change in an individual's life or health can trigger a relapse to irregular activity or even no activity. The commitment of long-term exercisers should not be taken for granted, as this behavior can change and relapse can occur on any given day. Behavioral change is truly a dynamic process and a CMES should never consider a client "locked in" at any of the stages of change.

EXPAND YOUR KNOWLEDGE

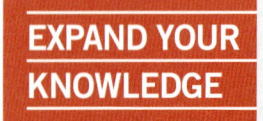

RELAPSE

Client relapse from program adherence is an inevitable part of the work of an exercise professional. The CMES must always remember that the lifestyle-modification program is only one part of the client's life, and priorities can shift at any moment so that a client is required to put time and energy into other areas. Whether it is illness, travel, work, or family, there are countless life variables that can interfere with a structured program. A CMES can help prepare clients to deal with relapse. The first step of this is the education that should be an integral part of the program from day one. If the CMES has been educating a client on how to make changes in their life, instead of just telling the client what to do, they will be better prepared to maintain certain program components during stressful, busy, or difficult times. Another key to dealing with relapse is support. Even if the CMES's contact with the client has decreased, letting the client know that the CMES understands their needs and is there to answer any questions or help in any way is critically important. Because relapse is often related to factors out of the client's control, being a constant and predictable source of support will be appreciated and will increase the likelihood of program re-adoption.

It can be frustrating to work with a client who exhibits a lack of commitment to their exercise training program. However, in the real world, this frustration will not help a CMES change people's lives. Being a supportive educator who understands not only that circumstances and priorities change, but also that adhering to an exercise training program is a difficult challenge that will have many ups and downs, is a key to being a successful CMES and building a successful business.

Processes of Change

The second component of the TTM consists of the processes of change that are used to pass from one stage to the next (see Table 4-1). Each transition has a unique set of processes and is based on specific individual decisions and mental states, such as individual readiness and motivation. Research has shown that the most effective change strategies are stage-matched interventions that target the natural processes people use as they move from one stage to the next (Spencer et al., 2006). It has also been suggested that the most effective technique is to use multiple strategies (e.g., print material, meetings, mass media, web-based information, and one-on-one communication) to promote progression.

Self-efficacy

Self-efficacy plays an important role in the TTM. It is a well-researched and commonly discussed topic that is defined (in the exercise context) as the belief in one's capabilities to be physically active (Bandura, 1986; Bandura, 1977). Self-efficacy is an important component of behavioral change because it is strongly related to program adoption and maintenance. A circular relationship exists between self-efficacy and behavioral change, such that self-efficacy is related to activity participation, and activity participation influences self-efficacy level. Therefore, self-efficacy acts as both a determinant and an outcome of behavioral change, making it a critical topic for a CMES to understand, assess, and apply. In terms of the TTM, there is a reliable relationship between self-efficacy for activity and stage of behavioral change, such that precontemplators and contemplators have significantly lower levels of self-efficacy than people in the action and maintenance stages. Additionally, self-efficacy levels differentiate people based on their stage of change (Marcus et al., 1992). This relationship makes intuitive sense, as those in the precontemplation and contemplation stages are not exercising, which may be reflective of the belief that they do not have the ability to be active, while those in the action and maintenance stages are engaged in a regular activity program, and thus demonstrating a belief in the ability to be active. It is important to note that the most important and powerful predictor of self-efficacy is past performance experience. Therefore, an individual who has had past success in adopting and maintaining a physical-activity program will be more effective in their ability to be active in the future.

The documented relationship between stage of change and self-efficacy also implies that if self-efficacy is improved, the client may be helped in progressing through the stages. This is especially important for the people in the contemplation and preparation stages, as they are thinking about being active, or want to be active, and are working toward the point where they can regularly participate in a physical-activity program. By helping such individuals increase their self-efficacy, the CMES may be able to move them through to the action stage more quickly. In other words, a CMES must never underestimate the importance of clients' belief in their own ability to succeed in the program.

PROMOTING SELF-EFFICACY BY CHOOSING THE RIGHT ASSESSMENTS

APPLY WHAT YOU KNOW

The vast majority of new clients seen by a CMES will come to the program with very low self-efficacy for exercise ability. Whether they are dealing with an injury or a health condition that creates unique activity challenges, most new clients will be apprehensive and uneasy about their capabilities. An important part of building rapport and client self-efficacy is to help new clients experience immediate success. The strongest predictor of self-efficacy is past performance experience, and if your new client has not exercised in many years or since before the occurrence of injury, it is your job to create a new and positive experience right away. As a CMES, you can help your clients feel excited and confident about their programs.

What does your first session look like with a new client? Are you doing an entire session of physical assessments? How are these assessments affecting the client?

When a client is deconditioned, post-rehabilitative, or dealing with a health condition, what is the likely result of the initial assessments? You certainly are not expecting your new clients to perform well on the tests, and what effect do you think this has on them? You want each new client to leave the first session feeling encouraged and optimistic, so it is essential to choose assessments that are appropriate for the client's conditioning and skill level. What information is absolutely critical to obtain for effective program design? Can you conduct these assessments in a way that your clients do not even realize that they are being assessed? There is no need to conduct every assessment you read about in a textbook. For example, most clients with obesity do not need to have their **body composition** assessed with skinfold calipers. Circumference measurements might be a better option. Put careful thought into what you are assessing and how you are collecting the needed data. Think about it from the client's point of view. The power of building self-efficacy from the first session trumps a file full of assessment data for a client who never comes back.

Decisional Balance

Another important behavior-change concept related to the TTM is decisional balance, which refers to the numbers of pros and cons an individual perceives regarding adopting and/or maintaining an activity program (Janis & Mann, 1979). When making any decision, people naturally weigh the pros and cons of each choice. The decision to be physically active has to be "worth it" to an individual and the CMES must remember that this is a difficult and complex decision for people to make. Precontemplators and contemplators perceive more cons (e.g., sweating, sore muscles, time, finances, and lack of ability) related to being regularly active than pros.

For a health and exercise professional who understands the physical and psychological benefits of an active lifestyle, it might be hard to understand that these cons would prevent someone from engaging in exercise. The reality is that the perceived cons do not have to be logical or realistic to prevent people from being active. The good news is that as people progress through the stages of change, the balance of pros and cons shifts naturally, such that people in the action and maintenance stages perceive more pros than cons related to engaging in exercise.

The shift in decisional balance that occurs as people progress through the stages of change suggests that influencing client perceptions about being active may encourage them to start an activity program. In other words, if a CMES is able to help people identify the relevant and meaningful benefits of engaging in activity, they may actually trigger more active behavior.

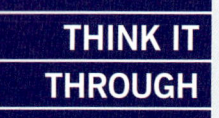

> **THINK IT THROUGH**
>
> A 48-year-old client was recently diagnosed with hypertension and elevated **cholesterol.** He does not engage in any regular activity, but plays golf a couple of times each month. He also tells you that he has not participated in a regular physical-activity program since before his children were born 17 years ago. He is scared by his recent diagnosis and knows that something needs to change, but he is clearly nervous about being in the gym environment and is not sure when he will find time for working out. However, he says he is up for the challenge and that his wife and children are supportive of him making some lifestyle changes. Based on this general information, you determine that this client is in the preparation stage, has low self-efficacy, and still perceives barriers to being active. What is your next step for getting this client started? What health information is important for program design? How will his perception of his diagnosis influence the program? What type of goals would you work with him to set? How prepared do you think he really is to make a lifestyle change?

HEALTH BELIEF MODEL

Examining readiness to change in relation to engagement in health behavior is only one approach to understanding and predicting outcomes. The relationship between people's beliefs about their health and how these beliefs influence the adoption or non-adoption of health behaviors has also been studied.

The **health belief model** predicts that people will engage in a health behavior based on the perceived threat they feel regarding a health problem, as well as the pros and cons of adopting that behavior (Becker, 1974). According to the model, perceived threat is the degree to which a person feels threatened or worried by the prospect of a particular health problem and it is influenced by three factors:

- The perceived severity of the health problem is defined as the feelings an individual has about the seriousness of contracting an illness or leaving it untreated. People take the severity of the potential consequences of the problem into consideration, and the more serious the consequences are perceived to be, the more likely people are to engage in a health behavior.
- The perceived susceptibility to the health problem is based on a person's subjective appraisal of the likelihood of developing the problem. People have a higher perceived threat and an increased likelihood to engage in a health behavior when they believe that they are vulnerable to a health problem.
- Cues to actions, or events, either bodily, such as physical symptoms, or environmental, such as health-promotion information, motivate people to make a change. The more people are reminded about a potential health problem, the more likely they are to take action and engage in a health behavior.

The pros and cons of engaging in a health behavior are examined by the health belief model in terms of perceived benefits and perceived barriers. In other words, people assess the benefits, such as getting healthier and preventing disease, along with the barriers, such as financial cost and time commitment, of engaging in a program. Research has shown that benefits and barriers are the strongest and most consistent predictors of behavior in the health belief model, such that if individuals perceive more barriers than benefits regarding a health behavior, they will be unlikely to make a behavioral change, and if the benefits outweigh the barriers, they will be more likely to change (Carpenter, 2010).

The model further predicts that if the perceived benefits outweigh the perceived barriers and the perceived threat of illness is high, people will be likely to take preventive action. It is likely that a CMES will have clients who fit this description, and it is important that the CMES is aware of the perceptions their clients have regarding illness and a healthy lifestyle, including their perceived benefits and barriers to program participation. If individuals perceive little threat of developing an illness related to their lifestyle choices, the lifestyle-modification program is going to be difficult to implement without making the seriousness of the illness more apparent and making the individual feel more susceptible to developing the condition. Research has demonstrated that the benefits-to-barriers ratio is the best predictor of behavior, with severity of the illness and susceptibility to the illness being very minor predictors, or even non-predictors, of behavior (Carpenter, 2010). For health and exercise professionals, this means that time should be spent helping potential clients identify quality benefits of program participation to create an increased likelihood of behavioral change.

CREATE HOPE, NOT FEAR

Educating clients about the seriousness of illness is not the same thing as scaring them about developing the illness. Fear is a very powerful motivator, but using it as a tactic to change behavior is not advised. Fear is a "negative motivator" and typically leads people to flee the situation in order to avoid the feelings that it elicits. Further, fear makes people uncomfortable, which typically does not lead to positive behavioral change. A more effective motivational strategy related to the principles of the health belief model is to educate clients about the facts of the disease state and how exercise can be used as a solution to aid in the treatment process. In other words, instead of providing stories of those suffering from different illnesses because they did not take care of themselves, the CMES can share stories of hope featuring people who have turned their health around because of healthy lifestyle choices.

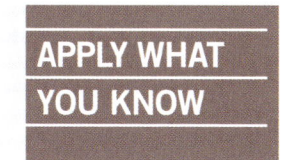

APPLY WHAT YOU KNOW

Self-efficacy

Self-efficacy is an important concept to understand when studying exercise and health behavior. As previously discussed, self-efficacy is the belief in one's own capabilities to successfully complete a task. Self-efficacy beliefs are believed to influence thought patterns, affective responses, and action. Self-efficacy is also positively related to motivation (Bandura, 1986). When working with post-rehabilitative populations or those with health issues, the CMES must be very aware of each client's self-efficacy regarding their ability to physically engage in a program. Physical limitations from an injury or illness can severely decrease one's perceived ability to be active and fit. Because of the importance of self-efficacy information, the CMES should understand where it comes from and directly attempt to increase it.

While there are several sources of self-efficacy, the most influential and practical source for a CMES to use is past performance experience. It is imperative to understand a client's past experience with an exercise program or physical activity in general, as this information influences how they feel about the current program. Even more importantly, the CMES needs to create new past performance information for the client. In other words, the CMES should create immediate success and positivity related to activity participation. This can serve as a powerful source of self-efficacy and can start to create excitement about a new program. This seems so intuitive, but many health and exercise professionals make the mistake of over-assessing and analyzing in the initial sessions with a new client. While assessment information is important, the purpose of assessments is often to identify weaknesses and generate fatigue, which means that they put a spotlight on the things that a client cannot do well. A CMES should instead guarantee success (even at the most basic levels) and create achievement opportunities right from the start.

Self-efficacy levels also influence behaviors and the quality of participation once a client has started a program. Specifically, self-efficacy predicts three important participation variables:
- *Task choice:* Individuals with high self-efficacy are more likely to choose challenging tasks, as compared to individuals with low self-efficacy, who are more likely to choose very easy, non-challenging tasks.
- *Effort:* Individuals with high self-efficacy are more likely to display maximal effort when engaged in a lifestyle-modification program.
- *Persistence:* Individuals with high self-efficacy are more likely to overcome obstacles and challenges and stick with a program. Those with low self-efficacy are more likely to drop out as soon as a challenge arises.

Based on these variables, it is clear that a CMES should work to build self-efficacy and not to dismiss feelings and perceptions of doubt or worry.

STRATEGIES FOR BEHAVIORAL CHANGE

Client education is a key component of every step of exercise program implementation, and this is particularly important for the populations who are clients of a CMES. People start an exercise program with a wide variety of previous knowledge (both accurate and inaccurate), and it is important to never assume what clients already, or should already, know.

Communication

Effective communication consists of both talking and listening. At the start of a client relationship, the role of the CMES will be to primarily listen. The more a CMES can learn about clients' history, past activity experiences, motivations, emotions, abilities, and apprehensions, the more they will understand client needs and the better prepared they will be to create effective programs.

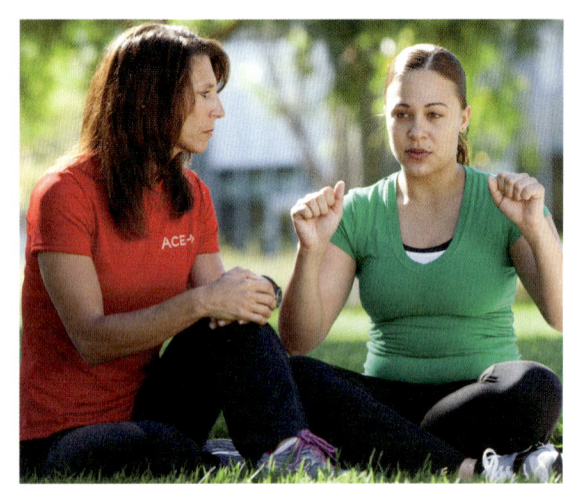

Program information should be communicated in a straightforward, basic, non-threatening, and consistent manner. Many people will not want to hear about the science of exercise programming, but instead are seeking basic information and strategies that are relevant to their situations and lives. Additionally, a CMES must only present small amounts of information at a time that is framed in a real-world, stepwise framework. A benefit of this approach is that if a client wants more information, they will typically ask. However, if a client is receiving information overload, they will likely tune it out and feel disconnected and misunderstood.

As part of effective communication with clients, a CMES should provide continuous information with regard to effective goal-setting techniques and self-monitoring strategies. It is the role of the CMES to empower clients to take their activity levels, and more importantly their health, into their own hands. Building autonomy through education and increased self-efficacy will create a foundation for success and long-term adherence. A CMES should always keep in mind that the ultimate goal of any program is a long-term commitment to change. The education aspect of a program should be an integral part of each program component and the CMES should continuously and consistently communicate, assess, and educate to maximize the likelihood of long-term adherence and successful behavioral change. Refer to *The Professional's Guide to Health and Wellness Coaching* for more information on how health and exercise professionals can use communication skills to improve the experience and success rates of their clients (ACE, 2019).

Avoid Making Assumptions

In any relationship, personal or professional, the majority of frustrations that occur are a result of miscommunication. The source of many of these issues in a professional context is when a CMES assumes that clients already know how to do something with which they are in fact unfamiliar. Whatever the topic may be, taking the time to educate clients is always the better choice and is always appreciated. If a client already has the information, they will likely let the CMES know.

Additionally, health and exercise professionals are influenced by the way they think and the assumptions that they make about themselves and others. These assumptions will directly impact the quality of client relationships and a CMES needs to build a strong sense of awareness of the types of thoughts they have. This includes making assumptions about people's motivations or capabilities to succeed. Any limits that the CMES places on people will likely come true. Therefore, the CMES must believe each and every individual has what it

WHAT IS SUCCESS?

Take a few minutes and ask your colleagues how they define a successful exercise/lifestyle-change program. You are almost certain to get a variety of responses, including "one that is safe," "one that helps a client reach his goals," or "one that is customized to meet individual client needs." There is no doubt that every answer you receive from your colleagues is valid and important, but it is also worthwhile to look at the bigger picture of your role as a CMES. Do you think that it is possible for a successful program to simply be one that a client adheres to over the long term? In other words, it is a valuable exercise for all health and exercise professionals to step back from the details of program design and remind themselves that the ultimate goal is always behavioral change. If you can help people make lasting changes in their lives, would you consider that the ultimate success?

APPLY WHAT YOU KNOW

Relapse Prevention

Once a program has started and a client is successfully following the program components, the CMES should start implementing a plan for relapse prevention. Relapse from regular physical-activity participation is a common occurrence, especially when clients are experiencing health and medical issues, and the more prepared a CMES is to deal with relapse, the more successful the client will be in avoiding it. The CMES should include the client in conversations about potential relapse and prepare them with coping strategies to deal with adherence challenges. These conversations should start early on in program participation so that clients are developing awareness and understanding about the likelihood of relapse and the factors associated with potential relapse. A basic, yet critical skill for a CMES to promote long-term program success is to be flexible and to understand each client's situation. Additionally, the CMES should be prepared to make program modifications at any time to facilitate changing health and medical conditions or concerns. Neglecting to do this will almost certainly lead to a program relapse. Programs can and should vary, because no one program is correct for all people or even for the same person over time, as interests, needs, goals, health, and fitness change.

DEALING WITH RELAPSE

Dealing with program relapse is an expected part of the role of a CMES. In fact, for most people, the question is not *if* they relapse, but *when* they relapse. Remember, a relapse does not have to be a permanent removal from program participation. The clients of a CMES are often dealing with complex health and medical issues that can change at any moment. Therefore, it is the role of the CMES to help prepare clients for dealing with relapse, and they should be prepared to make program modifications to overcome time, health, financial, and motivation constraints. Additionally, clients should be educated about the challenges of adherence so that they are prepared and do not feel like failures. The most important thing that a CMES can do from the start of a program is to empower the clients with autonomy in the program. If a CMES does not do this and simply tells the client what to do, the client is not learning anything about how to take control of their own program and health, and when circumstances change, the client is likely to withdraw from the program completely.

On the other hand, an autonomous person will have the knowledge and confidence to maintain some program components even during stressful times. Additionally, for many clients, the CMES is the core source of support for program participation. Even if the client is no longer actively engaged in the program, it is important for the CMES to continue to periodically reach out and express support. Relapse is often triggered by factors that are out of the client's direct control, and it is important for the client to know that the CMES is still supportive and encouraging of their behavior-change efforts, even during challenging times.

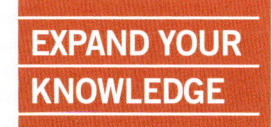

EXPAND YOUR KNOWLEDGE

Empowering the Client

During initial client meetings, the CMES should start to develop an understanding of clients' social-support networks related to activity participation. The more of this information that is learned in initial meetings, the better prepared the CMES will be to handle related issues throughout the program and to build support opportunities within the program. Oftentimes, even in the presence of serious health issues, people do not have support at home to make dramatic lifestyle changes. A CMES must be creative to build family buy-in to the program through education and opportunities for group involvement. Part of this process is helping family and friends see firsthand the commitment their loved one has made to living a healthy lifestyle. Furthermore, when the support from family and friends simply does not exist, the CMES must work to create opportunities for support within the program environment. Building a sense of connectedness with the program will create a perception of support and belonging, which is important for continued adherence.

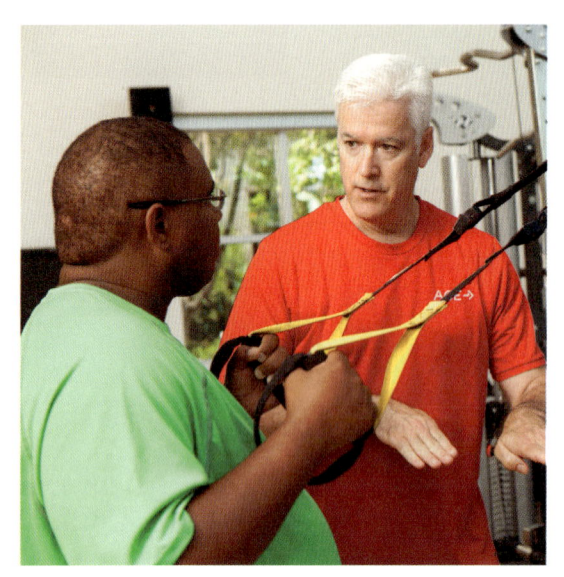

The CMES should consistently encourage clients to develop autonomy and a sense of control over their own health. The more effective clients become at self-regulating their behaviors, needs, schedules, and priorities, the more likely they will be to adhere to the program for the long term. One component of effective self-regulation is to encourage clients to be assertive. Assertiveness is a key trait for achieving success and is defined as the honest and straightforward expression of one's thoughts, feelings, and beliefs.

Typically, when individuals are not assertive, it is because they lack self-confidence or they feel vulnerable. The more assertive clients are regarding their progress, concerns, accomplishments, and struggles, the more likely they are to speak up and let others know what they need. They will be more willing and able to problem-solve and find solutions that will help them achieve long-term success.

No matter how much a CMES wants to control or to completely regulate and script clients' behavior, this is not an effective strategy for behavioral change and adherence. The CMES must remember the importance of education and teach clients to self-monitor and make behavioral changes on their own. Empowering clients with self-regulation strategies creates a sense of control over their own lives and provides the confidence they need to succeed. Once clients perceive control over their behavioral outcomes and believe they can do it, they are more able to deal with barriers and challenges as they arise. While this seems like a straightforward concept, health and exercise professionals often have a difficult time giving up control and teaching clients to take over, sometimes even doubting clients' ability to take on this task.

Self-monitoring can mean many different things in a behavior-modification program. A big part of it is having clients keep track of information regarding their activity participation. This tracking should include successes and challenges in adhering to the program. Not all clients will be ready for self-tracking, as it requires a great amount of client commitment and interest, but it is a very effective technique in identifying barriers and developing strategies for long-term adherence, so small steps should be made for clients to learn how to self-monitor.

In addition to promotion of long-term adherence, self-monitoring provides a source of up-to-date progress tracking. This can be rewarding and can also help clients develop self-correcting behaviors as they recognize small lapses in progress that can be easily corrected. There are countless technology tools and applications available to help clients self-monitor in real time. Implementing such tools can be a powerful learning opportunity and one that the CMES should encourage.

APPLY WHAT YOU KNOW

Have you ever wondered how much your clients know about program participation without your guidance? Could they guide themselves through a workout? Have you done an effective job explaining what you are doing and why? What happens when you are out of town? Do your clients still work out and engage in the program?

It is a valuable exercise to do a little test. Ask your long-term clients to identify exercises and explain the purpose of the exercise. Can they do it? Ask them if they know alternative ways to achieve the same result. You will quickly realize how effective you are at educating your clients about components of the program. You do not want your clients to be completely dependent on you in order for them to be active. Make it a priority to teach them how to do it on their own and build independence and confidence to help your clients help themselves.

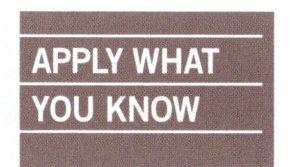

Managing High-risk Situations

Helping clients work through high-risk situations is an ongoing part of the work of a CMES. These situations, including changes to health status, vacations, work schedules, injuries, and holidays, are inevitable, and ignoring them will lead to relapse and drop-out. Instead, if a CMES can identify potential and known high-risk situations, they can work with clients to develop plans and strategies to succeed through these periods. It is also important for the CMES to identify clients who appear to be most at risk for program relapse. Those who do not handle change well or who have poor time-management skills, a lack of social support, low self-efficacy, or busy schedules are prime examples of people who will likely relapse. Extra education, support, and guidance for these people should be provided as they adopt their programs and approach challenging situations. It is also important to consistently observe clients' emotional states by watching for signs of being stressed, overwhelmed, and worn out. The CMES should not ignore cues that are pointing to such emotional states, but should instead take the time to address them, showing **empathy** and providing coping strategies and support. Additionally, the CMES should always be prepared to be flexible and to demonstrate to their clients that modifications are an expected part of the plan.

ADHERENCE

Behavioral Modification

Behavior-modification strategies can truly take any shape or form within a program. A CMES should be creative to meet individual needs and maximize success. Three common strategies that serve as a good place to start are written agreements, stimulus control, and **shaping.**

Written Agreements

Written agreements may sound very formal and rigid, but the CMES should view them as flexible educational tools that help build accountability. The written agreement itself can take any form and be a client–professional agreement or a self-agreement for the client. Regardless of its structure, the intent is to simply define program expectations, which should be straightforward and simple with the purpose of decreasing ambiguity and clarifying behaviors, commitments, and attitudes. These should include both self-expectations set by the client and also the CMES's expectations for the client. The purpose of written agreements is not to detail every aspect of the plan, as doing so will create a much too complex agreement that will not be followed. Additionally, written agreements are not successful if the client does not play an integral part in the creation of the document. Another beneficial use of written agreements is to clarify the role of the CMES in the program, which will generate an opportunity for discussion on this topic. As with all program components, the written agreement should be a "living document" that is modified as situations, needs, and expectations change.

Stimulus Control

Stimulus control is directly linked to the learning of new behaviors. Based on the principles of operant conditioning, stimulus control is the process of altering the environment to trigger healthy behaviors. When used in conjunction with an exercise program, the goal is to maximize program success. Stimulus-control strategies can also take any form and should be customized to each individual's life and habits. The ultimate goal of stimulus control is to build new habits and to make activity an "easier" choice throughout the day.

> **APPLY WHAT YOU KNOW**
>
> **STIMULUS-CONTROL STRATEGIES**
> The CMES can share the following stimulus-control strategies with clients:
> - Lay out everything you need (e.g., clothes, shoes, and water bottle) for early-morning workouts.
> - Keep a gym bag in the car with all necessary workout items.
> - Plan out meals in advance so that you are not scrambling at the last minute to make a healthy choice. Shop from a list and avoid purchasing non-listed items (if it is not in the house, it will not be eaten).
> - Wear comfortable shoes at work to maximize activity opportunities (if your feet hurt, you will not take the stairs).
> - Surround yourself with others who engage in physical activity (join a walking/running club or a hiking group).

Shaping

Shaping is a process of conditioning in which reinforcements are used to gradually work toward a target behavior. The idea is to positively reinforce or reward behaviors that are close to the target behavior. It is a long process, but over time the client will get closer and closer to the goal behavior. To use shaping, the CMES should start with the performance of a basic skill that the client is currently capable of doing. Over time, the demands of the skill are then gradually raised and reinforcement is given with each improvement. This consistent practice of continually increasing the demands at an appropriate rate and providing positive reinforcement will lead to the execution of the desired behavior and can serve as a powerful behavioral control and learning technique. One of the benefits of shaping is that it begins with the client executing a behavior at an appropriate skill level, so each individual can have their own starting point (Smith, 2010). Shaping is particularly effective in situations in which a client is apprehensive, uncomfortable, or even afraid to try something new. The most important thing for the CMES to remember as they use shaping with their clients is to truly start the process from the client's natural baseline level. If a CMES tries to use shaping and expect too much from a client at the start, the client will likely feel overwhelmed and incapable, which may lead to drop-out or regression.

> **APPLY WHAT YOU KNOW**
>
> **SHAPING**
> The use of shaping in an exercise environment involves creating basic exercise programming progressions. The CMES should use the pre-exercise screening and a client's readiness to change to identify target goal behaviors. Whether the goal is to increase range of motion, strength, or endurance, shaping is simply the process of starting with movements and exercises that are currently achievable for the client and then gradually increasing the challenges and demands over time to move closer to the goal movement or behavior. A simple example is building endurance to get through a 30-minute exercise session. Sessions may start out with only five minutes of actual activity and then slowly build to achieve the 30-minute activity goal. Small progressions and changes to programming prevent the client from becoming overwhelmed and also build self-efficacy for program participation. In reality, shaping can be used in each aspect of a program that is targeting the development of new skills and behaviors.

Cognitive Behavioral Techniques

Another approach to building lasting behavioral change is the use of cognitive behavioral techniques. This approach addresses behavioral change by altering people's thoughts and emotions. The general goal of cognitive behavioral techniques is to teach people to be able to easily identify problematic beliefs that are preventing them from making desired changes and to then be able to change those thoughts and feelings into something more positive and productive. Cognitive techniques can be used independently as intervention tools for behavioral change or in conjunction with other behavior-modification strategies (Dishman, 1991).

Goal Setting

Goal setting is the most commonly used cognitive behavioral technique, and most people are probably unaware that it even falls in this category. Goal setting is simple to understand and easy to use, and, when executed properly, is an extremely effective tool to help change a client's mindset and create action. The biggest problem with goal setting is that goals are often set at the start of a program, but are not integrated into the program on a daily basis. This type of goal-setting practice is not going to maximally benefit program adherence. Instead, goals need to be an integrated component of daily program participation. The first step of goal setting involves the actual setting of the goals. There are simple guidelines to follow for this process. Proper goals are SMART goals, meaning that they are specific, measurable, attainable, relevant, and time-bound. The CMES should take the time to educate clients about these guidelines to help them create appropriate goals, and the initial goal-setting process should be thoughtful and allow for enough time for communication about the client's needs and for education about proper goal setting (Table 4-2).

TABLE 4-2

TIPS FOR SETTING HEALTH AND FITNESS GOALS THAT MOTIVATE CLIENTS FOR LONG-TERM ADHERENCE

- Listen carefully to understand what clients hope to accomplish with an exercise program.
- Help them define measurable goals.
- Suggest additional goals that clients may not have thought of, such as feeling more energetic and less stressed.
- Break large goals (reachable in six months or more) into small goals (reachable in about eight to 10 weeks) and even weekly goals (e.g., completing a certain number of exercise sessions).
- Include many process goals, such as the completion of exercise sessions. That way, simply completing workouts accomplishes a goal.
- Record goals and set up a record-keeping system to record workouts and track progress toward goals.
- Be sure that clients understand what types of exercise will help them reach their health and fitness goals.
- Reevaluate and revise goals and exercise recommendations periodically to prevent discouragement if large goals are not being met.

Source: Brehm, B.A. (2004). *Successful Fitness Motivation Strategies.* Champaign, Ill.: Human Kinetics.

The CMES should also work with clients to help them follow other basic goal-setting guidelines. First, it is important to avoid setting too many goals. Keeping the number of goals manageable (e.g., fewer than three at a time) and attainable helps the client feel optimistic and in control. Having too many things to achieve can be overwhelming to the client. Next, avoid setting negative goals. If a client wants to set the goal to not miss any workouts, the goal should be reworded into a positive statement, such as, "Attend every scheduled workout session." Negative goals are ineffective because they focus clients' thoughts on the behavior they want to avoid, instead of promoting focus on the behavior they want to achieve.

Finally, both short- and long-term goals should be set along with outcome goals and performance goals. The goal of the CMES is for each client to achieve success in each workout. This can be done through implementing small goals that are achievable day to day. Once effective goals are set by the client—in collaboration with the CMES—the goals themselves should be a dynamic component of the program. They can be incorporated into the program in such a way that clients remember exactly what they are working for and what it will take to get there. Because of their dynamic nature, goals should be adjusted regularly to meet the changing needs and health and fitness levels of clients.

Most importantly, goals should not be set for the sake of setting goals, but should be used as a tool to direct attention and effort, and to promote persistence. As goals are reached, new ones should be set, and as challenges arise, goals should be modified. The CMES and clients want to avoid being too rigid and instead should be flexible and continue to modify goals so that they are relevant and purposeful in the program. Finally, the CMES must always remember that goals should be generated by the clients. As the expert, the CMES should provide input and guidance to ensure that the goals meet proper goal-setting guidelines, but the key component is that the clients are excited about the plan and the desired outcomes.

Feedback

Providing feedback is an integral part of what a CMES does on a daily basis. Whether giving encouragement, form correction, or motivation, or reviewing activity and food logs, health and exercise professionals are constantly providing information to their clients. Feedback is an interactive process that should be focused around the goals of the program. It is a powerful tool that, when used properly, can help build trust, credibility, and self-efficacy, and lead to proper execution of the program. The feedback that is generally utilized in a fitness setting is **extrinsic feedback**, which refers to verbal and nonverbal cues given by the CMES to the client about any aspect of program participation. Extrinsic feedback is critically important for initial program adoption. As a client becomes a regular program participant who is feeling comfortable and progressing properly, the extrinsic feedback from the CMES should actually decrease and the CMES should work to help clients provide themselves with information about their own progress, participation, and effort. This type of feedback is called **intrinsic feedback.** The ability to provide oneself with intrinsic feedback is a necessary skill for long-term program adherence. If the CMES is constantly providing feedback to clients, then clients have no reason to start generating their own feedback. Therefore, the CMES must gauge when it is appropriate to gradually taper down the amount of extrinsic feedback they provide and intentionally work with clients to create self-assessment information. This process is very similar to the relationship between extrinsic and intrinsic motivation. External motivators can be effective for short amounts of time (e.g., the first few months of a program) and can trigger initial change, but long-term adherence is dependent upon an intrinsic drive to engage and succeed in the program.

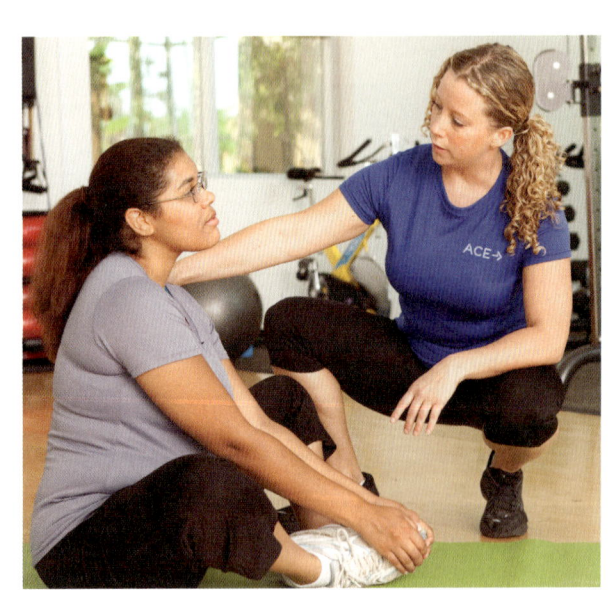

This process of gaining intrinsic control over a program is essential in developing the ability to self-monitor and self-correct, and the CMES has to allow clients the opportunity to learn and grow in this area. This is especially important with the populations that a CMES works with, as clients must be able to self-report and appropriately modify program components based on health and injury changes. Throughout the duration of the program, no matter how long a client has been participating, the CMES should be aware of the client's ability to provide intrinsic feedback and should be prepared to step in with extrinsic feedback whenever necessary. The main message of teaching and encouraging the use of intrinsic feedback is related to building autonomy and control. Clients will not succeed in making a long-term behavioral change if they are not playing an active role in all aspects of the program.

SUMMARY

In order for a program to be effectively integrated into a client's life and for a client to make lasting behavioral changes, a CMES needs to have an understanding of the principles of health psychology and behavioral change. The theoretical models should be understood and applied from a practitioner's perspective and the goal should always be to help the client better their life. The work of a CMES entails so much more than writing safe and effective exercise programs, as a CMES needs to be constantly aware of the social and psychological factors in their clients' lives that are influencing program adoption and adherence. The more that the CMES understands the concepts related to learning, exercise adoption, and adherence, the more successful they will be in developing programs that foster success.

REFERENCES

American Council on Exercise (2019). *The Professional's Guide to Health and Wellness Coaching*. San Diego, Calif.: American Council on Exercise.

Bandura, A. (1986). *Social Foundations of Thought and Action: A Social Cognitive Theory*. Englewood Cliffs, N.J.: Prentice-Hall.

Bandura, A. (1977). Self-efficacy: Toward a unifying theory of behavioral change. *Psychological Review*, 84, 191–215.

Becker, M.H. (1974). The health belief model and personal health behavior. *Health Education Monographs*, 2, 324–473.

Bogg, T. & Roberts, B.W. (2004). Conscientiousness and health-related behaviors: A meta-analysis of the leading contributors to mortality. *Psychological Bulletin*, 130, 887–919.

Brehm, B.A. (2004). *Successful Fitness Motivation Strategies*. Champaign, Ill.: Human Kinetics.

Camacho, E.M et al. (2013). Learned helplessness predicts functional disability, pain and fatigue in patients with recent-onset inflammatory polyarthritis. *Rheumatology*, 52, 1233–1238.

Carpenter, C.J. (2010). A meta-analysis of the effectiveness of health belief model variables in predicting behavior. *Health Communication*, 25, 661–669.

Centers for Disease Control and Prevention (2013). Adult participation in aerobic and muscle-strengthening physical activities—United States, 2011. *Morbidity and Mortality Weekly Reports*, 62, 17, 326–330.

Conner, M., Rodgers, W., & Murray, T. (2007). Conscientiousness and the intention-behavior relationship: Predicting exercise behavior. *Journal of Sport & Exercise Psychology*, 29, 518–533.

Deci, E.L. & Ryan, R.M. (2002). *Handbook of Self-Determination Research*. Rochester, N.Y.: University of Rochester Press.

Dishman, R.K. (1991). Increasing and maintaining exercise and physical activity. *Behavior Therapy*, 22, 345–378.

Dishman, R.K. (1982). Compliance/adherence in health-related exercise. *Health Psychology*, 1, 237–267.

Dishman, R.K. & Buckworth, J. (1997). Adherence to physical activity. In: Morgan, W.P. (Ed.). *Physical Activity & Mental Health* (pp. 63–80). Washington, D.C.: Taylor & Francis.

Duhigg, C. (2012). *The Power of Habit: Why We Do What We Do In Life and Business*. New York: Random House.

Duncan, T.E. & McAuley, E. (1993). Social support and efficacy cognitions in exercise adherence: A latent growth curve analysis. *Journal of Behavioral Medicine*, 16, 199–218.

Engel, G.L. (1977). The need for a new medical model: A challenge for biomedicine. *Science*, 196, 129–136.

Janis, I.L. & Mann, L. (1979). *Decision Making*. New York: Macmillan.

Kloek, G.C. et al. (2006). Stages of change for moderate-intensity physical activity in deprived neighborhoods. *Preventive Medicine*, 43, 4, 325–331.

Marcus, B.H. et al. (1992). Self-efficacy and the stages of exercise behavior change. *Research Quarterly for Exercise and Sport*, 63, 1.

Martin, G. & Pear, J. (2010). *Behavior Modification: What It Is and How to Do It* (9th ed.). Englewood Cliffs, N.J.: Prentice-Hall.

Prochaska, J.O. & DiClemente, C.C. (1984). *The Transtheoretical Approach: Crossing Traditional Boundaries of Therapy*. Homewood, Ill.: Dow Jones/Irwin.

Sarafino, E.P. & Smith, T.W. (2014). *Health Psychology: Biopsychosocial Interactions* (8th ed.). New York: John Wiley & Sons.

Skinner, B.F. (1938). *The Behavior of Organisms: An Experimental Analysis.* New York: Appleton-Century.

Skinner, J.S. (2005). General principles of exercise prescription. In: Skinner, J.S. (Ed.). *Exercise Testing and Exercise Prescription for Special Cases* (pp. 22–37). Philadelphia: Lippincott Williams & Wilkins.

Smith, R.E. (2010). A positive approach to coaching effectiveness and performance enhancement. In: Williams, J.M. (Ed.). *Applied Sport Psychology: Personal Growth to Peak Performance* (6th ed.). New York: McGraw-Hill.

Spencer, L. et al. (2006). Applying the transtheoretical model to exercise: A systematic and comprehensive review of the literature. *Health Promotion Practice,* 7, 4, 428–443.

Turk, D.C., Rudy, T.E., & Salovey, P. (1984). Health protection: Attitudes and behaviors of LPNs, teachers, and college students. *Health Psychology,* 3, 189–210.

Williams, G.C. et al. (2004). Motivation for behavior change in patients with chest pain. *Health Education,* 105, 4, 304–321.

SUGGESTED READING

American Council on Exercise (2019). *The Professional's Guide to Health and Wellness Coaching.* San Diego, Calif.: American Council on Exercise.

Bandura, A. (2001). Social cognitive theory: An agentive perspective. *Annual Review of Psychology,* 52, 1–26.

Bauman, A.E. et al. (2012). Correlates of physical activity: Why are some people physically active and others not? *Lancet,* 10, 258–271. DOI: 10.1016/S0140-6736(12)60735-1

Burke, L.E., Wang, J., & Sevick, M. (2011). Self-monitoring in weight loss: A systematic review of the literature. *Journal of the American Dietetic Association,* 111, 1, 92–102. DOI: 10.1016/j.jada.2010.10.008 PMCID: PMC3268700

Cowan, L.T. et al. (2013). Apps of steel: Are exercise apps providing consumers with realistic expectations? A content analysis of exercise apps for presence of behavior change theory. *Health Education & Behavior,* 40, 2, 133–139.

de Bruin, M. et al. (2012). Self-regulatory processes mediate the intention-behavior relation for adherence and exercise behaviors. *Health Psychology,* 31, 6, 695.

Prochaska, J.O. (2013). Transtheoretical model of behavior change. In: *Encyclopedia of Behavioral Medicine* (pp. 1997–2000). New York: Springer.

Williams S.L. & French, D.P. (2011). What are the most effective intervention techniques for changing physical activity self-efficacy and physical activity behaviour–and are they the same? *Health Education Research,* 10, 308–322. DOI: 10.1093/her/cyr005

5 COMMUNICATION STRATEGIES

IN THIS CHAPTER

COMMUNICATION GOALS
CREATING POSITIVE EMOTIONS AND OPTIMISM FOR CHANGE
ESTABLISHING FEELINGS OF CONNECTION AND TRUST
GATHERING INFORMATION AND SETTING THE AGENDA
COMMUNICATING BEHAVIOR-CHANGE RECOMMENDATIONS

UNDERSTANDING THE MEDICAL EXERCISE CLIENT
SEVERITY OF THE ILLNESS OR INJURY AND IMPACT ON QUALITY OF LIFE
EXPECTED OUTCOME
THE CLIENT'S PERSONAL RESOURCES
COMMUNICATING WITH CLIENTS IN DISTRESS

COMMUNICATION SKILLS BUILD POSITIVE AND PROFESSIONAL WORKING RELATIONSHIPS
FIRST IMPRESSIONS
VERBAL AND NONVERBAL COMMUNICATION

COMMUNICATION BASICS
DIRECTIVE AND GUIDING COMMUNICATION STYLES
IS EFFECTIVE COMMUNICATION MORE WORK FOR THE PROFESSIONAL?
BARRIERS TO EFFECTIVE COMMUNICATION

COMMUNICATION STRATEGIES AND MOTIVATION
ASSESSING READINESS TO CHANGE
CHANGE TALK: HELPING PRECONTEMPLATION AND CONTEMPLATION CLIENTS DECIDE TO CHANGE

COMMUNICATION STRATEGIES FOR EFFECTIVE EDUCATION
MOTOR LEARNING
COGNITIVE LEARNING

SUMMARY

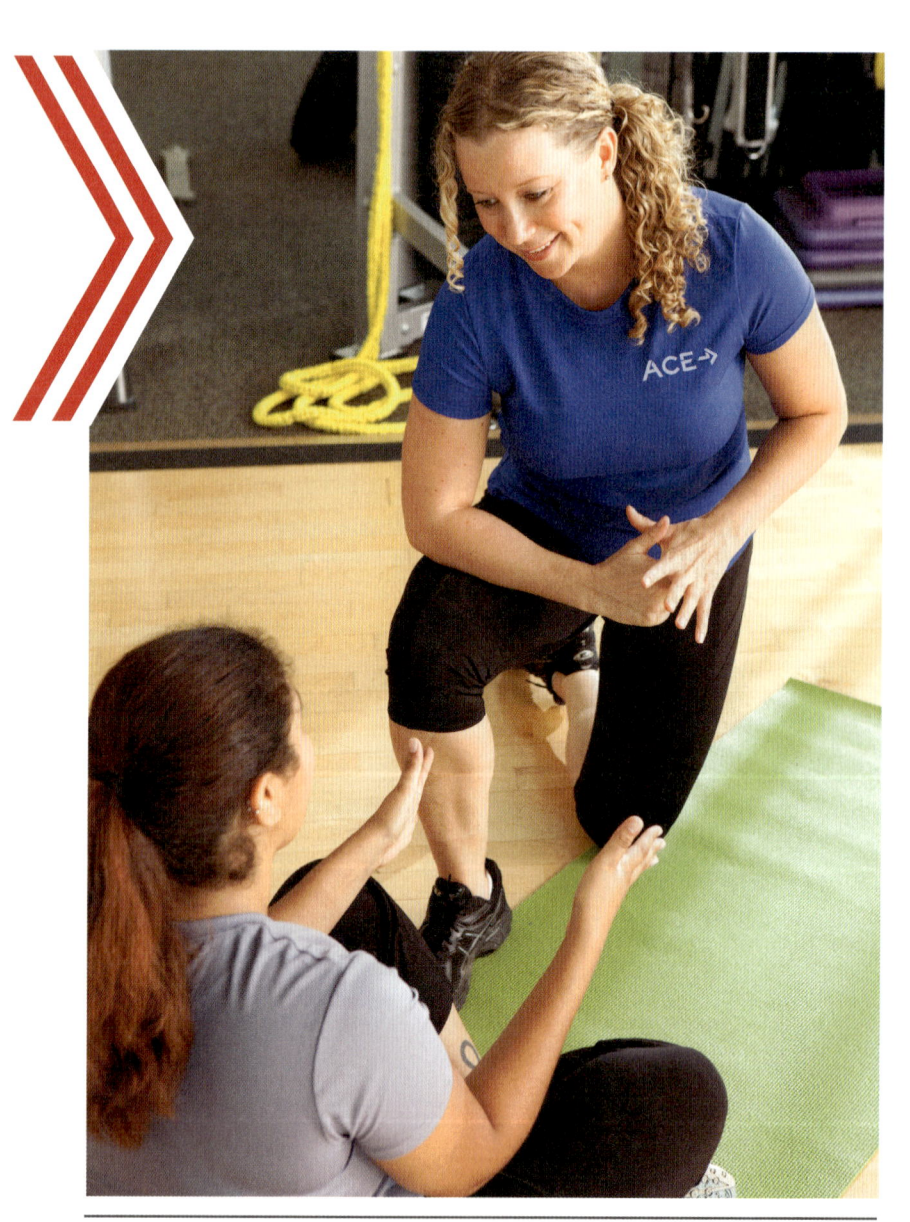

ABOUT THE AUTHOR
Barbara A. Brehm, Ed.D., is a professor of exercise and sport studies at Smith College, Northampton, Mass., where she teaches courses in nutrition, health behavior, and stress management. She is also director of the Smith Fitness Program for Faculty and Staff. Dr. Brehm is the author of several books, including *Successful Fitness Motivation Strategies* and *Psychology of Health and Fitness*.

By Barbara A. Brehm

EXCELLENT COMMUNICATION SKILLS ARE essential for the ACE® Certified Medical Exercise Specialist (CMES), who communicates closely with clients to design effective exercise and other behavior-change programs, and then support these clients in their efforts. Exercise professionals who are well-versed in exercise science and understand the intricacies of training principles will still lack effectiveness if they do not also have good communication skills, as this knowledge alone will be unlikely to result in positive behavioral change. Health and exercise professionals should use their communication skills in strategic ways to increase client understanding and motivation to follow exercise and other lifestyle-change recommendations. Good communication skills are also essential when working as part of a medical team and relating to supervisors and colleagues.

In the healthcare arena, interpersonal communication skills are strongly related to patient health outcomes (Ambady et al., 2002). Thus, curricula in many healthcare provider training programs, including those taking place at medical schools, have been expanded to include more training in effective communication skills (Rider & Keefer, 2006). Patient- and client-centered approaches are often based on **self-determination theory.** These approaches strive to strengthen the client's perceptions of autonomy, competence, and connection in provider settings and in the client's behavior-change programs. Whether behavioral change involves taking daily medication or a program of therapeutic exercises, a motivated client is more likely to stick to treatment recommendations. Client-centered approaches try to connect with clients' **intrinsic motivations** for treatment in order to maximize client willingness to address problems that occasionally arise. A CMES can learn to listen to clients' stories to uncover what is meaningful and motivational and then connect behavior-change recommendations to clients' meaningful goals. Research has shown that the quality of support provided by the health and exercise professional can enhance clients' adherence to behavior-change programs (Ryan et al., 2011).

A successful CMES must be skilled at working with all kinds of people.

LEARNING OBJECTIVES:

» Help clients improve health behaviors through creating positive emotions, establishing trust, gathering pertinent information, setting the client–CMES agenda, and communicating recommendations.

» Identify the impact that an illness or injury has on a client's life and offer support by understanding how to communicate with clients in distress.

» Build lasting professional working relationships through positive first impressions and the use of verbal and nonverbal communication.

» Use basic communication strategies for facilitating client goal achievement, enhancing motivation, and providing education.

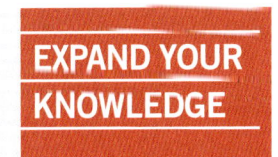

EXPAND YOUR KNOWLEDGE

SELF-DETERMINATION THEORY

Researchers Edward Deci and Richard Ryan (2008) study motivation and psychological well-being. They believe that people are naturally active and motivated to pursue activities and goals in which they are interested or from which they believe they will obtain some benefit. They have observed that people also act in response to external forces that put pressure on them to behave in certain ways. Deci and Ryan propose that there are different types of motivation that drive behavior and that some types of motivation are more likely to result in successful behavioral change than others. They talk specifically about two basic types of motivation: **autonomous motivation** and **controlled motivation.** Autonomous motivation means people feel like they are behaving of their own free will, in accordance with their own wishes. They are doing something because they want to do it. Controlled motivation means people do something because they feel pressured by demands from external forces. These types of motivation feel very different to people. The theory of motivation developed by Deci and Ryan is called the self-determination theory, which holds that the three most important factors that influence motivation are autonomy, competence, and connection.

Autonomy

People generally do not like to be told what to do, unless they have actively sought and asked for advice. People like to feel they have options and can make choices about behavior according to their own wishes, in accordance with their own values and goals. Autonomous motivation is stronger than controlled motivation for this reason: people like autonomy.

Competence

People like to feel competent at the activities in which they engage. They like to feel good about their performance and are pleased when their work goes well, when they receive good grades, or when they become proficient at skills they are working to develop. Competence is similar to **self-efficacy.** Both are specific to behavior. For example, a person may feel competent and have high self-efficacy for work situations but low competence in the fitness center—and thus low self-efficacy for following an exercise program. When people feel incompetent, they generally do not feel good, and they may lose motivation to continue in the area of incompetence. Feelings of competence are motivational and strengthen people's efforts.

Connection

People are social creatures and tend to seek relationships with other people. They like to feel understood, have the approval of others they respect, talk to one another, and reach out to others who need help. Connection means people feel they belong in a particular group or place. Positive connections make people feel good and reinforce motivation. The drive for feelings of connection helps to explain the strong role social support plays in people's lives.

As health and exercise professionals expand their clientele beyond the healthy, young exercise enthusiasts who walk into the fitness center, they often require more education and training in communication strategies to reach clients who find it difficult to incorporate regular physical activity into their lives. This chapter provides an overview of effective communication skills and presents basic information on how a CMES can most effectively motivate and support clients in their behavior-change efforts.

COMMUNICATION GOALS

The overarching goal of a CMES is to help clients improve health behaviors and stick to their behavior-change plans. Underlying this important goal are several other objectives that lay the groundwork for a productive working relationship with clients.

Creating Positive Emotions and Optimism for Change

The CMES should try to set a positive tone from the first contact with clients. Clients must begin their behavior-change journeys feeling as energetic and optimistic as possible. Positive emotions such as hope and anticipation of success give clients the energy they will need to stick to their programs. Positive emotions also help to create a more productive bond between the professional and the client. Clients who do not enjoy working with a health and exercise professional are likely to leave, either abandoning their behavior-change efforts or looking for other professionals with whom to work.

Establishing Feelings of Connection and Trust

Clients must feel that the CMES is trustworthy, since behavioral change often involves very personal issues. Clients often feel vulnerable discussing health issues, past behavior-change failures, and other information important in the behavior-change counseling process. A CMES will elicit the most trust and client buy-in if they convey a professional, unconditional positive regard for clients. Clients feel valued and ready to proceed with behavior-change programs when they feel the professional is interested in them and cares about the outcome of their work together. The positive regard and involvement must feel authentic. This creates a climate that allows clients to be more open and honest, giving the professional a better ability to design individualized behavior-change recommendations. A professional, trusting relationship contributes to feelings of connection that motivate people (Ryan et al., 2011).

Gathering Information and Setting the Agenda

Good communication skills and a caring demeanor allow the CMES to gather information from clients that helps set a productive direction. This information gives professionals a sense of clients' motivations for change, ideas about health and behavioral change, and past experiences with behavioral change. Using that information, the CMES can design the most effective behavior-change program for each client.

Communicating Behavior-change Recommendations

An effective CMES gives sound behavior-change advice, but tries to do so when clients are most receptive and motivated to change behaviors. Good communication skills help professionals find those moments when clients are open to advice and help them deliver advice in ways that are most likely to resonate with clients. Effective health and exercise professionals make behavior-change recommendations that build each client's sense of autonomous motivation in a way that matches their personal sense of self-efficacy for behavioral change.

UNDERSTANDING THE MEDICAL EXERCISE CLIENT

Clients' physical and psychological responses to illnesses and injuries are guiding considerations when designing safe and effective exercise programs. Health and exercise professionals must consider the impact that an illness or injury has had on a client's life. Depending upon the nature of the illness or injury, a client's psychological response to a diagnosis of an illness or serious injury may be similar to the process of grieving in response to a significant loss, such as the loss of a loved one. In general, grieving tends to begin with feelings of distress and shock, then move into feelings such as denial, anger, and sadness, and then eventually into resignation, acceptance, and hopefully some form of resolution (Maciejewski et al., 2007). People vary enormously in their responses to illness and injury, depending upon a number of factors.

Severity of the Illness or Injury and Impact on Quality of Life

The more serious the illness or injury, and the more it impacts daily activities, the more adjustment and coping are required from the client. Many medical treatments include therapies such as physical therapy and occupational therapy to help clients improve their ability to perform daily activities while coping with illness or injury. It is important to note that the client's *perception* of the illness or injury is more important than the actual physical nature of the illness or injury—and often is quite different (Brown, 2005). An illness or injury will obviously have different impacts depending on a client's personal situation. Disruptions in family life, work, school, the ability to produce income, and the ability to participate in fulfilling activities are associated with significant emotional distress.

Expected Outcome

If illness or disease outcome is expected to eventually be positive, clients will likely feel more optimistic and less stressed than when coping with an illness or injury that is not expected to significantly improve. Some clients will be living with an illness that may be expected to worsen and lead to significant disability and even premature death. Feeling uncertain about potential outcomes is often stressful.

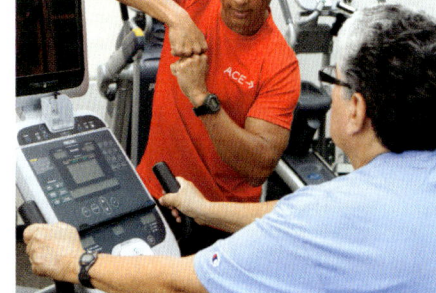

The Client's Personal Resources

Illness and injury can produce not only physical stress, but also financial and social stress. Medical care is expensive on many levels and places significant stress on the client and the client's family and friends. Clients with strong financial and social resources may be able to weather these stresses more easily than those with fewer resources. Personal resources also include individual capacities to adapt and cope with stress. Some people are more resilient than others and find hope in situations when others would give up.

Communicating With Clients in Distress

The CMES is likely to work with clients who have significant amounts of emotional distress because of illness and injury. Clients may or may not want to discuss their distress and personal situations. The professional should respect the client's need for privacy and not ask for details irrelevant to exercise program design. When clients share with the CMES that times are challenging, the professional can listen with **empathy** and acknowledge that life is really hard sometimes. The CMES need not try to "fix" everything, but, if appropriate, may recommend helpful resources available to the client. The following strategies may be useful in some situations.

Education

Clients need to understand the health issues and injuries they are coping with and be knowledgeable about rehabilitation and treatment recommendations. However, clients should not be overwhelmed with negative information. Education should focus on answering clients' questions and explaining the most productive ways of coping with the illness or injury. The CMES must encourage clients to hope for the best and to view regular physical activity as one of the ways to achieve the best possible outcome for post-rehabilitation and disease management, and for improving quality of life. Clients must believe in the efficacy of their exercise programs.

Goal Setting and Positive Outlook

Goal setting improves rehabilitation and treatment adherence. Small, achievable goals help clients feel they are making progress and taking control of their lives. The CMES should encourage clients to have as positive an outlook as possible. While not discounting fear and other negative emotions, the professional should help the client see positive progress. Positive progress may increase clients' feelings of self-efficacy. People with stronger self-efficacy are more likely to persist at trying to achieve their goals when obstacles arise.

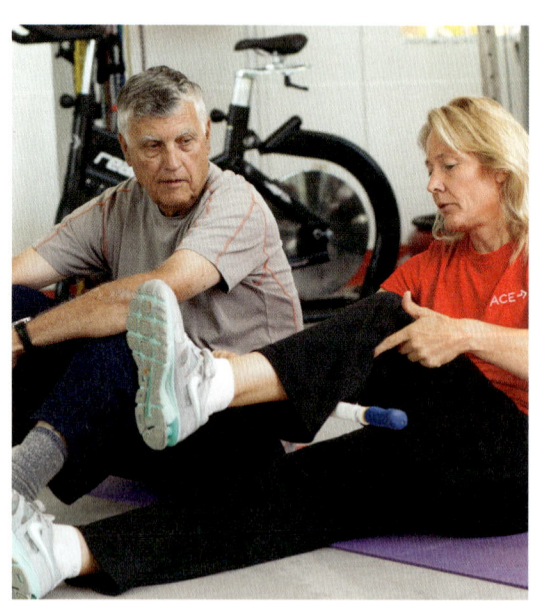

In addition to helping clients perceive progress as they meet goals, the CMES should reinforce positive emotions such as hope, confidence, and even enjoyment. Research in the field of positive psychology has demonstrated repeatedly that people who experience more positive emotions recover more quickly from illness, even very serious illness such as nonfatal **myocardial infarction** and **stroke** (Seligman, 2008).

Teaching behavior-change skills is best done in a positive way that generates hope and builds self-efficacy. A CMES should work with clients to connect behavior-change plans to clients' personal goals. When possible, professionals should present behavior-change skills as producing positive emotions. For example, instead of focusing only on how much exercise clients should perform, the professional should also focus on how regular activity may also help clients feel better, and that exercise may reduce feelings of **anxiety,** stress, and **depression.** One study found that messages promoting positive affect (i.e., exercise will help you feel good) were associated with higher levels of physical activity in subjects than cognitive messages that simply conveyed information about exercise benefits (i.e., exercise is good for you) (Conner et al., 2011). Good communication skills also create positive feelings, as clients feel respected and valued as they work with the CMES. If clients experience emotional health benefits with exercise, health and exercise professionals can encourage regular physical activity as part of behavior-change efforts.

Social Support

Support from family, friends, and medical staff enhances adherence and helps clients feel better. When possible, the CMES should welcome a family member or friend to participate with the client. Social support can be especially welcome, and even essential, for clients facing significant difficulties. Social support can help distressed clients in several ways:
- The soothing presence of a close friend or family member can help a distressed client feel more relaxed and less anxious.
- Friends and family can provide valuable feedback on clients' positive progress, cheering clients on. Verbal persuasion such as this can increase client self-efficacy.
- Social support enhances clients' planning efforts. Planning is a critical step in the behavior-change process.
- Friends, family members, and other acquaintances may provide instrumental support, such as giving clients rides to their appointments, helping with grocery shopping and meal preparation, or providing child care so that clients may exercise.
- Social support can reinforce positive social norms. People are swayed by the opinions of others. If friends and family agree that regular exercise is an important part of the client's post-rehabilitation program, this belief may be strengthened in the client.

Access to Exercise

Access to exercise opportunities is often limited for many people with health problems. Facilities, classes, and instructors may be inaccessible because of limitations in the physical environment, lack of qualified fitness specialists, or transportation difficulties.

Depression

Depression is more prevalent in people with severe chronic medical conditions than in those without. Some studies estimate that depression affects approximately 10% of individuals receiving medical treatment (Nease & Malouin, 2003). The special challenge of depression is that it often leads to feelings of lethargy and a lack of motivation to be active.

If clients tell the CMES that they are coping with depression, the professional should express empathy and acknowledge that dealing with depression can be very hard. The professional can also remind depressed clients that regular physical activity can help relieve depression symptoms. The CMES should also encourage clients to continue current depression treatments, however, and consult their healthcare providers regarding recommendations in this area.

Multiple Health Problems and Medication Side Effects

In addition to a client's primary medical focus, other illnesses and limitations may exist simultaneously. They may be related to the original problem, as when a person with **type 2 diabetes** also has **hypertension,** or unrelated, as when the same person also has **osteoarthritis.** Medication side effects, such as fatigue or dizziness, can also interfere with motivation to exercise.

Pain

Pain is associated with many medical problems. Pain is usually a warning to rest the affected area. Unfortunately, pain may be continuous in some medical conditions, such as many forms of arthritis, and people with such conditions may need to exercise with some level of pain. Rest and inactivity make some types of pain worse. The CMES will need to work closely with such clients and their medical teams to effectively address pain and to help clients understand their exercise capabilities and limits.

Fear of Harm

People coping with health problems and injury, especially those new to exercise, may feel fragile and vulnerable. Their bodies are already experiencing limitations, and they do not want to compromise their abilities further. For example, clients may fear falling or suffering another heart attack.

Of course, the CMES must do everything possible to ensure that clients' exercise programs are safe. When people voice concerns about the safety of their exercise programs, the CMES should address these concerns. The CMES might remind clients that their physicians recommended these exercises (when that is the case), and that exercise is an important part of the treatment program, emphasizing the substantial benefits that will be gained with regular exercise. Fearful clients should initially be given low levels of exercise to slowly strengthen confidence and improve exercise-specific self-efficacy.

COMMUNICATION SKILLS BUILD POSITIVE AND PROFESSIONAL WORKING RELATIONSHIPS

The first few meetings between a client and the CMES should establish good **rapport,** which refers to a relationship marked by mutual understanding and trust. Rapport begins with first impressions, so a CMES should do everything possible to present themself as professional and approachable. Rapport continues to build over time, and the longer professionals and clients work together, the more they come to understand one another. An early foundation of trust and respect increases the likelihood that a positive and productive relationship will develop.

First Impressions

Most people have a first impression, consisting of an initial judgment or emotional response, when meeting another person for the first time. People's first impressions of others are often fairly accurate (Biesanz et al., 2011). Many factors influence clients' first impressions of a health and exercise professional. Some of these factors are under the professional's control, such as attire and screening procedures. Exercise professionals have interacted, as clients or patients themselves, with health professionals and can likely recall both positive and negative first impressions. When people are asked to recall both negative and positive experiences with exercise professionals, many common themes emerge (Brehm, 2014a).

Negative experiences are marked by rudeness, indifference, ineptitude, neglect, and even malpractice. In describing negative experiences, people often report being left waiting a long time in environments that were dirty, disorganized, or dull. They describe professionals as appearing bored, uninterested in the client, uncaring, or distracted. They perceive communications with the professional as unclear, with clients saying they did not understand the information or the reasons for the treatments or recommendations. Questions were not encouraged or answered clearly.

Positive experiences are characterized by a sense of caring, respect, clear communication, and professionalism. Clients perceive that the professional takes their concerns seriously and that they are highly qualified, knowledgeable, and helpful. Questions are carefully considered and clearly answered, and the environment is clean and organized.

Positive first impressions provide a great start for the rapport-building process. Because first impressions are so important, a CMES must remember they may be contributing to a potential client's first impression before even meeting the client. For example, health and exercise professionals may exercise in the fitness facility where they work. This means they are always in the public eye. Their behavior in these settings may influence whether or not clients form a favorable impression of them. Similarly, a CMES often runs into clients in public places such as grocery stores, shopping malls, theaters, and so forth. Conduct in these environments can contribute to the impression the CMES makes on others and also to their reputation.

First impressions are also created by technologies such as telephone messages, websites, blogs, and other social networking tools. A CMES should consider what sort of professional image is projected when they employ these tools. New professionals and young people must be especially careful to avoid offensive images and text that could turn off potential employers and clients.

In emerging professions, such as personal training and health coaching, where credentialing is not always required or well understood by the public, it is especially important for professionals to establish credibility (George, 2008). A CMES should be sure that clients know about their education, training, certifications, other qualifications, and work experience. These can be highlighted in websites, business cards, and materials given to clients. A CMES should describe their experience and **scope of practice** when orienting new clients at the first meeting.

A CMES who has had little difficulty developing rapport with clients similar to themself may find that it takes a little longer to build trust with people who differ in age, gender, ethnicity, size, socioeconomic status, educational background, ability, or fitness level. Building rapport may take more effort when clients are reluctant to change their behavior, afraid of injury, or depressed and anxious about health issues. Some clients have had bad experiences that led them to develop prejudices against athletes, physical educators, dietitians, physical therapists, and other groups. They may have less trust of young people, old people, women, men, people who appear to have overweight, or people of a different ethnic background. Nevertheless, a CMES who consistently behaves professionally and employs good communication skills often win the hearts and trust of even the most reluctant clients.

THINK IT THROUGH

Think about the types of first impressions that clients might have regarding not only you personally, but your facility as well. Are they greeted professionally when they enter the building? Is everyone they meet dressed and behaving appropriately? What does your outgoing voicemail convey? Have a friend call the business to ask a series of questions and then provide feedback on their experience. Also, have a friend visit the facility during your busiest time and report back on how they are welcomed and treated by staff members. Health and exercise professionals should always be working hard to optimize the first impression they make on potential clients.

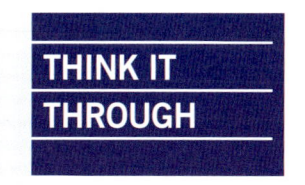

Verbal and Nonverbal Communication

Communication is influenced by the words that are spoken (or unspoken), the manner of speech, and many nonverbal details. People's verbal communications are only a small part of the messages they send. People pay attention to much more than words in their effort to decipher messages and understand social situations, including interactions with health and exercise professionals (Mast, 2007). While people hear each other's words, they seek to verify verbal content by evaluating the speaker's appearance, facial expressions, body language, and tone of voice. If someone's words ("I am glad to meet you") and body language (lack of eye contact, disinterested facial expression, body turned away, low energy) do not match, people generally trust body language over verbal content (Ambady & Weisbuch, 2010).

When talking with clients, the CMES should speak clearly and use language clients can easily understand, without speaking down to them. It is certainly appropriate to use exercise science and medical vocabulary, but health and exercise professionals should be sure to define terms that may be unfamiliar to clients. They can enhance verbal content with visual information, such as pictures, diagrams, and charts that illustrate concepts. Exercise demonstrations may accompany verbal explanations.

People often develop distracting habits that interfere with effective verbal communication. Peppering explanations with frequent fillers such as "um," "you know," and "like" gives a first impression that clients may perceive as uneducated and unprofessional. Older clients often complain that young people speak too quickly. To exacerbate matters, new professionals may have a tendency to speak even more quickly and add more fillers when nervous. Individuals who are new to professional–client interactions can benefit from conducting and then viewing and evaluating mock sessions that are filmed.

Nonverbal communication occurs in many ways, including:

- *Voice quality:* A weak, hesitant, or soft voice does not inspire client confidence. On the other hand, a loud, tense voice tends to make people nervous. A CMES should try to develop a voice that is firm, energetic, and confident to communicate professionalism. Some people end their sentences with a higher pitch, as though asking a question. This communicates indecisiveness and can detract from the confident impression the health and exercise professional should make.
- *Eye contact:* Direct, friendly eye contact shows clients they are the focus of attention. When a listener looks away while a person is speaking, the speaker does not feel heard. Similarly, when a speaker looks away, the listener does not feel important and thinks the speaker does not care about their reaction.
- *Facial expression:* Facial expressions convey emotion but work best when the emotion is sincere. Most clients can sense an artificial smile, so the CMES must reach deep to portray a genuine display of positive regard for clients. As professionals work with clients, their faces should display the concern, thoughtfulness, and/or enjoyment they are feeling.
- *Hand gestures:* Use of hand gestures varies from culture to culture. In general, people are most comfortable when a speaker uses relaxed, fluid hand gestures while explaining things. When listening, the CMES should refrain from hand gestures. Fidgeting hands, clenched fists, abrupt gestures, and finger pointing are distracting to many clients.
- *Body position:* An open, well-balanced, erect body position communicates confidence. Good posture is especially important for a CMES, whose body serves as a symbol of their professional expertise (Maguire, 2008). A body posture that is leaning or stooped suggests fatigue and boredom (not to mention poor health and physical fitness), while a rigid, hands-on-hips stance may be interpreted as aggressive. When the professional and client sit together talking, the professional should look attentive by leaning slightly forward and keeping arms uncrossed. They should eliminate distracting nervous activity such as foot or finger tapping or constantly shifting position.
- *Behavior:* Many behaviors serve as forms of communication. For example, when the CMES is late for an appointment or frequently reschedules appointments, this communicates a lack of respect for the client. Professionals communicate a lack of involvement when they interrupt an appointment to make a phone call or perform other tasks. A cell phone ringing in the middle of a discussion can throw conversation off track. Unless the meeting is explicitly taking place during a meal, eating while meeting with a client is distracting.

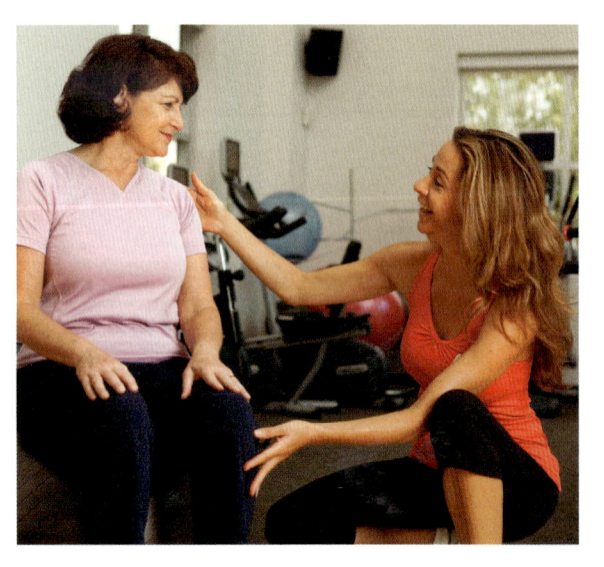

COMMUNICATION BASICS

Several communication skills form the foundation for effective communication strategies (Brehm, 2014b). This section describes and illustrates these skills. It should be noted that practicing these skills with peers and even family members will help the CMES master these communication techniques.

Directive and Guiding Communication Styles

A CMES utilizes both directive and guiding communication styles. Health and exercise professionals use directive communication styles when they give advice, design exercise programs, and tell clients what to do. Most clients value the CMES's knowledge and expertise; clients usually want direction on how to most effectively treat or cope with medical issues they are facing.

A CMES uses guiding communication styles when they sense ambivalence from clients that might interfere with the client's ability to follow through on exercise or other behavior-change recommendations. Rather than simply telling clients what to do, a CMES uses a variety of communication techniques to guide ambivalent clients to make a decision to change and to develop autonomous motivation to stick to their exercise programs.

The nature of the CMES's communication style during early sessions with a client depends upon the nature of the work and the client's commitment and motivation. Exercise professionals often see clients in the **preparation** stage of change, ready to take on a behavior-change program to improve health and fitness. Good communication skills are essential in these situations so that the professional can clearly understand client goals and use the information gathered to craft effective recommendations. In these situations, the CMES may use more of a directive style of communication, since clients are ready for advice, actively seeking the professional's opinion on what to do.

A CMES often sees clients or patients who are not even thinking of changing but want a quick fix for a health problem. In these cases, professionals may decide to communicate with more of a guiding style. A CMES must become skilled in communication strategies that help clients become open to thinking about behavioral change.

The best way to begin working with a new client in any setting is to ask good questions and listen mindfully to the answers. These answers will reveal how clients view behavioral change in terms of its importance to them, as well as their feelings of self-efficacy for changing. Answers will reveal clients' readiness to change and factors that will enhance the likelihood of behavior-change success. Effective communication tools for structuring information-gathering sessions come from **motivational interviewing (MI)** (Rollnick, Miller, & Butler, 2008). Using MI techniques requires training and practice. Developing skill in using MI begins with learning to listen mindfully and reflectively, the basis of the information-gathering practice described here. Many health and exercise professionals use modified MI procedures to engage with clients about behavioral change (Pfister-Minogue & Salveson, 2010). Modified procedures capture the collaborative, supportive spirit of MI. Learning to ask good questions and listen in an effective and mindful fashion is appropriate and helpful for a CMES discussing lifestyle change with clients, in order to gather information from the clients on their behavior-change goals and to design effective and motivational interventions.

EXPAND YOUR KNOWLEDGE

MOTIVATIONAL INTERVIEWING

MI is a counseling technique developed by William R. Miller and Stephen Rollnick (2013). While MI techniques were originally developed in the context of addiction treatment, they have been implemented and scientifically evaluated in many other health contexts and have become the basis for most evidence-based behavioral counseling. Miller, Rollnick, and colleagues helped to radically change the way addiction was viewed and the way therapists and health and exercise professionals work with clients trying to change addictions and negative health behaviors (Miller & Rollnick 2013; Miller & Rose, 2009).

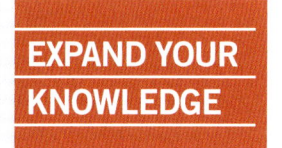

Miller and Rollnick believe that the harsh, confrontational methods formerly used to treat addiction actually reduced clients' motivation to change. It is natural for people to feel ambivalent about changing in the early stages of change. In these early stages, clients are weighing the pros and cons of changing behavior. When professionals try to convince clients they should change, a natural response is for clients to argue why they should not change, and instead sustain their current behaviors. MI practices empower a CMES to help clients voice and strengthen their reasons to change, increase their commitment to changing, and uncover autonomous motivation to change.

MI is both a philosophy and a set of strategies to help people increase their own internal drive to change. It is a way for the CMES to lead clients into forming their own decisions about the changes they need to make regarding their health behaviors. Health and exercise professionals work with clients to explore and resolve ambivalence about behavioral change. The professional and the client are collaborators. Ideally, MI helps clients develop autonomous motivation for behavioral change. The purpose of MI is to help clients feel autonomous, competent, and connected.

MI generally includes four broad processes:
- *Engaging:* Professionals work to establish a good rapport with clients using a communication style that is accepting, empathic, and compassionate.
- *Focusing:* Professionals and clients work together to clarify the goals of their work. For example, clients with diabetes may decide they want professionals to help them develop better eating habits in order to improve blood glucose control.
- *Evoking:* Professionals encourage clients to formulate their own reasons and motivations for changing. Throughout their work together, professionals help clients draw upon their personal motivations to support the behavior-change work.
- *Planning:* Planning can be woven into the behavior-change work, once clients are ready to change. Plans are not formulated by the professional, but created by the professional and client together in a collaborative manner.

For more information on motivational interviewing, refer to *The Professional's Guide to Health and Wellness Coaching* (ACE, 2019) and the Behavioral Change Specialist Program (www.acefitness.org/fitness-certifications/specialty-certifications/behavior-change.aspx).

APPLY WHAT YOU KNOW

SAMPLE CONVERSATIONS WITH CLIENTS IN THE CONTEMPLATION STAGE OF CHANGE

The following conversations illustrate a client's response to a CMES who uses (1) a standard directive style of communication and (2) a more guiding style of communication, using principles of MI.

Directive Style

CMES: I see from your forms that you are here because you have been diagnosed with type 2 diabetes. You'll be meeting with a dietitian tomorrow, and you are meeting with me to get started on an exercise program. Is this correct?

Client (C): I guess so. This is all happening so quickly, I am not really sure what I am supposed to do.

CMES: We've worked with lots of people newly diagnosed with diabetes at our center. Research shows that an exercise program that includes both aerobic and strength exercise can help improve blood sugar regulation. I can design an exercise program for you that uses both the aerobic exercise machines and the strength-training equipment. How does that sound?

C: Well, I'm not sure. I've never worked out in a fitness center like this before. The machines look awfully complicated...

CMES: Don't worry, I'll show you how they work; you'll pick it up in no time.

C: I'm not sure this will work. I have some arthritis in my knees...

CMES: Good news! Strength training can help reduce arthritis pain.

C: You don't think I might get injured? The last thing I need is more pain.

CMES: Studies show that people who perform exercises that strengthen the muscles around the knee joint often see an improvement in joint function, joint strength, and even a reduction in pain. I'm sure we can work together to come up with an exercise program that works for you.

C: How much time is this going to take? I'm really awfully busy at work these days…

The above scenario illustrates that often, the more the CMES tries to convince the client that change is a good idea, the more the client focuses on the reasons for not changing. Pushing clients who have not yet made a decision to change rarely leads to successful behavioral change.

Guiding Style

CMES: Come on in, have a seat. How can I help you?

C: I'm supposed to start exercising. My doctor told me I have diabetes, and that exercise will help get my sugar down.

CMES: Great. Exercise is very important for improving blood sugar control. What kinds of exercise did your doctor recommend for you?

C: I don't know. This is all happening so quickly, I didn't really understand what the doctor was saying, and I don't know what to do.

CMES: Would you like some information about what kinds of exercise work best for blood sugar control?

C: Well, there's not really much I can do. I mean, I have arthritis in my knees, and the last thing I need is more pain.

CMES: You must be worried that exercise will make your arthritis worse.

C: I guess so. I've tried walking before, but that didn't work.

CMES: So it would be really important to figure out a way to exercise that doesn't cause you any pain. Have you ever tried exercises to reduce the arthritis pain?

C: Well, no, I am not big on exercise. Like I said, I tried walking once for a few days, but that didn't work.

CMES: What if we started by trying exercises that might reduce your knee pain?

C: What kind of exercise can do that?

In this scenario, the CMES has attempted to listen to the client's concerns and address the issue of knee pain, which might be important to the client. Although the client has not necessarily decided to exercise yet, at least the client and the professional are still talking. In the first scenario, the client is not engaged, whereas in the second, they have at least not completely dismissed suggestions coming from the CMES.

Client-centered communication includes four important techniques: **open-ended questions, affirmations, reflective listening,** and **summarizing** (Miller & Rollnick, 2013). The **OARS model** (Figure 5-1) provides a mnemonic device that many individuals use to remember these techniques.

Open-ended Questions

Open-ended questions invite clients to give the CMES more information, tell their stories, and paint a broader picture. While **closed-ended questions** take the conversation in directions important for the CMES's agenda, open-ended questions allow information important to clients to surface. Examples of open questions include, "How can I help you?" "What does your typical weekday schedule look like?" and "What kinds of situations lead to overeating?" Closed-ended questions can be turned into open-ended questions very simply by responding to the answers with another question or request, such as "Can you tell me more about that?"

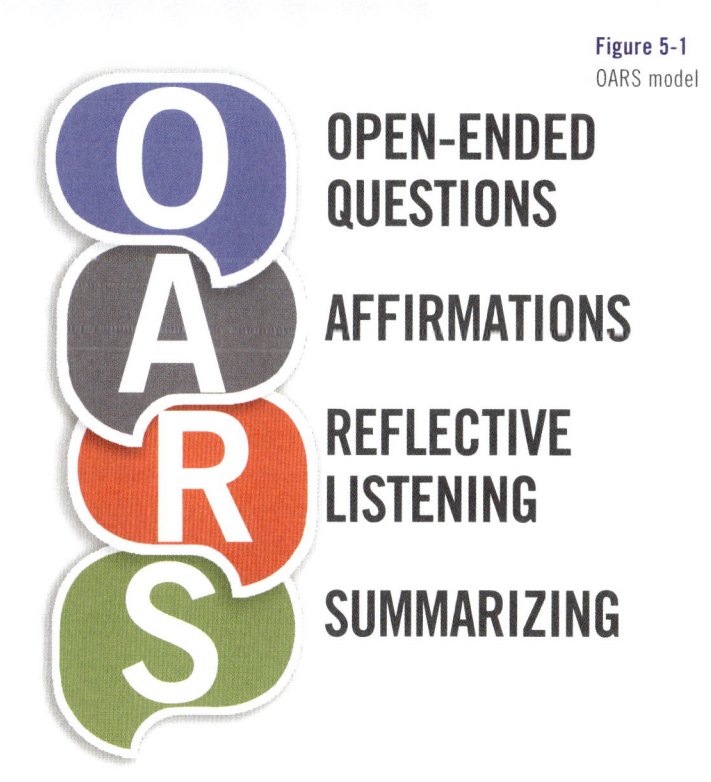

Figure 5-1
OARS model

OPEN-ENDED QUESTIONS

AFFIRMATIONS

REFLECTIVE LISTENING

SUMMARIZING

Skilled use of open-ended questions accomplishes several goals at once:
- *Break the ice of early meetings:* Open-ended questions asked during the first meeting get the conversation started in a client-centered fashion. Open-ended questions direct thinking in productive ways that get the discussion off to a good start.
- *Build rapport:* As clients sense the professional is interested in their situation, they feel more trusting.
- *Provide useful information:* Open-ended questions allow clients to provide information on their reasons for consulting the CMES and factors that may affect adherence to a behavior-change plan. The CMES learns about clients' strengths and positive characteristics to highlight in the future to build self-efficacy and motivation.
- *Nurture autonomous motivation in clients:* Asking open-ended questions temporarily hands the direction of the conversation to the client. It suggests the client is the focus not only of the information-gathering procedures but also of the direction the behavior-change program will take. Since the client is influencing recommendations, the result is more client buy-in and responsibility for results. Open-ended questions can lead to the development of goals and plans most relevant to and realistic for individual clients.
- *Increase client satisfaction:* Open-ended questions show clients that the CMES has their needs and interests at heart. Clients feel valued and empowered.

Closed-ended questions elicit brief answers and help to gather information on specific topics. Examples of closed questions include "Are you hoping to lose weight?" "Do you have time to exercise before work?" and "Does that exercise feel too difficult?" Closed-ended questions may often be answered with "yes" or "no" or a short sentence.

Affirmations

Affirmations are statements that reinforce clients' strengths and accomplishments or indicate that they are making progress. A CMES can use affirmations to build a client's self-efficacy for behavioral change. Affirmations must not be empty praise but should refer to specific situations and actions that showed character strengths and progress. Affirmations might be responses to a story the client tells: "That was a good strategy." Affirmations might be reminders to clients of past accomplishments that illustrate their ability to be successful: "You said last year you were able to continue walking several days a week by walking at the indoor track once it started getting dark early. That was a good idea."

Affirmations are designed to help clients build autonomous motivation, rather than changing in order to achieve praise from the health and exercise professional. Long-lasting lifestyle change is more likely to result from clients building the skills to make decisions and plan changes in their own lives, rather than changing to win recognition from the CMES. It is fine for the professional to indicate approval, but affirmations should help clients create a positive story about their abilities to succeed. "Look at how many more repetitions you are doing this week compared to last week," is a way to praise a client's efforts, show evidence of improvement, and build exercise self-efficacy.

Reflective Listening

Reflective listening refers to active listening combined with verbal and nonverbal responses to indicate interest and understanding and to encourage the speaker to continue. Reflective means that listeners reflect back to the speakers what they (the listeners) have heard to confirm accurate understanding. Reflective listening shows the speaker that the listener has heard not only the speaker's words but is also trying to perceive and understand the feelings that the words convey. Reflective listening helps speakers feel understood and valued and thus helps build connection and rapport.

Health and exercise professionals who work with people need to be good listeners. Unfortunately, many health and exercise professionals tend to believe that, because they get paid to give advice, the more they say, the better. They love to talk about exercise and health and equate information delivery with performance and giving clients their money's worth. Unfortunately, this focus on talking can interfere with good communication if the professional always dominates discussions with clients and interrupts clients before they are finished speaking.

Listening is important but difficult. Lives are busy and noisy, and it is not possible to listen mindfully to everything everyone says. Some of the time people pretend to listen but do not really pay attention. They may pretend to listen so that people will like them or not think them rude. People may hear only part of what the speaker is saying and tune out parts they find boring, offensive, or hard to understand. Instead of listening carefully to a speaker, listeners are often busy formulating arguments, forming judgments about the speaker, or thinking about what they will say next. They may simply be daydreaming about something else entirely. They might be preoccupied with themselves, perhaps distracted by their own problems.

Even if people try to listen, they may not hear what the speaker is saying. People often reconstruct messages to reflect their own beliefs and needs. They may have prejudices about the speaker and look for confirmation of these in the speaker's words. They may tend to hear what they expect to hear and neglect to take in other things the speaker is saying. Fortunately, listening skills can be learned, and reflective listening improves with practice.

Reflective listening occurs when the CMES listens carefully and empathetically to a client, with an open mind, trying to identify with the client's situation. When trying to listen, professionals should give clients their full attention. Effective communication occurs most easily in quiet, private spaces to limit distraction.

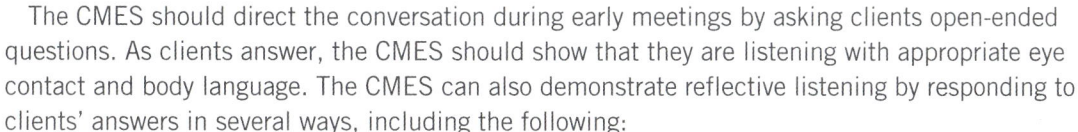

The CMES should direct the conversation during early meetings by asking clients open-ended questions. As clients answer, the CMES should show that they are listening with appropriate eye contact and body language. The CMES can also demonstrate reflective listening by responding to clients' answers in several ways, including the following:

- *Encouraging:* The CMES may use short words or phrases such as "I see," "Yes," and "That's interesting," that encourage the client to continue speaking when there is a natural pause in the client's speech. These phrases let the client know the CMES is listening carefully and following what is being said. Nodding and smiling can also indicate listening and encourage speakers to continue.
- *Paraphrasing:* The listener can demonstrate understanding by restating in a clear and concise way the essence of what the client has been saying. Paraphrasing may also extend the meaning of the client's answers. For example, the client may tell a story about how they maintained a lighter weight for several years. The CMES might paraphrase, "So that feels like it might be a realistic weight for you." If the paraphrase is not accurate, the speaker then has a chance to correct an erroneous impression.
- *Questioning:* Responding to a client's stories with more open-ended questions demonstrates good listening and directs the conversation, encouraging the client to continue sharing relevant information. The CMES might follow up a client's story with a comment such as, "You said you quit exercising last year. What made you stop?" A CMES should ask questions at appropriate times to clarify points they do not understand or to move the conversation in a more productive direction.
- *Reflecting emotional content:* The CMES should also find opportunities to confirm the emotional content of the client's story if appropriate and important. "That must have been upsetting." "You seem discouraged." "That sounds like fun."

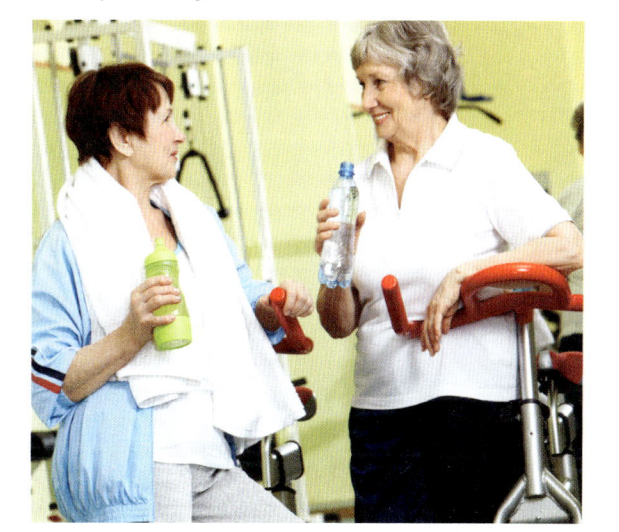

APPLY WHAT YOU KNOW

Practice reflective listening with coworkers, friends, or family members. Ask them to describe a problem they have had or are having in changing a health behavior. This might be a problem getting enough exercise or a problem with their diet. Maybe they are having difficulty quitting smoking or doing their back exercises regularly. It is best if you can get the person talking about a real problem that they want to discuss.

Once you have identified a helpful partner and a problem, your goal is simply to try to understand the problem, and the partner's situation, as clearly as possible. Do not try to solve the problem; simply try to listen and understand. Begin by asking open-ended questions to get your partner to describe the problem. Try to focus totally on listening. Try to paraphrase what the person is telling you and use appropriate nonverbal communication cues.

Notice how you felt during this exercise. Which paraphrasing attempts worked best? Which felt most awkward? How did the speaker respond? Did reflective listening feel different from how you usually interact with people? How could you further improve your reflective listening skills?

Summarizing

At appropriate points in the conversation, the CMES should try to summarize key points that have a bearing on the meeting objectives. After summarizing, the CMES should allow clients to comment on the summary to confirm its accuracy and correct misunderstandings. Summarizing not only demonstrates effective listening, but it gives the CMES an opportunity to guide a conversation that is wandering too far off topic or keep a meeting on track in terms of time. The summary also provides an opportunity for the CMES to emphasize certain parts of the conversation that are especially helpful and useful. Summaries can serve as a way to wrap up a topic before moving on to another.

Is Effective Communication More Work for the Professional?

A CMES who is accustomed to limiting client input and primarily giving advice may find that, like any form of behavioral change, changing communication habits is not easy at first. In fact, developing good communication skills takes a great deal of practice for anyone. People generally enjoy talking more than listening, and health and exercise professionals are no exception. However, once a CMES begins to practice reflective listening and a more mindful, present-moment awareness in their work, this approach can actually reduce work stress. Listening carefully is good for the listener. Listening with attention forces one to slow down and focus on the present moment, which can help reduce the stress people feel from trying to do too many things at the same time. In addition, by making conversations more productive, professionals feel better about their work.

Barriers to Effective Communication

Even when the CMES listens carefully and practices good communication skills, they may still find communication difficult. Sometimes the client is reluctant to participate fully, while other times the consultation environment is not conducive to productive conversation. With effort, most barriers to effective communication can be addressed. Some of the most common barriers encountered by the CMES include the following:
- *Cultural differences:* When the CMES and the client have significantly different backgrounds, the CMES must spend extra time and energy learning about the client. As they gain experience with a given population, the CMES will become more adept at establishing rapport with clients from that group. It is worth noting that while it is important to understand a client's cultural background, the CMES must never generalize or stereotype.
- *Emotional health problems:* Clients grappling with depression or anxiety may tend to focus on negative information, and not hear the positive. Research suggests that people look for information to justify their current mood and beliefs (Ambady & Gray, 2002), which

means that when working with clients with mood disorders, the CMES must be sure to phrase information in a positive, supportive way. Remember, the CMES cannot diagnose these disorders.
- *Too little/too much explanation:* The CMES should use language that clients can understand and try to meet clients' need for information.
- *Stress/feeling rushed:* By far the largest barrier to quality communication is a lack of effective listening, which is likely to occur when either party feels rushed and distracted, and does not pay attention to what the other person is saying. Cultivating the ability to focus one's attention mindfully is a good antidote to stress and improves communication.
- *Fitness center environment:* Initial meetings between the CMES and clients should occur in a comfortable, quiet, private space. Such space is not always readily available in fitness centers. In this case, fitness-center personnel should create a quiet space where clients do not feel like they will be overheard.

COMMUNICATION STRATEGIES AND MOTIVATION

The CMES should adapt their communication style and recommendations to a client's readiness to change (Brehm, 2014b). Clients ready to adopt the professional's recommendations may appreciate a more directive communication style; they are often hungry for good advice and clear direction. On the other hand, clients still reluctant or worried about exercise recommendations may not follow the professional's advice; time with these clients might be better spent helping them make a decision to change.

A client's level of motivation and readiness to exercise regularly is often difficult to measure. For one thing, motivation may change minute to minute, and a client who appears very motivated at a meeting with the CMES may still drop out early in the program. Clients may express the idea that they are motivated to increase the amount of exercise they are doing, perhaps wanting to say the right things, but then fail to follow through when challenges arise. Good communication skills can help the CMES assess a client's readiness to adhere to a behavior-change program. If clients do not yet seem committed to changing, the CMES can help them move toward a decision to change.

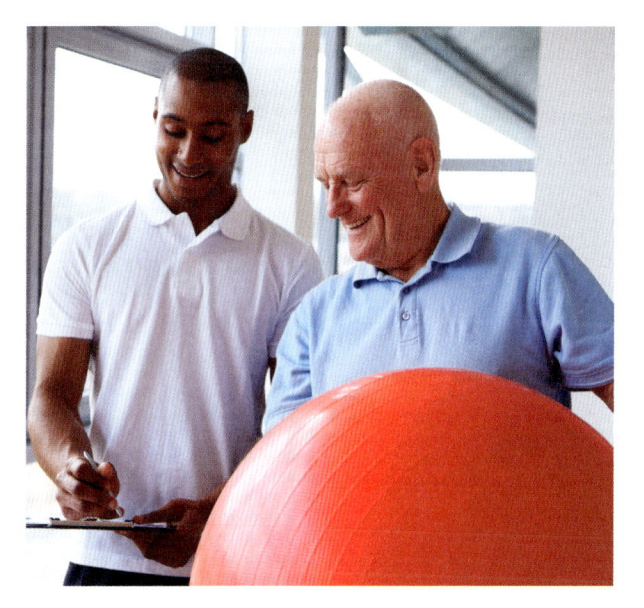

Assessing Readiness to Change

Usually, health and exercise professionals can get a sense of a client's stage of change by asking open-ended questions and listening to the client's answers. During early conversations with clients, health and exercise professionals can ask why they have sought to meet with the professional, how they view their health/behavior-change situations, how they feel about their ability to change, and how ready they are to change. Clients who are resistant to change may be in **precontemplation** or **contemplation** stages. Clients who have actively sought to meet with a health and exercise professional are likely contemplating or preparing for change. As discussed in Chapter 4, approaches for assisting clients would vary in these two situations.

When open-ended questions have not helped the CMES decide whether a client is ready to change, simply asking clients how they feel about changing can help. Questions might be placed in context. For example, "It seems like you are concerned about your diagnosis of diabetes. Diabetes is managed best if you can add some physical activity to your day. You are already walking twice a week for 20 minutes during your lunch hour. Do you think you could add another session of walking each week?" This closed-ended question might lead to more discussion and a better idea of a client's willingness to change.

Sometimes a CMES includes readiness-to-change questions on the paperwork that clients complete before their first visit. Answers to these questions can be helpful and may stimulate further discussion once professionals and clients begin working together.

The CMES can also use **scaling** to get a clearer idea of a client's readiness to change or any other variable of interest. Scaling refers to rating a variable on a numerical scale, for example, a scale from 0 to 10. "On a scale from 0 to 10, how confident are you that you will be able to exercise three days a week during your lunch hour?" The upper and lower limits of the scale should be defined. For example, "Let's say 0 represents no confidence, you think you will probably never do this, and 10 represents total confidence, you think you will have no problem doing this every week." If scaling suggests low confidence, the professional should work with the client to revise recommendations so that they are more in line with the client's self-efficacy.

Ryan and colleagues (2011) emphasize that categorizing clients into an exact stage may not always be helpful or necessary, as a person's stage can change from moment to moment. In the **stages-of-change model,** clients often move forward or backward in their stage. Movement from preparation to **action** is especially difficult to predict. Clients must be not only ready to change but also have the skills and energy required to follow through on their decisions. Many health and exercise professionals have stories about clients who appear totally committed to a behavior-change program but drop out after a few sessions. A CMES should still attempt to assess readiness but be somewhat flexible in their approach, listening carefully to clients' reasons for changing and adapting their interventions to best meet clients' needs.

Change Talk: Helping Precontemplation and Contemplation Clients Decide to Change

When a CMES finds themself working with clients who are not yet willing to change their behavior, it is important to refrain from arguing or bullying the client into changing. While it is tempting to forge ahead and tell clients what they should be doing, the CMES's advice may be wasted if clients have not yet made a commitment to change. Arguing and pressuring tend to alienate clients and create defensive resistance. Clients may eventually seem to agree, and even say they will follow recommendations, but may ignore the advice once they leave the CMES's office.

A more productive approach is to discuss with clients the reasons they feel unable or unwilling to change. Using the OARS model outlined earlier, the CMES can talk to clients in ways that show supportive concern for them while challenging their current behavior. The CMES's goal in behavior-change coaching situations with people not ready to change is to guide them to see that their current lifestyle is likely contributing to current or future problems. Using effective questions, the CMES tries to help clients see that good health is important and a healthful lifestyle will help them reach goals and engage in activities important to them. Helpful strategies include the following:

- *Ask open-ended questions:* The CMES may begin by asking clients open-ended questions about their health concerns and relevant lifestyle factors. The CMES should also ask clients questions about their families, work, and recreational pursuits. What do their days look like? What kinds of activities and hobbies do they enjoy?
- *Listen effectively:* The CMES should listen carefully to the client's answers. Listening effectively will help the the CMES understand the reasons a client feels, for example, unable to exercise, or does not feel the need to exercise. Listening carefully helps the CMES uncover valuable information and shows clients the the CMES respects them, even if they do not agree with them.
- *Guide clients to consider the importance of health:* Eventually, the CMES should move to questions that will hopefully help clients conclude that good health is important, so they can

continue to engage in those activities that are personally most meaningful and fulfilling. The CMES can then turn the discussion to the behavior-change issues at hand, trying to connect behavioral change with good health. For example, if clients have a family history of heart disease, the CMES could follow up by asking, "Did you know that regular physical activity helps to prevent heart disease?"

- *Keep the conversation friendly:* While a CMES may challenge statements made by clients ("I don't have a weight problem, so I don't need to exercise"), they should avoid heated arguments, since negative feelings may make clients defensive. If clients start to seem angry, the CMES should switch to a more neutral, information-gathering question. The CMES may also express empathy and respect for the difficulties the client faces. Experts in MI advise professionals to "roll with resistance" (Rollnick, Miller, & Butler, 2008), meaning that they should maintain an empathetic attitude toward the client, even if it means agreeing that change is too difficult right now. This prevents clients from shutting out the CMES and may even convince clients that the CMES is on their side and trying to help.
- *Keep listening and monitor client response:* The CMES should continually monitor clients' responses to questions. If the CMES senses the client has stopped listening, it's time to stop talking. Instead, the CMES can ask clients what they are thinking about or if they have any questions. These types of discussions can feel somewhat uncomfortable for professionals who tend to avoid conflict, but mild discomfort may help clients feel the need to change. If all else fails, try "How can I help you?"
- *Explore ambivalence:* It is human nature to feel ambivalent, which means having mixed or contradictory feelings about something. People often feel ambivalent about lifestyle change. On the one hand, a person might want to have more energy and might consider increasing physical activity to feel more energetic. On the other hand, that same person might find it difficult to summon the energy to actually get out and exercise. While recognizing that exercise helps them feel better, people might also feel that exercise takes too much energy to perform. As they speak with clients, the CMES should listen carefully to statements and stories that indicate ambivalent feelings about behavioral change. Sometimes, it is helpful to bring ambivalent issues to light for discussion. As clients explore their contradictory thoughts and feelings about the topic, over time they may be able to strengthen their resolve to change and to recognize the factors standing in the way of behavioral change. For example, they may learn to recognize a habit of starting to make excuses for why they cannot stick to their exercise program at this moment and be able to move forward with change and ignore "the little voice" making excuses. They may be able to come up with strategies to deal with perceived barriers and to increase their perceptions of the importance and feasibility of behavioral change.
- *Reinforce and support change talk:* Change talk refers to things clients say that favor positive behavioral change. The CMES tries to ask questions that elicit change talk from the client. For example, the CMES might ask, "Tell me more about the time two years ago when you enjoyed walking during your lunch hour." As the person describes their success, the CMES nods and smiles and remembers the points that seem to have contributed to success. When clients make statements such as, "I know I would feel better if I started exercising again," the CMES can agree with these statements and encourage clients to continue. When clients discuss the reasons they should not change, the CMES does not reinforce the reasons for not changing, but does not argue, either. The CMES must continually remind themself that it is the client who must decide to change and to find

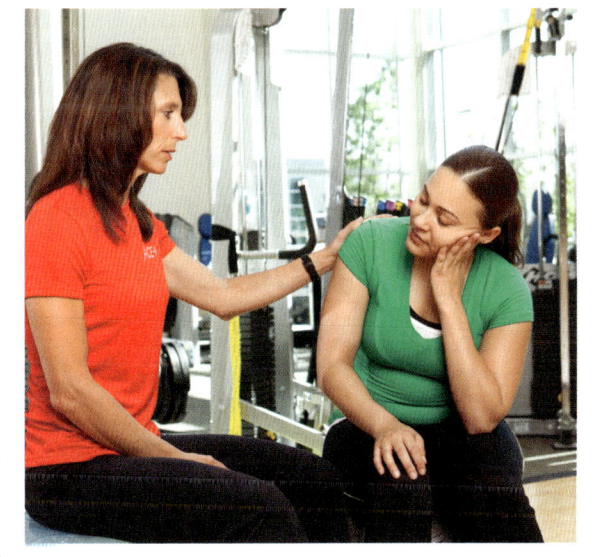

positive, motivational reasons for changing. Ryan and colleagues (2011) suggest that "truly reflective and person-centered techniques are effective only insofar as they are fostering autonomous change talk." If a CMES continues working with a client for a while, they can continue to mention and reinforce statements the client has made about positive, personally meaningful reasons for changing, guiding the client to pay more attention to productive ways of thinking and behaving.

- *Build self-confidence:* The CMES can help clients identify areas of success, no matter how small. For example, the CMES might praise a client who currently walks the dog twice a day for five minutes and then ask whether the client might consider increasing the walk time by a few minutes each week. The CMES can help clients identify personal strengths, based on stories clients have shared. "I admire the flexibility and persistence you showed when you were balancing your job and taking care of your children. Now that your children are older, I wonder if that same flexibility and persistence could be applied to fitting exercise into your day." Other strengths that the CMES might observe include an ability to organize and plan; manage stress effectively; use a sense of humor to cope with difficulty; cultivate and sustain social support; conduct web searches for helpful information; and solve problems creatively.
- *Encourage clients to generate ideas:* If clients seem willing to make even small changes, the CMES should let them take the lead in making suggestions that might work for them. The CMES should encourage clients to look for options that will work best in the context of clients' lives and abilities.
- *Ask permission before giving advice:* Clients only make use of advice to which they listen. Before launching into a lecture, a CMES should check to see whether clients are ready to listen. "Would you like more information on exercising to reduce high blood pressure?" If clients are ready to listen, the CMES should be prepared to provide helpful information. Attractive, readable handouts may help explain relevant issues about which the client desires more information.

COMMUNICATION STRATEGIES FOR EFFECTIVE EDUCATION

A CMES is often in the position of explaining and teaching material to their clients. They give instruction on the proper performance of exercises and other physical skills, and also explains cognitive material, such as describing the lifestyle factors that influence blood sugar regulation. Good communication strategies increase effective delivery of both types of information.

Motor Learning

Motor learning is the process of acquiring and improving motor skills. Many adult clients are quite self-conscious in the motor skill domain, especially if they have had little experience with sports and physical activity. Exercise professionals with a strong background in physical education and sports are often surprised at the lack of motor ability they see in many adult clients. Motor skills will be taught most effectively if the following communication strategies are kept in mind.

Remind Beginners That It Takes Time and Practice to Improve Motor Skills

Physical-education specialists have noted that many people tend to believe that good coordination and athletic ability are things with which a person is born (Rink, 2004). While ability in the motor-skills domain certainly varies from person to person, motor skills are more strongly related to practice and experience than to natural ability alone. It is important for people new to physical activity to understand that motor-skill improvement takes a great deal of practice; the people they see in exercise classes have often been performing similar movement patterns and choreography for years. The same holds true for athletes in every sport.

Many clients new to exercise feel self-conscious attending a new exercise class or participating in an exercise-training situation. They may feel out of place, awkward, and clumsy. The CMES must help new clients feel at home in the exercise environment and help new learners understand that most of the people they see working out have been performing these types of activities for months, years, or even decades.

It is also important to note that even clients with athletic experience may feel awkward when learning new motor skills. Such clients may believe that they should pick up new motor skills quickly, remembering how good they were at sports when they were younger. They may be frustrated if motor learning does not come quickly and easily (Rink, 2004). The CMES should reassure new clients that it is okay to be a beginner, and that with practice they will eventually look like fitness center regulars.

If clients appear to be self-conscious and nervous, the CMES should encourage them to relax and focus on the task at hand. If the CMES is demonstrating a skill, such as using a piece of exercise equipment, and a client does not appear to be watching, the CMES should draw the client's attention back to the demonstration and direct the client to focus on details of the motor skill.

Introduce a New Skill Slowly and Clearly

When introducing a new skill, the CMES should begin with a very short explanation of what they are going to do and why. Explanations should be clear and concise. Safety information should be emphasized, along with guidelines for preventing injury. A skill should be explained in terms of what it is accomplishing or why it is important.

When describing certain movements, the CMES should focus on the goal of the movement rather than giving distracting details about limb position (Marchant, Clough, & Cramshaw, 2005). For example, the CMES would not teach someone how to use an elliptical trainer by describing when to bend and straighten the knees. Instead, the CMES would emphasize moving the pedals around in a smooth, steady motion. The CMES should demonstrate the skill accurately and allow clients time to watch.

However, teaching strength-training exercises or exercise positions does require some explanation of limb position for safety and efficacy. For example, when teaching squats, the CMES might ask the client to focus on keeping their abdominals braced throughout the exercise movement. Descriptions should be brief and simple.

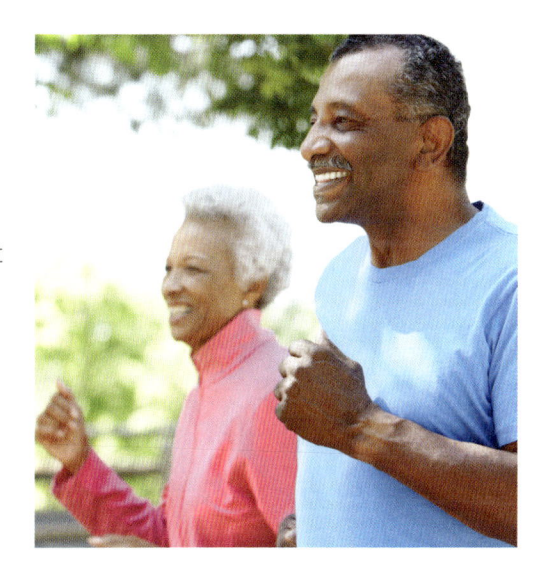

Adapt Teaching Methods to Each Client's Learning Style When Possible

Variations in the way people process and retain new information have been called learning style differences. Some clients like a lot of explanation and ask many questions (verbal learning style). Others learn better by watching and appreciate longer demonstrations with less talking (visual learning style), while others learn by doing, needing to feel the movement before catching on (kinesthetic learning style). Most people appreciate a blend of these three approaches. Once the CMES has been working with a particular client for a period of time, learning styles may become apparent. Clients may also be able to let the CMES know how they learn best, asking for longer demonstrations or more detailed explanations. The teaching pace should be comfortable for clients, allowing them to learn one skill before moving on to another.

Allow Clients the Opportunity for Focused Practice

People learn more quickly when they focus on performing the motor skill without being distracted by talking or listening. The CMES should not talk for a few minutes while the client is trying a new skill, and should encourage the client to give the skill a few tries without talking (except to interrupt the client to prevent an accident or injury) (Coker, Fischman, & Oxendine, 2006).

Give Helpful Feedback

Once clients have tried the skill, the CMES should give the following helpful feedback:
- Provide reinforcement for what was done well
- Correct errors
- Motivate clients to continue practicing and improving

Correcting errors, which may be seen as the more "negative" point, should be sandwiched between reinforcement and motivation (Coker, Fischman, & Oxendine, 2006). An example might be, "Your breathing and timing were just right on the first four lifts. Remember to keep breathing, even as the exercise starts to feel harder. You'll find the work easier now that you are learning how to breathe correctly."

The CMES should limit feedback to a few simple points, and decide which errors are the most important to correct first. Most important errors typically include those that involve safety, occur earliest in the movement sequence, or are fundamental in some other way. Feedback should be phrased positively, pointing out what clients should do: "Remember to breathe," rather than "Don't hold your breath."

Cognitive Learning

The CMES should also be able to provide effective instruction to clients about health- and exercise-related topics. Clients often ask health and exercise professionals to explain things like why exercise improves blood sugar regulation, what is meant by **overtraining,** or what is indicated by a pain in a certain area of the body. It is often enough to simply answer the question, giving clients the information they desire without launching into a detailed discussion filled with complex **exercise physiology** concepts. At other times, the CMES may need to teach clients information in a classroom or discussion setting on a particular topic. Guidelines for effective teaching in the cognitive domain are covered in the following sections.

Clarify Instructional Goals

A CMES may find themselves teaching material to clients for many reasons. Clarifying instructional goals can help the CMES decide on the most effective approach for a given situation.

In many cases, the CMES may need to give clients specific directions that should be followed as part of an exercise plan. In such cases, instructions should always be written as well as delivered verbally. Whenever material has an important bearing on the client's behavior, written explanations tailored to the client's educational level and language skills are essential.

Sometimes the CMES may wish to stimulate a client to make a change in their behavior, perhaps by convincing them of the importance of exercise. Many clients appreciate evidence that backs up the points the CMES is trying to make. Clients might like a list of helpful websites or well-written articles from respected experts.

Engage Learners

Readers who have spent time in classrooms know the sad truth: Dry factual information does not stick and the audience's attention will begin to wander after a very short period of lecturing. Only a very motivated audience learns much from a lecture composed solely of one person talking (Ennis, 2007).

To engage learners, the CMES must somehow make the material interesting, meaningful, and relevant to the learner. Pictures or slides promote engagement with the material, as do worksheets that get clients writing. The CMES can get clients involved by passing out a questionnaire that enables them to rate themselves on the topic of discussion, such as stress level or diet quality. Clients might interview each other about the topic and report results back to the larger group.

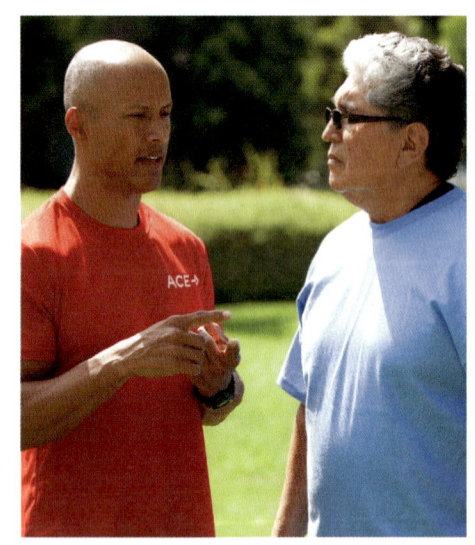

Use Instructional Media Wisely

Audiovisual aids enhance a presentation when used well. Many clients learn more effectively if visual images accompany a speaker's words. Music enhances learners' experiences, but only if learners find the music appealing.

Invite Motivational Guest Speakers

People love personal success stories. The CMES can invite role models of the behavior under discussion, such as a former client with diabetes who lost weight via a well-balanced diet and exercise program. Such speakers help build client self-efficacy, and thus enhance exercise adherence.

Entertain the Audience

Entertainment should be at the heart of many instructional sessions, since people can be entertained and learn at the same time. Entertainment can also be a motivator to return for more fun. Instructional material can be transmitted through personal stories and appropriately funny remarks.

SUMMARY

The CMES will be most effective when they are able to communicate effectively and build good rapport with clients. An understanding of communication strategies and practice of the OARS skills helps the CMES plan exercise recommendations and strategies that are most likely to motivate clients to adhere to their exercise programs. As the CMES works with clients in the realms of both motor and cognitive learning, good communication practices facilitate learning.

REFERENCES

Ambady, N. & Gray, H.M. (2002). On being sad and mistaken: Mood effects on the accuracy of thin-slice judgments. *Journal of Personality and Social Psychology*, 83, 4, 947–961.

Ambady, N. & Weisbuch, M. (2010). Nonverbal behavior. In: Fiske, S.T., Gilbert, D.T., & Lindzey, G. (Eds.). *Handbook of Social Psychology* (pp. 464–497). New York: McGraw-Hill.

Ambady, N. et al. (2002). Physical therapists' nonverbal communication predicts geriatric patients' health outcomes. *Psychology and Aging*, 17, 3, 443–452.

American Council on Exercise (2019). *The Professional's Guide to Health and Wellness Coaching.* San Diego: American Council on Exercise.

Biesanz, J.C. et al. (2011). Do we know when our impressions of others are valid? Evidence for realistic accuracy awareness in first impressions of personality. *Social Psychological and Personality Science*, 2, 5, 452–459.

Brehm, B.A. (2014a). Communication and teaching techniques. In: American Council on Exercise. *ACE Personal Trainer Manual* (5th ed.) (pp. 42–65). San Diego, Calif.: American Council on Exercise.

Brehm, B.A. (2014b). *Psychology of Health and Fitness.* Philadelphia: FA Davis.

Brown, C. (2005). Injuries: The psychology of recovery and rehab. In: Murphy, S. (Ed.) *The Sport Psych Handbook.* Champaign, Ill.: Human Kinetics.

Coker, C.A., Fischman, M.G., & Oxendine, J.B. (2006). Motor skill learning for effective coaching and performance. In: Williams, J.M. (Ed.) *Applied Sport Psychology.* New York: McGraw-Hill.

Conner, M. et al. (2011). Changing exercise through targeting affective or cognitive attitudes. *Psychology and Health*, 26, 2, 133–149.

Deci, E.L. & Ryan, R.M. (2008). Facilitating optimal motivation and psychological well-being across life's domains. *Canadian Psychology*, 49, 1, 14–23.

Ennis, C.D. (2007). Defining learning as conceptual change in physical education and physical activity settings. *Research Quarterly for Exercise and Sport*, 78, 3, 138–151.

George, M. (2008). Interactions in expert service work: Demonstrating professionalism in personal training. *Journal of Contemporary Ethnography*, 37, 1, 108–131.

Maciejewski, P.K. et al. (2007). An empirical examination of the stage theory of grief. *Journal of the American Medical Association*, 297, 7, 716–724.

Maguire, J.S. (2008). The personal is professional: Personal trainers as a case study of cultural intermediaries. *International Journal of Cultural Studies,* 11, 2, 211–229.

Marchant, D., Clough, P., & Cramshaw, M. (2005). Influence of attentional focusing strategies during practice and performance of a motor skill. *Journal of Sports Sciences,* 23, 11, 1258–1259.

Mast, M.S. (2007). On the importance of nonverbal communication in the physician-patient interaction. *Patient Education and Counseling,* 67, 3, 315–318.

Miller, W.R. & Rollnick, S. (2013). *Motivational Interviewing: Preparing People to Change* (3rd ed.). New York: Guilford Press.

Miller, W.R. & Rose, G.R. (2009). Toward a theory of motivational interviewing. *American Psychologist,* 64, 6, 527–537.

Nease, D.E. & Malouin, J.M. (2003). Depression screening: A practical strategy. *Journal of Family Practice,* 52, 2, 118–124.

Pfister-Minogue, K.A. & Salveson, C. (2010). Training and experience of public health nurses in using behavior change counseling. *Public Health Nursing,* 27, 6, 544–551.

Rider, E.A. & Keefer, C.H. (2006). Communication skills competencies: Definitions and a teaching toolbox. *Medical Education,* 40, 624–629.

Rink, J.E. (2004). It's okay to be a beginner: Teach a motor skill, and the skill may be learned. *Journal of Physical Education, Recreation, and Dance,* 75, 6, 31–35.

Rollnick, S., Miller, W.R., & Butler, C.C. (2008). *Motivational Interviewing in Health Care: Helping Patients Change Behavior.* New York: Guilford Press.

Ryan, R.M. et al. (2011). Motivation and autonomy in counseling, psychotherapy, and behavior change: A look at theory and practice. *The Counseling Psychologist,* 39, 2, 193–260.

Seligman, M.E.P. (2008). Positive health. *Applied Psychology,* 57, 3–18.

SUGGESTED READING

American Council on Exercise (2019). *The Professional's Guide to Health and Wellness Coaching.* San Diego: American Council on Exercise.

Brehm, B.A. (2014). *Psychology of Health and Fitness.* Philadelphia: F.A. Davis.

Miller, W.R. & Rollnick, S. (2013). *Motivational Interviewing: Preparing People to Change* (3rd ed.). New York: Guilford Press.

Ryan, R.M. et al. (2011). Motivation and autonomy in counseling, psychotherapy, and behavior change: A look at theory and practice. *The Counseling Psychologist,* 39, 2, 193–260.

6 PROFESSIONAL RELATIONSHIPS AND BUSINESS STRATEGIES

IN THIS CHAPTER

COMMUNICATING WITH ALLIED HEALTHCARE PROFESSIONALS

CONSULTATION NOTES

SOAP NOTES

CONFIDENTIALITY ISSUES

MARKETING THE BUSINESS FOR MEDICAL REFERRALS

BILLING AND PAYMENT POLICIES

LEGAL ISSUES, LIABILITIES, AND PROFESSIONAL RESPONSIBILITIES

ETHICS POLICY

LEGAL ISSUES AND LIABILITIES

AVOIDING LEGAL RISKS

EMPLOYMENT OPTIONS

BUSINESS PLANNING

EXECUTIVE SUMMARY

BUSINESS DESCRIPTION

MARKETING PLAN

OPERATIONAL PLAN

RISK ANALYSIS

DECISION-MAKING CRITERIA

SUMMARY

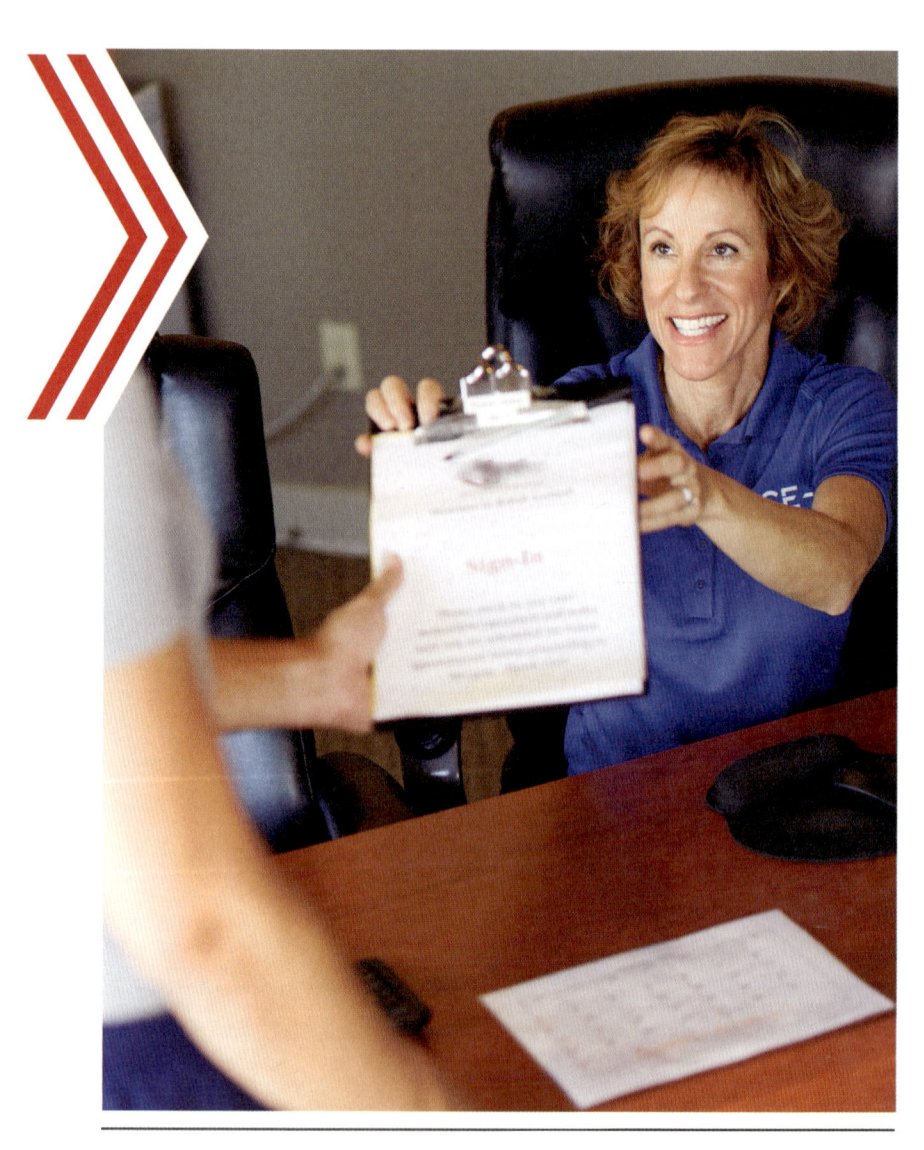

ABOUT THE AUTHOR

Lisa Coors, M.B.A., is the owner of Coors Core Fitness, LLC, a post-rehabilitation and sport-specific personal-training business located inside Wellington Orthopaedic and Sports Medicine in Cincinnati, Ohio, where she has developed a successful model partnering personal training with the local medical communities. In 2012, she started the Women's Fitness Association as a resource to mentor and educate women in the fitness industry. Coors is a two-time graduate of Xavier University, where she earned a Bachelor of Science degree in chemical science and her M.B.A. in general business. Coors is an ACE® Certified Medical Exercise Specialist. Coors is a national presenter in the fitness industry, was the 2006 first runner-up for ACE's Personal Trainer of the Year award, and serves as a subject matter expert for ACE.

By Lisa Coors

ONE OF THE MOST IMPORTANT ROLES OF an ACE® Certified Medical Exercise Specialist (CMES) is bridging the gap between the fitness industry and the allied healthcare professional field (e.g., physicians, physical therapists, occupational therapists, and athletic trainers). Networking is used to facilitate communication between multiple parties.

The establishment of this line of communication brings a win-win situation to everyone involved. By communicating with the CMES, allied healthcare professionals can get a better sense of the training progressions that may be used with one of their patients. Allied healthcare professionals also gain a sense of how working with an experienced and certified exercise professional can be an important next step for a patient. The CMES, meanwhile, can gain a referral base for new clients while learning more about the condition a particular client may have. Allied healthcare professionals are an excellent resource for the CMES.

Effective communication with a client's physician should be based on the following objectives:
- Obtaining medical clearance for a client
- Determining the physical limitations of a client
- Obtaining recommendations regarding exercise program design
- Introducing the CMES and their services
- Clarifying questions on the client's health/medical status
- Obtaining special considerations related to the client's health (e.g., a chronic disease such as **diabetes** or **hypertension**)
- Obtaining a list of medications with potential exercise-related side effects
- Providing progress reports on the exercise program, or receiving health status updates
- Establishing **rapport** with a potential referral source

COMMUNICATING WITH ALLIED HEALTHCARE PROFESSIONALS

There are many options for networking with allied healthcare professionals. The first step in the communication, however, should always be a completed medical release form (see Figure 3-7, page 85). This form provides the CMES with the client's medical information and explains physical-activity limitations and/or guidelines as outlined by the physicians. Any deviation from these guidelines must be approved by the client's personal physician. It is advised that the CMES send a medical release to all allied healthcare professionals that a particular patient/client may be seeing. An example would be a client who has **Parkinson's disease (PD),** had a hip replacement within the last year, and has obesity. A CMES should send a medical release to the movement disorder specialist (Parkinson's disease), orthopedic physician (hip replacement), physical therapist (hip replacement), and internal medicine doctor (general health and **obesity**). In this scenario, the CMES would gain four new contacts with allied healthcare professionals. The CMES should maintain a spreadsheet of all allied healthcare professionals with whom they have communicated for future reference.

LEARNING OBJECTIVES:

» Employ effective strategies for communicating with allied healthcare professionals and protecting confidential client information.

» Implement marketing, billing, and payment policies to foster a successful business for the CMES.

» Describe legal issues, liabilities, and professional responsibilities associated with doing business as a CMES.

» Develop a basic business plan based on established tools and resources for new and existing business owners.

There are five main options that can be used as means of communicating with a client's allied healthcare professionals: the medical release, progress notes, general communications (e.g., fax, email, or phone), visits, and promotional materials and events. The medical release is the first and most important tool in initiating allied healthcare professional communications. Once reviewed by an attorney, the medical release should abide by the **Health Insurance Portability and Accountability Act (HIPAA).** The medical release should include an area for the CMES to write in the conditions that are specific to that client. Line item examples would include **osteoporosis,** obesity, breast cancer, diabetes, and hypertension.

Next, a place is provided where the allied healthcare professional signs their name and dates the document. The most important component is the area where the allied healthcare professional is asked to write contraindications and/or restrictions to training this client/patient. Not all allied healthcare professionals will write in this area. It is up to the CMES to call the allied healthcare professionals and ask for more clarification, if necessary. A CMES, though trained to understand contraindications, should make no assumptions before talking to the allied healthcare professional.

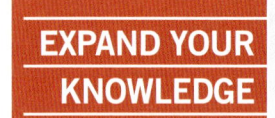

EXPAND YOUR KNOWLEDGE

HIPAA PRIVACY RULE HIGHLIGHTS

While exercise professionals are not technically bound by the HIPAA privacy rules, ACE encourages all of its certified professionals to adhere to these standards in an effort to display the utmost professionalism and be consistent with the standard of practice in the healthcare community.

- Health information protected by the law (i.e., "protected health information") includes all individually identifiable health information in any form, whether electronic, paper, or oral. Health information includes the individual's past, present, or future physical or mental health condition; the provision of healthcare to the individual; and the past, present, or future payment for the provision of healthcare to the individual.
- The Privacy Rule applies to any healthcare provider, including all "providers of medical or health services" as defined by Medicare, and any other person or organization that furnishes, bills, or is paid for healthcare.
- The Privacy Rule permits a covered entity to use and disclose protected health information for research purposes without an individual's authorization, provided the covered entity obtains necessary documentation of approval solely for the research from an Institutional Review Board or Privacy Board. Further, the researcher and/or covered entity must not remove any protected health information.
- A covered entity must obtain the individual's written authorization for any use or disclosure of protected health information that is not for treatment, payment, or healthcare operations.
- A covered entity must obtain an authorization to use or disclose protected health information for marketing.
- A covered entity must make reasonable efforts to use, disclose, and request only the minimum amount of protected health information needed to accomplish the intended purpose.
- Each covered entity must provide notice of its privacy practices.
- A covered entity must maintain reasonable and appropriate administrative, technical, and physical safeguards to prevent intentional or unintentional use or disclosure of protected health information, including shredding documents before discarding them, securing records with lock and key or passcode, and limiting access to keys or pass codes.

Source: U.S. Department of Health and Human Services (2014). *Summary of the HIPAA Privacy Rule.* www.hhs.gov/ocr/privacy/hipaa/understanding/summary/; retrieved March 3, 2014.

Note: This information serves exclusively to orient readers to the highlights of the HIPAA Privacy Rule and does not represent legal interpretation or advice.

An introductory letter or fax cover sheet should accompany the medical release and be used to introduce the CMES, present data or **SOAP notes** (subjective, objective, assessment, plan) on that particular client (see page 149), and present a possible training progression (Figure 6-1). The CMES may also wish to include a question regarding client contraindications or restrictions in the introductory letter to emphasize that this information is needed to appropriately train the client.

Professional Relationships and Business Strategies — CHAPTER 6

SAMPLE INTRODUCTORY LETTER

Dear Dr. Cox:

Sedentary lifestyle is considered to be a major health risk factor. Despite the proven benefits of physical activity, only approximately 20% of U.S. adults meet both aerobic activity and muscle-strengthening guidelines. Additionally, nearly 50% of those who begin exercising stop within the first six months. Exercise has been shown to improve medical outcomes in chronic diseases such as diabetes, hypertension, and coronary artery disease. However, few individuals know how to begin a safe, effective exercise program. I can help.

My name is Pedro Ruiz and I am a Certified Medical Exercise Specialist (CMES) at The Health and Fitness Institute in Baltimore. My certification is from the American Council on Exercise (ACE). As a CMES, I have a background in evaluating individuals referred to me by their physicians for design and supervision of a safe and effective exercise program. My evaluation includes:

- Exercise history
- Exercise likes and dislikes
- Aerobic power (METs)
- Body-composition analysis with impedance, anthropometric measurements, and body mass index calculations
- Muscular fitness assessment
- Range-of-motion evaluation

Once I have evaluated the client, with your specific instructions, I tailor an exercise program that usually includes both aerobic and resistance training. I monitor the client's progress and frequently provide you with progress reports and follow-up information.

Our facility provides a wide range of aerobic and resistance-training equipment, a pool for water aerobics, and professionally instructed and supervised group fitness classes.

I would like to offer my services to you and your patients. Enclosed is some material explaining the role of a CMES, as well as an article on exercise for special populations. Please feel free to use me as a resource for this type of information, as well as a referral source for your patients.

I would be happy to further discuss referrals at your convenience. My telephone number is 999-999-9999, and my email address is _____ @__.

I look forward to working with you to help improve your patients' health and overall quality of life.

Sincerely,
Pedro Ruiz
ACE Certified Medical Exercise Specialist

Figure 6-1
Sample introductory letter to a physician

Visit www.ACEfitness.org/CMESresources to download a free PDF of a sample introductory letter to a physician, as well as other forms and tools that you can use throughout your career as a CMES.

The introductory letter or fax cover sheet should also include the CMES's contact information so that the allied healthcare professional can return the signed release. This is an effective way for an allied healthcare professional to learn what the CMES is doing with the patient. It is also a great networking piece for the CMES.

The second channel in networking is the progress note, which should be typed and sent to each allied healthcare professional from whom the CMES has a medical release for a particular client. These progress notes are sent at the discretion of the CMES, but it is a good idea to send one every other month or right before a doctor's visit. Information presented may include details on the client's progress (e.g., weight loss, increased flexibility, decreased pain, or decreased blood pressure).

Information regarding a progression in exercise selection is also an effective means of showing how well a client is performing. Progress notes are essentially any written account of sessions with clients, and these notes can come in the form of SOAP notes.

General communications like faxes, emails, and phone calls are great for fine-tuning the communication channels with allied healthcare professionals. A CMES should have all physicians' contact information on the initial medical release and health-history forms. When working with physicians who are difficult to contact, finding out who their nurses are can help. Sometimes it is much easier to speak with a physician's nurse or medical assistant to communicate information about a client. It is important that the CMES is respectful and mindful of how busy most physicians are.

A surefire way to network with allied healthcare professionals is to make office visits. The easiest way to do this is to attend a visit with the client. Doing so gives the CMES higher credibility in that it shows that they truly care about the client. A CMES can also compile a list of all allied healthcare professionals from all clients and set goals of having one-on-one meetings with each of those professionals over the course of the year. Giving an allied healthcare professional a face to go with the name is a great way for the CMES to brand themself and the business.

The last channel of networking is through promotional events. Attending or speaking at a promotional event is a great opportunity for the CMES to meet other individuals who are also interested in health and fitness information. Furthermore, many clients with health challenges are aware of events pertaining to their particular condition, such as a "Race for the Cure" for Breast Cancer Awareness Month or the American Diabetes Association's Walk to Stop Diabetes. Local events, including symposiums, conferences, athletic events/races, support groups, and continuing education classes, are great places to meet local allied healthcare professionals.

Promotional campaigns within a health facility setting are another great idea for networking. A CMES and their fitness department can have "open houses" or "networking events" for allied healthcare professionals. This technique works well in that it brings allied healthcare professionals into the fitness facility to see first-hand where their patients will be trained. It also allows them to network with the actual trainers.

Networking with allied healthcare professionals is a great way to expand the awareness of the benefits that a CMES can provide to clients. Until recently, allied healthcare professionals and exercise professionals were not working as a team to help patients/clients, but the barriers between the two groups are breaking down and important relationships are being formed.

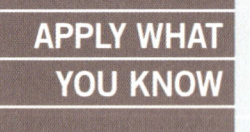

APPLY WHAT YOU KNOW

NETWORKING

For a CMES, building and retaining clientele is critical for success. Traditionally, the best tool in achieving this involves getting connected with networking groups, which allows the CMES to get the word out about the services offered in their fitness club or personal business. Networking groups also bring health and exercise professionals into the business world, increasing the professionalism of the fitness industry. Choosing a networking group may be as easy as opening the Sunday newspaper to find local groups. Anywhere from local Chamber of Commerce meetings to small business networking groups are great places to start. Prior to attending the meeting, prepare a short mission statement that describes who you are, what you do, and how you do it.

After going to a networking event, a CMES should send emails or personally written notes to each of the people with whom they connected at the event. After collecting business cards from individuals, the CMES should write on the back of the card the date, the name of the event, and a few words that can serve as reminders of any pertinent conversations.

Another increasingly valuable tool is the creation of a strong online presence through social media. Refer to pages 162–164 for a discussion of "Virtual Tools for the Certified Medical Exercise Specialist."

THINK IT THROUGH

How comfortable are you with the notion, and actual process, of networking? Many people struggle when introducing themselves to strangers, actively promoting their services, and making those all-important professional connections. If this is an area of concern for you, how might you address this potential weakness?

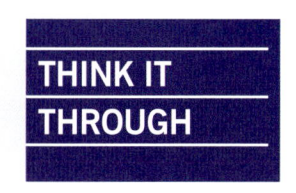

The client folder is an important item for the CMES to maintain. Client folders should include the following:
- Health history
- Medical releases
- Informed consent
- Liability waiver
- Training contracts
- Correspondence sheets
- Initial assessments
- Additional assessments
- Training progressions
- Consultation notes
- SOAP notes

A good way to start a professionally maintained client folder is to begin with the original documentation, which includes a health-history questionnaire (see Figure 3-4, page 79). The health-history form is the initial document used in each client's folder. The informed consent and training contract should be drawn up by a lawyer if the CMES is self-employed, or by the fitness facility's attorney. Once a CMES starts networking with their clients' allied healthcare professionals, all phone notes, emails, and faxes, as well as copies of any progress notes or other correspondence, should be included in the clients' folders. Other elements of the client folder are the initial assessment data, additional assessments, and the training progression sheet.

Consultation Notes

Medical clearance improves the safety margin from which a program may be created. For the CMES, having access to other professionals builds credibility and offers resources for consultation and reference. It also has the potential to build market share for the CMES's services. However, finding and maintaining relationships with other professionals can be a daunting experience for some individuals. It should be a relief to know that most potential team members are more than willing to network services.

When making contact with a physician or other healthcare practitioner, it may be advantageous to start with a physician with whom the CMES is already familiar. Meeting with a client's personal physician is an effective way to gain future referrals, though the CMES must be sure to obtain written permission from the client to meet their physician. A CMES may go to physician appointments with their clients, as this is the easiest way to meet with the physician. It also gives the CMES credibility when the client communicates having made progress in achieving their fitness goals. A client's success in working with a CMES is the best word-of-mouth marketing available.

The most difficult way to make initial contact is by "cold calling" an office to request an appointment. Once at the appointment, keep the presentation brief and collaborative in nature. Explain the concept of the CMES within a few minutes (no more than three), and describe the importance of having a place to refer patients with medical issues or special needs. Providing a brief written biography that includes education, credentials, and pertinent experience is beneficial, as are referral forms.

Physicians who might be the most open to a team relationship with a CMES include family practice and internal medicine specialists. Many of their patients are generally healthy, with controllable risk factors and/or manageable chronic medical conditions (e.g., hypertension, diabetes, or obesity). Members of these populations will benefit most from lifestyle changes. When a CMES collaborates with a primary care provider, the burden of compliance can be shared. Once an effective change has been made in one client, it is more likely that the physician will refer other patients to the CMES. There may also be the potential for the physician to refer colleagues, further expanding the team.

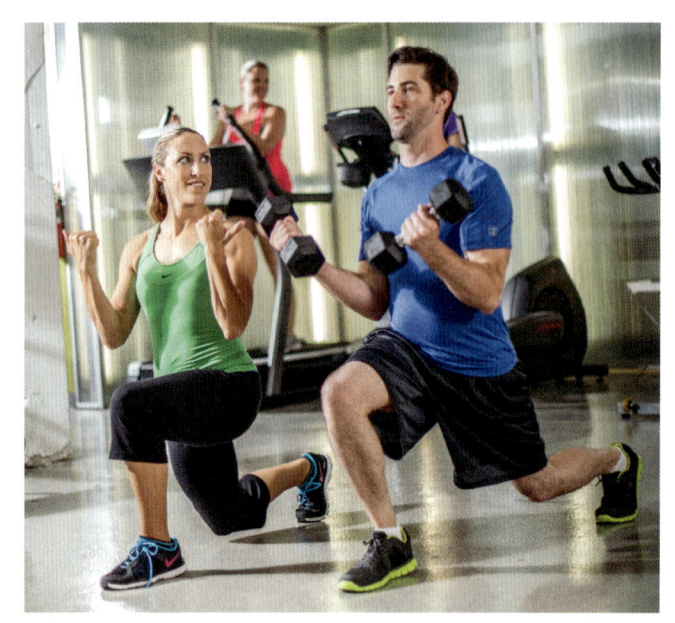

The CMES should send progress reports to a client's physicians every month or when goals have been achieved. The CMES should also send a progress report prior to a client's appointment with a particular physician. These reports can be faxed or emailed to the physician's office with a follow-up call to the physician or physician's nurse. The CMES should make sure all parties know their name and the reason for the call.

A CMES must get used to dealing with numerous types of physicians. Internal medicine and family practice physicians tend to be easier to contact. Specialists like neurologists, orthopedists, and cardiologists may be more difficult due to surgery schedules and hospital visits. Attending office visits with a client, as described above, is usually the easiest means to meet with these specialists.

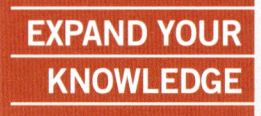

EXPAND YOUR KNOWLEDGE

MASTERING THE INITIAL CONSULTATION

The initial contact with a client typically involves gathering useful information. The key to establishing rapport and allowing an opportunity for the client to give the most useful information is the use of active listening. It is recommended that the CMES use an open-ended statement to allow the client to speak freely. Statements such as, "Tell me about yourself," delivered in a private setting, will most likely allow the client to give a more complete history of their challenges and successes. Allow the client to speak freely, and ask clarifying questions at regular intervals while maintaining good eye contact and mirroring the client's mood and body language. If notes are being taken, write down a few key words rather than transcribing entire sentences. Staying focused and actively engaged with the new client will assist with gathering the most useful and complete history.

Most consultation notes will have elements of the following:

- *Chief complaint:* Identify the challenges that the client is experiencing. It is recommended that dates and circumstances surrounding each of their health issues be elicited fully using open-ended, active questioning. Identify the client's feelings surrounding the challenges and barriers to change, as doing so will offer potential solutions in the planning stage. Employ the following strategies in active questioning:
  ✓ Explore needs, motivations, desires, skills, and thought processes. Facilitate the client's own thought processes in order to identify solutions and actions.
  ✓ Observe and listen actively to the client's description of their life circumstances.
  ✓ Maintain unconditional positive regard for the client. Be supportive and non-judgmental of the client's lifestyle and goals.
- *Past history:* How has the client attempted to work through this challenge in the past? What were successful strategies? What strategies did not work?
- *Current diet/medications/exercise program:* Inquire as to specifics regarding the client's eating habits and exercise program. The client may not have analyzed their eating, exercise, or behavior styles objectively. The CMES should strive to be unbiased and non-critical to promote honesty.

- *Social history:* Identify the client's environment, support structure, and sources of potential lifestyle stressors.
- *Physical assessment:* This involves the assessment of physical abilities, any biomechanical deficiencies or asymmetries, strength/flexibility/endurance factors, and so on. Use objective tests and measurements for future reference. It is important to note that there is no need to perform non-essential tests at the outset, as many clients are discouraged by the results, which can adversely affect motivation levels. List challenges and any correlation with identifiable stressors or barriers.
- *Plan:* Propose strategies to address each item listed under the assessment. Keep the following in mind when partnering with the client on a proposed plan:
  ✓ Identify realistic goals and objective means of assessing progress.
  ✓ Develop personal competencies and avoid dependency upon the CMES.
  ✓ Encourage personal choice to act positively toward each goal.
  ✓ Work within the framework of the client's competency to achieve change.
  ✓ Assist the individual in making real, lasting change by focusing on positive emotions.

THINK IT THROUGH

WRITING A CONSULTATION NOTE

A 35-year-old male accountant comes to you after being diagnosed with **multiple sclerosis (MS)**. MS lesions were detected in his lumbar spine. He plays soccer on an adult recreation team three days per week. He tore the **anterior cruciate ligament (ACL)** in his right knee 10 years ago and still experiences pain. His major symptoms are pain and occasional tingling in both of his legs when he plays soccer for more than two hours. He also swims two days per week for 45 minutes per workout.

The results of his physical from his family practice physician are as follows:
- Blood pressure: 115/65 mmHg
- Total blood cholesterol: 190 mg/dL
- Fasting blood sugar: 85 mg/dL
- He is 5'10" tall and weighs 175 lb

His goals are to decrease the pain in his right knee and perform exercises to decrease the pain and occasional tingling in his legs, which may be related to his MS. What would your consultation notes for this client look like?

SOAP Notes

In general, most professionals create value when they are engaged with client-related activities, even when not face-to-face. As such, time that is spent on client activities that do not involve direct contact with the client, however necessary, becomes administrative time. Most effective team leaders limit the amount of administrative work they must perform personally in order to optimize their schedules. Efficient methods of communicating with other professionals regarding mutual clients have been developed to best serve the client by minimizing the required administrative time.

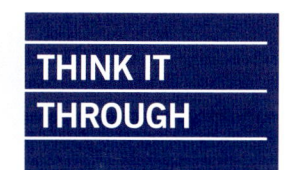

Recalling specific client information is paramount to team communication. A CMES typically has many clients, making it difficult to keep track of the details of each client's health status. For this reason, there should be some recordkeeping mechanism that allows for recall. When calling or meeting to discuss a mutual client, be ready to give their full name, age, gender, and some identifying information (e.g., birth date) to allow the other team member to pull up the documentation of the last visit. Be brief and direct when stating the nature of the discussion, keeping the purpose to two or three sentences at most. Having these details on hand will facilitate the discussion with other team members. Being concise in communications is a positive marker of a professional. It demonstrates that the caller has an appreciation for the value of time for both parties, while keeping the best interest of the mutual client in mind. Using the SOAP note format, the vital information about a client can be communicated very efficiently to a healthcare practitioner, typically within one minute. Being able to use this presentation skill with all team members decreases the amount of time performing non-compensated administrative activities, yet effectively harnesses the contributions of each member of the team. Some members of the healthcare team may prefer written updates.

The frequency of contact is somewhat established by those who interface with the particular professional on a regular basis. Typically, team members should expect to receive updates every four to six weeks. More frequent communication may be perceived by the team member as offering too much contact without being able to report on actual change. Communication that takes place less frequently than about every eight weeks runs the risk of being forgotten. For example, if a client is also seeing a **registered dietitian (RD)** or psychologist, four- to six-week intervals are typical, as this allows for measurable change that is used to assess the effectiveness of ongoing programs.

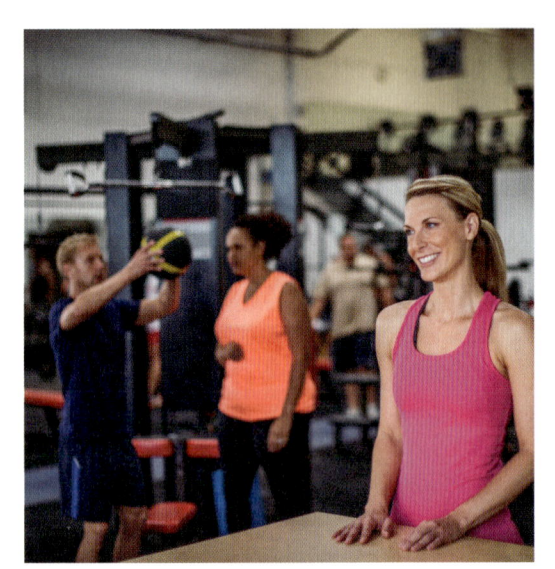

SOAP is an acronym for subjective, objective, assessment, and plan. A SOAP note is intended to improve communication among all those caring for a given client, communicate pertinent characteristics, and provide the assessment, problems, and plans in an organized format to facilitate the care of the client. Depending on the facility, SOAP notes may also be used for record review and quality control. Documentation of a client's characteristics, program concerns, and related plans must be consistent, concise, and comprehensive. As such, SOAP notes are commonly written by physicians and other licensed healthcare providers, such as a physician assistant, physical therapist, or licensed nurse practitioner. Many medical offices use the SOAP note format to standardize medical evaluation entries made in clinical records. Given this standard, SOAP notes provide an excellent method for the CMES to gather information and communicate client status during the referral process.

The components of a SOAP note are as follows:
- *Subjective:* The initial portion of the SOAP note consists of subjective observations. These are symptoms verbalized by the client or by a significant other. These subjective observations include the client's descriptions of pain or discomfort, the presence of shortness of breath or dizziness on exertion, or a multitude of other descriptions of any dysfunction, discomfort, or illness.
- *Objective:* The next portion is the objective observation, which includes symptoms that can actually be measured, seen, heard, touched, or felt. Objective observations include vital signs such as resting heart rate, blood pressure, body weight, percent body fat, waist circumference, and the results of any other related tests or evaluations.
- *Assessment:* The assessment follows the objective observations and is a statement of the client's condition. In some cases, this statement may be clear, such as "moderately obese." In other instances, an assessment may not be as clear and can include several possibilities. *Note:* The word "statement" is used quite intentionally in this description. In the medical field, the assessment is usually a "diagnosis," but the **scope of practice** for a CMES does not include making medical diagnoses. Therefore, any reference to a diagnosis should be avoided.
- *Plan:* The last part of the SOAP note is the plan. The plan may include further fitness testing or other diagnostic testing [e.g., **dual-energy x-ray absorptiometry (DXA)**]. This is where a referral to another healthcare professional would be noted. This is also the section where a CMES would record their appropriate plan in terms of exercise, nutrition, and adherence strategies.

Remember, the SOAP note is not supposed to be as detailed as a progress report. Complete sentences are not necessary and abbreviations are appropriate. However, the CMES should avoid using abbreviations until they have a thorough knowledge of how they are used. Abbreviations differ for each specialty and should be consistent within the facility in which the CMES works. The length of the note will differ depending on the use. SOAP notes that follow each client session will likely be shorter than ones that accompany a referral letter. SOAP notes can be flexible. Many health and exercise professionals often develop their own styles as they accommodate varied preferences.

SOAP NOTE CASE EXAMPLE

APPLY WHAT YOU KNOW

Peggy is a 55-year-old accountant who just completed her first month of exercise with a CMES. She sits at her desk all day and had not worked out for more than 10 years until one month ago. She was diagnosed with hypertension and has obesity. After initial assessment, it is noted that her height is 5'6" (1.7 m), her weight is 180 pounds (81 kg), and her body fat percentage is 40%. Her fitness goals are to lose weight while increasing flexibility and endurance. She was extremely intimidated to start a fitness program because of a fear of overexertion and having a heart attack. After the first month of training, she is experiencing sharp pain in her left hip that she feels while sitting or lying in bed. She does not feel the pain during exercise.

Associated SOAP Note

Patient Name: Peggy Jones   DOB: 09/17/58   Date: 04/27/14

S: Obese accountant with hypertension. Needs to lose significant weight, both lbs and body fat, while increasing flexibility and endurance. Was very intimidated to start exercising. Currently experiencing left hip pain while at rest.

O: 55 years old, height 5'6"(1.7 m), weight 180 lb (81 kg), and body fat 40%

A: 55-year-old sedentary woman needs a weight-loss program that will also help her manage her hypertension. She complains of left hip pain when she sits in a chair or lies down. She needs to see her physician prior to coming back for training.

P: CMES suggests that the client seek medical attention for left hip. CMES will not train client until she receives medical clearance.

Approach to Referring Peggy

The CMES explains to Peggy that working with individuals who are experiencing acute pain is outside the scope of practice for a CMES without first obtaining a medical evaluation and clearance from a client's physician. Therefore, the CMES informs Peggy that she needs to contact her physician to investigate her left hip pain.

The CMES must ask Peggy for permission to contact her primary care provider before proceeding any further. Permission must be in writing and kept in the client's file. When speaking with or writing to Peggy's physician, the CMES must outline their concerns, including the intensity of Peggy's program, her current response to exercise, and her stated goals. The CMES must ask Peggy's physician to send a letter providing medical clearance to continue exercise, along with any modifications related to the exercise program.

WRITING A SOAP NOTE

THINK IT THROUGH

Perla is a 20-year-old college student with obesity who is experiencing pain in her knees and hip joints. After a full physical exam from her internal medicine physician, her physician blames the pain on Perla's weight. She suggests Perla meet with a CMES to reduce her weight. Perla explains that she played soccer in high school but quit once she went to college. This is when she gained more than 50 pounds. She notes that she likes to exercise but needs a CMES to put together a workout schedule for her. She also needs motivation and is willing to see a CMES twice a week for an hour at a time.

Write a SOAP note for this client.

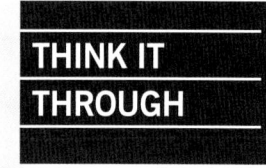

APPLY WHAT YOU KNOW

BARRIERS TO EFFECTIVE COMMUNICATION

Awareness of communication barriers can greatly facilitate the working relationship with healthcare providers and can lead to better coordinated client care. The CMES should use common courtesy, clarify expectations, and communicate clearly to avoid the following barriers to effective communication:

- *Timeliness of the communication:* Does the physician receive the referral letter within days, or within six weeks, of the initial session? Was the CMES able to call or send a letter before the physician had a follow-up visit with the client? Does the physician prefer calls or letters? Tardy communication places the physician in a position in which they are uninformed of what other team members are doing. This decreases the chance that the physician will send the CMES another referral. If the CMES knows the client has scheduled an appointment with the physician that will take place before they can send a letter, the CMES should consider contacting the physician via email or phone to give a brief report on any findings and recommendations. It is important to keep written notes in the client's file that detail any communications with the client or physician. The CMES should always be prompt and professional with all replies.
- *Lack of understanding of team member roles:* Physicians generally are unfamiliar with the role that the CMES can play in the healthcare team. Therefore, the CMES is in a position to educate physicians on what they have to offer. The method of doing so may include a communication to let the physician know that they can use the CMES as a resource for any fitness-related questions. Other means that the CMES can use to introduce themself to the physician include explaining their areas of expertise in all referral letters, personally visiting the physician's office, and sending pertinent articles on different aspects of exercise and health. As the CMES develops rapport with physicians, they will better understand their information needs.
- *Unclear expectations:* The root problem in many interpersonal and professional relationships is ambiguous or conflicting expectations (Covey, 2004). The CMES must be sure to understand what a physician expects, and then strive to deliver it. The CMES must be clear about what they have to offer the healthcare team and how to apply that expertise. It is important to let the physician know what kind of results clients can expect so that they may provide reinforcement when they see the client.
- *Reaching beyond the scope of practice:* If the CMES does not know an answer or cannot help an individual, they must be willing to refer the client to the appropriate member of the healthcare team. Refer to Chapter 1 and "Scope of Practice" on page 156 for more information.

CONFIDENTIALITY ISSUES

Because the CMES will keep track of confidential information on each client, it is absolutely essential that this information is kept in a locked file cabinet or be under password protection on a computer. The CMES should be the only one able to access these files. Clients expect that the CMES will keep all information private, which includes abstaining from sharing information with anyone but the client or any medical professionals from whom a medical release has been obtained (see Appendix A for the ACE Code of Ethics). Adherence to confidentiality policies is not only an ethical issue, but may also be a legal issue in some states or municipalities.

If any private information is communicated to someone other than the client or appropriate allied healthcare professional, the CMES and/or the facility can face legal action. To prevent a confidentiality breach, the CMES should adhere to the following guidelines:
- Client files should be stamped with "confidential" or "private."
- Client files should be kept in a locked file cabinet not accessible to the general public or other facility **employees.**
- Clients' folders should have all documentation papers clipped or stapled in so that papers are not lost.

- Fax machines should be in private areas not accessible to the general public. The CMES should be aware of when confidential fax transmittals are arriving so that the information stays private.
- All computer-based client information should be password protected. Firewalls should be used to ensure that no one steals client information.
- All employees working where confidential information is discussed with either another allied healthcare professional or the client should be made to sign a confidentiality policy developed by the company attorney. The policy should specify what legal consequences will occur if the policy is broken.
- All verbal discussion of client information should be done in private. This includes all phone calls and one-on-one client discussions.
- All transmittals such as faxes, email printouts, and written documentation should be put in client files. All other information should be shredded.
- The CMES should not talk to friends, family, employees, or coworkers about client information.

THINK IT THROUGH

What steps can be taken in your current business to better secure each client's confidentiality? Can you think of any behaviors in your daily practice that might compromise someone's confidentiality, such as placing a client's folder in a common area during a training session or leaving a client's information on a computer screen? As you perform your assessment, be sure to eliminate potential breaches if any are found.

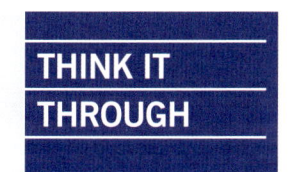

MARKETING THE BUSINESS FOR MEDICAL REFERRALS

Marketing is one of the most important business skills for the CMES. Marketing is defined as a group of activities designed to expedite transactions by creating, distributing, pricing, and promoting goods, services, and ideas (Ferrell, Hirt, & Ferrell, 2013).

Marketing health and fitness-training services to the medical community does not have to be an expensive endeavor for the CMES. Marketing will allow the CMES to better bridge exercise for special populations with the allied healthcare field. There are many different marketing channels that are effective means of educating allied healthcare professionals regarding the benefits of using the services of a CMES. Before marketing tactics can be discussed, the CMES needs to understand what it is that they are marketing. What is the competitive advantage? Competitive advantage refers to the way a business and/or individual tries to get consumers to purchase products and services over those offered by the competition (Bearden, Ingram, & LaForge, 2005). In other words, competitive advantage is what a business and/or individual does better than the competitors. Determining the competitive advantage allows the CMES to have selling points when communicating with the medical community. An example of a good selling point includes a CMES with specialty training in low-back post-rehabilitation.

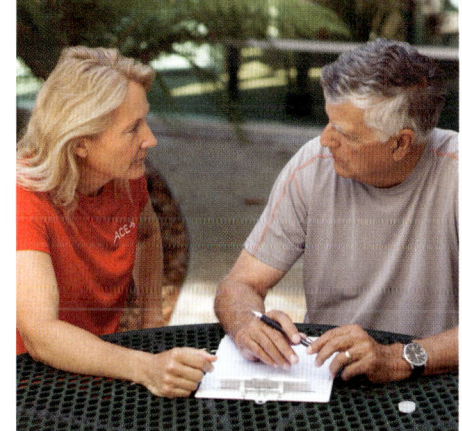

Once a competitive advantage is determined, the CMES can start researching the numerous marketing channels that provide links to the medical community. Some of the most popular channels include:
- Word of mouth from clients, employees, and physician offices
- Local schools and universities
- Orthopedic centers that employ physical therapists, athletic trainers, and occupational therapists
- Local businesses

Word of mouth is the most inexpensive, and often the most beneficial, form of marketing.

The easiest place for a CMES to start is with current clients. Providing clients with the highest quality and most professional experience can go a long way when it comes to marketing. Continuous quality checks in the form of verbal or written evaluations can also help a CMES to improve their service. This is truly an art, and for most exercise professionals, feedback and evaluations from clients can allow them to make changes that benefit their clients. Satisfied clients will make referrals to friends and family. Of course, word of mouth can be negative as well. If a CMES performs poorly, clients will quit and communicate their dissatisfaction to their friends, family, and coworkers. LeBoeuf (2000) noted that a typical dissatisfied customer will tell eight to 10 people about their problem, while one in five will tell 20. It takes 12 positive service incidents to make up for one negative incident.

Word of mouth can also come from non-clients. Employees who work at a fitness center can make referrals, as can a client's allied healthcare professional. A CMES can begin networking with fitness center employees by offering a free session to anyone interested. Whether training with the person working the front desk or the facility director, it is important to demonstrate the service provided.

A client's allied healthcare professionals may become impressed with the communication skills and professionalism of a particular CMES. If the allied healthcare professional has good rapport with a CMES and/or sees results, they may be more likely to promote that CMES. It is absolutely essential for a CMES to constantly work on cultivating these relationships. Of course, word-of-mouth marketing is not limited to these options.

It may also be productive for a CMES to network within their local community. An example of a simple way to network in this manner would be to offer a free fitness class or workout session at a local business. Another option is to provide instructional "lunch and learn" sessions on topics such as developing at-your-desk stretching techniques or 30-minute lunchtime workouts.

To do this, a CMES can call schools in their area and offer a simple one-time session or a series of after-school programs. One benefit of working with young children is that the CMES can give them brochures to take home to their parents, who may then become clients. High schools and universities are great places to find post-rehabilitation clients. Athletes coming out of physical therapy and transitioning back to their sports may need to learn skills like proper stretching, core training, balance training, and strength training to address muscle imbalances and strength deficiencies to decrease the chance of re-injury. The options for marketing to local schools are limitless and can allow the CMES to build their clientele while educating students on the importance of fitness.

Orthopedic centers are in a category of their own due to the high potential for prospective clients for a CMES. Physical therapists, athletic trainers, and occupational therapists rehabilitate patients after surgery or as a treatment for a particular condition. Once patients have completed their prescribed treatments, they are asked to continue exercising on their own. However, some patients are not educated on what to do aside from the exercises they performed in therapy. They may have a set of exercises that they performed with their physical or occupational therapist, but do not have any progressions for when they work out on their own. Post-rehabilitation exercise training is the logical next step for these patients. By building rapport with allied health professionals, a CMES may become a referral source. The best way to market the services of a CMES is to start with the orthopedic centers used by existing clients. Remember, the CMES must have a medical release from a client's physical therapist, occupational therapist, or athletic trainer before initiating a training program. The CMES can use these individuals as contacts. Doing a small presentation or meeting with a group of allied health professionals can be extremely beneficial to a CMES. Not only can the CMES help to decrease the chance of re-injury for a client, but they can also increase a client's quality of life, while simultaneously gaining new clientele.

A CMES can also market their services to local businesses. Athletic shoe stores, athletic apparel shops, and nutrition stores are just some of the places for a CMES to promote their services. Talking with the owner and/or manager about becoming a referral source is a good start. Offering employees a free session or doing a demonstration of a training session is a great way for a CMES to promote their services. A CMES must be professional in their approach and only leave brochures and business cards if permission is granted. Another way to market to local businesses is for a fitness department or studio to offer an open-house event for these vendors. At the open house, a CMES can network and demonstrate their training services.

Marketing is a critical business skill for any CMES. Countless marketing channels can be used to gain new clients. A CMES should always have marketing materials prepared, including business cards, portfolios, and/or personal brochures so that all networking opportunities can be maximized.

> **THINK IT THROUGH**
>
> Make a list of medical practices and businesses in your area that are potential sources of client referrals, as well as support groups for individuals with specific diseases or disorders. Which services offered in your community might also appeal to potential clients seeking improved health and fitness (e.g., hospital wellness centers, cosmetic surgery locations, and physical-therapy clinics)? Which special populations or health challenges do you feel most confident addressing in your practice? Brainstorm marketing pieces that might effectively reach out to these local organizations that highlight your areas of expertise. Be creative!

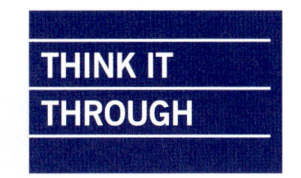

BILLING AND PAYMENT POLICIES

The following factors should be considered when determining the billing and payment procedures:

- *Pricing:* Pricing can be a little more challenging for a CMES who is self-employed or an **independent contractor** than for someone who is an employee for a facility. Facilities usually set a particular price per session for the CMES. Some facilities offer tiered systems that allow the CMES to increase prices and payouts as they graduate through the system. Self-employed individuals and independent contractors need to coordinate several factors in their pricing, including insurance, travel, certifications, experience, local market comparisons, and taxes. The CMES can also do research to determine what other professionals in the area are charging for their services.
- *Cash, check, or credit card:* This issue is simplified for an employee, as the facility takes care of this process. Independent contractors and self-employed individuals collect their own payments and need to be able to track payments for tax purposes. Credit card machines include a charge that needs to be agreed on by the CMES and the credit card machine company. A CMES who takes credit card payments provides convenience for clients, but has to weigh the costs of the processing fees. A CMES who takes cash for payment needs to record this income for tax purposes. Exercise professionals who do not claim cash payments place themselves at risk for tax-related legal issues should they be audited by the Internal Revenue Service (IRS).
- *Personal-training contract:* Employees of fitness facilities normally have a personal-training contract that is designed by the company's attorneys. These forms are handed to each client to sign and cover the following: liability, payment procedures, cancellation procedures, penalties, and late fees. Independent contractors and self-employed individuals need to get their own personal-training contracts designed by an attorney. These signed contracts legally bind clients to the CMES in case of missed payments, cancellations, and bounced checks.
- *Discounts and package plans:* Package plans are common incentives to get clients to sign up for training. A discount is often given per session in a package plan. Some facilities offer package plans that include five, 10, or even 20 or more sessions. For independent contractors and self-employed individuals, package plans offer the benefit of up-front payments. Most employees who sell packages get paid only when a session is actually used, whether or not it was part of a package. Sessions used from a package can be tracked using electronic or manual techniques.

In summary, the billing and payment procedures may be already set for the CMES if they are an employee of a fitness facility. Independent contractors and self-employed individuals have to design a system that is agreeable to their clients. It is important to have a written cancellation policy that is clearly communicated to clients. A client should understand the penalty for not showing up or canceling an appointment at the last minute. If a client cancels with sufficient notice (the industry standard is a 24-hour cancellation window), the CMES is usually able to schedule another client in that time slot. However, if a client cancels at the last minute or simply does not show up, they should be held accountable and charged for that session. Many fitness facilities have a policy of charging a client for a late cancellation, though this charge may be waived in the event of extenuating circumstances. As noted earlier, a CMES should always get legal assistance when drafting their billing and payment policies. Having legally reviewed documentation can give clients incentive to make timely payments and adhere to all billing policies.

LEGAL ISSUES, LIABILITIES, AND PROFESSIONAL RESPONSIBILITIES

Ethics Policy

To help ACE Certified Professionals understand the conduct expected from them as healthcare professionals in protecting the public from harm, ACE has developed the ACE Code of Ethics (Appendix A). This code of conduct serves as a guide for ethical and professional practices for all ACE Certified Professionals. This code is enforced through the ACE Professional Practices and Disciplinary Procedures (www.ACEfitness.org/getcertified/certified-code.aspx). All ACE Certified Professionals and candidates for ACE certification must be familiar with, and comply with, the ACE Code of Ethics and ACE Professional Practices and Disciplinary Procedures.

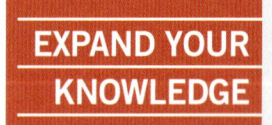

EXPAND YOUR KNOWLEDGE

ACE Code of Ethics

The ACE Code of Ethics governs the ethical and professional conduct of ACE Certified Professionals when working with clients, the public, or other health and exercise professionals. Every individual who registers for an ACE certification exam must agree to uphold the ACE Code of Ethics throughout the exam process and as a professional, should they earn an ACE certification. Exam candidates and ACE Certified Medical Exercise Specialists must have a comprehensive understanding of the code and the consequences and potential public harm that can come from violating each of its principles.

Legal Issues and Liabilities

There are several legal issues and liabilities that can be avoided if exercise professionals understand the appropriate standard of care. Training high-risk clients can bring about other issues not necessarily considered by health and exercise professionals who ordinarily work with the "apparently healthy" population. The three primary areas of concern are scope of practice, qualifications, and appropriate exercise selection and progression.

Scope of Practice

In collaboration with other healthcare professionals, a CMES will design, implement, and manage exercise, physical activity, and lifestyle programs for individuals following treatment or rehabilitation for clinically documented chronic disease, musculoskeletal injury, and/or disability. The CMES is *not* in the practice of providing the services of their profession to the immediate, primary, post-surgical, or post-trauma rehabilitation patient. Rather, the CMES provides a safe and effective bridge for the patient to cross from the structured clinical treatment and/or rehabilitation environment to mainstream community or home-based exercise.

Qualifications

Because the CMES will be receiving referrals from physicians, it is important for them to stay abreast of advancements in the health and fitness industry and complete all continuing education requirements. Times will arise when a client's needs will fall outside a CMES's scope of practice and area of expertise, in which case they should not hesitate to refer the client to an allied healthcare professional. For example, just because a CMES knows about a particular topic (e.g., post-rehabilitation after a knee injury), this does not mean that they are qualified to assume the role of a physical therapist.

Appropriate Exercise Selection and Progression

It is recommended that a CMES training high-risk clients base exercise selection and progression on the client's health-history data and the healthcare provider's recommendations, when available. The CMES should obtain a medical release from each of the physicians that a particular client is seeing. For example, a client who just finished chemotherapy from breast cancer should have two medical releases, one from the oncologist and one from the internal medicine physician. Along with these releases, a CMES can inform the physicians of the exercise progressions that will be used. Having those physicians sign the release allows for suitable exercises to be performed and the proper rate of progression followed, helping to lower injury risk for the client.

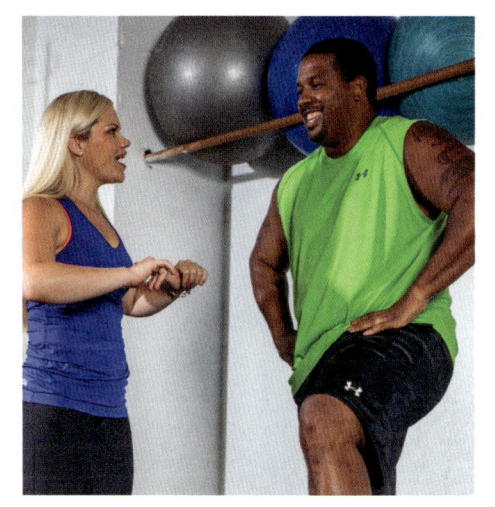

Avoiding Legal Risks

The following are ways that a CMES can protect themselves from legal disaster (Riley, 2006):
- Have legal professionals review all documentation used with clients.
- Allow clients to have appropriate time to read and sign all training documentation. Verbally answer questions when necessary.
- Store all documents securely for as long as is required by the state's **statute of limitations.**
- Be sure to carry sufficient **liability insurance** for ultimate protection against liability.
- Use a legally reviewed, standardized waiver form with all clients.

Employment Options

Employees

A fitness facility that hires a CMES as an employee can control when and how they train clients. Employees are required to sign an employment contract prior to working for the facility. They also receive a salary. Deductions such as withholding tax, social security, and payroll taxes are taken out for the employee by the company. Employees are also protected from discrimination and unfair hiring practices. Some employees are even offered benefits (e.g., medical, dental, and vision), 401K plans, paid vacation, and paid holidays. In the majority of facilities, the CMES would be covered under that facility's liability insurance. Despite this, it is advisable that health and exercise professionals have their own liability insurance as well. ACE encourages its certified professionals to educate themselves and work with legal professionals to determine the need for various types of insurance in their specific situations.

If a CMES works for a facility as an employee, in most cases the client will pay the facility, and the CMES will receive a paycheck based on how many sessions were produced during a particular pay period. Usually, a CMES will take a previously determined percentage of each session's revenue. Keep in mind that a CMES may be salaried and make the same amount of money no matter how many clients are seen during a particular pay period.

Independent Contractors

Many fitness facilities hire independent contractors, non-employees who pay their own taxes and insurance. The fitness facility sends a federal 1099 form for tax purposes if a CMES has earned $600 or more in a year. Fitness facilities do not have to pay benefits or taxes for the independent contractor, which saves the company money.

In many cases, independent contractors receive direct payment from their clients and then pay the facility certain set fees to rent the use of the facility. Some facilities require clients of independent contractors to pay the facility. In turn, the facility pays the independent contractor a fee that was previously agreed on by both parties.

Self-employed

A CMES may also choose to be self-employed by owning a facility, performing in-home training, or training in a facility. When choosing this option, a CMES must choose a business entity to file. A CMES should get legal advice before forming any business entity. There are three major options to choose from: **sole proprietorship, partnership,** and **corporation,** each of which has several subsets. No matter the business entity, clients will pay either the CMES or the business entity. In turn, the CMES pays taxes based on the type of business entity chosen. It is essential that the CMES consults with their tax professional for guidance in determining the best option.

- *Sole proprietorship:* This type of business is owned and operated by one individual. Such owners have total control over business activities, and forming a sole proprietorship is easy and inexpensive. Profits are considered personal income, which makes tax preparation simple. The disadvantage of a sole proprietorship is that the personal liability of the proprietor is not protected. If the business cannot pay its creditors, the CMES may be forced to use their own money to cover the debts. Personal and business funds are one account, not two different accounts. There is also a limited source of funds and individuals pay a higher marginal tax rate.
- *Partnership:* In a partnership, two or more people agree to operate a business and share profits and losses. A partnership is taxed like a sole proprietorship. There are two main types of partnerships: **general partnerships** and **limited partnerships**.
  ✓ *General partnership:* Each partner assumes management responsibility and unlimited liability and must have at least a 1% interest in profit and loss.
  ✓ *Limited partnership:* This is a hybrid organizational form, with both limited and general partners. A limited partner has no voice in management and is legally liable only for the amount of their capital contributions, plus any other debt obligations specifically accepted (Harvard Business Essentials, 2002).
- *Corporation:* A corporation is a legal entity recognized by the state, the assets and liabilities of which are separate from its owners. The advantages of a corporation are the limited liability, the ease of transfer of ownership, and the external sources of funds. Disadvantages of a corporation include double taxation, which means that both income and dividends are taxed. Other disadvantages are the costliness of formation and the disclosure of information. There are two primary subgroups of the corporation: the **S-Corp** and the **limited liability company (LLC).**
  ✓ *S-Corp:* An S-Corp is a form of business ownership taxed as though it were a partnership. It provides limited liability and is restricted to 75 shareholders and one class of stock. All shareholders must be U.S. citizens and cannot be corporations or partnerships.
  ✓ *LLC:* An LLC is a form of business ownership that provides limited liability and is taxed like a partnership. It is not limited to a certain number of shareholders and owners do not have to be U.S. citizens.

Refer to *The Exercise Professional's Guide to Personal Training* (ACE, 2020) to learn more about the various business structures.

> Visit www.ACEfitness.org/insurancecenter to learn more about your insurance options and to take advantage of discounted rates for ACE Certified Exercise Professionals.

BUSINESS PLANNING

To have a successful career, a CMES should take the time to perform an assessment of their own financial fitness and use that information to develop a business plan. The result of this organizational exercise will be a detailed plan of how to operate a successful business.

No one starting a business plans to fail; they simply fail to develop a systematic plan for effectively running a business. To run a successful fitness business, a CMES should take the time to create a detailed business plan that establishes definitive goals and a structure for achieving those goals. Any of the direct-employee, independent-contractor, or business-owner operating models will require a detailed business plan. A comprehensive business plan will serve as an operating guide for achieving specific objectives, such as yearly income and the number of clients needed to achieve that income, as well as a marketing plan for attracting new clients. The components of a business plan are as follows:
- Executive summary
- Business description
- Marketing plan
- Operational plan
- Risk analysis
- Decision-making criteria

Executive Summary

The executive summary is a brief outline of the business and an overview of how the business addresses a need within the marketplace. This should be a succinct synopsis of the business, with the rest of the business plan providing the exact specifications in greater detail. A well-written executive summary is one page and includes the following information:
- *Business concept:* A description of the business, the service it provides, the market for that service, and why this particular business holds a competitive advantage. A CMES interested in opening a studio would need to specify how their skills are different from what exists in the current marketplace.
- *Financial information:* The key financial points for the business, specifically the start-up costs for the first year of operation, the source of capital for the initial expenses, and the potential for sales revenue and profits, with an emphasis on the expected **return on investment (ROI).**
- *Current business position:* Relevant information about the owners of the business, their experiences in the industry, and the specific legal structure of the business. This section should highlight the CMES's experience in the field and identify the number of clients who plan on following them to the new location.
- *Major achievements:* Any awards received, or clients who have given written permission for their names to be used in marketing materials. This section should identify a specific protocol for exercise program design that is different from that of competitors, such as sport-specific training, or list any local or national celebrities who will provide an endorsement of the CMES's work.

Business Description

This section of the business plan provides the details for the business as outlined in the executive summary, including the mission statement, business model, current status of the market, how the business fills a need within the market, and the management team. It is important to develop a succinct mission statement that describes the benefit of using this particular service. When describing the business, the CMES should:
- Identify the operating model and how it is different or unique when compared to other training studios in the area

- Describe the fitness industry specific to the local market, including the present financial situation and the outlook for future growth
- Provide details such as the number and location of competitors, how many employees they have, and the number of clients to whom they provide services
- List the members of the management team, highlighting their knowledge, skills, and experience

The purpose of this section of the plan is to provide a description of the business, the market it will serve, and the people who will run it. Potential lenders or investors will want to see all of this information before making a decision about providing capital.

Marketing Plan

This section of the business plan specifies how prospective clients become paying clients. Whether working as an employee or as an independent contractor, a CMES will need to develop a comprehensive marketing plan to communicate with prospective clients. Marketing is the process of promoting a service by communicating the features, advantages, and benefits to potential clients. Marketing tools for a service such as personal training should tell a story about how that service can enhance a person's life. All marketing pieces should communicate the benefits of working with a CMES, specifically showing how they can help potential clients meet their health and fitness goals.

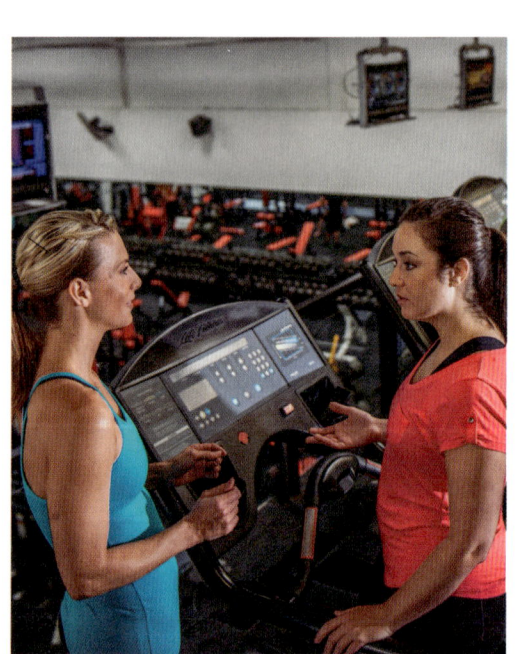

An effective marketing campaign will communicate how a specific product or service meets the needs of a potential client. Unfortunately, many people enter the fitness industry with the misperception that all they need to do is demonstrate their vast knowledge of exercise science and passion for fitness—when nothing could be further from the truth. In order to be successful, health and exercise professionals also need to develop marketing and business skills. The marketing plan should list the details on the demographics for the area around the training business, the demand for personal-training services, the specific type or brand of training services being offered, and the plan for communicating the benefits of the training services to potential customers.

To develop a full schedule, a CMES should take the time to first identify a target audience that can benefit from their services.

The marketing plan must match not only the professional's time availability, but also the potential audiences in the surrounding community. For example, if a CMES is working in a health club in a suburban location where a large percentage of the members are stay-at-home parents or retirees, they need to develop a plan to communicate with those specific audiences. Similarly, a CMES who is working in an urban location where a number of the facility's members are working professionals should identify the times of day that potential clients are available to train and should develop a plan to market their services to that audience to schedule those open time slots.

Operational Plan

This portion of a business plan describes the structure for how a business will operate, including an organizational chart that identifies key decision makers and the employees responsible for executing those decisions. A business plan for a CMES will not need a lengthy operational plan if they are working directly for an employer. However, if a CMES decides to follow the independent-contractor model, then they can make a decision about which operational model to use to create a business structure.

Risk Analysis

There are a number of risks involved in owning and operating a business. Risks can be categorized into one of the following general areas:

- *Barriers to entry:* The costs associated with starting a business, such as rental fees, equipment, employees, and marketing
- *Financial:* The access to the capital required to start or expand a business
- *Competitive:* Other players in the market who are competing for the same pool of potential clients (customers)
- *Staffing:* Issues associated with managing employees and budgeting for a consistent payroll

For a CMES who decides to work as a direct employee, most of the financial risks are covered by the employer. A CMES working as an employee in a health club or similar facility will experience limited risk, such as competition for clients from other health and exercise professionals in the facility, or from other facilities that open nearby.

An independent CMES will need to conduct an analysis to identify competitors and categorize the risks of competing in a specific marketplace. A simple tool for conducting a risk assessment is the **SWOT analysis,** which stands for strengths, weaknesses, opportunities, and threats (Figure 6-2).

Figure 6-2
Sample SWOT analysis

Strengths	Weaknesses
Four-year degree in kinesiology	Not confident when asking clients for money
ACE Medical Exercise Specialist certification	Need to learn more about marketing and sales
Like to help clients with chronic medical conditions; successful at helping clients adhere to exercise programs	Space to train clients when the club is crowded

Opportunities	Threats
Participate in a personal-training sales workshop	Competition from other trainers in the club and the four other facilities and training studios in the immediate area
Develop a talk on the health/medical benefits of leading a healthy lifestyle	
Work for the largest health facility in town, which attracts 100-plus new members per month	Consumer confidence in the current economic climate

A basic SWOT analysis is easy to perform. Begin by dividing a piece of paper into four squares. The upper-left square should be labeled "strengths"—under this heading, list all of the strengths and competitive advantages of the business. Examples might include location, the brand name of the fitness facility, or the education of the particular health and exercise professional.

The upper-right square should be labeled "weaknesses"—under this heading, identify all of the weaknesses of the business. Examples might include the limited visibility of a location or a lack of industry experience. It is important to be as honest and objective as possible about weaknesses, as this exercise will help turn any perceived weaknesses into new business opportunities.

The lower-left square should be labeled "opportunities"—under this heading, list all of the opportunities for attracting new clients or expanding the business. As just mentioned, weaknesses can be turned into opportunities for new business. For example, if limited location visibility is a weakness, then it is also an opportunity to develop new signage or create a new marketing campaign. Another example is a lack of education in a specific area or discipline of study, which could be turned into an opportunity to take a continuing education course or workshop to gain the necessary knowledge, skills, and training.

Finally, the lower-right square should be labeled "threats"—under this heading, list all of the threats that might impact the business. Examples are the general economic climate, adverse weather that might impact clients' abilities to make it to their appointments, or competitors who plan on entering or expanding in the marketplace.

Decision-making Criteria

This component of the business plan includes a detailed cost-benefit analysis that demonstrates that the expenses for operating the business are worth the financial risks involved with establishing operations. The CMES should highlight the specifics about the business plan that prove that it will be a successful business venture. A well-written plan will present all of the components of the business in such a way that the final section is simply a conclusion summarizing how the business will be a profitable venture. More time spent in the early planning stages detailing how the business will run will allow a business owner to focus their efforts on implementing the plan, attracting the clients, and providing the service once the business starts operating.

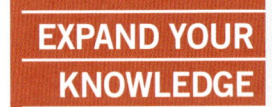

EXPAND YOUR KNOWLEDGE

VIRTUAL TOOLS FOR THE CERTIFIED MEDICAL EXERCISE SPECIALIST
By Ted Vickey, M.A.

Ted Vickey, Ph.D., is the Founder & President of FitWell, Inc., a San Diego–based consulting company specializing in entrepreneurship, innovation, and emerging technology within the fitness industry. He is also a professor at Point Loma University in the Master's program in the School of Kinesiology, teaching classes with research interests in fitness management, wellness entrepreneurship, disruptive health technologies, professional ethics, and fitness center design.

Imagine a training practice where your website ranks on page one of an internet search, where bills are paid, and fees are collected with the touch of a button. In addition, clients' nutrition and physical-activity achievements are wirelessly sent from their mobile phones to your email for tracking. That practice is readily available through the use of technology. There are two types of technology that a CMES should consider as part of the overall practice: business-management tools and connected health tools.

Business-management Tools

Training businesses can reap the benefits of various business-management tools, including the creation of a website, engagement with clients, professional relationship management, appointment scheduling, accounting, and online credit card processing.

It can be difficult to decide which platform is most suitable for a particular practice. Which platform allows for easy publishing of a site and can also grow with one's practice? Which platform drives engagement and leads to new clients and/or additional appointments? Which platform has reporting capabilities that can show a return on the initial investment? While the task may seem daunting at first, the reality is that with some trial runs, and even beta-testing with friends and family, creating an online business-management platform may offer tremendous return for very little time investment. No longer must a CMES hire an expensive design company to create a website, although for best results, consulting a website designer is never a bad idea.

Social media and online marketing are increasingly important for a CMES to get a practice noticed and utilized by potential clients on the web. There are a number of good reasons for a training practice to maintain an online presence, including the following:

- Connect and engage with current and potential clients
- Get discovered by people searching for your specific services
- Create an active and persuasive community around the practice
- Promote content such as webinars, blog articles, or health tips (visit www.ACEfitness.org for free tips you can use in your practice)
- Generate leads for the practice

Health and exercise professionals around the world are using Facebook as their primary website, not only to attract new business, but also to remain engaged with former and existing clients. On Facebook, "profiles" are meant for people, while "pages' are meant for businesses. To fully engage and leverage the power of

Facebook, be sure to create a page for your practice. Pages are public and are split into different categories, and are therefore searchable. These "branding" pages also allow anyone to become a fan of (or "like") the page without needing administrator approval. Facebook also provides flexible privacy settings to control who sees what parts of your page (*Source:* Hubspot). For additional information about setting up Facebook as your website, conduct an online search for "Facebook for Business."

Health and exercise professionals are also using Twitter to stay in touch with clients by sharing short, valuable health-related tips. Twitter is a free service that allows anyone to say anything in 140 characters or less. Twitter allows the CMES to promote particular services directed at a target market; connect with other professionals who share their views; get instant access to relevant, timely opinions; receive a steady stream of ideas, content, links, resources, and tips focused on their area of expertise; and monitor what is being said about the practice (*Source:* Duct Tape Marketing). Twitter is more than promotion; it is also about the sharing of valuable information. For every business/training promotion, consider sharing several health tips. For additional information about using Twitter in your coaching practice, search "Twitter for Business."

Another easy-to-use website that can add value to a CMES's practice is LinkedIn (www.linkedin.com). On LinkedIn, a CMES can connect not only with potential clients, but also with other health and wellness professionals in the area, state, and even around the world. The CMES should be sure to add all relevant information, include a professional picture, request the vanity URL (that can include your name in the URL), and use this resource to connect with other like-minded professionals with a click of the mouse. The LinkedIn help section provides tips to make a profile stand out from the rest. Once a member of LinkedIn, a CMES should join groups and be active by posting questions, providing answers, and engaging with the rest of the group. There are a number of ACE groups on LinkedIn that a CMES can join, all for free.

Other do-it-yourself websites include Tumblr (www.tumblr.com), Pinterest (www.pinterest.com), Instagram (www.instagram.com), and Tout (www.tout.com). Prior to committing to one site, spend some time planning an online strategy. It helps to have a checklist of features that are both user-friendly and useful. Review other professionals who are currently using these tools effectively.

For additional information about business tools for training practices, consider searching for these terms: social media, online marketing, online appointment scheduler, online accounting, and credit card processing. Also visit the ACE website (www.ACEfitness.org) for additional resources for building, marketing, and expanding a training practice.

Connected Health Tools

Former Surgeon General C. Evert Koop dreamed of a day where "…cutting-edge technology, especially in communication and information transfer, will enable the greatest advances yet in public health. Eventually, we will have access to health information 24 hours a day, 7 days a week, encouraging personal wellness and prevention, and leading to better informed decisions about health care" (Koop, 1995). That dream is now a reality, as personal trainers, nutritionists, health coaches, and certified medical exercise specialists are using the power of technology (the Internet, social networking services, and mobile phone applications) as persuasive tools to help clients lead healthier lives.

Specific to the exercise profession, connected health tools are small, inexpensive client-based mobile applications or websites that eliminate the four walls of a physical building and allow training to take place virtually in real time. These tools can transmit health data from the client to the CMES, such as heart rate, physical activity, meal logs, body weight, blood pressure, and sleep habits. This allows the CMES to not only hold clients accountable between appointments, but also allows for real-time immediate feedback and encouragement for daily behaviors. By using connected health technology, a CMES can provide a more personalized experience and potentially reach more individuals with effective health-related advice and information at a very low cost. Griffiths et al. (2006) suggest five reasons for using connected health tools for delivering web-based health, wellness, and fitness interventions:
- Reduced delivery costs
- Convenience to users

- Timeliness
- Reduction of stigma
- Reduction of time-based isolation barriers

Within the healthcare field, interactive technologies can be effectively deployed to take on multiple roles at the same time. For example, a simple online tool can measure calories while at the same time giving a reward upon attainment of a personal goal. This type of self-monitoring is a key ingredient in successful behavioral modification. The power of self-monitoring is not just between client and CMES. Research suggests that if several people are connected through the Internet, social support can be leveraged, which has been shown to impact motivation and behavioral change (Chatterjee & Price, 2009). A CMES should find ways to connect clients with friends, family, or other clients to create an "electronic bond." Accountability emails, online chats, Facebook posts, and Twitter messages can be powerful motivational tools.

Tracking of physical activity is moving away from the paper and pencil of a workout card and more toward digital tracking. Technology allows users to track progress, interact with a CMES who can suggest areas for improvement, and self-administer tests and measures. Blood pressure cuffs that connect to the web, body-weight scales that tweet a person's weight, and even sleep-monitoring systems are allowing people to track their personal health data from the comforts of their own homes (www.withings.com). Tracking tools such as BodyMedia (www.bodymedia.com) and FitBit (www.fitbit.com) empower users to collect and share exercise, nutrition, and sleep data. In-depth nutrition apps such as MyNetDiary (www.mynetdiary.com) and Foodzy (www.blog.foodzy.com) are modern, comprehensive diet services that help users track and monitor food intake while displaying a robust nutritional analysis based on personalized guidelines. These tools can be extremely useful for a client who needs that extra motivation to stay the course.

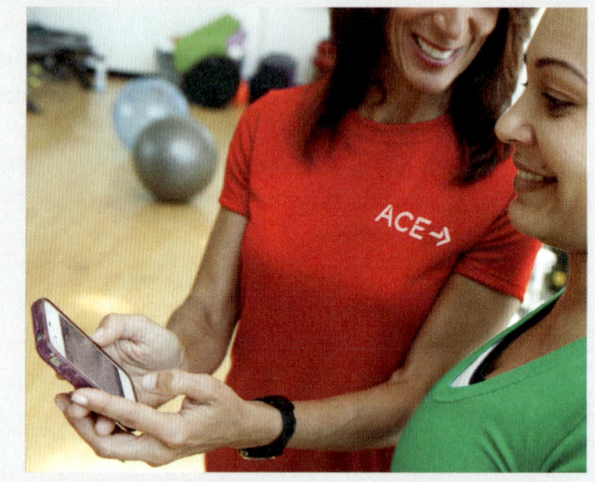

Mobile fitness applications can offer similar tracking options for a fraction of the cost. Apple and Android software provide data collection and motivational tools. The sharing of data within a private group, on Facebook, or on Twitter can provide additional accountability and support for clients. Health information data portals such as RunKeeper's HealthGraph (www.runkeeper.com) allow for health data to be collected, monitored, and shared not only with the client, but also with other members of the client's healthcare team, including physicians, nutritionists, personal trainers, and certified medical exercise specialists.

For more information about connected health tools that a CMES can implement in their practice, conduct an online search for mobile fitness applications (or "apps"), personal health-information management, Microsoft Health Vault, and mobile health apps.

SUMMARY

The role of the CMES is not only to train clients, but also to exemplify professional business skills in their everyday business practices. By working together with allied healthcare professionals, the CMES allows the client to receive the safest and most effective exercise training and lifestyle-modification programs. In terms of business development, networking provides a channel for the CMES to broaden their clientele and areas of expertise.

REFERENCES

American Council on Exercise (2020). *The Exercise Professional's Guide to Personal Training.* San Diego, Calif.: American Council on Exercise.

Bearden, W.O., Ingram, T.N., & LaForge, R.W. (2005). *Marketing Principles and Perspectives* (5th ed.). New York: McGraw Hill/Irwin.

Chatterjee, S. & Price, A. (2009). Healthy living with persuasive technologies: Framework, issues, and challenges. *Journal of the American Medical Informatics Association,* 16, 2, 171–178.

Covey, S.R. (2004). *The 7 Habits of Highly Effective People.* New York: Free Press.

Ferrell, O.C., Hirt, G., & Ferrell, L. (2013). *Business in a Changing World* (9th ed.). New York: McGraw Hill/Irwin.

Griffiths, F. et al. (2006). Why are health care interventions delivered over the internet? A systematic review of the published literature. *Journal of Medical Internet Research,* 8, 2, e10.

Harvard Business Essentials (2002). *Finance for Managers.* Boston: Harvard Business School Publishing.

Koop, C.E. (1995). A personal role in health care reform. *American Journal of Public Health,* 85, 6, 759–760. www.pubmedcentral.nih.gov/articlerender.fcgi?artid=1615490&tool=pmcentrez&rendertype=abstract

LeBoeuf, M. (2000). *How to Win Customers & Keep Them for Life* (revised edition). New York: Berkley Publishing Group.

Riley, S. (2006). The importance of protective legal documentation. *IDEA Trainer Success,* 3, 1, 10–12.

U.S. Department of Health and Human Services (2014). Summary of the HIPAA Privacy Rule. www.hhs.gov/ocr/privacy/hipaa/understanding/summary/

SUGGESTED READING

American Council on Exercise (2020). *The Exercise Professional's Guide to Personal Training.* San Diego, Calif.: American Council on Exercise.

Ferrell, O.C., Hirt, G., & Ferrell, L. (2013). *Business in a Changing World* (9th ed.). New York: McGraw Hill/Irwin.

Longenecker, J. P. et al. (2014). *Small Business Management* (17th ed.). Florence, Ky.: South-Western College Publishing.

Tharrett, S. & Peterson, J.A. (2012). *Fitness Management* (3rd ed.). Monterey, Calif.: Healthy Learning.

PART III
MAJOR CARDIOVASCULAR AND PULMONARY DISEASES AND DISORDERS

CHAPTER 7
CORONARY HEART DISEASE

CHAPTER 8
BLOOD LIPID DISORDERS

CHAPTER 9
HYPERTENSION

CHAPTER 10
PULMONARY DISEASE: ASTHMA AND CHRONIC OBSTRUCTIVE PULMONARY DISEASE

7 CORONARY HEART DISEASE

IN THIS CHAPTER

THE ROLE OF THE CMES
HIGH-RISK PRIMARY PREVENTION AND STABLE CHD

EPIDEMIOLOGY

OVERVIEW
ANGINA PECTORIS
CARDIAC DYSRHYTHMIAS
MYOCARDIAL INFARCTION
HEART FAILURE

DIAGNOSTIC TESTING AND CRITERIA
ELECTROCARDIOGRAM
ECG EXERCISE TESTING
RADIONUCLIDE STRESS TEST
STRESS ECHOCARDIOGRAPHY
CORONARY ANGIOGRAPHY (CARDIAC CATHETERIZATION)
VASCULAR IMAGING TECHNIQUES
CORONARY CALCIUM SCORING

TREATMENT OPTIONS

NUTRITIONAL CONSIDERATIONS
CARDIOVASCULAR DISEASE PREVENTION
CORONARY HEART DISEASE
CONGESTIVE HEART FAILURE
EATING PLANS TO SUPPORT OPTIMAL HEART HEALTH

EXERCISE TRAINING RECOMMENDATIONS FOR CLIENTS WITH STABLE CHD
APPROPRIATE PROGRAM CANDIDATES AND STABLE CHD
FITNESS TESTING CHD PATIENTS
CONTRAINDICATIONS TO EXERCISE TRAINING
EXERCISE TRAINING SUPERVISION CONSIDERATIONS
OVERALL WEEKLY EXERCISE ENERGY-EXPENDITURE GOALS
EXERCISE INTENSITY
EXERCISE FREQUENCY AND DURATION
MODE OF EXERCISE FOR CHD
INTERVAL/INTERMITTENT AEROBIC EXERCISE TRAINING
RESISTANCE TRAINING
MINDFUL EXERCISE AND THE CHD CLIENT

EXERCISE GUIDELINES SUMMARY FOR CLIENTS WITH STABLE CHD

CASE STUDY

SUMMARY

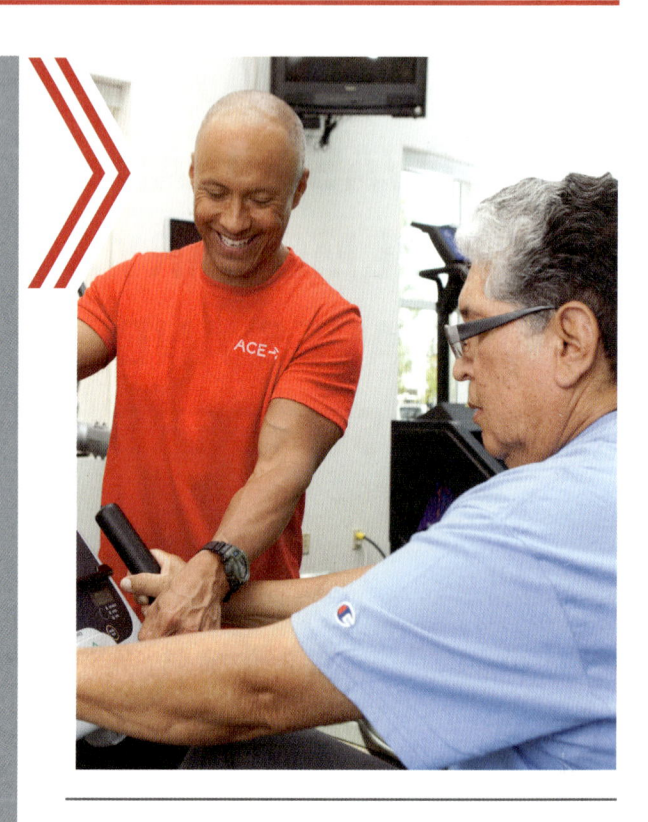

ABOUT THE AUTHOR

Ralph La Forge, M.S., is a physiologist and Accreditation Council on Clinical Lipidology–certified clinical lipid specialist and former managing director of the Cholesterol Disorder Physician Education Program at Duke University Medical Center, Endocrine Division in Durham, North Carolina. He was also managing director of preventive medicine and cardiac rehabilitation at Sharp Health Care in San Diego, where he also taught applied exercise physiology at the University of California at San Diego. Prior to that, La Forge was director of preventive cardiology and cardiac rehabilitation at the Lovelace Clinic in Albuquerque, New Mexico. He has helped more than 300 medical staff groups throughout North America organize and operate lipid disorder clinics and diabetes- and heart-disease-prevention programs. La Forge is the immediate past president of the Southeast Lipid Association and a clinical consultant to numerous healthcare institutions including the U.S. Indian Health Service Division of Diabetes Treatment and Prevention. He has published over 200 papers on clinical exercise science, lipidology, and preventive endocrinology.

By Ralph La Forge

ADULTS WITH STABLE AND WELL-MANAGED coronary heart disease (CHD) represent a key opportunity for competent and experienced personal trainers or ACE® Certified Medical Exercise Specialists (CMES). CHD (also called coronary disease, coronary artery disease, ischemic heart disease, and atherosclerotic heart disease) is a narrowing of the small blood vessels that supply blood and oxygen to the heart.

CHD is an important subset of the broader category of **cardiovascular disease (CVD),** which refers to any disease that affects the cardiovascular system, principally cardiac disease, vascular diseases of the brain and kidney, and **peripheral arterial disease.** Most people with CHD can feel healthy for years before they start experiencing symptoms. The most common symptom is a **myocardial infarction (MI)** (also called a heart attack). If CHD is not treated, some of the plaques in the coronary arteries can break away and block the blood flow to the heart. Coronary disease is the most common cause of sudden death. It is also the most common cause of death in people over 65 years old. Men are 10 times more likely to get coronary disease than women [Centers for Disease Control and Prevention (CDC), 2013].

The purpose of this chapter is to briefly acquaint the qualified CMES with CHD, describe its process, and provide appropriate exercise training recommendations. **Hypertension, diabetes, obesity,** and the **metabolic syndrome,** all of which impact the CHD process, are discussed elsewhere in this text. The CMES is strongly encouraged to partner the information in this chapter with *ACSM's Guidelines for Exercise Testing and Prescription* (11th edition) [American College of Sports Medicine (ACSM), 2022] and the American Association of Cardiovascular and Pulmonary Rehabilitation's (AACVPR) *Guidelines for Cardiac Rehabilitation Programs* (6th edition) (AACVPR, 2021). Both of these texts are good resources for the CMES who wishes to work with individuals with stable CHD. There is remarkable agreement between these and other guidelines (e.g., ACCF/AHA/ACP/AATS/PCNA/SCAI/STS, 2012), in terms of the recommended quantity and quality of exercise for those with CHD, although there are some minor differences. This chapter represents a diligent effort to maintain consistency to harmonize recommendations and eliminate discrepancies. Some recommendations from earlier guidelines have been updated as warranted by new evidence or a better understanding of earlier evidence. The CMES should see this chapter as a current synthesis of these guidelines, particularly those from ACSM and AACVPR.

THE ROLE OF THE CMES

Fundamentally, the role of the CMES who wishes to work with individuals with CHD is to work only with those clients who have stable CHD and are at low risk for exercise-related cardiovascular complications. The determination of stable CHD should only be made by the client's referring physician. Furthermore, the principal role of the CMES in this context is to design and allocate appropriate and

LEARNING OBJECTIVES:

» Explain the role of the CMES in the treatment of coronary heart disease (CHD).

» Describe the major forms of CHD (i.e., angina pectoris, cardiac dysrhythmias, myocardial infarction, and heart failure).

» Identify testing procedures and diagnostic criteria for the diagnosis of CHD.

» Describe how nutritional intake and physical activity influence a person's risk for, and management of, CHD.

» Identify treatment strategies for CHD, including medications and nutritional approaches.

» Explain how each major type of CHD affects a client's ability to perform physical activity and exercise.

» Design and implement appropriate exercise programs for clients with CHD, taking into account adherence to the clients' physicians' recommendations and limitations.

safe levels of physical activity to improve the client's functionality, favorably modify CHD risk factors, and further improve the function of the heart. It is strongly recommended that the clients with whom the CMES intends to work have successfully completed early phase cardiac rehabilitation (essentially phases I and II) by a formalized outpatient cardiac rehabilitation program when these programs are locally available. Fewer than 20% of eligible patients receive formalized cardiac rehabilitation exercise training, which would drastically narrow the population of individuals who could work with a CMES. Although there are no universally accepted guidelines for exercise specialists who work outside of the scope of formal cardiac rehabilitation programs, it is logical that these exercise professionals follow the same published standards of care (i.e., AACVPR and ACSM) as those working within cardiac rehabilitation programs. In cases where the client cannot participate in cardiac rehabilitation for various reasons, including program location and accessibility or work or personal schedules, the CMES can train the client with an appropriate physician referral and within the guidelines discussed in this chapter.

High-risk Primary Prevention and Stable CHD

An individual in need of a supervised exercise program may not have diagnosed CHD, but instead may merely be interested in preventing heart disease (primary prevention). Candidates for this program may also include those with multiple risk factors for CHD, but may never have had a cardiac event (secondary prevention). Those with documented CHD or unstable CHD are most appropriate for formalized and supervised cardiac rehabilitation. Ideally, the CHD client would have completed early phase cardiac rehabilitation prior to working with the CMES. An experienced CMES who wishes to work with CHD clients should work only with those who are under a physician's care and who have stable coronary disease.

For purposes of the CMES's **scope of practice,** stable CHD means that the individual's disease process is well managed [i.e., they do not have irregular, unpredictable symptoms, **unstable angina, heart failure (HF),** or malignant ventricular **arrhythmias**]. Stable also means that the individual is currently under the care of a physician and on appropriate medical therapy for their level of CHD. The CMES is not expected to discriminate between stable and unstable CHD, but should rely on the client's personal physician's clinical evaluation and judgment—a physician who is currently caring for the client's disease. This physician can be a cardiologist, internist, or, in some cases, a primary care physician such as a family practitioner. One means of confirming stable CHD is periodic exercise electrocardiographic stress testing [exercise **electrocardiogram (ECG)**] by a physician.

This chapter presents several tables illustrating and describing specific cautions and risk-stratification measures. Some of these overlap in intention, but it is imperative that the CMES keep in mind that CHD patients have a higher probability of cardiac symptoms and recurrent cardiovascular events (e.g., MI or **acute coronary syndrome**) and clearly require a more conservative approach to exercise training. This in no way should compromise the stable CHD patient's eventual ability to safely engage in higher levels of physical activity commensurate with those recommended for apparently healthy adults.

EPIDEMIOLOGY

In 2010, one in three deaths in American adults was caused by CVD, or approximately 2,150 deaths each day [American Heart Association (AHA), 2014]. To put these numbers in perspective, CVD took the life of one American every 40 seconds. However, the AHA (2014) report does provide some good news. From 2000 to 2010, the number of deaths attributable to CVD declined 31% and the number of CVD deaths per year declined 16.7%. In 2010, the number of deaths attributed to cardiovascular causes was 235.5 per 100,000 individuals. African-American males fared the worst, with 369.2 cardiovascular deaths per 100,000 individuals. The prevalence of CHD was greatest among persons aged ≥65 years (19.8%), followed by those aged 45–64 years (7.1%) and those aged 18–44 years (1.2%). CHD prevalence was greater among men (7.8%) than women (4.6%) (AHA, 2014). The decline in the mortality rate suggests that more persons are living with CHD, which should result in an increase in the prevalence of CHD. However, the decline in prevalence in this report was affected not only by CHD mortality but also by CHD incidence, which is decreased by the prevention and control of CHD risk factors, particularly a fall in **low-density lipoprotein (LDL),** with a greater percentage of adults taking statin drugs. Given that CHD mortality is declining, the observed decline in prevalence of CHD in this study suggests that CHD incidence also has declined. However, CHD remains the number-one killer of American adults. Every year approximately 715,000 Americans have a heart attack. Of these, 525,000 are a first heart attack and 190,000 happen in people who have already had a heart attack (CDC, 2013). These statistics are sobering and point to the likelihood that most health and exercise professionals will work with clients who suffer from a heart-related ailment.

OVERVIEW

CHD is the end result of the accumulation of lipid-rich plaques within the walls of the arteries that supply the **myocardium** (the muscle of the heart). CHD results from the development of **atherosclerosis** in the coronary arteries. Atherosclerosis is a disease affecting both large and small arterial blood vessels. It is a chronic inflammatory response in the walls of arteries, in large part due to the deposition of **lipoproteins** (plasma proteins that carry **cholesterol** and **triglycerides**). Atherosclerosis is essentially caused by the formation of multiple plaques within the arteries. Today, atherosclerosis is seen not as a disease of the **lumen** of the artery, but a disease of the vessel wall. **Atherogenesis** is the process of the development of these plaques, which involves the infiltration, retention, and oxidation of LDL cholesterol in the arterial intima, inflammation, development of fatty streaks, and the calcification of atherosclerotic plaques. Under normal circumstances, the vascular **endothelium** does not bind **leukocytes** (white blood cells) well. However, injury to the endothelium (innermost layer of the artery wall) causes inflammation that results in the expression of adhesion molecules that facilitate atherosclerosis. It is now understood that an acute coronary event (e.g., MI) is more often caused by rupture of a complex vulnerable atherosclerotic plaque than by a gradual closure of the coronary blood vessel (Figure 7-1). The **vulnerable plaque** is essentially characterized by adhesions with thin fibrous caps that predispose the plaque to rupture. Rupture of the plaque releases numerous thrombotic substances into the blood that usually stimulate a rapid sequence of events that results in a clot or coronary thrombosis. The formation, progression, and rupture of the vulnerable plaque are viewed as a process related directly to inflammation.

In recent years, **vascular inflammation** in atherogenesis and CHD has gained considerable support for its role in accelerating arterial narrowing and thrombosis. Experimental work has elucidated molecular and cellular pathways of vascular inflammation that promote atherosclerosis (Libby, 2012). It is now believed that systemic and local inflammatory events mediate all phases of plaque development, progression, and degeneration. Inflammatory **cytokines** [e.g., tumor necrosis factor-alpha, interleukin (IL)-6, and IL-18] are thought to accelerate the rate of atherogenesis even in the absence of traditional CHD risk factors. Inflammation also plays an important role in the recruitment of leukocytes at the endothelium to the atherosclerotic plaque rupture, causing the clinical symptoms of CHD (Figure 7-2). This new and expanding understanding of the participation of the inflammatory process in atherosclerosis in no way challenges the importance of traditional risk factors, such as high LDL levels and hypertension. Indeed, inflammation provides a pathway that mechanistically links alterations in traditional risk factors and modifications in the biology of the artery wall that give rise to atherosclerosis and its complications.

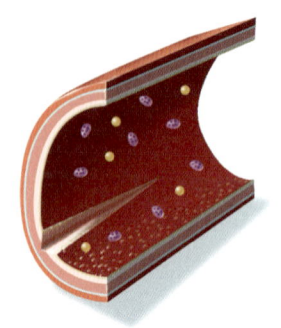

a A blood-borne irritant injures the arterial wall, disrupting the endothelial layer and exposing the underlying connective tissue.

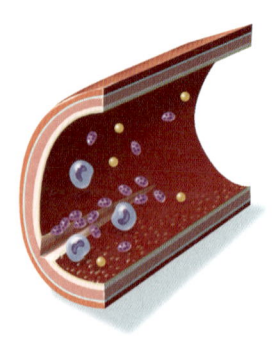

b Blood platelets and circulating immune cells known as monocytes are then attracted to the site of the injury and adhere to the exposed connective tissue. The platelets release a substance referred to as platelet-derived growth factor (PDGF) that promotes migration of smooth muscle cells from the media to the intima.

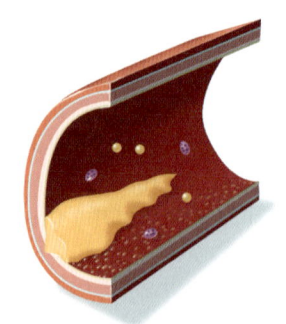

c A plaque, which is basically composed of smooth muscle cells, connective tissue, and debris, forms at the site of injury.

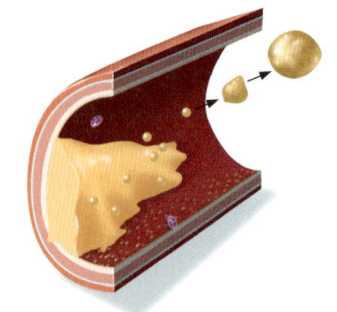

d As the plaque grows, it narrows the arterial opening and impedes blood flow. Lipids in the blood, specifically low-density lipoprotein cholesterol (LDL-C), are deposited in the plaque.

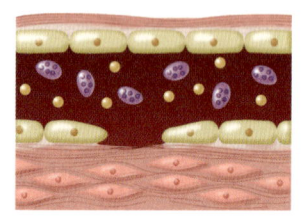

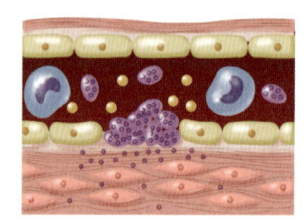

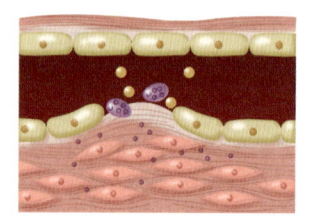

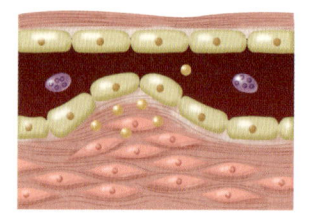

Figure 7-1
Sequence of progression of atherosclerosis

Reprinted with permission from Kenney, W.L., Wilmore, J.H., & Costill, D.L. (2012). *Physiology of Sport and Exercise* (5th ed.). Champaign, Ill.: Human Kinetics.

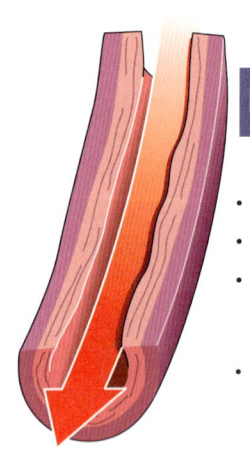

INFLAMMATION
- endothelium damage
- leukocytes chemotaxis
- cyotines, growth and adhesion factors synthesis
- free radicals induction, low-density lipoproteins oxidation

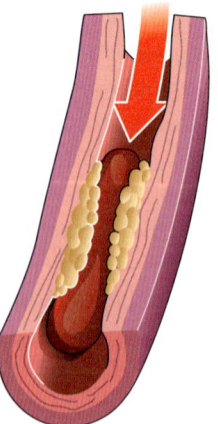

PROINFLAMMATORY FACTORS
- plaque destruction
- platelets activation
- clot formation

UNSTABLE ANGINA

MYOCARDIAL INFARCTION

STROKE

Figure 7-2
The arterial inflammation process

Angina Pectoris

Angina pectoris is the discomfort (and sometimes pain) in the chest, arms, shoulders, and even jaw that results from inadequate blood flow, and more specifically oxygen, to the heart. **Angina** that occurs regularly with activity, upon awakening, or at other *predictable* times is termed **stable angina** and is associated with high-grade narrowing of the coronary arteries. The typical level of physical effort–related angina is proportionate to the exercise intensity but can also be influenced by temperature (e.g., cold weather conditions) and altitude. Angina can be easily graded by the "Functional Classification of Angina Pectoris" guidelines presented in Table 7-1. When appropriate, this angina classification is a useful tool for documenting client chest discomfort or pain. The symptoms of angina are often treated with nitrate medicines such as nitroglycerin, which come in short-acting and long-acting forms, and may be self-administered transdermally, sublingually (i.e., under the tongue), or orally as needed. Unstable angina is angina that changes in intensity, character, or frequency. Unstable angina may precede MI and requires urgent medical attention. Individuals who have unstable angina are not appropriate clients for the CMES and should always be referred back to their physicians.

TABLE 7-1
CANADIAN CARDIOVASCULAR SOCIETY FUNCTIONAL CLASSIFICATION OF ANGINA PECTORIS

Class	Definition	Specific Activity Scale
I	Ordinary physical activity (e.g., walking and climbing stairs) does not cause angina; angina occurs with strenuous, rapid, or prolonged exertion at work or recreation	Ability to ski, play basketball, jog at 5 mph, or shovel snow without angina
II	Slight limitation of ordinary activity. Angina occurs when walking or climbing stairs rapidly, walking uphill, walking or stair climbing after meals, in cold, in wind, under emotional stress, or only during the few hours after awakening, when walking more than two blocks on level ground, or when climbing more than one flight of stairs at a normal pace and in normal conditions	Ability to garden, rake, roller skate, walk at 4 mph on level ground, or have sexual intercourse without stopping
III	Marked limitation of ordinary physical activity. Angina occurs on walking one or two blocks on level ground or climbing one flight of stairs at a normal pace in normal conditions	Ability to shower or dress without stopping, walk 2.5 mph, bowl, make a bed, or play golf
IV	Inability to perform any physical activity without discomfort	Anginal symptoms may be present at rest. Inability to perform activities requiring 2 or fewer metabolic equivalents without angina

Source: Goldman, L. et al. (1981). Comparative reproducibility and validity of systems for assessing cardiovascular functional class: Advantages of a new specific activity scale. *Circulation,* 64, 1227–1234.

Cardiac Dysrhythmias

Cardiac **dysrhythmias** are cardiac rhythm disturbances that can be of atrial, **atrioventricular node (AV node),** or ventricular origin. Many patients with CHD and/or who are post-MI or have had heart surgery have ventricular dysrhythmias. Some dysrhythmias are relatively benign, but some represent a high-risk state. For example, some rapid ventricular dysrhythmias can result in cardiac arrest. Cardiologists can prescribe several different classes of medicines or perform specific laboratory procedures (e.g., radiofrequency ablation or implantable defibrillators) that can reduce many types of cardiac dysrhythmias.

Cardiac dysrhythmias, especially ventricular arrhythmias, can be heart-rate and physical-effort related, and thus can be elicited by physical exercise. For this reason, the CMES should be particularly conscious of symptoms that are induced by exercise-generated ventricular dysrhythmias. Such rhythm disturbances can transpire during or after exercise and occasionally a delayed onset of one to two hours after exercise, particularly intense exercise, can occur. These symptoms include dizziness, lightheadedness, **palpitations,** and, in rare occurrences, **syncope** (fainting). Any individual with a history of exercise-induced dysrhythmias should be thoroughly evaluated by a cardiologist. Without physician clearance, these individuals should not be considered stable, although many are or can be well managed by their cardiologist. The four primary cautions if such clients are referred to a CMES are as follows:

- Always graduate the workload slowly, with no sudden onset or cessation of moderate or vigorous exercise. Always have the client gradually warm up and cool down.
- Monitor the client for at least 10 to 15 minutes after an exercise session has concluded.
- Avoid heavy resistance exercise or any exercise in which the client is exerting against either an **isometric** load or very high resistance, particularly if the client also holds their breath or executes a **Valsalva maneuver** (expiration against a closed glottis).
- Inverted **hatha yoga** poses (head below the level of the heart) or rapid changes in body position are also not advised.

Myocardial Infarction

Acute MI is a medical condition that occurs when the blood supply to the heart muscle is interrupted, most commonly due to the rupture of a lipid-rich, vulnerable plaque. The resulting oxygen shortage, or **ischemia,** causes damage and potential death of some of the heart muscle cells below the blockage. MI symptoms may include various combinations of pain in the chest, upper extremity, or jaw, or epigastric discomfort with exertion or at rest (i.e., mid-back pain). The discomfort associated with acute MI usually lasts at least 20 minutes. Frequently, the discomfort is diffuse, not localized, not positional, not affected by movement of the region, and may be accompanied by shortness of breath, **diaphoresis** (profuse sweating), nausea, or syncope. ECG and cardiac biomarkers (e.g., myocardial enzymes or cardiac troponin taken via blood test at the hospital) also help diagnose an MI. Patients frequently feel suddenly ill. Women often experience different symptoms than men. The most common symptoms of MI in women include shortness of breath, weakness, and fatigue. Approximately one-third of all MIs are "silent," without chest pain or other symptoms. Acute MI is a type of acute coronary syndrome, which is most frequently (but not always) a manifestation of CHD. In approximately half of all MIs, this is the individual's first indication of CHD. It is very important that the CMES be capable of recognizing the signs and symptoms of MI.

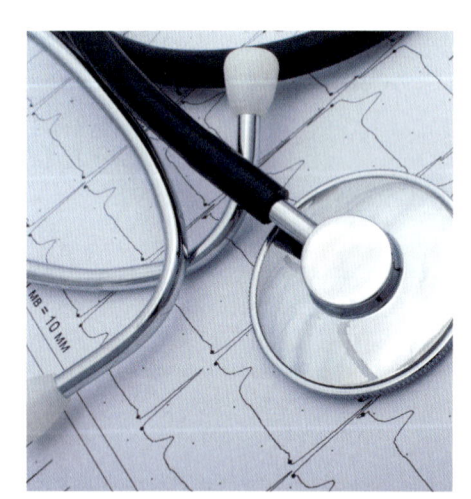

Training the post-MI client requires adherence to precautions very similar to those followed with the angina client. The CMES should never be in the position of training a client within four to six weeks of an MI and without direct written authorization and referral from the client's physician. Ideally, the client should have completed early phase cardiac rehabilitation or similarly supervised exercise therapy. It is important, however, to note that more than 70% of post-MI patients do not get referred to, or have access to, formal cardiac rehabilitation programs. In such cases, it is imperative that the CMES ensures that the individual has an appropriate physician evaluation prior to taking a referral. In all cases, clients should have a physician-supervised exercise ECG prior to working with the CMES. All post-MI clients, but especially those with an MI within the preceding eight to 12 weeks, should begin all exercise sessions with relatively low workloads [e.g., 3–5 **metabolic equivalents (METs)**] and progress very gradually. Most post-MI clients who have had symptom-free and negative exercise ECGs can progress to reasonably normal age- and gender-related aerobic and resistance work capacities over six to 12 months.

Heart Failure

One complication of CHD, particularly MI, is HF. More than 6.4 million Americans have HF, with more than 1 million new cases reported every year (AACVPR, 2021). An MI may compromise the function of the heart as a pump for the circulatory system, which can lead to HF. Essentially, HF is a condition characterized by a reduction in cardiac output sufficient to meet the body's metabolic demands, including many moderate-level physical activities. There are different types of HF. Left- or right-sided HF may occur depending on the affected part of the heart, which results in a low output. If one of the heart valves is affected, this may cause dysfunction, such as mitral valve regurgitation in the case of left-sided MI. The incidence of HF is particularly high in individuals with diabetes and requires special management strategies. These individuals, especially those who have poor **ventricular function** (i.e., the heart has a very poor pumping capacity), are at high risk for exercise-related complications. Some of the clinical manifestations of HF are listed in Table 7-2. Note that one key sign for the CMES is exercise intolerance (i.e., **dyspnea** at relatively low workloads).

The CMES should not train HF clients unless otherwise appropriately and specifically authorized by physician referral. Low-level progressive exercise (2 to 5 METs) can be helpful in early stages of training, but only with authorized supervision. Many restorative and easy yoga poses are also beneficial when appropriately taught by experienced and qualified yoga teachers. Higher-intensity (50 to 70+% of $\dot{V}O_2max$) interval or continuous exercise has been used with reasonable success in cardiac rehabilitation programs but only after the patient has successfully completed lower levels of exercise training. Ismail et al. (2013) reviewed 74 HF exercise studies and reported that higher levels of exercise training can improve aerobic power by an average of 16% compared to less than half of that with low-level training. These findings indicate that the magnitude of gain in cardiorespiratory fitness is greater with increasing exercise intensity and appears to be unrelated to baseline fitness level or exercise volume. Moreover, high and vigorous exercise intensities do not appear to increase the risk of cardiac death, adverse events, and hospitalization. The CMES should use great caution when introducing higher-intensity exercise as a training stimulus in HF patients without direct clinical supervision.

TABLE 7-2

CLINICAL MANIFESTATIONS OF HEART FAILURE

- Dyspnea (excessive shortness of breath) with physical effort
- Orthopnea (dyspnea at rest when lying flat)
- Elevated resting heart rate >100 bpm (tachycardia)
- Fluid retention, particularly in the extremities (peripheral edema)
- Weight gain
- Cold, pale, and possibly cyanotic extremities
- Exercise intolerance manifested by dyspnea and a rapid pulse

DIAGNOSTIC TESTING AND CRITERIA

There are a number of reasons for a physician to order a battery of diagnostic tests to confirm or rule out CVD. In many cases, those with mild to moderate CHD have no major complaints other than fatigue. As the disease progresses, they may develop angina pectoris during physical activity. This type of pain typically subsides with rest. It is not uncommon for these symptoms to be ignored. If a patient presents with complaints of periodic chest pain, a physician will likely be aggressive in their diagnostics. In some cases, the patient does not have any complaints signifying CHD, but due to their multiple risk factors, warrants a closer look. In addition to standard blood work assessing blood **lipids** and lipoproteins, **glucose,** and inflammatory markers, noninvasive and/or invasive diagnostic tests will be ordered to evaluate the likelihood of any clinically significant blockage.

Electrocardiogram

An ECG is a graphic produced by an electrocardiograph machine, which records the electrical activity of the heart over time. Analysis of the various ECG waveforms and of electrical depolarization and repolarization yields important diagnostic information. A typical ECG tracing of the cardiac cycle (heartbeat) consists of a P wave, a QRS complex, a T wave, and a U wave. One of the most important diagnostic waveform lines in the ECG is the S-T segment, which connects the QRS complex and the T wave and represents the period when the ventricles are electrically depolarized. Most modern ECG monitors incorporate computerized electrocardiography, which records and measures ECG waveforms and time intervals.

ECG Exercise Testing

An exercise ECG test is a graded (gradual increase in speed and grade) exercise treadmill or stationary bicycle test with electrocardiographic recording. The test is considered "positive" if there is a specific standard level of change in the S-T segment component of the ECG, suggesting that there is a delay in the recovery after the contraction of the ventricles associated with narrowing of the coronary arteries. The important diagnostic information that is recorded during a stress ECG is as follows: ECG response (S-T segment, S-T slope, and potential dysrhythmias), **heart rate (HR)** and **blood pressure (BP)** response, symptoms (angina, dyspnea, or dizziness), and the exercise level achieved (e.g., MET capacity). ECG stress testing can be employed for diagnostic or functional assessment. For functional assessment, the test is used primarily to evaluate the patient's symptomology, MET capacity, and training heart-rate response. The ECG stress test is not as effective of a diagnostic tool as a radionuclide (nuclear) stress test. It is important to note that standardized exercise ECG stress tests do have limitations in that they are not perfect for ruling in or out CHD. A well administered exercise ECG that stresses a patient to at least 90% of **maximal heart rate** will have a sensitivity of 73 to 90% and a specificity of 50 to 74% (Gibbons et al., 2002). Sensitivity is the percentage of sick people who are correctly identified as having the condition. Specificity indicates the percentage of healthy people who are correctly identified as not having the condition. Medical clearance is strongly recommended for clients with CHD or with signs and symptoms of CHD, regardless of disease status, before beginning a moderate-intensity exercise program, or prior to progressing to vigorous-intensity exercise if they are already exercising regularly. If signs and symptoms of CHD are present in clients who are already exercising regularly, exercise should be discontinued until medical clearance is provided (ACSM, 2022).

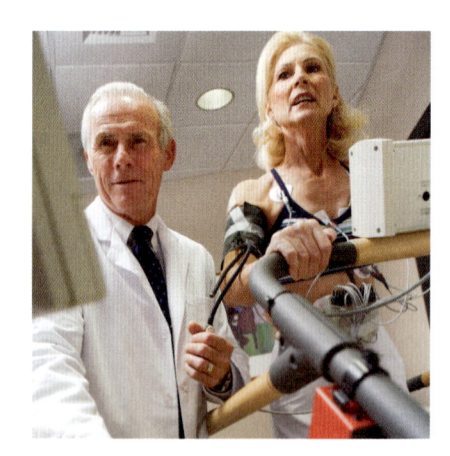

Radionuclide Stress Test

Radionuclide stress testing involves injecting a radioactive isotope (typically thallium or cardiolyte) into the person's vein, after which an image of the heart becomes visible with a special camera. The radioactive isotopes are absorbed by a healthy heart muscle. Nuclear images are obtained in the resting condition and again immediately following exercise. The two sets of images are then compared. During exercise, if a significant blockage in a coronary artery or arteries results in diminished blood flow to a part of the cardiac muscle, this region of the heart will appear as a relative "cold spot" on the nuclear scan, signifying reduced or diminished blood flow. This cold spot may not be visible on the images that are taken while the patient is at rest (when coronary flow is adequate). Radionuclide stress testing, while more time-consuming and expensive than a simple exercise ECG, greatly enhances the accuracy in diagnosing CHD.

Stress Echocardiography

Another supplement to the routine exercise ECG is **stress echocardiography** (cardiac ultrasound). During stress echocardiography, the sound waves of an ultrasound are used to produce images of the heart at rest and at the peak of exercise. In a heart with normal blood supply, all segments of the left ventricle exhibit enhanced contractions of the heart muscle during peak exercise. Conversely, in the setting of CHD, if a segment of the left ventricle does not receive optimal blood flow during exercise, that segment will demonstrate reduced contractions of the heart muscle relative to the rest of the heart on the exercise echocardiogram. Stress echocardiography is very useful in enhancing the interpretation of the exercise ECG, and can be used to exclude the presence of significant CHD in patients suspected of having a "false positive" stress ECG.

Coronary Angiography (Cardiac Catheterization)

Coronary angiography involves inserting a catheter into an artery in the groin area and routing it into the coronary arteries of the heart. This procedure is done for both diagnostic and interventional purposes. A radio contrast agent is passed into the catheter and is visualized on a fluoroscope to evaluate coronary blood flow in the major arteries of the heart. The benefit of this procedure is that while the catheter is inside the heart, the cardiologist can perform a **percutaneous transluminal coronary angioplasty (PTCA)**, a procedure that uses a small balloon at the tip of the heart catheter to push open plaques. Coronary angiography has several goals:
- To confirm the presence of a suspected blockage in a coronary artery
- To quantify the severity of the disease and its effect on the heart
- To seek the cause of a symptom such as angina, shortness of breath, or other signs of cardiac insufficiency
- To make a patient assessment prior to heart surgery

Vascular Imaging Techniques

Several invasive and noninvasive imaging techniques have been evaluated for use in characterizing atherosclerosis. Invasive coronary angiography has traditionally been the standard clinical tool for visualizing coronary arteries. Since its introduction more than 30 years ago, more than 2 million coronary angiograms have been performed annually in North America. Although coronary angiography is extremely useful in diagnosing obstructive atherosclerosis, it does not effectively define the extent of atherosclerosis in the vessel wall. Intravascular ultrasound is a newer invasive technique that allows for the direct observation of a vessel's plaque volume. The development of noninvasive cardiovascular techniques, such as **computed tomography (CT)** imaging of coronary artery calcium, CT angiographic imaging, B-mode ultrasound of carotid intima-media thickness (CIMT), and cardiovascular magnetic resonance imaging (CMRI), has enabled the more practical non-invasive evaluation of atherosclerosis at a preclinical stage.

Coronary Calcium Scoring

Coronary calcification is part of the pathogenesis of atherosclerosis and does not occur in normal vessels. Due to the association between coronary calcification and coronary plaque development, radiographically detected coronary artery calcium (CAC) can provide an estimate of total coronary plaque burden. Studies have reported that CAC scores are independently predictive of CHD outcomes, even after controlling for a variety of risk markers (Greenland et al., 2004). The primary methods for CAC measurement are electron-beam computed tomography (EBCT) and multi-detector computed tomography (MDCT).

EXPAND YOUR KNOWLEDGE

CORONARY CALCIUM CT SCAN

A cardiac CT scan for coronary calcium is a non-invasive way of obtaining information about the presence, location, and extent of calcified **plaque** in the coronary arteries. Calcified plaque results when there is a build-up of fat and other substances under the inner layer of the artery. This material can calcify, which signals the presence of atherosclerosis. The goal of a cardiac CT scan for calcium scoring is to determine if CHD is present and to what extent, even if there are no symptoms. It is a screening study that may be recommended by a physician for patients with risk factors for CHD, but no clinical symptoms.

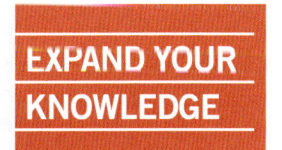

Calcified coronary plaque represents approximately 20% of the total coronary artery plaque burden, and thus, the more coronary calcium, the more atherosclerotic burden is present. The other 80% of the coronary plaque is fibrous plaque or lipid-rich (soft) plaque. Therefore, coronary calcium is a measure of a patient's atherosclerotic burden. After a coronary calcium scan, a calcium score called an **Agatston score** is generated. The score is based on the amount of calcium found in the coronary (heart) arteries. The client/patient may get an Agatston score for each major artery and a total score. The test is negative if no calcium deposits (calcifications) are found in the arteries. This means the individual's chance of having a **heart attack** in the next two to five years is low. The test is positive if calcifications are found in the arteries. The higher the Agatston score is, the more severe the atherosclerosis. It is important to note that although this test is used frequently to help predict CHD risk, it is not perfect and the scan does emit a small amount of radiation. Its best use in predicting CHD is when the score is combined with other CHD risk factors, particularly LDL level. Table 7-3 presents a general guide to the range of calcium scores (Agatston units) and their relationship to severity of atherosclerosis.

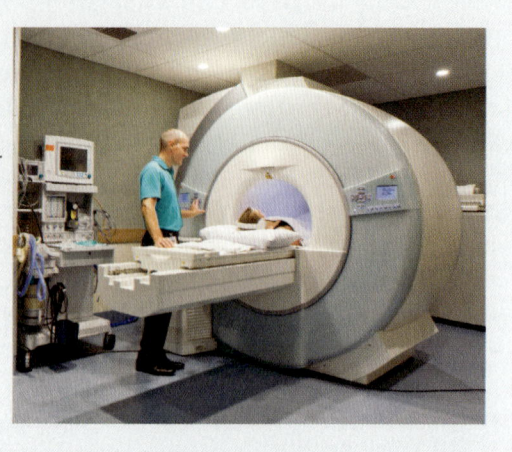

TABLE 7-3
CALCIUM SCORES AND THE SEVERITY OF ATHEROSCLEROSIS

0	No risk identified, negative test, low risk of CV event in next 5 years
1–10	Minimal risk, low risk of CV event in next 5 years
11–100	Mild risk, mild atherosclerosis is present, minimal coronary stenosis
101–400	Moderate calcium is detected, moderate risk of a CV event in next 5 years
>400	High calcium score, significant risk of a CV event in next 5 years

Note: CV = Cardiovascular

Source: National Cholesterol Education Program (2002). *Third Report of the National Cholesterol Education Program (NCEP) Expert Panel on Detection, Evaluation, and Treatment of High Blood Cholesterol in Adults (Adult Treatment Panel III)*. Final Report. National Heart, Lung, and Blood Institute National Institutes of Health NIH Publication No. 02-5215.

EXPAND YOUR KNOWLEDGE

OTHER VASCULAR IMAGING TECHNIQUES

Coronary CT Angiography

In CT angiography, computed tomography using a contrast material produces detailed pictures (a coronary CT angiogram). CT imaging uses special x-ray equipment to produce multiple images and a computer to join them together in cross-sectional views. This relatively new test is available to assess cholesterol plaque obstruction in the coronary arteries. Unlike a traditional coronary angiogram, CT angiograms do not use a catheter threaded through the blood vessels to the heart. Instead, a coronary CT angiogram relies on a powerful x-ray machine to produce images of the heart and heart vessels. In the past, noninvasive functional tests of the heart were used, such as treadmill tests and nuclear studies, to indirectly assess if there were blockages in the coronary arteries. The only way to directly look at the coronary arteries was via a cardiac catheterization and coronary angiogram.

CT scans have been used to look at various anatomic regions, but have not been useful for the heart because the heart is continuously in motion. Today, a new generation of CT scanners that can take 64 pictures a minute is available; with the use of medication to slow the HR to less than 64, CT images of the coronary arteries are now possible (Figure 7-3). There is some concern about the amount of radiation dosage used in CT angiography, which has given rise to a "micro-dose" CT angiography that provides a simplified procedure with one-tenth of the radiation dose and at a reduced cost.

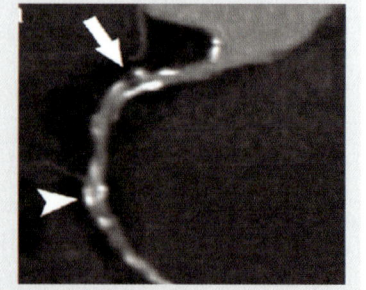

Figure 7-3
Computed tomography (CT) scan

High-resolution Magnetic Resonance Imaging

High-resolution cardiovascular magnetic resonance imaging of the arterial wall is emerging as a powerful research technology for characterizing atherosclerotic lesions within carotid arteries and other large vessels. High-resolution **magnetic resonance imaging (MRI)** is able to noninvasively characterize three important aspects of atherosclerotic lesions: size, composition, and biologic activity. It can quantify not only wall and lumen areas and volumes, but also plaque composition. For example, high-resolution MRI can assess cap thickness and distinguish ruptured plaque caps from thick and stable caps. This technique can also be used to characterize the composition of a plaque by differentiating lipid-free regions from lipid-rich and calcified regions. In addition, high-resolution MRI can identify recent intra-plaque hemorrhages using multi-contrast-weighted studies.

Intravascular Ultrasound

Intravascular ultrasound (IVUS) is a valuable adjunct to coronary angiography. While angiography provides only a two-dimensional assessment of the lumen of the target vessel, IVUS allows the tomographic measurement (the recording of internal body images at a predetermined plane) of artery lumen area, plaque size, plaque distribution, and to some extent, plaque composition.

IVUS involves invasively placing a specialized catheter with a miniaturized ultrasound probe attached to the distal end of the catheter. The proximal end of the catheter is attached to computerized ultrasound equipment. It allows the application of ultrasound technology to see from inside blood vessels out through the surrounding blood column, visualizing the endothelium (inner wall) of blood vessels. Because the arterial remodeling and plaque deposition that characterize the early stages of atherosclerotic progression occur without decreases in lumen area, IVUS may be able to detect atherosclerotic disease at an earlier state than coronary angiography. In many cases, IVUS may provide the ability to detect some "angiographically silent" **atheromas.**

B-mode Ultrasound Assessment

B-mode ultrasound is a noninvasive imaging modality that employs ultrasound to accurately image the walls of arteries and is a useful tool for evaluating carotid intima-media wall thickness (CIMT). The normal arterial wall consists of three layers: the tunica intima, tunica media, and tunica adventitia. The thickness of the two innermost layers in the carotid artery (the intima and media), or the CIMT, is increasingly used as a surrogate marker for early atherosclerosis. Carotid ultrasound measurements correlate well with histology, and increased CIMT is associated with the presence of vascular risk factors and more advanced atherosclerosis, including CHD. Large observational studies have established that CIMT is an independent marker of risk for cardiovascular events. A meta-analysis of eight studies reported that the relative risk per one 0.10-mm difference in common carotid artery CIMT was 1.15 for MI and 1.18 for **stroke,** adjusted for age and sex (Lorenz et al., 2007).

TREATMENT OPTIONS

Pharmacological therapy is usually first-step therapy for CHD and often used in conjunction with surgical therapy. The CMES should be familiar with each of these classes of medications and their principle indications. The principle classes of drug therapy for CHD are beta blockers, angiotensin-converting enzyme (ACE) inhibitors, angiotensin receptor blockers (ARBs), calcium channel blockers (CCBs), **diuretics, vasodilators,** cardiac glycosides, antiarrhythmic agents, blood modifiers (e.g., anticoagulants), and antilipemic agents (e.g., statins).

Aside from pharmacological therapy, the two interventions most often employed in CHD patients are **coronary artery bypass grafting (CABG)** and PTCA, also called percutaneous coronary intervention (PCI). PTCA will usually include intracoronary stenting (using a wire mesh device to open the artery). The CMES can work with all of these clients, as long as they have no complications and are stable from symptom, ventricular function, and ECG abnormality perspectives. Most often, these individuals require aggressive risk-factor control, especially blood lipid and BP management. The CMES should follow the exercise guidelines and precautions in this chapter for all CHD clients. The most important rule to remember for CABG clients, however, is to avoid traditional resistance-training programs with moderate to heavy weights for the first six weeks post-surgery. This will give the sternum sufficient time to heal from the CABG sternotomy (surgical opening of the sternum). Graduated upper-extremity range-of-motion exercises and many hatha yoga poses that do not place undue strain on the sternum or upper back are recommended for clients who have had CABG within the previous four to eight weeks. As with the post-MI client, the CMES should see these individuals only after physician evaluation and referral.

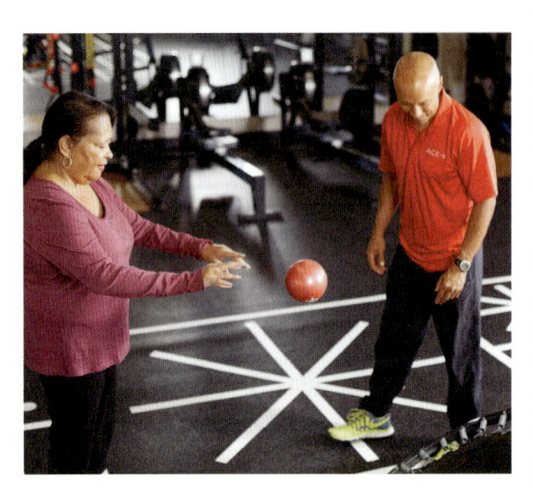

The success rate for CABG can reach beyond 10 years, but those with multiple risk factors may see coronary blockages in as little as six years post-CABG. Unfortunately, the success rates for angioplasty are not as promising. Up to 30% of post-PTCA clients will experience **restenosis** within the first six months of the procedure. PTCA is more effective than medical therapy in relieving angina, but it confers no greater survival benefit. Aggressive lipid-lowering therapy appears to be as effective as percutaneous coronary intervention plus usual medical care for preventing ischemic events (Boden et al., 2007).

A CMES working with clients who are post-PTCA or post-CABG should take notice of any of the following signs and symptoms of restenosis or worsening of the coronary atherosclerotic process:
- Complaints of general fatigue
- Reduced exercise tolerance or accelerated HR at customary workloads
- Any symptoms of chest discomfort or pain

Since CHD is common among the American population, an astute CMES may pick up on these subtle complaints in any of the populations they serve.

NUTRITIONAL CONSIDERATIONS

A foundational component of working with clients with CHD is knowledge of general nutrition recommendations for optimal heart health and how to best share them with clients to help facilitate adoption of the recommendations. It is also helpful to know when and how to refer to a **registered dietitian (RD)** for **medical nutrition therapy (MNT)** and to have a general understanding of the nutrition considerations the RD is likely to recommend.

This section will first outline foundational principles for nutrition and behavior change for CVD prevention and then provide an overview of nutrition considerations for individuals who have been diagnosed with CHD and who may have experienced complications from a cardiovascular event, such as **congestive heart failure (CHF).**

Cardiovascular Disease Prevention

While the CMES may work with clients who have already been diagnosed with CVD or are at very high risk of disease, knowledge and implementation of the guidelines to help prevent CVD are as valuable for secondary and tertiary prevention. In fact, the AHA states that preventive recommendations can be applied to the management of individuals with CVD, though in these cases the recommendations may have to be intensified (Eckel et al., 2013).

A critical component to the recommendations is consideration of the practicalities of implementing the guidelines, including behavior-change principles and the value of client-focused guidance, rather than simply sharing recommendations and adhering to the unrealistic expectation that the client will seamlessly convert recommendations into action. Table 7-4 highlights the AHA's major recommendations for lifestyle management.

In a follow-up to the release of these guidelines, the AHA published a paper on the best evidence to help implement the guidelines (Gidding et al., 2009). This paper placed heavy emphasis on recognizing the barriers and opportunities for implementation of change on multiple levels including the individual, family, community, and policy (the **socio-ecological model**) (Figure 7-4). The AHA statement reinforces ACE's strongly held belief that principles of behavioral change—including client-centered focus, readiness to change, goal setting, and repeated review and evaluation of the success and feasibility of the intervention—drive exercise and nutrition interventions. Communication strategies such as **motivational interviewing** (see Chapter 5) are helpful to facilitate this process. During lifestyle coaching sessions, the CMES may have an opportunity to share tips to help support healthy nutrition choices. When that opportunity occurs, the AHA advises targeting the behaviors shown in Table 7-5.

TABLE 7-4
SUMMARY OF RECOMMENDATIONS FOR LIFESTYLE MANAGEMENT

DIET

LDL-C—Advise adults who would benefit from LDL-C lowering to:

- Consume a dietary pattern that emphasizes intake of vegetables, fruits, and whole grains; includes low-fat dairy products, poultry, fish, legumes, nontropical vegetable oils, and nuts; and limit intake of sweets, sugar-sweetened beverages, and red meats.
    - ✓ Adapt this dietary pattern to appropriate calorie requirements, personal and cultural food preferences, and nutrition therapy for other medical conditions (including diabetes mellitus).
    - ✓ Achieve this pattern by following plans such as the DASH eating plan, the Healthy U.S.-Style Dietary Pattern, or the AHA diet.
- Aim for a dietary pattern that achieves 5 to 6% of calories from saturated fat.
- Reduce percent of calories from saturated fat.
- Reduce percent of calories from trans fat.

BP—Advise adults who would benefit from BP lowering to:

- Consume a dietary pattern that emphasizes intake of vegetables, fruits, and whole grains; includes low-fat dairy products, poultry, fish, legumes, nontropical vegetable oils, and nuts; and limit intake of sweets, sugar-sweetened beverages, and red meats.
    - ✓ Adapt this dietary pattern to appropriate calorie requirements, personal and cultural food preferences, and nutrition therapy for other medical conditions (including diabetes mellitus).
    - ✓ Achieve this pattern by following plans such as the DASH eating plan, the Healthy U.S.-Style Dietary Pattern, or the AHA diet.
- Lower sodium intake.
    - ✓ Consume no more than 2,300 mg of sodium/day.
    - ✓ Further reduction of sodium intake to 1,500 mg/day is desirable since it is associated with an even greater reduction in BP.
    - ✓ Reduce intake by at least 1,000 mg/day, since that will lower BP, even if the desired daily sodium intake is not yet achieved.
- Combine the DASH eating plan with lower sodium intake.

PHYSICAL ACTIVITY

Lipids
- In general, advise adults to engage in aerobic physical activity to reduce LDL-C and non-HDL-C: 3 to 4 sessions a week, lasting on average 40 minutes per session and involving moderate-to-vigorous intensity physical activity.

BP
- In general, advise adults to engage in aerobic physical activity to lower BP: 3 to 4 sessions a week, lasting on average 40 minutes per session and involving moderate-to-vigorous intensity physical activity.

Note: LDL-C = Low-density lipoprotein cholesterol; DASH = Dietary Approaches to Stop Hypertension; UDSA = U.S. Department of Agriculture; AHA = American Heart Association; BP = Blood pressure; non-HDL-C = non-high-density lipoprotein cholesterol

Source: Eckel, R.H. et al. (2013). 2013 AHA/ACC guideline on lifestyle management to reduce cardiovascular risk: A report of the American College of Cardiology/American Heart Association Task Force on Practice Guidelines. *Journal of the American College of Cardiology,* 63, 25. DOI: 10.1016/j.jacc.2013.11.003

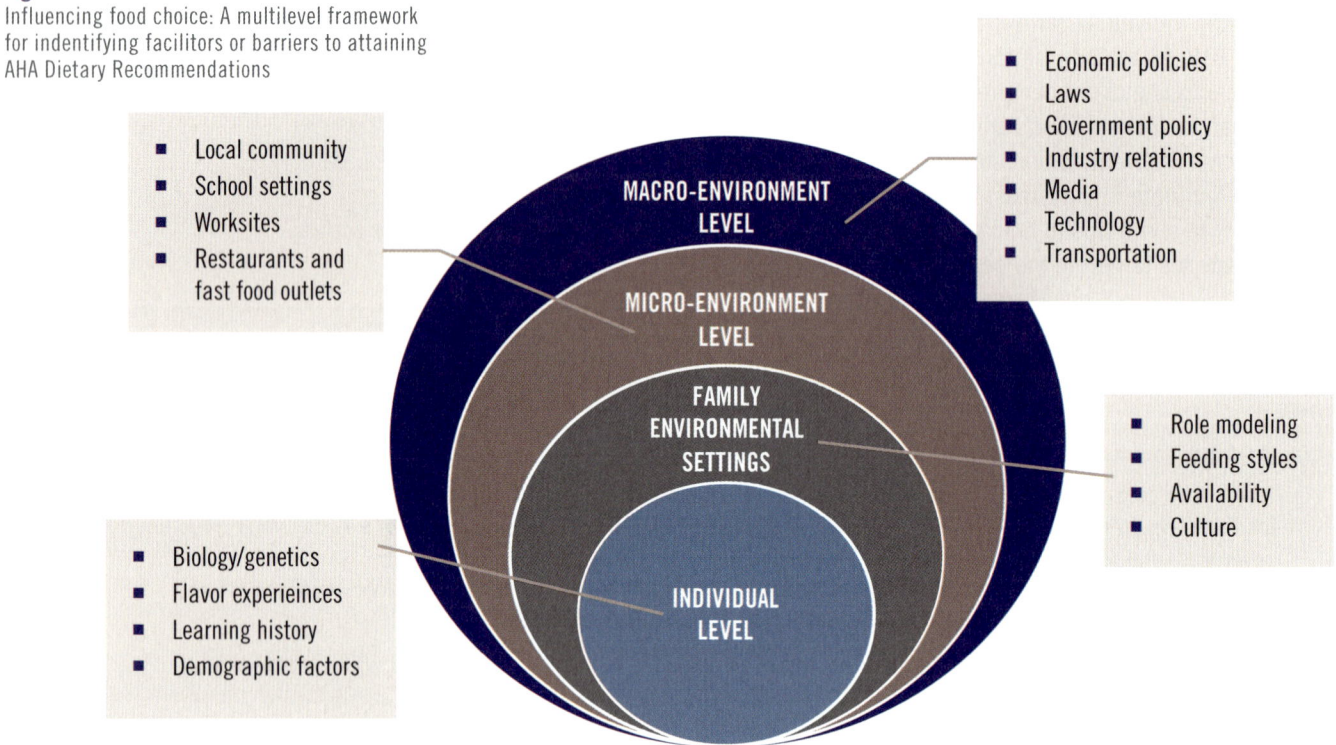

Figure 7-4
Influencing food choice: A multilevel framework for indentifying facilitators or barriers to attaining AHA Dietary Recommendations

- Local community
- School settings
- Worksites
- Restaurants and fast food outlets

- Economic policies
- Laws
- Government policy
- Industry relations
- Media
- Technology
- Transportation

- Role modeling
- Feeding styles
- Availability
- Culture

- Biology/genetics
- Flavor experieinces
- Learning history
- Demographic factors

MACRO-ENVIRONMENT LEVEL
MICRO-ENVIRONMENT LEVEL
FAMILY ENVIRONMENTAL SETTINGS
INDIVIDUAL LEVEL

Reprinted with permission from Gidding, S. et al. (2009). Implementing American Heart Association Pediatric and Adult Nutrition Guidelines: A Scientific Statement from the American Heart Association Nutrition Committee of the Council on Nutrition, Physical Activity and Metabolism, Council on Cardiovascular Disease in the Young, Council on Arteriosclerosis, Thrombosis and Vascular Biology, Council on Cardiovascular Nursing, Council on Epidemiology and Prevention, and Council for High Blood Pressure Research. *Circulation,* 119, 1161–1175.

TABLE 7-5
EXAMPLES OF EATING BEHAVIORS TO TARGET IN COACHING

Food selection	Food presentation
• Limiting sugar-containing beverages • Use of a simply structured diet table that categorizes foods into three easily identifiable groups (e.g., "go" for good foods and "slow" and "whoa" for poor foods)	• Eat more meals as a family • Reduce portion size • Choose healthy alternatives to poor food choices • Repeat presentation of foods not well liked
Food acquisition	**Self-monitoring**
• Make healthier choices on foods prepared and/or purchased outside the home • Shop for healthier foods • Control food availability in the home	• Routine weighing so that caloric intake adjustments can be made • Scheduled physical activity • Record of caloric intake

Additional strategies
- Praise for meeting goals from peers and others in the home must be provided
- Behavioral contracting with nonfood rewards; reinforcement should be social and not related to food, money, or gifts
- Removal of stimuli for undesired or inappropriate food choices
- Parents must model desired or appropriate behaviors

Reprinted with permission from Gidding, S. et al. (2009). Implementing American Heart Association Pediatric and Adult Nutrition Guidelines: A Scientific Statement from the American Heart Association Nutrition Committee of the Council on Nutrition, Physical Activity and Metabolism, Council on Cardiovascular Disease in the Young, Council on Arteriosclerosis, Thrombosis and Vascular Biology, Council on Cardiovascular Nursing, Council on Epidemiology and Prevention, and Council for High Blood Pressure Research. *Circulation,* 119, 1161–1175.

Coronary Heart Disease

CHD results from atherosclerotic narrowing of the coronary arteries likely to produce angina pectoris or MI. Thus, a major objective of nutrition therapy for individuals with CHD is to minimize atherosclerotic narrowing, or at least decrease the risk of an atherosclerotic lesion causing an MI.

Individuals with CHD are well served by an evaluation from an RD for MNT. Together the RD and client will develop an eating plan and lifestyle changes that are best suited to help prevent and treat CHD.

The Academy of Nutrition and Dietetics (A.N.D.) has established guidelines for optimal nutrition management for several cardiovascular conditions, including lipid disorders, hypertension, and CHF through its Evidence Analysis Library, a tool for RDs that synthesizes the nutrition research and offers evidence-based recommendations to help guide clinical decisions. The components of those guidelines that are most specific to CHD are included here. Further details for lipid disorders and hypertension are included within their respective chapters in this text (Chapters 8 and 9).

> **EXPAND YOUR KNOWLEDGE**
>
> **REGISTERED DIETITIANS AND MEDICAL NUTRITION THERAPY**
>
> A critical partner in the nutrition management of an individual with CHD is the RD, ideally one with specialized training in nutrition therapy for CVD.
>
> The A.N.D Evidence Analysis Library reports that patients who attend several visits with an RD over a period of six to 12 weeks effectively decrease dietary fat, **saturated fat,** and energy intake. Research suggests that these nutrition changes result in a 7 to 21% reduction in total cholesterol, a 7 to 22% reduction in LDL cholesterol, and an 11 to 31% reduction in triglycerides. The best results occur with at least three to six visits to an RD (A.N.D., 2013a).
>
> In these visits, the RD implements MNT, which includes:
> - A comprehensive nutrition assessment
> - Planning and implementation of an evidence-based nutrition intervention
> - Monitoring and evaluation of a client's progress
>
> Specifically, during the MNT visits, the RD assesses the client's current food and nutrition intake; related health history including medication, supplement use, labs, and anthropometrics; physical activity and sleep history; and current knowledge, attitudes, and beliefs about food and behavioral change. From there, the RD will determine the client's ideal energy and **macronutrient** needs, and compare needs with current intake. During the initial visit, the RD will recommend a meal plan based on the best evidence for optimal nutrition management of CHD, as well as the client's individual factors. Follow-up visits will gauge the client's adherence to recommendations, troubleshoot challenges, and acknowledge successes.
>
> In many cases for insured individuals, MNT is a reimbursable service for individuals diagnosed with CHD with referral from a physician.

Macronutrient Composition

Individuals with CHD are advised to consume 25 to 35% of calories from fat (with <7% of calories from saturated fat and as little **trans fatty acids** as possible). Total **protein** should comprise 15 to 20% of calories and 45 to 60% of calories should be from total **carbohydrates,** with emphasis on high-fiber sources and avoidance of refined carbohydrates. Individuals with baseline elevated saturated fat intake may benefit from replacing saturated fat calories with **unsaturated fats,** protein, or **complex carbohydrates** (fruits, vegetables, and whole grains). This substitution can decrease LDL cholesterol by up to 16%, subsequently decreasing the risk for a cardiovascular event (A.N.D., 2013a).

Specific Cardioprotective Nutrients

The A.N.D.'s Evidence Analysis Library (2013a; 2013b) also discusses nutrients thought to be cardioprotective. The main findings are highlighted here.

Omega-3 Fatty Acids

Knowledge of specific dietary components that help to optimize heart health continues to evolve. A fair body of evidence supports that individuals with CHD should consume two or more 4-oz servings of fatty fish per week, due to their high content of **omega-3 fatty acids.** These fatty acids, in particular docosahexaenoic acid (DHA) and eicosapentaenoic acid (EPA), have been shown to decrease risk of arrhythmias and fatal heart disease and decrease progression of coronary atherosclerosis in individuals with diagnosed CHD. High intake of plant-derived alpha-linolenic acid (ALA) (about 1.4 grams per day) is associated with decreased risk of cardiac death, non-fatal MI, and recurrent MI. **Adequate Intake (AI)** of ALA is 1.6 grams per day for men and 1.1 grams per day for women. No AI has been established for DHA or EPA, although the Institute of Medicine (IOM, 2005) suggests that 10% of the needed ALA could come from EPA or DHA, which suggests a daily intake of about 100 mg per day. Some expert panels have recommended much higher intakes of 250 and 500 mg per day due to the significant health benefits attributed to these fatty acids and the low risk of complications such as bleeding, even at this higher range (Harris, 2010).

Some RDs may advise clients with CHD but without angina or implantable cardioverter defibrillators (ICD) to supplement their diet with 850 mg per day of EPA and/or DHA to reduce risk of sudden death by 45%. (This is in contrast to individuals *without* CHD or those who have angina or ICD in which supplementation may be contraindicated.) Consumption of more than 3 grams per day of omega-3 fatty acids may cause gastrointestinal distress.

Antioxidants and Plant Stanols and Sterols

Antioxidant-rich whole foods, including fruits, vegetables, whole grains, and nuts high in vitamins E, C, and β-carotenoids (a form of vitamin A), appear to provide cardiovascular protection. However, supplementation of these antioxidants does not appear to provide benefit (Sesso et al., 2008; Cook et al., 2007). Plant **stanols** and **sterols** are cholesterol-mimicking substances that occur naturally in many whole grains, vegetables, fruits, legumes, nuts, and seeds. They also have been added to many common foods such as cereals and bars, margarine, and orange juice. Plant stanols and sterols so closely resemble cholesterol that they can bind to cholesterol receptors and prevent cholesterol from being absorbed into the bloodstream. Then, instead of eventually depositing into plaques in the arteries, they are excreted with the waste. Consumption of 2 to 3 grams per day of plant stanols and sterols appears to decrease total cholesterol with no documented adverse effects (see Chapter 8).

Nuts

Consumption of 5 ounces of unsalted and lower-saturated fat tree nuts (e.g., walnuts, almonds, pecans, and pistachios) per week decreases risk of CHD, mostly due to their omega-3-rich fatty acid profile, which helps to decrease total and LDL cholesterol. However, nuts have high caloric density (5 ounces of nuts is equivalent to approximately 900 kcal). It is essential that they serve as an isocaloric substitute, rather than an addition, to the diet.

Alcohol

Individuals with CHD may experience decreased risk of CVD from alcohol consumption (a maximum of one drink per day for women and up to two drinks per day for men) due to its effects on cholesterol composition. With that said, nondrinkers should never be encouraged to begin drinking in an effort to decrease CVD risk.

B Vitamins

High consumption of whole-food sources of B vitamins including **folate,** vitamin B6, and vitamin B12 provides cardioprotective benefit. However, supplementation of these vitamins does not appear to provide cardiovascular benefit.

Coronary Heart Disease

Fiber

Diets high in fiber (at least 25 to 30 grams per day), especially soluble fiber, provide substantial cardiovascular benefit, including a reduction in total and LDL cholesterol. Rich sources of soluble fiber include fruits, vegetables, and whole grains, especially high-fiber cereals, oatmeal, and legumes.

Congestive Heart Failure

As with other chronic conditions, referral to an RD for MNT of congestive heart failure is important. The RD will work with client to determine caloric, macronutrient, and **micronutrient** needs. RDs take several unique nutrition variables into consideration when developing a nutrition plan for a client with CHF, including protein to replace losses, fluid intake, specific micronutrient needs, and supplementation. A summary of recommendations from A.N.D.'s Evidence Analysis Library on Congestive Heart Failure (A.N.D., 2013b) are outlined here:

- *Protein:* Evidence suggests that individuals with CHF have higher protein needs than those without CHF. Protein needs vary considerably based on the extent of protein depletion as assessed by clinical and lab measures. On average, stable depleted clients need about 1.37 g/kg of protein per day, and adequately nourished need about 1.12 g/kg of protein per day.
- *Fluid intake:* Recommended fluid intake ranges from 1.4 to 1.9 liters per day (48 to 64 oz), with the actual advised amount within that range depending on clinical symptoms including **edema,** fatigue, and shortness of breath. Evidence supports that this fluid restriction helps to lessen symptoms and improve quality of life.
- *Sodium:* Recommended intake is less than 2 grams per day. As with fluid restriction, sodium restriction helps to lessen symptoms and improve quality of life.
- *Folate and Vitamin B12:* Consuming at least the **Dietary Reference Intake (DRI)** of folate and getting at least 200 to 500 mcg of vitamin B12 (whether through diet or supplementation) can improve clinical symptoms.
- *Thiamine:* Diuretic use is the standard of care for individuals with CHF. In some cases, diuretics can cause thiamine deficiency. For this reason, clients should be sure to consume (either through food or supplementation) at least the AI of 1.2 mg/day for men and 1.1 mg/day for women of thiamine (IOM, 2005).
- *Magnesium:* Individuals with CHF should be sure to consume at least the RDA of 320 mg/day for women >30 years and 420 mg/day for men >30 years, as low levels of magnesium can cause heart arrhythmias in those with CHF.
- *L-Arginine, Carnitine, Coenzyme Q10, and Hawthorn:* Insufficient evidence exists to confirm or deny the potential benefit of these supplements for individuals with CHF.

Eating Plans to Support Optimal Heart Health

An overall healthy, balanced eating plan to meet calorie needs is helpful in preventing and treating CHD. Many different eating plans and eating patterns have been studied, including very low-fat diets such as the Ornish plan to more moderate eating plans such as the Therapeutic Lifestyle Changes (TLC), *Dietary Guidelines for Americans* (U.S. Department of Agriculture, 2020), **Dietary Approaches to Stop Hypertension (DASH) eating plan,** and the **Healthy Mediterranean-Style Dietary Pattern.** (More information about the TLC eating plan is discussed in Chapter 8 and the DASH plan is included in the nutrition section of Chapter 9. The Ornish and Mediterranean eating plans are described here.)

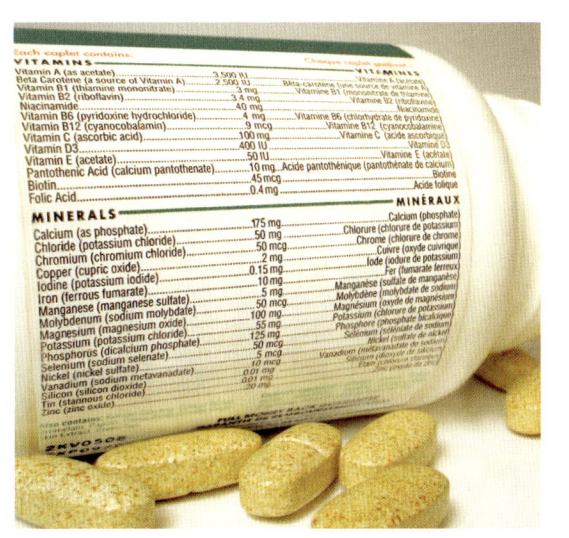

CHAPTER 7   Coronary Heart Disease

Each of these dietary approaches has demonstrated cardiovascular health benefits. In fact, these eating plans contain common elements, including: high in vegetables and fruits, high in whole grains, moderate amounts of protein-rich foods, limited added sugars, and emphasis on oils over solid fats. The plans are generally lower in sodium, saturated fat, and caloric density than the typical American diet and higher in fiber and potassium. In fact, the typical American diet is far from the recommendations in many of the dietary variables that best predict (or protect from) CVD. Figure 7-5 highlights the typical American diet compared to recommended intakes.

*NOTE: Recommended daily intake of whole grains is to be at least half of total grain consumption, and the limit for refined grains is to be no more than half of total grain consumption.

Data Source: Analysis of What We Eat in America, NHANES 2013-2016, ages 1 and older, 2 days dietary intake data, weighted. *Recommended Intake Ranges:* Healthy U.S.-Style Dietary Patterns (see **Appendix 3**).

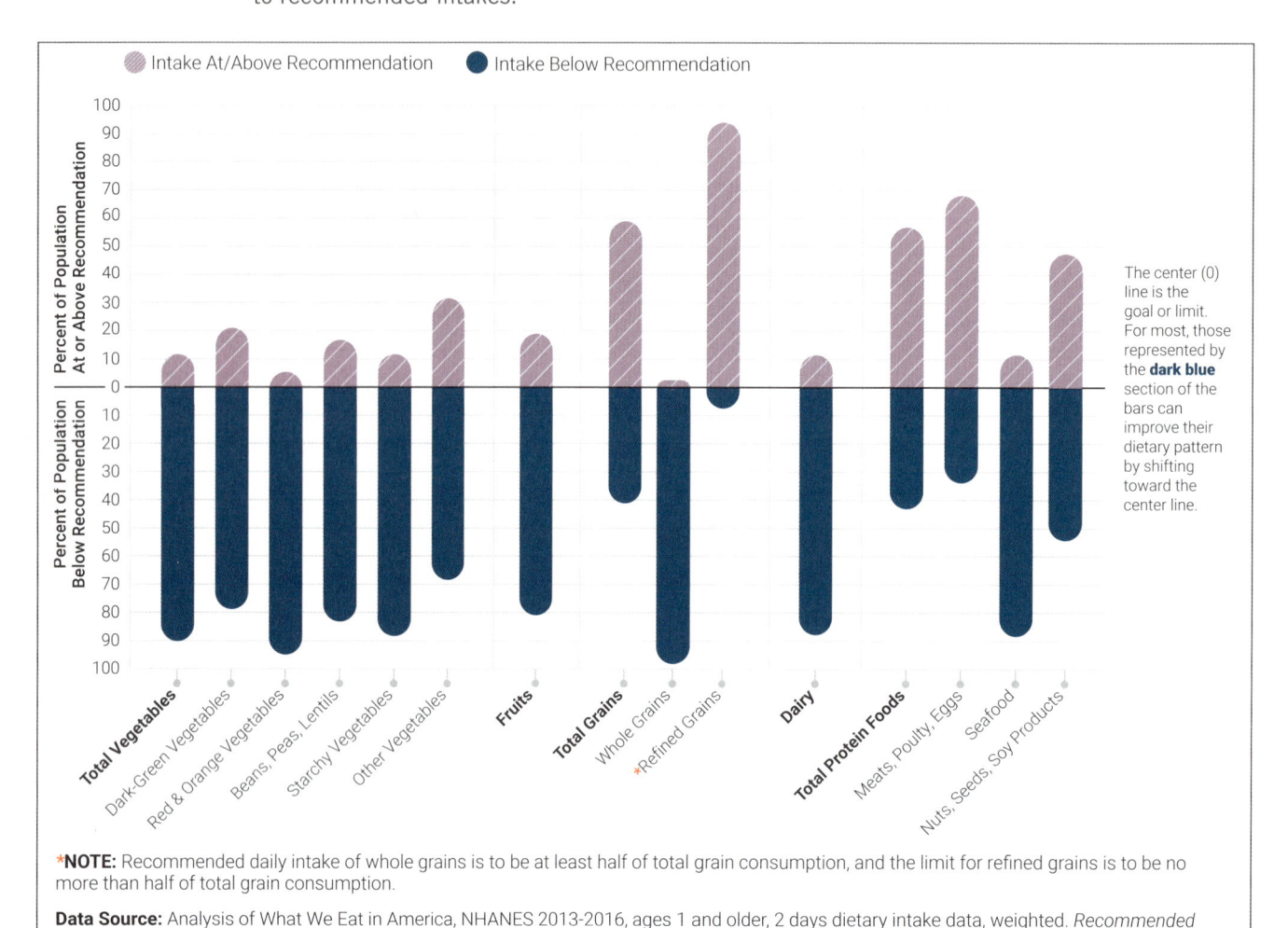

Figure 7-5
Dietary intakes compared to recommendations: Percent of the U.S. population ages 1 and older who are below and at or above each dietary goal
Reprinted from United States Department of Agriculture (2020). *2020-2025 Dietary Guidelines for Americans* (9th ed.). www.dietaryguidelines.gov

Ornish Diet and Lifestyle Spectrum Plan

Dean Ornish, a physician-researcher at the University of California-San Francisco and founder of the Preventive Medicine Research Institute was the first to demonstrate that nutrition, exercise, and stress management can *reverse* heart blockages. Ornish published a ground-breaking randomized-controlled study that first showed regression of disease after a one-year intensive lifestyle intervention (Ornish et al., 1990). A follow-up study found regression at both one and five years. In this intervention, 48 patients with moderate to severe CHD who were randomized to an intensive lifestyle change (consumption of a 10% fat, whole foods vegetarian diet, aerobic exercise, stress-management training, smoking cessation, and group psycho-social support) experienced reversal of their CVD (evidenced by decreased percent stenosis by 1.75 absolute percentage points by 1 year and 3.1 absolute percentage points after 5 years). The control group experienced a significant increase of stenosis and 45 cardiovascular events (compared to 28 in the experimental group) (Ornish et al., 1998). Numerous subsequent studies as part of this trial, coined the Lifestyle Heart Trial, have continued to validate these findings. The major challenge for the average person is adherence to such an eating plan. Recognizing this, Ornish has evolved his program to be more personalized through his Ornish Lifestyle Spectrum program (www.ornishspectrum.com).

Healthy Mediterranean-Style Dietary Pattern

Another particularly effective eating plan for individuals with, or at high risk of, CHD is the Healthy Mediterranean-Style Dietary Pattern. While there are many variations of the Mediterranean dietary pattern, it generally is high in vegetables, fruits, nuts, olive oils, and whole grains. Wine is included at most meals. Meats and full-fat milk products are limited. Overall, this eating plan is relatively high in **monounsaturated fat** and low in saturated fat. Many research studies evaluating Mediterranean dietary patterns use the following standards in determining how well a participant follows this type of dietary pattern (Trichopoulou et al., 2003):

- Vegetables (other than potatoes): 4 or more servings per day
- Fruits: 4 or more servings per day
- Whole grains: 2 or more servings per day
- Beans (legumes): 2 or more servings per week
- Nuts: 2 or more servings per week
- Fish: 2 or more servings per week
- Red and processed meat: 1 or fewer servings per day
- Dairy foods: 1 or fewer servings per day
- Alcohol: ½ to 1 drink per day for women, 1 to 2 for men

The body of research on the Healthy Mediterranean-Style Dietary Pattern continues to grow, with many studies demonstrating its efficacy in improving CVD markers such as weight, BP, fasting glucose, total cholesterol, C-reactive protein, stroke, and MI (Hoevenaar-Blom et al., 2012; Nordmann et al., 2011). Another study found a 73% lower risk of cardiac death and non-fatal MI compared to a prudent diet in study participants who had experienced a previous MI (de Lorgeril et al., 1999). Overall, greater adherence to a Mediterranean-style eating plan is associated with improved cardiovascular health (Sofi et al., 2010).

THINK IT THROUGH

How familiar are you with the Ornish eating plan and the Healthy Mediterranean-Style Dietary Pattern? Although it is outside the scope of practice for a CMES to provide eating plans to clients, it is important to understand the principles of eating a heart-healthy diet for those with CHD so that you can recognize when a client may need a referral to an RD for further support. Take the time to read the references provided for the Ornish and Mediterranean plans so that you have a good foundational understanding of how a supportive diet can influence heart health.

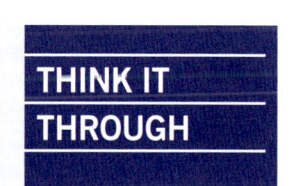

EXERCISE TRAINING RECOMMENDATIONS FOR CLIENTS WITH STABLE CHD

The last three decades have seen numerous published studies demonstrating the many benefits of cardiac rehabilitation, but particularly the exercise-training benefits in CHD clients (Table 7-6) (Lavie et al., 2009). These are essentially the same benefits realized by apparently healthy individuals without CHD, but are clearly more of a priority in those with CHD.

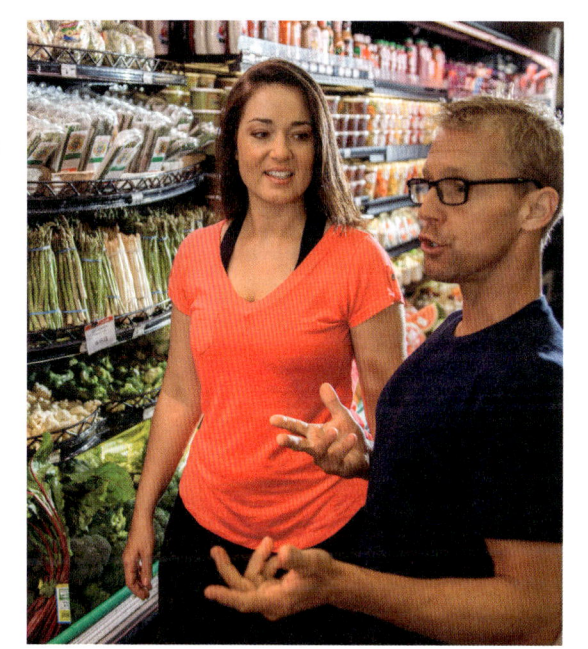

TABLE 7-6
KEY BENEFITS OF SYSTEMATIC EXERCISE TRAINING IN THOSE WITH CORONARY HEART DISEASE

- Improved exercise capacity and $\dot{V}O_2max$ (aerobic power)
- Increased muscular fitness (e.g., strength, endurance, and flexibility)
- Lessening of angina symptoms/raising of the ischemic threshold
- Modest decreases in body fat, blood pressure, total and LDL cholesterol, non-HDL cholesterol, triglycerides, and high-sensitivity c-reactive protein (hsCRP)
- Increased HDL cholesterol
- Improved endothelial (arterial) function
- Increased myocardial ischemia tolerance
- Increased myocardial capillary density
- Reduced adiposity and metabolic syndrome risk factors
- Reduced stress
- Control of diabetes mellitus
- Improved well-being and self-efficacy
- Improvement in behavioral characteristics (depression, anxiety, and hostility)
- Reduction in overall morbidity and mortality (especially that associated with depression and psychological distress)

Note: LDL = low-density lipoprotein; HDL = high-density lipoprotein

Appropriate Program Candidates and Stable CHD

Generally speaking, a CMES who wishes to work with individuals with CHD or those who are prone to CHD may see clients in one of two categories: those who do not have clinically documented CHD but who have elevated risk for CHD because of their CHD risk factors and those who have documented and stable CHD. Both groups require consideration for when a pre-program exercise ECG test is recommended. ACSM, along with the AACVPR, has published and updated guidelines for when a medical examination, exercise testing with ECG, and supervision of exercise testing is recommended. Refer to Chapter 3 for information on how to perform a pre-exercise health-risk assessment.

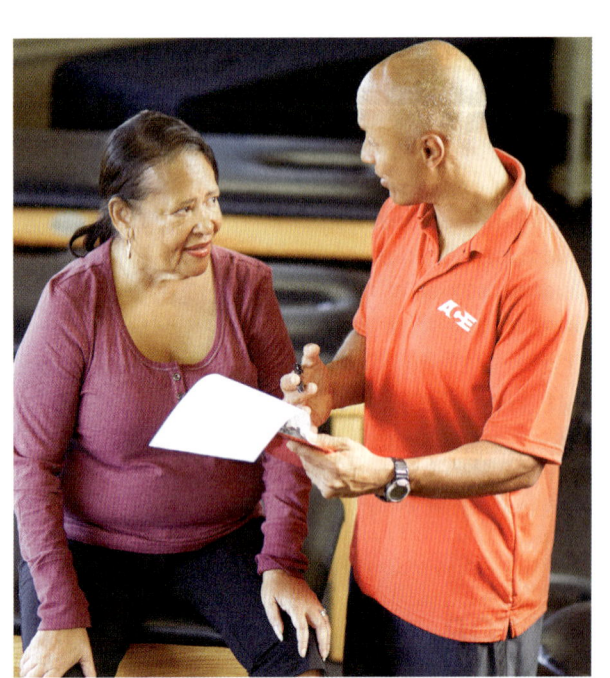

Note that exercise testing here should not be confused with "fitness testing," but instead refers to clinical exercise testing with ECG (i.e., exercise ECG) performed by a physician and/or a clinical exercise physiologist. It is imperative that the CMES understand the difference between pre-program clinical exercise ECG testing administered by clinical personnel and supervised by a physician and periodic submaximal fitness testing.

Although cardiovascular disease risk factors are no longer used to determine if medical clearance is required prior to initiating an exercise program, they should still be considered, as recognizing and controlling these risk factors is imperative for cardiovascular disease prevention and management (ACSM, 2022). The intended use for identifying risk factors is to aid in the identification of occult coronary artery disease and to then work together with clients on lifestyle behavioral change. Assessing CVD risk factors as part of a comprehensive health screening affords relevant information to be used not only for personalized exercise program design, but also for providing client education and collaborating on goals and next steps for lifestyle modification.

Coronary Heart Disease   CHAPTER 7

Fitness Testing CHD Patients

The CMES can administer most fitness tests to clients with stable CHD, provided that the client meets the overall considerations and recommendations in Table 7-7 and has no contraindications to resistance exercise. Appropriate fitness tests include flexibility, muscular endurance, and strength tests in which the client does not exert to muscular contraction "failure." Good cueing will prevent breath-holding (Valsalva maneuver). Inappropriate tests are those that push the client to a near-maximal perceived exertion, predicted HR, or $\dot{V}O_2$max. Submaximal aerobic endurance tests may be performed, but only when the client has had a recent physician-supervised negative exercise ECG and is free from exercise-related cardiac symptoms (e.g., angina and dysrhythmias).

TABLE 7-7
OVERALL RECOMMENDATIONS FOR TRAINING STABLE CORONARY HEART DISEASE (CHD) CLIENTS

- Perform a 5- to 10-minute warm-up and cool-down with each exercise session that includes static and dynamic stretching and light to very light aerobic activities.
- The aerobic portion of exercise sessions should emphasize increased caloric expenditure by using rhythmic large-muscle-group activities.
- Have clients perform conditioning for the upper and lower body using a variety of aerobic activities and exercise equipment.
- Consider all safety factors, including clinical status, risk stratification category, exercise capacity, adverse event/ischemic/angina threshold, cognitive/psychological impairment, and musculoskeletal limitations.
- Observe the presence of classic angina pectoris that is induced with exercise and relieved with rest or nitroglycerin, as this is evidence of myocardial ischemia.
- If an adverse event threshold has been established, exercise intensity should remain 10 bpm below that threshold HR.
- If peak HR is unknown, teach individuals to use RPE to guide exercise intensity.
- HIIT may be beneficial for this population.
- Individuals should use medications based on recommendations from their healthcare providers.
- If a change to beta-blocker medication has occurred without a new exercise test, monitor for signs and symptoms and note the RPE and HR most recently used during training as the new THR.
- If using diuretic therapy, emphasize and educate clients on proper hydration.
- Any amount of exercise is better than none, and multiple shorter daily bouts may be appropriate initially, with a gradual progression as tolerated.
- Perform an exercise test when there are clinical changes or symptoms that may indicate a compromised ability to exercise.
- Consider premorbid activity levels, the client's vocational and avocational goals and requirements, and personal health and fitness goals.

Note. bpm = Beats per minute; HR = Heart rate; RPE = Rating of perceived exertion; HIIT = High-intensity interval training; THR = Target heart rate
Source: American College of Sports Medicine (2022). *ACSM's Guidelines for Exercise Testing and Prescription* (11th ed.). Philadelphia: Wolters Kluwer.

Fitness testing protocols are discussed in more detail in *The Exercise Professional's Guide to Personal Training* (ACE, 2020) and will not be included here. The CMES must follow four rules when performing fitness assessments in patients with CHD:

- Avoid testing to maximal aerobic power (i.e., $\dot{V}O_2$max) or maximal heart-rate levels when assessing cardiorespiratory endurance.
- Always warm up prior to the fitness test with lower-level activity similar in nature to the fitness test protocol (i.e., do not allow the client to engage in sudden-onset intense exercise of any type), and always cool down after the test with low-level aerobic activity commensurate with the intensity of the primary conditioning activity.
- Ensure that the client is currently taking all of their prescription medicines, especially if they are on beta blockers, ACE inhibitors, and/or ARBs.

- Clearly understand and recognize signs and symptoms of inappropriate response to exercise (e.g., chest discomfort, dyspnea, unusual fatigue, confusion, dizziness or lightheadedness, and/or the reporting of palpitations prior to exercise).

The CMES should adhere to the general procedures for submaximal testing of cardiorespiratory fitness (Table 7-8).

TABLE 7-8
GENERAL PROCEDURES FOR SUBMAXIMAL TESTING OF CARDIORESPIRATORY FITNESS

- Obtain resting heart rate and blood pressure immediately prior to exercise in the exercise posture.
- The individual should be familiarized with the ergometer or treadmill. If using a cycle ergometer, properly position the individual on the ergometer (i.e., upright posture, ~25-degree bend in the knee at maximal leg extension, and hands in proper position on the handlebars).
- The exercise test should begin with a two- to three-minute warm-up to acquaint the individual with the cycle ergometer or treadmill and prepare him or her for the exercise intensity in the first stage of the test.
- A specific protocol should consist of two- or three-minute stages with appropriate increments in work rate.
- Heart rate should be monitored at least two times during each stage, near the end of the second and third minutes of each stage. If heart rate is >110 beats per minute (bpm), steady-state heart rate (i.e., two heart rates within 5 bpm) should be reached before the workload is increased.
- Blood pressure should be monitored in the last minute of each stage and repeated (verified) in the event of a hypotensive or hypertensive response.
- Rating of perceived exertion (using either the Borg category or category-ratio scale) and additional rating scales should be monitored near the end of the last minute of each stage.
- Individual's appearance and symptoms should be monitored and recorded regularly.
- The test should be terminated when the individual reaches 70% of heart-rate reserve (85% of age-predicted maximal heart rate), fails to conform to the exercise test protocol, experiences adverse signs or symptoms, requests to stop, or experiences an emergency situation.
- An appropriate cool-down/recovery period should be initiated consisting of either:
  ✓ Continued exercise at a work rate equivalent to that of the first stage of the exercise test protocol or lower or
  ✓ A passive cool-down if the individual experiences signs of discomfort or an emergency situation occurs
- All physiologic observations (e.g., heart rate, blood pressures, signs, symptoms) should be continued for at least five minutes of recovery unless abnormal responses occur, which would warrant a longer post-test surveillance period. Continue low-level exercise until heart rate and blood pressure stabilize, but not necessarily until they reach pre-exercise levels.

Reprinted with permission from American College of Sports Medicine (2022). *ACSM's Guidelines for Exercise Testing and Prescription* (11th ed.). Philadelphia: Wolters Kluwer.

Contraindications to Exercise Training

Similar to other clinical populations who present high risk for exercise-related complications, there are specific instances when the CMES should not train a CHD client. Table 7-9 includes standardized contraindications to exercise training that are consistent across nearly all of the professional organizations addressing cardiac rehabilitation physical activity. Exceptions should be considered based on the clinical judgment of the physician and qualified clinical exercise physiologists experienced in cardiac rehabilitation.

Exercise Training Supervision Considerations

Most patients/clients who have successfully completed 24 to 36 sessions of formalized early phase cardiac rehabilitation will not require direct supervision of every exercise session. This does not mean that they will not require specific supervised instruction by the CMES on exercise techniques and familiarization with new modes of exercise training. The AACVPR (2021) has

TABLE 7-9

INDICATIONS AND CONTRAINDICATIONS FOR INPATIENT AND OUTPATIENT CARDIAC REHABILITATION

Indications	Contraindications
• Medically stable postmyocardial infarction • Stable angina • Coronary artery bypass graft (surgery) • Percutaneous transluminal coronary angioplasty • Stable heart failure caused by either systolic or diastolic dysfunction (cardiomyopathy) • Heart transplantation • Valvular heart disease/surgery • Peripheral arterial disease • At risk for coronary artery disease with diagnoses of diabetes mellitus, dyslipidemia, hypertension, or obesity • Other patients who may benefit from structured exercise and/or patient education based on physician referral and consensus of the rehabilitation team	• Unstable angina • Uncontrolled hypertension (resting systolic blood pressure >180 mmHg and/or resting diastolic blood pressure >110 mmHg) • Orthostatic blood pressure drop of >20 mmHg with symptoms • Significant aortic stenosis (aortic valve area <1.0 cm^2) • Uncontrolled atrial or ventricular arrhythmias • Uncontrolled sinus tachycardia (>120 bpm) • Uncompensated heart failure • Third-degree atrioventricular block without pacemaker • Active pericarditis or myocarditis • Recent embolism (pulmonary or systemic) • Acute thrombophlebitis • Aortic dissection • Acute systemic illness or fever • Uncontrolled diabetes mellitus • Severe orthopedic conditions that would prohibit exercise • Other metabolic conditions, such as acute thyroiditis, hypokalemia, hyperkalemia, or hypovolemia (until adequately treated) • Severe psychological disorder

Source: Balady, G.J. et al. (2007). Core components of cardiac rehabilitation/secondary prevention programs: 2007 update: A scientific statement from the American Heart Association Exercise, Cardiac Rehabilitation, and Prevention Committee, the Council on Clinical Cardiology; the Councils on Cardiovascular Nursing, Epidemiology and Prevention, and Nutrition, Physical Activity, and Metabolism; and the American Association of Cardiovascular and Pulmonary Rehabilitation. *Circulation,* 115, 2675–2682.

Reprinted with permission from American College of Sports Medicine (2022). *ACSM's Guidelines for Exercise Testing and Prescription* (11th ed.). Philadelphia: Wolters Kluwer.

published recommendations on exercise supervision requirements based on the individual's risk of exercise-related cardiovascular complications. Those at the lowest, moderate, and highest risk for complications all require various levels of supervision (Table 7-10). The CMES can minimize risk by ensuring appropriate physician referral, requiring pre-program exercise ECG testing when necessary, and conservative application of progressive exercise training stimulus, particularly in the early stages of training. The CMES is also required to be currently certified in **cardiopulmonary resuscitation (CPR)** and proper use of an **automated external defibrillator (AED)** and must be fully knowledgeable of the 2020 AHA CPR guidelines (Merchant et al., 2020).

TABLE 7-10
STRATIFICATION OF RISK FOR CARDIAC EVENTS DURING EXERCISE PARTICIPATION

Characteristics of Patients at Lowest Risk	Characteristics of Patients at Moderate Risk	Characteristics of Patients at Highest Risk
• Absence of complex ventricular dysrhythmias during exercise testing and recovery • Absence of angina or other significant symptoms (e.g., unusual shortness of breath, lightheadedness, or dizziness during exercise testing and recovery) • Normal heart rate and blood pressure response to exercise and recovery • Functional capacity ≥7 METs	• Presence of stable angina or other significant symptoms (e.g., unusual shortness of breath, lightheadedness, or dizziness) occurring only at high levels of exertion (≥7 METs) • Functional capacity <5 METs	• Presence of complex ventricular arrhythmias during exercise testing or recovery • Presence of angina or other significant symptoms [e.g., unusual shortness of breath, lightheadedness, or dizziness at low levels of exertion (e.g., <5 METs) or during recovery] • Abnormal clinical exercise ECG (e.g., ST-segment abnormalities) during exercise testing or recovery • Abnormal heart rate or blood pressure response to exercise and recovery • Functional capacity ≤3 METs

Note: MET = Metabolic equivalent; ECG = Electrocardiogram

Sources: American Association of Cardiovascular and Pulmonary Rehabilitation (2021). *Guidelines for Cardiac Rehabilitation Programs* (6th ed.). Champaign, Ill.: Human Kinetics; Williams, M.A. (2001). Exercise testing in cardiac rehabilitation: Exercise prescription and beyond. *Cardiology Clinics,* 19, 3, 415–431.

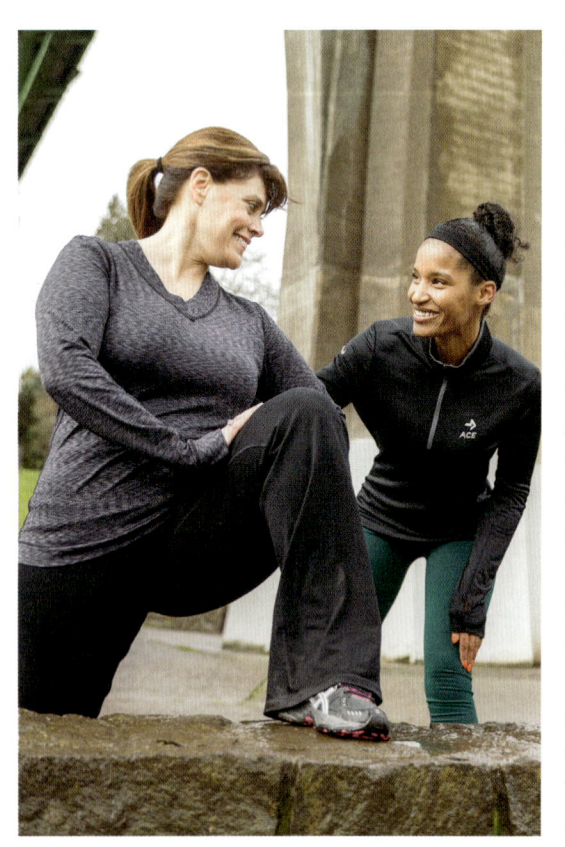

Overall Weekly Exercise Energy-expenditure Goals

All Americans, including those with stable and symptom-free CHD, should participate in an amount of energy expenditure equivalent to 150 minutes per week of moderate-intensity aerobic physical activity or 75 minutes per week of vigorous-intensity aerobic physical activity or a combination of both that generates energy equivalency for substantial overall health benefits including cardiovascular health (U.S. Department of Health & Human Services, 2018). This seems to be an acceptable goal for most CHD patients who successfully complete graduated cardiac rehabilitation physical-activity programs. This volume includes systematic workouts, recreational activities, and **activities of daily living (ADL).** Considering that most CHD patients have one or more CHD and/or metabolic syndrome risk factors that are related to increased adiposity, it seems reasonable to consider *at least* 2,000 kcal per week of moderate physical activity as an optimal goal, which is the overall ACSM recommendation for individuals who have overweight or obesity (Donnelly et al., 2009). This volume of activity approximates 250 to 300 minutes per week of moderate-level exercise. The CMES must understand how to estimate the energy cost of various physical activities in terms of kcal per session, per day, and per week (Howley, 2012; Ainsworth et al., 2011). The CMES should adhere to the overall recommendations for exercise in clients with stable CHD (see Table 7-7).

CLINICAL PEDOMETRY AND THE CHD PATIENT

Clinical pedometry [the process of employing well-engineered reliable step-counters (pedometers) in clinical disease prevention and management programs] can be helpful, particularly in the maintenance stages of CHD exercise programming. Note that walking for 30 minutes equates to 3,000 to 4,000 steps, whereas a 1-mile walk equates to approximately 2,000 steps.

Research has indicated that approximately 8,000 steps a day approximates 30 minutes of moderate to vigorous physical activity (i.e., approximately 8,000 steps a day of walking is an acceptable proxy for 30 minutes of moderate to vigorous physical activity) (Tudor-Locke et al., 2011). This does not mean that 8,000 walking steps (approximately 3 to 4 miles of walking) can or should be done in 30 minutes; however, keeping up a moderate pace (rather than a more leisurely cadence) is required to derive the benefits of higher-intensity aerobic activities. This level of daily walking appears to be what would be required for CHD patients who wish to maintain at least a minimum level of cardiovascular health. There is evidence that targeting 7,500 to 8,000 steps daily may be efficient to maintain waist circumference and to improve lipid profile during the year following a MI or acute coronary syndrome (Houle et al., 2013). This could be considered a starting target point to initiate changes in physical-activity behavior. Considerably more steps per day are generally required for weight loss. It is important to note that the CMES should use the step count (daily, weekly, or monthly) as the principal outcomes measure versus projected estimates of caloric expenditure or distance.

There is also evidence that the walking speed of ≥100 steps/minute represents the lower boundary of moderate-intensity walking for most adults. Indeed, to meet current U.S. public health physical-activity guidelines, individuals are encouraged to walk a minimum of 3,000 steps in 30 minutes (approximately 3 mph for most adults) on five days each week (Marshall et al., 2009). Three bouts of 1,000 steps in 10 minutes each day can also be used to meet the recommended goal. This walking speed, when maintained, is sufficient to stimulate insulin sensitization among other cardiometabolic mechanisms that are important in diabetes- and CHD-prevention programs. Does this mean that anything slower than 3,000 steps in 30 minutes is not clinically effective? Absolutely not, but at higher muscle contraction frequencies (i.e., walking speeds) there is greater regulation of lipid and glucose metabolism, which are key mechanisms that underscore cardiometabolic risk reduction in both diabetes- and CHD-prevention programs. It is also important to note that the 3 mph speed threshold would be faster than necessary for shorter individuals (e.g., <5'7", or perhaps slower than optimal for those taller than 6'2"), so height and gait mechanics should be taken into consideration.

New Lifestyles, Yamax, and Accusplit are three companies selling reliable pedometers. The CMES should choose pedometers that have been validated to accurately measure steps, are inexpensive, and have step filters, such as the Accusplit AX 2720 and 120 XLM series pedometers. Step filters are built into the pedometer's electronics and reduce the recording of spontaneous and fidgety movements. These Yamax-Digiwalker and Accusplit pedometers have been used in many studies and are generally inexpensive and well-engineered. Most reliable pedometers have relatively long-term memories (i.e., ≥99,999 step memory does not need resetting more than once a week or even once a month in some models). The 2720 and XLE models also record the number of minutes over the course of a day that the individual is actively moving. The interested CMESs can obtain a practical detailed instruction document with references (LaForge, 2013).

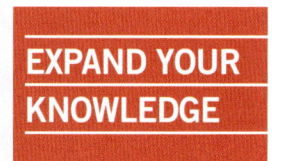

Figure 7-6 illustrates a formal method of creating pedometry programs for those with CHD by using Rx forms to both instruct and demonstrate the formality of the systematic clinical use of pedometers. It is important to note that this is an example of a form that a client would receive from a physician or clinician, not from the CMES.

EXPAND YOUR KNOWLEDGE

Figure 7-6
Sample outpatient pedometry prescription form for CHD clients. It is important to note that this is an example of a form that a client would receive from a physician or clinician, not from the CMES.

Rx for Outpatient Pedometry

Patient name: Date:

Therapuetic code:

Order for following patient physical activity pedometer:

☐ Pedometer: e.g., AX 2720 pedometer

    Rx: steps/day___   steps/week/month: ___/___

    Other Rx:

Patient instructions: See attached physical activity and pedometer guidelines

_____

Referring Certified Medical Exercise Specialist

Exercise Intensity

Exercise intensity or exercise workload is perhaps the most important and modifiable component of the exercise program. Work intensity most directly relates to the workload placed on the heart and the coronary arteries. Exercise speed, movement velocity, and resistance load all increase the workload of the heart, primarily through increased HR and BP. The two most practical intensity-monitoring strategies for the CMES are the client's volitional response to the exercise workload [e.g., **rating of perceived exertion (RPE)**] and exercise HR. In some cases, HR response may be blunted due to medications (e.g., beta blockers). Recognizing signs and symptoms of excessive physical effort is essential whether the individual is performing yard work or engaging in structured fitness activity (Table 7-11).

TABLE 7-11
SIGNS AND SYMPTOMS OF EXCESSIVE EFFORT IN CORONARY HEART DISEASE (CHD) PATIENTS

- Chest discomfort or chest pain that intensifies with increasing physical effort
- Dyspnea (excessive shortness of breath) at relatively low work levels
- Palpitations (e.g., palpable ventricular arrhythmias)
- A drop in systolic blood pressure with increasing work loads
- Inappropriate heart-rate response to exercise (chronotropic incompetence)
- Sudden onset fatigue at rest or low-levels of physical activity

The CMES should understand the principles of cardiorespiratory endurance exercise programming, particularly the relationship between **heart-rate reserve (HRR)** and **$\dot{V}O_2$ reserve ($\dot{V}O_2R$)** (i.e., HRR is more closely aligned with percent $\dot{V}O_2R$ versus percent $\dot{V}O_2$max and this is true for nearly all conventional forms of aerobic exercise, including stationary exercise machine work) (ACSM, 2022; Dalleck & Kravitz, 2006).

ACSM (2022) recommends that the *initial* stages of aerobic-conditioning cardiac rehabilitation programs for low-risk and stable CHD clients have an exercise intensity of 20 (for patients with myocardial infarction) to 30 (for patients recovering from heart surgery) beats per minute above seated or standing resting heart rate to a maximum of ≤120 beats per minute. This corresponds to an RPE of ≤13 on the 6 to 20 scale. However, it should be assumed that in most cases the CMES will be working with clients who are not in the early phases of cardiac rehabilitation (e.g., two to four weeks post-MI or -hospitalization), but who are in the improvement or maintenance stage of conditioning, in which case a moderate to vigorous intensity is used, ranging from 40 to 80% of HRR and $\dot{V}O_2R$ is more appropriate. The majority of work in this stage should be in the 45 to 65% $\dot{V}O_2R$ range, with higher intensities reserved for those who have safely and asymptomatically performed at the lower range. The majority of CHD clients will do well with 20 to 60 minutes of exercise per session. For durations of 45 minutes or longer, exercise intensity should be in the moderate range (i.e., 40 to 59% of HRR and $\dot{V}O_2R$). It is important to understand that some CHD clients fail to achieve predicted maximal heart rates even in the absence of medications that reduce HR (e.g., beta-blocking agents). This phenomenon is known as **chronotropic incompetence**. These individuals are at higher risk for CVD complications and are not within the CMES scope of practice.

A good but simple estimate of cardiac workload intensity can be determined using the following formula:

The Double Product
Myocardial (heart muscle) work =
Heart rate (in beats per minute) x Systolic blood pressure (mmHg) / 100
For example: 150 beats/minute x 150 mmHg/100 = 225

Coronary Heart Disease   CHAPTER 7

This expression is known as the **double product,** but is also sometimes referred to as the **rate-pressure product** and often corresponds to the threshold for cardiac-related symptoms (e.g., angina). Intensive aerobic activities significantly increase HR but moderately increase **systolic blood pressure (SBP),** whereas intensive resistance workloads (e.g., resistance training) moderately increase HR but cause a more significant rise in SBP. Both forms of exercise can dramatically raise the double product and therefore increase cardiac workload. Cardiac symptoms and heart-muscle dysfunction are directly related to exertional HR and BP. It is not practical for the CMES to calculate the double product for each exercise session, but they should thoroughly understand the consequences of various aerobic, resistance, and even mindful exercise modalities (e.g., hatha yoga styles and **Pilates**) and how they influence cardiac work.

It is important to understand which physical activities and exercises can rapidly increase SBP. For example, during heavy resistance exercise where an individual is exerting at ≥80% of maximal voluntary contraction (MVC) levels, SBP increases quickly along with the **diastolic blood pressure (DBP).** Additionally, when a person exerts to muscular failure during resistance exercise (which is not recommended), the CMES can assume a peak or near-peak BP response. Even for individuals with relatively stable CHD, this level of arterial pressure (also called "afterload"), which the heart has to work against, can be dramatic and deserves serious caution.

Exercise Frequency and Duration

Exercise should be performed at least every other day, but preferably on most days of the week. Frequency of exercise depends on several factors including disease status, baseline exercise tolerance, exercise intensity, musculoskeletal health, and other health goals. For clients with very limited exercise capacities, multiple short (1- to 10-minute) daily sessions may be appropriate.

Exercise duration for most CHD clients in the maintenance stage of conditioning is usually set between 30 and 60 minutes per day. However, as mentioned previously, many clients will require 60 or more minutes per day to adequately manage body weight, **dyslipidemia,** and associated risk factors. CHD, diabetes, and metabolic syndrome clients should have exercise programming dosed by daily or weekly energy expenditure rather than separately quantifying only frequency, intensity, and duration. The total accumulated energy expenditure of the exercise sessions is perhaps the single most important program feature associated with risk-factor reduction.

In most cases, the CHD client will require an activity program that uses *at least* 1,000 kcal/week but preferably (at least eventually) 2,000 kcal or more per week. In the case of a CHD client with the metabolic syndrome, **atherogenic dyslipidemia,** and obesity, the physical-activity program's energy expenditure should be ≥2,000 kcal per week (gross kcal cost) to meaningfully alter these risk factors. Of course, these energy expenditures are a function of activity mode, frequency, duration, and intensity, and therein lies an opportunity for the CMES and the client to work together to design a creative and productive activity program. Once again, to constructively do this, the CMES will need a good working knowledge of the energy costs of a broad range of physical activities (Ainsworth et al., 2011).

Mode of Exercise for CHD

As with apparently healthy adults, cardiorespiratory endurance exercise is the principal focus of exercise programming for those with CHD, and should include rhythmic, large muscle group activities with an emphasis on increased caloric expenditure for maintenance of a healthy body weight and its many other associated health benefits. Cardiorespiratory endurance exercise programs should promote whole-body physical activity, feature conditioning that includes the upper and lower extremities, and include multiple forms of aerobic activities and exercise equipment.

Stationary Exercise Machines and CHD Exercise Training

Stationary exercise machines (e.g., treadmills, cycles, and elliptical machines) all provide a reasonable cardiorespiratory endurance stimulus for the CHD client. Remember that in the case of motor-driven treadmills, the "motivation" to keep up with high workloads is provided by the self-selected speed and grade, which can be an incentive for some clients and problematic in others who attempt to keep pace with workloads beyond their work capacity. Three considerations should be kept in mind for advising stationary equipment exercise:

- Use a fan for cross-ventilation and to help with evaporative heat loss, which can help reduce cardiac work (i.e., the double-product).
- Some stationary cycles generate a significantly higher blood pressure response than others, particularly in deconditioned adults (Kim, Chun, & Kim, 2013).
- Always warm up and cool down with lower speeds and resistances, which is particularly important in those who have active CHD.

The different types of exercise equipment may include the following:
- Arm ergometer
- Combination of upper and lower (dual action) extremity cycle ergometer
- Upright and recumbent cycle ergometer
- Recumbent stepper
- Rower
- Elliptical
- Stair climber
- Treadmill for walking

Interval/Intermittent Aerobic Exercise Training

Early stages of CHD client training should appropriately use intermittent bouts of aerobic training and progressively elongate the time so that the client can eventually maintain 30 or more minutes of continuous exercise without symptoms. In recent years, there have been programs that have judiciously and cautiously incorporated higher-intensity aerobic training, including high-intensity interval training (HIIT) in stable CHD patients with reasonable improvements in aerobic power without an increase in cardiovascular complications (Rognmo et al., 2012; Guiraud et al., 2011). HIIT, for example, involves alternating three- to four-minute periods of exercise at high intensity (80 to 90% HRR) with exercise at a lower intensity (60 to 70% HRR). Such training for approximately 40 minutes, three times per week has been shown to increase $\dot{V}O_2$peak in patients with HF and produce greater long-term improvements in $\dot{V}O_2$peak in patients after CABG compared to standard continuous moderate-intensity exercise (Guiraud et al., 2011). The CMES should be well acquainted with the relationships among $\dot{V}O_2$max, $\dot{V}O_2$peak, $\dot{V}O_2$R, and HRR, particularly when advising and monitoring exercise intensities.

> **Understanding $\dot{V}O_2$max, $\dot{V}O_2$peak, $\dot{V}O_2$R, and HRR Relationships**
> $\dot{V}O_2$max = Highest personal oxygen uptake capacity possible
> $\dot{V}O_2$peak = Highest value of oxygen uptake attained (measured or estimated) in an exercise test
> $\dot{V}O_2$reserve ($\dot{V}O_2$R) = The difference between $\dot{V}O_2$max and $\dot{V}O_2$ (% $\dot{V}O_2$R ≈ % Heart-rate reserve)
> Heart-rate reserve = The difference between maximal and resting heart rate

HIIT should not be used as an initial training stimulus, particularly in the first eight to 10 weeks of CHD exercise training. The CMES is strongly advised to ensure that the client has a preprogram negative exercise ECG test with physician clearance and consider the aforementioned recommendations on CHD exercise training, particularly the information discussed in Tables 7-7, 7-9 and 7-11.

EXERCISE GUIDELINES FOR STABLE ANGINA

The CMES should ensure that any client with exercise-induced angina or angina equivalent (e.g., reproducible shortness of breath or extreme fatigue) are medically cleared and are stable. Such clients would not be specifically targeted by the CMES but may occasionally be referred by a physician or a discharge referral after completing formalized cardiac rehabilitation. Angina is a primary manifestation of **myocardial ischemia** (i.e., insufficient blood supply to the heart muscle) and is relatively high risk within the category of all CHD patients. Any individual who experiences angina with physical workloads ≤3 METs (i.e., low physical exertion levels such as walking at 2 mph) should not be trained by the CMES.

- Progressive aerobic endurance exercise is recommended, as long as it is within the individual's exercise tolerance as indicated by the most recent exercise ECG, or is just below the **anginal threshold** or physician-recommended percent of $\dot{V}O_2max$.
- Intermittent, shorter-duration exercise on a more frequent basis [e.g., three to five sets of five- to 10-minutes of low- to moderate-intensity aerobic exercise bouts (e.g., cycling or treadmill walking)] may be most appropriate in the initial stages of training. Upper-extremity aerobic training (e.g., rowing or arm cranking) may initially exacerbate angina because of a higher HR and/or SBP.
- Avoid breath holding, isometric exercises, or activities where the individual physically exerts to muscular contraction failure (i.e., very high-resistance exercise).
- Keep close observation of anginal symptoms and ensure that the individual understands when to take angina-resolving medications (e.g., nitroglycerin, such as nitrostat). Instances when the client uses angina-resolving medications should be documented for the client's physician.

Nitroglycerin Administration

Nitroglycerin should be administered by the individual exactly as directed by their physician. Nitroglycerin is available as two types of products that are used for different reasons. The extended-release capsules are used every day on a specific schedule to prevent angina attacks. The oral spray and sublingual tablets work quickly to stop an angina attack that has already started or they can be used to prevent angina if the person plans to exercise or expects a stressful event.

For clients experiencing angina pectoris and who have been prescribed nitroglycerin PRN (as needed), the typical protocol is as follows:

- Discontinue activity and incorporate rest to see if chest discomfort/pain resolves on its own.
- If there is no relief, the client will self-administer one dose of nitroglycerin, either in tablet or spray form. A tablet will be placed sublingually or between the cheek and gums. If a spray is used, it would be delivered in the same locations.
- The client will then wait five minutes to see if the chest pain is resolved. If not, a second dose will be administered. They will then wait five more minutes and then repeat one more time before calling 9-1-1.

Nitroglycerin is a vasodilator and dilates coronary arteries by relaxing vascular smooth muscle, allowing for a greater oxygen delivery to the heart. Side effects of nitroglycerin administration include severe headache and a drop in BP.

EXPAND YOUR KNOWLEDGE

THINK IT THROUGH

Do you have a plan in the event of an acute onset of angina while training a client who has been diagnosed with stable angina? Visualize the steps you would take during a training session if a client expresses the onset of angina pain, including what you would say to the individual and how you would encourage them to take nitroglycerin medication as prescribed by their physician. As the occurrence of anginal episodes that require the administration of medication should be documented and reported to the client's physician, think about how you will do this (e.g., create a specialized form and phone the physician's office for further direction).

Resistance Training

Resistance-training modalities can clearly improve the client's muscular fitness and functionality. Because there are so many types of resistance training and associated protocols, certain precautions are important to note. The primary consideration for the CMES in this context is the amount and rate of force delivered to the client's muscles relative to their capacity and cardiac ventricular function. Table 7-12 denotes criteria for the resistance training of CHD clients. In this instance, resistance training applies to the use of free weights, machines, or other resistive devices that deliver a resistive force ≥40% of the client's MVC. As long as the client is not straining to concentrically or eccentrically contract a muscle group or performing breath-holding, resistance training can be very beneficial. The contraindications for resistance training, as well as more intense forms of hatha yoga (e.g., Bikram or "hot" yoga and Ashtanga or "power" yoga), are essentially the same (see Table 7-9). There are no contraindications to Pilates exercises, provided that the same guidelines are adhered to as previously stated. One caution, however, would be to avoid resistance-training regimens in clients who have maximal exercise capacities of <6 METs. The CMES should not place themselves in the position to recognize these clinical contraindications, but should ensure physician clearance for these contraindications.

TABLE 7-12

CRITERIA FOR RESISTANCE-TRAINING PROGRAMS*

- Low- to moderate-risk clients and possibly higher-risk clients with supervision

- Those who require strength for work or recreational activities, particularly in their upper extremities

- Initiate a minimum of 6 to 10 weeks after date of myocardial infarction or cardiac surgery, including 4 weeks of consistent participation in a supervised cardiac rehabilitation endurance training program

- Initiate a minimum of 3 weeks following transcatheter procedure (i.e., PCI or other), including 2 weeks of consistent participation in a supervised cardiac rehabilitation endurance training program

- No evidence of acute congestive heart failure, uncontrolled dysrhythmias, severe valvular disease, uncontrolled hypertension, and unstable symptoms

*In this table, a resistance-training program is defined as one in which clients lift weight >50% of one-repetition maximum (1-RM). The use of elastic bands, 1- to 3-lb (0.45–1.36 kg) hand weights, and light free weights may be initiated in a progressive fashion at outpatient program entry provided no other contraindications exist.

Note: PCI = Percutaneous coronary intervention

Source: American Association of Cardiovascular and Pulmonary Rehabilitation (2021). *Guidelines for Cardiac Rehabilitation Programs* (6th ed.). Champaign, Ill.: Human Kinetics..

Recommendations for the Initial Resistance-training Program

While BP certainly may rise excessively during resistance training, the actual rise depends on a variety of controllable factors, including magnitude of the isometric component, the load intensity, the amount of muscle mass involved, and the number of repetitions and/or the load duration. Intra-arterial BP measurements in cardiac patients have demonstrated that during low-intensity resistance training (40 to 60% MVC) with 15 to 20 repetitions, only modest elevations in BP are revealed, similar to those seen during moderate-intensity endurance training (Bjarnason-Wehrens et al., 2004). For CHD patients, the use of elastic bands and/or small weights is very suitable. More precise training with less risk of overloading can be achieved through the use of training machines, whereby the load dose can be individually adjusted and the execution of the movement is predetermined.

Mindful Exercise and the CHD Client

Select forms and styles of mindful exercise modalities are most often appropriate or can be easily adapted for clients with CHD. This is particularly true for yogic-based breathwork therapy (Pal et al., 2014). Table 7-13 provides examples of forms of mindful exercise that are appropriate for the majority of individuals with CHD.

Mindful exercise programs can range from those requiring very low energy expenditure and deep relaxation qualities to those that require considerable muscular strength and impose considerable myocardial work. Thus, several considerations are important when choosing particular mindful exercise modalities. Many styles of hatha yoga, for example, involve acute dynamic changes in body position (i.e., the relationship of the head, chest, and lower limbs to each other). It is therefore important to fundamentally understand the **hemodynamic** and cardiac ventricular responses to such exercise and how these may alter cardiac function in individuals with CHD, including clients with hypertension, metabolic syndrome, or diabetes.

Inverted poses where the head is below the heart (e.g., downward facing dog or headstands), or situations in which such a position is alternated with a "head-up" pose, should be avoided. In most cases, those who are initially deconditioned and/or have CHD should minimize acute changes in body position that require the head to be below the level of the heart in early stages of hatha yoga training and use slower transitions from one yoga pose to the next. Because Ashtanga and traditional Iyengar yoga poses and sequences generally require considerable strength, flexibility, and mental concentration, they should be reserved for higher-functioning individuals (i.e., clients with a >10 MET exercise capacity). Some yoga poses significantly increase BP and may also be inappropriate for older adults with stage II or higher hypertension (i.e., BP ≥160/100 mmHg). One study on intermediate and advanced yoga practitioners showed that some Iyengar poses can rapidly and significantly increase mean and peak systolic BP particularly with back arch poses (Blank, 2006). Systolic, mean, and diastolic BP can increase significantly during yoga practice. At least one report has indicated that the magnitude of these increases in BP was greatest with standing postures (Miles et al., 2013). This should not be a deterrent to stable CHD clients safely practicing various hatha yoga asanas. The CMES should be aware, however, that this level of BP can impose significant double-product stress on the heart of some CHD clients, particularly if the stress is a sudden increase in SBP rather than the gradual workload increase seen with graduated aerobic exercise work levels. It is strongly recommended that the CMES start the client with restorative yoga poses prior to engaging in a full complement of Iyengar or equivalent yoga poses.

TABLE 7-13
EXAMPLES OF APPROPRIATE FORMS OF MINDFUL EXERCISE FOR CLIENTS WITH CHD

• Restorative yoga	• Tai chi chih
• Kripalu yoga	• Meditation walking
• Viniyoga	• Chi walking
• Integral yoga	• Yogic breathwork
• Select Iyengar and yoga poses	• Pilates mat and reformer work
• Tai chi chuan (moderate pace)	• NIA at low-to-moderate level

Note: NIA = Neuromuscular integrative action

YOGIC BREATHING

Perhaps most useful in those with any level of CHD is yogic breathing. Although there are many styles of yogic breathing, the breath is generally drawn through the nose during both inhalation and exhalation. Each breath is intentionally slow and deep with an even distribution, or smoothness, of effort. Lengthening exhalations by using the abdominal muscles to expire more air while breathing through the nose will cause a relaxation response. In addition to reduced stress and mental tension, cardiovascular benefits result from yogic breathing. One of the mechanisms responsible for the mental quiescence experienced with yogic breathing is its stimulation of the **parasympathetic nervous system.** When fully stimulated by adequate yogic inspiration and expiration, mechanical receptors in pulmonary tissue (e.g., alveoli) activate parasympathetic nerves, which transiently reduces mental tension and elicits a relaxation response (Pal, Velkumary, & Madanmohan, 2004). A suitable inhalation/exhalation ratio is to inhale for a 2-count, exhale for a 4-count, and then work up to inhaling for an 8-count and exhaling for a 16-count. To test this relaxation response, the client can feel their pulse during this breathing exercise. They may notice a reduced pulse rate with prolonged exhalation. This slight slowing of HR includes a reciprocal slight increase in HR variability—a process called respiratory sinus arrhythmia. Acute reductions in BP also have resulted from yogic breathing training (Pal et al., 2014; Adhana et al., 2013).

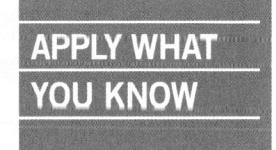

APPLY WHAT YOU KNOW

EXPAND YOUR KNOWLEDGE

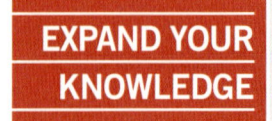

THE 2012 ACCF PHYSICAL-ACTIVITY RECOMMENDATIONS FOR CHD PATIENTS

In 2012, the American College of Cardiology Foundation, in collaboration with six other health care organizations (ACCF/AHA/ACP/AATS/PCNA/SCAI/STS, 2012), advanced their recommendations for physical activity in patients with CHD. Although these are quite generalized, they are in synergy with ACSM and AACVPR's CHD guidelines. The ACCF CHD physical-activity guidelines are summarized as follows:

- For all CHD patients, the CMES should encourage 30 to 60 minutes of moderate-intensity aerobic activity, such as brisk walking, at least five days and preferably seven days per week, supplemented by an increase in daily lifestyle activities (e.g., walking breaks at work, gardening, and household work) to improve cardiorespiratory fitness and move clients out of the least-fit, least-active, high-risk cohort (bottom 20%).
- For all clients, risk assessment with a physical-activity history and/or an exercise test is recommended to guide exercise programming.
- Medically supervised programs (cardiac rehabilitation) and physician-directed, home-based programs are recommended for at-risk patients at first diagnosis.

EXERCISE GUIDELINES SUMMARY FOR CLIENTS WITH CARDIOVASCULAR DISEASE

Given the aforementioned synergy of physical-activity guidelines for individuals with CHD, the following summarizes the recommendations made in this chapter:

CARDIORESPIRATORY TRAINING	
Frequency	• At least 3, but preferably up to 5 days of the week • Current guidelines suggest that any amount of exercise is better than none.

Intensity	• Moderate to vigorous intensity*
	• Intensity may be determined through the following methods:
	  ✓ With an exercise test, use 40–80% HRR or $\dot{V}O_2R$ or $\dot{V}O_2$ peak
	  ✓ Without an exercise test, use RPE of 12–16 (6–20 scale) or add 20–30 bpm to RHR
	  ✓ HR should remain at least 10 bpm below the HR associated with the ischemic threshold (if exercise ischemic threshold has been determined)
	• High-intensity interval training may be a safe and effective method for enhancing cardiorespiratory fitness for individuals with stable disease and a base level of conditioning.

Time	• Eventual goal of 20–60 minutes for cardiorespiratory training • Warm-up and cool-down activities lasting 5–10 minutes should be included in each exercise session.

Type	• Rhythmic, large muscle group exercise that emphasizes increased caloric expenditure and utilizes multiple activities and pieces of equipment, such as:
	  ✓ Arm ergometer
	  ✓ Upright and recumbent cycle ergometer
	  ✓ Recumbent stepper
	  ✓ Rower
	  ✓ Elliptical
	  ✓ Treadmill for walking

Progression	• Progress following the ACE Integrated Fitness Training® Model based on client goals and availability. • Sessions may include continuous or intermittent exercise.

Coronary Heart Disease CHAPTER 7

	MUSCULAR TRAINING
Frequency	• 2–3 days per week with a minimum of 48 hours separating exercise for the same muscle group
Intensity	• 40–60% 1-RM, or a load that can be lifted 10–15 repetitions without straining • RPE of 11–13 (6–20 scale)
Time	• 1–3 sets of 8–10 different exercises focused on major muscle groups

Type	• Select equipment that is safe and comfortable, including:
	  ✓ Elastic resistance
	  ✓ Free weights
	  ✓ Pulleys
	  ✓ Selectorized machines
	• Each major muscle group should be trained initially with one set
	• Multiple-set routines may be introduced later, as tolerated

Progression	• Progress following the ACE Integrated Fitness Training Model based on client goals and availability. • Progression can be introduced through increases in resistance, number of repetitions or sets, or decreasing rest periods between sets. • Progression should be slow and dependent on tolerance. ✓ Volume can be increased 2–10% once clients comfortably complete 1–2 repetitions beyond the target range on two consecutive training sessions.

*Moderate intensity = Heart rates <VT1 where speech remains comfortable and is not affected by breathing; Vigorous intensity = Heart rates from ≥VT1 to <VT2 where clients feel unsure if speech is comfortable.

Note: HRR = Heart-rate reserve; $\dot{V}O_2R$ = Oxygen uptake reserve; RPE = Rating of perceived exertion; bpm = Beats per minute; HR = Heart rate; RHR = Resting heart rate; 1-RM = One-repetition maximum; VT1 = First ventilatory threshold; VT2 = Second ventilatory threshold

CMES FOCUS

Aerobic exercise and resistance training are safe and effective for most clients with CHD. However, all clients with CHD should be clinically evaluated and classified according to future risk for the occurrence of cardiac-related events during exercise. Exercise programs will be highly individualized and dependent on the client's unique needs and exercise tolerance.

Source: American College of Sports Medicine (2022). *ACSM's Guidelines for Exercise Testing and Prescription* (11th ed.). Philadelphia: Wolters Kluwer.

CASE STUDY

Client Information

Jerome is a 59-year-old engineer who is sedentary and has a history of CHD, dyslipidemia (LDL cholesterol = 182 mg/dL, HDL cholesterol = 39 mg/dL, triglycerides = 175 mg/dL), and stage I hypertension (162/100 mmHg). He is referred to the CMES by an internist. His CHD was documented after a positive treadmill ECG and an angiogram confirming two-vessel coronary disease. Jerome has not had an MI or significant history of angina and had no reportable angina-like symptoms on his treadmill ECG. His treadmill ECG was positive beginning at a HR of 155 to 160 bpm and he was capable of achieving an 11 MET exercise capacity. After prescribing a beta blocker, a statin, and an ACE inhibitor for his risk factors, Jerome's doctor decided to refer him to a CMES rather than a formalized cardiac rehabilitation program. Up to this point, the patient was minimally physically active, walking the equivalent of 1 mile a day. Upon referral to the CMES, his baseline numbers are as follows (on his new medications):

- Weight: 190 lb (86 kg)
- Height: 5'9" (1.75 m)
- Body mass index (BMI): 29 kg/m^2
- Waist circumference: 39 inches (99 cm)
- LDL cholesterol: 98 mg/dL
- HDL cholesterol: 44 mg/dL
- Triglycerides: 129 mg/dL
- BP: 134/84 mmHg
- Exercise capacity: 11 METs

Medications: Carvedilol (6.25 mg), rosuvastatin (20 mg), Lisinopril (10 mg), and sublingual nitroglycerin if needed

CMES Approach

Exercise plan: The initial exercise plan would build on the client's current activity of walking 1 mile per day, progressing his home walking program to 2 miles per day performed five or more days per week. In addition, the CMES adds the following: 1,000 kcal/week of a combination of three sessions/week of elliptical trainer exercise (starting with two 10-minute sessions at low-to-moderate level stride rate and progressing to one continuous 30-minute session over a six-week period, keeping exercise HR between 130 and 145 bpm) to expend 1,000 kcal/week for the three sessions combined. An effort is made to ensure that he is remaining compliant with his medications and the Healthy Mediterranean-Style Dietary Pattern. Total weekly physical activity energy-expenditure goal is 1,900 to 2,000 kcal.

Follow-up: At three months, he has lost 7 pounds (3 kg) and his follow-up labs are as follows:

- Weight: 183 lb (83 kg)
- BMI: 27.5 kg/m^2
- Waist circumference: 38 inches (96 cm)
- LDL cholesterol: 92 mg/dL
- HDL cholesterol: 51 mg/dL
- Triglycerides: 118 mg/dL
- BP: 130/84 mmHg
- Exercise capacity: 13.5 METs

One 60-minute variable-terrain walk per week was added, along with two circuit resistance-training sessions/week (one or two sets of 10 exercises at 15 RM) focused on proper movement patterns and exercises using body weight and light resistance to build muscular endurance. Total weekly energy expenditure, including existing walking/elliptical program, is now 2,500 to 2,700 kcal.

This client's six-month goals are as follows:
- Weight: <165 lb (74 kg)
- BMI: <26 kg/m^2
- Waist circumference: <35 inches (88 cm)
- LDL cholesterol: <70 mg/dL

ACE IFT® MODEL AT A GLANCE

Cardiorespiratory Training

This client's initial exercise program is focused on consistently performing moderate-intensity cardiorespiratory exercise in the Base Training phase.

ACE IFT® MODEL AT A GLANCE

Cardiorespiratory Training

At three months, the client has progressed to the Fitness Training phase.

Muscular Training

He is also performing a circuit resistance-training workout that is focused primarily on Movement Training.

Coronary Heart Disease

- HDL cholesterol: >50 mg/dL
- Triglycerides: <150 mg/dL
- Exercise capacity: >15 METs

In the absence of significant further reduction in LDL cholesterol, his physician may choose to increase the rosuvastatin dose to 40 mg. Note that with documented CHD, his ideal therapeutic LDL cholesterol goal is 70 mg/dL. Intensive statin therapy (i.e., high-dose rosuvastatin or atorvastatin) (ACC/AHA, 2013; International Atherosclerosis Society, 2017) may also need to be implemented.

SUMMARY

Exercise therapy for the prevention and treatment of CHD works well beyond its moderate lipid-lowering effects by improving functional capacity, antioxidant defenses, arterial endothelial function, insulin sensitization, glucose transport, fibrinolytic capacity, and psychological well-being, and by reducing BP and body-fat stores. Ideally, the CHD client would have completed early phase cardiac rehabilitation (i.e., phase I and II cardiac rehabilitation) prior to working with the CMES. An experienced CMES who wishes to work with CHD clients should work only with those who are under a physician's care and who have stable coronary disease. To optimize the potential for improvement of CHD risk factors and stabilize the disease process, clients should achieve a total volume of moderate physical activity of 1,500 to 2,000 kcal or more per week. This volume includes systematic workouts (including aerobic, resistance, and select mindful exercise training), recreational activities, and activities of daily living.

REFERENCES

Academy of Nutrition and Dietetics Evidence Analysis Library 1 (2013a). *Disorders of Lipid Metabolism Evidence Analysis Project.* Retrieved November 10, 2013. http://andevidencelibrary.com/topic.cfm?cat=4527

Academy of Nutrition and Dietetics Evidence Analysis Library 2 (2013b). *Heart Failure Evidence-based Nutrition Practice Guidelines.* Retrieved November 10, 2013. http://andevidencelibrary.com/topic.cfm?cat=4527

ACCF/AHA/ACP/AATS/PCNA/SCAI/STS (2012). Guideline for the diagnosis and management of patients with stable ischemic heart disease: A report of the American College of Cardiology Foundation/American Heart Association Task Force on Practice Guidelines, and the American College of Physicians, American Association for Thoracic Surgery, Preventive Cardiovascular Nurses Association, Society for Stephan D. Fihn, MD, MPH, Chair. *Circulation,* 126, e354–e471.

Adhana, R. et al. (2013). The influence of the 2:1 yogic breathing technique on essential hypertension. *Indian Journal of Physiology and Pharmacology,* 57, 1, 38–44.

Ainsworth, B.E. et al. (2011). (2011), Compendium of physical activities: A second update of codes and MET values. *Medicine & Science in Sports & Exercise,* 43, 8, 1575–1581.

American Association of Cardiovascular and Pulmonary Rehabilitation (2021). *Guidelines for Cardiac Rehabilitation Programs* (6th ed.). Champaign, Ill.: Human Kinetics.

American College of Cardiology/American Heart Association (2013). Guidelines on the treatment of blood cholesterol to reduce atherosclerotic cardiovascular risk in adults: A report of the American College of Cardiology/American Heart Association Task Force on Practice Guidelines. *Circulation,* published online November 12, 2013.

American College of Sports Medicine (2022). *ACSM's Guidelines for Exercise Testing and Prescription* (11th ed.). Philadelphia: Wolters Kluwer.

American Council on Exercise (2020). *The Exercise Professional's Guide to Personal Training.* San Diego, Calif.: American Council on Exercise.

American Heart Association (2014). AHA statistical update: Heart disease and stroke statistics—2014 update: A report from the American Heart Association. *Circulation,* published online December 18, 2013. http://circ.ahajournals.org/content/early/2013/12/18/01.cir.0000441139.02102.80.citation

Balady, G.J. et al. (2007). Core components of cardiac rehabilitation/secondary prevention programs: 2007 update: A scientific statement from the American Heart Association Exercise, Cardiac Rehabilitation, and Prevention

Committee, the Council on Clinical Cardiology; the Councils on Cardiovascular Nursing, Epidemiology and Prevention, and Nutrition, Physical Activity, and Metabolism; and the American Association of Cardiovascular and Pulmonary Rehabilitation. *Circulation,* 115, 2675–2682.

Bjarnason-Wehrens, B. et al. (2004). Recommendations for resistance exercise in cardiac rehabilitation: Recommendations of the German Federation for Cardiovascular Prevention and Rehabilitation. *European Journal of Cardiovascular Prevention and Rehabilitation,* 11, 4, 352–361.

Blank, S. (2006). Physiological responses to Iyengar yoga poses performed by trained practitioners. *Journal of Exercise Physiology,* 9, 7–23.

Boden, W.E. et al. (2007). Optimal medical therapy with or without PCI for stable coronary disease. *New England Journal of Medicine*, 12, 356, 1503–1516.

Centers for Disease Control and Prevention (2013). Surveillance for certain health behaviors among states and selected local areas—United States, 2010. *Morbidity and Mortality Weekly Report: Surveillance Summaries,* 62(ss01), 1–247.

Cook, N.R. et al. (2007). A randomized factorial trial of vitamins C and E and beta carotene in the secondary prevention of cardiovascular events in women: Results from the Women's Antioxidant Cardiovascular Study. *Archives of Internal Medicine*, 167, 15, 1610–1618.

Dalleck, L.C. & Kravitz, L. (2006). Relationship between percent heart rate reserve and percent VO_2 reserve during elliptical crosstrainer exercise. *Journal of Sports Science and Medicine,* 25, 662–671.

de Lorgeril, M. et al. (1999). Mediterranean diet, traditional risk factors, and the rate of cardiovascular complications after myocardial infarction: Final report of the Lyon Diet Heart Study. *Circulation*, 99, 779–785.

Donnelly, J.E. et al. (2009). Appropriate physical activity intervention strategies for weight loss and prevention of weight regain for adults. *Medicine & Science in Sports & Exercise,* 41, 2, 459–471.

Eckel, R.H. et al. (2013). 2013 AHA/ACC guideline on lifestyle management to reduce cardiovascular risk: A report of the American College of Cardiology/American Heart Association Task Force on Practice Guidelines. *Journal of the American College of Cardiology*, 63, 25. DOI: 10.1016/j.jacc.2013.11.003

Gibbons, R. et al. (2002). ACC/AHA 2002 guideline update for exercise testing: Summary article—A report of the American College of Cardiology/American Heart Association Task Force on Practice Guidelines. *Circulation,* 106, 1883–1892.

Gidding, S. et al. (2009). Implementing American Heart Association Pediatric and Adult Nutrition Guidelines: A Scientific Statement from the American Heart Association Nutrition Committee of the Council on Nutrition, Physical Activity and Metabolism, Council on Cardiovascular Disease in the Young, Council on Arteriosclerosis, Thrombosis and Vascular Biology, Council on Cardiovascular Nursing, Council on Epidemiology and Prevention, and Council for High Blood Pressure Research. *Circulation,* 119, 1161–1175.

Goldman, L. et al. (1981). Comparative reproducibility and validity of systems for assessing cardiovascular functional class: Advantages of a new specific activity scale. *Circulation,* 64, 1227–1234.

Greenland, P. et al. (2004). Coronary artery calcium score combined with Framingham score for risk prediction in asymptomatic individuals. *Journal of the American Medical Association,* 291, 210–215.

Guiraud, T. et al. (2011). Acute responses to high-intensity intermittent exercise in CHD patients. *Medicine & Science in Sports & Exercise,* 43, 2, 211–217.

Harris, W.S. (2010). Omega-6 and omega-3 fatty acids: Partners in prevention. *Current Opinions in Clinical Nutrition and Metabolic Care,* 13, 2, 125–129.

Hoevenaar-Blom, M.P. et al. (2012). Mediterranean style diet and 12-year incidence of cardiovascular diseases: The EPIC-NL cohort study. *PloS One,* 7, 9, e45458.

Houle, J. et al. (2013). Daily steps threshold to improve cardiovascular disease risk factors during the year after an acute coronary syndrome. *Journal of Cardiopulmonary Rehabilitation and Prevention,* 33, 6, 406–410.

Howley, E. (2012). Energy costs of physical activity. In: Howley, E. & Franks, B.D. (Eds.) *Health and Fitness Instructor's Manual* (6th ed.). Champaign, Ill.: Human Kinetics.

Institute of Medicine, Food and Nutrition Board (2005). *Dietary Reference Intakes: Energy, Carbohydrates, Fiber, Fat, Fatty Acids, Cholesterol, Protein and Amino Acids.* Washington, D.C.: National Academies Press.

International Atherosclerosis Society (2017). *An International Atherosclerosis Society Position Paper: Global Recommendations for the Management of Dyslipidemia—Full Report.* www.lipidjournal.com/article/S1933-2874(13)00354-1/fulltext

Ismail, H. et al. (2013). Clinical outcomes and cardiovascular responses to different exercise training intensities in patients with heart failure: A systematic review and meta-analysis. *Journal of the American College of Cardiology,* 1, 6, 514–522.

Kenney, W.L., Wilmore, J.H., & Costill, D.L. (2012). *Physiology of Sport and Exercise* (5th ed.). Champaign, Ill.: Human Kinetics.

Kim, Y.J., Chun, H., & Kim, C.H. (2013). Exaggerated response of systolic blood pressure to cycle ergometer. *Annals of Rehabilitation Medicine,* 37, 3, 364–372.

LaForge, R. (2013). *Clinical Pedometry: A Brief Overview and Instructions for Health Care Providers.* Jacksonville, Fla.: National Lipid Association.

Lavie, C.J. et al. (2009). Exercise training and cardiac rehabilitation in primary and secondary prevention of coronary heart disease. *Mayo Clinic Proceedings, 84,* 4, 373–383.

Libby, P. (2012). Inflammation in atherosclerosis. *Arteriosclerosis, Thrombosis, and Vascular Biology,* 32, 2045–2051.

Lorenz, M.W. et al. (2007). Prediction of clinical cardiovascular events with carotid intima-media thickness: A systematic review and meta-analysis. *Circulation,* 115, 459–467.

Marshall, S.J. et al. (2009).Translating physical activity recommendations into a pedometer-based step goal: 3000 steps in 30 minutes. *American Journal of Preventive Medicine,* 36, 410.

Merchant, R.M. et al. (2020). 2020 American Heart Association guidelines for cardiopulmonary resuscitation and emergency cardiovascular care. *Circulation,* 142, 16, S337–S357.

Miles, S.C. et al. (2013). Arterial blood pressure and cardiovascular responses to yoga practice. *Alternative Therapies in Health and Medicine,* 19, 1, 38–45.

National Cholesterol Education Program (2002). *Third Report of the National Cholesterol Education Program (NCEP) Expert Panel on Detection, Evaluation, and Treatment of High Blood Cholesterol in Adults (Adult Treatment Panel III).* Final Report. National Heart, Lung, and Blood Institute National Institutes of Health NIH Publication No. 02-5215.

Nordmann, A.J. et al. (2011). Meta-analysis comparing Mediterranean to low-fat diets for modification of cardiovascular risk factors. *American Journal of Medicine*, 124, 841–851, e842.

Ornish, D. et al. (1998). Intensive lifestyle changes for reversal of coronary heart disease. *Journal of the American Medical Association*, 280, 2001–2007.

Ornish, D. et al. (1990). Can lifestyle changes reverse coronary heart disease? *Lancet*, 336, 129–133.

Pal, G.K., Velkumary, S., & Madanmohan (2004). Effect of short-term practice of breathing exercises on autonomic functions in normal human volunteers. *Indian Journal of Medical Research,* 120, 115–121.

Pal, G.K. et al. (2014). Slow yogic breathing through right and left nostril influences sympathovagal balance, heart rate variability, and cardiovascular risks in young adults. *North American Journal of Medical Sciences*, 6, 3, 145–151.

Rognmo, Ø. et al. (2012). Cardiovascular risk of high- versus moderate-intensity aerobic exercise in coronary heart disease patients. *Circulation,* 126, 12, 1436–1440.

Sesso, H.D. et al. (2008). Vitamins E and C in the prevention of cardiovascular disease in men: The Physicians' Health Study II randomized controlled trial. *Journal of the American Medical Association*, 300, 18, 2123–2133.

Sofi, F. et al. (2010). Review accruing evidence on benefits of adherence to the Mediterranean diet on health: An updated systemic review and meta-analysis. *American Journal of Clinical Nutrition*, 92, 5, 1189–1196.

Trichopoulou, A. et al. (2003). Adherence to a Mediterranean diet and survival in a Greek population. *New England Journal of Medicine,* 348, 2599–2608.

Tudor-Locke, C. et al. (2011). Accelerometer steps/day translation of moderate-to-vigorous activity. *Preventive Medicine,* 53, 1–2, 31–33.

U.S. Department of Agriculture (2020). *2020-2025 Dietary Guidelines for Americans* (9th ed.) www.dietaryguidelines.gov

U.S. Department of Health & Human Services (2018). *Physical Activity Guidelines for Americans* (2nd ed.). www.health.gov/paguidelines/

Williams, M.A. (2001). Exercise testing in cardiac rehabilitation: Exercise prescription and beyond. *Cardiology Clinics,* 19, 3, 415–431.

SUGGESTED READING

ACCF/AHA/ACP/AATS/PCNA/SCAI/STS (2012). Guideline for the diagnosis and management of patients with stable ischemic heart disease: A report of the American College of Cardiology Foundation/American Heart Association Task Force on Practice Guidelines, and the American College of Physicians, American Association for Thoracic Surgery, Preventive Cardiovascular Nurses Association, Society for Stephan D. Fihn, MD, MPH, Chair. *Circulation,* 126, e354–e471.

American College of Cardiology/American Heart Association (2013). Guidelines on the treatment of blood cholesterol to reduce atherosclerotic cardiovascular risk in adults: A report of the American College of Cardiology/American Heart Association Task Force on Practice Guidelines. *Circulation,* published online November 12, 2013.

American Association of Cardiovascular and Pulmonary Rehabilitation (2021). *Guidelines for Cardiac Rehabilitation Programs* (6th ed.). Champaign, Ill.: Human Kinetics.

American College of Sports Medicine (2022). *ACSM's Guidelines for Exercise Testing and Prescription* (11th ed.). Philadelphia: Wolters Kluwer.

American Heart Association (2014). AHA statistical update: Heart disease and stroke statistics—2014 update: A report from the American Heart Association. *Circulation,* published online December 18, 2013. http://circ.ahajournals.org/content/early/2013/12/18/01.cir.0000441139.02102.80.citation

8 BLOOD LIPID DISORDERS

IN THIS CHAPTER

EPIDEMIOLOGY

OVERVIEW
LIPIDS, LIPOPROTEINS, AND ATHEROSCLEROSIS

BACKGROUND ON CONSENSUS CHOLESTEROL GUIDELINES

RECOMMENDED LIPID AND LIPOPROTEIN THERAPEUTIC GOALS

DIAGNOSTIC CRITERIA
FRAMINGHAM 10-YEAR RISK ALGORITHM

NATIONAL LIPID ASSOCIATION ASCVD RISK ASSESSMENT AND TREATMENT GOALS

ACC/AHA POOLED COHORT 10-YEAR ASCVD RISK ASSESSMENT

LONG-TERM AND LIFETIME RISK ASSESSMENT

TREATMENT OPTIONS
NON-PHARMACOLOGICAL TREATMENT

PHARMACOLOGICAL TREATMENT

EXERCISE TREATMENT

NUTRITIONAL CONSIDERATIONS
IMPROVING THE CHOLESTEROL PROFILE

IMPROVING BLOOD TRIGLYCERIDES

EATING PLANS TO SUPPORT OPTIMAL BLOOD LIPID PROFILE

EXERCISE RECOMMENDATIONS
ACSM EXERCISE AND DYSLIPIDEMIA GUIDELINES

EXERCISE GUIDELINES SUMMARY FOR CLIENTS WITH DYSLIPIDEMIA

CASE STUDY

SUMMARY

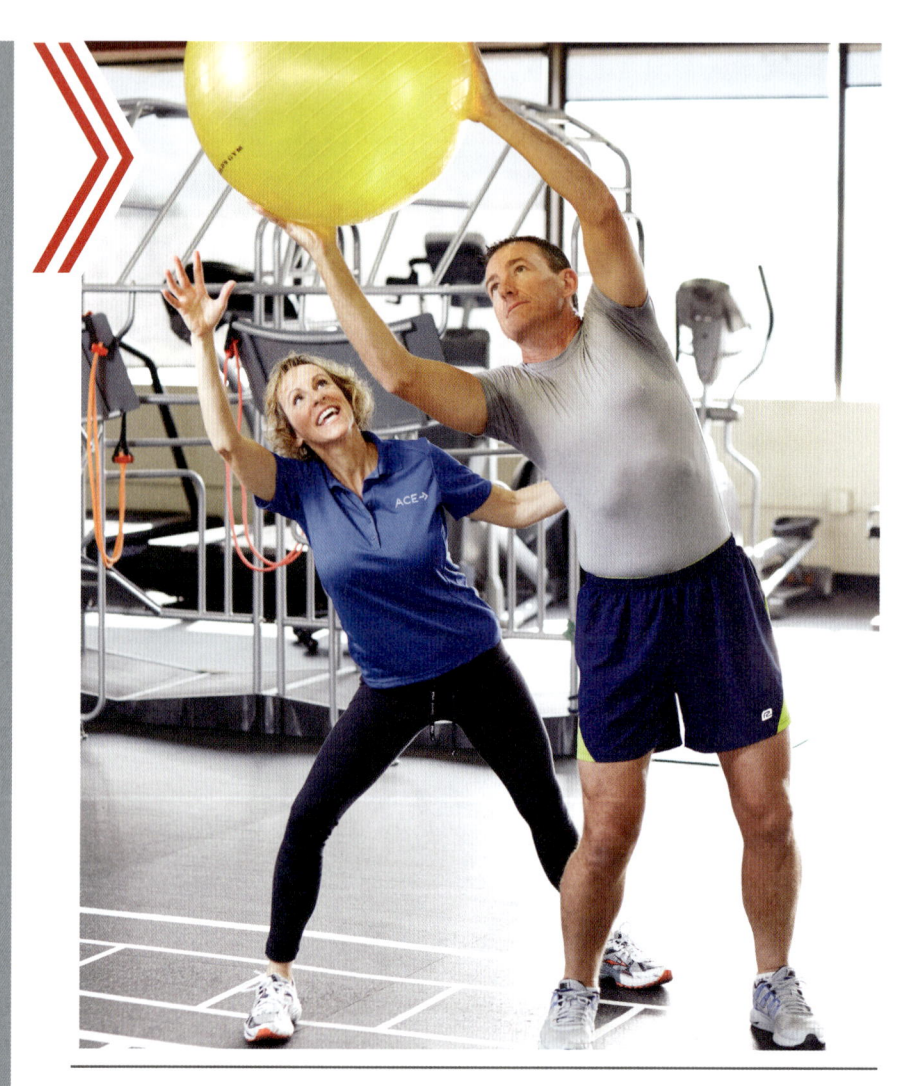

ABOUT THE AUTHOR
Ralph La Forge, M.S., is a physiologist and Accreditation Council on Clinical Lipidology–certified clinical lipid specialist and former managing director of the Cholesterol Disorder Physician Education Program at Duke University Medical Center, Endocrine Division in Durham, North Carolina. He was also managing director of preventive medicine and cardiac rehabilitation at Sharp Health Care in San Diego, where he also taught applied exercise physiology at the University of California at San Diego. Prior to that, La Forge was director of preventive cardiology and cardiac rehabilitation at the Lovelace Clinic in Albuquerque, New Mexico. He has helped more than 300 medical staff groups throughout North America organize and operate lipid disorder clinics and diabetes- and heart-disease-prevention programs. La Forge is the immediate past president of the Southeast Lipid Association and a clinical consultant to numerous healthcare institutions including the U.S. Indian Health Service Division of Diabetes Treatment and Prevention. He has published more than 200 papers on clinical exercise science, lipidology, and preventive endocrinology.

By Ralph La Forge

IT IS IMPERATIVE THAT THE ACE® CERTIFIED MEDICAL Exercise Specialist (CMES) understand the principal **coronary heart disease (CHD)** risk factors, as most of these are favorably altered by physical activity. The principal risk factors for CHD include elevated **low-density lipoprotein (LDL)** cholesterol, low **high-density lipoprotein (HDL)** cholesterol, elevated **non-HDL cholesterol,** high **blood pressure,** smoking, and **diabetes.** Of course, **obesity,** age, gender, family history, and stress all play a role, but the central focus of both lifestyle and pharmacological therapy is on the principal risk factors. Physical activity, weight loss, smoking cessation, dietary behavior changes, and reduction in stress play key behavioral roles in the modification of these principal atherosclerotic risk factors. Other **lipids** (**fatty acids**) and biomarkers of atherosclerotic risk have also been identified, including: elevated **triglycerides,** LDL cholesterol particle number (LDL-P), and apolipoprotein B levels (apo B); low apolipoprotein A-1 levels; elevated lipoprotein(a) [Lp(a)]; and high C-reactive protein (CRP), coronary calcium, and lipoprotein-associated phospholipase A_2 (Lp-PLA_2). This chapter addresses the importance of managing blood lipid disorders (**dyslipidemia**) in the prevention and management of CHD. The increasing use of **cholesterol**-lowering drug therapy, particularly in primary **cardiovascular disease (CVD)** prevention, continues to present challenges to those healthcare professionals who teach and coach lifestyle therapy—the value of physical activity is well established in CVD prevention and as both primary and adjunct therapy for many clients diagnosed with dyslipidemia.

In this chapter, the term CVD will be mostly stated as **atherosclerotic cardiovascular disease (ASCVD),** as this disease description is now used within the framework of guidelines for dyslipidemia diagnosis and therapy. ASCVD is more comprehensive in that it includes CHD, as well as acute coronary syndromes, **myocardial infarction (MI),** stable or unstable **angina,** coronary or other arterial revascularization, **stroke, transient ischemic attacks,** and **peripheral arterial disease** presumed to be of atherosclerotic origin. There are instances in this chapter that discuss dyslipidemia to manage total ASCVD risk, but also instances that will illustrate the efficacy of managing dyslipidemia, particularly elevated LDL, in clients with CHD.

EPIDEMIOLOGY

A large body of data has established that **serum cholesterol** and associated **lipoproteins** are crucial risk factors for **atherosclerosis** and ultimately clinical events such as MI and strokes. Blood lipid disorders (also called dyslipidemia and **dyslipoproteinemia**) represent an important modifiable risk factor for the development and progression of CHD. In recent years, lipid levels have improved, mostly owing to the growing use of prescription lipid-lowering medications, particularly statin drugs (Table 8-1).

The CMES can play an important role in **clinical lipidology** (the diagnosis and management of lipid disorders) by working directly with physicians in the management of lipid disorders. The CMES should prioritize a systematic approach to physical activity for the CHD client, while also helping them achieve optimal blood lipid control—ideally through therapeutic lifestyle changes but frequently in concert with lipid-lowering drug therapy. Therefore, the CMES should also understand the role of pharmacotherapy in treating lipid disorders.

LEARNING OBJECTIVES:

» Identify the various factors that are taken into account when considering an individual's risk for dyslipidemia, including lipids, lipoproteins, chylomicrons, triglycerides, and atherosclerosis.

» Briefly describe the background on consensus cholesterol guidelines and recommended lipid and lipoprotein therapeutic goals from established organizations (e.g., American College of Cardiology, American Heart Association, and National Lipid Association).

» Describe the available treatment options for dyslipidemia, including an emphasis on the role of physical activity and structured exercise.

» Explain nutrition-related strategies for the treatment and management of dyslipidemia.

» Design and implement safe and effective exercise programs for clients who have been diagnosed with dyslipidemia.

TABLE 8-1
TRENDS IN CHOLESTEROL LEVELS IN THE UNITED STATES

National Health and Nutrition Examination Survey: Cholesterol levels improve among U.S. adults ~1990–2010

Total cholesterol	Decreased from 206 mg/dL in 1988–1994 to 196 mg/dL in 2007–2010
Low-density lipoprotein (LDL)	Decreased from 129 mg/dL to 116 mg/dL
High-density lipoprotein (HDL)	Increased from 50.7 mg/dL to 52.5 mg/dL
Non-HDL	Decreased from 155 mg/dL to 114 mg/dL
Triglycerides	Increased from 118 mg/dL in 1988–1994 to 123 mg/dL in 1999–2002, but then decreased to 100 mg/dL in 2007–2010
Patients taking lipid-lowering medications	Increased from 3.4% to 15.5%

Data from: National Health and Nutrition Examination Survey (2012). Cholesterol levels improve among U.S. adults. *Journal of the American Medical Association,* 308, 1545–1554.

OVERVIEW

Dyslipidemia and its related condition, the **metabolic syndrome (MetS),** are influenced by lipids, cholesterol, and other lipoproteins. This section covers contributing factors for these conditions, as well as how these factors combine to put an individual at greater risk for developing CHD.

Lipids, Lipoproteins, and Atherosclerosis

Cholesterol is a fatty substance that travels in the blood in distinct particles that contain both lipids and proteins. These particles are called lipoproteins. The cholesterol level in the blood is determined partly by genetics and partly by lifestyle factors such as diet, body fat, physical activity, and even psychological stress. There are six major classes of lipoproteins found in the blood of a fasting individual:

- Chylomicrons
- **Very-low-density lipoprotein (VLDL)**
- **Intermediate-density lipoprotein (IDL)**
- Low-density lipoprotein (LDL)
- High-density lipoprotein (HDL)
- Non-HDL cholesterol

Chylomicrons

Chylomicrons are the largest and least dense of the lipoproteins (Figure 8-1). These 1,000-nanometer particles originate in the intestinal mucosa. Their function is to transport dietary triglycerides and cholesterol absorbed by the intestinal epithelial cells. The lymphatic system transports chylomicrons to the **plasma** where they acquire additional **apolipoproteins** from HDL. Triglycerides contained in chylomicrons are hydrolyzed in the tissues and the chylomicron particle remnants are processed by the liver.

Figure 8-1
Relative sizes of lipoproteins

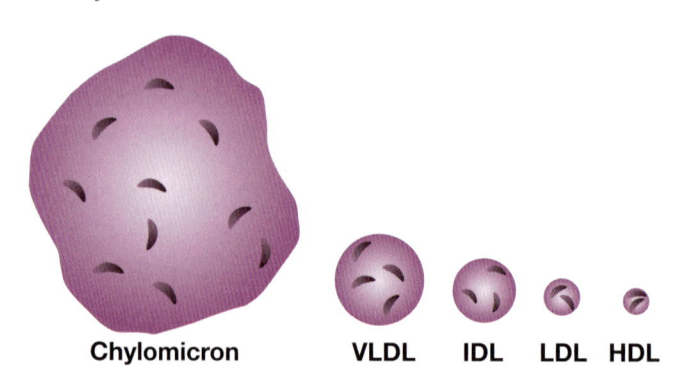

Chylomicron   VLDL   IDL   LDL   HDL

Note: VLDL = Very-low-density lipoprotein; IDL = Intermediate-density lipoprotein; LDL = Low-density lipoprotein; HDL = High-density lipoprotein

Triglycerides and Very-low-density Lipoprotein Cholesterol

VLDL is a major carrier of triglycerides in the plasma. Triglyceride is a major form of **fat**. A triglyceride consists of three molecules of fatty acid combined with a molecule of **glycerol.** Synthesized in the liver, triglyceride-rich VLDL carries endogenously synthesized (i.e., produced by the body) triglycerides and cholesterol to their sites of utilization. VLDL also contains 10 to 15% of the body's total serum cholesterol. Increased concentrations of VLDL are associated with a number of lipoprotein disorders, such as **familial hypertriglyceridemia,** obesity, diabetes, and **nephrotic syndrome.** Strong evidence points to VLDL as being atherogenic like LDL. Combining LDL and VLDL makes non-HDL, which is an alternate target of therapy in patients with hypertriglyceridemia in whom VLDL is elevated [Varbo et al., 2013; National Cholesterol Education Program (NCEP), 2002].

High levels of triglycerides in the blood (**hypertriglyceridemia**) frequently is a marker of high **atherogenic** particle burden and apo B levels in excess of that reflected by more traditional measures such as LDL. Triglycerides do not accumulate in the vessel wall. Their atherogenicity is based on their association with other particles in the blood, including VLDL, IDL, and/or increased small and large LDL particles. Therefore, the risk of having elevated triglycerides is based primarily on its association with other lipoproteins.

Intermediate-density Lipoprotein

IDL belongs to the lipoprotein particle family and is formed from the degradation of VLDL. The native IDL particle consists of protein that encircles various fatty acids, enabling, as a water-soluble particle, these fatty acids to travel in the aqueous blood environment as part of the fat transport system within the body. They are cleared from the plasma into the liver by receptor-mediated endocytosis, or further degraded to form LDL particles. IDL and cholesterol-rich VLDL combine to contribute to the development of **atherogenesis,** the early stages of atherosclerosis, and CHD.

Low-density Lipoprotein Cholesterol

LDL is the major carrier of cholesterol in the circulation. It contains 60 to 70% of the body's total serum cholesterol and is directly correlated with the risk for CHD. LDL and LDL-P play a pivotal role in atherogenesis. This role is illustrated in Figures 8-2 and 8-3, which show LDL infiltration into the arterial endothelium and fatty streak and plaque formation. Although all blood lipids play a role in the development of atherosclerosis, epidemiologic studies suggest that LDL is the most significant blood lipid. LDL is also the primary focus of most blood-lipid-lowering therapies. Plasma LDL concentrations are regulated by specialized LDL receptors (LDLR) in the liver and on the arterial endothelium. Many patients have mutations in the LDLR gene that encodes the LDL receptor protein, which normally removes LDL from the circulation In such cases, plasma LDL concentrations increase dramatically, as seen in individuals with **familial hypercholesterolemia.** Table 8-2 depicts various LDL-lowering strategies and their respective efficacy. LDL management is the cornerstone of blood lipid control and the reduction in risk for CVD, most specifically CHD [Grundy et al., 2018; Jacobson et al., 2014; International Atherosclerosis Society (IAS), 2013].

High-density Lipoprotein Cholesterol

HDL is formed in the intestine and liver. HDL normally contains 20 to 30% of the body's total cholesterol, and HDL levels are inversely correlated with CHD risk. HDL has grown to be understood in recent years to be a very complex lipoprotein with at least a dozen functions. HDL plays an important role in reverse cholesterol transport (i.e., removal of cholesterol from cells and transporting it back to the liver), but it also has **antioxidant** and anti-inflammatory functions. By removing excess cholesterol from the circulation, HDL may provide a protective mechanism against the development of atherosclerosis. Research has shown that each mg/dL increase in plasma HDL cholesterol concentration is associated with approximately 3% reduction in CHD risk. However, targeting HDL with anything beyond lifestyle therapy (e.g., exercise and weight

Figure 8-2
Impact of LDL cholesterol infiltration on coronary artery inflammation

Reprinted with permission from Hansson, G.K. (2005). Mechanisms of disease: Inflammation, atherosclerosis, and coronary artery disease. *New England Journal of Medicine*, 352, 1685–1695.

Copyright ©2005. Massachusetts Medical Society. All rights reserved.

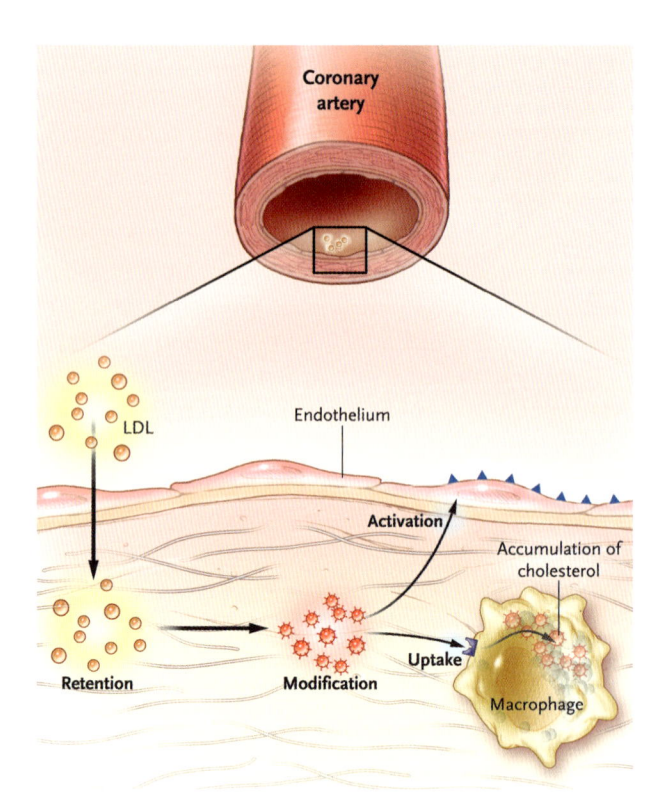

Figure 8-3
Fatty streak formation in atherosclerosis

Reprinted with permission from Ross, R. (1999). Atherosclerosis: An inflammatory disease. *New England Journal of Medicine*, 340, 115–126.

Copyright ©1999. Massachusetts Medical Society. All rights reserved.

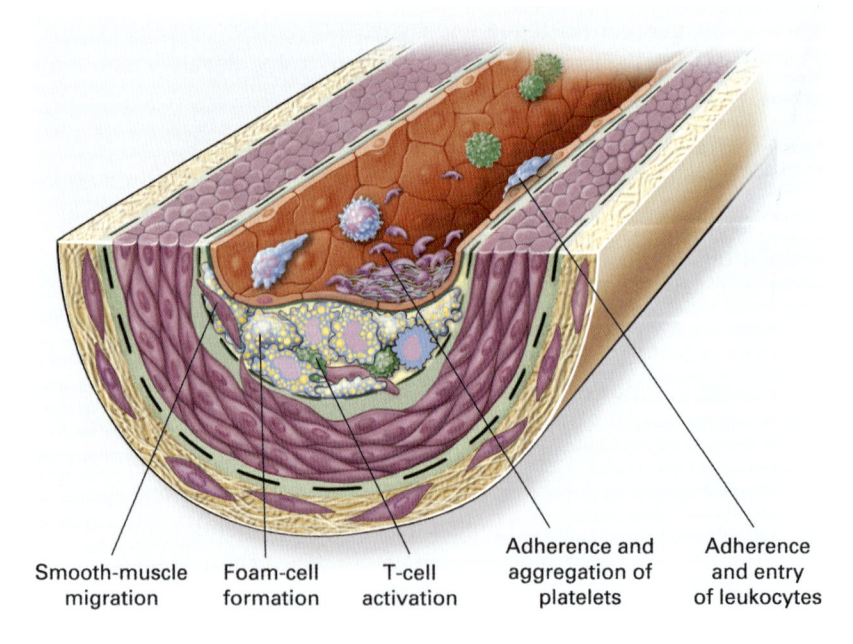

TABLE 8-2	
GENERALIZED COMPARISONS OF LOW-DENSITY LIPOPROTEIN CHOLESTEROL REDUCTION STRATEGIES	
	% Reduction
Dietary modification (e.g., 10–25% reduction in total fat)	8–35%
Weight loss (e.g., 3–10+% weight loss)	5–20%
Physical activity	4–7+%
Drug therapy (e.g., moderate to intense statin therapy)	20–65%

loss) does not appear to reduce CHD risk—at least thus far. There is also evidence that some individuals have a "dysfunctional" form of HDL, owing to the oxidation of HDL's major structural apoprotein—apo A1. This "dysfunctional" form of HDL is apparently not cardioprotective (Huang et al., 2014). Currently, there is no readily available method to assess if one has an abundance of "dysfunctional" HDL.

Although epidemiological studies clearly defined a link between HDL levels and CHD, more recent clinical trials aimed at raising HDL levels have either been terminated early because of futility or even led to negative results in terms of causing an increase in cardiovascular events (HPS2-THRIVE Collaborative Group, 2013; AIM-HIGH Investigators, 2011). Niacin, one of the most effective drugs for raising HDL, showed lack of efficacy in the AIM-HIGH (2011) trial, although this has been attributed to the trial design. Likewise, the HPS2-THRIVE trial found that extended-release niacin with laropiprant, an agent to reduce flushing caused by niacin, did not improve cardiovascular health or decrease cardiovascular events compared with statin-only therapy (HPS2-THRIVE Collaborative Group, 2013). Importantly, current treatment guidelines do not make a low HDL concentration a primary target of drug therapy. They do however support maximizing lifestyle therapies in an effort to raise HDL. What the CMES should understand is that HDL is a very complex lipoprotein and research is in a state of flux on how to manage it pharmacologically. HDL is clearly an important CHD risk predictor and is used in nearly all algorithms to score ASCVD risk, including CHD risk, but at this point it is unclear whether pharmacologically raising HDL independently reduces the risk of CHD (Jacobson et al., 2014; IAS, 2013). Table 8-3 lists factors that influence HDL levels.

TABLE 8-3

FACTORS THAT INFLUENCE HIGH-DENSITY LIPOPROTEIN (HDL) LEVELS

Factors That Decrease HDL Levels	Factors That Increase HDL Levels*
Overweight and obesity	Alcohol
Smoking	Estrogens, fibrates, and nicotinic acid
Physical inactivity	Diet
Androgenic and anabolic drugs	Exercise
Type 2 diabetes, hypertriglyceridemia, infections, and cachexia	

Non-HDL Cholesterol and Apolipoprotein B

Non-HDL cholesterol is a very important lipid measure that is strongly associated with CHD, as well as the ever-increasing prevalence of obesity, MetS, and **type 2 diabetes (T2DM),** and thus should be of special therapeutic interest to health and exercise professionals, particularly the CMES and health coach.

Non-HDL cholesterol is calculated as follows:

> Non-HDL cholesterol = Total cholesterol − HDL cholesterol

The goal for non-HDL cholesterol is the same as for LDL, plus 30 mg/dL. For example, someone with diabetes or CHD might have an LDL goal of <100 mg/dL. Therefore, their non-HDL goal would be <130 mg/dL. LDL is still the principal target of therapy for most patients with, or at high risk for, CHD and for all patients with T2DM. In contrast to LDL, non-HDL cholesterol values can be calculated in non-fasting patients without measuring triglycerides.

Why is non-HDL so important? Non-HDL cholesterol is inclusive of all atherogenic lipoproteins, including LDL, and thus is a more comprehensive measure of atherogenic particles than LDL alone (Figure 8-4).

Figure 8-4

Non-HDL cholesterol

Note: The yellow box includes all non-HDL; HDL = High-density lipoprotein; apo B = Apolipoprotein B; LDL = Low-density lipoprotein; LDL-P = LDL cholesterol particle number; IDL = Intermediate-density lipoprotein; VLDL = Very low-density lipoprotein; Lp(a) = Lipoprotein(a); HDL_2 = Larger HDL subspecies; HDL_3 = Smaller HDL subspecies

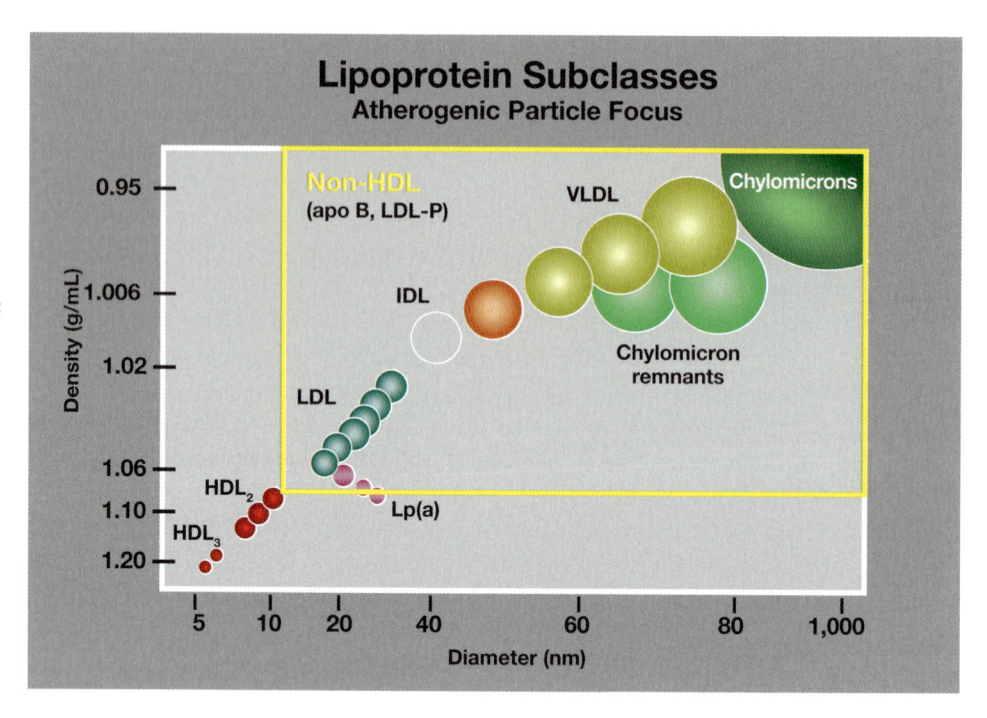

Available data suggest that using non-HDL cholesterol level is as good as, or better than, LDL for predicting CHD, especially in individuals who have elevated triglycerides (e.g., those with MetS and/or diabetes) (Boekholdt et al., 2012; Bittner, 2004). An analysis of contemporary statin trials moreover demonstrated that on-treatment levels of non-HDL are more strongly associated with future risk of ASCVD events than either apo B or LDL (Boekholdt et al., 2012). In the same analysis, non-HDL explained a larger proportion of the atheroprotective effects of statin therapy than either apo B or LDL (Boekholdt et al., 2012).

Since LDL is the major atherogenic lipoprotein, LDL is accepted as the major target of lipid-lowering therapy. Non-HDL should now be considered at least as important as LDL as the primary focus of lipid-lowering therapy (Jacobson et al., 2014; IAS, 2013). It is expected that in future guidelines non-HDL will replace LDL as the better target of treatment (Jacobson et al., 2014; IAS, 2013). Non-HDL cholesterol is also a good surrogate for apo B, which may be somewhat more atherogenic than the calculated non-HDL. Apo B is a measure of total atherogenic particle load and includes a measure of both triglyceride-rich lipoproteins and LDL (i.e., there is one apo B particle attached on the surface of each of these atherogenic lipoproteins).

Other Lipoproteins and Associated Biomarkers of CVD Risk

There are other lipoproteins, apoproteins, and lipoprotein fractions such as lipoprotein (a) [Lp(a)]; apoproteins A, B, C, D, and E; and various subfractions of VLDL, LDL, and HDL [e.g., large- and small-dense LDL cholesterol (also designated as LDL phenotype A and B, respectively)].

These lipoproteins are largely used to more definitively diagnose more complex forms of dyslipidemia and to provide additional CVD risk prediction. For example, Lp(a) is structurally similar to LDL both in protein and lipid composition and is related to thrombotic (blood coagulation) risk. When significantly elevated (>30 mg/dL), Lp(a) can also help define CHD risk, but screening for Lp(a) in the general population is not suggested at this time. European guidelines recommend that a desirable level for Lp(a) should be below the 80th percentile (<50 mg/dL) (Nordestgaard et al., 2010).

Lipoprotein subfractions (smaller LDL-particle size) can also help further predict CVD risk, but their measurement requires more advanced laboratory technology [e.g., **nuclear magnetic resonance (NMR)** instrumentation] and LDL particle *number* has reproducibly been shown to be more related to CHD risk than LDL particle *size* (Cromwell & Otvos, 2007; Cromwell et al., 2007).

Blood Lipid Disorders — CHAPTER 8

Apolipoproteins lie on the surface of the larger lipoproteins and act as **ligands** (points that attach to various target receptors) that help provide structural integrity of lipoproteins, but more importantly can activate and regulate lipoprotein metabolism. Their measurement can help determine the cause of a particular lipid disorder, which is often genetic.

LDL Particle Number Analysis

The use of a NMR imaging spectroscopy assay to assess lipoproteins has demonstrated that measuring the number of LDL cholesterol particles has shown much promise. There is evidence that the LDL particles themselves, not just LDL cholesterol, are the atherogenic culprits in CHD. Cromwell and others have convincingly shown that in a number of patient populations, but especially in those with the MetS, LDL particle number is a better predictor of CVD incidence than LDL cholesterol (Cromwell et al., 2007). LDL-P has a relationship with LDL (e.g., 100 mg/dL of LDL cholesterol is equal to ~1,100 nm/L of LDL particles). Rosenson and Underberg (2013) reviewed 36 studies and established that different lipid-lowering drugs can lead to discordance between LDL-P and LDL. Therefore, basing LDL-lowering therapy only on the achievement of cholesterol goals may result in a treatment gap. Therefore, the use of LDL-P for monitoring lipid-lowering therapy, particularly for statins, can provide a more accurate assessment of residual cardiovascular risk (Rosenson & Underberg, 2013). Interestingly, Kraus and others also demonstrated this trend, with NMR-measured LDL-P being a more sensitive measure of aerobic exercise training responsiveness (Kraus et al., 2002).

Background on Consensus Cholesterol Guidelines

In order for the CMES to have a frame of reference on what constitutes appropriate cholesterol goals and lipid-management therapy, they should have some understanding of the changes and advances in consensus recommendations, including some of the divergence of expert opinion. This will be particularly helpful when working with healthcare provider referrals, as this is one of the fundamental responsibilities of a CMES.

For the past 25 years and under the expert leadership of Dr. Scott Grundy, the National Cholesterol Education Program (NCEP) from the National Institutes of Health (NIH) contributed the authoritative guidelines on dyslipidemia diagnosis and management. The IAS (2013), National Lipid Association (NLA) (Jacobson et al., 2014), and the European Atherosclerosis Society in conjunction with the European Cardiology Society (Reiner et al., 2011) published their dyslipidemia guidelines. There is much consensus of agreement in all of these guideline documents. The 2018 AHA/ACC/AACVPR/AAPA/ABC/ACPM/ADA/AGS/APhA/ASPC/NLA/PCNA Guidelines on the Management of Blood Cholesterol, for example, recommend a heart healthy lifestyle across the life course. This includes addressing elevated blood pressure, cigarette smoking, and elevated blood sugar levels, if indicated, using pharmacological therapy to reduce LDL cholesterol based on current cholesterol measurements, 10-year ASCVD risk, and risk-enhancing factors such as family history of premature ASCVD, metabolic syndrome, and the presence of chronic inflammatory disorders (Grundy et al., 2018).

Recommended Lipid and Lipoprotein Therapeutic Goals

The major innovations/updates from earlier NCEP recommendations in the IAS and NLA guidelines are the following:
- Guidelines were based on multiple lines of evidence (epidemiological studies, genetic studies, and clinical trials)
- Identification of non-HDL as a major form of atherogenic cholesterol
- Definition of atherogenic cholesterol as either LDL or non-HDL
- Definition of optimal levels of atherogenic cholesterol (both LDL and non-HDL) for primary and secondary prevention

- Assigning priority to long-term risk categories over short-term risk
- Adjustment of risk estimation according to baseline risk of different nations or regions
- Primary emphasis on lifestyle intervention; secondary emphasis on drug therapy

2018 ACC/AHA Cholesterol Guidelines

The AHA/ACC/AACVPR/AAPA/ABC/ACPM/ADA/AGS/APhA/ASPC/NLA/PCNA cholesterol guidelines (Grundy et al., 2018) do not recommend target laboratory lipid and lipoprotein goals, but argue that a percentage reduction should be used to estimate the efficacy of statin therapy, since lowering LDL cholesterol levels by 1% produces an approximate 1% reduction in ASCVD risk. ASCVD risk is reduced by using statin therapy and the absolute response is dependent upon baseline LDL concentrations, with a given dose of statins producing a similar percentage reduction in LDL levels across a wide range of initial LDL values. In addition to the use of lipid-lowering drugs, the following lifestyle therapies are also recommended:

- Diet composition: Emphasizing vegetables, fruits, whole grains, healthy proteins, beans, peas, lentils, and nontropical vegetable oils, and limiting sweets and beverages with added sugar
- Weight control to avoid weight gain and promote weight loss in those with overweight or obesity
- Cardiorespiratory physical activity three to four times per week for an average of 40 minutes per session at a moderate to vigorous intensity

It is important that the CMES be familiar with the key recommendations from the ACC/AHA cholesterol guidelines and those set forth by other organizations. From a day-to-day client care perspective, the NLA guidelines (Jacobson et al., 2014) are much more comprehensive (not just LDL) and appropriate because they give some relative target numbers to consider and are consistent with prior NCEP guidelines in format and focus.

Recommended Lipid and Lipoprotein Goals in Children

According to the National Heart, Lung, and Blood Institute (NHLBI) (2012), a major increase in the prevalence of obesity has led to a much larger population of children with dyslipidemia. The predominant dyslipidemic pattern in childhood is a combined pattern associated with obesity, with moderate to severe elevation in triglycerides, normal to mild elevation in LDL, and reduced HDL. Each of these dyslipidemic patterns has been shown to be associated with the initiation and progression of atherosclerotic lesions in children and adolescents, as demonstrated by pathology and imaging studies (NHLBI, 2012). See Tables 8-4 and 8-5 for plasma lipid and lipoprotein goals in children and adolescents.

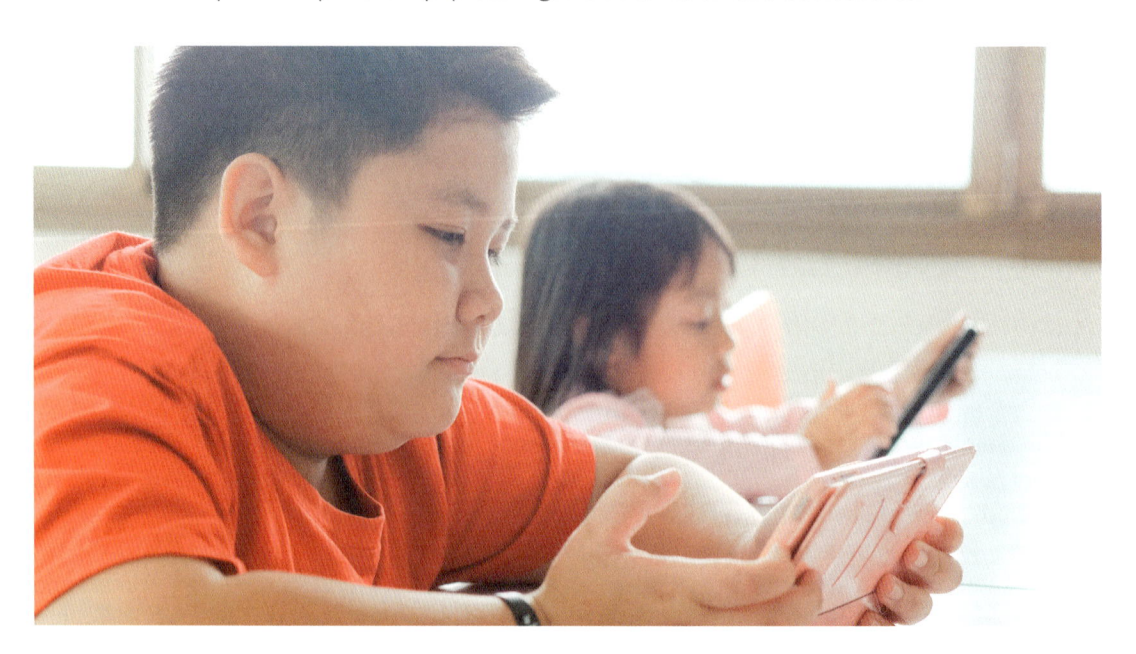

Blood Lipid Disorders   CHAPTER 8

TABLE 8-4
ACCEPTABLE, BORDERLINE-HIGH, AND HIGH PLASMA LIPID, AND LIPOPROTEIN CONCENTRATIONS (MG/DL) FOR CHILDREN AND ADOLESCENTS*

Category	Acceptable	Borderline	High[†]
Total cholesterol	<170	170–199	≥200
LDL	<110	110–129	≥130
Non-HDL	<120	120–144	≥145
Triglycerides 0–9 years 10–19 years	 <75 <90	 75–99 90–129	 ≥100 ≥130
Category	**Acceptable**	**Borderline**	**Low[†]**
HDL	>45	40–45	<40

Note: LDL = Low-density lipoprotein; HDL = High-density lipoprotein

Note: Values given are in mg/dL; to convert to SI units, divide the results for total cholesterol, LDL, HDL, and non-HDL by 38.6; for triglycerides, divide by 88.6.

*Values for plasma lipid and lipoprotein levels are from the National Cholesterol Education Program (NCEP) Expert Panel on Cholesterol Levels in Children. Non-HDL values are from the Bogalusa Heart Study and are equivalent to the NCEP Pediatric Panel cut points for LDL.

[†] The cut points for high and borderline-high represent approximately the 95th and 75th percentiles, respectively. Low cut points for HDL represent approximately the 10th percentile.

Source: National Heart, Lung, and Blood Institute (2012). *Expert Panel on Integrated Guidelines for Cardiovascular Health and Risk Reduction in Children and Adolescents Summary Report.* NIH Publication No. 12-7486A.

TABLE 8-5
RECOMMENDED CUT POINTS FOR LIPID AND LIPOPROTEIN LEVELS (MG/DL) FOR YOUNG ADULTS*

Category	Acceptable	Borderline High	High
Total cholesterol	<190	190–224	≥225
LDL	<120	120–159	≥160
Non-HDL	<150	150–189	≥190
Triglycerides	<115	115–149	≥150
Category	**Acceptable**	**Borderline Low**	**Low**
HDL	>45	40–44	<40

Note: LDL = Low-density lipoprotein; HDL = High-density lipoprotein

* Values provided are from the Lipid Research Clinics Prevalence Study. The cut points for total cholesterol, LDL, and non-HDL represent the 95th percentile for 20–24 year old subjects and are not identical with the cut points used in the most recent NHLBI adult guidelines, ATP III, which are derived from combined data on adults of all ages. The age-specific cut points given here are provided for pediatric care providers to use in managing this young adult age group. For total cholesterol, LDL, and non-HDL, borderline high values are between the 75th and 94th percentile, while acceptable are <75th percentile. The high triglyceride cut point represents approximately the 90th percentile, with borderline high between the 75th and 89th percentile and acceptable <75th percentile. The low HDL cut point represents roughly the 25th percentile, with borderline low between the 26th and 50th percentile and acceptable >the 50th percentile.

Source: National Heart, Lung, and Blood Institute (2012). *Expert Panel on Integrated Guidelines for Cardiovascular Health and Risk Reduction in Children and Adolescents Summary Report.* NIH Publication No. 12-7486A.

DIAGNOSTIC CRITERIA

There are several ASCVD risk-scoring tools that healthcare professionals can use to determine cholesterol treatment goals. These tools are essentially for those who do not have CHD and are used to estimate low, moderate, and high risk for CHD and ASCVD, and thus the LDL goal and/or the intensity of LDL reduction therapy. Those clients who have existing CHD, stroke, or **peripheral vascular disease** histories are automatically high risk and warrant more aggressive LDL reduction therapy—and of course intensive lifestyle therapy. All of these risk-assessment tools are for determining CHD and ASCVD risk, but more specifically for determining LDL and non-HDL goals, which are the principal targets of therapy based on many lines of clinical evidence and consensus guidelines. Each assessment tool uses traditional risk factors to score risk [e.g., **systolic blood pressure (SBP)**, HDL, total cholesterol, smoking, age, and gender]. The four assessment tools are:

- The Framingham 10-year CHD Risk Assessment
- The National Lipid Association ASCVD Risk Assessment
- New ACC/AHA Pooled Cohort 10-year ASCVD Risk Assessment (Caucasians and African Americans only)
- Long-term (Lifetime) Risk Assessment

What is important to understand when comparing these four assessment tools is that whereas the Framingham risk assessment is used to make a judgment if the patient has sufficient risk to recommend that LDL be <100 mg/dL (moderate-high risk) or <70 mg/dL (high risk for CVD). The ACC/AHA 10-year risk assessment tool is used strictly to recommend low, moderate, and intensive doses of statin therapy, ignoring actual LDL target levels. Obviously, the application and use of the ACC/AHA assessment is a complete departure from targeting specific LDL goals and has been the subject of considerable criticism. The ACC/AHA's justification is based on a comprehensive review of large clinical trials that in their view supports monitoring reductions in percentage of LDL cholesterol to monitor the response of LDL cholesterol to statin therapy for determining efficacy.

The CMES does not need to understand all of these guideline differences in any great detail because it will not have a meaningful impact on the recommended level of physical activity for dyslipidemic clients. However, some familiarity with the different assessment philosophies will help the CMES appreciate some of the current issues in evaluating risk in clinical lipidology and patient-management styles among healthcare providers referring individuals to the CMES.

Framingham 10-year Risk Algorithm

The National Institutes of Health's NCEP ATP III cholesterol guidelines (NCEP, 2002) define the risk categories as follows:
- High risk: 10-year risk for CHD >20%
- Intermediate risk: 10-year risk for CHD 5 to 20%
  ✓ Moderately high risk: 10 to 20%
  ✓ Moderate risk: two or more risk factors, or ~5 to 9%
- Low risk: 10-year risk for CHD <5%

The risk-assessment tool can be found at www.nhlbi.nih.gov/guidelines/cholesterol/atglance.pdf.

National Lipid Association ASCVD Risk Assessment and Treatment Goals

The National Lipid Association recommends the strategy presented in Figure 8-5 for determining ASCVD risk (Jacobson et al., 2014). Table 8-6 lists the treatment goals and drug therapy recommendations according to risk category.

ACC/AHA Pooled Cohort 10-year ASCVD Risk Assessment

The ACC/AHA Pooled Cohort 10-year ASCVD Risk Assessment tool (Goff et al., 2013) incorporates race- and sex-specific pooled cohort equations to predict 30-year risk for a first nonfatal MI, CHD death, or stroke. This assessment is for use *only* in non-Hispanic African Americans and non-Hispanic whites, 40 to 79 years of age.

The predicted risk of ASCVD is categorized into one of the following graded levels of 10-year risk (probability of hard ASCVD): <2.5%, 2.5 to 4.9%, 5.0 to 7.4%, 7.5 to 9.9%, and ≥10%. Low risk is considered risk below 7.5%, with a score >7.5% being high risk. The 7.5% threshold is important because LDL therapy decision making is based on this level, such that moderate to intensive statin therapy is recommended. The ACC/AHA guidelines clearly describe statin doses (all seven statins) commensurate with their potency to generate low, moderate, and intensive statin therapy.

The risk assessment tool can be found at http://clincalc.com/Cardiology/ASCVD/PooledCohort.aspx. A screen shot of the assessment is presented in Figure 8-6.

Long-term and Lifetime Risk Assessment

Long-term and lifetime risk estimation may be less valuable for individuals who are found to be at high short-term (10-year) risk based on multivariable equations and for whom decisions regarding prevention efforts may be clear. However, an understanding of long-term risk may provide a means for encouraging adherence to lifestyle or pharmacological therapies, especially for patients

Blood Lipid Disorders — CHAPTER 8

STEPS IN ASCVD RISK ASSESSMENT

Identify patients with *very high-risk* conditions.*
- ASCVD
- Diabetes mellitus with ≥2 other major ASCVD risk factors or end organ damage

Identify patients with *high-risk* conditions
- Diabetes mellitus with 0–1 other major ASCVD risk factors
- Chronic kidney disease Stage 3 or 4
- LDL ≥190 mg/dL

*Further risk assessment is not required in those with very high-risk conditions.

Note: LDL = Low-density lipoprotein; CHD = Coronary heart disease

Count **major ASCVD risk factors**
- If 0–1 and no other indicators of higher risk, assign to *low-risk* category. Consider assigning to a higher risk category based on other risk factors, if known.
- If ≥3 major ASCVD risk factors are present, assign to *high-risk* category.

If 2 major ASCVD risk factors, ***risk scoring*** is recommended and additional testing may be useful for some patients.
- If <10% 10-year hard CHD risk, assign to *moderate-risk* category.
- If ≥10% 10-year hard CHD risk, assign to *high-risk* category.
- Assign as above, or consider assigning to *high* or *very high-risk* category, as appropriate, if other risk indicators are present based on additional testing.

Figure 8-5
Steps in atherosclerotic cardiovascular disease (ASCVD) risk assessment

Source: Jacobson, T.A. et al. (2014). National Lipid Association recommendations for patient-centered management of dyslipidemia: Part 1 – executive summary. *Journal of Clinical Lipidology,* 8, 473–488.

TABLE 8-6
TREATMENT GOALS AND LEVELS TO CONSIDER DRUG THERAPY ACCORDING TO RISK CATEGORY

Risk Category	Treatment Goal Non-HDL mg/dL	Treatment Goal LDL mg/dL	Consider Drug Therapy Non-HDL mg/dL	Consider Drug Therapy LDL mg/dL
Low	<130	<100	≥190	≥160
Moderate	<130	<100	≥160	≥130
High	<130	<100	≥160	≥100
Very High	<100	<70	≥100	≥70

Note: For patients with atherosclerotic cardiovascular disease (ASCVD) or diabetes mellitus, consideration should be given to use of moderate- or high-intensity statin therapy, irrespective of baseline atherogenic cholesterol levels. HDL = High-density lipoprotein; LDL = Low-density lipoprotein

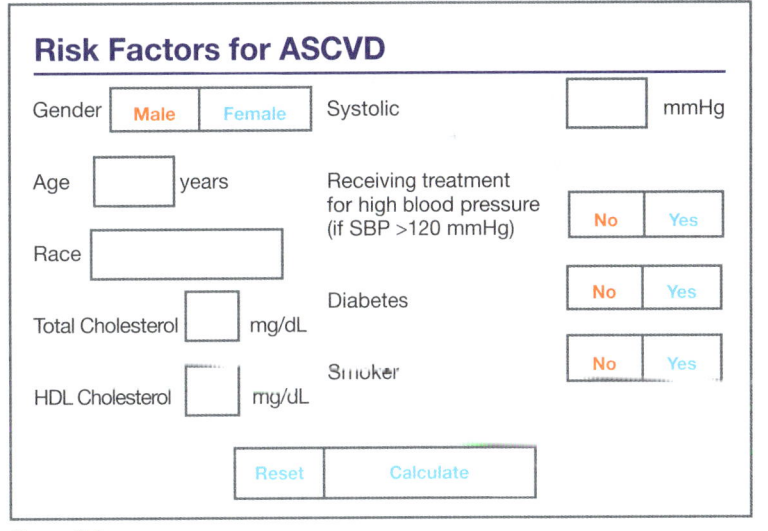

Risk Factors for ASCVD

Gender: Male / Female
Age: ___ years
Race: ___
Total Cholesterol: ___ mg/dL
HDL Cholesterol: ___ mg/dL
Systolic: ___ mmHg
Receiving treatment for high blood pressure (if SBP >120 mmHg): No / Yes
Diabetes: No / Yes
Smoker: No / Yes

[Reset] [Calculate]

Figure 8-6
Screen shot of the ACC/AHA pooled cohort 10-year atherosclerotic cardiovascular disease (ASCVD) risk assessment. http://clincalc.com/Cardiology/ASCVD/PooledCohort.aspx. Reprinted with permission.

who might have difficulty understanding the importance of their short-term risk. Long-term or lifetime risk estimation is recommended for all persons who are between 20 to 39 years of age and for those between 40 to 59 years of age who are determined to be at low 10-year risk by ACC/AHA risk assessment guidelines (<7.5%) (Goff et al., 2013). Long-term (lifetime) risk estimates can be determined by one of two resources: QRisk (www.qrisk.org/lifetime) or the ACC/AHA assessment tool, which estimates both 10-year and long-term risk (http://clincalc.com/Cardiology/ASCVD/PooledCohort.aspx).

> **EXPAND YOUR KNOWLEDGE**
>
> **THE METABOLIC SYNDROME AND CARDIOMETABOLIC RISK**
>
> MetS refers to a cluster of risk factors for CVD and T2DM (see Chapter 12). Although several different definitions for MetS have been proposed, the International Diabetes Federation, NHLBI, AHA, and others proposed a harmonized definition for MetS (Alberti et al., 2009; Grundy, 2007). By this definition, MetS is diagnosed when three or more of the following five risk factors are present (most, but not all, people with diabetes will be classified as having MetS by this definition):
>
> - Abdominal obesity indicated by a waist circumference ≥40 inches (102 cm) in men and ≥35 inches (88 cm) in women
> - Levels of triglycerides ≥150 mg/dL (1.7 mmol/L)
> - HDL levels <40 and <50 mg/dL (1.0 and 1.3 mmol/L) in men and women, respectively
> - Blood pressure levels ≥130/85 mmHg
> - Fasting glucose levels ≥100 mg/dL (5.6 mmol/L)
>
> The main purpose of identifying individuals with MetS is not to predict CHD, but to get healthcare providers to pay more attention to the medical aspects of obesity and its complications and to prioritize lifestyle therapy, especially physical activity and healthier dietary behavior.
>
> From 1999–2000 to 2009–2010, there were decreases in the age-adjusted prevalence of MetS, hypertriglyceridemia, and elevated blood pressure, while the prevalence of hyperglycemia and waist circumference increased. These trends varied considerably by sex and race/ethnicity. Mexican Americans, particularly female adults, have a higher MetS prevalence than other subgroups. Decreases in elevated blood pressure, suboptimal triglycerides, and low HDL prevalence are due in part to increases in anti-hypertensive and lipid-modifying drug therapy. Even with this small decline in MetS prevalence, approximately one-fifth of the adult U.S. population would be classified as having MetS, living with suboptimal measures for at least three of the five MetS components (Beltran-Sanchez et al., 2013). Of all of the lipid disorders that are responsive to exercise therapy, high triglycerides and low HDL are prime targets for the CMES, with reducing abdominal fat being an important goal. A review of nine studies employing dynamic aerobic endurance training on MetS patients indicated significant increases in HDL, along with significant reductions in waist circumference and blood pressure (Pattyn et al., 2013).
>
> The CMES should also note that the term **cardiometabolic risk** has been used to describe a broadened view of MetS. Cardiometabolic risk is essentially defined by an integration of the traditional Framingham CHD risk factors (e.g., smoking, cholesterol, and diabetes) and the MetS risk factors. Cardiometabolic risk extends beyond MetS. It encompasses a cluster of modifiable risk factors and markers that identify individuals at increased risk of CVD (MI, stroke, peripheral arterial disease) and T2DM. That said, one important utility of MetS itself is that it is a better predictor of persons at high risk for T2DM than traditional Framingham CHD risk factors (Stern, Williams, & Haffner, 2002). Prospective population studies have shown that MetS confers a twofold relative risk for atherosclerotic cardiovascular events (e.g., heart attack) and a fivefold increase in risk compared with people who do not have the syndrome (Grundy et al., 2005). A more thorough description and management strategy for MetS is discussed in Chapter 12.

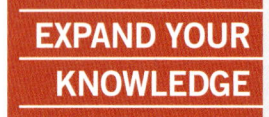

TREATMENT OPTIONS

Exercise, dietary modification, and drug therapy are treatment options for dyslipidemia.

Non-pharmacological Treatment

As indicated in the NCEP and IAS guidelines, drug therapy should be considered only after patients have received at least three to six months of non-pharmacological therapy, specifically intensive dietary and exercise therapy. Exceptions may include those who are high risk for ASCVD, including CHD patients who have suboptimal LDL levels where both intensive lifestyle and drug therapy would be recommended.

Blood Lipid Disorders

Pharmacological Treatment

It is important for the CMES to recognize these drugs and understand their effects on blood lipids and lipoproteins. The drug classes and drugs most commonly prescribed for patients with lipid disorders include the following:

- *Bile acid sequestrants (cholestyramine, colestipol, colesevelam):* These agents bind bile acids in the small intestine and cause decreased bile acid absorption, in turn lowering total and LDL cholesterol. The agents are available as dry powders in bulk or individual packets, and are usually consumed within one hour of eating and/or are taken with the evening meal. The bile acid sequestrants are quite effective for patients younger than age 55 who have LDL between 160 and 220 mg/dL. Side effects are primarily gastrointestinal, with constipation being the most common.

- *Nicotinic acid (niacin, niaspan, niacor):* Niacin is a water-soluble B vitamin that is very effective in lowering LDL and triglycerides, but is especially utilized to increase HDL when used in high doses (>1,500 mg/day). Nicotinic acid is relatively inexpensive, making it an attractive choice as either single therapy or in combination with other drugs, such as statins. Its chief side effects include significant cutaneous flushing and vasodilatation. Niacin must be used with caution in patients with liver disease, diabetes, or gout and those at risk for peptic ulcer disease. It is important to note that many over-the-counter (OTC) forms of "niacin" consist of inositol hexanicotinate (often termed "no-flush niacin") and are relatively void of sufficient free nicotinic acid, and therefore do very little for LDL, triglycerides, or HDL.

- *HMG-CoA reductase inhibitors (also known as statins, which include: lovastatin, pravastatin, simvastatin, fluvastatin, atorvastatin, rosuvastatin, and pitavastatin):* These drugs effectively lower LDL by interfering with cholesterol synthesis. They are competitive inhibitors of HMG-CoA reductase, the enzyme responsible for the rate-limiting step in the cholesterol biosynthetic pathway. They also block the formation of mevalonic acid and decrease intracellular cholesterol synthesis. These drugs are the most effective and expensive class of medications available for lowering LDL. Statins as a drug class have substantial clinical trial support for reducing cardiovascular **morbidity** and **mortality,** as well as clinical events and the need for cardiovascular intervention procedures. While no direct comparison exists, all statins appear effective regardless of potency or degree of cholesterol reduction (Tonelli et al., 2011).

- *Combination nicotinic acid and statin drugs:* Advicor and Simcor are combination drugs that combine in one pill various combinations of niaspan and lovastatin (Advicor) and niaspan and simvastatin (Simcor).

- *Cholesterol transport inhibitors (Ezetimibe):* Ezetimibe lowers plasma cholesterol levels by decreasing cholesterol absorption in the small intestine. It may be used alone (marketed as Zetia for example), when other cholesterol-lowering medications are not tolerated, or together with statins (e.g., ezetimibe/simvastatin, marketed as Vytorin) when statins alone do not control cholesterol. In the summer of 2013, the U.S. Food and Drug Administration (FDA) approved Liptruzet, a single tablet combining atorvastatin and ezetimibe.

- *Fibrates (gemfibrozil, fenofibrate, trilipix):* Gemfibrozil and fenofibrate primarily lower triglycerides and, to a lesser extent, increase HDL by reducing VLDL (triglyceride) synthesis and increase VLDL clearance by increasing lipoprotein lipase activity. Fibrates are used in accessory therapy in many forms of hypercholesterolemia, usually in combination with statins.

- *Omega-3 fatty acids (select OTC brands or Lovaza, Vascepa, Epanova):* Marine **omega-3 fatty acid** therapy (fish oil capsules) is prescribed for individuals with high or very high triglycerides. The prescription may be for 1 to 4 grams per day of omega-3 fatty acids in the presence of high or very high triglycerides (200 to 500 mg/dL or higher). It is important to understand that only at the higher intakes of omega-3 fatty acids (≥2 grams/day) are there significant reductions in triglycerides, whereas the lower dosages have other benefits not directly related

to triglyceride lowering. Prescription omega-3 fatty acids come in two forms: ethyl-esters (Lovaza and Vascepa) and triglyceride formulations (Epanova).
- *Antisense ApoB inhibitors (Kynamro):* These injectable drugs target the production of apo B-100 containing lipoproteins (e.g.,VLDL and LDL) by inhibiting the synthesis of these lipoproteins. Mipomersen has been shown to decrease apo B, LDL, and lipoprotein(a) in patients with heterozygous and homozygous familial hypercholesterolemia for which this drug is indicated.
- *Microsomal triglyceride transfer protein inhibitor (Lomitapide, Juxtapid):* This drug decreases lipoprotein production, specifically VLDL assembly in the liver. It is approved as an adjunct to diet and other lipid-lowering treatments to reduce LDL, apo B, and non-HDL in homozygous familial hypercholesterolemia.
- *Other agents (non-FDA-approved):* A variety of other nutritive and herbal OTC agents are available to consumers. Many of these agents (e.g., "natural cholesterol-lowering products") will be accompanied by ad campaigns claiming the power to lower blood cholesterol. For example, several red yeast rice (RYR)–based supplements claim on their package inserts that they can lower LDL by 13 to 22%. The active ingredient in RYR is monacolin K, which is lovastatin, usually at the 10 mg dose. There are at least 30 brands of RYR. The FDA warns that the safety of RYR products has not been established. The same holds true for policosanol nutrient products (a sugar-cane extract). While not particularly harmful, these products have claims of 15 to 25% reductions in LDL. Guggulipid and green tea extract product campaigns also promote lipid lowering and may have some promise in select individuals, but lack controlled clinical trials substantiating their benefit. Consideration must also be given to the potential adverse interaction that these supplements may have when combined with prescription medications. Until better-controlled research is conducted and published, these supplements should not be considered primary modes of therapy in lipid management, and any client considering these supplements should first consult a licensed practitioner.
- *Investigational drugs:* There are a number of promising drugs that are in relatively late stages of clinical investigation that may be approved by the FDA in the near future. Among these are the PCSK9 and the CETP inhibitors. PCSK9 is an enzyme that in humans is encoded by the PCSK9 gene. Some individuals have a variant of this gene that leads to increased LDL receptor destruction and increases in total cholesterol and LDL. There are a number of promising investigational drugs that inhibit this enzyme, which will help in the treatment of familial hypercholesterolemia, particularly when used in combination with statin therapy. Cholesterol ester transport protein (CETP) inhibitors form another relatively promising new drug class that dramatically increases HDL by perhaps 60 to 100% and provides respectable decreases in LDL. Early results with this drug class were not promising, but several drug companies have since made significant strides in improving the efficacy and safety of CETP inhibitors (e.g., evacetrapib and anacetrapib). New investigational agents that lower triglycerides, including omega-3 fatty acid drugs with improved efficacy and **bioavailability,** are also likely to be approved in the next few years.

LDL and the Primary Prevention of CHD

ASCVD is ranked as the number-one cause of mortality and is a major cause of morbidity worldwide. Lowering LDL is the principle target of therapy for ASCVD compared to the other lipoproteins. Statins have been shown in nearly all major clinical trials to be first-choice treatments, particularly in high-risk patients. This is particularly noteworthy because rosuvastatin, a statin, is the number-one branded drug in the world (Lowes, 2013).

Since the early statin RCTs were reported in the 1990s, several reviews of the effects of statins have been published highlighting their benefits, particularly in people with a past history of ASCVD. Benefits include a reduction in CHD events, including strokes. Statins have also been shown to reduce the risk of a first event in otherwise healthy individuals at high risk of ASCVD (primary prevention), but information on possible hazards has not been reported fully. There are hundreds of published statin-related clinical trials, but rather than going through all of the key trials it may serve the CMES best to review the most respected and influential systematic published review of the best-controlled major statin trials in primary prevention (i.e., statin use in those who do not have clinically documented ASCVD) [Taylor, Huffman, & Ebrahim, 2013; Cholesterol Treatment Trialists' (CTT) Collaboration, 2010].

The incidence of cancers, **myalgia, rhabdomyolysis** (the breakdown of muscle tissue that leads to the release of myoglobin into the bloodstream, which often results in kidney damage), liver enzyme elevation, renal dysfunction, or arthritis did not differ between the groups, although not all trials reported fully on these outcomes. Rates of adverse events (17%) and stopping treatment (12%) were similar in statin and placebo/control groups. An increased risk of incident diabetes was found in one of the two trials reporting this outcome. Overall, results suggest that the benefits of statin therapy outweigh serious life-threatening hazards (Taylor, Huffman, & Ebrahim, 2013). *Note:* The incidence of new-onset diabetes with statin therapy—particularly more intensive statin therapy—has been shown; in individuals with diabetic susceptibility however, the probability of this occurrence is very low (Grundy et al., 2018; Jacobson et al., 2014).

Intensive Versus Moderate Statin Therapy

The 2010 CTT Collaboration reviewing 26 statin trials demonstrated greater benefit with intensive versus lower statin therapy (Table 8-7) (CTT, 2010).

Further reductions in LDL safely produce definite further reductions in the incidence of heart attack, revascularisation, and **ischemic stroke**. In other words, the size of the proportional reduction in major vascular events is directly proportional to the absolute LDL reduction that is achieved, with further benefit from more intensive statin therapy. This is important for the CMES to know because when working with individuals with dyslipidemia, statin therapy, particularly intensive statin therapy, is very likely to be part of your client's medical therapy.

LDL and the Secondary Prevention of ASCVD

Secondary prevention extends to all individuals with established ASCVD. These conditions include a history of CHD, stroke, peripheral arterial disease, carotid artery disease, and other forms of atherosclerotic vascular disease. Evidence supporting a lower level for optimal LDL in secondary prevention comes from key major clinical trials in ASCVD patients and their subgroup analyses reviewed in the IAS (2013) and NLA (Jacobson et al., 2014) guideline documents. The IAS and NLA guideline panels found convincing evidence from the randomized controlled trials (RCTs) that they reviewed for an optimal LDL in the range of 70 mg/dL or lower in high-risk secondary prevention (Jacobson et al., 2014; IAS, 2013). Future RCTs utilizing highly efficacious LDL-lowering drugs could uncover a still lower optimal range. In the meantime, an optimal LDL in the range of <70 mg/dL seems acceptable for high-CHD-risk patients. The IAS and NLA panels further identified an optimal non-HDL as being <100 mg/dL in secondary prevention, a view shared by the European Society of Cardiology and European Cardiology Society.

TABLE 8-7
INTENSIVE STATIN OUTCOMES
• Atherosclerotic plaque regression
• Slowed progression of atherosclerosis
• Decreased risk of myocardial infarction and stroke
• Decreased risk of all vascular events
• Decreased cardiovascular mortality
• Decreased need for CABG surgery
• Increased arterial function
• Decreased hospitalization for unstable angina
• Decreased venous thromboembolism

Note: CABG = Coronary artery bypass graft

Source: Cholesterol Treatment Trialists' (CTT) Collaboration (2010). Efficacy and safety of more intensive lowering of LDL cholesterol: A meta-analysis of data from 170,000 participants in 26 randomized trials. *Lancet,* 376, 1670–1681.

Exercise Treatment

Exercise of appropriate quality and quantity not only clearly reduces CHD and metabolic risk through nonlipid mechanisms, but also induces significant favorable changes in the lipid and lipoprotein profile, in part as a result of reductions in **adiposity.**

Lipids are an important substrate for the aerobic production of energy in human skeletal muscle during low- and moderate-intensity dynamic exercise and even with high-intensity dynamic exercise in well-trained individuals. Fatty acids mobilized from adipose tissue and transported to contracting muscles are a major source of fuel during exercise—particularly aerobic endurance exercise. Most authorities agree that the exercise-generated reduction in adipose tissue is directly and biologically related to the concomitant but modest reduction in blood triglycerides, total cholesterol, and LDL seen in many trials involving exercise training (Gordon, Chen, & Durstine, 2014; Durstine et al., 2002).

Weekly physical activity of sufficient energy expenditure can improve various elements of dyslipidemia, although it should be understood that studies of exercise training on lipid parameters have been confounded by a number of variables that independently exert effects on lipid parameters:

- Sex
- Total net energy expenditure of the activity
- Length of training period (e.g., 1 month, 6 months, or 18 months)
- The lipid/lipoprotein disorder, (e.g., hypertriglyceridemia or hypercholesterolemia)
- Baseline lipid values (i.e., magnitude of the lipid disorder)
- Corresponding body-fat loss
- Corresponding dietary changes
- Concomitant alcohol intake
- Plasma volume changes
- Menopausal status
- Race/ethnicity
- Genetic factors (e.g., apolipoprotein E and C isoforms or perilipin genotype)
- Biologic variation (seasonal and diurnal changes)

LDL Response

Perhaps the most important key concept when educating clients on exercise and LDL reduction is to understand that unlike fatty acids and triglycerides, cholesterol and LDL cannot be hydrolyzed to generate **adenosine triphosphate (ATP)** (i.e., cholesterol is a **sterol** and cannot be oxidized for energy production). Although exercise programs have the best chance of reducing LDL when there is associated body-weight reduction, such programs can also favorably alter lipoproteins in the absence of body-weight reduction (Eckel et al., 2013). Most studies evaluating the total cholesterol and/or LDL response to exercise training have found very little to only moderate decreases in these lipids and lipoproteins. Many studies used inadequate exercise volumes and/or energy expenditure or failed to control for confounding variables such as training-induced changes in plasma volume, dietary habits, or seasonal variation in cholesterol and lipoproteins.

An often quoted meta-analysis of 13 studies by Kelley, Kelley, and Tran (2005a) found a non-significant decrease of less than 1% in LDL independent of changes in body weight. The tendency to segregate exercise-LDL changes from body-weight alterations is problematic here, as both require integrated exercise and lifestyle programming. The other issue with this meta-analytic trial, which is often the case in interpreting meta-analysis findings, is that there was a wide range of training modalities (e.g., running, swimming, stationary cycling, and dancing) and there was an average training stimulus of ~40 minutes per session, 3.9 times a week, of moderate-intensity exercise. This weekly volume of exercise, approximately 1,600 to 1,800 kcal/week, is insufficient according to current recommendations (≥2,000 kcal/week) to demonstrate meaningful reductions in LDL. Of course, at that volume of physical activity, most adults are likely to lose some body weight and will certainly see a reduction in adiposity.

There is a wide variation in the lipoprotein response to exercise training. On average, exercise training by itself will reduce LDL by 4 to 7% depending on baseline lipid values and total exercise volume (i.e., added weekly energy expenditure) (Bays et al., 2013; Mestek, 2009). Very few controlled exercise trials have been conducted on patients with dyslipidemia, with most evaluating those with normal or modestly elevated triglycerides and/or LDL.

As previously stated, fat weight reduction is required for the most favorable blood lipid response in those who have elevated total and LDL. This volume of exercise (150 minutes or more per week, optimally 200 to 300 minutes per week or >2,000 kcal per week) is similar to that recommended for long-term weight control (Donnelly et al., 2009). If exercise is of sufficient volume, exercise intensity is not of primary importance in improving the lipid profile, although most research supports a minimum intensity of at least 40% of peak work capacity. Any effect on lipids and lipoproteins of the intensity of exercise is small compared to that of the volume of exercise (e.g., kcal expended per week) (Kraus et al., 2002). This is one reason why many of the resistance-training studies, despite confirmed metabolic benefits, have shown little if any reduction LDL and or triglycerides—because of inadequate energy expenditure for the resistance-training session. Some resistance-training studies have reported slight-to-moderate reductions in total and LDL levels, with others reporting no change (Kelley & Kelley, 2009; Trejo-Gutierrez & Fletcher, 2007). It is likely that the blood lipid response to strength training is related to total net energy expenditure of the session (kcal per workout), as it is with aerobic endurance exercise. One example of a relatively high energy expenditure resistance-training session involves low-resistance, high-repetition circuit weight training performed for extended periods and approaching 300 kcal or more per session, which is similar to 35 to 40 minutes of moderate-intensity aerobic exercise.

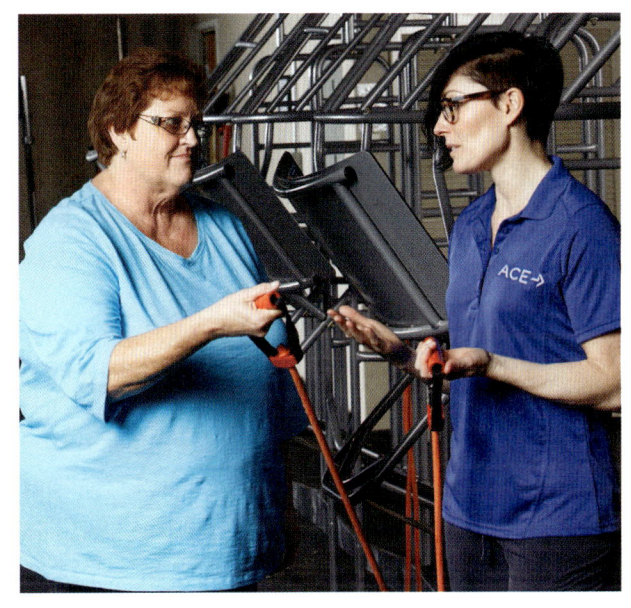

HDL Response

The HDL response to exercise training is under considerable genetic influence, with underlying genetic polymorphisms (e.g., lipoprotein and hepatic lipase) explaining up to 50% of the variation in HDL (Blazek et al., 2013; Teslovich et al., 2010). The CMES should be cautious in predicting the HDL response in clients, as there is a considerable variation in the magnitude of changes in HDL. There are also individuals with genetic variants of very-low-HDL cholesterol (**hypoalphalipoproteinemia,** defined as HDL levels <30 mg/dL) and, in general, they will respond minimally to even high volumes of exercise training. There are several forms of familial hypoalphalipoproteinemia and the prevalence is approximately 2%.

On average, exercise training by itself can increase HDL by 4 to 25% depending on baseline lipid values and total exercise volume (i.e., added weekly energy expenditure). As a rule, the HDL response to training is quite moderate (Mestek, 2009). Most exercise trials support between 700 and nearly 2,000 kcal of exercise per week to significantly alter HDL (Bays et al., 2013). Kodama and colleagues performed a large meta-analysis of 25 randomized controlled trials of exercise alone, without diet or drug therapy, and found that aerobic exercise of ~5.3 METs (65% of maximal aerobic power) significantly increased HDL by 2.53 mg/dL. Among exercise variables, exercise duration was found to be the most important determinant of the increase in HDL on multivariate analysis (Kodama et al., 2011). Minimal weekly exercise volume for increasing HDL level was estimated to be 900 kcal of energy expenditure or 120 minutes of exercise per week. There have been mixed findings among studies investigating the relationship between exercise intensity and increases in HDL, with some studies reporting the necessity for more vigorous exercise intensities (Paoli, Pacelli, & Moro, 2013). Inactive subjects may not increase HDL through energy expenditure as easily as physically active subjects (Durstine & Moore, 1997).

Baseline fasting triglycerides also may contribute to the HDL-raising effects of exercise training. Couillard and others (2005) studied 200 men enrolled in the HERITAGE Family Study and demonstrated that regular endurance exercise training may be particularly helpful in men with low HDL, elevated triglycerides, and abdominal obesity. Slentz and colleagues (2007) have shown that higher versus moderate volumes of exercise may in some cases be required for significant HDL increases.

Resistance training may also generate increases in HDL. There are reports that six to nine weeks of resistance training three times per week (eight to 10 exercises) can significantly increase HDL by 4 to 9% in men and women (Costa et al., 2011; Sheikholeslami et al., 2011). At least one study demonstrated greater HDL increases with higher-intensity resistance training [80 to 90% **one-repetition maximum (1-RM)**] compared to moderate-intensity training (Sheikholeslami et al., 2011). Not all studies demonstrate significant increases, however (Wooten et al., 2011).

Non-HDL Response

Surprisingly, considering the importance of non-HDL as a major player in the development of CHD, there has been very little research that exclusively evaluated the response of non-HDL to exercise training. One meta-analysis of 22 studies (Kelley, Kelley, & Tran, 2005b) that retrospectively looked at walking and non-HDL responsivity found a decrease of approximately 6 mg/dL in response to training programs that lasted 10 to 104 weeks. The greatest non-HDL response apparently is observed when dietary and exercise interventions were combined. The same investigators published a meta-analysis of 26 studies retrospectively looking at non-HDL and resistance exercise and found an average 9 mg/dL reduction in non-HDL independent of body-weight changes (Kelley & Kelley, 2009). Again, one must be cautious in over-interpreting findings from large meta-analytic trials.

Triglyceride Response

Compared to other lipids, such as LDL, individuals with elevated baseline triglycerides (e.g. >150 mg/dL) are generally more responsive to exercise training of sufficient volume. Triglyceride mobilization and utilization appears to be in direct proportion to exercise energy expenditure. Unlike LDL, triglycerides generally decrease immediately after a session of high-volume endurance exercise (e.g., greater than 45 to 50 minutes of sustained effort), and remain lower for up to 48 hours after the session. Exercise training programs have also been shown to decrease fasting triglycerides by 4 to 37% (approximate mean change of 24%) (Trejo-Gutierrez & Fletcher, 2007). Overall, exercise is most effective in lowering triglycerides when baseline levels are elevated (i.e., >150 mg/dL), activity is moderate to intensive, and total caloric intake is reduced (Durstine et al., 2002).

A study of 176 adults with MetS demonstrated a 12% reduction in fasting triglycerides after 24 weeks of walking one hour a day, five days a week, but like so many other studies, the triglyceride reduction correlated strongly with decreases in **body mass index (BMI),** body weight, and waist circumference (Di Raimondo et al., 2013). Higher baseline triglyceride levels (mean 197 mg/dL) also translated into significant triglyceride reductions (26%) in a six-month trial of subjects with overweight who walked 12 miles weekly at 40 to 55% of peak oxygen uptake (Kraus et al., 2002).

Those who have familial hypertriglyceridemia (e.g., lipoprotein lipase or apo C-II deficiencies) will have fasting triglycerides well above 500 mg/dL and often greater than 1,000 mg/dL. While there is very little published research on this population's response to exercise training, it is important to note that a relatively high volume of exercise in addition to drug therapy will be the most appropriate combination. Overall, several facts stand out after reviewing scores of exercise-triglyceride metabolism trials (Magkos, 2009):

Blood Lipid Disorders   CHAPTER 8

- Exercise-induced triglyceride-lowering is acute, in that it manifests after just a single bout of exercise and is not the result of repeated exercise sessions (i.e., training), and short-lived, as it is readily reversed when exercise is withdrawn (i.e., detraining).
- Numerous studies have confirmed this initial hypothesis: the magnitude of the decrease in plasma triglyceride concentration after a single exercise session and after training is the same (i.e., 15 to 50%).
- These observations suggest that chronic exercise does not have an equally sustainable effect on plasma triglyceride concentration (i.e., beyond that attributed to acute exercise; hence exercise should be performed on a regular and uninterrupted basis to maintain lower triglycerides).

Exercise + Statin Combination Therapy

Combining statin therapy and exercise training generates additional benefits over statin therapy alone. Coen et al. (2009) demonstrated that combining 10 mg of rosuvastatin a day and aerobic and resistance exercise for 20 weeks in hypercholesterolemic adults generated a greater reduction in oxidized-LDL (the intracellular LDL that readily forms obstructive arterial plaques) and triglycerides than rosuvastatin alone. HDL was also more favorably altered. There was no abnormal sustained increase in creatine kinase (CK) or reports of myalgia after the addition of exercise training to rosuvastatin treatment. From a mortality risk perspective, Kokkinos et al. (2013) demonstrated in a large cohort of veterans (N = 10,043) that statin treatment and increased fitness together are independently associated with low mortality among dyslipidemic individuals. The combination of statin treatment and increased **metabolic equivalent (MET)** capacity achieved on a treadmill exercise tolerance test resulted in substantially lower mortality risk than either alone, reinforcing the importance of physical activity for individuals with dyslipidemia (Kokkinos et al., 2013).

Inactivity and Lipids

Sedentary lifestyles, particularly sitting time, have been associated with elevated triglycerides and decreased HDL, as well as other cardiometabolic risk factors (Staiano et al., 2014). A modest amount of exercise training can prevent a deterioration of the lipid profile that is seen with inactivity (Slentz et al., 2007). This is particularly true for LDL and HDL size, LDL-P, and total HDL cholesterol. In fact, it appears that only 7 to 10 miles (11 to 16 km) of walking per week will prevent inactivity-associated deterioration in these lipid parameters. Moderate-intensity but not vigorous-intensity aerobic exercise of sufficient quantity can elicit sustained reductions in VLDL-triglycerides for up to two weeks even after exercise training has stopped ($P<0.05$) (Slentz et al., 2007).

EXERCISE AND POSTPRANDIAL LIPEMIA

EXPAND YOUR KNOWLEDGE

Postprandial lipemia is essentially the acute blood lipid, particularly triglyceride, response to a meal, particularly a fatty meal. Depending on how much fat or sugar is consumed in a meal, a person with normal fasting triglycerides will increase their triglycerides by 120 to 300+ mg/dL for two to six hours after the meal. Those with **visceral obesity,** MetS, or T2DM can have much larger increases in post-meal triglycerides. The problem with prolonged elevated postprandial triglyceride states is that for the amount of time triglycerides are elevated much above 250 to 300 mg/dL, there is diminished arterial function, lower HDL, and exposure of the arterial wall to atherogenic lipoprotein particles (e.g., IDL and VLDL remnant particles). Over the past 15 years, there has been abundant research supporting the finding that sufficient exercise timed anywhere from one to 12 hours before a fat-rich meal will reduce postprandial lipemia by 25 to 40% (Malkova & Gill, 2006). This observation was also found in men with baseline hypertriglyceridemia, with a

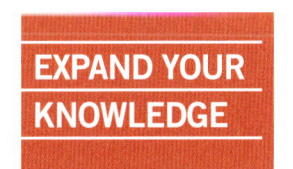

30 to 39% reduction in postprandial triglycerides with moderate and vigorous exercise, respectively (Zhang, 2006). The relative suppression of triglycerides can last up to 36 hours after a significant bout of exercise (e.g., >400 kcal). Some investigators report that women may be more responsive to reducing postprandial triglycerides with exercise than men (Henderson et al., 2010). This somewhat blunted triglyceride response to high-fat or high-glycemic meals is one of the benefits of engaging in aerobic physical activity every day.

Researchers have also studied the effects of aerobic exercise conducted before a meal compared to the same exercise after a meal. Plaisance and Fisher (2014) reported that aerobic exercise conducted one hour following a high-fat meal produced only modest reductions in postprandial lipemia, suggesting that prior exercise is superior to exercise conducted after a meal.

There are also reports that higher-intensity exercise can be more effective in reducing postprandial triglycerides than moderate-intensity exercise, even when both are matched for the same total energy expenditure (Trombold et al., 2013). Having clients exercise *at least* every other day is an excellent way to keep triglycerides reasonably low.

THINK IT THROUGH

Clients often hire exercise professionals because they are concerned about improving their health. Many potential clients have learned about the role of physical activity in the treatment of medical conditions and seek out exercise professionals who have expertise in working with individuals who have health problems. It is not unusual for an exercise professional to encounter a client who is intent on pursuing exercise as a treatment or "cure" for their health condition, sometimes as an alternative to seeking a medical evaluation. The CMES should understand that in those instances where a defined exercise regimen is personally recommended for a client with a specific medical condition (e.g., diabetes or dyslipidemia), exercise becomes a liable prescriptive intervention. How would you handle a client who is reluctant to follow up with their healthcare provider under the assumption that an exercise program is all that is needed to "treat" the condition? Or a client who stops their medication(s) without disclosing this to the primary care physician?

APPLY WHAT YOU KNOW

PEDOMETER STEP COUNTS, ENERGY EXPENDITURE, AND DYSLIPIDEMIA

Systematic use of pedometers (pedometry) or walking step counts have been employed as an acceptable estimate of walking energy expenditure. For blood lipid changes or weight loss, the minimal weekly physical-activity goals should be *at least* 1,500 kcal more than entry level physical activity (entry level being evaluated on the first visit). As a rule, this weekly energy expenditure would be equivalent to about 30,000 or more walking step counts *beyond* the client's weekly baseline step count. The CMES is encouraged to recommend reliable well-engineered pedometers to estimate walking energy expenditure. Perhaps most applicable would be the use of pedometer models that have a step filter, which is incorporated software that minimizes the recording of meaningless spontaneous movements. Optimal goals are ≥2,000 kcal per week, 200+ minutes per week, and/or ≥70,000 total steps per week. As a general rule, about 2,000 steps (plus or minus approximately 150 steps) with a step-only pedometer is equivalent to roughly one mile, or about 100 kcal of gross energy expenditure for individuals who are within 10 to 20 pounds of their **ideal body weight**. Of course, for those individuals who have a significantly higher BMI (e.g., >35 kg/m^2), the gross caloric cost of walking per mile is greater (about 120 to 150 kcal per mile) and in proportion to their body weight.

Resistance Training and Lipid Disorders

As mentioned earlier, resistance training has shown some promise as a means to improve the blood lipid profile, but the effect is modest at best. It is not recommended as the primary form of exercise therapy for individuals with blood lipid disorders, but certainly should play a supportive role. The lipid and lipoprotein response to resistance training depends on the energy expenditure of the sessions, which essentially means that each session (e.g., 30+ minutes) includes an abundance of repetitions versus just three sets of 10 to 12 repetitions of four or five exercises. In a review of 13 published resistance training and lipid response trials, Mann, Beedie, and Jimenez (2014) reinforced the requirement of higher-repetition resistance-training doses for a sufficient stimulus lipid and lipoprotein response. Their review concluded it has been shown consistently that the increased volume of movement via increased numbers of sets and/or repetitions has a greater impact upon the lipid profile than increased intensity (e.g., via high-weight, low-repetition training), a view supported by other studies (Lira et al., 2010).

EXPAND YOUR KNOWLEDGE

EXERCISE, STATINS, AND MYALGIA

Muscle complaints represent the most frequent adverse reports among patients treated with statins. These complaints occur in a population that often has musculoskeletal pain and dysfunction in the absence of statins (Rosenson & Underberg, 2014). Clients on statins, particularly on higher-dose statin therapy, who are exercising at relatively high intensities or volumes, are somewhat more susceptible to exercise-associated muscle symptoms [e.g., myalgia (muscle pain) or **myopathy** (muscle weakness)] (Rosenson & Underberg, 2014). Although statins are usually well-tolerated, they have sometimes been associated with myalgia and myopathy and with increases in creatine kinase. There is a fair chance that this situation could be exacerbated with exercise, as intensive aerobic or resistance exercise has been evidenced in a number of reports (Mansi et al., 2013; Mikus et al., 2013; Cham et al., 2010). Statin-induced myalgia and myopathy is rapidly reversible if diagnosed early by a physician and treated with discontinuance of drug and improvements in hydration. Although the occasional occurrence of statin-related myalgia/myopathy should not alarm the CMES, it does reinforce the need for the CMES to keep reasonably close track of any acute and/or recovery musculoskeletal symptoms through at least the early stages of the exercise program and after statin dose increases. The CMES should not unintentionally program the client to expect statin-exercise associated muscle symptoms, as the vast majority will not experience any of these muscle-related symptoms. There are reports that supplemental coenzyme Q (coQ) and/or vitamin D3 supplementation may help decrease statin-related muscle symptoms, but there are mixed reviews on this practice (Rosenson & Underberg, 2014; Reinhart & Woods, 2012; Caso et al., 2007). The client with statin-induced muscle symptoms should discuss adding CoQ or vitamin D to their supplement regimen with a physician.

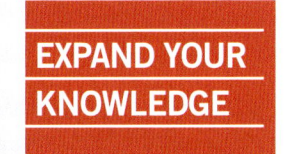

NUTRITIONAL CONSIDERATIONS

Elevated LDL cholesterol is one of the most potent risk factors for CVD. As such, physicians aggressively treat cholesterol, most often with statins and recommendations to improve one's lifestyle. In some cases, individuals with elevated cholesterol will be referred by the physician to a **registered dietitian (RD).** However, in many cases, the individual may be left with a medication prescription and vague advice to "eat better."

The Academy of Nutrition and Dietetics (A.N.D.) has compiled the most valid scientific research on foods and nutrients that help to improve cholesterol profile through its Evidence Analysis Library. While this information is geared toward helping RDs make evidence-based decisions when providing **medical nutrition therapy (MNT),** many of the recommendations are general enough that they can be shared with clients by the CMES. In addition, a large body of evidence supporting the role of a few specific eating plans in improving cholesterol is available to help guide clients in making nutrition choices.

This section will first outline the A.N.D. Evidence Analysis Library guidelines for optimizing cholesterol levels and then will describe several foods and eating plans that have been shown to decrease LDL cholesterol ("bad cholesterol") and/or increase HDL cholesterol ("good cholesterol").

Improving the Cholesterol Profile

All of the nutrition recommendations described in Chapter 7 for individuals with CHD apply to those with elevated cholesterol. Additionally, several nutrition choices to specifically target decreasing LDL cholesterol and increasing HDL cholesterol may be implemented.

For instance, plant **stanols** and sterols have been heavily investigated for their role in affecting blood lipids. Plant stanols and sterols are cholesterol-mimicking substances that occur naturally in many whole grains, vegetables, fruits, legumes, nuts, and seeds. They also have been added to many common foods, such as cereals and cereal bars, margarine, and orange juice. (Those used in food products are usually extracted from soybean and tall pine-tree oils.) Plant stanols and sterols so closely resemble cholesterol that they can bind to cholesterol receptors and prevent cholesterol from being absorbed into the bloodstream. Then, instead of eventually depositing into plaques in the arteries, they are excreted as waste.

The A.N.D. Evidence Analysis Library suggests that clients may consider consuming plant stanols and sterols two to three times per day, for a total consumption of two to three grams per day. Evidence supports that this regimen decreases total cholesterol by 4 to 11% and LDL cholesterol by 7 to 15% (A.N.D. Evidence Analysis Library, 2013). In fact, the benefits of plant stanols and sterols on cholesterol are so clear and widely endorsed in the scientific community that the FDA has approved the health claim that allows manufacturers to advertise the cholesterol-lowering, heart-healthy properties of plant stanols and sterols. Of note, daily doses above three grams per day do not provide additional benefit. There have been no documented adverse events from use of plant stanols and sterols (A.N.D. Evidence Analysis Library, 2013).

In addition to plant stanols, several other foods improve total and LDL cholesterol, including foods high in fiber and soluble fiber and nuts, soy, and other food items (Table 8-8). Few food items have been found to substantially improve HDL cholesterol levels, though moderate alcohol consumption (one to three drinks per day) increases HDL cholesterol levels by about 12% (Gaziano et al., 1993). (Of note, public health guidelines recommend that men drink no more than two and women drink no more than one alcoholic drink per day.) Diets rich in **polyunsaturated fats** improve HDL's anti-inflammatory properties, with particular benefit from omega-3 fatty acids which also increase overall concentration of HDL, especially when used as a replacement of dietary **carbohydrate** (Siri-Tarino, 2011; Nicholls et al., 2006).

Improving Blood Triglycerides

Clients with elevated triglycerides will benefit from the nutrition considerations for individuals with CHD and blood lipid disorders. Additionally, clients should discuss with their physician if high-dose supplemental EPA and DHA (2 to 4 grams) would be advisable. This dose of supplementation has been shown to reduce triglyceride levels in individuals with baseline triglycerides >200 mg/dL (A.N.D. Evidence Analysis Library, 2013).

Eating Plans to Support Optimal Blood Lipid Profile

Several eating plans have shown benefit in improving lipid profile, including both the Ornish and Mediterranean eating plans described in Chapter 7 and the DASH eating plan described in Chapter 9, as well as the **Therapeutic Lifestyle Change (TLC) eating plan** described here. In fact, a 2013 Cochrane Review of the effectiveness of dietary advice for reducing cardiovascular risk found that dietary advice to decrease consumption of one or more of fat, **saturated fatty acids,** cholesterol, or salt; or increase consumption of one or more of fruit, vegetables, polyunsaturated fatty acids, **monounsaturated fatty acids,** fish, fiber, or potassium; or both contributed to a decrease in total cholesterol of 0.15 mmol/L (5.8 mg/dL) and LDL by 0.16 mmol/L (6.2 mg/dL) after three to 24 months. Mean HDL cholesterol and triglyceride levels were unchanged. The authors concluded that dietary changes are apparently effective in modestly improving CVD risk over a period of about one year, but longer-term benefits have not been well established (Rees et al., 2013).

The TLC Eating Plan

The TLC eating plan from the National Heart, Lung, and Blood Institute (NHLBI) was developed specifically to improve cholesterol levels. It consists of three components: (1) dietary changes, specifically a decrease in saturated fat, trans fat, and cholesterol and an increase of soluble fiber and inclusion of plant stanols and sterols; (2) physical activity; and (3) weight management. The TLC dietary recommendations advise:

- Decrease saturated fat to <7% of calories (8 to 10% reduction in LDL)
- Decrease cholesterol to <200 mg/day (3 to 5% reduction in LDL)

Blood Lipid Disorders

CHAPTER 8

TABLE 8-8
THE INFLUENCE OF DIETARY ELEMENTS TO TOTAL CHOLESTEROL

	CHANGE IN CHOLESTEROL			
	LDL	**HDL**	**Total cholesterol**	**Level of Evidence**
Red yeast rice[1]	↓ 42.9–46.0 mg/dL (1.11–1.19 mmol/L)	Unaffected	40.2 mg/dL (1.04 mmol/L)	B
Guggulipid[2]	↓ 6.6 mg/dL (0.17 mmol/L)	Unaffected	Unaffected	C
Almond consumption[3]	↑ 5.8 mg/dL (0.15 mmol/L)	Unaffected	↑ 7.0 mg/dL (0.18 mmol/L)	B
Garlic[4]	Unaffected	Unaffected	Unaffected	B
Green tea catechins[5]	↑ 5.4 mg/dL (0.14 mmol/L)	Unaffected	↑ 5.4 mg/dL (0.14 mmol/L)	A
Chitosan[6]	Unaffected	Unaffected	↑ 11.6 mg/dL (0.30 mmol/L)	A
Plant sterols/stanols[7]	↑ 13.5 mg/dL (0.35 mmol/L)	↑ 13.9 mg/dL (0.36 mmol/L)	↑ 3.9 mg/dL (0.1 mmol/L)	A
Virgin olive oil[8]	↑ 3.1 mg/dL (0.08 mmol/L)	↓ 1.7 mg/dL (0.045 mmol/L	↑ [phenol]–*	B
Mediterranean diet[9]	↑ 3.5 mg/dL (0.09 mmol/L) **	↓ 1.2 mg/dL (0.03 mmol/L)	↑ 7.3 mg/dL (0.19 mmol/L)	A
Cocoa[10]	↑ 5.8 mg/dL (0.15 mmol/L)	Unaffected	↑ 5.8 mg/dL (0.15 mmol/L)+	A
Soy protein isoflavones[11]	↑ 8.1 mg/dL (0.21 mmol/L)	↓ 1.5 mg/dL (0.04 mmol/L)	↑ 8.5 mg/dL (0.22 mmol/L)	A

Note: For references associated with the following notes, visit www.ncbi.nlm.nih.gov/pmc/articles/PMC3584303/

Note: LDL = Low-density lipoprotein; HDL = High-density lipoprotein

[1] 41 patients were given capsules containing either rice powder placebo vs. 42 patients given 2.4 g red yeast rice daily with serum measurements at 8 and 12 weeks. A further randomized trial involved giving 1,800 mg to 31 patients with 12–24 week follow-up.

[2] Data based on a double-blind, randomized, placebo-controlled trial using a parallel design. However, conflicting data available from older studies.

[3] 25 to 168 g/day significantly lowered total cholesterol. However, insufficient body of evidence to promote almond ingestion as lipid-lowering regimen.

[4] Data from parallel-design randomized clinical trial involving 192 adults.

[5] Data from meta-analysis from 20 trials of GTCs at doses ranging from 145 to 3,000 mg/day taken for 3 to 24 weeks (N=1,415).

[6] Data from meta-analysis from six randomized, placebo-controlled trials of chitosan in hypercholesterolemic patients (n = 416 patients).

[7] Data from a systematic review with meta-analysis of 20 studies showing foods enriched with 2.0 g of phytosterols/stanols per day had a significant cholesterol lowering effect. There is no significant difference between plant sterols and stanols in their cholesterol lowering ability.

[8] Data based on a multicenter randomized, crossover, controlled trial conducted at 6 research centers from 5 European countries. 200 healthy male participants were randomly assigned to 3 sequences of daily administration of 25 ml of 3 olive oils of varying phenolic content at 3 weeks intervals preceded by 2-week washout periods.

*Decrease in total cholesterol linearly dependent on phenol concentration of olive oil consumed.

[9] Data obtained from meta-analysis that identified 6 trials, including 2,650 individuals. A further meta-analysis included 50 original research studies (35 clinical trials, 2 prospective and 13 cross-sectional), with 534,906 participants.

**Widely quoted but statistically not significant

[10] Data obtained from meta-analysis involving eight trials (215 participants). [+ = total cholesterol lowered by 0.15 (mmol/L)], however statistically insignificant at p=0.08.

[11] Data obtained from meta-analysis involving 23 eligible randomized controlled trials published from 1995 to 2002.

Level of Evidence: A = Systematic review, B = Randomized control trials, C = A large degree of conflicting data between studies

Reprinted with permission from Mannu, G.S. et al. (2013). Evidence of lifestyle modification in the management of hypercholesterolemia. *Current Cardiology Reviews,* 9, 2–14.

- Lose 10 pounds (4.5 kg) if overweight (5 to 8% reduction in LDL)
- Add 5 to 10 grams per day of soluble fiber (3 to 5% reduction in LDL) (Table 8-9 shows the amount of soluble fiber in various high-fiber foods)
- Add 2 grams per day of plant stanols and sterols (5 to 15% reduction in LDL)

Together, these five changes lead to a 20–30% reduction in LDL, on par with the lipid-lowering seen with many cholesterol-lowering medications. A typical TLC eating plan is shown in Figure 8-7. For more information on the complete plan, visit the NHLBI website (www.nhlbi.nih.gov) and search "TLC program."

TABLE 8-9
A SAMPLING OF HIGH-FIBER FOODS

	Soluble Fiber	Total Fiber		Soluble Fiber	Total Fiber
Whole-grain cereals – ½ cup cooked (except where noted)			**Vegetable (½ cup cooked)**		
Barley	1	4	Broccoli	1	1.5
Oatmeal	1	2	Brussels sprouts	3	4.5
Oatbran	1	3	Carrots	1	2.5
Psyllium seeds, ground (1 Tbsp)	5	6			
Fruit – 1 medium (except where noted)			**Legumes – ½ cup cooked**		
Apple	1	4	Black beans	2	5.5
Banana	1	3	Kidney beans	3	6
Blackberries (½ cup)	1	4	Lima beans	3.5	6.5
Citrus (orange, grapefruit)	2	2–3	Navy beans	2	6
Nectarine	1	2	Northern beans	1.5	5.5
Peach	1	2	Pinto beans	2	7
Pear	2	4	Lentils (yellow, green, orange)	1	8
Plum	1	1.5	Chickpeas	1	6
Prunes (¼ cup)	1.5	3	Black-eyed peas	1	5.5

Source: National Heart, Lung, and Blood Institute (2005). *Your Guide to Lowering Your Cholesterol with TLC.* NIH Publication No. 06-5235.

Figure 8-7
A TLC eating plan

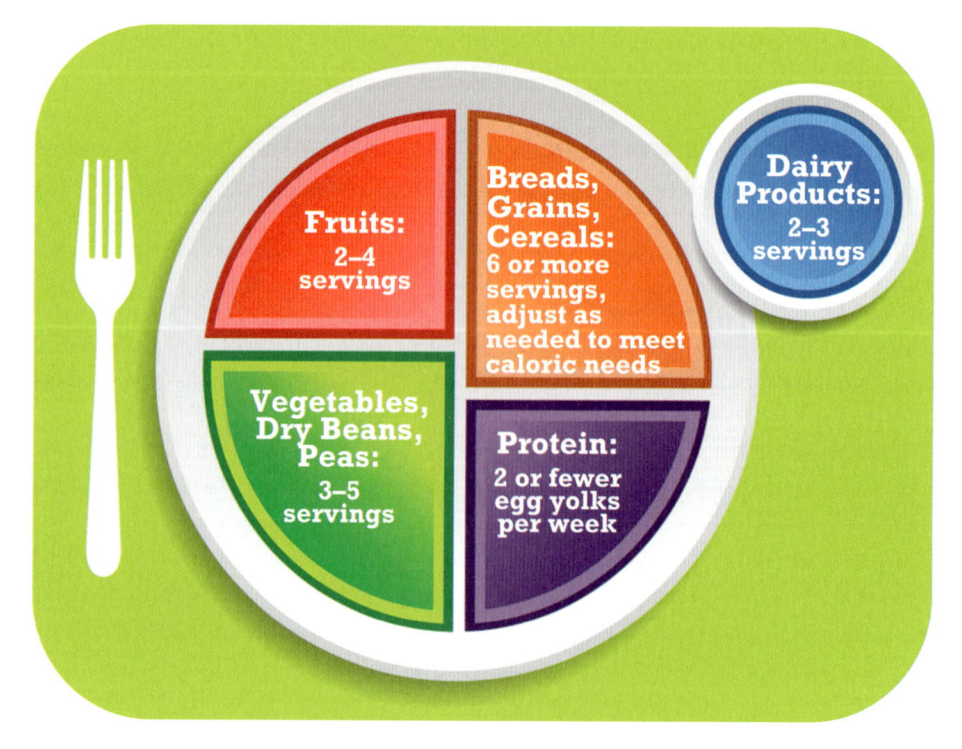

Ultimately, healthful dietary changes can have substantial effects on cholesterol levels, in particular total and LDL cholesterol. While most clients with a diagnosis of high cholesterol will be prescribed anti-cholesterol medications by their physicians, making meaningful dietary changes combined with an appropriate physical-activity program can serve as a potent adjunct to pharmacological management, and may even help the client to need a smaller dosage of the medication, or in some cases, none at all.

EXERCISE RECOMMENDATIONS

Although there will be significant individual variation, it appears that to improve overall lipoprotein status (LDL, HDL, non-HDL, and triglycerides), an exercise volume of at least 1,500+ kcal per week (e.g., running 15 miles or walking 20+ miles per week) may be the minimum necessary based on available research. Optimally, 2,000 kcal/week or more is recommended. The American College of Sports Medicine (ACSM, 2022) guidelines state that the exercise volume to reduce dyslipidemia should be consistent with the same guidelines for healthy weight loss and maintenance.

Table 8-10 depicts example exercise plans with approximate weekly energy expenditures ranging from 600 to 3,000+ kcal per week. This may provide a frame of reference for what approximates higher weekly energy expenditures most often required for significant reductions in LDL and non-HDL. Note that this table states approximate gross energy costs of weight-bearing physical activity. The gross energy cost per walking mile is greater, for example, for individuals who have higher body weight.

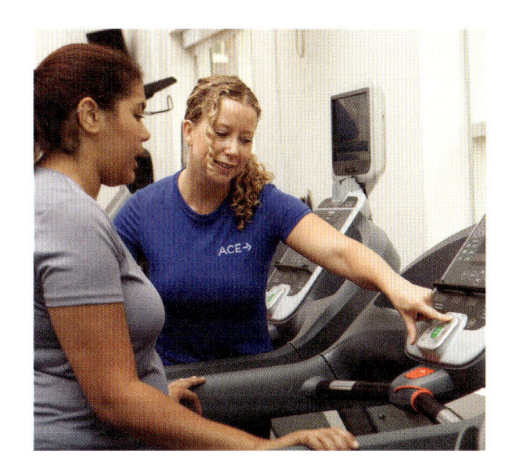

TABLE 8-10

EXAMPLE WEEKLY EXERCISE ENERGY EXPENDITURES*

Protocol A (600–800 kcal/week)
Monday, Wednesday, Friday: Walk 2 miles/day[†] = 600 kcal
Sunday: 20 minutes of low-level stationary cycling = 100 kcal

Protocol B (1,000–1,200 kcal/week)
Monday, Wednesday, Friday: Walk 2 miles/day[†] = 600 kcal
Tuesday: Walk 3 miles[†] = 300 kcal
Sunday: Nine holes of golf or 30 minutes of singles tennis = 300 kcal

Protocol C (1,500–1,800 kcal/week)
Monday, Wednesday, Friday: Walk 3 miles/day[†] = 900 kcal
Tuesday, Thursday: 30 min of cycling (50–60% $\dot{V}O_2max$) = 300 kcal
Sunday: 60 minutes of singles tennis plus 2-mile walk[†] = 500 kcal

Protocol D (2,000+ kcal/week)
5 days per week, average 300 kcal workout (e.g., 30- to 45-minute aerobic session) = 1,500 kcal/week; 1 day/week perform a long slow-distance workout (e.g., 2-hour moderate- to fast-pace variable-terrain walk) = 600+ kcal

Protocol E (2,500–3,000+ kcal/week)
5 days per week, 400 kcal/session (~45 minutes of walk-run or 90 minutes of walking ~3mph) = 2,000 kcal/week
1 day/week 2-hour variable terrain hike = 500–1,000 kcal

* Assumes 160–180 pound (72–81 kg) body weight (values are expressed in estimated gross energy expenditure costs)
[†] Walking at moderate pace (2.5–3 mph)

ACSM Exercise and Dyslipidemia Guidelines

Although there will be significant individual variation, it appears that to improve overall lipoprotein status, the following general guidelines are appropriate: Aerobic exercise performed five or more days a week, for 30 to 60 minutes per day (50 to 60 minutes or more per day is recommended to promote or maintain weight loss), at 40 to 75% of $\dot{V}O_2$ reserve ($\dot{V}O_2R$) or **heart-rate reserve (HRR)** (ACSM, 2022; Jacobson et al., 2014; IAS, 2013).

Although this guideline is somewhat nonspecific, it is helpful to know that this amount of physical activity is consistent with recommendations for long-term weight control (i.e., 200 to 300 minutes/week of moderate physical activity or ≥2,000 kcal/week of activity). This volume may be accumulated with repeated exercise bouts of ≥10 minutes.

A Word About the 2013 AHA/ACC Lifestyle Guidelines to Reduce ASCVD

In December 2013, the AHA and ACC released lifestyle guidelines to reduce CVD risk, including those for physical activity and dyslipidemia (Eckel et al., 2013). This report was based on systematic reviews and meta-analyses of randomized controlled trials or individual controlled clinical trials in adults published from 2001 to 2011. More importantly, their physical activity and dyslipidemia guidelines were based only on studies supporting the use of physical-activity *alone* (i.e., not in combination with other interventions, such as dietary interventions or weight loss) versus no physical activity or other type of intervention for improvements in selected blood lipids (HDL, LDL, triglycerides, and non-HDL). Given these restrictions (i.e., no other lifestyle interventions), their findings were:

- Among adults, aerobic physical activity, as compared to control interventions, reduces LDL by 3.0 to 6.0 mg/dL on average.
- Among adults, aerobic physical activity alone, as compared to control interventions, has no consistent effect on triglycerides.
- Among adults, aerobic physical activity alone, as compared to control interventions, has no consistent effect on HDL.
- Among adults, resistance training, as compared to control interventions, reduces LDL, triglycerides, and non-HDL by 6 to 9 mg/dL on average and has no effect on HDL. Typical interventions shown to reduce LDL, triglycerides, and non-HDL and having no effect on HDL include resistance physical-activity programs that average 24 weeks in duration and include three or more days per week, nine exercises performed for three sets, and 11 repetitions at an average intensity of 70% of 1-RM.
- AHA/ACC recommendations for physical activity and dyslipidemia: In general, advise adults to engage in aerobic physical activity to reduce LDL and non-HDL: three or four sessions a week, lasting on average of 40 minutes per session, and involving moderate-to-vigorous intensity physical activity.

These guidelines should be interpreted with caution, not because they are not evidence-based by well-controlled trials, but because of potentially basing an exercise plan solely on a conservative requirement of using physical activity alone *without* any dietary or adiposity reduction intervention. Of course, this is not a practical or realistic approach for the CMES educating clients in the context of advising physical activity without concomitant changes in diet and **body composition.**

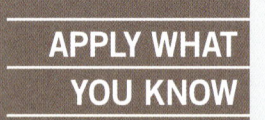

APPLY WHAT YOU KNOW

ESSENTIAL EXERCISE-PROGRAMMING STEPS FOR INDIVIDUALS WITH DYSLIPIDEMIA

Step 1: Evaluate Health and Lifestyle History
- Relevant comorbidities
- Blood lipid history and current blood lipid profile
- Exercise treadmill test history if at high CVD risk

- Medications, especially lipid-altering medications
- Diet and exercise history

Clients with documented or suspected dyslipidemia frequently have other related clinical conditions (i.e., comorbidities) that also may influence exercise programming. Prolonged elevations in LDL, for example, can increase the likelihood of CHD. Other conditions, such as diabetes, especially T2DM, and obesity, often coexist with lipid disorders and can influence the exercise-lipid response. Although many individuals who have primary lipid disorders do not have associated comorbidities, they should have a thorough health history conducted by the CMES for the following conditions or comorbidities:

- Coronary heart disease
- Previous myocardial infarction
- Angina
- Diabetes
- Insulin resistance
- Hypertension
- Obesity
- MetS
- Peripheral vascular disease
- Renal disease
- Chronic obstructive pulmonary disease

Some of these conditions may necessitate a thorough examination by a physician and an exercise **electrocardiogram (ECG).** It is important in these instances that the CMES obtain this medical information and use it to help establish the recommended mode, frequency, duration, intensity, and progression of exercise.

Step 2: Determine the Necessity for Medical Clearance

In general, asymptomatic individuals with dyslipidemia will not require medical clearance and exercise testing prior to beginning a light-to-moderate intensity exercise program (ACSM, 2022). However, if it is determined that an exercise test is warranted, it is acceptable to follow standard methods and protocols. Because individuals with dyslipidemia often present with other chronic diseases and health conditions, it may be necessary to receive medical clearance prior to exercise testing and the initiation of an exercise program. The need for medical clearance will be determined during the preparticipation health screening process and be based on the presence of cardiovascular, metabolic, or renal disease, or the presence of signs and symptoms indicative of such diseases, current levels of exercise participation, and the desired exercise intensity. In the presence of other diseases or conditions, it may be necessary to modify exercise testing protocols (ACSM, 2022).

Step 3: Perform Anthropometric Measures

Many lipid disorders are sensitive to changes in body-fat stores. For this reason, it is essential that a CMES initially and serially assess valid measures of body fat. Body weight, abdominal girth (measured at the level just above the iliac crest, a measure of central visceral fat stores), and/or upper-body skinfolds (e.g., triceps or subscapular), as assessed by Lange or equivalent skinfold calipers, should be recorded during the client's initial visit and at four- to six-week intervals throughout the course of exercise training. It is important to focus on the change in waist circumference, BMI, and anthropometric measures rather than their relationship to normative body-fat data. Total cholesterol, LDL, non-HDL, and triglycerides usually decrease with a diminution in body fat, especially abdominal or visceral fat reduction. HDL may or may not directly correlate with fat-weight changes.

Step 4: Set a Realistic Target Lipid Goal for Exercise Therapy

It is important to emphasize that exercise-lipid responses vary among people and that the volume of exercise required for significant changes in blood lipids is generally at a higher weekly energy expenditure threshold than that for reducing blood pressure or improving psychological well-being. For this reason, it may take more time to realize the clinical benefits. The CMES must be conservative with short-term lipid-reduction goals, especially with total and LDL reductions. A 5 to 8% LDL reduction or a 6 to 12% reduction in non-HDL is generally a realistic goal for the first 12 to 16 weeks of exercise training, assuming sufficient weekly exercise energy expenditure. Because non-HDL includes more atherogenic triglyceride-rich particles than LDL, it may be a better target of exercise therapy. Many clients may take six months or longer to show significant decreases in non-HDL and LDL. This is not unusual, as there are a considerable variety of lipid disorders and blood lipid phenotypes. When possible, the CMES should incorporate other co-variants of lipid reduction, such as valid anthropometric measures of obesity and abdominal-visceral fat, to demonstrate progress toward predetermined goals.

Laboratory analysis of lipid and lipoprotein values characteristically vary by 8 to 12%, based on biological variation, lab bias, and analytic factors. This is important to consider when interpreting serial blood lipid values. Examples of variation in LDL and HDL concentration include hospitalization, **estrogen** replacement therapy, pregnancy, T2DM, smoking, acute infection, posture, venous occlusion, and seasonal and circadian biological variation. The NHLBI published a comprehensive set of recommendations for laboratories and healthcare providers on ensuring valid lipoprotein measurement and interpretation (NHLBI, 2012).

Step 5: Determine the Exercise Plan from Prior Health History, Level of Fitness, and Current Lipid Profile

The exercise plan should be written clearly and concisely and include exercise mode, frequency, duration, intensity, progression plan, and safety precautions. The client's health history and initial fitness level are integral to formulating the weekly volume. For example, for clients with stable CHD who have had a recent exercise ECG, it will be important to review exercise electrocardiographic and **hemodynamic** data to appropriately set the exercise intensity and duration range. The individual's exercise capacity in METs or measured $\dot{V}O_2$ will also be helpful in determining initial exercise work levels.

Overall, it may be most straightforward to program exercise by energy expenditure or total weekly caloric expenditure with pedometry (i.e., weekly step counts), or simply by duration and intensity. Initial weekly exercise volumes should be set realistically according to the client's initial level of fitness, body composition, and existing comorbidities. See Table 8-10 for a sample set of exercise energy-expenditure protocols. Since many clients may be significantly deconditioned and have overweight, it may be most appropriate to start on a progressive walking program. In this case, walking distance, speed, and the difficulty of the terrain should be gradually increased over the course of the program to generate higher energy expenditures. Since overall blood lipid improvement is responsive to weekly exercise volumes (total physical activity energy expenditures) and exercise-generated fat-weight loss, it is imperative that the CMES knows how to reliably estimate session, daily, and weekly exercise energy expenditures in kcal. The following are examples of gross energy-expenditure target goals by lipid and lipoprotein:

- *Elevated LDL and/or non-HDL:* ≥2,000 kcal per week or the same exercise volume as that required for long-term weight loss
- *Low HDL:* ≥1,500 kcal per week
- *Elevated triglycerides:* ≥1,500 kcal per week
- *Combined dyslipidemia (elevated LDL and triglycerides with low HDL):* ≥2,000 kcal per week

Step 6: Keep Track of the Client's Lipid-lowering Drugs and Other Medications, if Applicable

If a client is on lipid-lowering drugs, it is wise to know which drug or combination of drugs they are taking and any associated dosage changes. The combined use of exercise and lipid-lowering drug therapy can significantly reduce the time needed to achieve the lipid goal. As a group, lipid-lowering drugs have little, if any, effect on exercise hemodynamics. Beta-blocking medications, with the exception of the few that have intrinsic **sympathomimetic** activity (e.g., acebutolol and pindolol), will have a tendency to increase triglycerides and decrease HDL cholesterol. Individuals on significant dosages of niacin therapy (e.g., >1,500 mg/day) may have a greater tendency to experience a drop in blood pressures after exercise in warm weather. Niacin can also cause flushing and headaches in early stages of this form of pharmacotherapy. As a final note, many lipid-lowering drugs (e.g., statins, fibrates, and niacin) require periodic liver-function tests to assess the possibility of liver toxicity.

Step 7: Follow Up

Encourage follow-up blood lipid profile laboratory evaluations in accordance with the referring physician or the lipid clinic's follow-up protocol. Follow-up would ideally be executed in conjunction with the routine lipid clinic follow-up visit,

Blood Lipid Disorders   CHAPTER 8

or at six- or eight-week intervals. The exercise plan should be revised as needed, with documentation of weekly energy expenditures and exercise mode(s). Anthropometric measures should be assessed at every clinic evaluation or at the follow-up visit. Dietary and medication compliance should also be routinely assessed at each session.

Step 8: Maintain a Working Knowledge of Other Evidence-based Non-pharmacological Interventions That Can Help Manage Lipid Disorders

For optimal results, it will often be important to use exercise as a complement to other non-pharmacological (and pharmacological) measures. For example, exercise stands the best chance of helping a client reach their lipid goal if it is combined with dietary therapy (Jacobson et al., 2014; Eckel et al., 2013). Supplemental antioxidant vitamin intake (e.g., vitamin E) may be of value in reducing LDL oxidation, although these supplements do not directly affect blood lipid levels (Rimm & Stampfer, 1997). **Folic acid,** vitamin B6, and vitamin B12 supplementation may also be of help in reducing serum **homocysteine** levels. Homocysteine is an **amino acid** that contributes to the build-up of lipids in **arteries** and increases blood clotting tendency (Wald et al., 1998). The client should discuss adding any of the aforementioned supplements with their physician.

Stress- and anger-management interventions, when applicable, should also be included in a comprehensive lipid-management plan. The rationale for such behavioral programs stems from stress-related **catecholamine** production and its putative relationship with LDL oxidation, LDL receptor regulation, and macrophage activation, all of which are integral in the development of atherosclerosis (Muldoon et al., 1999; Williams et al., 1991).

Step 9: Partner With Healthcare Professionals

In some cases, the CMES will be collaborating with a physician-directed lipid clinic or diabetes care team in providing therapy. In this sense, the CMES is a member of a medical team and may be required to provide progress reports to the patient record. A helpful description of lipid clinic operations and referral affiliations is available through the NLA. In other instances, the CMES may act independently through self-referral. In this case, it will be necessary to communicate exercise progress to the client's physician and to discuss the relevance of additional tests. Becoming a member of the NLA (www.lipid.org) is an essential first step.

EXPAND YOUR KNOWLEDGE

THE ACCREDITATION COUNCIL FOR CLINICAL LIPIDOLOGY

The Accreditation Council for Clinical Lipidology (ACCL) (www.lipidspecialist.org) is an independent certifying organization that has developed standards and an examination in the field of clinical lipidology for the growing number of mid- and advanced-level nonphysician healthcare practitioners who manage individuals with lipid and other related disorders. This organization was developed in association with the National Lipid Association specifically for non-physician advanced-practice clinical professionals, including clinical exercise specialists, registered clinical exercise physiologists, and certified medical exercise specialists. A CMES can qualify, prepare for, and sit for the ACCL board exam, which is offered online during a variety of testing windows throughout the year. This is an academically and clinically robust exam that is administered by computer through Krytorion Testing Centers throughout the U.S. The requirements for sitting for this exam are on the www.lipidspecialist.org website. The board credential is "certified clinical lipid specialist." Professional knowledge and skill competencies for this credential include the following:

- Metabolism of lipids and lipoproteins and the pathophysiology of atherosclerosis
- Genetics, diagnosis, and management of dyslipidemia and the metabolic syndrome
- Cardiovascular risk assessment
- Pharmacology, safety, and efficacy of lipid-altering drugs
- Fundamentals of non-pharmacological therapy: nutrition, exercise, and behavior and compliance

The ACCL also offers a more basic competency exam and certificate: the Basic Competency in Clinical Lipidology (BCCL). This is a more basic written exam open to anyone with a general involvement in the field of lipidology, which of course can include interested certified medical exercise specialists. Information about the BCCL is also on the www.lipidspecialist.org website.

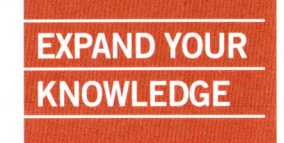

EXERCISE GUIDELINES SUMMARY FOR CLIENTS WITH DYSLIPIDEMIA

CARDIORESPIRATORY TRAINING	
Frequency	• 5 or more days per week to maximize caloric expenditure
Intensity	• Below, at, and above VT1, but below VT2 • 40–75% HRR or $\dot{V}O_2R$
Time	• 30–60 minutes per day • However, a minimum of 50–60 minutes per day is recommended to promote or maintain weight loss
Type	• A variety of rhythmic large-muscle-group exercise
Progression	• Progress following the ACE Integrated Fitness Training® Model based on client goals and availability.
MUSCULAR TRAINING	
Frequency	• 2–3 days per week
Intensity	• 50–85% 1-RM to improve muscular strength
Time	• 2–4 sets of 8–12 repetitions for muscular strength or 1–2 sets of 12–20 repetitions for muscular endurance
Type	• Resistance machines, free weights, and body weight
Progression	• Progress following the ACE Integrated Fitness Training Model based on client goals and availability.

Note: VT1 = First ventilatory threshold; VT2 = Second ventilatory threshold; $\dot{V}O_2R$ = Oxygen uptake reserve; HRR = Heart-rate reserve; 1-RM = One-repetition maximum

Source: American College of Sports Medicine (2022). *ACSM's Guidelines for Exercise Testing and Prescription* (11th ed.). Philadelphia: Wolters Kluwer.

CMES FOCUS

Clients with dyslipidemia who have no comorbidities (e.g., MetS, obesity, or hypertension) should engage in exercise programming that emphasizes weight loss and weight-loss maintenance [e.g., > 250 minutes of aerobic exercise per week (see Chapter 11 for more information)]. Furthermore, resistance training and flexibility exercise recommendations for healthy adults can be followed by clients with dyslipidemia with no comorbidities. Clients with comorbidities may need to be provided with a modified exercise program based on their other health limitations. Exercise professionals should encourage their clients with dyslipidemia who are taking lipid-lowering medications (i.e., HMG-CoA reductase inhibitors or statins and fibric acid) to report any unusual muscle weakness or soreness and consult their physicians if this occurs when exercising.

CASE STUDY

Client Information

Kevin is a 58-year-old male computer programmer with a family history of CHD (mother had a MI at age 51), a 12-year history of obesity, elevated LDL (ranging from 168 to 185 mg/dL), non-HDL 150 to 165 mg/dL, HDL ranging from 42 to 49 mg/dL, and triglycerides ranging from 170 to 184 mg/dL. He is 5'6" (1.7 m) tall, weighs 175 pounds (79 kg), and has a waist circumference of 35 inches (89 cm). He had an exercise ECG, which was normal. Kevin's initial physical activity consisted of several recreational activities, including participation in a bowling league for two hours a week and a 30- to 40-minute walk at a moderate intensity performed twice a week.

- *Minimal lipid goal (provided by his physician):* <130 mg/dL LDL, <160 non-HDL, and <35 inches (89 cm) waist circumference
- *Optimal lipid goal (provided by his physician):* <100 mg/dL LDL, <130 mg/dL non-HDL

Kevin was put on 10 mg/day of rosuvastatin almost three years ago, but during the first two years on this medication he failed to consistently take the dose every day. He was also prescribed a therapeutic lifestyle dietary program (focusing on saturated and trans fat reduction). Subsequently, he decreased his LDL to 119 mg/dL after complying with 10 mg of rosuvastatin every day, but his body weight has remained at 175 pounds (79 kg) and his waist circumference is still 35 inches (89 cm). Six months ago, Kevin was encouraged to continue to comply with 10 mg of rosuvastatin once a day, every day, and to work with a CMES, who implemented the following exercise program.

CMES Approach

Exercise program: This 12-week program is designed to progress Kevin to weekly energy expenditure from exercise totaling 2,000+ kcal/week. Variable-terrain walking four times per week at approximately 50 to 60% of peak heart rate as determined from his exercise ECG; the walking duration began at 20 minutes per session and progressed to 50 minutes per session after 12 weeks. He also performed two 50-minute total cardiorespiratory (combination stationary bike, treadmill, elliptical trainer) exercise sessions a week at a local fitness center, where his average exercise intensity is 65 to 70% of peak heart rate (50 to 65% of HRR).

Follow-up: His six-month follow-up (while on the 10 mg rosuvastatin and ~2,000 kcal exercise program) showed that he decreased his LDL to 102 mg/dL, non-HDL to 135 mg/dL, and triglycerides to 118 mg/dL, and had an HDL of 52 mg/dL. His body weight and waist circumference decreased to 164 pounds (74 kg) and 32 inches (81 cm), respectively.

ACE IFT® MODEL AT A GLANCE

Cardiorespiratory Training

The progressive program designed by the CMES starts with Base Training and progresses to Fitness Training.

Muscular Training

This client's initial program does not include Muscular Training, as all exercise is focused on cardiorespiratory exercise to improve his blood lipid profile. Modifications after the six-month follow-up can include the addition of movement screens and fitness assessments to help build this client's Muscular Training program, focused initially on establishing postural stability and kinetic-chain mobility.

SUMMARY

Depending on the type of blood lipid disorder and baseline lipids, exercise training of sufficient volume can quite favorably alter blood lipids. Further reductions in LDL and non-HDL can be realized with concomitant dietary restrictions of saturated and trans fats and reduction in body fat. With the exception of those who have existing ASCVD, especially CHD and/or diabetes, the essential first steps of therapy should be dietary and systematic exercise therapy. Epidemiologic studies have clearly demonstrated that for every 1% reduction in LDL, there is a 2 to 3% reduction in the incidence of CHD (NCEP, 2002).

Dyslipidemia management represents a most worthwhile opportunity for the CMES, given the growth of supportive clinical trials justifying intensive LDL therapy in dyslipidemic patients and the burgeoning growth of physician-directed lipid and cardiometabolic risk-reduction programs. Currently, the majority of these programs do not adequately address exercise in any meaningful systematic manner. Any CMES who is interested in helping clients manage dyslipidemia should find this a welcome challenge and seek to forge strong alliances with these outpatient healthcare provider teams.

REFERENCES

Academy of Nutrition and Dietetics Evidence Analysis Library 1 (2013). *Disorders of Lipid Metabolism Evidence Analysis Project.* http://andevidencelibrary.com/topic.cfm?cat=4527

AIM-HIGH Investigators (2011). Niacin in patients with low HDL cholesterol levels receiving intensive statin therapy. *New England Journal of Medicine,* 365, 2255–2267.

CHAPTER 8

Alberti, K.G. et al. (2009). Harmonizing the metabolic syndrome: A joint interim statement of the International Diabetes Federation Task Force on Epidemiology and Prevention; National Heart, Lung, and Blood Institute; American Heart Association; World Heart Federation; International Atherosclerosis Society; and International Association for the Study of Obesity. *Circulation,* 120, 1640–1645

American College of Sports Medicine (2022). *ACSM'S Guidelines for Exercise Testing and Prescription* (11th ed.). Philadelphia: Wolters Kluwer.

Bays, H. et al. (2013). Obesity, adiposity, and dyslipidemia: A consensus statement from the National Lipid Association. *Journal of Clinical Lipidology,* 7, 304–383.

Beltran-Sanchez, H. et al. (2013) Prevalence and trends of metabolic syndrome in the U.S. population 1999–2010. *Journal of the American College of Cardiology,* 62, 8, 697–703.

Bittner, V. (2004). Non-high-density lipoprotein cholesterol: An alternate target for lipid-lowering therapy. *Preventive Cardiology,* 7, 3, 122–126.

Blazek, A. et al. (2013). Exercise-mediated changes in high-density lipoprotein: Impact on form and function. *American Heart Journal,* 166, 392–400.

Boekholdt, S.M. et al. (2012). Association of LDL cholesterol, non-HDL cholesterol, and apolipoprotein B Levels with risk of cardiovascular events among patients treated with statins. *Journal of the American Medical Association,* 307, 1302–1309.

Caso, G. et al. (2007). Effect of coenzyme-Q10 on myopathic symptoms in patients treated with statins. *American Journal of Cardiology,* 99, 1409–1412.

Cham, S. et al. (2010). Statin-associated muscle-related adverse effects: A case series of 354 patients. *Pharmacotherapy,* 30, 6, 541–553.

Cholesterol Treatment Trialists' (CTT) Collaboration (2010). Efficacy and safety of more intensive lowering of LDL cholesterol: A meta-analysis of data from 170,000 participants in 26 randomised trials. *Lancet,* 376, 1670–1681.

Coen, P.M. et al. (2009). Adding exercise training to rosuvastatin treatment: Influence on serum lipids and biomarkers of muscle and liver damage. *Metabolism–Clinical and Experimental,* 58, 1030–1038.

Costa, R.R. et al. (2011). Effects of resistance training on the lipid profile in obese women. *Journal of Sports Medicine and Physical Fitness,* 51, 1, 169–177.

Couillard, C. et al. (2005). Effects of endurance exercise training on plasma HDL cholesterol levels depend on levels of triglycerides. *Arteriosclerosis, Thrombosis, and Vascular Biology,* 21, 1226–1235.

Cromwell, W. & Otvos, J. (2007). Utilization of lipoprotein subfractions. In: Davidson, M., Toth, P., & Maki, H. (Eds.) *Therapeutic Lipidology.* Totowa, N.J.: Humana Press.

Cromwell, W.C. et al. (2007). LDL particle number and the risk of future cardiovascular disease in the Framingham Offspring study: Implications for LDL-C management. *Journal of Clinical Lipidology,* 1, 583–592.

Di Raimondo D. et al. (2013). Metabolic and anti-inflammatory effects of a home-based programme of aerobic physical exercise. *International Journal of Clinical Practice,* 67, 12, 1247–1253.

Donnelly, J.E. et al. (2009). Appropriate physical activity intervention strategies for weight loss and prevention of weight regain for adults: American College of Sports Medicine position stand. *Medicine & Science in Sports & Exercise,* 41, 2, 459–471.

Durstine, J.L. & Moore, G.E. (1997). Hyperlipidemia. In: Durstine, J.L. (Ed.) *ACSM's Exercise Management for Persons with Chronic Diseases and Disabilities.* Champaign, Ill.: Human Kinetics.

Durstine J.L. et al. (2002). Lipids, lipoproteins, and exercise. *Journal of Cardiopulmonary Rehabilitation,* 22, 385–398.

Eckel, R.H. et al. (2013). 2013 AHA/ACC guideline on lifestyle management to reduce cardiovascular risk: A report of the American College of Cardiology/American Heart Association Task Force on Practice Guidelines. *Journal of the American College of Cardiology,* 63, 25. DOI: 10.1016/j.jacc.2013.11.003

Gaziano, J.M. et al. (1993). Moderate alcohol intake, increased levels of high-density lipoproteins and its subfractions, and decreased risk of myocardial infarction. *New England Journal of Medicine,* 329, 25, 1829–1834.

Goff, D.C. et al. (2013). ACC/AHA guideline on the assessment of cardiovascular risk: A report of the American College of Cardiology/American Heart Association Task Force on practice guidelines. *Circulation,* published online November 12, 2013. http://circ.ahajournals.org/content/early/2013/11/11/01.cir.0000437741.48606.98.citation

Gordon, D., Chen, S., & Durstine L. (2014). The effects of exercise training on the traditional lipid profile and beyond. *Current Sports Medicine and Reports,* 13, 4, 253–259.

Grundy, S.M. (2007). Cardiovascular and metabolic risk factors: How can we improve outcomes in the high-risk patient? *The American Journal of Medicine,* 120, 9, Suppl. 1, S3.

Grundy, S.M. et al. (2018). 2018 AHA/ACC/AACVPR/AAPA/ABC/ACPM/ADA/AGS/APhA/ASPC/NLA/PCNA guideline on the management of blood cholesterol: A report of the American College of Cardiology/American Heart Association Task Force on Clinical Practice Guidelines. *Circulation,* 139, 25, e1082–e1143.

Grundy, S.M. et al. (2005). Diagnosis and management of the metabolic syndrome: An American Heart Association/National Heart, Lung and Blood Institute Scientific Statement. *Circulation,* 112, 2735–2752.

Hansson, G.K. (2005). Mechanisms of disease: Inflammation, atherosclerosis, and coronary artery disease. *New England Journal of Medicine,* 352, 1685–1695.

Henderson, G.C. et al. (2010). Plasma triglyceride concentrations are rapidly reduced followingindividual bouts of endurance exercise in women. *European Journal of Applied Physiology,* 109, 721–730.

HPS2-THRIVE Collaborative Group (2013). HPS2-THRIVE randomized placebo-controlled trial in 25,673 high-risk patients of ER niacin/laropiprant: Trial design, pre-specified muscle and liver outcomes, and reasons for stopping study treatment. *European Heart Journal,* 34, 17, 1279–1291.

Huang, Y. et al. (2014). An abundant dysfunctional apolipoprotein A1 in human atheroma. *Nature Medicine,* 20, 193–203. DOI:10.1038/nm.3459

International Atherosclerosis Society (2013). *An International Atherosclerosis Society Position Paper: Global Recommendations for the Management of Dyslipidemia.* www.atherosclerosis-journal.com/article/S0021-9150(13)00681-3/fulltext

Jacobson, T.A. et al. (2014). National Lipid Association recommendations for patient-centered management of dyslipidemia: Part 1 – executive summary. *Journal of Clinical Lipidology,* 8, 473–488.

Kelley, G.A. & Kelley, K.S. (2009). Impact of progressive resistance training on lipids and lipoproteins in adults: A meta-analysis of randomized controlled trials. *Preventive Medicine,* 48, 9–19.

Kelley, G.A., Kelley, K.S., & Tran, Z.V. (2005a). Aerobic exercise, lipids and lipoproteins in 24 overweight and obese adults: A meta-analysis of randomized controlled trials. *International Journal of Obesity (London),* 29, 881–893.

Kelley, G.A., Kelley, K.S., & Tran, Z.V. (2005b). Walking and non-HDL-C in adults: A meta-analysis of randomized controlled trials. *Preventive Cardiology,* 8, 102–107.

Kodama, S., et al. (2011). Effect of aerobic exercise training on serum levels of high-density lipoprotein cholesterol: A meta-analysis. *Archives of Internal Medicine,* 167, 999–1008.

Kokkinos, P.K. et al. (2013). Interactive effects of fitness and statin treatment on mortality risk in veterans with dyslipidaemia: A cohort study. *The Lancet,* 381.

Kraus, W. et al. (2002). Effects of the amount and intensity of exercise on plasma lipoproteins. *New England Journal of Medicine,* 347, 19, 1522–1524.

Lira, F. et al. (2010). Low and moderate, rather than high intensity strength exercise induces benefit regarding plasma lipid profile. *Diabetology and Metabolic Syndrome,* 2, 31.

Lowes, R. (2013). *Crestor Tops List of Best-Selling Drugs.* www.webmd.com/cholesterol-management/news/20131101/crestor-is-top-selling-drug

Magkos, F. (2009). Basal very low-density lipoprotein metabolism in response to exercise: Mechanisms of hypotriacylglycerolemia. *Progress in Lipid Research,* 48, 171–190.

Malkova, D. & Gill, J. (2006). Effects of exercise on postprandial metabolism. *Future Lipidology,* 1, 743–755.

Mann, S., Beedie, C., & Jimenez, A. (2014). Differential effects of aerobic exercise, resistance training and combined exercise modalities on cholesterol and the lipid profile: Review, synthesis and recommendations. *Sports Medicine,* 44, 2, 211–221.

Mannu, G.S. et al. (2013). Evidence of lifestyle modification in the management of hypercholesterolemia. *Current Cardiology Reviews,* 9, 2–14.

Mansi, I. et al. (2013). Statins and musculoskeletal conditions, arthropathies, and injuries. *Journal of Internal Medicine,* 173, 1–9.

Mestek, M.L. (2009). Physical activity, blood lipids, and lipoproteins. *American Journal of Lifestyle Medicine,* 3, 279–283.

Mikus, C.R. et al. (2013). Simvastatin impairs exercise training adaptations. *Journal of the American College of Cardiology,* 62, 709–714.

Muldoon, M.F. et al. (1999). Acute cholesterol responses to mental stress and change in posture. *Archives of Internal Medicine,* 152, 775–780.

National Cholesterol Education Program (2002). Expert panel on detection, evaluation and treatment of high blood cholesterol in adults: Summary of the 2nd report of NCEP expert panel on detection, evaluation and treatment of high blood cholesterol in adults (Adult Treatment Panel III). NIH Publication 02-5213. *Journal of the American Medical Association,* 285, 2486–2497.

National Health and Nutrition Examination Survey (2012). Cholesterol levels improve among U.S. adults. *Journal of the American Medical Association,* 308, 1545–1554.

National Heart, Lung, and Blood Institute (2012). *Expert Panel on Integrated Guidelines for Cardiovascular Health and Risk Reduction in Children and Adolescents Summary Report.* NIH Publication No. 12-7486A.

National Heart, Lung, and Blood Institute (2005). *Your Guide to Lowering Your Cholesterol with TLC.* NIH Publication No. 06-5235.

Nicholls, S.J. et al. (2006). Consumption of saturated fat impairs the anti-inflammatory properties of high-density lipoproteins and endothelial function. *Journal of the American College of Cardiology,* 48, 4, 715–720.

Nordestgaard, B.G. et al. (2010). Lipoprotein(a) as a cardiovascular risk factor: Current status. *European Heart Journal,* 31, 23, 2844–2853.

Paoli, A., Pacelli, Q., & Moro, T. (2013). Effects of high-intensity circuit training, low-intensity circuit training and endurance training on blood pressure and lipoproteins in middle-aged overweight men. *Lipids in Health and Disease,* 12, 131.

Pattyn, N. et al. (2013). The effect of exercise on the cardiovascular risk factors constituting the metabolic syndrome: A meta-analysis of controlled trials. *Sports Medicine,* 43, 121–133.

Plaisance, E.P. & Fisher, G. (2014). Exercise and dietary-mediated reductions in postprandial lipemia. *Journal of Nutrition and Metabolism,* 902065. DOI: 10.1155/2014/902065

Rees, K. et al. (2013). Dietary advice for reducing cardiovascular risk. *Cochrane Database of Systematic Reviews,* 3, CD002128. DOI: 10.1002/14651858.CD002128.pub4

Reiner, Z. et al. (2011). ESC/EAS guidelines for the management of dyslipidaemias: The task force for the management of dyslipidaemias of the European Society of Cardiology (ESC) and the European Atherosclerosis Society (EAS). *European Heart Journal,* 32, 1769–1818.

Reinhart, K.M. & Woods, J.A. (2012). Strategies to preserve the use of statins in patients with previous muscular adverse effects. *American Journal of Health-System Pharmacy,* 69, 4, 291–300.

Rimm, E.B. & Stampfer, M.J. (1997). The role of antioxidants in preventive cardiology. *Current Opinion in Cardiology,* 12, 188–194.

Rosenson, R.S. & Underberg, J.A. (2013). Systematic review: Evaluating the effect of lipid-lowering therapy on lipoprotein and lipid values. *Cardiovascular Drugs and Therapy,* 27, 5, 465–479.

Ross, R. (1999). Atherosclerosis: An inflammatory disease. *New England Journal of Medicine,* 340, 115–126.

Sheikholeslami, V.D. et al. (2011). Changes in cardiovascular risk factors and inflammatory markers of young, healthy, men after six weeks of moderate or high intensity resistance training. *Journal of Sports Medicine and Physical Fitness,* 51, 4, 695–700.

Siri-Tarino, P.W. (2011). Effects of diet on high-density lipoprotein cholesterol. *Current Atherosclerosis Reports,* 13, 6, 453–460.

Slentz, C.A. et al. (2007). Inactivity, exercise training and detraining, and plasma lipoproteins. *Journal of Applied Physiology,* 103, 432–442.

Staiano, A. et al. (2014). Sitting time and cardiometabolic risk in US adults: Associations by sex, race, socioeconomic status and activity level. *British Journal of Sports Medicine,* 48, 213–219.

Stern, M., Williams, K., & Haffner, S.M. (2002). Identification of persons at high risk for type 2 diabetes mellitus: Do we need the glucose tolerance test? *Annals of Internal Medicine,* 136, 575–581.

Taylor, F.C., Huffman, M., & Ebrahim, S. (2013). Statin therapy for primary prevention of cardiovascular disease.

Journal of the American Medical Association, 310, 22, 2451–2452.

Teslovich, T.M. et al. (2010). Biological, clinical and population relevance of 95 loci for blood lipids. *Nature,* 466, 707–713.

Tonelli, M. et al. (2011). Efficacy of statins for primary prevention in people at low cardiovascular risk: A meta-analysis. *Canadian Medical Association Journal,* 183, 16, E1189–E1202.

Trejo-Gutierrez, J.F. & Fletcher, G. (2007). Impact of exercise on blood lipids and lipoproteins. *Journal of Clinical Lipidology,* 1, 175–181.

Trombold, J.R. et al. (2013). Acute high-intensity endurance exercise is more effective than moderate-intensity exercise for attenuation of postprandial triglyceride elevation. *Journal of Applied Physiology,* 114, 792–800.

Varbo, A. et al. (2013). Remnant cholesterol as a causal risk factor for ischemic heart disease. *Journal of the American College of Cardiology,* 61, 4, 427–436.

Wald, N. et al. (1998). Homocysteine and ischemic heart disease. *Archives of Internal Medicine,* 158, 862–867.

Williams, R.B. et al. (1991). Biobehavioral basis of coronary-prone behavior in middle-aged men. Part I: Evidence for chronic SNS activiation in type A's. *Psychosomatic Medicine,* 53, 517–527.

Wooten, J.S. et al. (2011). Resistance exercise and lipoproteins in postmenopausal women. *International Journal of Sports Medicine,* 32, 1, 7–13.

Zhang, J.Q. (2006). Effect of exercise on postprandial lipemia in men with hypertriglyceridemia. *European Journal of Applied Physiology,* 98, 575–582.

SUGGESTED READING

Gleeson, R. & Davidson, M. (2010). *Lipidology, a Primer: The What, Why, and How of Better Lipid Management.* Prevent CVD Publishing.

Eckel, R.H. et al. (2013). 2013 AHA/ACC guideline on lifestyle management to reduce cardiovascular risk: A report of the American College of Cardiology/American Heart Association Task Force on Practice Guidelines. *Journal of the American College of Cardiology,* 63, 25. DOI: 10.1016/j.jacc.2013.11.003

Goff, D.C. et al. (2013). ACC/AHA guideline on the assessment of cardiovascular risk: A report of the American College of Cardiology/American Heart Association Task Force on practice guidelines. *Circulation,* published online November 12, 2013. http://circ.ahajournals.org/content/early/2013/11/11/01.cir.0000437741.48606.98.citation

Grundy, S.M. et al. (2018). 2018 AHA/ACC/AACVPR/AAPA/ABC/ACPM/ADA/AGS/APhA/ASPC/NLA/PCNA guideline on the management of blood cholesterol: A report of the American College of Cardiology/American Heart Association Task Force on Clinical Practice Guidelines. *Circulation,* 139, 25, e1082–e1143.

International Atherosclerosis Society (2013). *An International Atherosclerosis Society Position Paper: Global Recommendations for the Management of Dyslipidemia.* www.atherosclerosis-journal.com/article/S0021-9150(13)00681-3/fulltext

Jacobson, T.A. et al. (2014). National Lipid Association recommendations for patient-centered management of dyslipidemia: Part 1 – executive summary. *Journal of Clinical Lipidology,* 8, 473–488.

9 HYPERTENSION

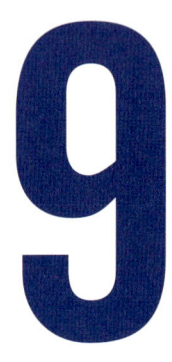

IN THIS CHAPTER

EPIDEMIOLOGY

OVERVIEW
CONTROL OF BLOOD PRESSURE
PHYSIOLOGY OF HYPERTENSION

DIAGNOSTIC CRITERIA

TREATMENT OPTIONS
NON-PHARMACOLOGICAL TREATMENT
PHARMACOLOGICAL TREATMENT
SURGICAL TREATMENT
EXERCISE TREATMENT

NUTRITIONAL CONSIDERATIONS
NUTRITION GUIDELINES
NUTRIENTS THAT AFFECT BLOOD PRESSURE
THE DASH EATING PLAN

EXERCISE RECOMMENDATIONS
CARDIOVASCULAR RESPONSES TO AEROBIC EXERCISE TRAINING
PROGRAMMING AND PROGRESSION GUIDELINES AND CONSIDERATIONS
CARDIORESPIRATORY TRAINING
RESISTANCE TRAINING

EXERCISE GUIDELINES SUMMARY FOR CLIENTS WITH HYPERTENSION

CASE STUDIES

SUMMARY

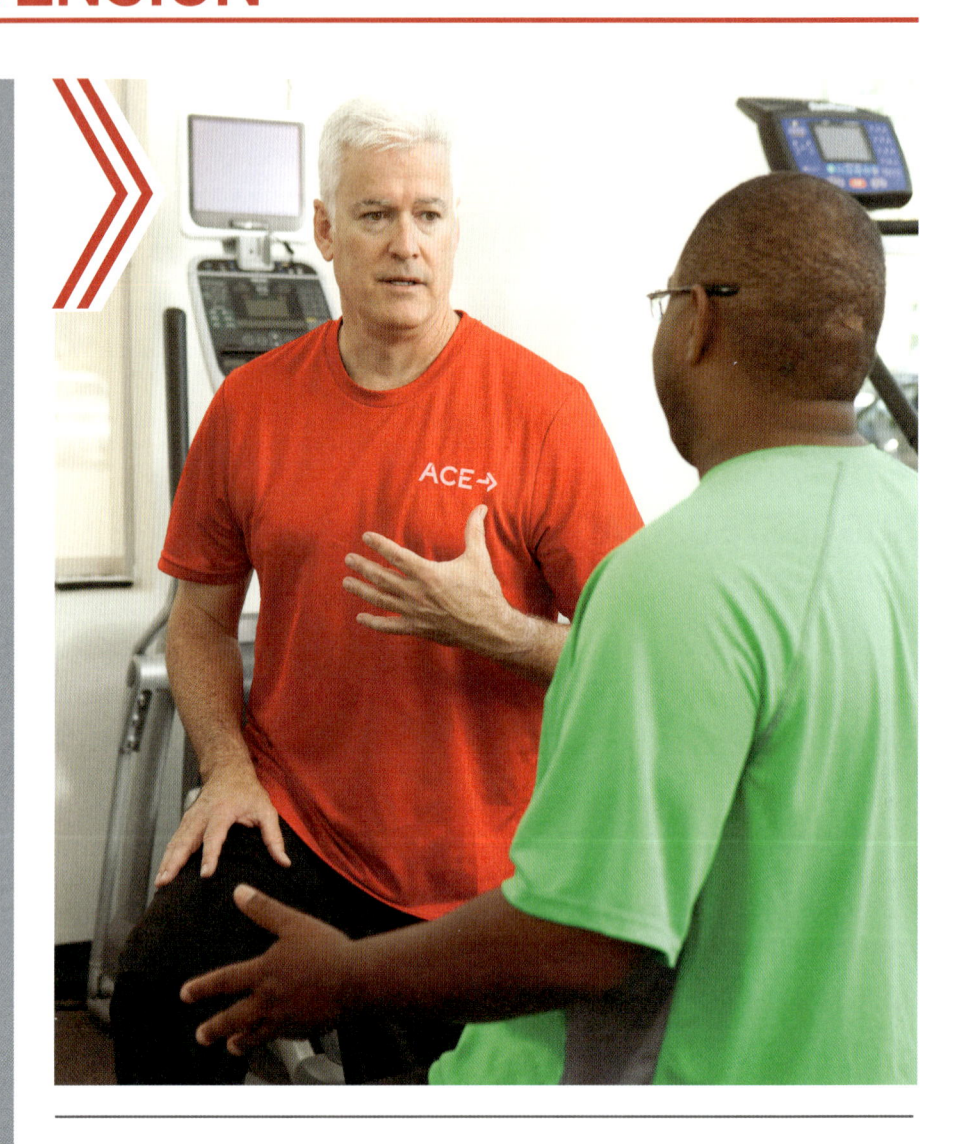

ABOUT THE AUTHORS

W. Larry Kenney, Ph.D., is a professor of kinesiology and physiology at Pennsylvania State University, and former president of the American College of Sports Medicine. His research focuses on thermal physiology and the biophysics of heat transfer, including the effect of aging and hypertension on human skin blood flow. Dr. Kenney has published more than 150 papers and has been continually funded by that National Institutes of Health since 1985.

Lacy M. Alexander, Ph.D, is a research associate professor of kinesiology at Pennsylvania State University. Dr. Alexander is a fellow of the American College of Sports Medicine and has received the young investigator award from the American Physiological Society. Her research interests include the mechanisms underlying microvascular dysfunction in humans with essential hypertension. Dr. Alexander is funded by the National Institutes of Health and has contributed more than 55 papers to the scientific literature.

By W. Larry Kenney & Lacy M. Alexander

AN INDEPENDENT PREDICTOR OF MORTALITY, hypertension (HTN) affects nearly 108 million adults in the United States [Centers for Disease Control and Prevention (CDC), 2020a]. Exercise is a cornerstone therapy in the prevention and treatment of this disease. It is important for an ACE® Certified Medical Exercise Specialist (CMES) to know the role of regular exercise therapy in the management of HTN and how physical activity produces a decrease in **blood pressure (BP)**. Because most hypertensive individuals will take two or more antihypertensive medications to control their BP, it is also important to know the potential effects and interactions of antihypertensive medications on the cardiovascular system during exercise.

LEARNING OBJECTIVES:

» Define hypertension and discuss how having high blood pressure adversely affects health and places individuals at risk for other conditions, such as heart disease and stroke.

» Identify the diagnostic criteria for elevated blood pressure and hypertension.

» Explain nutrition considerations for individuals with high blood pressure and identify eating approaches that may help improve blood pressure.

» Identify treatment strategies for hypertension, including common antihypertensive medications and how those medications affect an individual's exercise response.

» Explain how hypertension may affect a client's ability to perform physical activity and exercise.

» Design and implement appropriate exercise programs for clients with hypertension, taking into account the potential risk for complications related to obesity, target organ disease, and/or cardiovascular disease that may occur in clients with this condition.

EPIDEMIOLOGY

HTN is an independent risk factor for **coronary artery disease, stroke,** and **renal failure.** The relationship between BP and adverse cardiovascular events is direct—the higher the BP, the greater the chance of heart attack, heart failure, stroke, and kidney disease. HTN is defined as having a **systolic blood pressure (SBP)** ≥130 mmHg, a **diastolic blood pressure (DBP)** ≥80 mmHg (Whelton et al., 2017). According to these criteria, approximately 1.13 billion individuals worldwide have HTN (World Health Organization, 2019).

The incidence of HTN increases with advancing age, with approximately 70% of Americans over the age of 75 having some form (Fleg et al., 2013). The relationship between BP and age is complex. After age 50, SBP steadily increases, whereas DBP plateaus around the sixth decade of life and decreases thereafter. Accordingly, the incidence of isolated systolic HTN (SBP ≥160 mmHg and a DBP of 90 mmHg or lower) or combined systolic-diastolic HTN (SBP ≥120 mmHg and DBP ≥80 mmHg) increases with age, while the incidence of isolated diastolic HTN (SBP <130 mmHg with DBP ≥80 mmHg) decreases with age. The longitudinal Framingham Heart Study has estimated that the lifetime risk for developing HTN is 90% (Roger et al., 2012).

With the increased mortality risk associated with HTN, combined with the age-related increase in BP, the early identification and treatment of individuals who will likely become hypertensive has become increasingly important. These individuals are categorized as having elevated blood pressure—an SBP of 120 to 129 mmHg and a DBP of <80 mmHg. The risk for **cardiovascular disease (CVD)** increases in a linear fashion beginning at 115/75 mmHg and the risk of death from heart disease, stroke, or other vascular disease doubles for each 20/10 mmHg increase (Whelton et al., 2017). Thus, effective diet, exercise, lifestyle modifications, and pharmacological (drug) therapy to lower BP in individuals with elevated and high blood pressure is vital to decreasing their total cardiovascular risk.

Even though the benefit of reducing and controlling BP in individuals with elevated and high blood pressure is clear, only about 24% of adults with hypertension have their condition under control and one in four adults in the U.S. are unaware they have hypertension (CDC, 2020a; CDC, 2020b).

OVERVIEW

Cardiac output is the product of **heart rate (HR)** and **stroke volume (SV),** the volume of blood the heart pumps in one beat. BP is the product of cardiac output, the amount of blood the heart pumps out in one minute, and **total peripheral resistance (TPR),** the resistance to blood flow that the blood vessels provide.

> Cardiac output = Heart rate x Stroke volume
> Blood pressure = Cardiac output x Total peripheral resistance

SV is altered by the amount of blood filling the heart (preload), the pressure the heart must pump against (afterload), and the force of cardiac **contractility.** Therefore, alterations in these variables resulting in an increase in either cardiac output or TPR can cause HTN.

Control of Blood Pressure

Short-term Reflex Control of Blood Pressure

Maintaining an adequate BP to ensure sufficient blood flow to the brain is one of the main priorities of the cardiovascular system. Blood pressure is integratively controlled by cardiovascular, neural, renal, and hormonal networks. Like many other controlled variables in physiology, BP is controlled via negative feedback with sensors, a defended set point, and effector responses. The sensors that regulate BP regulation are **baroreceptors** (pressure receptors) and they are located in the aortic arch and the carotid artery walls. Baroreceptors send neural signals to the cardiovascular control centers in the brain regarding the current BP. The cardiovascular control centers in the brain set a predetermined set point and integrate the incoming signals from the baroreceptors regarding the current BP. Depending on what the current BP is and how it compares to this predetermined set point, signals are sent out to the heart, blood vessels, and kidneys via the **autonomic nervous system** to cause a change in BP to bring it closer to the set point. When BP is low or below the set point, there is little stretch on the baroreceptors, resulting in a reduction in the **afferent nervous system** signal going to the brain. The cardiovascular control centers integrate the signal from the baroreceptors and send out signals to the heart and blood vessels in an attempt to increase BP. These efferent signals are carried through the autonomic nervous system (**parasympathetic** and **sympathetic nervous systems**). During a low-BP state, parasympathetic activity to the heart is quickly decreased, which serves to rapidly increase HR. In addition, sympathetic nervous system activity increases, which also increases HR and cardiac contractility. The actions of the parasympathetic and the sympathetic nervous systems on the heart increase cardiac output. Increased sympathetic activity also causes **vasoconstriction** in the blood vessels, which increases total peripheral TPR.

When BP is high, the baroreceptors are stretched and the afferent signal to the cardiovascular control centers in the brain is increased. The resulting efferent response is to increase parasympathetic activity to the heart to slow HR and to inhibit sympathetic activity to cause a passive **vasodilation** of the peripheral blood vessels. This decreases BP, bringing it closer to the set point.

Long-term Neural-hormonal Control of Blood Pressure

In addition to the short-term mechanisms that alter BP, increased sympathetic nervous system activity has prolonged effects through its action on the kidneys and the release of **hormones** to increase blood volume. During a drop in BP, when there is decreased stretch on the baroreceptors, the hormone **vasopressin** (antidiuretic hormone) is released to help increase blood volume. This hormone causes water to be reabsorbed in the kidneys. In addition to vasopressin release, increased sympathetic nerve activity activates the **beta receptors** in the kidneys, which results in a decrease in blood flow to the kidneys, causing the release of another hormone called **renin.** Renin, in turn, activates a cascade of hormonal events to cause further vasoconstriction in the peripheral blood vessels and an increase in salt and water reabsorption in the kidney to enhance blood volume. Figure 9-1 illustrates the **renin-angiotensin-aldosterone system (RAAS).** Renin is an enzyme released from the kidneys that activates the hormone angiotensinogen by cleaving off part of the protein to form angiotensin I. Angiotensin I is then converted to angiotensin II through another enzyme called angiotensin converting enzyme (ACE). Angiotensin II is a potent vasoconstrictor that binds to receptors on peripheral blood vessels, causing the vascular smooth muscle in the blood vessels to contract. Angiotensin II also causes the mineral corticoid hormone **aldosterone** to be released from the adrenal cortex. Aldosterone causes sodium and water to be reabsorbed in the kidneys. Overall, the actions of aldosterone serve to increase blood volume. The RAAS system is extremely important for the long-term regulation of BP (Takahashi et al., 2011), and in the pathogenesis of HTN.

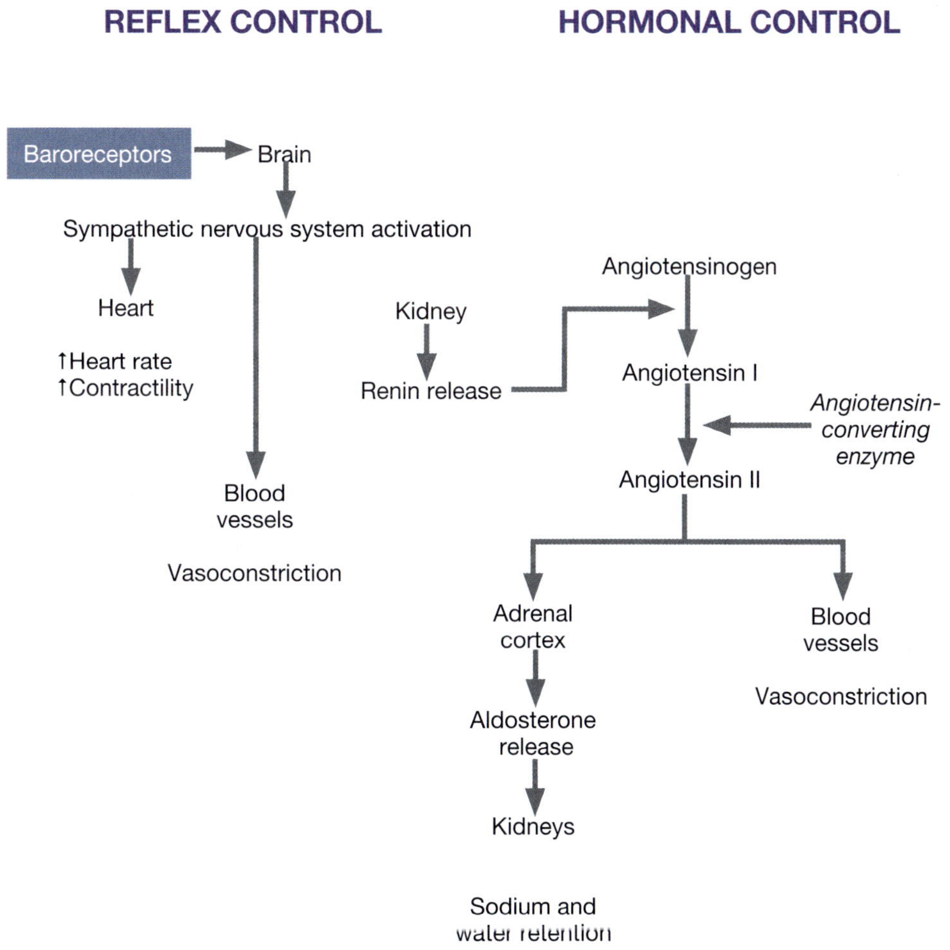

Figure 9-1
The renin-angiotensin-aldosterone system

Source: Kester, M. et al. (2007) *Elsevier's Integrated Pharmacology.* Philadelphia: Elsevier.

Physiology of Hypertension

Any disturbance in the normal negative feedback control of BP between the cardiovascular, neural, renal, or hormonal systems can result in HTN. There are several identifiable causes of HTN that are summarized in Table 9-1. When there is an identifiable cause of HTN, this is termed **secondary hypertension,** because it is secondary to a disease state. In these cases, correcting the underlying pathology can sometimes cure the HTN. However, in greater than 90% of cases of HTN, there is no single identifiable cause [American Heart Association (AHA), 2011]. HTN without an identifiable cause is clinically termed **essential** or **primary hypertension.** While the etiology of essential HTN is unclear, in general, central cardiovascular control centers and the baroreceptors in patients with HTN acquire a new elevated set point and become less sensitive,

TABLE 9-1
CAUSES OF SECONDARY HYPERTENSION\

COMMON CAUSES	PREVALENCE
Obstructive sleep apnea	25–50%
Renovascular disease	5–34%
Primary aldosteronism	8–20%
Drug or alcohol induced	2–4%
Renal parenchymal disease	1–2%
UNCOMMON CAUSES	**PREVALENCE**
Hypothyroidism	<1%
Hyperthyroidism	<1%
Pheochromocytoma/paraganglioma	0.1–0.6%
Aortic coarctation (undiagnosed or repaired)	0.1%
Cushing's syndrome	<0.1%
Primary hyperparathyroidism	Rare
Congenital adrenal hyperplasia	Rare
Mineralocorticoid excess syndromes other than primary aldosteronism	Rare
Acromegaly	Rare

Source: Whelton, P.K. et al. (2017). 2017 ACC/AHA/AAPA/ABC/ACPM/AGS/ PhA/ASH/ASPC/NMA/PCNA guideline for the prevention, detection, evaluation, and management of high blood pressure in adults: A report of the American College of Cardiology/American Heart Association Task Force on Clinical Practice Guidelines. *Journal of the American College of Cardiology,* Nov 7. pii: S0735-1097 (17) 41519-1.

meaning that it takes a larger change in BP for the system to respond and correct that change. As a result of the elevated set point, there is a decrease in parasympathetic nerve activity to the heart and an increase in resting sympathetic nerve activity to the heart, vasculature, and kidneys. This situation causes an increase in HR and cardiac contractility via stimulation of the beta receptors in the myocardium, as well as an increase in peripheral vasoconstriction via the action of the sympathetic nervous system **neurotransmitters** (e.g., **norepinephrine**) on the blood vessels. Furthermore, in the kidneys, increased sympathetic stimulation causes renin to be released, which activates the RAAS. RAAS activation increases peripheral vasoconstriction through the actions of angiotensin II on the vasculature and increases salt and water reabsorption in the proximal tubules of the kidneys. The resulting increase in total body extracellular volume increases preload on the heart, which serves to further increase cardiac contractility. Thus, feedback regulation in this tightly controlled BP regulatory system is impaired and results in HTN (Takahashi et al., 2011).

Because the control of BP involves many different organ systems, there can be various mechanisms that ultimately lead to HTN. There are several common pathophysiological findings associated with high BP. There appears to be a change in the BP set point, an overall increase in sympathetic nervous system activity, and a decrease in the sensitivity of the baroreceptors to a change in BP (Kougias et al., 2010; Hesse et al., 2007). In addition, there are alterations in the local control of peripheral blood vessels. To help control blood flow, blood vessels release substances called vasodilators, which cause the blood vessels to open wider, and vasoconstrictors, which cause the blood vessels to narrow. With HTN, there is a shift from locally released vasodilators to vasoconstrictors. This change is associated with an increase in **free radical** (**oxidant**) stress in the blood vessels. This pro-vasoconstrictor state, along with the elevated pressure on the blood vessels themselves, causes remodeling of the blood vessel walls. This remodeling makes the blood vessel walls **hypertrophy** and become stiff.

Hypertension

CHAPTER 9

Long-term elevations in BP can also induce changes in the heart itself. Just like in the blood vessels, the heart muscle begins to hypertrophy. This is not an advantageous hypertrophy like the changes that are induced in the myocardium during endurance-exercise training. Instead, with HTN, the heart muscle becomes thicker through concentric hypertrophy and less efficient as a pump. This is referred to as left ventricular hypertrophy and can be detected on an **electrocardiogram.**

Prolonged uncontrolled HTN has many deleterious effects on the cardiovascular system, including remodeling of the myocardium and vascular smooth muscle. This type of remodeling can cause target organ damage in the heart, brain, kidneys, and peripheral blood vessels. Table 9-2 lists the major pathologies caused by HTN-induced target organ damage.

TABLE 9-2
SELECT PATHOLOGIES CAUSED BY HYPERTENSION-INDUCED TARGET ORGAN DAMAGE

Heart • Left ventricular hypertrophy • Angina or prior myocardial infarction • Prior coronary revascularization • Heart failure
Brain • Stroke or transient ischemic attack
Chronic kidney disease
Peripheral arterial disease
Retinopathy

Source: Schmieder, R.E. (2010). End organ damage in hypertension. *Deutsches Arzteblatt International,* 107, 49, 866–873.

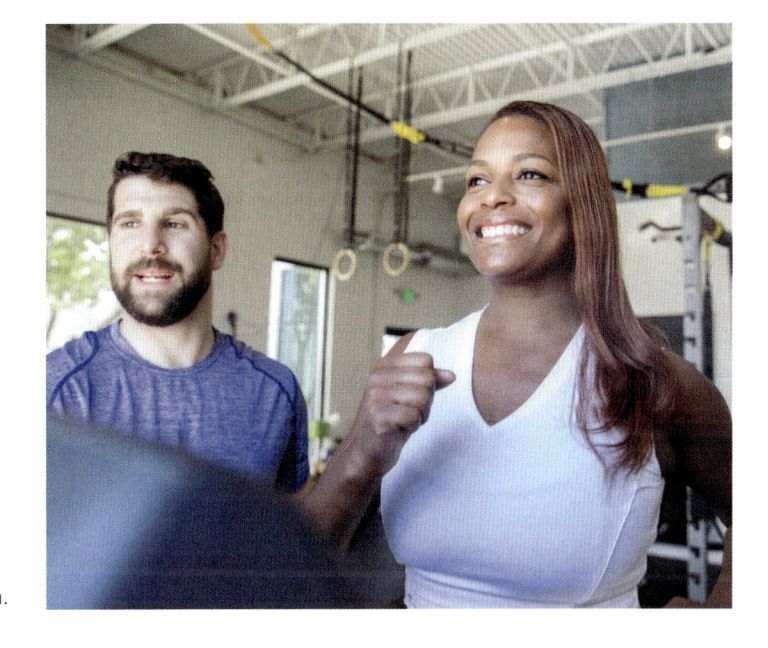

GENETICS AND HYPERTENSION

The underlying genetic and pathophysiological mechanisms contributing to essential HTN vary widely and depend on individual characteristics and environmental interactions. Genetic studies in humans to identify the genes that cause essential HTN are in their infancy. Essential HTN is genetically encoded on multiple genes and has several phenotypic (outward physical manifestations of disease) and genotypic (genetic code) subtypes. Therefore, each gene that encodes for HTN only has a small effect on BP (Weder, 2008). However, the genetic predisposition for HTN is permissive, meaning that environmental influences are necessary for HTN to ultimately develop.

Considering the genetic and environmental contributing factors in the development of HTN, it is not surprising that there are many different physiological mechanisms responsible for high BP. The mechanisms that cause HTN and the individual responses to treatment can differ depending on several variables, including race and age. For example, the incidence of HTN is greater among African Americans than it is among other ethnic groups. Furthermore, it has also been demonstrated that blood pressure control is lower for non-Hispanic black adults among those recommended to take blood pressure medication (CDC, 2020a). Certainly, the data suggest that there are physiological differences in the mechanisms of HTN depending on genetics, but there are also many environmental and socioeconomic explanations for some of these findings. One additional example to illustrate different causes and physiological mechanisms of HTN involves individuals who develop high BP at a young age versus those who develop it later in life. In younger individuals, the onset of HTN is associated with an increase in salt and water retention that results in an increase in cardiac output. In contrast, HTN in older patients is more commonly associated with an increase in peripheral vascular resistance. These different mechanisms and contributing factors to high BP should be considered, especially when selecting suitable pharmacological and non-pharmacological interventions to treat high BP.

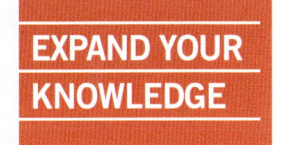

EXPAND YOUR KNOWLEDGE

DIAGNOSTIC CRITERIA

BP is measured within the arterial system. Pressures in that system will vary depending on where they are taken. When a person is standing, the pressure at the feet is higher because of gravity (i.e., the weight of the blood is greatest at the lowest level and there is more blood in the lower arteries). Likewise, the pressure at the head is lower. Because one wants to know the pressures in the heart, BP is measured at a location that is on the same level as the heart itself. The standard site of measurement is the brachial artery (Figure 9-2), given its easy accessibility and proximity to the heart.

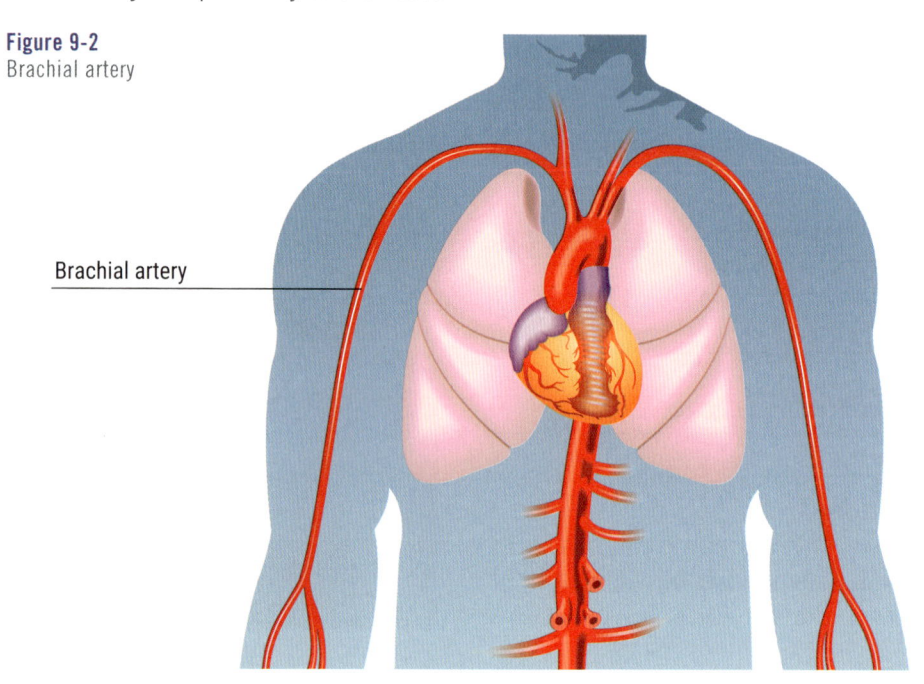

Figure 9-2
Brachial artery

It is important to note that BP cuffs come in a variety of sizes (Table 9-3). It is important to ensure the correct size is used, as clients who are muscular or have obesity may have falsely elevated BP readings, while individuals who are thin or have small frames my have falsely low BP readings, with a standard-sized cuffs.

TABLE 9-3

BLOOD-PRESSURE CUFF SIZES BASED ON ARM CIRCUMFERENCE

ARM CIRCUMFERENCE	SIZE	LABEL
22 to 26 cm	12 × 22 cm	Small adult
27 to 34 cm	16 × 30 cm	Adult
35 to 44 cm	16 × 36 cm	Large adult

Source: Kaplan, N.M. & Victor, R.G. (2014). *Kaplan's Clinical Hypertension* (11th ed.). Philadelphia: Wolters Kluwer/Lippincott Williams & Wilkins.

BP is measured indirectly by listening to the **Korotkoff sounds**; these are sounds made from vibrations as blood moves along the walls of the vessel. These sounds are present only when there is some degree of wall deformation. If the vessel has unimpeded blood flow, no vibrations are heard. However, under pressure of a BP cuff, vessel deformity facilitates hearing these sounds. This deformity is created as the air bladder within the cuff is inflated, restricting the flow of blood.

When the pressure in the cuff is higher than the pressure in the heart during contractions, the brachial artery collapses and blood flow through the cuff is blocked. As the air is slowly released from the bladder, blood begins to flow past the compressed area, creating turbulent flow and vibration along the vascular wall, producing the onset of tapping Korotkoff sounds, corresponding to SBP.

As the pressure in the cuff is reduced to the point where there is no deformation of the arterial wall, this represents the pressure in the arteries during relaxation or diastole. This is the DBP. DBP is indicated by a significant muffling of sound and the disappearance of sound (Figure 9-3). Typically, in adults with normal BP, the disappearance of sound is recorded as DBP. In children and adults with the disappearance of sound occurring below 40 mmHg, but who appear healthy, the first sign of significant muffling may be used.

The classification of BP for adults is presented in Table 9-4.

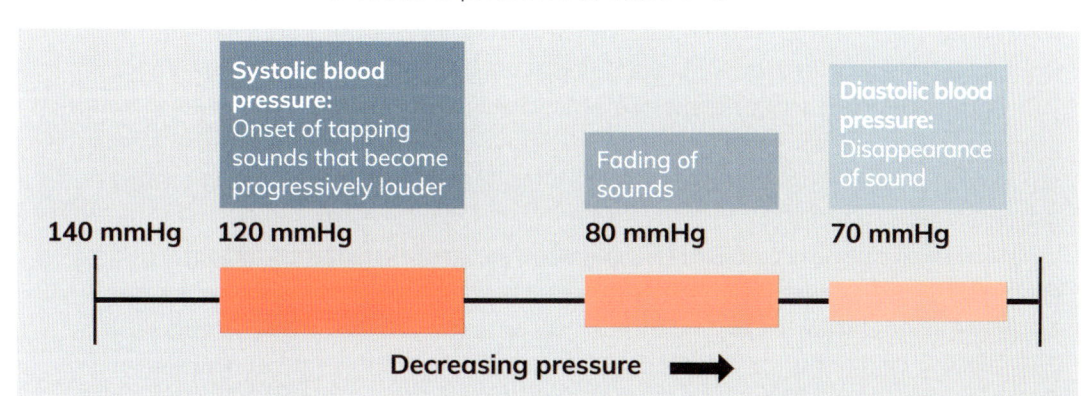

Figure 9-3
Korotkoff sounds

TABLE 9-4
CATEGORIES OF BLOOD PRESSURE IN ADULTS*

CATEGORY	SBP		DBP
Normal	<120 mmHg	and	<80 mmHg
Elevated	120–129 mmHg	and	<80 mmHg
Hypertension			
Stage 1	130–139 mmHg	or	80–89 mmHg
Stage 2	≥140 mmHg	or	≥90 mmHg

Note: SBP = Systolic blood pressure; DBP = Diastolic blood pressure

*Individuals with SBP and DBP in two different categories should be designated to the higher BP category. BP is based on an average of two or more careful readings obtained on two or more occasions.

Reprinted with permission from Whelton, P.K. et al. (2017). 2017 ACC/AHA/AAPA/ABC/ACPM/AGS/APhA/ASH/ASPC/NMA/PCNA guideline for the prevention, detection, evaluation, and management of high blood pressure in adults: A report of the American College of Cardiology/American Heart Association Task Force on Clinical Practice Guidelines. *Journal of the American College of Cardiology,* Nov 7. pii: S0735-1097 (17) 41519-1.

ACCURACY OF BLOOD PRESSURE MACHINES

EXPAND YOUR KNOWLEDGE

Clients sometimes ask about the BP machines found at pharmacies and personal BP monitors used at home. While these monitors can provide useful information, the results may not be accurate. As an example, readings obtained from wrist BP monitors are usually higher and less accurate than readings from the arm. Compared to readings obtained by auscultation, one study (Ringrose et al., 2017) found that home monitors provided SBP or DBP readings that were not accurate within 5 mmHg 69% of the time. Inaccurate readings within 10 mmHg and 15 mmHg were found 29% and 7% of the time, respectively.

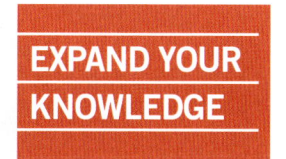

> **EXPAND YOUR KNOWLEDGE**

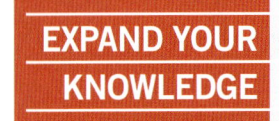

ACC/AHA GUIDELINES

In 2017, the American College of Cardiology (ACC) and the American Heart Association (AHA) partnered with nine other professional organizations to provide new guidelines for the prevention, detection, evaluation, and management of high BP in adults (Whelton et al., 2017). These guidelines are based on a systematic review of research studies and are meant to inform regulatory and payer decisions, as well as improve the quality of patient care and align with patients' interests. Taking a collaborative approach among patients and practitioners about treatment options and interventions based on patient preferences, individual values, associated comorbidities, and conditions may enhance adherence to recommendations.

One of the key elements of the ACC/AHA report was the inclusion of new categories for BP in adults (see Table 9-4). As part of this update, there are now only four categories, as the "prehypertension" category has been removed. The rationale for the changes is based on observational data related to SBP/DBP levels and CVD risk, randomized, controlled trials (RCTs) featuring the use of lifestyle modification to lower BP, and RCTs focused on the use of antihypertensive medications to prevent CVD. Primarily, these updates were made because the risk of heart attack, stroke, cardiovascular diseases, and other BP-related consequences begin to increase as BP readings increase to and above 120/80 mmHg and the risk doubles by the time stage 1 hypertension levels are reached.

There is also an increased emphasis on the importance of accurate BP-measurement techniques and lifestyle modification, as well as on prescribing medication for those with stage 1 hypertension only if the patient is at an elevated risk of stroke or heart attack, has had a cardiovascular event, or presents with chronic kidney disease or diabetes. A goal of lowering the threshold for a HTN diagnosis is to increase awareness and promote intervention at an earlier stage to minimize or avoid further increases in BP and minimize BP-related complications. The guidelines set forth by the ACC and AHA also emphasize the importance of targeting modifiable risk factors for CVD including dyslipidemia, cigarette smoke/tobacco smoke exposure, diabetes, physical inactivity, overweight/obesity, and an unhealthy diet. The CMES plays a key educational and motivational role in supporting individuals with elevated and high BP. Nonpharmacological treatment can be beneficial, and the most effective interventions are weight loss, adherence to the **Dietary Approaches to Stop Hypertension (DASH) eating plan,** reduced sodium intake, potassium supplementation, increased physical activity, and reduced alcohol intake.

Table 9-5 lists the recommended lifestyle modifications and the resulting average decrease in SBP.

TABLE 9-5
BEST PROVEN NONPHARMACOLOGICAL INTERVENTIONS FOR PREVENTION AND TREATMENT OF HYPERTENSION*

INTERVENTION	DOSE	APPROXIMATE IMPACT ON SBP
Weight and body-fat loss	• Ideal body weight is the best goal • At least 1 kg reduction in body weight for most adults who have overweight • Expect about 1 mmHg for every 1 kg reduction in body weight	Hypertension: –5 mmHg Normotension: –2/3 mmHg
DASH eating plan	• Diet rich in fruits, vegetables, whole grains, and low-fat dairy products with reduced content of saturated and trans fat	Hypertension: –11 mmHg Normotension: –3 mmHg
Reduced intake of dietary sodium	• <1,500 mg/day is optimal, but at least 1,000 mg/day reduction in most adults	Hypertension: –5/6 mmHg Normotension: –2/3 mmHg

TABLE 9-5 *(continued)*		
INTERVENTION	DOSE	APPROXIMATE IMPACT ON SBP
Enhanced intake of dietary potassium	• 3,500–5,000 mg/day, preferably by consumption of a diet rich in potassium	Hypertension: –4/5 mmHg Normotension: –2 mmHg
Aerobic activity	• 90–150 minutes/week • 65–75% heart-rate reserve	Hypertension: –5/8 mmHg Normotension: –2/4 mmHg
Dynamic resistance training	• 90–150 minutes/week • 50–80% 1-repetition maximum • 6 exercises, 3 sets/exercise, 10 repetitions/set	Hypertension: –4 mmHg Normotension: –2 mmHg
Isometric resistance training	• 4 x 2 minutes (hand grip), 1-minute rest between exercises, 30–40% maximum voluntary contraction, 3 sessions/week • 8–10 weeks	Hypertension: –5 mmHg Normotension: –4 mmHg

Moderation in alcohol intake	• In individuals who drink alcohol, reduce alcohol[†] to:
	  ✓ Men: ≤2 drinks daily
	  ✓ Women: ≤1 drink daily
		Hypertension: –4 mmHg
		Normotension: –3 mmHg

* Type, dose, and expected impact on blood pressure in adults with a normal blood pressure and with hypertension.

[†] In the United States, one "standard" drink contains roughly 14 g of pure alcohol, which is typically found in 12 oz of regular beer (usually around 5% alcohol), 5 oz of wine (usually about 12% alcohol), and 1.5 oz of distilled spirits (usually about 40% alcohol).

Note: DASH = Dietary Approaches to Stop Hypertension; SBP = Systolic blood pressure

Source: Whelton, P.K. et al. (2017). 2017 ACC/AHA/AAPA/ABC/ACPM/AGS/ PhA/ASH/ASPC/NMA/PCNA guideline for the prevention, detection, evaluation, and management of high blood pressure in adults: A report of the American College of Cardiology/American Heart Association Task Force on Clinical Practice Guidelines *Journal of the American College of Cardiology*, Nov 7. pii: S0735-1097 (17) 41519-1.

The most significant decrease in BP with lifestyle modification comes as the result of following a healthy diet using the DASH eating plan. Because physical activity is a key component of weight loss and results in a significant decrease in BP, appropriate exercise programs following the ACE Integrated Fitness Training® (ACE IFT®) Model should be incorporated into the treatment plan for clients with elevated and high BP. Lifestyle modifications, including exercise and weight reduction, can prevent a progressive rise in BP and CVD, especially in individuals with elevated BP or HTN. If the target BP is not achieved by adopting healthy lifestyle changes, then pharmacotherapy is necessary.

Depending on the initial BP category, the need for pharmacological treatment in addition to lifestyle modification will be determined. For initial drug treatment, long-acting thiazide-type agents may be an optimal choice for first-step drug therapy. This type of drug works on the kidneys to decrease salt and water load, thereby decreasing excess extracellular volume. Alternatively, other BP-lowering drugs may be prescribed based on specific individual variables and the primary mechanisms causing the HTN.

Figure 9-4 is the algorithm that healthcare providers use for the treatment of HTN. The primary goal of any treatment (non-pharmacological and pharmacological) is to decrease BP to reduce CVD risk. For individuals with diabetes or existing chronic kidney disease, the goal of BP treatment is to attain a BP of <130/80 mmHg, as these populations are at an increased risk of further target organ damage and cardiovascular events. The majority of individuals with HTN will require two or more medications, in addition to lifestyle modifications, to reach their target BP. However, the first line of defense in treating elevated BP is to adopt a healthy lifestyle that includes the DASH eating plan, weight loss, and regular physical activity.

Figure 9-4
Blood pressure (BP) thresholds and recommendations for treatment and follow-up

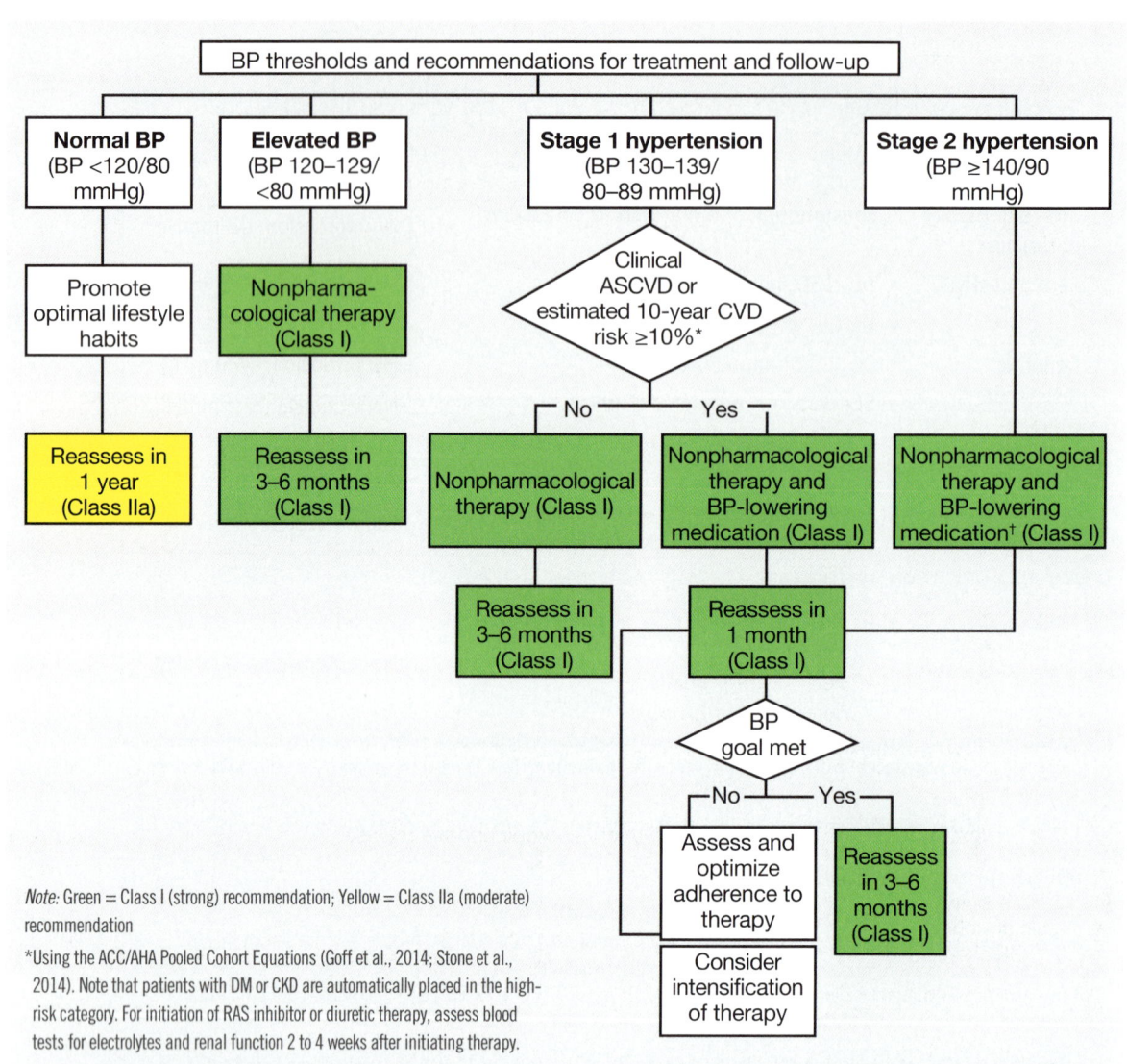

BP thresholds and recommendations for treatment and follow-up

- **Normal BP** (BP <120/80 mmHg) → Promote optimal lifestyle habits → Reassess in 1 year (Class IIa)
- **Elevated BP** (BP 120–129/<80 mmHg) → Nonpharmacological therapy (Class I) → Reassess in 3–6 months (Class I)
- **Stage 1 hypertension** (BP 130–139/80–89 mmHg) → Clinical ASCVD or estimated 10-year CVD risk ≥10%*
  - No → Nonpharmacological therapy (Class I) → Reassess in 3–6 months (Class I)
  - Yes → Nonpharmacological therapy and BP-lowering medication (Class I) → Reassess in 1 month (Class I) → BP goal met
    - No → Assess and optimize adherence to therapy; Consider intensification of therapy
    - Yes → Reassess in 3–6 months (Class I)
- **Stage 2 hypertension** (BP ≥140/90 mmHg) → Nonpharmacological therapy and BP-lowering medication† (Class I)

Note: Green = Class I (strong) recommendation; Yellow = Class IIa (moderate) recommendation

*Using the ACC/AHA Pooled Cohort Equations (Goff et al., 2014; Stone et al., 2014). Note that patients with DM or CKD are automatically placed in the high-risk category. For initiation of RAS inhibitor or diuretic therapy, assess blood tests for electrolytes and renal function 2 to 4 weeks after initiating therapy.

†Consider initiation of pharmacological therapy for stage 2 hypertension with 2 antihypertensive agents of different classes. Patients with stage 2 hypertension and BP ≥160/100 mmHg should be promptly treated, carefully monitored, and subject to upward medication dose adjustment as necessary to control BP. Reassessment includes BP measurement, detection of orthostatic hypotension in selected patients (e.g., older or with postural symptoms), identification of white coat hypertension or a white coat effect, documentation of adherence, monitoring of the response to therapy, reinforcement of the importance of adherence, reinforcement of the importance of treatment, and assistance with treatment to achieve BP target.

Note: ACC = American College of Cardiology; AHA = American Heart Association; ASCVD = Atherosclerotic cardiovascular disease; BP = Blood pressure; CKD = Chronic kidney disease; DM = Diabetes mellitus; RAS = Renin-angiotensin system.

Reprinted with permission from Whelton, P.K. et al. (2017). 2017 ACC/AHA/AAPA/ABC/ACPM/AGS/ PhA/ASH/ASPC/NMA/PCNA guideline for the prevention, detection, evaluation, and management of high blood pressure in adults: A report of the American College of Cardiology/American Heart Association Task Force on Clinical Practice Guidelines. *Journal of the American College of Cardiology*, Nov 7. pii: S0735-1097 (17) 41519-1.

TREATMENT OPTIONS

It is important for health and exercise professionals to work in collaboration with clinicians and nutritionists to optimize the BP-lowering potential of lifestyle modifications with pharmacotherapy. This collaborative relationship creates a support network for clients with HTN, thereby improving adherence to treatment.

Non-pharmacological Treatment

Non-pharmacological treatments for HTN include significant lifestyle modifications. These lifestyle modifications, along with the corresponding decrease in systolic BP, are detailed in

Hypertension

CHAPTER 9

Table 9-5. Evidence suggests that individuals with overweight and/or obesity can decrease blood pressure by 1 mmHg for every 1-kg reduction in body weight (Whelton et al., 2017). Refer to "Nutritional Considerations" on page 260 for more information.

Pharmacological Treatment

There are many pharmacological options available to treat HTN. Treatment options depend on other diseases and confounding pathologies that are unique to the individual. Considering that there are many potential contributing mechanisms to the development of HTN, the optimal pharmacotherapy will differ for each individual. In general, the following drug classes are used:

- Diuretics
- Beta blockers
- Angiotensin-converting enzyme (ACE) inhibitors
- Angiotensin receptor blockers (ARBs)
- Aldosterone receptor antagonists
- Alpha 1 blockers
- Calcium channel blockers
- Centrally acting alpha 2 agonists
- Peripheral vasodilators

Figure 9-5 illustrates where each of the antihypertensive drug classes alters the physiological mechanisms that control BP. The different classes of antihypertensive medications exert their effect on one or more of the organ systems that control BP.

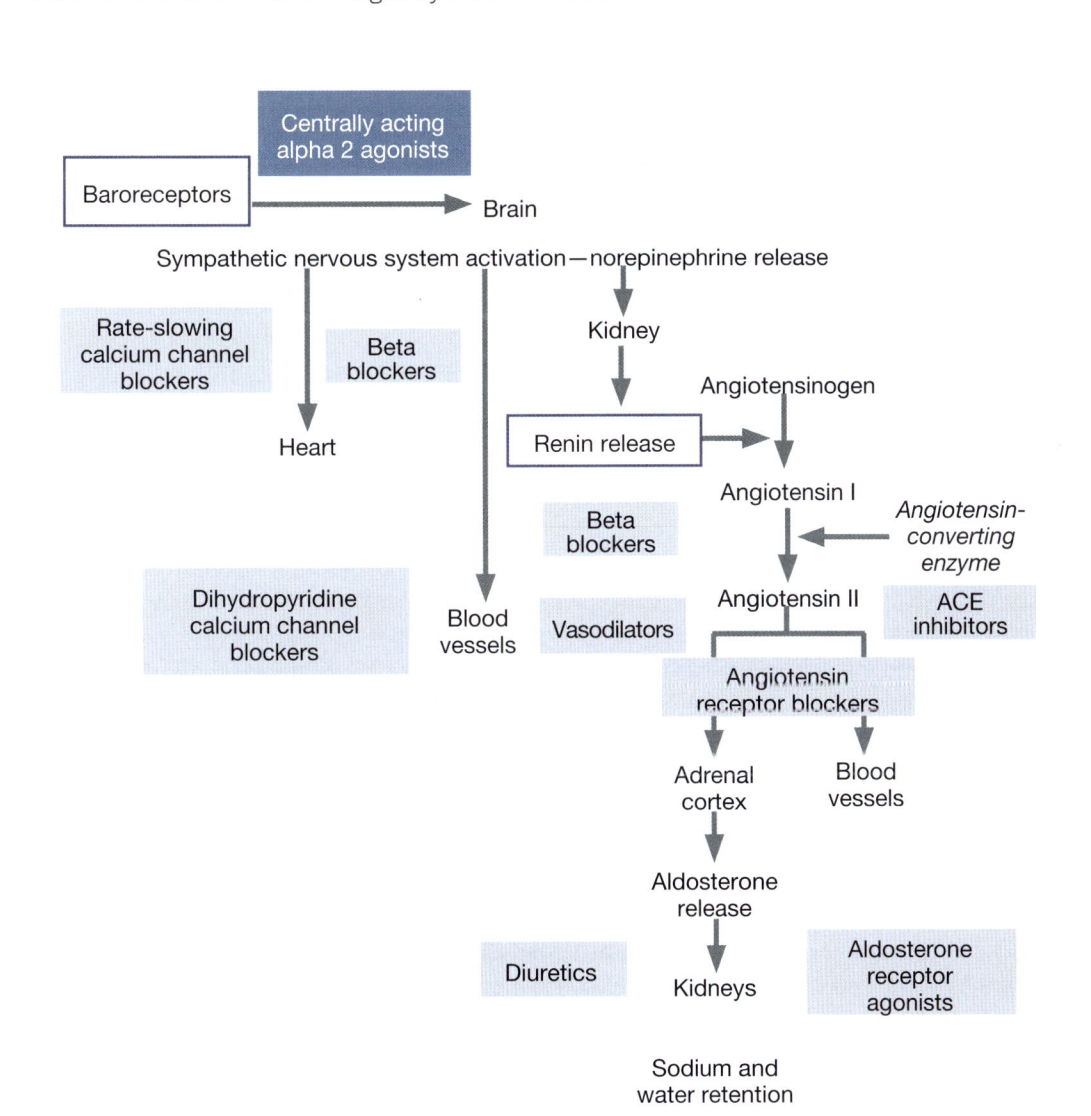

Figure 9-5
The effect of antihypertensive drug classes on the physiological mechanisms that control blood pressure

Source: Kester, M. et al. (2007) *Elsevier's Integrated Pharmacology.* Philadelphia: Elsevier.

Antihypertensive Medications and Cardiovascular Response

There are a number of classes of antihypertensive medications. Although lifestyle modification is a cornerstone therapy for treatment of elevated blood pressure and HTN, most hypertensive individuals will require two or more medications to reach their target BP. It is important that a CMES knows the medications their clients are taking, how they act on the cardiovascular system to lower BP, and any effects they have on the cardiovascular responses to exercise.

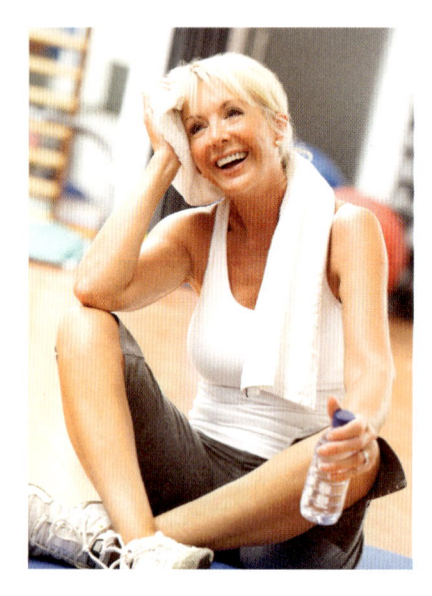

Diuretics

Diuretics are the most commonly prescribed BP-lowering drugs and are typically the first-line antihypertensive drugs prescribed for hypertensive patients. This drug class has been used for many years and is very effective at lowering BP, especially in cases in which the HTN is caused by excess extracellular fluid volume. Diuretics initially work to decrease BP by stimulating the excretion of sodium in the proximal tubule of the nephron (the functional unit of the kidneys). To maintain osmotic balance, water follows the sodium, resulting in a loss of extracellular fluid volume. It is hypothesized that the excess sodium contributes to the peripheral blood vessels' rigidity, thus promoting an increase in peripheral vascular resistance. The long-term BP-lowering capabilities of diuretics may be a result of decreasing sodium and indirectly lowering blood vessel rigidity (Kester et al., 2007).

Clients taking diuretics to manage their HTN should be instructed to pay particular attention to hydration during exercise, especially when exercising in warm environments. Because diuretics decrease plasma volume, hypertensive clients can easily become dehydrated during exercise. Clients should be instructed to drink fluids throughout exercise to replace the fluid that they are losing through sweat. The volume of sweat lost can be calculated by taking pre- and post-exercise body weights (accounting for fluid intake or loss via urine). The timing of exercise may also be important, as frequent trips to the restroom can be frustrating to the most avid exercisers.

Beta Blockers

There are many different types of beta blockers with different specificities and mechanisms of action. In general, beta blockers primarily work to lower BP by antagonizing the beta receptors in the heart and the kidneys. In the heart, normal stimulation of beta receptors by epinephrine increases HR and increases calcium entry into the myocardial cells, thereby increasing contractility. Stimulation of these receptors causes an increase in cardiac output. Blocking the beta receptors therefore decreases HR and contractility, collectively causing a decreased cardiac output. Initially, the antihypertensive effect of beta blockers is due to this decrease in cardiac output.

Beta blockers also inhibit renin release as a result of sympathetic nerve stimulation to the kidney. Recall that the release of renin stimulates a cascade of events that cause peripheral vasoconstriction through angiotensin II, as well as salt and water retention in the kidneys through the RAAS (see Figure 9-1). Thus, blocking the beta receptors in the kidneys inhibits this cascade of events and results in a passive vasodilation of the peripheral vasculature, thereby lowering peripheral vascular resistance.

Beta blockers blunt the normal elevation in HR that is observed during exercise. Therefore, gauging exercise intensity via target HR when working with hypertensive clients who are taking beta blockers is not appropriate. Instead, **rating of perceived exertion (RPE)** (6 to 20 scale), should be used to evaluate exercise intensity. This perceived exertion correlates well with exercise intensity in the absence of an appropriate exercise heart-rate response due to the beta-blocker effect.

In addition to the heart-rate response, there are additional precautions that a CMES should be aware of with this class of drugs. First, beta blockers can sometimes mask the symptoms of **hypoglycemia** (low blood sugar). Because exercise also decreases blood sugar, significant hypoglycemia during exercise can sometimes occur in clients taking beta blockers. Second, some clients taking beta blockers may complain of exercise intolerance due to the blunted heart-rate response. If this occurs, it is important that the client sees their healthcare provider to adjust the dosage of medication. The client must not abruptly stop taking their medication, as doing so can result in rebound HTN. Lastly, beta blockers can cause fatigue, sedation, **depression,** and sexual dysfunction. If a client complains of these symptoms, it is important that they see their healthcare provider.

Angiotensin-converting Enzyme (ACE) Inhibitors

ACE inhibitors block the conversion of angiotensin I to angiotensin II in the RAAS (see Figure 9-1), which results in an inhibition of peripheral vasoconstriction mediated by angiotensin II in the vasculature. It also results in an inhibition of aldosterone release from the adrenal cortex, thus preventing sodium and water reabsorption in the kidney. Recall that BP is integratively controlled by many physiological systems working in concert. In some cases, when one component of a body system is altered by pharmacology (such as causing a reduction in peripheral vascular resistance), there is a compensatory response by the other systems (increased cardiac output and sympathetic nerve activity) in an attempt to return to a homeostatic balance. However, in the case of HTN, the desired effect of the drug treatment is to lower BP, avoiding the compensatory changes that may occur in other systems that regulate BP. One of the advantages of ACE inhibitors is that they cause vasodilation of the peripheral vasculature without inducing a compensatory increase in sympathetic nerve activity.

Angiotensin Receptor Blockers (ARBs)

ARBs are similar to ACE inhibitors in the way that they lower BP. However, instead of inhibiting the production of angiotensin II, they block the receptor on which angiotensin II acts. ARBs cause a decrease in peripheral vasoconstriction, resulting in a decrease in peripheral vascular resistance. Furthermore, ARBs also inhibit the release of aldosterone from the adrenal cortex, which ultimately inhibits sodium and water reabsorption in the kidneys.

Aldosterone Receptor Antagonists

Aldosterone-receptor blockers inhibit the effect of aldosterone on the kidney. Thus, sodium and water are not reabsorbed and plasma volume is decreased.

Aldosterone-receptor antagonists can cause **hyperkalemia** (increase in serum potassium levels). When clients are taking these medications, it is important that the CMES monitors them for signs and symptoms of hyperkalemia, which can include a general feeling of fatigue, muscle weakness, nausea, tingling sensations, and, most seriously, slow heart beat and a weak pulse.

Alpha Blockers

This class of drugs works by inhibiting the alpha 1 receptors in the peripheral blood vessels, leading to a reduction in vasoconstriction and reduced peripheral vascular resistance. However, when the alpha 1 receptors are blocked, there is a compensatory increase in HR in an attempt to increase BP to achieve homeostatic balance. The baroreceptors send signals to the cardiovascular control centers that BP is low and a response ensues through the parasympathetic and sympathetic nervous systems to increase HR. However, the effect of the increased sympathetic activity on the peripheral vasculature is blocked by the drug. Alpha 1 blockers are no longer routinely used to manage HTN.

A common side effect of alpha 1 blockers is **orthostatic hypotension** (low BP upon standing). If clients are taking this drug class, they should be reminded to change body positions slowly and to not abruptly stop exercising. In addition, clients should be instructed to do an extended cool-down to limit the potential for a rapid decrease in BP with the cessation of exercise.

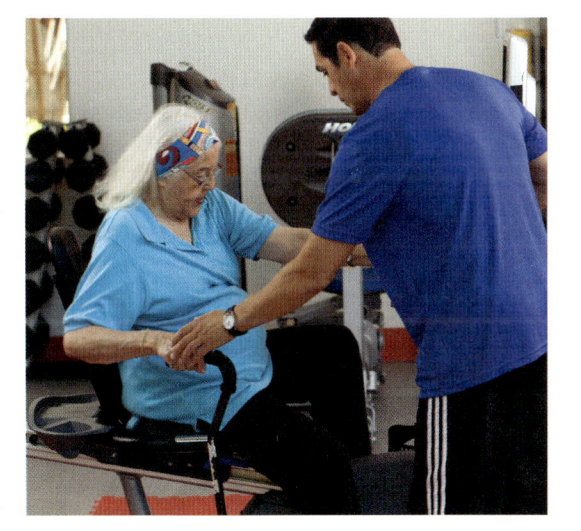

Calcium Channel Blockers

Calcium channel blockers prevent calcium from entering the cardiac and vascular smooth muscle cells. This in turn causes a decrease in cardiac contractility, a decrease in conduction of the electrical signal that controls HR, and a decrease in peripheral blood vessel vasoconstriction. The BP-lowering action of calcium channel blockers is therefore twofold, in that they reduce both cardiac output (decreased SV and HR) and peripheral vascular resistance (decreased vasoconstriction). However, some types of calcium channel blockers have a greater effect on the heart and others have a greater effect on the peripheral blood vessels.

In relation to exercise training, similar to beta blockers, these drugs cause HR to be slowed (**bradycardia**) and can cause a substantial drop in BP upon standing. Clients taking these drugs should be advised to use RPE to monitor exercise intensity instead of a target HR, prolong the cool-down, and change body positions slowly.

Centrally Acting Alpha 2 Agonists

Centrally acting alpha 2 agonists work in the BP control centers in the brain to reset and lower the BP set point; this reduces sympathetic activity to the heart and increases parasympathetic activity, resulting in a slowing of the HR. In addition, the reduction in sympathetic activity to the peripheral blood vessels and kidneys decreases vasoconstriction and the release of renin, resulting in decreased peripheral vascular resistance.

This class of antihypertensive drugs is rarely used in cases of essential HTN. They have several side effects, including severe sedation. Orthostatic hypotension is also common with centrally acting alpha 2 agonists, so caution should be used when changing body positions if clients are taking this class of antihypertensive drugs.

Peripheral Vasodilators

These drugs cause vasodilation and reduce BP by relaxing the vascular smooth muscle in the peripheral blood vessels. Typically, peripheral vasodilators are only used in combination with other antihypertensive drugs in cases of resistant HTN or a hypertensive crisis.

Surgical Treatment

There is no surgical treatment option for essential HTN. In cases of secondary HTN (see Table 9-1), surgery can be used to correct the underlying cause of HTN. For example, renal artery stenosis decreases blood flow to the kidney. This condition occurs as a result of congenital defects in the renal artery or as a result of **atherosclerosis.** BP can return to normal if the blockage can be surgically repaired or through removal of the affected kidney.

Another cause of secondary HTN is an epinephrine-secreting tumor on the adrenal gland called a **pheochromocytoma.** The excess epinephrine caused by the tumor increases HR and contractility to increase cardiac output. Treatment for this condition includes surgical removal of the tumor, which normally corrects the HTN.

Exercise Treatment

For the CMES, it is important that clients have appropriate medical clearance from their healthcare providers when necessary prior to beginning an exercise program or increasing the intensity of an existing exercise program. Incorporation of exercise and a healthy lifestyle is a cornerstone therapy in the treatment of HTN. However, proper medical clearance may be necessary to ensure that exercise is appropriate and will not lead to potential cardiovascular events in unstable hypertensive clients. After a diagnosis of HTN is made, further medical evaluation may be necessary to assess lifestyle, identify other cardiovascular risk factors, and reveal potential identifiable causes of HTN (see Table 9-1). Medical evaluation is also necessary to assess the presence or absence of target organ damage and CVD. In addition to a thorough physical examination, the following routine laboratory tests are recommended:

- An electrocardiogram to assess rate, rhythm, and structural changes in the heart

- Fasting blood glucose measurements to examine the presence or absence of diabetes
- Serum potassium, creatinine, or other measure of glomerular filtration rate to assess kidney function
- A lipid profile that includes the breakdown of high- and low-density lipoprotein concentrations

These laboratory tests help to identify additional risk factors for CVD and potential contributing factors to HTN. If warranted, clinicians may want clients to undergo supervised exercise testing to ensure that it is safe for them to engage in a regular exercise program. Furthermore, these tests are helpful for clinicians to prescribe the appropriate individualized pharmacological and non-pharmacological treatments for HTN. Table 9-6 lists the major cardiovascular risk factors and associated diseases caused by HTN-induced target organ damage.

Aerobic exercise training is a cornerstone in the prevention and treatment of HTN. Exercise training induces many physiological adaptations that lower BP both acutely and chronically. In uncomplicated cases of elevated blood pressure or HTN, aerobic exercise training along with dietary modification may be sufficient to lower BP to reach the target BP without the addition of pharmacotherapy. In more complicated cases of HTN, the addition of regular aerobic exercise to pharmacotherapy has an additive effect on BP reduction. Exercise training also improves other cardiovascular risk factors, including blood lipoprotein profile, **insulin** sensitivity, and body composition.

Acute Effects of Exercise

Dynamic exercise induces an acute post-exercise reduction in both SBP and DBP. This response is known as **post-exercise hypotension (PEH).** The PEH cardiovascular response is characterized by a reduction in peripheral vascular resistance that is not compensated for by an increase in cardiac output, resulting in a decrease in BP (Anunciação & Polito, 2011). On average, the magnitude of the effect of PEH on BP in hypertensive individuals is approximately 15 and 4 mmHg on SBP and DBP, respectively, and can persist for up to 22 hours following an exercise bout (Pescatello et al., 2004). The PEH response occurs in normotensive and hypertensive men and women of all ages, although the largest reductions in BP occur in hypertensive individuals. This acute exercise-induced reduction in BP is clinically significant. It is unknown whether there is a dose-response effect of exercise duration and intensity on PEH, with longer duration or higher intensity of exercise resulting in a greater reduction in BP. It is known that PEH occurs with relatively short-duration bouts of exercise (as little as three minutes) at low intensities (40% $\dot{V}O_2max$).

TABLE 9-6
CARDIOVASCULAR DISEASE (CVD) RISK FACTORS COMMON IN PATIENTS WITH HYPERTENSION

MODIFIABLE RISK FACTORS*	RELATIVELY FIXED RISK FACTORS†
Current cigarette smoking, secondhand smoking	Chronic kidney disease (CKD)
Diabetes mellitus	Family history
Dyslipidemia/hypercholesterolemia	Increased age
Overweight/obesity	Low socioeconomic/educational status
Physical inactivity/low fitness	Male sex
Unhealthy diet	Obstructive sleep apnea
	Psychosocial stress

*Factors that can be changed and, if changed, may reduce CVD risk.

†Factors that are difficult to change (CKD), low socioeconomic/educational status, obstructive sleep apnea), cannot be changed (family history, increased age, male sex) or, if changed through the use of current intervention techniques, may not reduce CVD risk (psychosocial stress).

Reprinted with permission from Whelton, P.K. et al. (2017). 2017 ACC/AHA/AAPA/ABC/ACPM/AGS/PhA/ASH/ASPC/NMA/PCNA guideline for the prevention, detection, evaluation, and management of high blood pressure in adults: A report of the American College of Cardiology/American Heart Association Task Force on Clinical Practice Guidelines. *Journal f the American College of Cardiology*, Nov 7. pii: S0735-1097 (17) 41519-1.

Chronic Effects of Exercise

In addition to the acute effects of dynamic exercise on post-exercise BP, there are significant long-term (chronic) effects of exercise on BP. Epidemiological studies show that there is an inverse relationship between physical activity and BP. Analysis of studies examining the effects of exercise on BP show that 150 minutes of aerobic exercise weekly reduces SBP by 2 to 6 mmHg (Simons-Morton, 2008a). Furthermore, physical activity lowers BP in all populations studied, with the greatest reductions in BP occurring in hypertensive individuals. It is recommended that all prehypertensive and hypertensive individuals engage in regular moderate-intensity physical activity.

At a minimum, prehypertensive and hypertensive individuals should participate in 90 to 150 minutes of cumulative exercise, such as brisk walking, per week (Whelton et al., 2017). As stated previously, exercise alone is sometimes sufficient to reduce BP in prehypertensive individuals and ward off the manifestation of clinically significant HTN. Furthermore, exercise causes an additional reduction in BP in individuals being treated with antihypertensive medication.

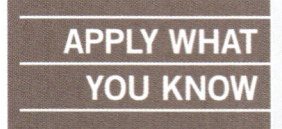

APPLY WHAT YOU KNOW

ORTHOSTATIC HYPOTENSION

Specific safety issues are associated with working with hypertensive clients that a CMES must consider. First, because dynamic exercise does induce a clinically significant drop in BP through PEH, the CMES should remind clients to get up slowly from **supine** and/or seated positions to avoid a sudden drop in BP (orthostatic hypotension). Secondly, many of the drug treatments for HTN limit peripheral vascular vasoconstriction. Therefore, the hypotensive response upon abruptly ceasing exercise may be greater in clients taking these medications. Clients should extend their cool-down periods. If orthostatic hypotension is a chronic problem, clients should be referred to their healthcare providers to have the dosage or class of antihypertensive medication changed.

NUTRITIONAL CONSIDERATIONS

Nutrition plays an important role in the development, treatment, and reversal of HTN. The Academy of Nutrition and Dietetics (A.N.D., 2013) has compiled the most valid scientific research on foods and nutrients that help to improve blood pressure through its Evidence Analysis Library (EAL). While this information is geared toward helping **registered dietitians (RDs)** make evidence-based decisions when providing **medical nutrition therapy,** many of the recommendations are general enough that they can be shared with clients by the CMES. Other resources include the AHA and American College of Cardiology (ACC) guidelines on the lifestyle management to reduce HTN (Eckel et al., 2013) and a large body of evidence supporting the role of the DASH eating plan in improving blood pressure (summarized in Eckel et al., 2013).

Nutrition Guidelines

The EAL advises that individuals with HTN follow several nutrition recommendations, including the following:
- Carefully assess any potential food or nutrient/medication interactions in individuals taking BP-lowering medications. For the CMES, referral to an RD or physician to help clients complete this evaluation is advisable.
- Adopt the DASH eating plan. Details of the DASH eating plan are discussed later in this section. In general, this eating plan is high in vegetables, fruits, and whole grains and low in sodium and saturated and trans fats.
- Limit sodium intake to no more than 2,300 mg per day, and as little as 1,600 mg or less for some individuals.
- Aim to achieve a healthy **body mass index (BMI)** of 18.5 to 24.9 kg/m^2. For individuals who are above a healthy weight, every 22 pounds (10 kg) of weight lost results in a decrease in SBP of 5 to 20 mmHg.

The AHA/ACC recommendations (Whelton et al., 2017) are in alignment with the EAL guidelines, with a few exceptions. The AHA/ACC guidelines advise consuming no more than 1,500 mg per day for most people with HTN. At the least, the organizations advise a 1,000 mg decrease in sodium intake from baseline, even if the goal level of sodium has not been met. This decrease in sodium decreases CVD events by 30% (Eckel et al., 2013). Strong evidence supports this recommendation, showing that in adults aged 25 to 80 years with a blood pressure of 120–159/80–95 mmHg, reducing sodium intake decreases SBP by 2 to 6 mmHg and DBP by 1 to 3 mmHg. Decreasing sodium intake lowers blood pressure across various ages and ethnicities, even those individuals without HTN (Eckel et al., 2013).

The relationship between sodium and blood pressure has been a source of some controversy and conflicting results from scientific studies, with some even suggesting that there is a J-shaped association between sodium intake and CVD risk, indicating that those with the lowest sodium consumption and those with the highest consumption both are at increased risk (Whelton et al., 2012). However, in a 2012 AHA Presidential Advisory, the AHA strongly refuted this research and further emphasized the important role of sodium reduction in achieving and maintaining heart health. The report notes that most U.S. adults consume far more sodium than guideline recommendations or is physiologically needed, mostly due to added sodium with food processing (Whelton et al., 2012).

Nutrients That Affect Blood Pressure

In addition to sodium, the effects of several other nutrients on blood pressure have been studied with mixed results. In most cases, the strength of evidence is too weak to make any definitive conclusions or recommendations. Table 9-7 highlights these foods/nutrients and their effect on blood pressure, if any, based on the evidence to date.

TABLE 9-7
FOODS AND NUTRIENTS PROPOSED TO AFFECT BLOOD PRESSURE

FOOD/NUTRIENT	EFFECT ON BLOOD PRESSURE	STRENGTH OF THE EVIDENCE
Sodium	Increases	Strong
Omega-3 fatty acids	None	Fair
Dietary protein	Unclear	Weak
Soluble fiber	Unclear	Weak
Potassium	If inadequate, may increase	Fair
Vitamin C	Unclear	Weak
Vitamin E	Unclear	Weak
Magnesium	If inadequate, may increase	Fair
Calcium	If inadequate, may increase	Fair
Fruits and vegetables	When at least 5–10 servings per day, decreases	Strong
Soy foods	Unclear	Weak
Garlic	Inconclusive	Weak
Cocoa and chocolate	Inconclusive	Weak
Caffeine	Acute intake increases, effect of chronic intake unclear	Weak
Alcohol	Decreased intake decreases blood pressure	Consensus

Data from: Academy of Nutrition and Dietetics Evidence Analysis Library (2013). *Hypertension Nutrition Evidence Analysis Project.* Retrieved December 4, 2013: http://andevidencelibrary.com/topic.cfm?cat=1405&auth=1

The DASH Eating Plan

The AHA/ACC advise consuming a diet high in vegetables, fruits, and whole grains; including low-fat dairy products, poultry, fish, beans, peas, lentils, nontropical vegetable oils and nuts; and limiting sweets, sugar-sweetened beverages, and red meats. Several eating patterns such as the **Healthy U.S.-Style Dietary Pattern** (*Dietary Guidelines*), AHA Diet, and **Healthy Mediterranean-Style Dietary Pattern** fit this profile; however, the DASH eating plan has been the most studied and has the most profound effects on blood pressure.

The DASH eating plan, while developed to reduce BP, is an overall healthy eating plan that can be adopted by anyone regardless of whether they have elevated BP. In fact, some studies suggest that the DASH eating plan may also reduce CVD risk by lowering total cholesterol and LDL cholesterol in addition to lowering BP (Eckel et al., 2013). The DASH eating plan is low in saturated fat, cholesterol, and total fat. The staples are fruits, vegetables, and low-fat dairy products. Fish, poultry, nuts, and other unsaturated fats as well as whole grains are also encouraged. Consequently, it is rich in potassium, magnesium, calcium, protein, and fiber. Red meat, sweets, and sugar-containing beverages are very limited. The DASH eating plan recommends that men drink 2 or fewer and women drink 1 or fewer alcoholic beverages per day. One drink is equivalent to 12 ounces of beer, 5 ounces of wine, or 1.5 ounces of hard liquor. The DASH eating plan is outlined in Table 9-8.

TABLE 9-8
DASH EATING PLAN BY CALORIE LEVEL

THE NUMBER OF DAILY SERVINGS IN A FOOD GROUP VARY DEPENDING ON CALORIC NEEDS*

Food Group[†]	1,200 calories	1,400 calories	1,600 calories	1,800 calories	2,000 calories	2,600 calories	3,100 calories	Serving Sizes
Grains	4–5	5–6	6	6	6–8	10–11	12–13	1 slice bread 1 oz dry cereal[‡] ½ cup cooked rice, pasta, or cereal[‡]
Vegetables	3–4	3–4	3–4	4–5	4–5	5–6	6	1 cup raw leafy vegetable ½ cup cut-up raw or cooked vegetable ½ cup vegetable juice
Fruits	3–4	4	4	4–5	4–5	5–6	6	1 medium fruit ¼ cup dried fruit ½ cup fresh, frozen, or canned fruit ½ cup fruit juice
Fat-free or low-fat milk and milk products	2–3	2–3	2–3	2–3	2–3	3	3–4	1 cup milk or yogurt 1½ oz cheese
Lean meats, poultry, and fish	3 or less	3–4 or less	3–4 or less	6 or less	6 or less	6 or less	6–9	1 oz cooked meats, poultry, or fish 1 egg
Nuts, seeds, and legumes	3 per week	3 per week	3–4 per week	4 per week	4–5 per week	1	1	⅓ cup or 1½ oz nuts 2 Tbsp peanut butter 2 Tbsp or ½ oz seeds ½ cup cooked legumes (dried beans, peas)

Hypertension CHAPTER 9

TABLE 9-8 *(continued)*

Fats and oils	1	1	2	2–3	2–3	3	4	1 tsp soft margarine 1 tsp vegetable oil 1 Tbsp mayonnaise 1 Tbsp salad dressing
Sweets and added sugars	3 or less per week	3 or less per week	3 or less per week	5 or less per week	5 or less per week	≤2	≤2	1 Tbsp sugar 1 Tbsp jelly or jam ½ cup sorbet, gelatin dessert 1 cup lemonade
Maximum sodium limit**	2,300 mg/day	2,300 mg/day	2,300 mg/day	2,300 mg/day	2,300 mg/day	2,300 mg/day	2,300 mg/day	

* The DASH eating plan from 1,200 to 1,800 calories meet the nutritional needs of children 4 to 8 years old. Patterns from 1,600 to 3,100 calories meet the nutritional needs of children 9 years and older and adults.

† Significance to DASH eating plan, selection notes, and examples of foods in each food group.

- Grains: Major sources of energy and fiber. Whole grains are recommended for most grain servings as a good source of fiber and nutrients. Examples: Whole-wheat bread and rolls; whole-wheat pasta, English muffin, pita bread, bagel, cereals; grits, oatmeal, brown rice; unsalted pretzels and popcorn.
- Vegetables: Rich sources of potassium, magnesium, and fiber. Examples: Broccoli, carrots, collards, green beans, green peas, kale, lima beans, potatoes, spinach, squash, sweet potatoes, tomatoes.
- Fruits: Important sources of potassium, magnesium, and fiber. Examples: Apples, apricots, bananas, dates, grapes, oranges, grapefruit, grapefruit juice, mangoes, melons, peaches, pineapples, raisins, strawberries, tangerines.
- Fat-free or low-fat milk and milk products: Major sources of calcium and protein. Examples: Fat-free milk or buttermilk; fat-free, low-fat, or reduced-fat cheese; fat-free/low-fat regular or frozen yogurt.
- Lean meats, poultry, and fish: Rich sources of protein and magnesium. Select only lean; trim away visible fats; broil, roast, or poach; remove skin from poultry. Since eggs are high in cholesterol, limit egg yolk intake to no more than four per week; two egg whites have the same protein content as 1 oz meat.
- Nuts, seeds, and legumes: Rich sources of energy, magnesium, protein, and fiber. Examples: Almonds, filberts, mixed nuts, peanuts, walnuts, sunflower seeds, peanut butter, kidney beans, lentils, split peas.
- Fats and oils: DASH study had 27% of calories as fat, including fat in or added to foods. Fat content changes serving amount for fats and oils. For example, 1 Tbsp regular salad dressing = one serving; 2 Tbsp low-fat dressing = one serving; 1 Tbsp fat-free dressing = zero servings. Examples: Soft margarine, vegetable oil (canola, corn, olive, safflower), low-fat mayonnaise, light salad dressing.
- Sweets and added sugars: Sweets should be low in fat. Examples: Fruit-flavored gelatin, fruit punch, hard candy, jelly, maple syrup, sorbet and ices, sugar.

‡ Serving sizes vary between ½ cup and 1¼ cups, depending on cereal type. Check product's Nutrition Facts label.

** The DASH Eating Plan consists of patterns with a sodium limit of 2,300 mg and 1,500 mg per day.

Source: National Heart, Lung, and Blood Institute (2021). *DASH Eating Plan.* www.nhlbi.nih.gov/health-topics/dash-eating-plan

The DASH eating plan lowers SBP by about 3 to 11 mmHg in adults with and without hypertension. This effect on BP holds true across ages, gender, and ethnicity and is especially effective in black persons (Whelton et al., 2017).

Several variations of the DASH eating plan have been studied, with even more pronounced results. For example, when 10% of calories from carbohydrates were replaced with an equal number of calories from protein or unsaturated fat, SBP decreased by an additional 1 mmHg compared to the standard eating plan in both hypertensive and nonhypertensive individuals. When looking at only hypertensive individuals, SBP decreases by 3 mmHg compared to the standard DASH eating plan (Eckel et al., 2013).

EXERCISE RECOMMENDATIONS

Unequivocally, regular physical activity and exercise training are associated with a lower incidence of CVD. In broad survey-based epidemiological studies, there is a negative association between exercise training and the development of HTN. Individuals with the highest levels of physical activity or who participate in vigorous sporting activities show the lowest incidence of HTN. Furthermore, a higher fitness level is also associated with a lower risk for developing HTN. People with a low fitness level have a higher relative risk of developing HTN compared with highly fit people (Pal, Radavelli-Bagatini, & Ho, 2013).

While exercise training is pivotal for the prevention and treatment of HTN, HTN is a multifaceted pathology and is caused by an interaction of genes and environmental factors. There are certain populations with a strong genetic propensity for HTN, and exercise training may delay the onset of HTN and/or decrease the severity of the disease.

Cardiovascular Responses to Aerobic Exercise Training

There are many cardiovascular adaptations that cause a reduction in BP as a result of exercise training. Many of these adaptations positively affect BP both at rest and during acute bouts of exercise. An examination of the determinants of mean arterial pressure reveals that for BP to be reduced, a decrease in either cardiac output or total peripheral resistance must occur. With exercise training, there are alterations in the determinants of cardiac output, but the primary mechanism for the decrease in BP is through a decrease in peripheral vascular resistance. The BP-lowering effects of exercise training occur as a result of changes to the systems that integratively control BP.

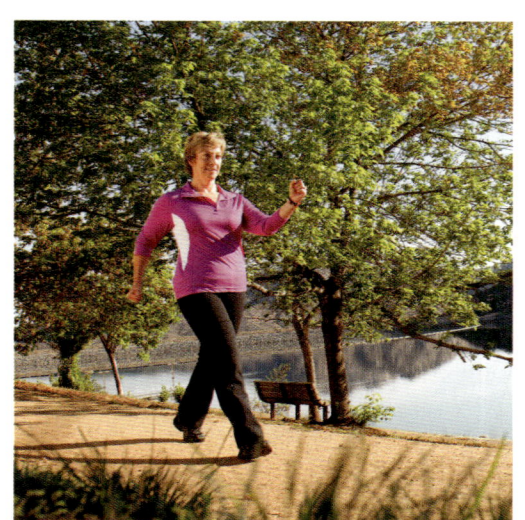

Changes to the Sympathetic Nervous System

One of the changes that occur as a result of exercise training takes place in the sympathetic nervous system. Essential HTN is associated with an increase in the nerve traffic from the sympathetic nervous system to the heart and the peripheral blood vessels. In general, there is a decrease in sympathetic nerve traffic with exercise training. Some studies have shown that direct measures of sympathetic nerve traffic at rest decrease after exercise training, though not all studies have been able to consistently replicate this finding (Dick et al., 2010).

An additional way to indirectly measure globalized systemic changes in sympathetic nerve activity is to measure the concentration of norepinephrine (the sympathetic adrenergic neurotransmitter) in the blood. Recall that the sympathetic nerves release norepinephrine, which binds to receptors on blood vessels and causes the peripheral blood vessels to vasoconstrict. Measuring the amount of norepinephrine in the blood is an indirect assessment of sympathetic nerve activity, because the absolute concentration is influenced by how much norepinephrine is released and how well it is cleared. In individuals with HTN, norepinephrine concentration in the blood has been shown to decrease after exercise training (Edwards et al., 2011).

Changes to the Renin-Angiotensin-Aldosterone System

The RAAS is involved in the long-term regulation of BP. It would be expected that changes to this system would contribute to the reduction in BP observed with exercise training. Decreases in renin and angiotensin II are observed in normotensive individuals after exercise training and contribute to the reduction in BP. However, this response is not observed in hypertensive subjects after exercise training (Pescatello et al., 2004).

Changes to the Peripheral Blood Vessels

One prominent change induced by exercise training in hypertensive individuals takes place in the peripheral blood vessels. Exercise training reduces the amount of vasoconstriction that occurs when norepinephrine binds to the receptors on the blood vessels. In addition, there are changes in the locally produced vasoconstrictors and vasodilators in the blood vessels. The two most prominent changes are to a vasoconstrictor called endothelin 1 and the vasodilator nitric oxide. After exercise training, endothelin 1 is reduced and nitric oxide is increased (Pescatello et al., 2004). Long-term exercise training can also cause beneficial adaptations of the structure of the blood vessels themselves, increasing their elasticity. Together, reduced responsiveness to norepinephrine, decreased endothelin 1, increased nitric oxide, and structural adaptations in the blood vessels result in decreased vascular resistance and contribute to the reduction in BP.

Finally, just as there is a complex interaction among genetic and environmental factors in the development of HTN, there is significant variation in the response to exercise training. Certain genetic profiles may respond more favorably to exercise training. It has been suggested that genetic factors can explain some of the reduction in SBP after exercise training (Pescatello et al., 2004).

HYPERTENSION AND THERMOREGULATION

EXPAND YOUR KNOWLEDGE

Individuals with HTN have a diminished ability to dissipate body heat to the environment during heat stress (Charkoudian, 2010). Thermal heat stress occurs during exercise, passive exposure to hot and humid environments, or the combination that comes with exercising in the heat. The normal physiological response to rising body core temperature during heat stress includes activation of the sympathetic nervous system, which causes an integrated cardiovascular response in an effort to increase blood flow to the skin for **thermoregulation.** Increased skin blood flow allows warm blood from the body core to flow through the cooler skin circulation, where heat is lost through convection. In addition, the evaporation of sweat from the skin cools the skin and serves as a major avenue of heat loss. The integrated cardiovascular response to heat stress includes an increase in HR and cardiac contractility, which together increase cardiac output and vasoconstriction in the renal and the splanchnic circulations, thereby allowing the redistribution of blood flow to the skin (Charkoudian, 2010).

Heat stress significantly challenges the cardiovascular system, especially in individuals with cardiovascular pathologies like HTN. Most heat-related injuries and deaths occur in individuals with cardiovascular pathology (Ye et al., 2012; McGeehin & Mirabelli, 2001). There are several underlying factors contributing to this increased risk, including impairments in the cardiovascular response to heat stress directly caused by the hypertensive disease, as well as the inability of the cardiovascular system to respond appropriately during heat stress caused by the pharmacology used to treat HTN.

Hypertensive individuals have a reduction in skin blood flow during heat stress, which results in a decreased ability to transfer body heat to the environment (Charkoudian, 2010) and a significant increase in body core temperature. This significant reduction in skin blood flow in hypertensive individuals is related to structural alteration in the skin blood vessels and to changes in the locally produced signaling molecules in the skin that allow the skin blood vessels to vasodilate during heat stress (Holowatz & Kenney, 2007). In hypertensive individuals, the increase in cardiac work during heat stress is especially dangerous in individuals with cardiac or other end organ damage (left ventricular hypertrophy or coronary artery disease).

In addition to the HTN-induced physiological changes that occur with heat stress, many of the pharmacological treatments for HTN also blunt the integrated cardiovascular response to heat stress. It should be noted that diuretics, vasodilators, and beta blockers may significantly reduce heat tolerance when combined with exercise and warm ambient conditions (Glen et al., 2010). Diuretics decrease plasma volume. Individuals taking diuretics can easily become dehydrated during heat stress, and dehydration alone decreases blood flow to the skin and impairs thermoregulation. Other drugs that adversely affect the cardiovascular response to heat stress include beta blockers, calcium channel blockers, and alpha blockers. These drugs impair the central cardiovascular and peripheral blood flow responses that occur during heat stress.

Exercise training has beneficial thermoregulatory effects in hypertensive individuals. Exercise training sufficient to increase $\dot{V}O_2$max strengthens the central cardiovascular system. The amount of cardiac work during exercise at the same absolute workload will be less after exercise training. In addition, peripheral sweating and blood vessel changes allow individuals to start sweating and vasodilating their skin blood vessels at lower body core temperatures. Together, these adaptations confer positive benefits on thermoregulation.

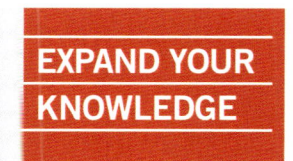

> **THINK IT THROUGH**
>
> Individuals with HTN have many exercise-related issues with which to contend, including orthostatic hypotension, impaired thermoregulation, and medication side effects. If you plan on training clients with HTN, you should have a thorough understanding of how exercise programming will affect those dealing with high BP. How will you address these important concerns with hypertensive clients? For example, will you ensure that the exercise environment is maintained at a relatively cool temperature to reduce the risk of heat illness? Will you plan to educate the client about the importance of hydration and exercise, especially if they are taking a diuretic? Spend some time thinking about how you can communicate your program-specific approaches to a hypertensive client so that they will trust in your professional expertise.

Programming and Progression Guidelines and Considerations

Prior to beginning a new exercise program with a hypertensive client, several important safety issues should be addressed. In normal healthy individuals, the initiation of exercise acutely increases SBP. This acute increase in SBP is normal and necessary to increase blood flow to the exercising muscle to deliver oxygen and clear metabolic by-products. However, some hypertensive individuals experience an exaggerated increase in SBP and/or DBP during dynamic exercise, which is predictive of future morbidity from CVD. Depending on the initial resting BP and whether the client has target organ damage or additional cardiovascular risk factors, a medically supervised exercise-tolerance test should be conducted. Furthermore, these high-risk clients may benefit from a medically supervised cardiac rehabilitation program. Clients may be unaware that they may qualify for such programs.

Table 9-9 lists the general indications set forth by ACSM for terminating exercise. A relative contraindication to exercise is if resting SBP is >200 mmHg or if DBP is >110 mmHg.

Exercise programming guidelines following the FITT principle (frequency, intensity, time, and type) are suitable for individuals with HTN. Dynamic endurance training, dynamic resistance training, and combined training (i.e., programs including both endurance and

TABLE 9-9

GENERAL INDICATIONS FOR STOPPING AN EXERCISE TEST*

Onset of angina or angina-like symptoms	Failure of HR to increase with increased exercise intensity
Drop in SBP of ≥10 mmHg with an increase in work rate or if SBP decreases below the value obtained in the same position prior to testing	Noticeable change in heart rhythm by palpation or auscultation
Excessive rise in BP: SBP >250 mmHg and/or DBP >115 mmHg	Subject requests to stop
Shortness of breath, wheezing, leg cramps, or claudication	Physical or verbal manifestations of severe fatigue
Signs of poor perfusion: lightheadedness, confusion, ataxia, pallor, cyanosis, nausea, or cold and clammy skin	Failure of the testing equipment

*Assumes that testing is nondiagnostic and is being performed without direct physician involvement or ECG monitoring.

Note: SBP = Systolic blood pressure; BP = Blood pressure; DBP = Diastolic blood pressure; HR = Heart rate; ECG = Electrocardiogram

Reprinted with permission of American College of Sports Medicine (2022). *ACSM's Guidelines for Exercise Testing and Prescription* (11th ed.). Philadelphia: Wolters Kluwer.

Hypertension

resistance training) have each been associated with decreases in SBP and DBP (Cornelissen & Smart, 2013). The AHA and the ACC have reported that among adults at all BP levels, including individuals with HTN, interventions shown to be effective for lowering BP include aerobic physical activity of, on average, 90 to 150 minutes per week at 65 to 75% of HRR (Whelton et al., 2017).

Cardiorespiratory Training

To a certain extent, the dose of exercise needed to observe a reduction in BP is related to initial fitness level. In sedentary individuals, clinically significant reductions in BP can be observed with relatively modest increases in physical activity. Researchers have found that significant reductions in resting SBP and DBP can occur with as little as 60 minutes of exercise at an intensity of approximately 50% of $\dot{V}O_2max$ per week (Ishikawa-Takata, Ohta, & Tanaka, 2003). There is an even greater reduction when the exercise duration is increased to 90 minutes.

Frequency

Studies have consistently shown that training frequencies between three and five days a week will cause a significant reduction in BP. However, increasing the frequency of exercise training to most days of the week may confer additional BP-lowering benefits for hypertensive individuals. These additional benefits are likely due to the acute BP-lowering effects of exercise (i.e., post-exercise hypotension).

Intensity

The intensity of aerobic exercise for hypertensive clients should be moderate (ACSM, 2022). Significant reductions in BP are observed with exercise intensities between 40 and 70% of $\dot{V}O_2max$. Exercise intensities higher than 70% of $\dot{V}O_2max$ do not cause greater reductions in BP and may in fact blunt the BP-lowering effect of exercise (Hagberg, Park, & Brown, 2000). Thus, hypertensive clients experience the beneficial effects of exercise at an intensity of 40 to 59% of $\dot{V}O_2reserve$. This exercise intensity corresponds to a rating of approximately 12 to 13 on the Borg RPE scale (6 to 20 scale). Using the RPE scale to gauge exercise intensity is beneficial, especially when clients are taking antihypertensive medications that alter the cardiovascular responses to exercise (e.g., beta blockers).

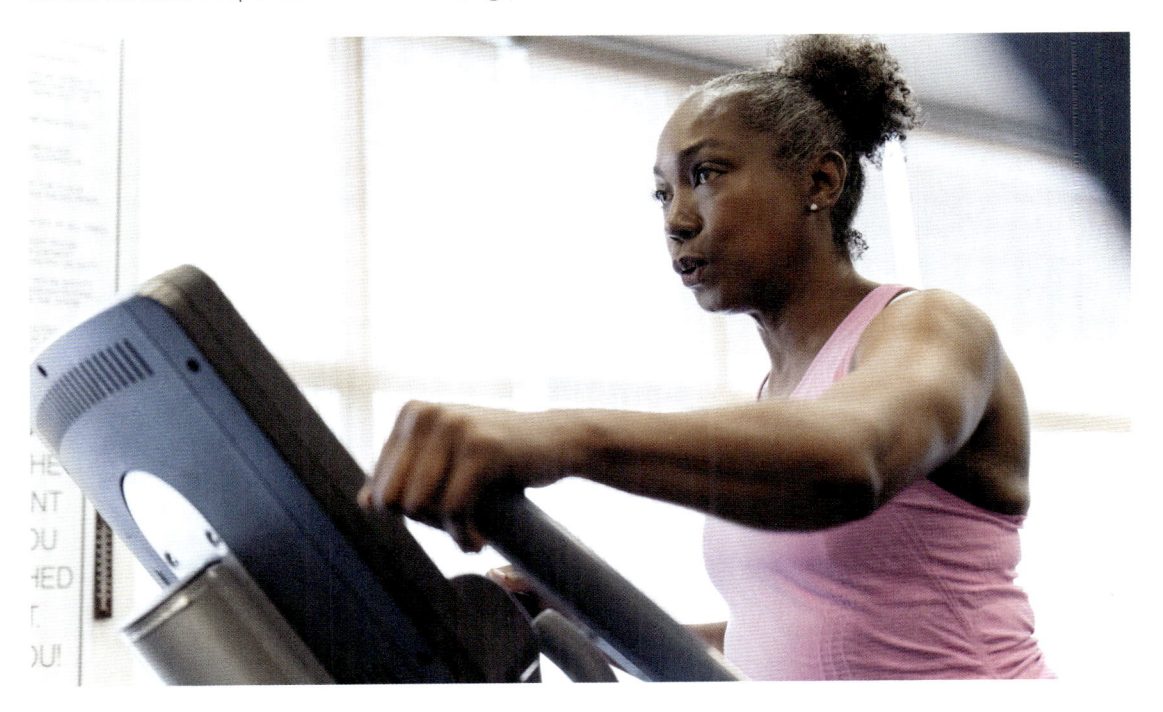

Time

The duration of daily exercise should be at least 30 minutes to have a beneficial effect on cardiovascular health. This 30-minute duration can be continuous or intermittent, as any amount of exercise contributes to the health benefits associated with the accumulated volume of activity. This can also be expressed in terms of calories burned (700 kcal/week is a good initial goal, progressing to 2,000 kcal/week).

Type

Prolonged, rhythmic aerobic endurance-type exercise such as walking, jogging, running, swimming, and cycling is recommended. Walking is one of the easiest exercise modalities to start with, especially in previously sedentary clients. Any physical activity that engages the large muscle groups and is rhythmic and aerobic will be beneficial. The type of exercise performed should be individualized so that clients do what they enjoy and are more likely to adhere to their programs. Thus, the exercises should be relatively simple and offer some variety.

Progression

The progression of exercise training in clients with hypertension can follow the same basic principles of progression as those for healthy adults, as long as it is gradual and avoids any large increases in any of the FITT components, especially intensity (ACSM, 2022). The program should be tailored to the client's initial fitness level and to attain the client's specific fitness goals. In general, clients with hypertension should progress to exercising five to seven days per week, for 30 minutes or more, at an intensity of 40 to 59% of $\dot{V}O_2$ reserve. The initial conditioning stage should include a moderate level of aerobic exercise that causes minimal muscle soreness or discomfort. For clients with hypertension, this may include walking for two 10-minute bouts twice a week (Simons-Morton, 2008b). This stage may last up to four weeks depending on the adaptation of the individual to the training program. The duration of an exercise session during this initial stage may begin at 15 to 20 minutes and progress to 30 minutes five to seven days per week. During the improvement stage, the intensity of exercise is progressively increased every two to three weeks until the client is able to exercise at a moderate intensity for 20 to 30 minutes. During the maintenance stage, the exercise frequency, intensity, and time are maintained while program goals are reviewed and new goals are set.

Resistance Training

There has been significant controversy surrounding the safety of resistance training for hypertensive clients. During **isometric** resistance exercise, both SBP and DBP increase. The magnitude of the increase in BP with resistance exercise is related to the intensity of exercise and the amount of muscle mass involved. This increase in BP is potentially dangerous for hypertensive clients because heavy resistance training can cause large increases in both SBP and DBP. In general, moderate resistance training is beneficial and safe for this population, as long as the HTN is controlled. According to the guidelines from the AHA, resistance training is contraindicated in individuals with unstable **angina** (chest pain), uncontrolled HTN (systolic BP ≥160 mmHg and/or diastolic BP ≥100 mmHg), uncontrolled cardiac arrhythmias, a recent history of **congestive heart failure**, significant heart valve disease, or pathological enlargement of the heart (**hypertrophic cardiomyopathy**) (Braith & Stewart, 2006). While aerobic exercise is the mainstay in the treatment of HTN, it can be safely supplemented with resistance training.

Resistance training offers several beneficial physiological effects. It increases muscular strength, endurance, and mass. The increase in muscle mass causes an increased **basal metabolic rate (BMR).** Perhaps one of the most beneficial effects of resistance training on BP results from the positive effects on insulin sensitivity. There is a significant link between decreased insulin sensitivity and HTN. Because consistent and long-term resistance training increases insulin sensitivity, this may be one of the mechanisms mediating the reduction in BP. Resistance training also attenuates the **rate-pressure product** (an index of cardiac work) when lifting any given load, which decreases the demand on the heart when performing **activities of daily living (ADL)** and various work- and recreation-related tasks:

Rate-pressure product = Heart rate x Systolic blood pressure

In addition, resistance training is beneficial for the prevention and management of other chronic conditions, such as low-back pain, **osteoporosis, obesity, sarcopenia** (the loss of skeletal muscle mass that may accompany aging), and diabetes, as well as the susceptibility to falls. Resistance training of the major muscle groups decreases resting SBP and DBP in hypertensive individuals by approximately 3 mmHg (Braith & Stewart, 2006). In studies examining different types of resistance training (circuit training vs. conventional), no difference in BP reduction was found among modalities. However, because circuit training uses lighter weights with limited rest periods between exercises, thereby introducing an aerobic component, it is the type of resistance training recommended for hypertensive clients.

A preliminary orientation with clients should establish appropriate weight loads, and the CMES should instruct the client on proper lifting techniques and correct breathing patterns to avoid straining or performing the **Valsalva maneuver.** Straining during resistance training causes significant and potentially dangerous increases in BP.

SAMPLE RESISTANCE-TRAINING PROGRAM

At minimum, clients with HTN should perform one exercise per major muscle group. For example, a resistance-training program for a hypertensive client might include eight to 12 repetitions of the following exercises performed two to three days per week:

- Chest press
- Seated row
- Shoulder press
- Lower-back extension
- Triceps extension
- Biceps curl
- Abdominal crunch/curl-up
- Quadriceps extension or leg press
- Leg curls (hamstrings)
- Heel raises

Older or frailer clients should initially perform 10 to 15 repetitions at a lower relative resistance to prevent injury. The CMES can slowly increase the number of sets until clients are performing three sets two to three days per week.

MIND-BODY EXERCISE

Mind-body exercises such as **yoga** and **tai chi** are increasingly being incorporated into exercise training programs to promote flexibility, strength, and relaxation. There are few randomized controlled studies examining the effects of these alternative exercise programs specifically on high BP. The few studies that have been conducted suggest a beneficial reduction in BP attributable to both physical activity and relaxation (La Forge, 2014; Santaella et al., 2006).

Randomized clinical studies on the effects of **hatha yoga** on BP demonstrate a large reduction in SBP with regular yoga therapy. These studies showed a 33 mmHg and 26 mmHg reduction in SBP after practicing yoga and biofeedback, respectively, for six hours a week for 11 weeks (Murugesan, Govindarajulu, & Bera, 2000; Patel & North, 1975). The combined effects on BP of physical activity and relaxation, as practiced through mind-body exercise, appear to be synergistic, meaning that the combined effect is greater than the individual BP-lowering capabilities of either physical activity or relaxation alone (Cohen & Townsend, 2007). More recently, investigators reviewed the available research on yoga's effects on BP among individuals with elevated blood pressure or HTN. Overall, the practice of yoga was associated with a significant reduction in BP (~4 mmHg, SBP and DBP) in this population (Hagins et al., 2013). Mind-body exercise practiced regularly (three times per week for 60 minutes) also improves balance and upper- and lower-body muscular strength and endurance (Taylor-Piliae et al., 2006). Further, these mind-body exercises improve proprioceptive awareness.

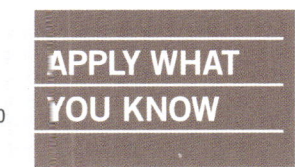

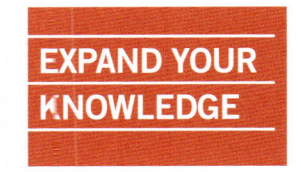

Several general precautions should be used when recommending mind-body exercise to hypertensive clients. First, many styles of hatha yoga involve isometric muscle contractions combined with dynamic movement of the body into different positions. This work should be done with caution, because isometric muscle contractions cause significant increases in BP. In addition, hypertensive clients taking certain antihypertensive medications may experience dramatic decreases in BP when changing body position. Specifically, diuretics, alpha blockers, calcium channel blockers, and beta blockers can cause orthostatic hypotension. Hypertensive clients should avoid holding strenuous poses, avoid inverted poses (e.g., downward-facing dog and shoulder stands), and be encouraged to transition slowly between poses. Caution should be used when practicing yoga with stage I and II hypertensive clients. Bikram yoga (rapidly paced yoga in very hot environments) should be avoided altogether because of the impaired thermoregulatory mechanisms seen in hypertensive clients.

EXERCISE GUIDELINES SUMMARY FOR CLIENTS WITH HYPERTENSION

	CARDIORESPIRATORY TRAINING
Frequency	• Most, but preferably all, days of the week
Intensity	• Intensity may be determined through the following methods: ✓ 40–59% HRR or $\dot{V}O_2R$ ✓ RPE of 12–13 (6–20 scale) ✓ Below VT1 HR; can talk comfortably
Time	• Eventual goal of at least 30 minutes of continuous or accumulated exercise • Bouts of any length contribute to the health benefits linked with the accumulated volume
Type	• Emphasis should be placed on rhythmic, large-muscle-group activities: ✓ Walking ✓ Jogging ✓ Cycling ✓ Swimming
Progression	• Progress following the ACE Integrated Fitness Training Model based on client goals and availability. • Progression should be personalized dependent on tolerance, client goals, and consideration of the following factors: ✓ Recent changes in antihypertensive drug therapy ✓ Medication-related adverse effects ✓ The presence of target-organ disease and/or other comorbidities ✓ Level of blood pressure control ✓ Age
	MUSCULAR TRAINING
Frequency	• At least 2–3 days per week with a minimum of 48 hours separating exercise for the same muscle group
Intensity	• 60–80% 1-RM • 40–50% 1-RM for older adults and novice exercisers
Time	• 2–4 sets of 8–12 repetitions • Each major muscle group should be trained. • Session duration should be a minimum of 20 minutes
Type	• Machines, free weights, resistance bands, and body-weight exercises • Avoid the Valsalva maneuver during resistance training.
Progression	• Progress following the ACE Integrated Fitness Training Model based on client goals and availability.

Note: HRR = Heart-rate reserve; $\dot{V}O_2R$ = Oxygen uptake reserve; RPE = Rating of perceived exertion; VT1 = First ventilatory threshold; HR = Heart rate; 1-RM = One-repetition maximum

CMES FOCUS

Evolving research suggests that dynamic muscular training confers a similar or greater reduction in blood pressure compared to those experienced during cardiorespiratory exercise. For this reason, emphasis should not be placed on cardiorespiratory exercise alone, but rather on multimodal training programs that take client preferences into consideration. Cardiorespiratory and muscular training may be combined (concurrent exercise) or each training type can be completed separately. The CMES must consider the blood-pressure response to exercise, optimize the benefit-to-risk ratio when making decisions about exercise intensity, and focus on caloric expenditure to facilitate weight reduction. Thus, exercise programs will be highly individualized and dependent on the client's unique needs and exercise tolerance.

Source: American College of Sports Medicine (2022). *ACSM's Guidelines for Exercise Testing and Prescription* (11th ed.). Philadelphia: Wolters Kluwer.

CASE STUDIES

Case Study 1

Client Information

Edith is a 45-year-old woman who would like to start an exercise program to lose weight. She is 5'4" tall (1.6 m) and weighs 150 pounds (68 kg). Her physician has also told her that she has high total cholesterol, with an HDL cholesterol of 68 mg/dL and an LDL cholesterol of 140 mg/dL. She has been diagnosed with HTN in the past, but admits that she gets very nervous when she visits her doctor's office. She is currently not involved in a regular exercise program but is motivated to start an exercise program to lose weight. Edith's diet is high in total calories, saturated fat, cholesterol, and sodium and low in fruits, vegetables, and fiber. After being seated in a quiet consulting room with both feet on the floor for five minutes, her resting BP is 138/86 mmHg. After an additional five minutes of sitting quietly, her BP drops to 130/82 mmHg. Edith's BMI is 26.6 kg/m^2 [68 kg ÷ (1.6 m)^2].

CMES Approach

Edith has been diagnosed with HTN in the past. However, her current BP measurements indicate that she is within the elevated range, as her readings fall within the 120 to 129 SBP and less than 80 DBP mmHg range. Edith should begin with a cardiorespiratory training following the basic principles of an initial conditioning stage, an improvement stage, and a maintenance stage. In general, she should progress to exercising five to seven days per week, for 30 minutes or more, at an intensity of 40 to 59% of $\dot{V}O_2R$. The initial conditioning stage should include a moderate level of aerobic exercise that causes minimal muscle soreness or discomfort. This stage may last up to four weeks, depending on her adaptation to the training program. The duration of an exercise session during this initial stage may begin at 15 to 20 minutes and progress to 30 minutes five to seven days per week. During the improvement stage, the intensity of exercise is progressively increased every two to three weeks until Edith is able to exercise at a moderate intensity for 20 to 30 minutes. During the maintenance stage, the exercise frequency, intensity, and time are maintained while program goals are reviewed and new goals are set.

In general, moderate resistance training should be safe for Edith, as long as her HTN is controlled. While cardiorespiratory exercise is the mainstay in the treatment of HTN, it can be safely supplemented with resistance training. Circuit training using lighter

ACE IFT® MODEL AT A GLANCE

Cardiorespiratory Training

This client is beginning in the Base Training phase, where the program focus is on moving more consistently and establishing basic cardiorespiratory endurance. As she progresses exercise duration to 20 minutes or more, and exercise intensity to at and above VT1, she would be advancing to Fitness Training.

Muscular Training

Circuit training with lighter weights and limited recovery periods, with a focus on proper movement patterns and exercise techniques, would be part of Movement Training. A circuit-training program of this nature should be introduced only after the client has demonstrated postural stability and kinetic-chain mobility and can perform movement patterns without compromising postural or joint stability.

weights with limited rest periods between exercises would be an appropriate initial resistance-training program for this client, providing an additional moderate-intensity exercise component to her workouts. However, she should be instructed on proper movement patterns and exercise techniques and correct breathing patterns to avoid straining or performing the Valsalva maneuver. Additionally, mind-body exercises such as yoga and tai chi may be incorporated into Edith's exercise training program to promote flexibility, strength, and relaxation.

Edith can make the following lifestyle modifications (in addition to her exercise program) to help control her BP:
- Weight reduction of as little as 10 pounds (4.5 kg)
- Limiting dietary sodium intake to less than 2,300 mg per day
- Adopting a healthy eating plan that includes fresh fruits and vegetables, low-fat dairy products, and reduced saturated and total fat content (DASH eating plan)
- Avoiding or limiting alcohol consumption to no more than one drink per day

Case Study 2

Client Information

Harry is a 60-year-old man who takes a diuretic and a beta blocker to control his BP. His resting BP with his medication is not very well controlled and today his BP reading is 144/88 mmHg. Harry is relatively healthy, with the exception of his BP, but he does have a strong family history of heart disease (his father died at age 44 from a heart attack). Harry has recently retired from his job and has found that his level of regular physical activity has decreased substantially. Because Harry had a physically demanding job, he has never engaged in a regular exercise program. Harry's age, high BP, family history of heart disease, and current sedentary lifestyle give him four cardiovascular risk factors.

CMES Approach

Harry does not need medical clearance prior to participating in a new low-to-moderate intensity (40 to 59% of $\dot{V}O_2R$) exercise program. It may, however, be beneficial to conduct an exercise test if he plans to engage in vigorous-intensity exercise (≥60% of $\dot{V}O_2R$).

In general, an exercise program for Harry should follow the FITT principle and take place on five to seven days of the week, at a moderate intensity (40 to 59% $\dot{V}O_2R$), and be primarily endurance-type activities. Low-resistance, high-repetition resistance training and mind/body activity such as yoga or Pilates can supplement Harry's regular endurance training. The CMES should be prepared to assess Harry's BP before, during, and after exercise or as recommended by his physician.

ACE IFT® MODEL AT A GLANCE

Cardiorespiratory Training

This client's exercise program should focus initially on Base Training to build cardiorespiratory endurance. Initial progressions would move the client to the upper levels of Base Training until he can perform 20 minutes or more of continuous moderate-intensity exercise, before progressing to Fitness Training.

Muscular Resistance Training

His resistance-training program, using low resistance and high repetitions, should focus first on establishing or reestablishing postural stability and kinetic-chain mobility, and then progress to Movement Training. Load/Speed Training can be introduced as appropriate once the client has demonstrated adequate joint and postural stability and mobility, good movement patterns, and sufficient muscular fitness.

SUMMARY

Exercise is a cornerstone therapy for the treatment and prevention of HTN. Exercise combined with dietary modification can prevent the development of HTN in prehypertensive clients, and can have an additive effect with antihypertensive drugs in reducing BP. Exercise for all hypertensive clients should follow the FITT principle and take place on most, preferably all, days of the week, at a moderate intensity (40 to 59% $\dot{V}O_2R$), and be primarily endurance-type activity. Low-resistance, high-repetition muscular training and mind-body exercise activities can also supplement regular endurance exercise in hypertensive clients.

REFERENCES

Academy of Nutrition and Dietetics Evidence Analysis Library (2013). *Hypertension Nutrition Evidence Analysis Project*. Retrieved December 4, 2013: http://andevidencelibrary.com/topic.cfm?cat=1405&auth=1

American College of Sports Medicine (2022). *ACSM's Guidelines for Exercise Testing and Prescription* (11th ed.). Philadelphia: Wolters Kluwer.

American Heart Association (2011). Heart disease and stroke statistics—2011 update: A report from the American Heart Association. *Circulation,* 123, e18–e209.

Anunciação, P.G. & Polito, M.D. (2011). A review on post-exercise hypotension in hypertensive individuals. *Arquivos Brasileiros de Cardiologia,* 96, e100–e109.

Braith, R.W. & Stewart, K.J. (2006). Resistance exercise training: Its role in the prevention of cardiovascular disease. *Circulation,* 113, 2642–2650.

Centers for Disease Control and Prevention (2020a). *Facts About Hypertension.* www.cdc.gov/bloodpressure/facts.htm

Centers for Disease Control and Prevention (2020b). *5 Surprising Facts About High Blood Pressure.* www.cdc.gov/bloodpressure/5_surprising_facts.htm#:~:text=About%201%20in%203%20U.S.,to%20control%20their%20blood%20pressure.&text=Even%20though%20most%20people%20with,condition%20is%20often%20not%20diagnosed

Charkoudian, N. (2010). Mechanisms and modifiers of reflex induced cutaneous vasodilation and vasoconstriction in humans. *Journal of Applied Physiology,* 109, 4, 1221–1228. DOI: 10.1152/japplphysiol.00298.2010

Cohen, D. & Townsend, R.R. (2007). Yoga and hypertension. *Journal of Clinical Hypertension,* 9, 800–801.

Cornelissen, V.A. & Smart, N.A. (2013). Exercise training for blood pressure: A systematic review and meta-analysis. *Journal of the American Heart Association,* 1, 2, 1, e004473. DOI: 10.1161/JAHA.112.004473

Dick H.J. et al. (2010). Impact of inactivity and exercise on the vasculature in humans. *European Journal of Applied Physiology,* 108, 5, 845–875. DOI: 10.1007/s00421-009-1260-x

Eckel, R.H. et al. (2103). AHA/ACC guideline on lifestyle management to reduce cardiovascular risk: A report of the American College of Cardiology/American Heart Association Task Force on Practice Guidelines. *Journal of the American College of Cardiology,* DOI:10.1016/j.jacc.2013.11.003

Edwards, K.M. et al. (2011). Effects on blood pressure and autonomic nervous system function of a 12-week exercise or exercise plus DASH-diet intervention in individuals with elevated blood pressure. *Acta Physiol (Oxf),* 203, 3, 343–350. DOI: 10.1111/j.1748-1716.2011.02329.x

Fleg, J.L. et al. (2013). Secondary prevention of atherosclerotic cardiovascular disease in older adults: A scientific statement from the American Heart Association. *Circulation,* DOI: 10.1161/01.cir.0000436752.99896.22

Glen, P. et al. (2010). Heat stress in older individuals and patients with common chronic diseases. *Canadian Medical Association Journal,* 13, 182, 10, 1053–1060. DOI: 10.1503/cmaj.081050

Goff, D.C. et al. (2014). ACC/AHA guideline on the assessment of cardiovascular risk: A report of the American College of Cardiology/American Heart Association Task Force on Practice Guidelines. *Circulation,* 129, Suppl. 2, S49–S73.

Hagberg, J.M., Park, J.J., & Brown, M.D. (2000). The role of exercise training in the treatment of hypertension: An update. *Sports Medicine,* 30, 193–206.

Hagins, M. et al. (2013). Effectiveness of yoga for hypertension: Systematic review and meta-analysis. *Evidence-Based Complementary and Alternative Medicine,* Article ID: 649836. DOI: 10.1155/2013/649836

Hesse, C. et al. (2007). Baroreflex sensitivity inversely correlates with ambulatory blood pressure in healthy normotensive humans. *Hypertension,* 50, 41–46.

Holowatz, L.A. & Kenney, W.L. (2007). Up-regulation of arginase activity contributes to attenuated reflex cutaneous vasodilatation in hypertensive humans. *The Journal of Physiology,* 581, 863–872.

Ishikawa-Takata, K., Ohta, T., & Tanaka, H. (2003). How much exercise is required to reduce blood pressure in essential hypertensives: A dose-response study. *American Journal of Hypertension,* 16, 629–633.

Kaplan, N.M. & Victor, R.G. (2014). *Kaplan's Clinical Hypertension* (11th ed.). Philadelphia: Wolters Kluwer/Lippincott Williams & Wilkins.

Kester, M.V. et al. (2007). *Elsevier's Integrated Pharmacology.* Philadelphia: Mosby, Inc.

Kougias, P. et al. (2010). Arterial baroreceptors in the management of systemic hypertension. *Medical Science Monitor,* 16, 1, RA1–RA8.

La Forge, R. (2014). Mind-body exercise In: American Council on Exercise. *ACE Personal Trainer Manual* (5th ed.). San Diego: American Council on Exercise.

McGeehin, M.A. & Mirabelli, M. (2001). The potential impacts of climate variability and change on temperature-related morbidity and mortality in the United States. *Environmental Health Perspectives,* 109, Suppl. 2, 185–189.

Murugesan, R., Govindarajulu, N., & Bera, T.K. (2000). Effect of selected yogic practices on the management of hypertension. *Indian Journal of Physiology and Pharmacology,* 44, 207–210.

National Heart, Lung, and Blood Institute (2021). *DASH Eating Plan.* www.nhlbi.nih.gov/health-topics/dash-eating-plan

Pal, S., Radavelli-Bagatini, S., & Ho, S. (2013). Potential benefits of exercise on blood pressure and vascular function. *Journal of the American Society of Hypertension,* 7, 6, 494–506. DOI: 10.1016/j.jash.2013.07.004

Patel, C. & North, W.R. (1975). Randomised controlled trial of yoga and bio-feedback in management of hypertension. *Lancet,* 2, 93–95.

Pescatello, L.S. et al. (2004). American College of Sports Medicine position stand: Exercise and hypertension. *Medicine & Science in Sports & Exercise,* 36, 533–553.

Ringrose, J. et al. (2017). An assessment of the accuracy of home blood pressure monitors when used in device owners. *American Journal of Hypertension,* 30, 7, 683–689.

Roger, V.L. et al. (2012). Heart disease and stroke statistics – 2012 update: A report from the American Heart Association. *Circulation,* 125, e12–e230.

Santaella, D.F. et al. (2006). Aftereffects of exercise and relaxation on blood pressure. *Clinical Journal of Sports Medicine,* 16, 341–347.

Schmieder, R.E. (2010). End organ damage in hypertension. *Deutsches Arzteblatt International,* 107, 49, 866–873.

Simons-Morton, D.G. (2008a). Physical activity and blood pressure. In: Izzo, J.L. et al. (Eds.) *Hypertension Primer: The Essentials of High Blood Pressure: Basic Science, Population Science, and Clinical Management* (4th ed.). Philadelphia: Lippincott Williams & Williams.

Simons-Morton, D.G. (2008b). Exercise therapy. In: Izzo, J.L. et al. (Eds.) *Hypertension Primer: The Essentials of High Blood Pressure: Basic Science, Population Science, and Clinical Management* (4th ed.). Philadelphia: Lippincott Williams & Williams.

Stone, N.J. et al. (2014). ACC/AHA guideline on the treatment of blood cholesterol to reduce atherosclerotic cardiovascular risk in adults: A report of the American College of Cardiology/American Heart Association Task Force on Practice Guidelines. *Circulation,* 129, Suppl. 2, S1–S45.

Takahashi, H. et al. (2011). The central mechanism underlying hypertension: A review of the roles of sodium ions, epithelial sodium channels, the renin-angiotensin-aldosterone system, oxidative stress and endogenous digitalis in the brain. *Hypertension Research,* 34, 11, 1147–1160.

Taylor-Piliae, R.E. et al. (2006). Improvement in balance, strength, and flexibility after 12 weeks of tai chi exercise in ethnic Chinese adults with cardiovascular disease risk factors. *Alternative Therapies in Health and Medicine,* 12, 50–58.

Weder, A.B. (2008). Genetics of hypertension. In: Izzo, J.L. et al. (Eds.) *Hypertension Primer: The Essentials of High Blood Pressure: Basic Science, Population Science, and Clinical Management* (4th ed.). Philadelphia: Lippincott Williams & Williams.

Whelton, P.K. et al. (2017). 2017 ACC/AHA/AAPA/ABC/ACPM/AGS/ PhA/ASH/ASPC/NMA/PCNA guideline for the prevention, detection, evaluation, and management of high blood pressure in adults: A report of the American College of Cardiology/American Heart Association Task Force on Clinical Practice Guidelines. *Journal of the American College of Cardiology,* Nov 7. pii: S0735-1097 (17) 41519-1.

Whelton, P.K. et al. (2012). Sodium, blood pressure, and cardiovascular disease: Further evidence supporting the American Heart Association sodium reduction recommendations. *Circulation,* 126, 2880–2889.

World Health Organization (2019). *Hypertension.* www.who.int/news-room/fact-sheets/detail/hypertension

Ye, X. et al. (2012). Ambient temperature and morbidity: A review of epidemiological evidence. *Environmental Health Perspectives,* 120, 1, 19–28. DOI: 10.1289/ehp.1003198

SUGGESTED READING

American College of Sports Medicine (2022). *ACSM's Guidelines for Exercise Testing and Prescription* (11th ed.). Philadelphia: Wolters Kluwer.

Cohen, D. & Townsend, R.R. (2007). Yoga and hypertension. *Journal of Clinical Hypertension,* 9, 800–801.

Cornelissen, V.A. & Smart, N.A. (2013). Exercise training for blood pressure: A systematic review and meta-analysis. *Journal of the American Heart Association,* 1, 2, 1, e004473. DOI: 10.1161/JAHA.112.004473

Hagins, M. et al. (2013). Effectiveness of yoga for hypertension: Systematic review and meta-analysis. *Evidence-Based Complementary and Alternative Medicine*, Article ID: 649836. DOI: 10.1155/2013/649836

Pescatello, L.S. et al. (2004). American College of Sports Medicine position stand: Exercise and hypertension. *Medicine & Science in Sports & Exercise*, 36, 533–553.

Whelton, P.K. et al. (2017). 2017 ACC/AHA/AAPA/ABC/ACPM/AGS/ PhA/ASH/ASPC/NMA/PCNA guideline for the prevention, detection, evaluation, and management of high blood pressure in adults: A report of the American College of Cardiology/American Heart Association Task Force on Clinical Practice Guidelines. *Journal of the American College of Cardiology*, Nov 7. pii: S0735-1097 (17) 41519-1.

10 PULMONARY DISEASE: ASTHMA AND CHRONIC OBSTRUCTIVE PULMONARY DISEASE

IN THIS CHAPTER

ASTHMA

EPIDEMIOLOGY

OVERVIEW
ASTHMA TRIGGERS

DIAGNOSTIC TESTING AND CRITERIA
SPIROMETRY
PEAK EXPIRATORY FLOW
ALLERGY TESTING

TREATMENT OPTIONS
EDUCATION
MANAGEMENT OF ASTHMA EXACERBATION

NUTRITIONAL CONSIDERATIONS
NUTRITIONAL CONSIDERATIONS IN THE MANAGEMENT AND TREATMENT OF ASTHMA
NUTRITIONAL CONSIDERATIONS TO MANAGE COMORBIDITIES ASSOCIATED WITH ASTHMA

EXERCISE RECOMMENDATIONS
PULMONARY RESPONSES TO EXERCISE TRAINING
PROGRAMMING AND PROGRESSION GUIDELINES AND CONSIDERATIONS

EXERCISE GUIDELINES SUMMARY FOR CLIENTS WITH ASTHMA

CASE STUDIES

CHRONIC OBSTRUCTIVE PULMONARY DISEASE

EPIDEMIOLOGY

OVERVIEW

DIAGNOSTIC TESTING AND CRITERIA

TREATMENT OPTIONS
IMPROVE QUALITY OF LIFE
REDUCE RISK

NUTRITIONAL CONSIDERATIONS

EXERCISE RECOMMENDATIONS
CARDIOVASCULAR AND PULMONARY RESPONSES TO EXERCISE TRAINING
THE CMES IN THE CONTINUUM OF CARE
PROGRAMMING AND PROGRESSION GUIDELINES AND CONSIDERATIONS
EXERCISE TESTING

EXERCISE GUIDELINES SUMMARY FOR CLIENTS WITH COPD

CASE STUDY

SUMMARY

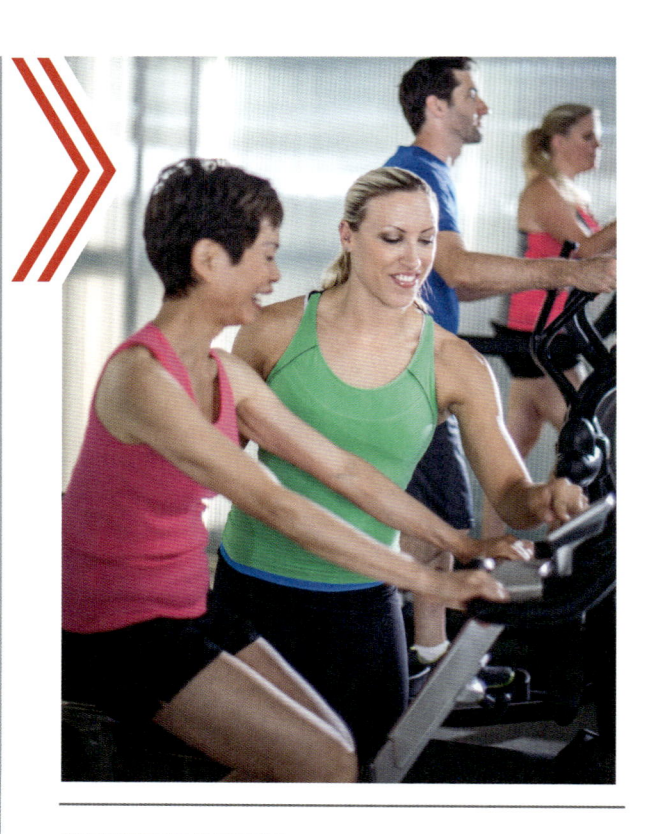

ABOUT THE AUTHOR

Natalie Digate Muth, M.D., M.P.H., R.D., FAAP, is a pediatrician in North County San Diego and ACE Senior Advisor for Healthcare Solutions. She is dual board-certified in pediatrics and obesity medicine and is a Diplomate of the American Board of Obesity Medicine. She also serves on the Executive Committee of the Section on Obesity for the American Academy of Pediatrics. She holds credentials as a registered dietitian, Certified-Specialist in Sports Dietetics, and ACE® Certified Health Coach. She is author of nearly 100 articles, books, and book chapters, including the *ACE Fitness Nutrition Manual* (ACE, 2013), *"Eat Your Vegetables!" and Other Mistakes Parents Make: Redefining How to Raise Healthy Eaters* (Healthy Learning, 2012), the textbook *Sports Nutrition for Allied Health Professionals* (F.A. Davis, 2014), and several chapters in *The Professional's Guide to Health and Wellness Coaching*. She holds a Bachelor of Science degree in Psychology and Physiological Science from UCLA, and a Master of Public Health and Medical Doctor degree from the University of North Carolina-Chapel Hill.

By Natalie Digate Muth

PULMONARY DISORDERS, INCLUDING **ASTHMA** and **chronic obstructive pulmonary disease (COPD)**, are among the most prevalent **chronic** diseases that an ACE® Certified Medical Exercise Specialist (CMES) will encounter. This chapter arms the CMES with the basic knowledge and resources necessary to recommend the highest-quality and safest exercise programs for clients with these pulmonary conditions.

ASTHMA

Asthma is a chronic inflammatory disorder of the airways that causes varying degrees of difficulty breathing, wheezing, coughing, and chest tightness. Asthma affects people differently depending on various genetic and environmental factors, though asthma onset begins in childhood for most people. In some individuals, exercise and physical activity can induce an asthmatic response. However, with appropriate medical management and precautions, most severe exercise-related and non-exercise-related asthma responses can be avoided. Furthermore, in many cases, a well-designed and effectively implemented exercise program can help to minimize asthma symptoms and exacerbations.

EPIDEMIOLOGY

Asthma affects more than 25 million children and adults in the United States [Moorman et al., 2012; National Asthma Education and Prevention Program (NAEPP), 2007]. The disorder is responsible for nearly 500,000 hospitalizations, 2 million emergency room visits, and 3,400 deaths in the United States each year. Among children, boys have higher prevalence than girls (11.1% compared with 7.8%) whereas among adults, men have lower prevalence than women (5.7% compared with 9.7%) (Moorman et al., 2012). Of note, research has established an increased risk for asthma in people with **obesity** (Rasmussen & Hancox, 2013).

OVERVIEW

Asthma is a chronic inflammatory disorder of the airways that affects genetically susceptible individuals in response to various environmental triggers such as **allergens,** viral infections, exercise, cold, and stress. The inflammation leads to narrowing of the airways and **bronchospasm,** making it more difficult to transfer inhaled oxygen through the respiratory system and to the rest of the body. These inflammation-induced airway changes contribute to the severity and frequency of the attacks and are responsible for symptoms such as shortness of breath, wheezing, coughing, and chest tightness. The flow diagram in Figure 10-1 shows the relationships among airway inflammation, airway hyperresponsiveness, airway obstruction, and asthma symptoms. These symptoms are usually worse at night and in the early morning. For some people, chronic inflammation leads to permanent changes in airway structure. Figure 10-2 compares a normal bronchus to an inflamed bronchus.

LEARNING OBJECTIVES:

» Explain the difference between chronic asthma and exercise-induced bronchoconstriction.

» Identify triggers for an asthma episode and explain strategies for avoiding those triggers when possible.

» Briefly describe the diagnostic testing and criteria for asthma and COPD, as well as the available treatment options for both.

» Explain how the use of asthma medications affects the performance of exercise and best practices for administering short-acting asthma medications around the time of exercise.

» Describe nutrition-related strategies for the treatment and management of asthma, asthma-related comorbidities, and COPD.

» Design and implement safe and effective exercise programs for clients with asthma and COPD.

Figure 10-1
Relationships among airway inflammation, airway hyperresponsiveness, airway obstruction, and asthma symptoms

Source: United States Department of Health & Human Services & National Institutes of Health (2003). *Making a Difference in the Management of Asthma: A Guide for Respiratory Therapists.* Pub. No. 02-1064.

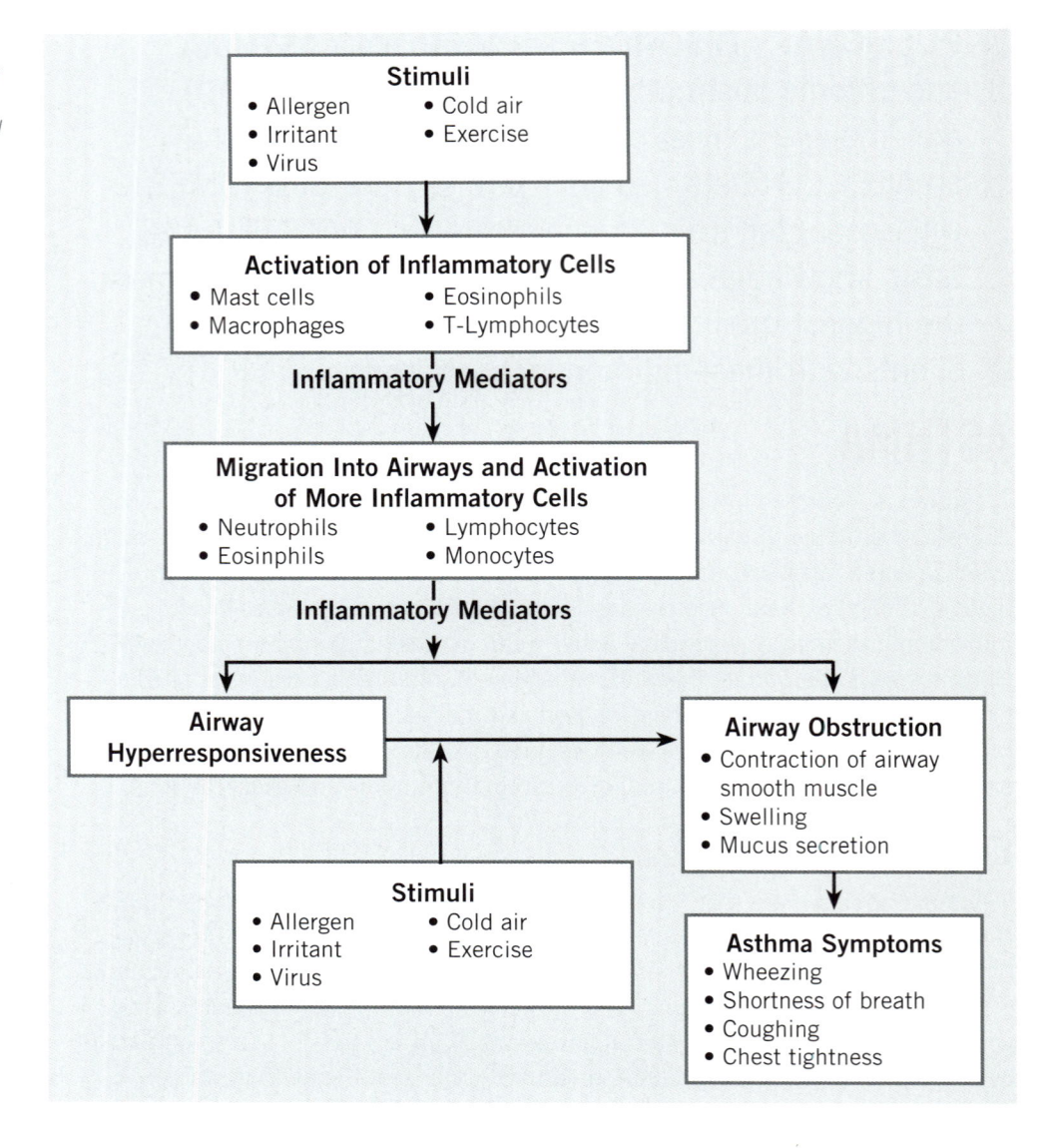

Figure 10-2
Asthma

Source: National Heart, Lung, and Blood Institute (2012). *What Is Asthma?* www.nhlbi.nih.gov/health/health-topics/topics/asthma/

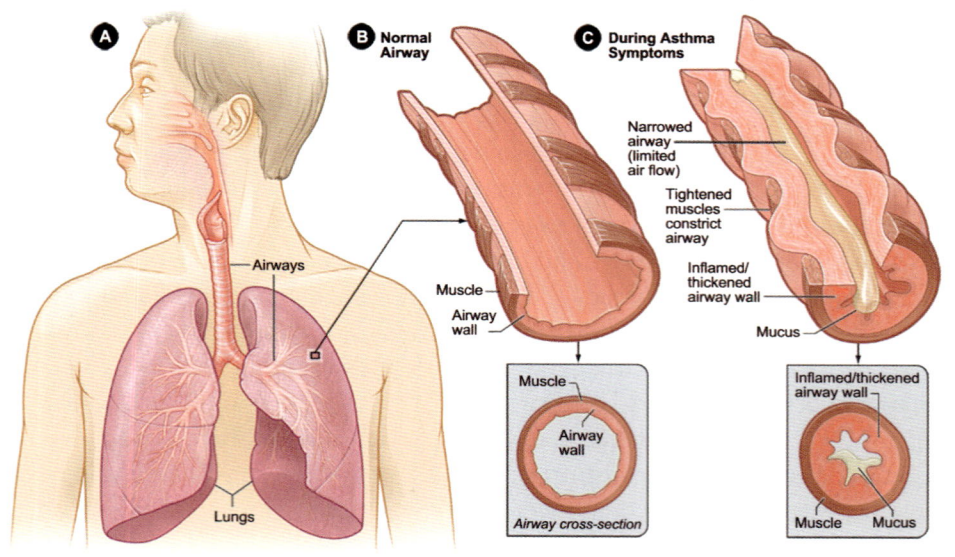

Pulmonary Disease: Asthma and Chronic Obstructive Pulmonary Disease   CHAPTER 10

Asthma severity at the time of initial diagnosis is categorized based on the frequency of symptoms and the results from **pulmonary function tests (PFTs)** (Table 10-1). The disease categorization determines the medical treatment and the individual's susceptibility to a severe attack, though it is important to note that asthma severity changes—both for better and worse—over time and even someone with mild intermittent disease can suffer a severe life-threatening **asthma exacerbation.** At each follow-up visit after initial diagnosis, the physician will assess how well controlled the asthma is, and make necessary medication changes, based upon the components of severity described in Table 10-1.

The reason why some individuals develop airway inflammation, and subsequently an asthma diagnosis, is uncertain. Asthma usually begins in childhood in response to various gene–environment interactions. As described earlier, asthma is more prevalent in boys, but at puberty the sex ratio shifts and asthma becomes more common in women (Horwood, Fergusson, & Shannon, 1985). **Hormones** likely play an important role in this shift, though the precise mechanism is unknown.

TABLE 10-1
CLASSIFYING ASTHMA SEVERITY IN INDIVIDUALS ≥12 YEARS

Components of Severity		Classification of Asthma Severity			
		INTERMITTENT	PERSISTENT		
			Mild	Moderate	Severe
Impairment Normal FEV1/FVC: 8–19 years: 85% 20–39 years: 80% 40–59 years: 75% 60–80 years: 70%	Symptoms	≤2 days/week	>2 days/week but not daily	Daily	Throughout the day
	Nighttime awakenings	≤2x/month	3–4x/month	>1x/week but not nightly	Often 7x/week
	Short-acting beta-agonist use for symptom control (not prevention of EIB)	≤2 days/week	>2 days/week but not >1x/day	Daily	Several times/day
	Interference with normal activity	None	Minor limitation	Some limitation	Extremely limited
	Lung function	Normal FEV1 between exacerbations FEV1 >80% predicted FEV1/FVC normal	FEV1 >80% predicted FEV1/FVC normal	FEV1 >60% but <80% predicted FEV1/FVC reduced 5%	FEV1 <60% predicted FEV1/FVC reduced >5%
Risk	Exacerbations requiring oral systemic corticosteroids	0–1/year	≥2/year*	≥2/year*	≥2/year*
		Consider severity and interval since last exacerbation. Frequency and severity may fluctuate over time for patients in any severity category.			
		Relative annual risk of exacerbations may be related to FEV1.			

*At present, there are inadequate data to correspond frequencies of exacerbations with different levels of asthma severity. In general, more frequent and intense exacerbations (e.g., requiring urgent, unscheduled care, hospitalization, or ICU admission) indicate greater underlying disease severity. For treatment purposes, patients who had ≥2 exacerbations requiring oral systemic corticosteroids in the past year may be considered the same as patients who have persistent asthma, even in the absence of impairment levels consistent with persistent asthma.

Note: EIB = Exercise-induced bronchoconstriction; FEV1 = Forced expiratory volume in one second; FVC = Forced vital capacity

Source: National Asthma Education and Prevention Program (2007). *Expert Panel Report 3: Guidelines for the Diagnosis and Management of Asthma.* Bethesda, Md.: U.S. Department of Health & Human Services, Public Health Service, National Institutes of Health, National Heart, Lung, and Blood Institute. NIH publication number 08-4051.

Asthma Triggers

Not all genetically susceptible individuals develop asthma. Rather, a gene–environment interaction occurs in some individuals in response to exposure to environmental triggers. The two most important triggers are allergens and viral respiratory infections. Exposure to house-dust mites and cockroaches in early life increases the risk of asthma in susceptible children. Some studies have shown that exposure to dog and cat dander also increases the risk of asthma, but others have found that exposure to dogs and cats in childhood may actually protect against asthma (NAEPP, 2007). Likewise, exposure to **respiratory syncytial virus (RSV)** as an infant seems to increase the risk of asthma in later childhood, with about 13% of all cases of asthma attributable to prior RSV infection (James et al., 2013). However, according to the "hygiene hypothesis," exposure to various viral infections, including RSV, in early life decreases the risk of developing asthma by promoting the development of a child's immune system along a "nonallergic" pathway (NAEPP, 2007). Gaining a clearer understanding of the relationship among allergens, viral infections, and the development of asthma is a priority for asthma researchers.

Other environmental factors that may predispose an individual to asthma development include tobacco smoke, certain occupational exposures, possibly a low intake of **antioxidants** and **omega-3 fatty acids,** and air pollution (NAEPP, 2007). Notably, an epidemiologic study found that heavy outdoor exercise (three or more team sports) in communities with high levels of air pollution was associated with an increased risk of developing asthma in school-age children (McConnell et al., 2002). Individuals with asthma often experience a worsening of symptoms in response to a variety of triggers (Table 10-2).

TABLE 10-2
COMMON ASTHMA TRIGGERS

• Exercise	• Mold	• Airborne chemicals or dusts
• Cold air	• Smoke (tobacco, wood)	• Menstrual cycles
• Viral infection	• Pollen	• Stress
• Animals with fur or hair	• Changes in weather	• Comorbid conditions such as sinusitis, rhinitis, gastroesophageal reflux disease (GERD), and obstructive sleep apnea (OSA)
• House-dust mites (in mattresses, pillows, upholstered furniture, carpets)	• Strong emotional expressions (intense laughing or crying)	

APPLY WHAT YOU KNOW

The CMES should share this information with clients with asthma and let them know that their doctors can help them develop a plan to cope with the disorder.

HOW TO CONTROL THINGS THAT MAKE YOUR ASTHMA WORSE

You can help prevent asthma attacks by staying away from things that make your asthma worse. This guide suggests many ways to help you do this.

You need to find out what makes your asthma worse. Some things that make asthma worse for some people are not a problem for others. You do not need to do all of the things listed in this guide.

Look at the things listed in dark print below. Put a check next to the ones that you know make your asthma worse. Ask your doctor to help you find out what else makes your asthma worse. Then, decide with your doctor what steps you will take. Start with the things in your bedroom that bother your asthma. Try something simple first.

■ **TOBACCO SMOKE**
- ❑ If you smoke, ask your doctor for ways to help you quit. Ask family members to quit smoking, too.
- ❑ Do not allow smoking in your home or around you.
- ❑ Be sure no one smokes at a child's day care center.

■ **DUST MITES**
- ❑ Many people with asthma are allergic to dust mites. Dust mites are like tiny "bugs" you cannot see that live in cloth or carpet.

Things that will help the most:
- ❑ Encase your mattress in a special dust-proof cover.*
- ❑ Encase your pillow in a special dust-proof cover* or wash the pillow each week in hot water. Water must be hotter than 130° F (54° C) to kill the mites.
- ❑ Wash the sheets and blankets on your bed each week in hot water.

Pulmonary Disease: Asthma and Chronic Obstructive Pulmonary Disease — CHAPTER 10

Other things that can help:
- Reduce indoor humidity to less than 50%. Dehumidifiers or central air conditioners can do this.
- Try not to sleep or lie on cloth-covered cushions or furniture.
- Remove carpets from your bedroom and those laid on concrete, if you can.
- Keep stuffed toys out of the bed or wash the toys weekly in hot water.

■ ANIMAL DANDER
- Some people are allergic to the flakes of skin or dried saliva from animals with fur or feathers.

The best thing to do:
- Keep furred or feathered pets out of your home.

If you can't keep the pet outdoors, then:
- Keep the pet out of your bedroom and keep the bedroom door closed.
- Cover the air vents in your bedroom with heavy material to filter the air.*
- Remove carpets and furniture covered with cloth from your home. If that is not possible, keep the pet out of the rooms where these are.

■ COCKROACH
- Many people with asthma are allergic to the dried droppings and remains of cockroaches.
- Keep all food out of your bedroom.
- Keep food and garbage in closed containers (never leave food out).
- Use poison baits, powders, gels, or paste (for example, boric acid). You can also use traps.
- If a spray is used to kill roaches, stay out of the room until the odor goes away.

■ VACUUM CLEANING
- Try to get someone else to vacuum for you once or twice a week, if you can. Stay out of rooms while they are being vacuumed and for a short while afterward.
- If you vacuum, use a dust mask (from a hardware store), a double-layered or microfilter vacuum cleaner bag,* or a vacuum cleaner with a HEPA filter.*

■ INDOOR MOLD
- Fix leaky faucets, pipes, or other sources of water.
- Clean moldy surfaces with a cleaner that has bleach in it.

■ POLLEN AND OUTDOOR MOLD

What to do during your allergy season (when pollen or mold spore counts are high):
- Try to keep your windows closed.
- Stay indoors with windows closed during the midday and afternoon, if you can. Pollen and some mold spore counts are highest at that time.
- Ask your doctor whether you need to take or increase anti-inflammatory medicine before your allergy season starts.

■ SMOKE, STRONG ODORS, AND SPRAYS
- If possible, do not use a wood-burning stove, kerosene heater, or fireplace.
- Try to stay away from strong odors and sprays, such as perfume, talcum powder, hair spray, and paints.

■ EXERCISE, SPORTS, WORK, OR PLAY
- You should be able to be active without symptoms. See your doctor if you have asthma symptoms when you are active—like when you exercise, do sports, play, or work hard.
- Ask your doctor about taking medicine before you exercise to prevent symptoms.
- Warm up for about 6 to 10 minutes before you exercise.
- Try not to work or play hard outside when the air pollution or pollen levels (if you are allergic to the pollen) are high.

Other Things That Can Make Asthma Worse
- **Flu:** Get a flu shot.
- **Sulfites in foods:** Do not drink beer or wine or eat shrimp, dried fruit, or processed potatoes if they cause asthma symptoms.
- **Cold air:** Cover your nose and mouth with a scarf on cold or windy days.
- **Other medicines:** Tell your doctor about all the medicines you may take. Include cold medicines, aspirin, and even eye drops.

*To find out where to get products mentioned in this guide, visit:
- Asthma and Allergy Foundation of America (www.aafa.org)
- Allergy and Asthma Network/Mothers of Asthmatics, Inc. (www.aanma.org)
- American Academy of Allergy, Asthma, and Immunology (www.aaaai.org)
- National Jewish Medical and Research Center (Lung Line) (www.nationaljewish.org)

Source: National Heart, Lung, and Blood Institute (1997). *Facts About Controlling Asthma.* Bethesda, Md.: National Asthma Education and Prevention Program, National Heart, Lung, and Blood Institute, NIH Publication No. 97-2339. A Reproducible Handout.

THINK IT THROUGH

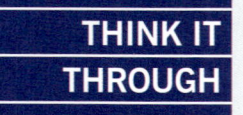

Spend some time looking around your home or workplace, identifying things that may trigger or worsen a person's asthma. Open garbage containers and a little animal hair on the couch may be harmless to you, but are potential triggers for people with asthma. This exercise will help you teach clients what to look out for in their own homes.

DIAGNOSTIC TESTING AND CRITERIA

A combination of patient history, physical examination, and objective tests is important for physicians to diagnose asthma, as well as assess severity and control of the disease. Patient history often reveals the occurrence of symptoms characteristic of asthma (e.g., shortness of breath, wheezing, coughing, and chest tightness, usually worse in the early morning and at night). Common physical findings in individuals with asthma include the following:
- Use of accessory muscles to breathe
- Appearance of hunched shoulders and/or chest deformity
- Sounds of wheezing during normal breathing or prolonged forced exhalation
- Increased nasal secretion, mucosal swelling, and/or nasal polyp
- Eczema and other signs of an allergic skin condition

Importantly, not all individuals with asthma have these physical findings, and in some people such findings may indicate another medical condition and not asthma (e.g., **congestive heart failure** or a cough secondary to medication). The objective test most often used to diagnose asthma and assess risk of a future asthma event is **spirometry,** a type of PFT.

Spirometry

Spirometry measures lung function by assessing the amount (volume) and/or speed (flow) of air that can be maximally inhaled and exhaled. Spirometry helps to determine if there is airflow obstruction, its severity, and whether it is reversible. In obstructive lung disease (discussed later in this chapter), a narrowing or blockage of the airways causes a decrease in exhaled air flow. In asthma, the narrowing is due to inflammation-induced swelling and sometimes mucus build-up. In spirometric testing, the patient takes a deep breath and blows into a mouthpiece attached to the spirometer. The patient is then instructed to exhale as hard and fast as possible until the lungs feel completely empty (Figure 10-3). This sequence is repeated until two to three good measurements are recorded. A computerized sensor in the spirometer calculates and graphs the results. The patient is then given a short-acting bronchodilator or nebulizer and the sequence is repeated. A decrease in airflow in people with asthma usually can be partially reversed with short-acting bronchodilators or nebulizers. Spirometry is performed at the time of initial assessment; after treatment is initiated and symptoms and **peak expiratory flow (PEF)** have stabilized; during a period of poorly controlled symptoms; and at least every one to two years to assess maintenance of airway function.

Figure 10-3
Spirometry

Source: Fotosearch
www.fotosearch.com

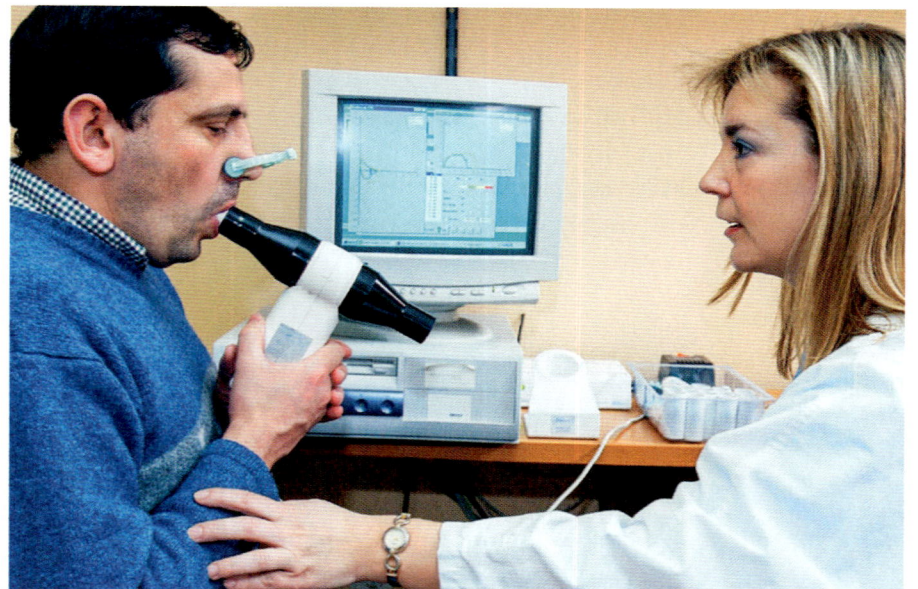

Pulmonary Disease: Asthma and Chronic Obstructive Pulmonary Disease — CHAPTER 10

SPIROMETRY INTERPRETATION

A sample spirometry reading in a person with asthma is depicted in Figure 10-4. Note that the person's age, height, and gender are used to determine reference, or predicted, values. The sample patient completed three trials pre-bronchodilator and three trials post-bronchodilator, with the best value used to analyze test results. Refer to the pre-bronchodilator **forced vital capacity (FVC)** and **forced expiratory volume in one second (FEV1)**. FVC is the total amount of air that can be forcibly exhaled after a maximal inhalation, compared to predicted value. Sometimes FEV6 (the amount of air exhaled in the first six seconds of maximal exhalation) is used instead of FVC for older adults who may be unable to complete a maximal expiratory effort to exhale their entire vital capacity. An obstructive lung pattern reveals a reduced FEV1 and a reduced FEV1/FVC ratio. The sample patient in Figure 10-4 has 79.7% of FEV1 and 73.8% of predicted FEV1/FVC. In general, an FEV1 or FEV1/FVC of ≥80% of predicted is normal, while 60 to 79% of predicted indicates mild obstruction; 40 to 59% of predicted indicates moderate obstruction; and <40% indicates severe obstruction, though values vary somewhat with age.

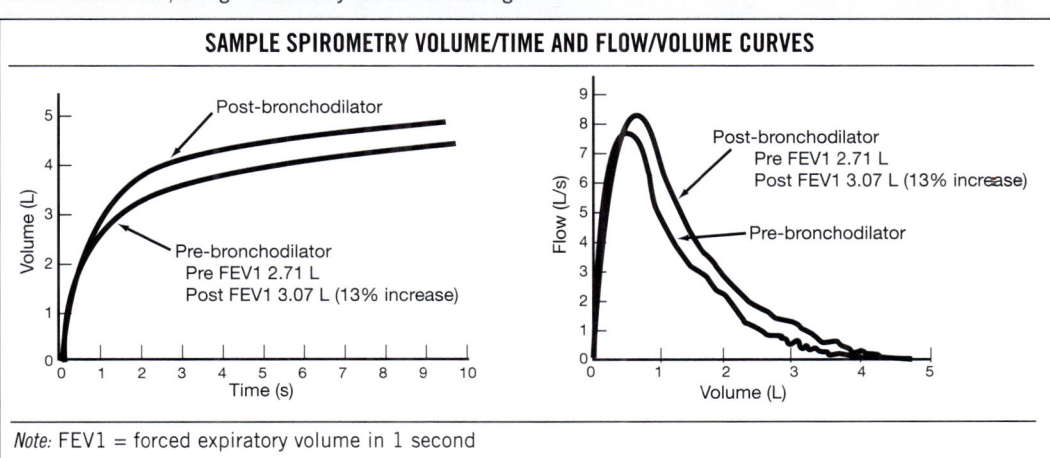

EXPAND YOUR KNOWLEDGE

SAMPLE SPIROMETRY VOLUME/TIME AND FLOW/VOLUME CURVES

Post-bronchodilator
Pre-bronchodilator
Pre FEV1 2.71 L
Post FEV1 3.07 L (13% increase)

Post-bronchodilator
Pre FEV1 2.71 L
Post FEV1 3.07 L (13% increase)
Pre-bronchodilator

Note: FEV1 = forced expiratory volume in 1 second

Figure 10-4
Sample spirometry curves in an individual with asthma

Source: Chobanian, A.V. et al. (2003). *JNC 7 Express: The Seventh Report of the Joint National Committee on Prevention, Detection, Evaluation, and Treatment of High Blood Pressure.* NIH Publication No. 03-5233. Washington, D.C.: National Institutes of Health & National Heart, Lung, and Blood Institute.

REPORT OF SPIROMETRY FINDINGS PRE- AND POST-BRONCHODILATOR

Pre-bronchodilator
Study: bronch
Age 59
ID:
Height: 175 cm
Test date: 8/7/14
Sex: M
Time: 9:38 a.m.
System: 7 20 17

Trial	FVC	FEV1	FEV1/FVC (%)
1	4.34	2.68	61.8%
2	4.44	2.62	58.9%
3	4.56	2.71	59.4%
Best values	4.56	2.71	59.4%
Predicted values*	4.23	3.40	80.5%
Percent predicted	107.8%	79.7%	73.8%

Post-bronchodilator
Study: bronch
Age 59
ID:
Height: 175 cm
Test date: 8/7/14
Sex: M
Time: 9:58 a.m.
System: 7 20 17

Trial	FVC	FEV1	FEV1/FVC (%)
1	4.73	2.94	62.2%
2	4.76	3.07	64.5%
3	4.78	3.04	63.5%
Best values	4.78	3.07	64.3%
Reference values	4.56	2.71	
Difference (L)	0.22	0.36	
Difference (%)	4.8%	13.4%	

Interpretations:
FEV1 and FEV1/FVC are below normal range. The reduced rate at which air is exhaled indicates obstruction to airflow.
*Predicted values from Knudson, R.J. et al. (1983). Changes in the normal maximal expiratory flow-volume curve with growth and aging. *American Review of Respiratory Diseases*, 127, 6, 725–734.

Interpretations:
Significant increases in FEV1 with bronchodilator (≥12% increase after bronchodilator indicates a significant change).

Note: FEV1 = Forced expiratory volume in 1 second; FVC = Forced vital capacity

Figure 10-5
How to use a peak flow meter:
1. Take a deep breath
2. Blow out hard and fast
3. Record the reading on the meter

Source: Fotosearch
www.fotosearch.com

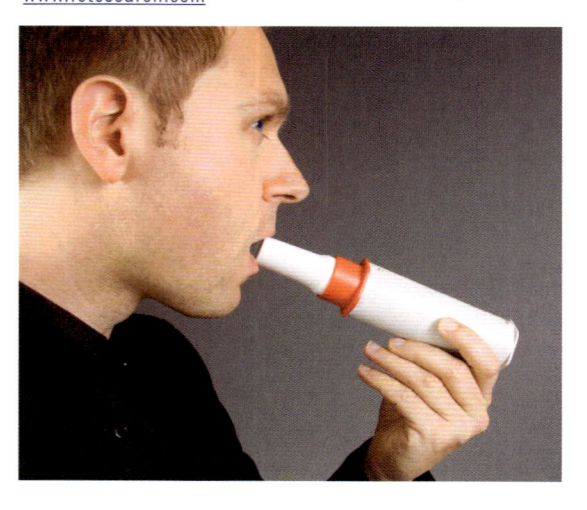

In individuals with an asthma diagnosis, the reduced FEV1 is improved by at least 12% from baseline or 10% of predicted FEV1 after inhalation of a short-acting bronchodilator. For the sample patient in Figure 10-4, the best value from the post-bronchodilator trials showed a 13.4% increase in FEV1 following bronchodilation.

The spirometry volume time and flow volume curves show improved function following bronchodilation, with a greater volume of air expired in the first second of expiration as well as overall (figure on left); and increased maximal flow, area under the curve, and total volume expired (figure on right).

Peak Expiratory Flow

While spirometry is the most useful method for monitoring lung function and asthma control, some individuals and their physicians prefer to also use a peak flow meter to measure how well air moves out of the lungs. Peak flow is used to monitor asthma, not for asthma diagnosis. A peak flow meter is a handheld mechanical or electronic device that provides a simple, reproducible, and quantitative way to measure exhalation capacity (Figure 10-5). When PEF is used, the individual's personal best peak flow should be used as the reference value. When a patient senses a worsening of symptoms or wants to monitor the response to treatment, they compare peak flow to the established reference value. The patient and physician then work together based on the personal best peak flow to set up zones (see Figure 10-7, page 288) (NAEPP, 2007):

- Green zone (>80% of personal best) signals good control. No asthma symptoms are present. The individual should take medications as usual.
- Yellow zone (50 to 80% of personal best) signals caution. Measure peak flow several times. If measurements remain in this zone, the individual should take an inhaled short-acting beta agonist. If peak flows continue to be in the yellow zone, this may signal that asthma is not under good control. The client should consult with their physician to change or increase daily medications.
- Red zone (<50% of personal best) signals a medical alert. The individual must take a short-acting beta-agonist immediately. The CMES should call the client's physician or the emergency room and ask what to do, or take the client directly to the emergency room. If the client is alone, they should call 9-1-1.

A CMES should ask clients with asthma if they use a peak flow meter to monitor symptoms and if they have set up zones to help them decide how to manage PEF results. The CMES may find this information beneficial should a client develop symptoms during exercise.

Allergy Testing

A strong relationship exists between asthma and **atopy,** or allergic hypersensitivity. For some individuals with persistent asthma, a thorough evaluation to determine the contributing role of allergens helps to better characterize asthma triggers and aggressively avoid them. After attaining a complete exposure and medical history, a physician may order skin testing or *in vitro* testing to determine the presence of specific **IgE antibodies** to indoor allergens, such as dust mites and animal dander. Importantly, the individual should only be tested for those allergens to which they are exposed, as it can be difficult to determine whether a specific IgE is responsible for the patient's symptoms.

TREATMENT OPTIONS

Once an asthma diagnosis has been established, the next step is for the physician to assess the severity of the asthma based on spirometry results and the patient's recall of symptoms over the past two to four weeks. A critically important non-pharmacological treatment is for the patient to aggressively avoid asthma triggers and control comorbid conditions, many of which are listed in Table 10-2.

Medical management consists of a regimen of long-term-control medications and quick-relief medications, depending on asthma classification and severity. Long-term-control medications prevent symptoms, usually by reducing inflammation. These medications must be taken daily and do not typically provide quick relief. Quick-relief medications are short-acting beta-agonists that act to relax muscles around the airway and provide rapid improvement of symptoms. Quick-relief medications should only be used when symptoms occur. The need for these medications on a regular basis may indicate insufficiently controlled asthma and the need to start or increase long-term control medications. Table 10-3 provides a basic overview of the long- and short-term medications used in asthma treatment. Note that the typical response and possible side effects of medication use are included in Table 10-3 as well. Importantly, short-acting beta-agonists, the medications used most often during an exercise-induced asthma exacerbation, also affect the **sympathetic nervous system,** leading to elevated heart rate. Figure 10-6 describes in more detail the evidence-based treatment regimens that physicians use to help an individual best manage asthma symptoms. Some physicians also may recommend sinus surgery for people who have asthma and chronic rhinosinusitis, though results are mixed as to whether surgery improves asthma symptoms.

TABLE 10-3
ASTHMA MEDICATIONS

Long-term-control Medications

- *Corticosteroids:* The most potent and effective anti-inflammatory medications currently available. Inhaled corticosteroids are used in the long-term control of asthma. Possible side effects include hoarseness, headache, and mouth infection. A short course of oral corticosteroids is used to gain prompt control of the disease when initiating long-term therapy. Long-term use of systemic steroids is reserved for severe, persistent asthma. Short-term use of oral corticosteroids can cause weight gain, fluid retention, mood changes, and high blood pressure, while long-term use can cause hyperglycemia, osteoporosis, cataracts, muscle weakness, and immune suppression.

- *Long-acting beta agonists (salmeterol and formoterol):* Bronchodilators that relax or open airways in the lungs and that work for at least 12 hours. They are used in combination with inhaled corticosteroids for long-term control and prevention of symptoms in moderate or severe persistent asthma, and are the preferred therapy in combination with inhaled corticosteroids for individuals ≥12 years. Possible cardiopulmonary side effects include tremor, rapid heartbeat, elevated blood pressure, and upper airway irritation.

- *Cromolyn sodium and nedocromil:* Used as an alternative, not preferred, medication for treatment of mild persistent asthma. They can also be used as preventive treatment prior to exercise or unavoidable exposure to known allergens. Dry cough is a possible side effect.

- *Immunomodulators (omalizumab):* Adjunctive therapy for individuals ≥12 years who have allergies and severe persistent asthma. Note that anaphylaxis may occur.

- *Leukotriene modifiers (montelukast, zafirlukast, 5-lipoxygenase inhibitor):* Alternative therapy for mild persistent asthma. Note that anaphylaxis may occur.

- *Methylxanthines (theophylline):* Mild to moderate bronchodilator used as an alternative adjunctive therapy with inhaled corticosteroids.

Quick-relief Medications

- *Short-acting beta agonists (albuterol, levalbuterol, pirbuterol):* Bronchodilators that relax or open airways in the lungs. They are the therapy of choice for relief of acute symptoms and prevention of exercise-induced bronchoconstriction. Bronchodilators activate the sympathetic nervous system and may cause rapid heartbeat, tremors, anxiety, and nausea.

- *Anticholinergics (ipratropium bromide):* Reduce vagal tone of the airway leading to dilation. They provide additive benefit to short-acting-bronchodilators in moderate-to-severe asthma exacerbation. Possible side effects include dizziness, nausea, heartburn, and dry mouth.

- *Oral corticosteroids:* Though not short-acting, they can be used for moderate and severe exacerbations, in addition to short-acting bronchodilators to speed recovery and prevent recurrence of exacerbations.

Figure 10-6
Stepwise approach for managing asthma in individuals ≥12 years

Note: Step 1 treatment corresponds to intermittent asthma, step 2 treatment corresponds to mild persistent asthma, step 3 and step 4 treatment correspond to moderate persistent asthma, and step 5 and step 6 treatment correspond to severe persistent asthma.

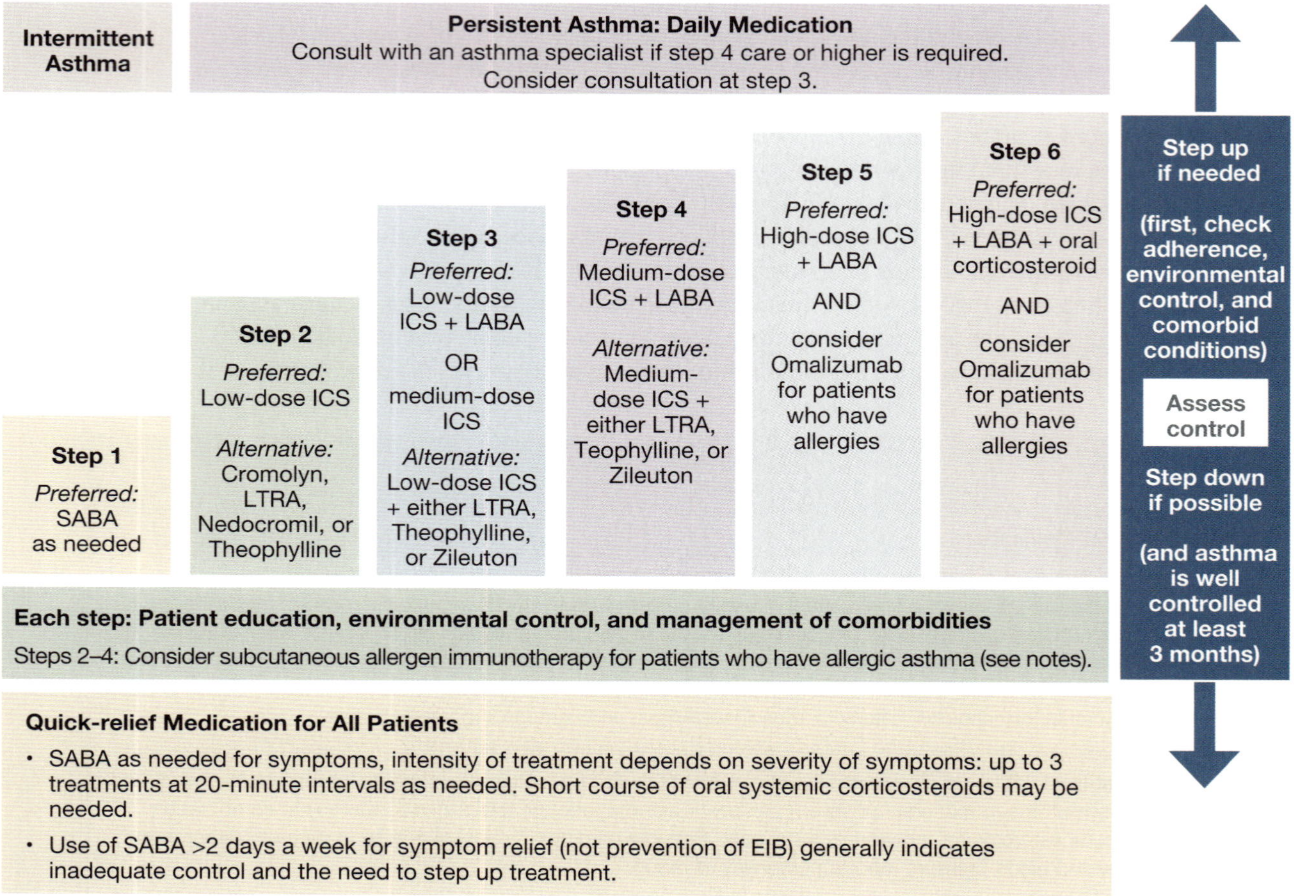

Intermittent Asthma

Persistent Asthma: Daily Medication
Consult with an asthma specialist if step 4 care or higher is required.
Consider consultation at step 3.

Step 1
Preferred: SABA as needed

Step 2
Preferred: Low-dose ICS
Alternative: Cromolyn, LTRA, Nedocromil, or Theophylline

Step 3
Preferred: Low-dose ICS + LABA OR medium-dose ICS
Alternative: Low-dose ICS + either LTRA, Theophylline, or Zileuton

Step 4
Preferred: Medium-dose ICS + LABA
Alternative: Medium-dose ICS + either LTRA, Teophylline, or Zileuton

Step 5
Preferred: High-dose ICS + LABA
AND consider Omalizumab for patients who have allergies

Step 6
Preferred: High-dose ICS + LABA + oral corticosteroid
AND consider Omalizumab for patients who have allergies

Step up if needed (first, check adherence, environmental control, and comorbid conditions)

Assess control

Step down if possible (and asthma is well controlled at least 3 months)

Each step: Patient education, environmental control, and management of comorbidities
Steps 2–4: Consider subcutaneous allergen immunotherapy for patients who have allergic asthma (see notes).

Quick-relief Medication for All Patients
- SABA as needed for symptoms, intensity of treatment depends on severity of symptoms: up to 3 treatments at 20-minute intervals as needed. Short course of oral systemic corticosteroids may be needed.
- Use of SABA >2 days a week for symptom relief (not prevention of EIB) generally indicates inadequate control and the need to step up treatment.

Note: Alphabetical order is used when more than one treatment option is listed within either preferred or alternative therapy. EIB = Exercise-induced bronchoconstriction; ICS = Inhaled corticosteroid; LABA = Inhaled long-acting beta-2 agonist; LTRA = Leukotriene antagonist; SABA = Inhaled short-acting beta-2 agonist

Source: National Asthma Education and Prevention Program (2007). *Expert Panel Report 3: Guidelines for the Diagnosis and Management of Asthma.* Bethesda, Md.: U.S. Department of Health & Human Services, Public Health Service, National Institutes of Health, National Heart, Lung, and Blood Institute. NIH publication number 08-4051.

Notes:
- The stepwise approach is meant to assist, not replace, the clinical decision making required to meet individual patient needs.
- If alternative treatment is used and response is inadequate, discontinue it and use the preferred treatment before stepping up.
- Zileuton is a less desirable alternative due to limited studies as adjunctive therapy and the need to monitor liver function. Theophylline requires monitoring of serum concentration levels.
- In step 6, before oral systemic corticosteroids are introduced, a trial of high-dose ICS + LABA + either LTRA, theophylline, or zileuton may be considered, although this approach has not been studied in clinical trials.
- Step 1, 2, and 3 preferred therapies are based on Evidence A; step 3 alternative therapy is based on Evidence A for LTRA, Evidence B for theophylline, and Evidence D for zileuton. Step 4 preferred therapy is based on Evidence B, and alternative therapy is based on Evidence B for LTRA and theophylline and Evidence D for zileuton. Step 5 preferred therapy is based on Evidence B. Step 6 preferred therapy is based on (EPR–2 1997) and Evidence B for omalizumab.
- Immunotherapy for steps 2–4 is based on Evidence B for house-dust mites, animal danders, and pollens; evidence is weak or lacking for molds and cockroaches. Evidence is strongest for immunotherapy with single allergens. The role of allergy in asthma is greater in children than in adults.
- Clinicians who administer immunotherapy or omalizumab should be prepared and equipped to identify and treat anaphylaxis that may occur.

Education

While a CMES cannot prescribe medications or treatment regimens, recognition of the complexity of asthma management will help them better understand clients' disease- and asthma-related challenges. Furthermore, the CMES can play an important role in helping to reinforce the physician's recommendations, help a client effectively self-monitor, and provide asthma education. Education is a critical component of a successful asthma-management program, as it empowers individuals to effectively carry out complex medication regimens, implement environmental control strategies, detect and self-treat most exacerbations, and communicate effectively with healthcare providers. The CMES should ask clients the following questions about their asthma:
- What are your triggers?
- What medications do you take (including those prescribed by a physician and any over-the-counter or alternative therapies)?
- When was your last asthma exacerbation?
- When was the last time you saw your physician?
- Is your physician aware of everything that you have disclosed to me?

The process of answering these questions will force clients to acknowledge and understand their illness, and perhaps identify discussion points for their next physician visit. The CMES can also remind clients to carefully monitor symptoms and adhere to their asthma action plan, which all people with asthma should have developed and discussed with their physicians (Figure 10-7). The asthma action plan will be particularly important should a client develop symptoms during exercise. All people, especially pregnant women and adults with infants and young children, can be encouraged to not smoke or be referred to a smoking cessation program.

Management of Asthma Exacerbation

An asthma exacerbation, or asthma attack, is defined as an episode of progressively worsening shortness of breath, cough, wheezing, and/or chest tightness that results in decreases in expiratory airflow. An asthma exacerbation can be triggered by any of the exposures noted in Table 10-2 or by other unknown factors. The intensity of an exacerbation can range from mild to life-threatening. Individuals at highest risk of asthma exacerbation include those who:
- Have had an exacerbation in the past year requiring an emergency room visit, hospitalization, or intensive care unit admission
- Have severe airflow obstruction based on spirometry
- Report feeling in danger or frightened by their asthma
- Have certain demographic and psychosocial characteristics such as female, non-white, non-users of inhaled corticosteroids, current smoking, depression, and stress

People who have had good control of asthma symptoms with inhaled corticosteroid treatment have a decreased risk of an exacerbation. Importantly, individuals who currently may have few symptoms and little impairment of quality of life still are at risk for a potentially life-threatening exacerbation.

Early treatment of an asthma exacerbation is important. Most exacerbations can be managed at home with appropriate advanced planning. Everyone with asthma should have a written asthma action plan to guide self-management. People with asthma should be able to recognize early signs of worsening asthma and promptly take action. Some may find that use of the modified 0 to 10 Borg scale for assessing **dyspnea** is helpful to characterize the severity of the exacerbation (Table 10-4). When necessary, a person with asthma can intensify therapy by increasing inhaled short-acting beta agonist and, if needed, adding a short course of oral systemic steroids, under their physician's guidance. It is also critical to remove the environmental trigger contributing to the exacerbation and promptly communicate with the individual's physician should symptoms not improve (NAEPP, 2007).

TABLE 10-4	
MODIFIED BORG DYSPNEA SCALE	
0	No breathlessness at all
0.5	Very, very slight (just noticeable)
1	Very slight
2	Slight breathlessness
3	Moderate
4	Somewhat severe
5	Severe breathlessness
6	
7	Very severe breathlessness
8	
9	Very, very severe (almost maximal)
10	Maximal

ASTHMA ACTION PLAN

For: _____ Doctor: _____ Date: _____

Doctor's Phone Number: _____ Hospital/Emergency Department Phone Number: _____

GREEN ZONE

Doing Well
- No cough, wheeze, chest tightness, or shortness of breath during the day or night
- Can do usual activities

And, if a peak flow meter is used,

Peak flow: more than _____
(80% or more of my best peak flow)

My best peak flow is: _____

Take these long-term control medicines each day (include an anti-inflammatory).

Medicine	How much to take	When to take it
_____	_____	_____
_____	_____	_____
_____	_____	_____
_____	_____	_____
_____	_____	_____

Before exercise ❑ _____ ❑ 2 or ❑ 4 puffs _____ 5 to 60 minutes before exercise

YELLOW ZONE

Asthma Is Getting Worse
- Cough, wheeze, chest tightness, or shortness of breath or
- Waking at night due to asthma, or
- Can do some, but not all, usual activities

-Or-

Peak flow: _____ to _____
(50 to 80% of my best peak flow)

First → Add: quick-relief medicine ___ and keep taking your GREEN ZONE medicine.
_____ ❑ 2 or ❑ 4 puffs every 20 minutes for up to 1 hour
(short-acting beta-2 agonist) ❑ Nebulizer, once

Second → If your symptoms (and peak flow, if used) return to GREEN ZONE after 1 hour of above treatment:
❑ Continue monitoring to be sure you stay in the green zone.

-Or-

If your symptoms (and peak flow, if used) do not return to GREEN ZONE after 1 hour of above treatment:
❑ Take:_____ ❑ 2 or ❑ 4 puffs or ❑ Nebulizer
(short-acting beta-2 agonist)
❑ Add:_____ mg per day For _____ (3–10) days
(oral steroid)
❑ Call the doctor ❑ before/ ❑ within _____ hours after taking the oral steroid

RED ZONE

Medical Alert!
- Very short of breath, or
- Quick-relief medicines have not helped, or
- Cannot do usual activities, or
- Symptoms are same or get worse after 24 hours in Yellow Zone

-Or-

Peak flow: less than _____
(50% of my best peak flow)

Take this medicine:

❑ _____ ❑ 4 or ❑ 6 puffs or ❑ Nebulizer
(short-acting beta-2 agonist)
❑ _____ mg
(oral steroid)

Then call your doctor NOW.
Go to the hospital or call an ambulance if:
- You are still in the red zone after 15 minutes AND
- You have not reached your doctor.

DANGER SIGNS
- Trouble walking and talking due to shortness of breath
- Lips or fingernails are blue

→ • Take ❑ 4 or ❑ 6 puffs of your quick-relief medicine AND
• Go to the hospital or call for an ambulance _____ NOW
(phone)

Source: National Heart, Lung, and Blood Institute (1997). *Facts About Controlling Asthma.* Bethesda, Md.: National Asthma Education and Prevention Program, National Heart, Lung, and Blood Institute, NIH Publication No. 97-2339.

Figure 10-7
Asthma action plan

In the case of an exacerbation that does not improve with home management, the individual should promptly report to urgent care or the emergency room or call 9-1-1. At that time, the individual will receive some combination of oxygen, a short-acting beta agonist plus ipratropium bromide, systemic corticosteroids, serial lung-function measurements, consideration of other adjunct treatment in severe cases, and a discharge plan that includes follow-up in one to four weeks, medication instructions, review of inhaler techniques, and consideration of initiating inhaled corticosteroids. Evidence suggests that methylxanthines, antibiotics (unless necessary for comorbid conditions), aggressive hydration, chest physical therapy, mucolytics, and sedation are not necessary (NAEPP, 2007). Refer to Table 10-5 for a summary of what a CMES should do when a client has an asthma exacerbation during exercise.

TABLE 10-5
WHAT TO DO WHEN A CLIENT HAS AN ASTHMA EXACERBATION DURING EXERCISE

- Reduce exercise intensity so that the client can easily administer rescue medication according to their asthma action plan. Do not encourage the client to "push through" an attack or stop the exercise abruptly.
- Remove the client from any environmental allergens or irritants, such as cold or polluted air, that may be contributing to the symptoms.
- Provide calm support and coach the client to use diaphragmatic breathing, taking deep breaths in through the nose and extending through the abdomen, and out through the mouth and drawing in the abdomen.
- If symptoms persist, discontinue exercise and seek immediate medical attention.
- Follow the gym or business protocol to document the incident and the actions taken.

NUTRITIONAL CONSIDERATIONS

Asthma is characterized by inflammation and narrowing of the airways. As there are few foods and no established eating plans that effectively decrease airway inflammation or narrowing, unlike many other chronic diseases, there is no specific nutrition plan recommended to prevent or treat asthma. That is, there is no "asthma diet." However, the relationship between nutrition and asthma is an area of active investigation, and some relationships between nutritional factors and the prevention and treatment of asthma have been identified.

Nutritional Considerations in the Management and Treatment of Asthma

In a discussion of asthma and nutrition, three groups of foods and **nutrients** deserve special mention for their role in mitigating disease: caffeine, fruits and vegetables, and fatty acids.

Caffeine
Very few foods have been shown to directly affect the airway narrowing and inflammation of asthma. The most notable of these is caffeine. A Cochrane Review concluded that caffeine, even at modest doses of less than 5 mg/kg of body weight [that is about 1.5 cups of coffee, or 150 mg of caffeine for a 150 lb (68 kg) adult], improves lung function for up to two to four hours after consumption (Welsh et al., 2010). Of note, the effect is modest and is much weaker than the airway response to bronchodilators, such as albuterol. The mechanism of this response is due mostly to the molecular structure of caffeine, which closely resembles theophylline, a standard medication in the treatment of asthma. Because of the similarity in structure between caffeine and theophylline, side effects of theophylline can be compounded in individuals who take the medication and also consume caffeine. Thus, clients who take theophylline need to monitor their caffeine intake. Clients should not attempt to substitute caffeine for their prescribed asthma medications.

Fruits and Vegetables
A diet high in fruits and vegetables has shown promise in not only helping to prevent asthma, but also into lessening its severity. In several epidemiologic studies (which by their design can only

determine relationships and not causation), a diet high in antioxidants (which are found naturally in fruits and vegetables) has been associated with decreased prevalence of asthma; however, in many cases these benefits occur only when several antioxidants are consumed together (such as when consuming a whole fruit or vegetables), rather than in isolation (as an extract or through supplementation) (reviewed in McKeever & Britton, 2004). In a randomized controlled trial (which *can* establish causation) of adults with diagnosed asthma, a higher intake of beta-carotene, a type of antioxidant, led to a higher FEV1 and percentage predicted FVC, decreased plasma c-reactive protein (a marker of inflammation), and decreased risk of, and longer time to, asthma exacerbation than was found with the low antioxidant group. This improvement occurred only when the beta-carotene was obtained from whole produce, and not with supplementation, suggesting that consumption of vegetables and fruits is of more value than taking an antioxidant supplement (Wood et al., 2012).

The importance of attaining antioxidants from whole fruits and vegetables (rather than supplementation) was highlighted in a classic review of the role of nutrition and asthma (McKeever & Britton, 2004). While there has been speculation of the potential role of various specific nutrients in the prevalence and severity of asthma (Table 10-6), in many cases the evidence to validate these claims is limited and weak. In fact, the review authors noted that attention may be better spent focusing on the whole eating plan and foods rather than specific nutrients. Whether for asthma or for overall general health, a diet high in whole fruits and vegetables—which contains a large variety of **vitamins, minerals,** and other nutrients thought to play a role in asthma—clearly provides health benefits and should be supported and encouraged with all clients.

Fatty Acids

Omega-3 fatty acids may provide benefit for individuals with asthma due to their anti-inflammatory effects. However, research to verify this is limited and mixed. A 2004 review from the Agency for Healthcare Research and Quality (AHRQ) concluded that a lack of evidence is available to make any definitive conclusion of the role of omega-3 fatty acids in asthma (U.S. Department of Health & Human Services, 2004). Though this report was published more than 10 years ago, a 2013 review came to essentially the same conclusion (Yang et al., 2013). **Omega-6 fatty acids** may be harmful to individuals with asthma due to their proinflammatory effects, though this remains an area of active investigation. There is consensus that high intake of omega-6 fatty acids does not benefit asthma.

TABLE 10-6
NUTRIENTS OR NUTRIENT GROUPS IMPLICATED IN ETIOLOGY OF ASTHMA AND THEIR POSTULATED MECHANISM OF EFFECT

NUTRIENT(S)	ACTIVITY AND POTENTIAL MECHANISMS OF EFFECT
Vitamins A, C, E	Antioxidants; protection against endogenous and exogenous oxidant inflammation
Vitamin C	Prostaglandin inhibition
Vitamin E	Membrane stabilization; inhibition of IgE production
Flavones and flavonoids	Antioxidant; mast cell stabilization
Magnesium	Smooth muscle relaxation; mast cell stabilization
Selenium	Antioxidant cofactor in glutathione peroxidase
Copper, zinc	Antioxidant cofactors in superoxide dismutase
Omega-3 fatty acids	Leukotriene substitution; stabilization of inflammatory cell membranes
Omega-6 polyunsaturated/trans fatty acids	Increased eicosanoid production
Sodium	Increased smooth muscle contraction

Reprinted with permission from the American Thoracic Society. Copyright © 2014 American Thoracic Society McKeever, T.M. & Britton, J. (2004). Diet and asthma. *American Journal of Respiratory and Critical Care Medicine*, 170, 7, 725–729. Official Journal of the American Thoracic Society.

Nutritional Considerations to Manage Comorbidities Associated With Asthma

Ultimately, individuals with asthma will benefit from following the same type of overall healthy eating plan as for the prevention and treatment of other chronic diseases. Several conditions commonly occur with asthma, including obesity, food allergies, and **gastroesophageal reflux disease (GERD)**. Individuals with asthma and any of these conditions should take special measures to help improve their asthma control.

Obesity

Obesity is associated with the prevalence and (poor) control of asthma. While the precise mechanisms have not been well defined, the relationship is probably due to obesity-induced inflammatory changes that contribute to airway hyperresponsiveness. These effects are reversed with bariatric surgery (Sideleva et al., 2012). Even moderate amounts of weight loss contribute to improved asthma control and symptomatic relief (Juel et al., 2012). Clients with concurrent asthma and obesity will benefit from an eating plan that contributes to sustained weight loss.

> **EXPAND YOUR KNOWLEDGE**
>
> **INDIVIDUALS WITH OBESITY REDUCE ASTHMA SYMPTOMS WITH WEIGHT LOSS**
>
> Obesity is associated with a high incidence of asthma and poor asthma control. Estimates demonstrate that approximately 30% of adults with asthma have **overweight** and an additional 30% have obesity (McHugh et al., 2009), with similar prevalence among youth with asthma (Kattan et al., 2010). With the dramatic increase in obesity over recent decades, obesity has been recognized as an important risk factor for a diagnosis of asthma (Juel et al., 2012). There is even evidence that suggests a probable shared genetic link between obesity and asthma (Farzan, 2013; Beuther, Weiss, & Sutherland, 2006). Thus, obesity may be a potentially modifiable risk factor for asthma, and weight loss may be expected to improve the clinical status of individuals suffering from asthma.
>
> In their literature review of asthma and obesity, Juel and colleagues (2012) found that weight loss in individuals with obesity with doctor-diagnosed asthma is associated with a 48 to 100% remission of asthma symptoms and use of asthma medication. In fact, all papers identified for their study reported some positive effect of weight loss on asthma control. Interestingly, the positive effects of weight loss on asthma-related health outcomes did not seem to be related to improvements in airway inflammation. The authors reported that the improvements were more likely related to changes in lung mechanics instead of being caused by asthmatic airway inflammation. Increased **body mass index (BMI)** is associated with a number of physiologic changes in the airways, independent of asthma, such as reductions in functional residual capacity and expiratory reserve volume. Modest reductions in total lung capacity, vital capacity, and residual volume have also been observed when comparing normal-weight individuals to those with a BMI of 30 kg/m^2 or greater (Farzan, 2013).
>
> These findings support the role of health and exercise professionals aiding individuals with overweight and obesity with asthma so that they can achieve safe and effective weight loss for improved asthma symptoms. Although the positive effects of weight loss on asthma do not seem to be related to improvements in airway inflammation, they have important implications with regard to the overall burden of asthma and health status of the individual.

Food Allergies

Many people with asthma also have food allergies. For these people, it is important to avoid these foods, as an allergic reaction can trigger an asthma exacerbation. (The eight most allergenic foods are cow's milk, eggs, fish, peanuts, shellfish, soy, tree nuts, and wheat.) However, avoidance of highly allergenic food in individuals with asthma who do not also have a food allergy is unlikely to provide benefit in asthma control.

Gastroesophageal Reflux Disease

GERD and asthma often coexist. While treatment of asymptomatic reflux is unlikely to benefit asthma, efforts to keep reflux well managed with efforts such as moderating intake of alcohol, caffeine, spicy foods, and other reflux triggers, while also avoiding eating before bedtime, will also help to improve asthma control.

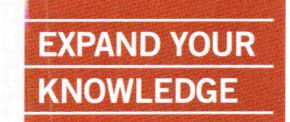

EXERCISE RECOMMENDATIONS

For many active individuals of all ages, sports, and levels of competition, exercise can trigger an asthmatic response, known as **exercise-induced bronchoconstriction (EIB)** or **exercise-induced asthma (EIA),** in which the airways transiently and reversibly narrow, causing symptoms such as cough, shortness of breath, chest pain or tightness, wheezing, or unexpected endurance problems. Up to 80% of people with classic asthma may experience symptoms with exercise (Butcher, 2006). For other individuals, exercise is the only asthma trigger.

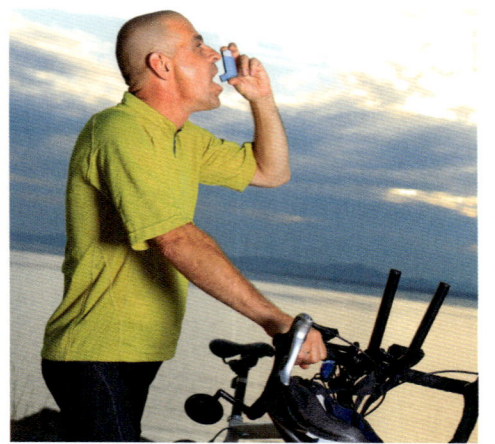

EIB results from a loss of heat, water, or both from the lungs during exercise due to hyperventilation of air that is cooler and drier than the air of the respiratory tree. Most studies suggest that inflammation plays a role in the cause of EIB, but the precise mechanisms behind EIB are not fully understood.

EIB typically occurs during or shortly after vigorous activity, reaching its peak five to 10 minutes after stopping activity and lasting for 20 to 30 minutes. The individual may also develop a hacking cough two to 12 hours after exercise cessation. The cough may last for one to two days and often is mistaken for an upper respiratory infection. A CMES should suspect EIB in a client who experiences asthma symptoms during exercise, especially if this individual has a history of asthma or has been exercising at a vigorous intensity in cold or dry air. The CMES should encourage clients to follow their asthma action plan if they have one. Otherwise, the best way to control acute symptoms is usually to markedly decrease or discontinue activity and use a rescue inhaler to open the airways. Clients should seek immediate medical assistance if symptoms persist or worsen. In most cases, symptoms will quickly improve. In those situations, the client can resume exercise as long as the event was not triggered by environmental contaminants such as pollution, cold air, and pollens.

In fact, the client may be least likely to experience asthma symptoms up to one hour following an acute exercise-induced asthma attack. Following the exercise bout, the CMES should refer the client to a physician who can then arrange an exercise challenge in which the client engages in sufficiently strenuous activity to increase heart rate to 80% of **maximal heart rate (MHR)** for four to six minutes. A 15% decrease in PEF or FEV1 confirms a diagnosis of EIB.

APPLY WHAT YOU KNOW

GENERAL ACTIVITY GUIDELINES FOR INDIVIDUALS WITH ASTHMA
- Avoid asthma triggers during exercise.
- Always have rescue medication nearby for use in the event of an attack.
- Establish a flexible program that can accommodate fluctuations in exercise capacity due to asthma symptoms.
- Utilize an extended warm-up and cool-down.
- Emphasize hydration before, during, and after exercise.
- Have the client practice diaphragmatic breathing.
- Determine exercise intensity according to the client's state of deconditioning, psychological preparedness for exercise, and asthma severity.
- Encourage clients to work at or just below their **first ventilatory threshold (VT1),** or the intensity of exercise at which ventilation starts to increase in a non-linear fashion.
- Incorporate intervals for high-intensity training.
- Closely monitor the client for early signs of an asthma attack and respond immediately. Get medical help if symptoms do not subside.
- Use **rating of perceived exertion (RPE)** and the dyspnea scale to communicate with the client regarding symptoms.
- Choose exercise testing methods that accommodate a warm-up period.

Pulmonary Responses to Exercise Training

While the precise mechanisms behind EIB are not fully understood, knowledge of the pulmonary responses to exercise training can help a CMES understand why EIB may occur for some people. During physical activity, **minute ventilation ($\dot{V}_E$)**, calculated as the **tidal volume** (the volume of air inspired per breath) multiplied by the **ventilatory rate** (the number of breaths per minute), increases.

> Minute ventilation = Tidal volume x Ventilatory rate

Thus, the respiratory system experiences increased demand. The large amounts of relatively cool and dry inspired air must be warmed and humidified by the tracheobronchial mucosa. When the air is warmed and humidified, water evaporates from the epithelial surface of the airway, leading to cooling. One theory is that this process of increased airway cooling provokes bronchoconstriction in individuals with hyperreactive airways. However, research has suggested that perhaps humidity, not air temperature, plays a more important role in causing EIB (Evans et al., 2005), leading to a theory that high $\dot{V}_E$ in relatively low humidity results in water loss in the airway. The airway drying may then lead to osmotic changes in the epithelium, which causes a release of inflammatory mediators and subsequent bronchospasm (Butcher, 2006).

Because the severity of bronchoconstriction in EIB is related to the ventilatory rate, the risk of EIB increases with increased exercise intensity. EIB generally occurs at ≥80% of $\dot{V}O_2$**max,** though people who suffer from severe asthma may experience symptoms at much lower intensities. Due to the discomfort that may occur with exercise for people with asthma and other pulmonary diseases, many avoid exercise and become deconditioned. Research suggests that while exercise may not decrease the incidence of EIB or improve pulmonary function, aerobic conditioning decreases risk of an asthma attack in general by reducing the ventilatory requirement for any given activity (NAEPP, 2007). Thus, people with asthma are strongly encouraged to engage in a regular physical-activity program.

While individuals who are susceptible to EIB should use caution when performing high-intensity exercise or prolonged exercise durations, they otherwise can follow the general FITT recommendations for healthy individuals from the American College of Sports Medicine (ACSM, 2022) for comprehensive exercise, including resistance training, in healthy adults. For some clients, upper-body exercises such as arm cranking, rowing, and cross-country skiing may not be appropriate because of the higher ventilation demands. Some research suggests that certain relaxation techniques, particularly muscle relaxation, may help to improve lung function (NAEPP, 2007). While some people anticipate that yoga may also provide unique benefits for individuals with asthma, little research is available to confirm or reject this hypothesis (NAEPP, 2007).

Programming and Progression Guidelines and Considerations

Individuals with asthma often exhibit low physical-activity levels because they typically avoid exercise (Williams et al., 2008). Exercise training is thought to be beneficial in asthma management, but it has not been extensively studied. Although the effectiveness of exercise on airway inflammation is yet unproven, there is some evidence to suggest that regular exercise may reduce inflammation in an asthmatic airway (Pakhale et al., 2013).

Clients with known asthma and/or EIB should receive medical clearance from a physician before beginning an exercise program. The client and their physician can discuss what to do in case of an asthmatic episode during exercise and how to best control the underlying asthma to prevent a symptomatic exercise bout. While exercise may be the only asthma trigger for many people, these individuals should still be evaluated by a physician prior to beginning an exercise program.

Individuals with well-controlled asthma who experience few or no symptoms during exercise can follow exercise guidelines for the general population. However, people with poorly controlled asthma or those who experience EIB should follow certain precautions to minimize symptoms and the risk of an exacerbation. First, the client and their physician should develop a treatment plan, which may include long-term-control therapy and/or pretreatment before exercise, if necessary. Long-term-control therapy reduces airway responsiveness and thus decreases the frequency and severity of EIB. Pretreatment usually includes use of a short-acting bronchodilator (albuterol or pirbuterol) or, less commonly, a long-acting bronchodilator (salmeterol). For mild symptoms, the short-acting bronchodilators are administered as two puffs of an inhaler spaced five to 10 minutes apart, 20 to 40 minutes before exercise. For maximal benefit from the inhaled medications, clients should be sure to consume water after using inhalers to help clear the back of the throat of the medicine. To minimize the risk of EIB, people with asthma should also engage in a prolonged warm-up and cool-down, remain indoors when air pollution or pollen levels are high, exercise with a mask or scarf over the mouth when exercising in cold weather, and avoid dehydration. Avoiding dehydration is especially important because mucus plugging can result from inadequate fluid intake. In practice, the prolonged warm-up and cool-down decrease the risk of EIB, though the mechanisms are speculative. Some believe a prolonged warm-up induces a milder bronchoconstriction, which leads to a refractory period in the hour or so after the warm-up, during which an attack is less likely to occur, and thus the exercise bout can be completed with a lower level of risk. The prolonged cool-down gradually decreases body temperature, which may decrease the risk for EIB that tends to occur immediately following cessation of exercise.

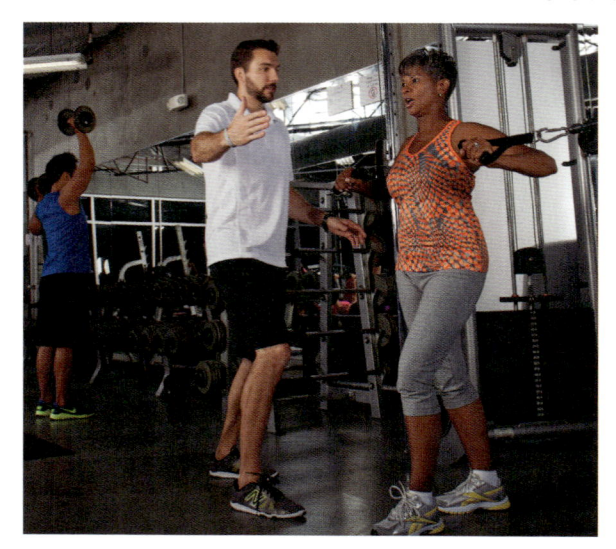

ACSM recommends that people with asthma engage in aerobic exercise three to five days per week beginning at a moderate intensity and progressively increasing duration to at least 30 to 40 minutes (ACSM, 2022). They can then progress to exercising five days per week for 40 minutes after the first month if the exercise has been well tolerated. Clients may use RPE to monitor intensity and the Borg dyspnea scale (see Table 10-4) to characterize the extent of breathlessness during exercise and to guide exercise-progression decisions. Swimming (preferably in a nonchlorinated pool) is often considered the mode of choice for people with asthma and those with a tendency toward bronchospasm because of its many positive factors: a warm, humid atmosphere; year-round availability; and the way the horizontal position may help mobilize mucus from the bottom of the lungs. Land-based exercise such as walking, leisure biking, and hiking are also good choices, as they are less likely to provoke EIB than other more intense fitness modalities.

Fitness Testing

Fitness-testing protocols may need to be modified to accommodate clients with EIB. Extended stages, smaller increments, and slower progressions in graded exercise tests may be necessary for individuals with functional limitations or early-onset dyspnea. Typically, exercise testing is performed on an electronically braked cycle ergometer or on a motor-driven treadmill. Targets for high heart rates and ventilation are better assessed on a treadmill, while sport-specific modes of assessment may be more appropriate for athletes. Six-minute walk testing may be used for clients with moderate-to-severe persistent asthma when other testing equipment is not available (ACSM, 2022). Exercise testing should be performed in the environment least likely to cause symptoms; therefore, indoor testing is preferred to outdoor testing, as outdoor triggers are more difficult to control. Fitness testing should always be preceded by an extended warm-up and a short-acting medication if the client usually uses medication prior to exercise.

6-MINUTE WALK TEST

The 6-minute walk test (6MWT) is a practical, simple test that measures the distance that a client can quickly walk on a flat, hard surface in a period of 6 minutes. It evaluates the global and integrated responses of all the systems involved during exercise, including the pulmonary and cardiovascular systems, systemic circulation, peripheral circulation, blood, neuromuscular units, and muscle metabolism [American Thoracic Society (ATS), 2002]. The self-paced 6MWT assesses the submaximal level of **functional capacity,** as clients choose their own intensity of exercise and are allowed to stop and rest during the test. However, because most **activities of daily living (ADL)** are performed at submaximal levels of exertion, the 6MWT may better reflect the functional exercise level for daily physical activities.

The following protocol was developed by Rikli and Jones (2013) as part of their Senior Fitness Test for community-dwelling older adults, but it is appropriate for a CMES to administer to most of their clients.

Equipment:
- Four cones
- Stopwatch

Protocol:
- Place four cones on a flat surface so that they create a rectangle measuring 20 x 5 yards (18.3 x 4.6 m) (Figure 10-8).
- Place a mark with masking tape on the floor at every 5-yard (4.57-m) increment to make scoring easier.
- Demonstrate the correct path around the rectangle using proper heel-to-toe walking keeping one foot in contact with the floor at all times (to ensure no running).
- Ask the client to stand at the starting line.
- Start the stopwatch and simultaneously give the instruction to "Go."
- Have the client walk continuously around the 50-yard (45.7-m) rectangular course for 6 minutes, or until the client decides to stop walking, whichever comes first.

The score is the number of laps walked multiplied by 50 yards (45.7 m), plus the number of extra yards or meters [indicated by the closest 5-yard (4.57-m) marker].

Because of the high variability of results for the 6-minute walk test, standardized norms for test scores are unavailable. The ATS recommends using the difference between the distances covered from the pre- and post-intervention assessment as a marker for changes made in functional capacity (ATS, 2002).

Contraindications

This type of testing is not recommended for:
- Individuals with unstable **angina** and **myocardial infarction** during the previous month
- Individuals with a **resting heart rate (RHR)** >120 bpm
- Individuals with **systolic blood pressure (SBP)** >180 mmHg and **diastolic blood pressure (DBP)** >100 mmHg

Note: Clients with any of these findings should be referred to their physicians for further evaluation.

Visit www.ACEfitness.org/CMESresources to download a free PDF of the 6MWT protocol, as well as other forms and tools that you can use throughout your career as a CMES.

Figure 10-8
6-minute walk test cone placement

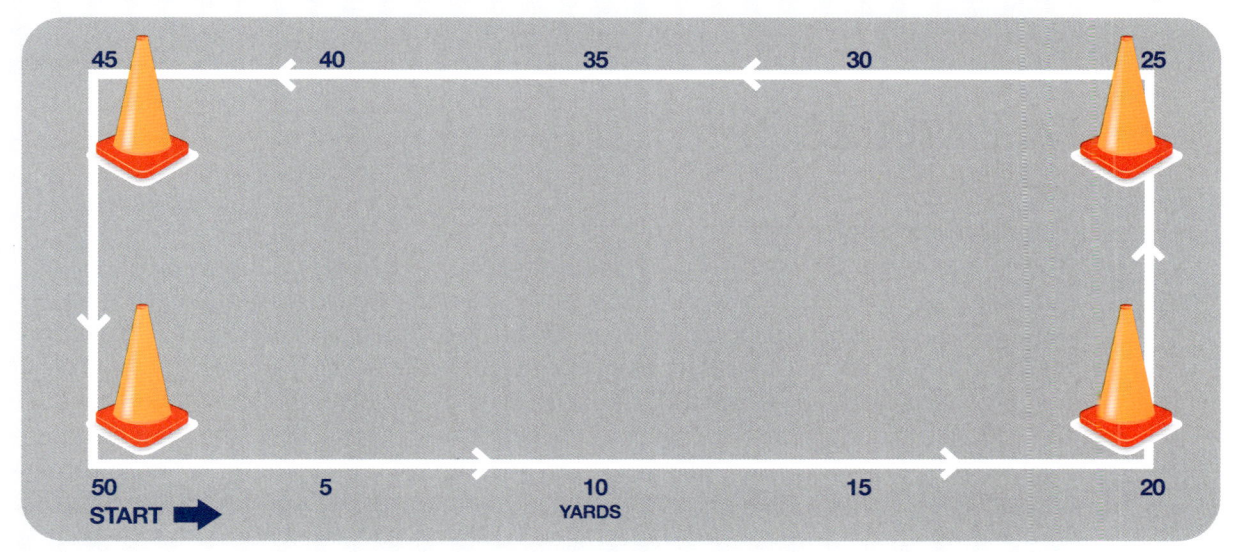

EXERCISE GUIDELINES SUMMARY FOR CLIENTS WITH ASTHMA

	CARDIORESPIRATORY TRAINING
Frequency	• 3–5 days per week
Intensity	• Initially, below VT1
	• 40–59% HRR or $\dot{V}O_2R$. If well tolerated, progress to 60–70% HRR or $\dot{V}O_2R$ after 1 month.
	• RPE 12–13 (6–20 scale)
Time	• Progressively increase to at least 30–40 minutes per day
Type	• Rhythmic large-muscle-group exercise such as: ✓ Walking ✓ Cycling ✓ Running ✓ Swimming or pool exercises in a nonchlorinated pool
Progression	• Progress following the ACE Integrated Fitness Training® Model based on client goals and availability.
	MUSCULAR TRAINING
Frequency	• A minimum of 2 nonconsecutive days per week
Intensity	• <50% 1-RM for muscular endurance
	• 60–70% 1-RM for muscular strength for beginners and ≥80% 1-RM for experienced weight lifters
Time	• 2–4 sets of 8–12 repetitions for muscular strength
	• 1–2 sets of 15–20 repetitions for muscular endurance
Type	• All major muscle groups
	• Resistance machines, free weights, or body-weight exercises
Progression	• Progress following the ACE Integrated Fitness Training Model based on client goals and availability.

Note: VT1 = First ventilatory threshold; $\dot{V}O_2R$ = Oxygen uptake reserve; HRR = Heart-rate reserve; RPE = Rating of perceived exertion; 1-RM = One-repetition maximum

CMES FOCUS

Clients with asthma may have reduced physical activity and sports participation levels as a result of their breathing symptoms and a tendency to be inactive to avoid symptoms. As such, the CMES should take a conservative approach to exercise program design for clients with asthma who are new to exercise, as they likely have very low cardiorespiratory fitness. Clients with an asthma exacerbation should postpone exercise until the symptoms have improved. The CMES should avoid recommending exercise in cold environments or in areas with airborne allergens or pollutants to limits clients' exposure to potential asthma triggers. Further, clients with EIB are more susceptible to an exacerbation of symptoms with long-duration and high-intensity exercise sessions.

Source: American College of Sports Medicine (2022). *ACSM's Guidelines for Exercise Testing and Prescription* (11th ed.). Philadelphia: Wolters Kluwer.

CASE STUDIES

Case Study 1

Client Information

Sarah is a 55-year-old woman who has overweight and has struggled with asthma since childhood. She asks the CMES to help her begin an exercise program for weight loss. Sarah has never enjoyed exercise, as it caused her some breathing difficulty in the past and she feared that she might have an asthma attack. However, after her physician strongly encouraged her to begin exercising to control her weight and achieve other benefits, she contacted the CMES for help. On further questioning, Sarah reveals that she experiences shortness of breath and chest tightness when climbing stairs and playing with her grandchildren (*Note:* Her physician has ruled out any cardiovascular disorder as being responsible for her symptoms.) She is allergic to pollen, mold, dust, and cats. Sarah takes inhaled corticosteroids daily and uses an albuterol inhaler when she experiences symptoms. Her physician ordered spirometry testing, which showed a FEV1 of 75% that was increased to 89% following inhalation of a short-acting bronchodilator.

Pulmonary Disease: Asthma and Chronic Obstructive Pulmonary Disease — CHAPTER 10

CMES Approach

The CMES should begin by reassuring Sarah that they will design an exercise program for her that is least likely to cause asthma symptoms and that every effort will be made for her to have a comfortable and enjoyable experience. It is important for the CMES to encourage Sarah to discuss any symptoms that she experiences, such as an unusual shortness of breath, chest tightness, coughing, or wheezing. The CMES should introduce the RPE and dyspnea scales to provide a communication tool and help Sarah differentiate between exercise-related and asthma-related breathlessness. The CMES should also ask Sarah if she has an asthma action plan in place and if she has discussed pre-exercise medication with her physician and what to do should she have an exercise-induced asthma attack. Also, the CMES must ask Sarah for permission to contact her physician for medical clearance prior to beginning the exercise program. The CMES should perform fitness tests to identify the threshold at which Sarah starts displaying symptoms, and then use this threshold as a baseline. When designing Sarah's exercise program, the CMES should start with low-intensity indoor exercise such as treadmill walking, stationary cycling, or indoor aquatic classes, complemented by Functional Training, including exercises that improve muscular endurance, core function, static and dynamic balance, and flexibility. It is important to gradually progress Sarah's program based on her comfort level and her initial response to exercise, with the ultimate goal of safely increasing caloric expenditure for weight loss. It may also be a good idea to have Sarah meet with a dietitian.

Case Study 2

Client Information

Josh is a 19-year-old college student and avid runner who was recently diagnosed with exercise-induced bronchoconstriction. During the past several months, Josh has noticed increased difficulty breathing during his vigorous training days and his athletic performance has suffered. His physician prescribed a cromolyn sodium inhaler for use three times per day (one time is 20 minutes prior to running) in combination with an albuterol inhaler. While this regimen has helped, he consults the CMES to help him maximize his performance for the New York City Marathon in November.

CMES Approach

The CMES should start by asking Josh more about the symptoms he experiences during his vigorous training days. In addition to difficulty breathing, he may also have chest tightness, wheezing, and cough. The CMES should encourage Josh to pay attention to these symptoms so that he can quickly recognize and respond to them by modifying his training and using his rescue inhaler. Also, the CMES should inquire whether other triggers such as pollution, cold air, pollens, or other environmental contaminants cause him to experience symptoms. The CMES may want to encourage Josh

---

ACE IFT® MODEL AT A GLANCE

Cardiorespiratory Training

This client is starting Base Training, as she needs to develop an aerobic base before progressing. Special attention is given to her asthma triggers and the exercise intensity at which her symptoms begin to appear.

Muscular Training

Sarah's initial program includes Functional Training to establish postural stability and kinetic-chain mobility with exercises to improve joint and core function, balance, and flexibility.

ACE IFT® MODEL AT A GLANCE

Cardiorespiratory Training

Josh is already performing some of his training at vigorous intensities. Following his physician's recommendations for medication and training, and incorporating the results of his fitness assessment and the training steps included in this case study, the CMES should develop an initial program that begins with Fitness Training. If he responds well to the medication and training, his program can progress to intervals performed slightly below VT2. If he responds well to this progression, the CMES can develop a Performance Training program to help him "peak" for the marathon. Josh's combined response to his medication and training will guide this progression.

Muscular Training

While this case study does not include a specific Muscular Training program, his warm-up and cool-down may include Functional and Movement Training exercises that help improve postural stability (e.g., planks), joint mobility (e.g., glute bridges and cat-cow), and movement patterns (e.g., lunge matrix). Progression to a Load/Speed Training program can be introduced as he becomes accustomed to his new medications and demonstrates good movement patterns without compromising postural and joint stability.

to keep a workout log, noting the environmental conditions and his symptoms to help him and his physician identify other triggers.

Prior to designing an exercise program or working with Josh to set marathon goals, the CMES should arrange for Josh to complete fitness testing to assess his cardiorespiratory fitness level. The CMES must remember to choose an indoor test (preferably a running test performed on a treadmill since Josh is preparing for a marathon), incorporate a prolonged warm-up prior to beginning the test, and gradually increase the intensity if a graded exercise test is being utilized. The CMES can use these results to program exercise intensities based on his heart rate at VT1 and the **second ventilatory threshold (VT2)** and evaluate Josh's response to the training program. If the data are available, the CMES should examine the ventilatory and heart-rate response relationship to determine the heart rate at which Josh's ventilatory response begins to increase disproportionately. With practice, a prolonged warm-up, and medication use, Josh should be able to train at high intensities and progress his training program with few difficulties. However, if Josh experiences repeated asthma exacerbations during his workouts, with exercise performance fluctuating from day to day, he should consult his physician to assess his overall and pre-exercise medication regimen and possible environmental triggers. On the other hand, if Josh consistently cannot tolerate the exercise program, it may be that the program is too difficult, insufficient recovery time has been programmed, or he has reached a training plateau, and the CMES should reassess his program and make similar modifications as would be made for a healthy runner.

When preparing Josh for race day, the CMES should remind him of the importance of the following:
- Performing a prolonged warm-up
- Covering his mouth with a scarf or mask if the temperature outside is cold
- Taking his medication 20 minutes before the race and keeping it with him in case he experiences symptoms
- Using a spacer to ensure that the medicine inhaled reaches the lungs and does not simply coat the roof of the mouth or the back of the throat
- Staying well hydrated
- Breathing through the nose as much as possible while running
- Avoiding hyperventilation by using a controlled breathing pattern
- Avoiding any foods known to trigger an attack, as some foods may precipitate an asthma attack in certain individuals (e.g., celery, carrots, peanuts, egg whites, bananas, and shrimp)
- Always listening to his body for signs that he should modify his intensity

CHRONIC OBSTRUCTIVE PULMONARY DISEASE

COPD is a progressive lung disease characterized by difficulty breathing, lung airflow limitations causing wheezing and cough, sputum production, and exercise intolerance. COPD is strongly associated with cigarette smoking and is the main cause of death due to chronic lower respiratory disease (Kosacz et al., 2012).

EPIDEMIOLOGY

COPD is the third leading cause of death in the United States (Kosacz et al., 2012). It affects about 15 million Americans and is responsible for about 8 million physician visits, 1.5 million emergency department visits, and 726,000 hospitalizations annually (Mannino et al., 2002). COPD results from exposure to damaging particulates, most notably cigarette smoke but also outdoor, occupational, and indoor pollutants. While smoking is the strongest risk factor for COPD, occupational exposures account for nearly 20% of cases (Balmes et al., 2003). Other risk factors for COPD include asthma, chronic **bronchitis,** severe childhood respiratory infections, and tuberculosis. Older adults are commonly affected. Some people develop COPD as a result of a genetic deficiency of alpha-1-antitrypsin. COPD used to disproportionately affect men, but currently it kills roughly equal numbers of men and women each year (Mannino et al., 2002).

OVERVIEW

COPD is characterized by a combination of small airway disease, airway inflammation increased airway resistance (chronic bronchitis), parenchymal destruction (**emphysema**), loss of alveolar attachments, and decrease of elastic recoil (Figure 10-9). Together, these changes lead to respiratory compromise, causing air trapping and hyperinflation of the lungs. Ultimately, inadequate oxygen is delivered to the bloodstream and working tissues and too much carbon dioxide accumulates in the bloodstream. This results in many harmful effects on the body, including shortness of breath and exercise intolerance, the chief symptoms reported by people with COPD.

While COPD primarily affects lung function, it also negatively affects other organs and tissues, most notably skeletal muscle. Histologic studies of leg muscle tissue in people with COPD have found that the muscle tissues to have decreased aerobic enzyme activity, decreased proportion of **type I muscle fibers,** decreased capillary concentration, increased inflammatory cells, and increased apoptosis (cell death) compared to normal leg muscle fibers (Casaburi & ZuWallack, 2009). This skeletal muscle dysfunction leads to diminished aerobic power and early muscle fatigue. In fact, for a large portion of individuals with COPD, muscle fatigue is more limiting to physical activity than shortness of breath.

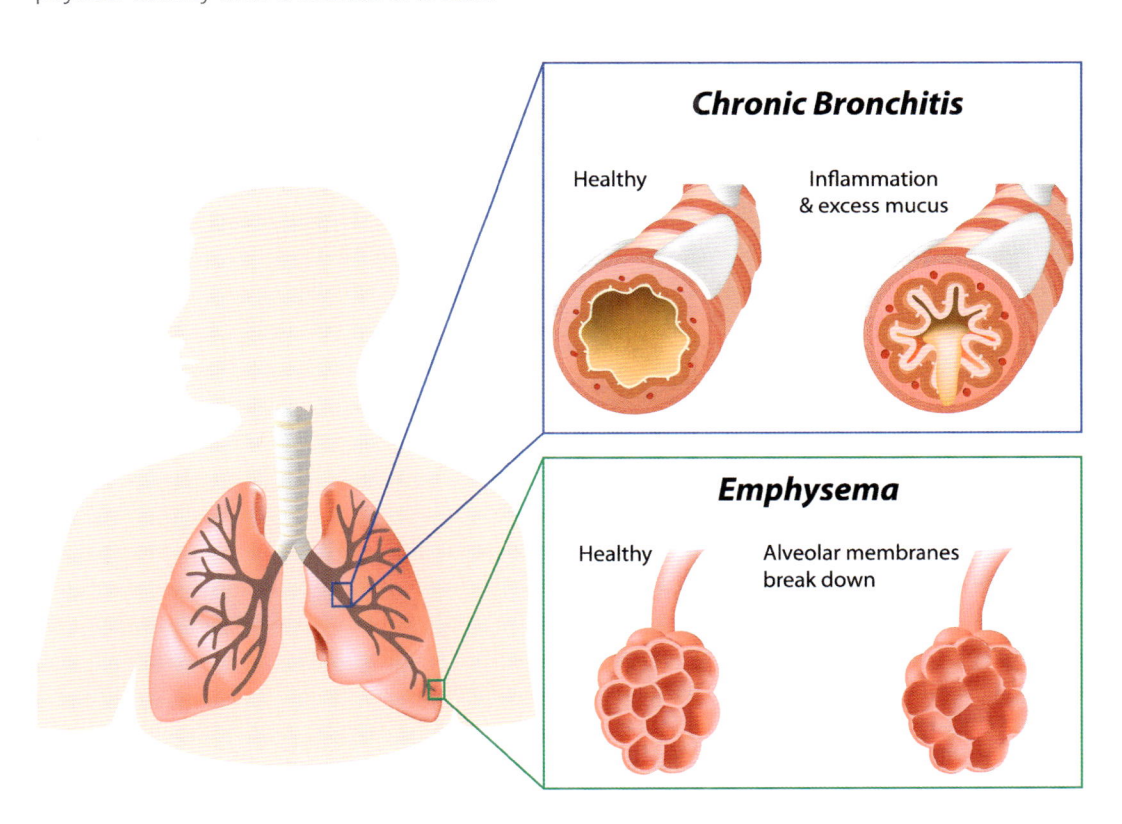

Figure 10-9
COPD
© Fotosearch
www.fotosearch.com

DIAGNOSTIC TESTING AND CRITERIA

COPD is a disease of older adults, best diagnosed by the primary care physician when faced with a series of complaints, including progressive or persistent shortness of breath that is worse with exercise; chronic cough or sputum production or wheezing; and a history of exposure to risk factors including tobacco smoke, smoke from home cooking and heating fuels, and/or occupational dusts and chemicals. Signs of severe disease include fatigue, weight loss, and **anorexia.** In many cases, COPD and asthma present to the physician with similar symptoms and it is through careful questioning and evaluation that the physician arrives to the correct diagnosis.

TABLE 10-7	
SPIROMETRY CLASSIFICATION OF COPD SEVERITY	
STAGE AND SEVERITY	**DEFINITION**
I - Mild	FEV1/FVC <0.70; FEV1 ≥80% predicted
II - Moderate	FEV1/FVC <0.70; FEV1 50 to <80% of predicted
III - Severe	FEV1/FVC <0.70; FEV1 30 to <50% of predicted
IV - Very severe	FEV1/FVC <0.70; FEV1<30% of predicted; FEV1 <50% of predicted plus chronic respiratory failure

As with asthma, spirometry is used to confirm the diagnosis. A diagnosis of COPD is characterized by a decrease in FEV1 due to inflammation and narrowing of the peripheral airways. Specifically, an FEV1/FVC <0.7 is characteristic of COPD. Spirometry results are used to determine severity of disease (Table 10-7). Unlike asthma, the airflow limitation does not improve with administration of a bronchodilator.

TREATMENT OPTIONS

Treatment of COPD includes two aims: (1) improve quality of life through symptom relief, improved exercise tolerance, and improved health status and (2) reduce risk through prevention and management of exacerbations and strategies to slow progression of disease and reduce mortality [Global Initiative for Chronic Obstructive Lung Disease (GOLD), 2013]. COPD is not curable or reversible.

Improve Quality of Life
Smoking Cessation

To slow disease progression, and optimize chances at preserving a reasonable quality of life, the most critical step to treatment of COPD is smoking cessation. Though this appears obvious, quitting proves extremely challenging for many people. The entire healthcare team for a person with COPD should aim to reinforce the need to quit and to work in partnership with the client to be successful. A commonly recommended strategy for smoking cessation is the use of the "5 A's," which will help guide the healthcare professional coach a client who is willing to make this lifestyle change. A CMES who is skilled in communication and facilitating behavior change can prove to be a key asset on the client's care team. Efforts to reduce exposure to other harmful substances such as occupational exposures and indoor and outdoor pollution are also beneficial. The 5 A's are as follows (GOLD, 2013):

- *Step 1–Ask:* At each session, ask the client about tobacco use, and ask for permission to discuss quitting. If the client smokes and provides permission to discuss further, proceed to step 2.
- *Step 2–Advise:* Urge the client to quit smoking. Use clear, strong, and personalized language.
- *Step 3–Assess:* Ask the client if they are willing to make a quit attempt now or within the next 30 days. If yes, establish a quit date and proceed to step 4.
- *Step 4–Assist:* For the client willing to make a quit attempt, use **motivational interviewing** and referral to other resources and medications to help the client succeed. Clients can be encouraged to visit www.smokefree.gov for information about exploring ways to quit, managing withdrawal symptoms, and developing a customized plan for smoking cessation.
- *Step 5–Arrange:* Schedule follow-up contact, in person or by telephone, email, or text message within the first week after the quit date.

APPLY WHAT YOU KNOW

Considering that smoking is the leading cause of COPD, a CMES can be an important encourager and supporter of smoking cessation. How will you support clients who are dealing with the challenges of quitting smoking? Practice or role-play how you would approach the 5 A's with a client who is working toward smoking cessation.

Physical Activity and Rehabilitation

Physical activity is recommended for all individuals diagnosed with COPD to help improve symptoms (GOLD, 2013). Physical activity and pulmonary rehabilitation recommendations are described in detail later in this chapter.

Medications

Medications used for COPD aim to decrease symptoms, decrease frequency and severity of exacerbations, and improve overall health status and exercise tolerance. The treatment regimen for an individual with COPD is based on FEV1, a very good predictor of disease severity. Inhaled bronchodilators including short- and long-acting beta-agonists (such as albuterol and salmetero) and anticholinergics (such as ipratropium bromide) are the mainstays of therapy.

Bronchodilators are of particular importance as they act on peripheral airways and reduce air trapping, which helps to reduce hyperinflation, lessens dyspnea, and improves exercise capacity. Methylxanthines (e.g., theophylline), inhaled steroids (e.g., budesonide or fluticasone), and/or systemic steroids (e.g., prednisone) may also be used.

Other Therapies

Other therapies for COPD include oxygen therapy in those with severe resting hypoxemia, ventilator support for those with very severe but stable COPD, a variety of surgical treatments including lung transplantation, and palliative care for some with advanced disease.

Reduce Risk

Efforts to reduce risk include prevention and quick treatment of exacerbations and monitoring and management of comorbidities.

Exacerbations

Similar to asthma, individuals with COPD experience exacerbations, often incited by infection, environmental factors, and other poorly defined triggers. Signs of exacerbation include an acute change in degree of dyspnea, cough, and/or sputum production. Most COPD exacerbations can be prevented with smoking cessation, flu and pneumonia vaccines, knowledge of current therapy and proper inhaler technique, and treatment with long-acting inhaled bronchodilators with or without inhaled steroids (GOLD, 2013). However, the reality is that many exacerbations are not prevented and can lead to life-threatening complications. If a person with COPD develops accessory respiratory muscle use, paradoxical chest wall movements (portion of chest moves in with inspiration; this is also known as "flail chest"), worsening or new onset central **cyanosis,** peripheral **edema,** hemodynamic instability, or altered mental status, immediate medical attention is essential.

Typically, short-acting beta agonists (e.g., albuterol) with or without a short-acting anticholinergic (e.g., iptratropium bromide), oral steroids, and antibiotics are the mainstay treatments for an exacerbation, though in many cases hospital admission is required.

Comorbidities

Given that the majority of individuals with COPD are older adults and that most cases of COPD result from smoking, which is responsible for myriad health problems, comorbidities are common in individuals with COPD. The most common of these health problems include **ischemic heart disease,** heart failure, atrial fibrillation, **hypertension, osteoporosis, anxiety** and depression, lung cancer, serious infections, **metabolic syndrome,** and **diabetes** (GOLD, 2013). These coexisting illnesses increase the complexity of management of COPD and amplify its disability. Further, due to weakness as a result of muscle wasting and fatigue, clients with COPD will begin to hyperventilate at lower power outputs. This may cause them to avoid exercise, leading to further physiological declines. While the client's physician(s) will be responsible for overseeing the management of these conditions, the CMES should aim to gain a full health history for the client and take comorbidities into consideration when developing exercise programs.

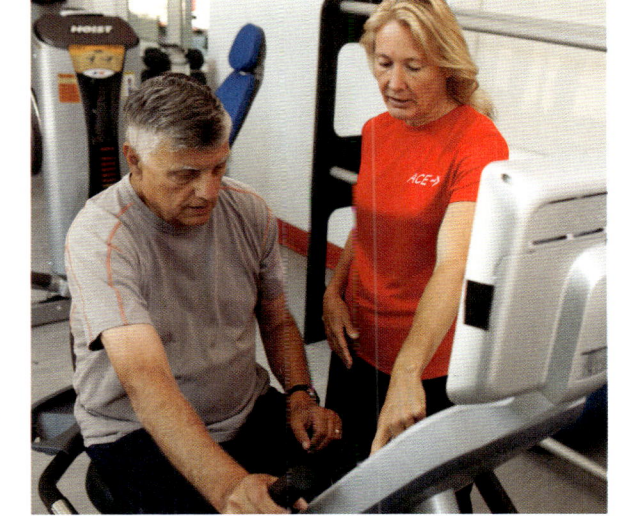

NUTRITIONAL CONSIDERATIONS

Many clients with COPD find it difficult to meet nutritional needs, in part due to the trouble with feeding that can accompany the disease, including difficulty swallowing and chewing due to shortness of breath, altered taste sensation, fatigue, anorexia, depression, medication side effects, altered mental activity due to **hypercapnia** (elevated blood carbon dioxide), and other factors. The goal of nutrition therapy is to provide adequate energy to avoid weight loss and prevent malnutrition. Several strategies to help clients do this are highlighted in Table 10-8.

The Academy of Nutrition and Dietetics (A.N.D., 2008) has compiled the most valid scientific research on foods and nutrients that help to improve the nutritional management of COPD through its Evidence Analysis Library (EAL). While this information is geared toward helping **registered dietitians (RDs)** make evidence-based decisions when providing **medical nutrition therapy,** knowledge of best practices in nutritional management of COPD is important for the CMES. However, nutritional care for clients with COPD should be overseen by an appropriately qualified RD.

During the initial intake and in follow-up sessions, the RD will assess and monitor the client's quality of life, weight status, and **body composition.** These factors greatly influence nutrition management. Quality of life for individuals with COPD affects their ability to obtain, prepare, and consume foods to meet nutritional needs. Up to 30% of people with COPD suffer from low BMI (<20 kg/m^2) which is associated with **sarcopenia** due to disease and inactivity, lower lung function measurements, more difficulty breathing, poorer nutritional status, and a twofold increase in COPD-related death. Many people with COPD also have lower-than-normal levels of fat-free mass and **bone mineral density** (A.N.D., 2008).

Nutrition recommendations are based on a determination of energy needs in stable COPD as well as during exacerbations and with physical activity, as both increase needs. In cases in which BMI is <20 kg/m^2, or where there is concern for malnutrition, the RD will initiate oral supplementation to meet nutritional needs. A Cochrane review found that in malnourished people with COPD, this nutritional supplementation promotes weight gain and improvement in fat-free mass, performance on the 6MWT, skinfold thickness, respiratory muscle strength, and health-related quality of life (Ferreira et al., 2012).

TABLE 10-8
STRATEGIES TO HELP CLIENTS WITH COPD ATTAIN NUTRITIONAL NEEDS

- Make mealtimes pleasant. Choose foods you enjoy. Invite others to share in mealtimes and allow them to help with shopping, preparation, and clean up.
- Be sure to eat when energy is the highest. Sometimes the first meal in the morning works best. Sometimes late afternoon or early evening is best.
- Divide your daily foods into 5–6 small meals, or into 5–6 large snacks.
- Drink enough fluids, including water, throughout the day and evening. This helps to keep mucus loose and easier to cough up.
- Drink high-calorie, high-nutrient beverages such as milkshakes, whole milk, flavored milk, and commercial nutritional products. The milk does not contribute to thickened secretion and can help to ensure adequate calcium intake.
- Choose foods high in calories. Increase calories by adding healthy oils, cream cheese, margarine, butter, cheese, salad dressing, and yogurt and cottage cheese made from whole milk to foods.
- Choose foods high in protein. Some examples are eggs, milk, cheese, yogurt, meats, poultry, fish, nuts, and beans.
- Choose foods with fiber, like whole grains and vegetables and fruits with skins or seeds, such as apples, blueberries, tomatoes, and sweet potatoes.
- Choose foods with vitamins and minerals, like colorful, fresh fruits and vegetables and fortified or enriched products, such as cereals and nutritional supplements.
- Avoid foods low in nutrients and calories, like diet foods and drinks and clear soups.

Source: American Dietetic Association (2008). *Nutrition Therapy for Chronic Obstructive Pulmonary Disease (COPD).* www.adancm.com/vault/editor/Docs/COPDNutritionTherapy_FINAL.pdf

The EAL advises that clients have the opportunity to choose these supplements based on their own personal preferences, more so than the substance's percentage of calories from fat or carbohydrate. These should be consumed frequently and in small amounts to avoid **postprandial dyspnea** and to promote **satiety** (A.N.D., 2008).

The EAL also advises that RDs ensure that clients meet the **Recommended Dietary Allowances (RDAs)** for vitamins A, C, and E and the **Adequate Intake (AI)** for omega-3 fatty acids, as these nutrients are low in many individuals with COPD. Additionally, the EAL notes that RDs should share with individuals with COPD that consumption of milk and milk products is unrelated to mucus production (A.N.D., 2008).

EXERCISE RECOMMENDATIONS

Due to its overall health benefits and improvement to quality of life, physical activity is strongly encouraged for all individuals with COPD (GOLD, 2013).

Cardiovascular and Pulmonary Responses to Exercise Training

While physical activity and structured exercise programs do not directly improve lung function, they do lead to other positive effects in multiple body systems, which helps to improve quality of life for people with COPD. Exercise helps to increase the brain's response to chronic elevation in carbon dioxide so that respiratory drive is improved. Exercise improves mood and reduces anxiety and depression. Exercise helps to decrease hyperinflation and make breathing easier. Exercise also improves skeletal muscle function, making ADL, such as walking from one side of the room to another, more manageable (Casaburi & ZuWallack, 2009). A pictorial representation of these benefits is shown in Figure 10-10.

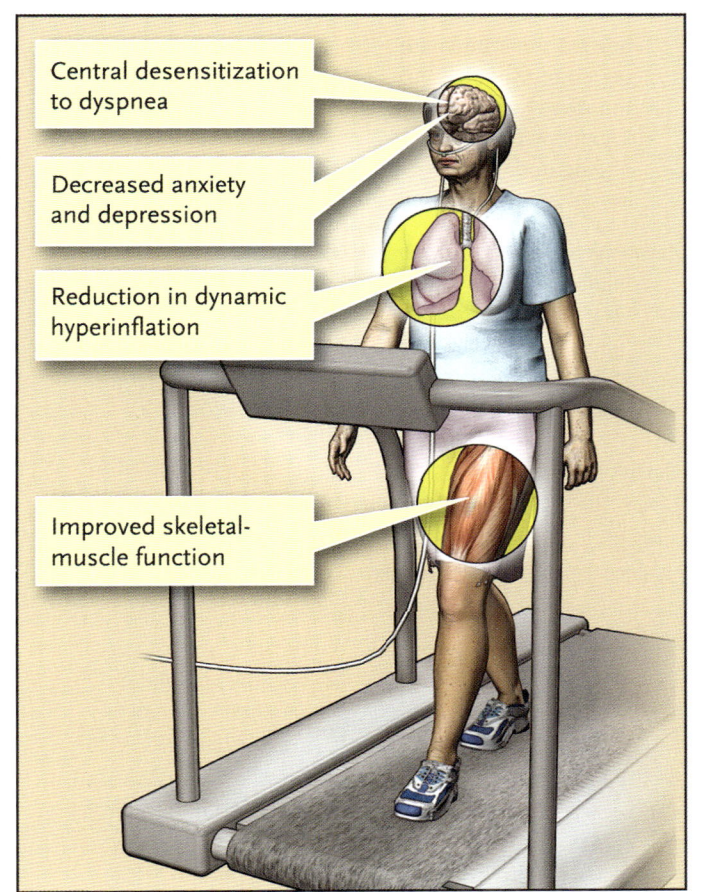

Figure 10-10
Targets of exercise training as part of pulmonary rehabilitation program for patients with COPD

- Central desensitization to dyspnea
- Decreased anxiety and depression
- Reduction in dynamic hyperinflation
- Improved skeletal-muscle function

Exercise training does not improve lung function, but it does ease other manifestations of COPD, increasing exercise tolerance, reducing dyspnea, and improving quality of life. Improved skeletal-muscle function is related, in part, to a reversal of deconditioning. Exercise training improves aerobic function of the muscles of ambulation. Dyspnea is mitigated by the reduction in dynamic hyperinflation that occurs when exercise-induced increases in the rate and depth of breathing result in inadequate time for full expiration, given the high expiratory airflow resistance. End-expiratory lung volume rises, and exercise is terminated when end-inspiratory lung volume approaches levels at which the high elastic work of breathing causes severe dyspnea. Exercise training reduces the ventilatory requirement and respiratory rate during heavy exercise, prolonging the time allowed for expiration and reducing dynamic hyperinflation. Desensitization to dyspnea occurs centrally as a result of exercise training; the underlying mechanism is uncertain. Decreased anxiety and depression are thought to result from increased exercise capacity and consequent increases in activities of daily living, coupled with feelings of mastery.

Reprinted with permission from Casaburi, R. & ZuWallack, R. (2009). Pulmonary rehabilitation for management of chronic obstructive pulmonary disease. *New England Journal of Medicine, 360,* 1329–1335.

EXPAND YOUR KNOWLEDGE

PULMONARY REHABILITATION

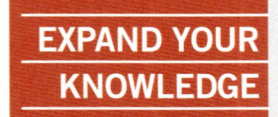

Physical activity and exercise therapy can come in various forms for people with COPD. The most well studied and clearly proven to provide significant benefit is a supervised pulmonary rehabilitation program. The five areas of focus of pulmonary rehabilitation typically include exercise conditioning, socialization, mood (and protection from depression), muscle strengthening, and weight management. This focus is intended to offset the exercise deconditioning, social isolation, depression, muscle wasting, and weight loss that often accompany COPD (GOLD, 2013).

Most programs emphasize exercise training, but also include nutrition coaching and education. Note that education is very important in a rehabilitation program to help the client improve understanding of disease and treatment and to facilitate goal setting and client ownership. Education topics include smoking cessation, incorporation of exercise and physical activity in the home setting, adherence to therapy, and an action plan for identification and treatment of exacerbation. A strong marker of a rehabilitation program's success is how well it has helped to not only increase knowledge of these areas, but also how it has helped to translate the knowledge into lasting behavioral change that will continue even once the client graduates from the program. In fact, while benefits from pulmonary rehabilitation are substantial, they reverse within months of the program end date if activities are not continued outside of rehabilitation (GOLD, 2013; Casaburi & ZuWallack, 2009). Table 10-9 highlights the demonstrated benefits of pulmonary rehabilitation.

TABLE 10-9
BENEFITS OF PULMONARY REHABILITATION IN COPD

EVIDENCE A	EVIDENCE B	EVIDENCE C
• Improves exercise capacity • Reduces perceived intensity of breathlessness • Improves health-related quality of life • Reduces the number of hospitalizations and days in the hospital • Reduces anxiety and depression associated with COPD • Improves recovery after hospitalization for an exacerbation	• Strength and endurance training of the upper limbs improves arm function • Benefits extend well beyond the immediate period of training • Improves survival • Enhances the effect of long-acting bronchodilators	• Respiratory muscle training can be beneficial, especially when combined with general exercise training

Key: Evidence A: Evidence is from randomized controlled trials and rich body of data; Evidence B: Evidence is from randomized controlled trials with limited body of data; Evidence C: Evidence is from nonrandomized trials and observational studies.

Source: Global Initiative for Chronic Obstructive Lung Disease (GOLD) (2013). *The Global Strategy for the Diagnosis, Management, and Prevention of COPD.* www.goldcopd.org

The best candidates for a pulmonary rehabilitation program have stage 3 disease, though those with either less severe and more severe disease may also benefit. The problem is that resources are limited, with variability in availability, costs, and financing of such programs, which cost approximately $2,200 per patient for an eight-week program. Pulmonary rehabilitation is not recommended for people who are unable to walk, have unstable cardiac disease, or have cognitive or psychiatric problems that would prevent adherence to the treatment plan. Some programs refuse to enroll active smokers (Casaburi & ZuWallack, 2009).

While programs vary somewhat, in general a pulmonary rehabilitation program consists of three sessions per week, each lasting three to four hours, including exercise, education, coaching, and nutrition support. The sessions are generally supervised by a pulmonologist and led by a rehabilitation coordinator, who is typically an allied health professional with training in nursing, respiratory therapy, or physical therapy. The most successful coordinators are also effective coaches, helping a client to continue the program, although it is typically very unpleasant initially due to baseline exercise intolerance and deconditioning.

Most programs last from six to 12 weeks, with longer programs showing greater benefit. In fact, programs with fewer than 28 sessions show inferior results to longer programs. The main focus of pulmonary rehabilitation is endurance exercise for the lower-leg muscles through walking, stationary cycling, and treadmill exercise. In most programs, the client is encouraged to walk to a symptom-limited maximum, rest, and then continue walking until 20 minutes of exercise have been completed. The typical goal is that a client is able to achieve 60 to 80% of symptom-limited maximal endurance training, as either continuous training or interval training, with bouts of higher-intensity exercise preferred. Wheeled walking devices may be helpful for some.

A robust body of evidence supports that pulmonary rehabilitation improves peak workload, peak oxygen uptake, and endurance. Benefits result whether rehabilitation occurs in an inpatient, outpatient, or home setting. While there are many benefits, there are also risks to pulmonary rehabilitation, including musculoskeletal injury, exercise-induced bronchoconstriction and cardiovascular events. A physician-supervised stress test is advisable prior to beginning rehabilitation (Casaburi & ZuWallack, 2009).

Some programs include upper-limb exercises, usually involving an upper-limb ergometer or resistance training with weights. No randomized clinical trial data are available to confirm its helpfulness, but presumably stronger upper-body muscles help with performance of ADL. Inclusion of upper-limb exercises seems to improve strength, but does not improve quality of life or exercise tolerance (Casaburi & ZuWallack, 2009).

Some programs use additional measures to help improve the benefits of an exercise program, including bronchodilation during exercise and supplemental oxygen, noninvasive ventilator support, heliox (a gaseous combination of helium and oxygen), ventilator-pattern feedback, and anabolic steroids.

The CMES in the Continuum of Care

There is widespread consensus that physical activity is good for the vast majority of individuals with COPD (GOLD, 2013). While not all have access to pulmonary rehabilitation, most are encouraged to participate in some degree of activity, even if it means a self-directed program of walking for 20 minutes per day, or use of various physical-activity recording devices. Some pulmonary rehabilitation programs have integrated group activity classes into their programs for rehabilitation "graduates."

A currently underutilized but potentially highly valuable member of the healthcare team for a person with COPD is an exercise professional not only with expertise in developing and overseeing an exercise program for someone with COPD, but also with the communication and coaching skills to help a client adopt a program that can be maintained for the long term. The CMES can play an important role both for those who have completed a pulmonary rehabilitation program as well as those who do not have access or resources to participate in a structured pulmonary rehabilitation program, but may have the resources to work with a qualified exercise professional either one-on-one or in a group setting.

Programming and Progression Guidelines and Considerations

Prior to beginning an exercise program for a client with COPD, it is important that the client undergo a medically monitored exercise evaluation for risk stratification. The client may also benefit from medically supervised training at the beginning of the program.

A primary goal of an exercise program for a client with COPD is to attain a higher level of physical activity. Studies support that these individuals have better exercise tolerance, experience have less dyspnea, have lower rates of hospitalizations, use fewer healthcare resources, and have lower risk of death (GOLD, 2013). Thus, the primary objective is to ensure that the activity occurs and ideally, that it is something that the client comes to enjoy.

For many, this is an uphill battle. Clients may feel anxiety about beginning a program. Teaching a client how to use pursed lip breathing can help to reduce this anxiety. The CMES can also play a key role in supporting and reinforcing physician and RD recommendations to help the client adhere to the medication and nutritional regimen, especially as they pertain to physical activity.

APPLY WHAT YOU KNOW

PURSED-LIP BREATHING

Pursed-lip breathing has been shown to increase tidal volume and reduce respiratory rate in patients with COPD. Additionally, pursed-lip breathing can lead to increased rib cage movement and accessory muscle recruitment during inspiration and expiration in patients with COPD (Kim et al., 2012). The following pursed-lip breathing technique can be used to ease shortness of breath:

- Relax the neck and shoulder muscles.
- Breathe in for two seconds through the nose, keeping your mouth closed.
- Breathe out for four seconds through pursed lips. If this is too long, simply breathe out twice as long as you breathe in.

People with COPD should engage in physical activity daily for 20 to 60 minutes per day, either continuously or in intervals (ACSM, 2022). Clients should use RPE and the Borg dyspnea scale (see Table 10-4) to characterize the extent of breathlessness during exercise and to guide exercise-progression decisions. In most rehabilitation programs, goal intensity is 50 to 80% of peak work rate. For most clients, the minimum amount of activity to attain exercise benefits is 20 minutes of moderate-intensity activity three days per week. Regardless of COPD severity, exercise is a potent and effective intervention that can decrease functional impairment and disability, and improve symptoms and quality of life (ACSM, 2022). Inclusion of flexibility training can provide additional benefits related to postural impairments, thoracic mobility, and lung function. ACSM (2022) also recommends two to four sets of eight to 12 repetitions of resistance exercise for each of the major muscle groups.

As with all exercisers, clients with COPD should stop exercising if they experience pressure or pain in the chest, arm, or jaw, or nausea, lightheadedness, dizziness, or headache. Increased work of breathing should be transient. However, if labored breathing above baseline persists, the client should stop and rest.

EXERCISE GUIDELINES SUMMARY FOR CLIENTS WITH COPD

	CARDIORESPIRATORY TRAINING
Frequency	• 3–5 days per week
Intensity	• Moderate to vigorous
	• Below, at, and above VT1 but below VT2 HR
	• 50–80% peak work rate
	• RPE 4–6 (0–10 scale)
Time	• 20–60 minutes per day
	• Intermittent exercise (i.e., interval training) may be used if continuous training is not achievable
Type	• Walking or cycling, upper-body endurance activities to help improve activities of daily living
Progression	• Progress following the ACE Integrated Fitness Training Model based on client goals and availability.
	MUSCULAR TRAINING
Frequency	• At least 2 days per week on nonconsecutive days
Intensity	• 60–70% of 1-RM for beginners' muscular strength
	• ≥80% of 1-RM for experienced weight trainers' muscular strength
	• <50% of 1-RM for muscular endurance
Time	• 2–4 sets of 8–12 repetitions for muscular strength
	• 1–2 sets of 15–20 repetitions for muscular endurance
Type	• Weight machines, free weights, or body-weight exercise
Progression	• Progress following the ACE Integrated Fitness Training Model based on client goals and availability.

Note: VT1 = First ventilatory threshold; VT2 = Second ventilatory threshold; HR = Heart rate; RPE = Rating of perceived exertion; 1-RM = One-repetition maximum; Peak work rate measured in watts

> **CMES FOCUS**
>
> Both cardiorespiratory and resistance-training exercise are important modes of activity to include in programming for a client with COPD. Aerobic exercise helps to condition the lungs and respiratory muscles, while resistance exercise helps improve strength in the skeletal muscles. Muscular training is the most potent intervention for addressing the muscle dysfunction that may occur as result of pulmonary diseases and their treatments. Also, lower-extremity muscular and balance training are important in addressing the common occurrence of falls in people with COPD. Regardless of prescribed exercise intensity for clients with COPD, the CMES should closely monitor clients in each exercise session for symptoms associated with the disease and adjust intensity accordingly. That is, the presence of symptoms, particularly dyspnea/breathlessness, supersedes any prescribed objective measures for exercise.
>
> *Source:* American College of Sports Medicine (2022). *ACSM's Guidelines for Exercise Testing and Prescription* (11th ed.). Philadelphia: Wolters Kluwer.

Exercise Testing

Individuals with COPD who participate in a rehabilitation program will likely have had exercise testing. This exercise testing is also something that a CMES can oversee. The most practical exercise test for individuals with COPD in a community-based program is the 6MWT (see page 295).

CASE STUDY

Client Information

Shaila is a 63-year-old female diagnosed with COPD four months ago. She smoked one pack of cigarettes per day for 25 years, but quit two years ago after her husband died of lung cancer. For the past 18 months, she has experienced worsening shortness of breath, especially while walking or doing even light-intensity activity. She is currently being treated with inhaled medications to control her COPD. She is sedentary and her BMI is 28 kg/m^2. Her daughter comes to visit about twice a month, but otherwise her only social activity is going to church once per week. Shaila's doctor referred her to a pulmonary rehabilitation program, but the closest facility is about a 30-minute drive. She told her doctor that the drive is too far for her, but that she is highly motivated to improve her symptoms and would like to begin a regular physical-activity program, even though she knows that it will be difficult. Her doctor referred her to the local wellness center where she has signed up for 14 hours of training with a CMES.

Prior to referral to the wellness center, Shaila's primary care physician referred her to a cardiologist for an exercise stress test to ensure that she would be able to safely begin an exercise program. Her primary care physician also discussed her case with a pulmonary specialist who agreed that beginning an exercise program would be beneficial for Shaila, and that it would be acceptable for her to attend a community-based program since pulmonary rehabilitation was not feasible for her.

ACE IFT® MODEL AT A GLANCE

Cardiorespiratory Training

This client is starting Base Training, as she needs to develop an aerobic base before progressing. Due to her COPD, this client may continue to with Base Training for an extended period before progressing to other phases of Cardiorespiratory Training.

Muscular Training

After demonstrating good postural stability and kinetic-chain mobility, the client can progress to Movement Training with a focus on improved movement patterns and muscular endurance. This Movement Training workout that can transition to Load/Speed Training focusing on increased muscular endurance once she has developed adequate stability and movement.

CMES Approach

At the initial consultation, the CMES took extra care to develop **rapport** with Shaila and congratulated her on successfully quitting smoking. The CMES arranged for Shaila to complete a 6MWT for baseline functional status. This walking test occurred in the wellness center at a time during which it could be medically supervised. The CMES then developed a nine-week program for Shaila consisting of two 60-minute sessions per week for the first three weeks followed by one 60-minute session per week for the next eight weeks. The CMES advised Shaila to purchase an inexpensive activity monitor to track her activity during the days that she is not working with the CMES, and to provide the CMES with data from the monitor at each training session, with an ultimate goal of building up to five to seven days per week of physical activity. Initially, Shaila engages in 10 to 20 minutes of relatively low- to moderate-intensity treadmill walking as her initial cardiorespiratory-training program. After demonstrating that Shaila has adequate postural stability and joint mobility, the CMES designs a Muscular Training program focused on improving movement patterns and developing initial muscular endurance. The initial Muscular Training program consists of one set of low-intensity resistance-training exercises for each of the major muscle groups. As she progresses in her program, the CMES focuses on helping Shaila to internalize the program and feel successful and empowered so that she can continue it once the 14 hours of training with the CMES are completed. The CMES also shares information with her about a local support group for people with COPD, in case she is interested in attending. At the end of the program, Shaila completes a follow-up 6MWT, where her test results show that she has experienced substantial improvements. She makes a plan to check in with the CMES once every two weeks over the next several months to continue progressing with her program. She also schedules a follow-up visit with her physician, who notices her improvement in mood and strength and notes that there has not been any progression of her disease.

SUMMARY

Asthma is a common pulmonary disease that can interfere not only with establishing and adhering to a regular exercise program, but also with the individual's quality of life. Individuals with asthma often exhibit low physical-activity levels because they typically avoid exercise. However, with appropriate precautions and asthma-related education, most people with asthma can effectively control their disease and enjoy a regular and vigorous activity program. Clients with known asthma and/or EIB should receive medical clearance from a physician before beginning an exercise program. While exercise may be the only asthma trigger for many people, these individuals should still be evaluated by a physician prior to beginning an exercise program.

COPD is a serious, incurable pulmonary disease that negatively impacts a person's quality and quantity of life. Though it is not reversible, early detection and intervention can be life-changing. Prior to beginning an exercise program for a client with COPD, it is important that they undergo a medically monitored exercise evaluation for risk stratification. The client may also benefit from medically supervised training at the beginning of the program. One of the most important components of therapy for a person with COPD is physical activity and exercise, as individuals with COPD who are physically active have better exercise tolerance, experience less dyspnea, have lower rates of hospitalizations, use fewer healthcare resources, and have lower risk of death. An appropriately qualified and trained CMES is positioned to play an important role in helping individuals with COPD substantially improve their quality of life.

REFERENCES

Academy of Nutrition and Dietetics Evidence Analysis Library (2008). *Chronic Obstructive Pulmonary Disease Guideline.* www.andeal.org/topic.cfm?cat=3708

American College of Sports Medicine (2022). *ACSM's Guidelines for Exercise Testing and Prescription* (11th ed.). Philadelphia: Wolters Kluwer.

American Dietetic Association (2008). *Nutrition Therapy for Chronic Obstructive Pulmonary Disease (COPD).* www.adancm.com/vault/editor/Docs/COPDNutritionTherapy_FINAL.pdf

American Thoracic Society (2002). ATS Statement: Guidelines for the six-minute walk test. *American Journal of Respiratory and Critical Care Medicine,* 166, 111–117.

Balmes, J., et al. (2003). American Thoracic Society Statement: Occupational contribution to the burden of airway disease. *American Journal of Respiratory and Critical Care Medicine,* 167, 787–797.

Beuther, D.A., Weiss, S.T., & Sutherland, E.R. (2006). Obesity and asthma. *American Journal of Respiratory and Critical Care Medicine,* 174, 112–119.

Butcher, J.D. (2006). Exercise-induced asthma in the competitive cold weather athlete. *Current Sports Medicine Reports,* 5, 284–288.

Casaburi, R. & ZuWallack, R. (2009). Pulmonary rehabilitation for management of chronic obstructive pulmonary disease. *New England Journal of Medicine,* 360, 1329–1335.

Chobanian, A.V. et al. (2003). *JNC 7 Express: The Seventh Report of the Joint National Committee on Prevention, Detection, Evaluation, and Treatment of High Blood Pressure. NIH Publication No. 03-5233.* Washington, D.C.: National Institutes of Health & National Heart, Lung, and Blood Institute.

Evans, T.M. et al. (2005). Cold air inhalation does not affect the severity of EIB after exercise or eucapnic voluntary hyperventilation. *Medicine & Science in Sports & Exercise,* 37, 544–549.

Farzan, S. (2013). The asthma phenotype in the obese: Distinct or otherwise? *Journal of Allergy,* DOI: 10.1155/2013/602908 PMCID: PMC3708411

Ferreira, I.M. et al. (2012). Nutritional supplementation for stable chronic obstructive pulmonary disease. *Cochrane Database System Reviews,* 12:CD000998. DOI: 10.1002/14651858.CD000998.pub.3

Global Initiative for Chronic Obstructive Lung Disease (GOLD) (2013). *The Global Strategy for the Diagnosis, Management, and Prevention of COPD.* www.goldcopd.org

Horwood, L.J., Fergusson, D.M., & Shannon, F.T. (1985). Social and familial factors in the development of early childhood asthma. *Pediatrics,* 75, 5, 859–868.

James, K.M. et al. (2013). Risk of childhood asthma following infant bronchiolitis during the respiratory syncytial virus season. *The Journal of Allergy and Clinical Immunology,* 132, 1, 227–229.

Juel, CT-B. et al. (2012). Asthma and obesity: Does weight loss improve asthma control? A systematic review. *Journal of Asthma and Allergy,* 5, 21–26.

Kattan, M. et al. (2010). Asthma control, adiposity, and adipokines among inner-city adolescents. *Journal of Allergy and Clinical Immunology,* 125, 3, 584–592.

Kim, K-S. et al. (2012). Effects of breathing maneuver and sitting posture on muscle activity in inspiratory accessory muscles in patients with chronic obstructive pulmonary disease. *Multidisciplinary Respiratory Medicine,* 7, 1, 9.

Knudson, R.J. et al. (1983). Changes in the normal maximal expiratory flow-volume curve with growth and aging. *American Review of Respiratory Diseases,* 127, 6, 725–734.

Kosacz, N.M. et al. (2012). Chronic obstructive pulmonary disease among adults—United States, 2011. *Morbidity and Mortality Weekly Report,* 61, 46, 938–943.

Mannino, D.M. et al. (2002). Chronic obstructive pulmonary disease surveillance—United States, 1971–2000. *Morbidity and Mortality Weekly Report Surveillance Summary,* 51, SS-6, 1–16.

McConnell, R. et al. (2002). Asthma in exercising children exposed to ozone: A cohort study. *Lancet,* 359, 9304, 386–391.

McHugh, M.K. et al. (2009). Prevalence of asthma among adult females and males in the United States: Results from the National Health and Nutrition Examination Survey (NHANES), 2001–2004. *Journal of Asthma,* 46, 8, 759–766.

McKeever, T.M. & Britton, J. (2004). Diet and asthma. *American Journal of Respiratory and Critical Care Medicine,* 170, 7, 725–729.

Moorman, J.E. et al. (2012). National surveillance for asthma—United States 2001–2010. National Center for Health Statistics. *Vital Health Statistics,* 3, 35.

National Asthma Education and Prevention Program (2007). *Expert Panel Report 3: Guidelines for the Diagnosis and Management of Asthma.* Bethesda, Md.: U.S. Department of Health & Human Services, Public Health Service, National Institutes of Health, National Heart, Lung, and Blood Institute; NIH publication number 08-4051.

National Heart, Lung, and Blood Institute (2012). *What Is Asthma?* www.nhlbi.nih.gov/health/health-topics/topics/asthma/

National Heart, Lung, and Blood Institute (1997). *Facts About Controlling Asthma.* Bethesda, Md.: National Asthma Education and Prevention Program, National Heart, Lung, and Blood Institute, NIH Publication No. 97-2339.

Pakhale, S. et al. (2013). Effects of physical training on airway inflammation in bronchial asthma: A systematic review. *BMC Pulmonary Medicine,* 13, 38, 1–21.

Rasmussen, F. & Hancox, R.J. (2013). Mechanisms of obesity in asthma. *Current Opinion in Allergy and Clinical Immunology*, 2013, Dec 2. [Epub ahead of print]

Rikli, R.E. & Jones, J.C. (2013). *Senior Fitness Test Manual* (2nd ed.). Champaign, Ill.: Human Kinetics.

Sideleva, O. et al. (2012). Obesity and asthma. *American Journal of Respiratory and Critical Care Medicine*, 186, 7, 598–605.

United States Department of Health & Human Services, Agency for Healthcare Research & Quality (2004). Evidence Report/Technology Assessment No. 91, *Health Effects of Omega-3 Fatty Acids on Asthma*. Retrieved December 27, 2013: http://archive.ahrq.gov/clinic/tp/o3asthmtp.htm

United States Department of Health & Human Services & National Institutes of Health (2003). *Making a Difference in the Management of Asthma: A Guide for Respiratory Therapists*. Pub. No. 02-1064.

Welsh, E.J. et al. (2010). Caffeine for asthma. *Cochrane Database of Systematic Reviews.* Issue 1, Artical No.: CD001112. DOI: 10.1002/14651858.CD001112.pub2

Williams, B. et al. (2008). Exploring and explaining low participation in physical activity among children and young people with asthma: A review. *BMC Family Practice,* 13, 1, 40.

Wood, L.G. et al. (2012). Manipulating antioxidant intake in asthma: A randomized controlled trial. *American Journal of Clinical Nutrition,* 96, 3, 534–543.

Yang, H. et al. (2013). Fish and fish oil intake in relation to risk of asthma: A systematic review and meta-analysis. *PLoS One,* 12, 8, 11:e80048. DOI: 10.1371/journal.pone.0080048

SUGGESTED READING

Global Initiative for Chronic Obstructive Lung Disease (GOLD) (2013). *The Global Strategy for the Diagnosis, Management, and Prevention of COPD.* www.goldcopd.org

National Asthma Education and Prevention Program (2007). *Expert Panel Report 3: Guidelines for the Diagnosis and Management of Asthma.* Bethesda, Md.: U.S. Department of Health & Human Services, Public Health Service, National Institutes of Health, National Heart, Lung, and Blood Institute; NIH publication number 08-4051.

Pakhale, S. et al. (2013). Effects of physical training on airway inflammation in bronchial asthma: A systematic review. *BMC Pulmonary Medicine,* 13, 38, 1–21.

Rasmussen, F. & Hancox, R.J. (2013). Mechanisms of obesity in asthma. *Current Opinion in Allergy and Clinical Immunology,* 2013, Dec 2. [Epub ahead of print]

PART IV
METABOLIC DISEASES AND DISORDERS

CHAPTER 11
OVERWEIGHT AND OBESITY

CHAPTER 12
THE METABOLIC SYNDROME

CHAPTER 13
DIABETES MELLITUS

11 OVERWEIGHT AND OBESITY

IN THIS CHAPTER

EPIDEMIOLOGY

OVERVIEW
THE BIOLOGY OF OVERWEIGHT AND OBESITY

DIAGNOSTIC TESTING AND CRITERIA

TREATMENT OPTIONS
NON-PHARMACOLOGICAL TREATMENT
PHARMACOLOGICAL TREATMENT
SURGICAL TREATMENT
EXERCISE TREATMENT

NUTRITIONAL CONSIDERATIONS
POPULAR DIETS
NUTRITIONAL CONSIDERATIONS FOR CLIENTS BEFORE AND AFTER BARIATRIC SURGERY

EXERCISE RECOMMENDATIONS FOR CLIENTS WITH OBESITY
THE ROLE OF EXERCISE IN WEIGHT LOSS AND WEIGHT-GAIN PREVENTION
PROGRAMMING AND PROGRESSIVE EXERCISE GUIDELINES FOR OVERWEIGHT AND OBESITY
CARDIORESPIRATORY EXERCISE CONSIDERATIONS
RESISTANCE-TRAINING CONSIDERATIONS

EXERCISE GUIDELINES SUMMARY FOR CLIENTS WITH OBESITY

CASE STUDIES

SUMMARY

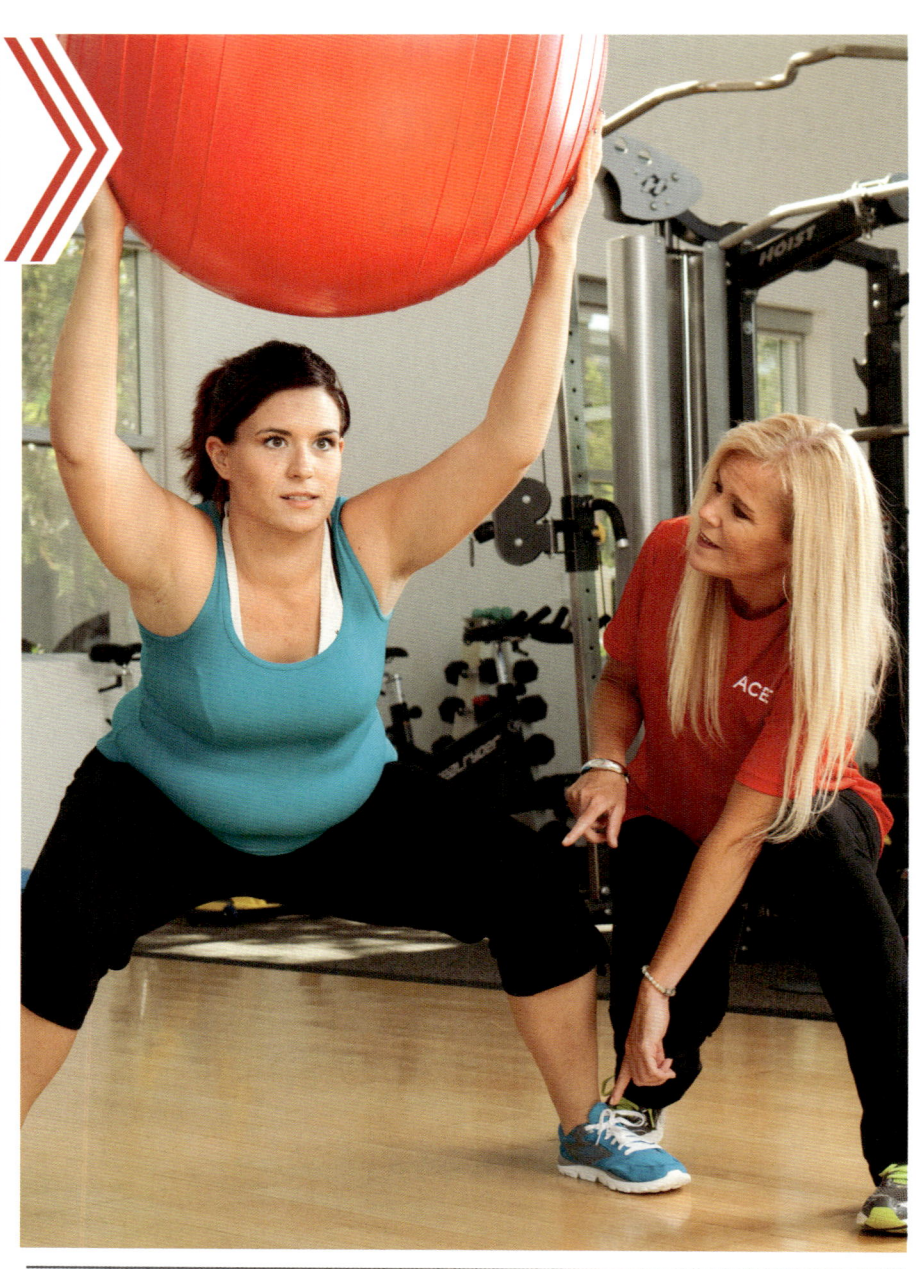

ABOUT THE AUTHOR
Len Kravitz, Ph.D., is the Program Coordinator of Exercise Science and Researcher at the University of New Mexico where he won the "Outstanding Teacher of the Year" award. Dr. Kravitz was honored with the 2009 Canadian Fitness Professional "Specialty Presenter of the Year" award and chosen as the American Council on Exercise 2006 "Fitness Educator of the Year." He also has received the prestigious Canadian Fitness Professional "Lifetime Achievement Award" and the "Global Award" from the Aquatic Exercise Association.

By Len Kravitz

IN MOST CASES, **OVERWEIGHT** AND **OBESITY** ARE the result of an imbalance between calories consumed and calories expended. An increased consumption of high-calorie foods, without an equal increase in physical activity, leads to an unhealthy increase in weight. Decreased levels of physical activity will also result in an energy imbalance and lead to weight gain. Supportive environments are absolutely necessary in shaping people's choices and preventing obesity. Individual responsibility can only have its full effect where people have access to a healthy lifestyle and are supported to make healthy choices. With knowledge and skill in effective exercise techniques and healthy nutrition strategies, an ACE® Certified Medical Exercise Specialist (CMES) is in a unique position to offer much needed education and support in the fight against obesity. This chapter covers current concepts related to the causes of, and potential treatments for, the obesity epidemic.

EPIDEMIOLOGY

Once associated with high-income countries, obesity is now also prevalent in low- and middle-income countries. Worldwide projections by the World Health Organization (WHO, 2020) indicate that 1.9 billion people aged 18 years or older have overweight, with approximately 650 million of them having obesity. Some contributing factors to this epidemic can be credited largely to the progression from a rural lifestyle to a highly technological urban existence, and the tempting capacity of the modern environment to encourage individuals to eat more and move less. Almost all countries are experiencing this dramatic increase in overweight and obesity.

Excess body weight is associated with an increased likelihood to develop heart disease, **hypertension, type 2 diabetes mellitus (T2DM),** gallstones, breathing problems, musculoskeletal disabilities, and certain forms of cancer (endometrial, breast, and colon) [National Institutes of Health (NIH), 2012; American College of Sports Medicine (ACSM), 2022]. In addition, obesity has a deleterious effect on the economy of all countries, as it increases the associated costs for treating the related diseases.

MISCONCEPTIONS AND FACTS ABOUT OBESITY

Casazza and colleagues (2013) set out to study numerous beliefs about obesity that persist despite contradicting evidence (myths), as well as those that persist in the absence of supporting scientific evidence (presumptions). The researchers used internet searches of popular media and scientific literature to identify, review, and classify obesity-related myths and presumptions. What they found were seven obesity-related myths and six presumptions. Lastly, the authors reported nine evidence-supported facts that are relevant for the formulation of sound public health, policy, or clinical recommendations.

The following myths of obesity were found to persist, even though there are contradictory data:
- Small, sustained changes in energy intake or expenditure result in significant, long-term weight changes. Changes in energy intake and output often result in compensatory adjustments that inhibit continual weight loss.

LEARNING OBJECTIVES:

» Explain the difference between overweight and obesity and the diagnostic criteria for each.

» Describe the available treatment options for obesity, including an emphasis on the role of physical activity and structured exercise, as well as behavioral interventions.

» Explain nutrition-related strategies for the treatment and management of obesity, including evidence-based information on popular diets and considerations for clients before and after bariatric surgery.

» Design and implement safe and effective exercise programs for clients who have overweight or obesity.

EXPAND YOUR KNOWLEDGE

- Setting realistic weight-loss goals is important so that individuals with obesity do not become frustrated and therefore lose less weight. The research does not show any undesirable outcomes from clients having more ambitious weight-loss goals.
- Large, rapid weight loss results in poorer long-term weight outcomes than slow, gradual weight loss. Some research suggests that rapid initial weight loss (via low-energy diets) may actually be favorable for long-term outcomes with some individuals with overweight/obesity.
- Assessing the stage of change or diet readiness is important in helping patients who seek weight-loss treatment. In fact, that readiness to change is not always a predictor of weight loss achieved.
- The way physical education classes are taught today plays an important role in preventing or reducing childhood obesity. It does not appear that the dose response in most physical education classes meaningfully results in significant changes in the prevalence of obesity.
- Breast-feeding protects against obesity. Some well-designed current studies do not show evidence of an anti-obesity effect from breast-feeding.
- The calorie expenditure of one bout of sexual activity equates to 100 to 300 kcal for each person involved. This energy expenditure estimate from sexual activity appears to be inflated.

The following presumptions about obesity were reported, even though there is a lack of evidence to support them:

- Regularly eating (rather than skipping) breakfast protects against obesity.
- The exercise and eating patterns that we learn in early childhood become habits that influence our weight throughout life.
- Eating more fruits and vegetables protects against obesity, regardless of whether any other intentional behavioral or environmental changes are made.
- Weight cycling (e.g., yo-yo dieting) is associated with increased mortality.
- Snacking contributes to weight gain and obesity.
- The built environment (e.g., accessibility to sidewalks and parks) influences obesity.

Lastly, the following list presents obesity-related facts that are supported by sufficient evidence to consider them empirically proved:

- Although genetic factors play a large role in one's weight status, genes do not fully dictate a person's destiny.
- Diets very effectively reduce weight, but they generally do not work well in the long-term.
- Exercise increases health levels, regardless of body weight or weight loss.
- Sufficient doses of physical activity or exercise aids in long-term weight maintenance.
- Continuation of conditions that promote weight loss promotes maintenance of lower weight.
- Greater weight loss or maintenance is achieved for children with overweight in programs that involve the parents and the home setting.
- Provision of meals and use of meal-replacement products promote greater weight loss.
- The continued use of some pharmaceutical agents can help patients achieve clinically meaningful weight loss and maintain the reduction.
- In appropriate patients, bariatric surgery results in long-term weight loss and reductions in the rate of incident diabetes and mortality.

Health and exercise professionals are encouraged to read the entire manuscript of this study, as it sheds light on the numerous myths and presumptions about obesity that reflect unsupported beliefs held by many people, including academics and the general public. The authors of this study were careful to conclude that any of the aforementioned myths and presumptions might one day be justifiably proved correct with appropriate scientific research.

OVERVIEW

Ultimately, weight management is dependent on **energy balance,** wherein if energy intake (EI) (via calories consumed from food and beverages) is greater than expenditure energy (EE) from resting metabolism, physical activity, and exercise, a **positive energy balance** is created. In contrast, a **negative energy balance** occurs when EE exceeds EI (ACSM, 2022). Human existence has evolved from times when shelter and food were in short supply and famine was a constant threat to life. In addition, major amounts of physical exertion were once necessary to obtain food and cope with harsh living environments. Therefore, humans have evolved an outstanding ability to biologically function with great energy efficiency by storing large amounts of excess **fat** as **adipose tissue.** In modern society, many people spend hours every day watching TV, playing video games, using computers, doing schoolwork, and adopting other **sedentary** leisure behaviors. In fact, more than two hours a day of regular TV viewing has been linked to overweight and obesity (NIH, 2012). It is important to also note the existence of obesity disorders such as hypothyroidism, Prader-Willi syndrome, and Cushing's syndrome. With these diseases, metabolic and/or hormonal dysfunctions or impairment contribute to obesity.

An abundance of food may be a by-product of the success of a society, but it clearly creates the conditions for a positive energy balance in the modern lifestyle. Other environmental factors contributing to obesity include not having enough sidewalks, trails, parks, and affordable fitness facilities for all people. Restaurants, fast-food chains, and movie theaters compete for business by offering very large food **portions.** In addition, healthy food choices are more expensive, making access to these foods less of an option for the financially challenged, while food companies that encourage people of all ages to select high-calorie, high-fat snacks and sugary drinks dominate food advertising.

FAMILIAL CONNECTIONS TO OBESITY

EXPAND YOUR KNOWLEDGE

Currently, obesity in children is in excess of 17% in the United States, and approximately 70% of adolescents with obesity grow up to become adults with obesity, which in turn increases their overall mortality later in life (Xia & Grant, 2013). Overweight and obesity tend to run in families (NIH, 2012). A person's genes may affect the amount of fat they store in the body, as well as where the fat is stored (NIH, 2012). It is well established that fat-site deposition is highly linked to a person's relative health risk. Fat deposited in the hips and thighs, referred to as gluteofemoral or **gynoid** fat (more often observed in females), appears to be quite benign and metabolically inactive. On the other hand, fat found in the trunk area around the internal organs of the abdomen (often observed in men) is referred to as **android** or **visceral fat.** Excess visceral fat is correlated with hypertension, diabetes, high blood **triglycerides,** and **coronary heart disease (CHD).** It is interesting to observe that with exercise, it is the visceral fat that is often the first to disappear.

Familial factors also contribute to the prevalence of overweight and obesity. For example, families commonly share eating and physical-activity habits. Children tend to adopt the habits of their parents and live-in relatives, at least in part because parents and other family members tend to serve as the primary role models for dietary intake and physical activity. It has been estimated that foods prepared at home contribute to more than 65% of daily energy intake, potentially resulting in the majority of daily calories consumed with, or in the presence of, other household members (Swanson et al., 2011). Therefore, a child with parents who are overweight, inactive, and eat high-calorie meals may later have overweight as well. However, if a family adopts healthful food and physical-activity habits, the child's chance of becoming overweight are reduced (NIH, 2012).

THINK IT THROUGH

You are working with a teenager who has obesity at the request of his parents, who are concerned about their son's health. The teenager clearly shares a sedentary lifestyle and a tendency to make poor nutrition choices with his parents, both of whom have substantial overweight. How might you approach this topic in a way that avoids insulting the boy and his parents, but instead inspires them to improve their lifestyle as a family?

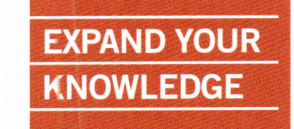

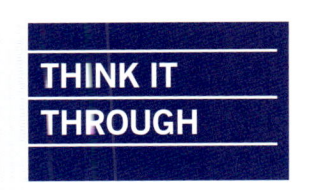

The Biology of Overweight and Obesity

Fat tissue, for the most part, was once understood to be an extra layer of cushioning with few metabolic responsibilities. It was viewed and described like a balloon that inflates when a person eats more food and/or expends fewer calories, and deflates when there is greater physical activity and/or less food consumption. Research has revealed that fat tissue (composed of **adipocyte** cells that specialize in fat storage) functions like other **endocrine** organs (i.e., glands that secrete **hormones**) in the body, sending signals to the brain that affect several intricate physiological mechanisms of energy-expenditure regulation, **insulin** sensitivity, and fat and **carbohydrate** metabolism (Townsend & Tseng, 2012). Two key hormones related to energy metabolism regulation are **leptin** and **adiponectin,** while a host of other hormones are involved in immune reactions in the body.

EXPAND YOUR KNOWLEDGE

BROWN ADIPOSE TISSUE

Brown adipose tissue was first described in small mammals and infants as an important thermogenesis adaptation to defend against the cold. Found near the scapulae, it was originally referred to as the "hibernating gland" due to its function in maintaining body temperature in hibernating animals (Rasmussen, 1923). Since then, several studies have demonstrated that brown fat is present and active in adult humans. Since it was first noted for its ability to protect animals from hypothermia, research over the past several decades has produced evidence that brown fat has an anti-obesity role. More recently, researchers have described inducible thermogenic adipose tissue, also referred to as beige fat, that can emerge in white fat depots under certain conditions (Wu, Cohen, & Spiegelman, 2013).

Energy-providing adipocytes stored in adipose tissue are not passive structures. They act as endocrine organs, secreting molecules like leptin that can regulate appetite and whole-body metabolism. Adipocytes can also transform chemical energy into heat. Brown adipocytes, which get their name from a high number of **mitochondria** (which are lacking in their white adipocyte counterparts), are specialized to dissipate energy in the form of heat, a process called **nonshivering thermogenesis.** There also appears to be an extensive vascular and nerve supply to adipose tissue where brown adipocytes are found. Brown and beige fat cells can increase whole-body energy expenditure and therefore can protect against obesity and its **comorbidities.** In humans, it has been estimated that as little as 50 grams of brown adipose tissue (less than 0.1% of body weight) could utilize up to 20% of basal caloric needs if maximally stimulated (Townsend & Tseng, 2012). This role of brown (and more recently beige) adipose cells in increasing metabolic rates has driven much of the research interest in these cell types, as finding ways to activate this tissue could result in prevention and treatment strategies for obesity (Wu, Cohen, & Spiegelman, 2013).

Interestingly, there appears to be more active brown/beige fat in women than in men, which has been explained by some researchers as a result of hormonal differences (Pfannenberg et al., 2010). Further, brown/beige fat activity correlates inversely with age (from 50% activity in subjects in their 20s, down to 10% for subjects in their 50s and 60s) (Ouellet et al., 2011; Yoneshiro et al., 2011), is rather low in subjects with obesity, and is increased after weight loss from bariatric surgery (Vijgen et al., 2012; Vijgen et al., 2011).

Given the global epidemic of obesity and the projection for epidemic rates of comorbidities like diabetes, research into brown/beige fat as a potential therapeutic agent is becoming more common. For example, transplantation of as little as 0.1 to 0.4 grams of brown adipose tissue into the visceral cavity of rodents is able to prevent weight gain and improve **glucose** homeostasis in mice with obesity (Stanford et al., 2013). Although the potential for this type of therapy in humans is still uncertain, the CMES should be alert to new research efforts in this area.

Leptin

Leptin, which resides in all fat cells, communicates directly with the hypothalamus in the brain, providing information about how much energy is currently stored in the body's fat cells. Leptin functions in what is referred to in biology as a **negative feedback loop.** For example, when fat cells decrease in size, leptin decreases, sending a message to the hypothalamus to direct the body to eat more. Similarly, when fat cells increase in size, leptin increases and the message sent to the hypothalamus is to instruct the body to eat less. However, it appears that the primary biological role of leptin is to facilitate energy intake when energy storage is low, as opposed to slowing down overconsumption when energy storage is high (Mantzoros et al., 2011). Scientific attempts to take leptin as a pill have not shown any benefit for individuals who have overweight, possibly because the digestion process changes the synthetic form of leptin's structure and function.

Adiponectin

Another specialized hormone secreted by fat is adiponectin, which helps insulin by sending blood glucose into the body's cells for storage or use as fuel, thus increasing the cells' insulin sensitivity or glucose metabolism. It also helps decrease blood levels of triglycerides by working with insulin to stimulate fat breakdown. If a person has a lot of body fat, then they typically will have lower levels of adiponectin, which is predictably low with all individuals with overweight and especially low in individuals with **insulin resistance,** which occurs when the normal amount of insulin secreted by the pancreas is not able to transport glucose into cells. To maintain a normal blood glucose level, the pancreas secretes additional insulin. In some people, when the body cells resist, or do not respond to even high levels of insulin, glucose builds up in the blood, resulting in high blood glucose, which may lead to T2DM. Even people with diabetes who take medications to control their blood glucose levels can have higher than normal blood insulin levels due to insulin resistance. Healthy lifestyle interventions have been shown to increase circulating adiponectin levels.

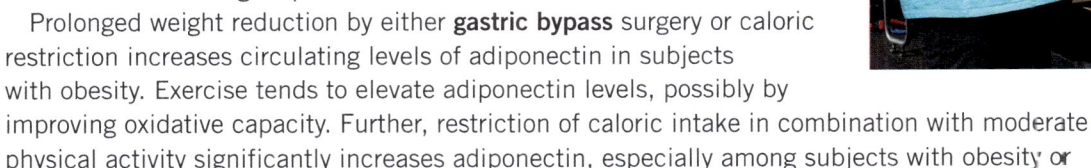

Prolonged weight reduction by either **gastric bypass** surgery or caloric restriction increases circulating levels of adiponectin in subjects with obesity. Exercise tends to elevate adiponectin levels, possibly by improving oxidative capacity. Further, restriction of caloric intake in combination with moderate physical activity significantly increases adiponectin, especially among subjects with obesity or diabetes (Hui et al., 2012).

Immune Hormones

It is known that fat tissue produces a number of immune-system hormones, such as tumor necrosis factor-alpha, interleukin-6, plasminogen activator inhibitor 1, angiotensin II, and other **cytokines** (Federico et al., 2010). Cytokines, which are hormone-like **proteins**, function largely as inflammatory proteins, reacting to areas of infection or injury in the body. However, persons with excess fat appear to have an overreaction in terms of the release of these inflammatory proteins. The concept of **inflammation** is one of the most critical in obesity biology. Both obesity and diabetes are associated with chronic low-grade inflammation (Wang et al., 2013). In addition, inflammation is understood to be a key facet in heart disease (see Chapter 7). The release of these proteins may inflame arterial plaque, causing the plaque to rupture and thus lead to a heart attack or **stroke** (Kaptoge et al., 2010). With weight loss, there is a corresponding decrease in the circulating levels of these inflammatory proteins. There is also evidence that these fat tissue–derived inflammatory hormones may play a causal role in the development of insulin resistance (Mazza, Pratley, & Smith, 2011).

Ghrelin

Another component of the energy reserve regulation in the body involves some of the hormones that control feeding and appetite, which are located in the gastrointestinal tract. Specific hunger signals trigger eating, while **satiety** messages reduce appetite. These distinctive hormones are often referred to as the "gut hormones," one of which—**ghrelin**—has been proposed to be particularly associated with obesity (Koliaki et al., 2010). Ghrelin, secreted by the stomach, plays a chief role in appetite regulation. It is recognized as the "hunger hormone" and has garnered much attention in the research due to its role in the prevalence of obesity.

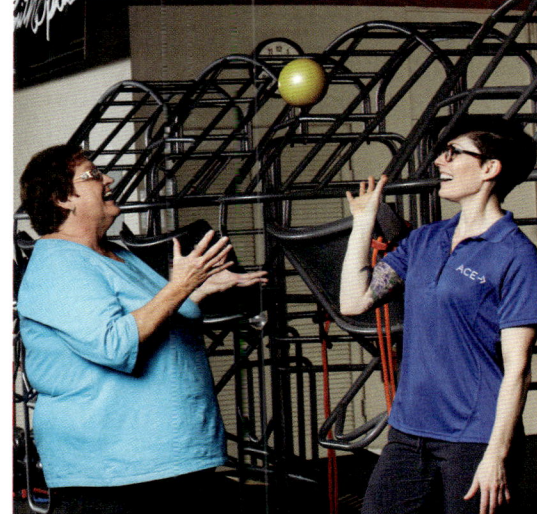

Working in a **positive feedback loop,** high levels of ghrelin during a fasted state promote increased food intake, while lower levels of ghrelin are observed after eating a meal. However, when individuals with obesity lose weight, it often results in an elevation of ghrelin, thereby promoting food intake, which may be a physiological reason why dieters have so much difficulty maintaining their newfound weight. In addition, it appears that food consumption does not suppress ghrelin levels in people with obesity, again contributing to overeating.

Peptide YY

In response to food intake, the hormone **peptide YY** (and other satiety hormones, such as cholecystokinin and glucagon-like peptide-1) is released from the intestines. It is particularly stimulated by lipids and carbohydrates. This gut hormone is thought to work with the **central nervous system** to regulate the cessation of appetite. Thus, when released, it provides a feeling of satiety. Research is ongoing related to the effectiveness of treating individuals with obesity with gut hormones, such as peptide YY, to help regulate food intake and energy homeostasis (Karra, Chandarana, & Batterham, 2009).

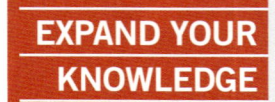

EXPAND YOUR KNOWLEDGE

THE SLEEP–OBESITY CONNECTION

It appears that less sleep is highly associated with weight gain, especially in children and young adults (Magee & Hale, 2012). People who report regularly sleeping less than seven hours a night, for example, are more likely to gain weight compared to people who sleep seven to eight hours a night. Those persons who sleep less tend to eat foods that are higher in calories and get less physical activity. Chronic sleep deprivation leads to feelings of fatigue, which may lead to reductions in physical activity. In fact, cross-sectional studies in children have found short sleep durations to be associated with increased television viewing and reduced participation in organized sports (Patel & Hu, 2008).

Appetite-regulating hormones, such as leptin, insulin, and ghrelin, may also be affected by sleep. For example, insulin controls the rise and fall of blood sugar levels during sleep. People who do not get enough sleep have insulin and blood sugar levels that are similar to those in people who are likely to have diabetes. Several cross-sectional studies have shown that short sleep duration (fewer than five to six hours) is associated with the development of insulin resistance and diabetes (Lucassen, Rother, & Cizza, 2012). Although the research on the association between sleep duration and leptin and ghrelin is still emerging, it appears that people who do not get enough sleep on a regular basis seem to have high levels of ghrelin (causing hunger) and low levels of leptin (increasing eating) (St-Onge, 2013).

Further, there is evidence that links sleep deprivation to an increase in the hedonic value of food. Sleep loss causes a constellation of metabolic and endocrine changes, including an increase in circulating ghrelin (and thus increase in appetite). Studies on sleep deprivation have revealed that it increases overall brain response to palatable food images (Chapman et al., 2012). That is, sleep loss has been shown to activate areas in the brain involved in reward processing that encourage eating.

There is also evidence that having obesity puts a person at risk for not getting a good night's sleep. A form of disordered breathing known as obstructive sleep apnea (OSA) is common in individuals with obesity. Obesity, in particular central obesity, is the most important risk factor for OSA. In general, OSA with complaints of excessive sleepiness affects 4% of middle-aged men and 2% of middle-aged women, but these percentages are much higher among subjects with obesity. OSA prevalence in subjects with morbid obesity who require bariatric surgery has been found to be between 40% and 94% (Arnardottir et al., 2009).

OSA refers to momentary disruptions in breathing rhythm sufficient to cause significant arterial hypoxemia (low blood-oxygen level) and **hypercapnia** (excess blood–carbon dioxide level). One of the mechanisms by which this occurs is due to upper airway narrowing, especially during sleep, because lung volumes are markedly reduced by a combination of increased abdominal fat mass and the recumbent posture (Dempsey et al., 2010). These ventilatory inadequacies and their accompanying intermittent hypoxemia often lead to arousals from sleep and sleep fragmentation throughout the night. As previously described, disruptions in normal sleep can set off a cascade of hormonal and cognitive problems that could lead to behaviors that encourage obesity.

Overweight and Obesity CHAPTER 11

For the CMES, the strong association between chronic short-duration sleep, disordered sleep, and obesity is worth keeping in mind. Informing clients about the importance of regular, good-quality sleep as it relates to potentially preventing obesity is a good practice for promoting weight-loss efforts. Further, recommending that clients with obesity who report disordered sleeping visit their healthcare providers for evaluation could be an important first step in alleviating sleep-related problems.

THINK IT THROUGH

Poor-quality and short-duration sleep (i.e., fewer than seven hours) is associated with many adverse health effects, including obesity. Therefore, it behooves the CMES to educate clients with obesity about the importance of good-quality, habitual sleep patterns. Create a short list of strategies to help your clients create the best environment for sound sleep. Visit the National Sleep Foundation's website (www.sleepfoundation.org) for helpful tips you can share.

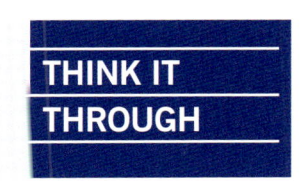

DIAGNOSTIC TESTING AND CRITERIA

Body mass index (BMI) is a simple height–weight index that is commonly used for classifying overweight and obesity in adult populations and individuals. However, BMI should only be considered as a useful guide, because it may not correspond to the same degree of fatness in different individuals. For example, BMI does not discriminate between lean mass and fat mass and therefore tends to overestimate body fatness in athletic, heavily muscled individuals.

Online calculators are available where an individual can simply key in their height and weight and be given the BMI, including one on ACE's website (www.ACEfitness.org/calculators). The Centers for Disease Control and Prevention (CDC) website has a BMI calculator specifically for children and teens (www.cdc.gov/healthyweight/bmi/calculator.html). BMI calculations are presented here, though Table 11-1 can be used as a quick reference.

$$BMI = Weight\ (kg)/Height^2\ (m) \quad \text{or} \quad \frac{Weight\ (lb)}{Height^2\ (in)} \times 703$$

The WHO defines overweight as a BMI $\geq 25\ kg/m^2$ and obesity as a BMI $\geq 30\ kg/m^2$ (WHO 2020). These cutoff points provide a benchmark for individual assessment (Table 11-2).

A CMES can also utilize **waist circumference** to establish health risk. This is a horizontal measurement taken at the narrowest part of the torso above the umbilicus and below the xiphoid process.

Another tool for health-risk assessment is the **waist-to-hip ratio,** which is the circumference of the waist divided by the circumference of the hips. This measurement can be taken in inches or centimeters. To determine if a client has a healthy waist-to-hip ratio, the CMES can use a measuring tape to determine the smallest part of the waist (usually above the belly button and below the rib cage) and the largest part of the hips (Figures 11-1 and 11-2). The measuring tape must be horizontal all the way around the body when taking a measurement. When measuring the hip circumference, the CMES should have the client stand with their feet together and in a relaxed posture, breathing normally (not holding the breath and not sucking in the abdomen). The standards for risk vary with sex (Table 11-3).

There are also a variety of assessment methods that can be used to determine a person's body fatness, such as skinfold testing, **hydrostatic weighing, bioelectrical impedance analysis, infrared interactance, computed tomography, magnetic resonance imaging,** and **dual-energy x-ray absorptiometry.**

TABLE 11-1
BODY MASS INDEX

Height (inches)	19	20	21	22	23	24	25	26	27	28	29	30	35	40
									Weight (pounds)					
58	91	95	100	105	110	115	119	124	129	134	138	143	167	191
59	94	99	104	109	114	119	124	128	133	138	143	148	173	198
60	97	102	107	112	118	123	128	133	138	143	148	153	179	204
61	100	106	111	116	121	127	132	137	143	148	153	158	185	211
62	104	109	115	120	125	131	136	142	147	153	158	164	191	218
63	107	113	118	124	130	135	141	146	152	158	163	169	197	225
64	110	116	122	128	134	140	145	151	157	163	169	174	203	233
65	114	120	126	132	138	144	150	156	162	168	174	180	210	240
66	117	124	130	136	142	148	155	161	167	173	179	185	216	247
67	121	127	134	140	147	153	159	166	172	178	185	191	223	255
68	125	131	138	144	151	158	164	171	177	184	190	197	230	263
69	128	135	142	149	155	162	169	176	182	189	196	203	237	270
70	132	139	146	153	160	167	174	181	188	195	202	209	243	278
71	136	143	150	157	165	172	179	186	193	200	207	215	250	286
72	140	147	155	162	169	177	184	191	199	206	213	221	258	294
73	144	151	159	166	174	182	189	197	204	212	219	227	265	303
74	148	155	163	171	179	187	194	202	210	218	225	233	272	311
75	152	160	168	176	184	192	200	208	216	224	232	240	279	319
76	156	164	172	180	189	197	205	213	221	230	238	246	287	328

Note: Find your client's height in the far left column and move across the row to the weight that is closest to the client's weight. Their body mass index will be at the top of that column.

TABLE 11-2
CLASSIFICATION OF OVERWEIGHT AND OBESITY BY BODY MASS INDEX (BMI)

	BMI Category (kg/m^2)	Obesity Class
Underweight	<18.5	—
Normal	18.5–24.9	—
Overweight	25.0–29.9	—
Obesity	30.0–34.9	I
	35.0–39.9	II
Extreme Obesity	>40	III

Note: Increased waist circumference also can be a marker for increased risk, even in persons of normal weight.

Source: National Heart, Lung, and Blood Institute (2019). *Classification of Overweight and Obesity by BMI, Waist Circumference, and Associated Disease Risks.* www.nhlbi.nih.gov/health/educational/lose_wt/BMI/bmi_dis.htm

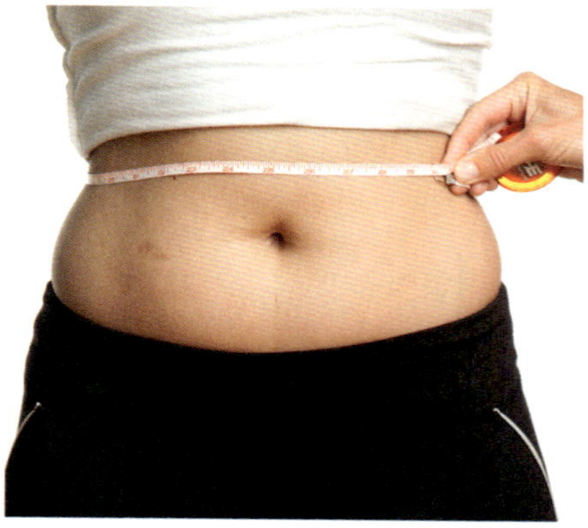

Figure 11-1
Waist circumference

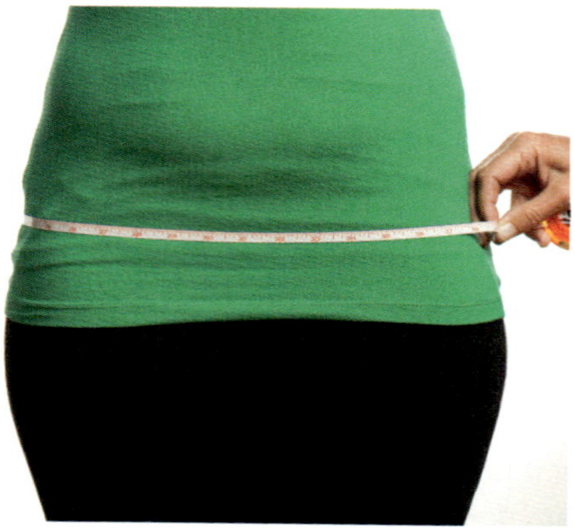

Figure 11-2
Hip circumference

TABLE 11-3
WAIST-TO-HIP CIRCUMFERENCE RATIO NORMS FOR MEN AND WOMEN

			RISK		
	Age	Low	Moderate	High	Very High
Men	20–29	<0.83	0.83–0.88	0.89–0.94	>0.94
	30–39	<0.84	0.84–0.91	0.92–0.96	>0.96
	40–49	<0.88	0.88–0.95	0.96–1.00	>1.00
	50–59	<0.90	0.90–0.96	0.97–1.02	>1.02
	60–69	<0.91	0.91–0.98	0.99–1.03	>1.03
Women	20–29	<0.71	0.71–0.77	0.78–0.82	>0.82
	30–39	<0.72	0.72–0.78	0.79–0.84	>0.84
	40–49	<0.73	0.73–0.79	0.80–0.87	>0.87
	50–59	<0.74	0.74–0.81	0.82–0.88	>0.88
	60–69	<0.76	0.76–0.83	0.84–0.90	>0.90

Reprinted with permission from Gibson, A.L., Wagner, D.R., & Hayward, V.H. (2019). *Advanced Fitness Assessment and Exercise Prescription* (8th ed.). Champaign, Ill.: Human Kinetics.

TREATMENT OPTIONS

Losing weight, and then maintaining the weight loss, is often very difficult due to the multifactorial nature of obesity. It is compelling to point out that small changes in body weight result in health benefits. Studies show that a 5 to 10% loss of initial body weight is associated with meaningful improvements in CVD risk factors, including **cholesterol** and triglyceride levels, hypertension, and glucose metabolism (Wing et al., 2011). Further, the odds of having a clinically meaningful improvement in CVD risk factors also are strongly related to the total amount of weight loss achieved. In an observational analysis of participants in the Look AHEAD (Action for Health in Diabetes) study, Wing and colleagues (2011) found that, compared with those who remained weight-stable, individuals who lost 2 to 5% of their body weight had increased odds of having significant improvements in **systolic blood pressure (SBP),** glucose, and triglycerides, and those who lost 5 to <10% of their body weight had increased odds of significant improvement in all CVD risk factors. The analysis also revealed that the odds of clinically significant improvements in CVD risk factors were increased even more with greater weight losses, such that those who lost 5 to 10% had greater odds of improvements than those who lost 2 to 5%, and those who lost 10 to 15% had greater odds of improvement than those who lost 5 to 10% (Wing et al., 2011). These results provide empirical support for the assertion that modest weight losses of 5 to 10% of initial weight are sufficient to produce significant, clinically relevant improvements in CVD risk factors in individuals with overweight and obesity who also have T2DM.

Non-pharmacological Treatment

Lifestyle modification refers to changes being made that represent an overall change in the way a person lives their life. All too often, individuals view a weight-loss program as an isolated period of time during which a person goes on a diet, takes exercise classes, or employs a personal trainer to get in shape. Others may attempt diet strategies with very unrealistic expectations for weight loss, and then give up when these hopes are not met. It is important to remind clients that they are truly establishing a new way of life, not just a temporary quick fix for some loss of weight. In addition, it is important to emphasize to clients the overall health benefits of increasing physical activity and incorporating a balanced approach to eating and meal planning. These changes can improve the quality of their lives and reduce the risks of developing CHD, hypertension, certain cancers, and diabetes, while also improving their mental well-being and musculoskeletal function in **activities of daily living (ADL)** (Kravitz, 2007).

Behavioral Therapy

The behavioral approaches to weight loss are multifaceted. Behavioral-therapy evidence suggests the following techniques can be successfully incorporated to help clients attain long-term weight control:

- *Properly attempt to assess the client's readiness to change:* Weight-loss achievement and maintenance in the long term is associated with an individual being ready and able to build new attitudes and behaviors into their daily life.
- *Teach accurate self-monitoring of food consumption:* The systematic recording of target behaviors is a cornerstone of behavioral treatment. Self-monitoring is strongly associated with weight-loss success, such that individuals who monitor their food intake and body weight most consistently have the largest weight losses (Butryn, Webb, & Wadden, 2011). Therefore, a focus on accurate self-monitoring is vital for long-term success of the weight-management intervention.
- *Set SMART goals:* **SMART goals** are specific, measurable, attainable, relevant, and time-bound (see Chapter 4). This goal-setting process should be followed with a written and personalized action plan. For enhanced motivation, the CMES and client can together establish rewards along the way for desired outcomes. SMART goals are best set for process goals (e.g., walk five days per week) instead of body-weight goals.
- *Incorporate sound dietary change:* See "Nutritional Considerations" on page 328.
- *Increase physical activity:* See "Exercise Recommendations for Clients With Obesity" on page 333.
- *Utilize stimulus control:* **Stimulus control** involves learning how to avoid **triggers** such as the sight of food and dealing with cravings for food (see Chapter 4). Since food cravings are not fully understood, a few different strategies may need to be attempted. Most importantly, it is essential that clients not adopt a strict diet based on specific food deprivation. In fact, eating craved foods in moderation may quell the craving and prevent overeating. In addition, creating workable diversions to food cravings may be a viable solution.
- *Utilize cognitive restructuring:* **Cognitive restructuring** is a behavioral technique that involves learning how to replace unhealthy or negative thoughts and self-talk regarding weight loss with positive affirmations (see Chapter 4). Examples of cognitive traps include all-or-nothing thinking (e.g., "I blew my diet last night, so I might as well blow it again today") and discounting the positive (e.g., "I lost only 1 pound this week instead of 2").
- *Utilize relapse management:* **Relapse** management attempts to make clients aware that **lapses** and relapses are a normal part of behavior change (see Chapter 4). This strategy helps to relieve the stress of "being a diet failure" that some individuals experience when they miss an exercise session or overindulge in a meal.
- *Establish ongoing support:* Ongoing support involves creatively utilizing communication techniques such as email, phone, and websites that provide maintenance support to clients in an effort to sustain the lifestyle changes that have been made.

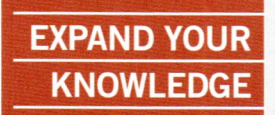

EXPAND YOUR KNOWLEDGE

THE FORCE OF HABIT

Research on people who have successfully lost weight supports the idea that modifying lifestyle is a crucial component of successful weight-management efforts. Some of the most interesting data on successful lifestyle-modification practices come from research work done by Wing, Hill, and colleagues at the National Weight Control Registry (NWCR). The NWCR was created in 1994, and follows individuals who have lost at least 30 pounds (13.6 kg) and maintained the weight loss for one year or more. Data from the NWCR have found the following lifestyle-modification strategies to be most commonly used among people who have been successful in their weight-management efforts (Wing & Phelan, 2005):

- Engaging in high levels of physical activity, at least one hour each day
- Eating a low-calorie, low-fat diet

- Eating breakfast daily
- Self-monitoring body weight regularly
- Maintaining a consistent eating pattern every day, on both weekdays and weekends

Participants in the NWCR who maintained their weight loss for more than two years had greater long-term success rates, suggesting that lifestyles had become modified, with the force of habit supporting weight maintenance. Data from this study also support the **health belief model,** in that a medical incentive for weight loss (e.g., treatment of hypertension) was associated with long-term success.

Pharmacological Treatment

Between 2003 and 2007, the U.S. patent office received more than 1,700 submissions with the word "obesity" in them (Hickey & Israel, 2007). Hickey and Israel (2007) also noted that at the time there were nearly 300 clinical trials currently researching some aspect of obesity. Currently, there is only one drug that has been FDA-approved for long-term treatment of obesity—orlistat (marketed under the trade name Xenical or over-the-counter as Alli). Sibutramine (trade name is Meridia) is another antiobesity drug that was approved by the U.S. Food and Drug Administration (FDA), but has been subsequently removed from the market for health reasons.

Orlistat's primary function is preventing the intestinal absorption of fats from the diet, thereby reducing the caloric impact of food consumed. It is intended for use in combination with a physician-supervised reduced-calorie diet. Orlistat is successful at blocking absorption of approximately 30% of dietary fat (Hickey & Israel, 2007). Over the course of a year, the use of orlistat creates approximately 6.5 pounds (2.9 kg) greater weight loss as compared to a placebo (Hickey & Israel, 2007). However, the researchers also note that orlistat has been shown to have considerable gastrointestinal side effects, including abdominal pain, diarrhea, flatulence, bloating, and upset stomach. In a review of the literature on pharmaceutical interventions for weight loss, Zhou and colleagues (2012) found that orlistat may play an important role in reducing SBP, DBP, total cholesterol, **low-density lipoprotein (LDL),** and fasting glucose in subjects with obesity.

Clearly, a great deal more needs to be learned about the interplay of food intake and the complex biological, neuroendocrine, and physiological mechanisms of the human body. Although much research is going on in this area of study, simple solutions do not appear to be forthcoming in the near future. In addition, Hickey and Israel (2007) note that the **pathogenesis** (i.e., disease development) of obesity is multifaceted and likely to vary among individuals. This suggests that the idea of one "super pill" for overweight and obesity treatment is unlikely. Thus, any obesity medications should be administered along with lifestyle changes that involve behavior modification, exercise, and healthy food consumption. Further, given the expected rates of weight regain and the high costs of medication, some researchers have suggested that the implementation of pharmaceutical interventions for the primary prevention of obesity is not cost effective, owing to the evidence that the overall effect of these pharmaceuticals on the obesity-related burden of disease is negligible (Veerman et al., 2011).

Surgical Treatment

Bariatrics is the branch of medicine that deals with the causes, prevention, and treatment of obesity. The term bariatrics comes from the Greek root *baro* (weight) and the suffix *iatrics* (a branch of medicine). Compared with non-surgical treatment of obesity, bariatric surgery leads to greater body weight loss and higher remission rates of T2DM and **metabolic syndrome.** The most common reported adverse events after bariatric surgery have been iron-deficiency anemia (15% of individuals undergoing malabsorptive bariatric surgery) and reoperations (8%) (Gloy et al., 2013).

Current guidelines recommend evaluation of bariatric surgery for individuals with a BMI ≥40 kg/m² or a BMI ≥35 kg/m² in the presence of comorbid risk factors (one or more disorders or diseases in addition to a primary disease—in this case, obesity) (ACSM, 2022). The most commonly used bariatric surgery techniques are Roux-en-Y gastric bypass, sleeve gastrectomy, and laparoscopic adjustable gastric banding (Gloy et al., 2013). These procedures involve separating a small pouch of stomach with a line of staples to dramatically limit food intake. Bariatric surgery results in a 30% (gastric bypass) and 25% (vertical banded gastroplasty) average reduction of initial weight. Improvements in quality of life, decreased waist circumference, and reductions in the use of antidiabetic, antihypertensive, and lipid-lowering drugs have also been observed (Gloy et al., 2013). Clinical trials suggest that gastric bypass surgery is associated with much better weight-loss maintenance than vertical banded gastroplasty, because patients who have undergone gastric bypass surgery and then eat high-fat or high-sugar meals tend to experience stomach cramping and gastrointestinal distress and thus avoid these foods to evade this discomfort. Naturally, before any type of bariatric procedure, individuals need to be rigorously screened to determine if there are any medical or behavioral contraindications to the surgery.

EXPAND YOUR KNOWLEDGE

POST-SURGERY EXERCISE PROGRAMMING

Comprehensive treatment following surgery includes exercise, though this has not yet been studied adequately. Exercise will likely help post-surgery clients achieve and maintain energy balance. Once individuals are are cleared for exercise by their physician, the CMES can develop a progressive exercise program using the FITT principle guidelines for healthy adults (see Table 2-2, page 29 and Table 2-5, page 47).

Because of the weight placed on joints, coupled with the fact that these clients likely performed very low levels of exercise prior to surgery, intermittent or non-weight-bearing exercise may be part of the initial exercise program. Clients should progress so that continuous, weight-bearing exercise (e.g., walking) makes up a great portion of the exercise program. ACSM (2022) recommends ≥250 minutes per week of moderate-to-vigorous intensity exercise for promoting long-term weight-loss maintenance.

Exercise Treatment

Although there are various evidence-based physical-activity and exercise approaches to weight control, such as the 10,000-steps-a-day model or the >2,000 kilocalories per week target goal, the "accumulated time" approach will be highlighted here for designing weight-management programs because of its simplicity and its varied utility for all different forms of exercise (e.g., walking, elliptical training, water exercise, rowing, and cycling). The accumulated time approach addresses the fact that energy expenditure is actually a cumulative phenomenon, including both low-intensity ADL, such as walking and recreational dancing, and more vigorous exercise like swimming, elliptical training, and cycling. When pursuing weight-management goals, the evidence suggests that persons who have overweight or obesity should gradually progress to 60 minutes per day of accumulated exercise. There appears to be an optimal dose of maintaining an average of greater than 250 minutes/week (ACSM, 2022). These greater weekly volumes of exercise tend to lead to less food consumption in individuals, and the combined exercise and decreased food consumption facilitate weight loss.

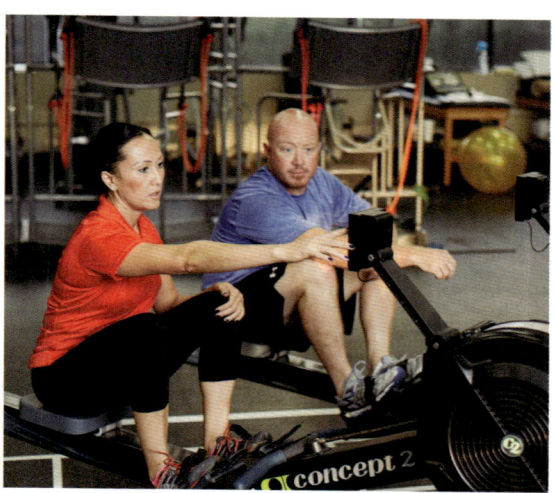

It is important to note that although resistance exercises are highly recommended for enhanced muscular strength, muscular endurance, physical function, and a host of other

Overweight and Obesity   CHAPTER 11

health benefits, it is cardiovascular exercise that elicits the needed energy-expenditure deficits for weight loss and the prevention of weight regain (Jakicic et al., 2009). Resistance training may enhance muscular strength and improve physical function in individuals who have overweight or obesity but it does not result in clinically significant weight loss, prevent the loss of fat-free mass, or cause a reduction in resting energy expenditure (ACSM, 2022).

Therefore, any resistance-training program designed for individuals with overweight or obesity should be considered an adjunct to the cardiovascular program for weight loss. Initially, the exercise intensity should be moderate—approximately 40 to 59% of $\dot{V}O_2$ **reserve ($\dot{V}O_2R$) or heart-rate reserve (HRR)** (ACSM, 2022) or a rating of 12 to 13 ("fairly light" to "somewhat hard") on the Borg **rating of perceived exertion (RPE)** scale (6 to 20 scale) (Table 11-4).

TABLE 11-4
RATING OF PERCEIVED EXERTION (RPE)

RPE	Category Ratio Scale
6	0 Nothing at all
7 Very, very light	0.5 Very, very weak
8	1 Very weak
9 Very light	2 Weak
10	3 Moderate
11 Fairly light	4 Somewhat strong
12	5 Strong
13 Somewhat hard	6
14	7 Very strong
15 Hard	8
16	9
17 Very hard	10 Very, very strong
18	* Maximal
19 Very, very hard	
20	

Source: Borg, G. (1998). *Borg's Perceived Exertion and Pain Scales*. Champaign, Ill.: Human Kinetics.

PHYSICAL ACTIVITY: UNSTRUCTURED EXERCISE

Researchers have been investigating the impact that standing, walking, and fidgeting play on weight gain and obesity. As such, a relatively newly discovered component of energy expenditure is **non-exercise activity thermogenesis (NEAT)** (physiological processes that produce heat). Innovative research in this area has revealed surprising and beneficial information (Garland et al., 2011).

NEAT comprises the energy expenditure of daily activities that are not considered planned physical activity or exercise of a person's daily life. NEAT is measured with sensitive physical-activity monitoring inclinometers and triaxial accelerometers, which are worn on the hips and legs (similar to a pedometer). These devices capture data on body position through all planes of movement 120 times a minute. The combination of this information with other laboratory measurements of energy expenditure leads to a calculation of NEAT. Findings indicate that changes in NEAT accompany changes in energy balance, which are very meaningful in affecting weight loss (Levine et al., 2005). For example, NEAT has been shown to vary between two people of similar size by 2,000 calories per day due to individuals' different occupations and leisure-time activities. Not surprisingly, individuals with obesity score lower for NEAT compared with lean individuals (Levine, 2007).

Levine and colleagues (2005) recruited 20 healthy, sedentary volunteers who were self-proclaimed "couch potatoes." Of the 20 volunteers, five men and five women had BMI measurements of 23 ± 2 kg/m^2 (classifying them as lean) and five men and five women had BMI measurements of 33 ± 2 kg/m^2 (classifying them as having mild obesity). A population with mild obesity was selected because these individuals were less likely to have medical impediments and orthopedic troubles as compared to a group with morbid obesity. With each subject wearing an inclinometer and triaxial accelerometer, the researchers collected data every half-second for 10 days.

The investigators were searching for posture and movement clues of how the 10 lean non-exercisers were different from 10 non-exercisers who had mild obesity. They found that the subjects with obesity were seated for 164 minutes longer each day than the lean participants. In addition, the lean participants were upright for 153 minutes longer per day than the subjects with obesity.

Importantly, sleep times between the groups did not vary at all. The lean subjects had significantly more total-body ambulatory movement, which consisted of standing and walking. In essence, the extra movement by the lean subjects averaged 352 ± 65 calories per day, which is equivalent to 36.5 pounds (16.6 kg) in one year.

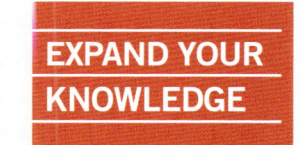

EXPAND YOUR KNOWLEDGE

APPLY WHAT YOU KNOW

SMALL CONTINUAL CHANGES CAN ADD UP TO BIG RESULTS

A very important way to help clients achieve their weight-loss goals is to find ways for them to be more active in their daily lives (Table 11-5). Encouraging and educating clients to make small continual movement changes in their daily lives, in addition to their structured exercise plan, may very well contribute to profound weight-management success.

TABLE 11-5
SUGGESTIONS TO HELP CLIENTS BE MORE ACTIVE DURING THE DAY

• Walk to work.	• Walk to a coworker's desk instead of emailing or calling.
• Walk during your lunch hour.	• Make time in your day for physical activity.
• Walk instead of drive whenever you can.	• Bike to the barbershop or beauty salon instead of driving.
• Take a family walk after dinner.	• If you find it difficult to be active after work, try it before work.
• Skate to work instead of drive.	• Take a walk break instead of a coffee break.
• Mow the lawn with a push mower.	• Perform gardening and/or home-repair activities.
• Walk to your place of worship instead of driving.	• Avoid labor-saving devices.
• Walk your dog.	• Take small trips on foot to get your body moving.
• Replace the Sunday drive with a Sunday walk.	• Play with your kids 30 minutes a day.
• Get off the bus or subway a stop early and walk.	• Dance to music.
• Work and walk around the house.	• Walk briskly in the mall.
• Take your dog to the park.	• Take the long way to the water cooler.
• Wash the car by hand.	• Take the stairs instead of the escalator.
• Run or walk fast when doing errands.	• Go for a hike.
• Pace the sidelines at your kids' athletic games.	
• Take the wheels off your luggage.	

NUTRITIONAL CONSIDERATIONS

To successfully lose a sizeable amount of weight, a client needs to make significant long-term lifestyle changes. The goal is to create a caloric deficit so that fewer calories are eaten than are expended. With about 3,500 calories in a pound of fat, a 500- to 1,000-calorie deficit each day through decreased food intake and/or increased physical activity leads to about a 1- to 2-pound weight loss per week. By making meaningful lifestyle changes, such as drinking water rather than a 20-oz bottle of soda (250 calories) and taking a 45-minute, 2.5-mile walk each day (about 250 calories), a client could begin to lose weight. But after a few weeks or months, continued weight loss becomes much more difficult. While predicting weight loss based on the equation of 3,500 calories per pound of fat (approximately) is useful early on in weight loss, as an individual loses weight, metabolism (and thus energy expenditure) changes and the equation becomes less accurate and overpredicts weight loss.

A group of scientists at the National Institutes of Health developed a mathematical model to more accurately account for these metabolic changes. They approximate that for every 10-calorie decrease in daily intake, the average adult with overweight will lose about 1 pound, with half of the weight lost by one year and 95% of the weight change by three years (Hall et al., 2011). For example, a person who decreased their daily caloric consumption from 2,200 calories to 2,000

Overweight and Obesity   CHAPTER 11

calories would lose about 10 pounds after one year of the lowered caloric intake, and about 10 more pounds by the end of three years. If they had created a 500 kcal deficit each day, they would lose 25 pounds in the first year and about 25 more pounds by the end of three years.

A WEIGHT-LOSS SIMULATOR

EXPAND YOUR KNOWLEDGE

Scientists at the National Institutes of Health developed an online simulation to help determine how long and how much change in physical activity and caloric intake is necessary to achieve various weight-loss goals (Hall et al., 2011). The simulator can be accessed at bwsimulator.niddk.nih.gov.

Based on this simulation, a 30-year-old female weighing 150 lb (68 kg) and measuring 5'4" tall (162.6 cm) who is classified in the "light work physical activity level, active leisure time physical activity level" could achieve a weight goal of 130 lb (59.1 kg) in 20 weeks.

The simulator divides weight change into two stages: weight-change phase and weight-maintenance phase. It shows that an individual needs to consume fewer calories to lose weight than to maintain weight loss. The calories are lower in the beginning to expedite the weight loss, and the calories during the maintenance phase are what are required to maintain the goal weight. If the maintenance calories were consumed the entire period, it would take longer to lose the desired amount of weight.

The scientists who developed this simulation are adamant that the commonly held belief that "there are 3,500 calories in a pound of fat" is somewhat flawed. The rationale of why many people say there are 3,500 calories comes from the fact that there are approximately 9 calories per gram of fat. One pound of fat is 454 grams; however, it is not stored as 100% lipid. Rather, it is approximately 85 to 90% lipid and 10 to 15% water. Therefore, 1 pound of "fat" is approximately 400 grams of lipid x 9 calories/gram = 3,600 calories/pound. To make it simple, the value is commonly rounded to 3,500 calories per gram of fat. As such, the rationale is that for every 3,500 calories you cut from your diet, you can lose 1 pound of fat. These scientists challenge this premise because their data indicate that the body changes as a person is gradually losing weight. Therefore, weight loss from calorie restriction is somewhat imprecise (due to energy-expenditure changes) and will also vary from person to person. The scientists also found that "the fatter you get, the easier it is to gain weight. An extra 10 calories a day puts more weight onto an obese person than on a thinner one" (Hall et al., 2011).

For background on this simulation, refer to "A Mathematical Challenge to Obesity" by Claudia Dreifus (2012) of *The New York Times*: www.nytimes.com/2012/05/15/science/a-mathematical-challenge-to-obesity.html.
Source: Muth, N.D. (2014). *Nutrition for Health Professionals.* Philadelphia: F.A. Davis.

The American Heart Association (AHA), American College of Cardiology (ACC), and The Obesity Society (TOS) published a comprehensive guideline on the management of obesity, including nutritional considerations. The following are highlights from this report (Jensen et al., 2013):
Dietary approaches to weight loss may include:
- Prescription of a 1,200 to 1,500 kcal/day for women and 1,500 to 1,800 kcal/day eating plan for men, with calorie level adjustments made based on body weight. Note that the dietary prescription should come from a physician or **registered dietitian (RD)**; diet prescription is outside the **scope of practice** for a CMES.
  ✓ Prescription of an eating plan that will create a 500 to 750 kcal/day energy deficit
  ✓ Prescription of an evidence-based eating plan that restricts certain food (such as high-carbohydrate foods, low-fiber foods, or high-fat foods) in order to create a caloric deficit.
  ✓ A comprehensive weight-management program should include behavioral therapy in addition to dietary and activity changes. The best programs last at least six months and feature a weight-maintenance intervention afterward, which should include monthly or more frequent contact and an emphasis on physical activity, regular body-weight monitoring, and consumption of a reduced-calorie diet.

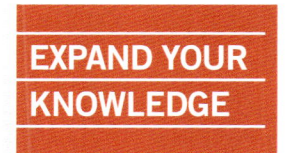

- **Adherence** to a very low-calorie diet (<800 kcal per day) results in significant weight loss and varying degrees of weight-loss maintenance. However, this type of diet is contraindicated for certain populations and should be followed only under the supervision of a physician and/or RD due to the rapid weight loss and potential for complications.

In its position statement on adult weight management, the Academy of Nutrition and Dietetics advises these additional considerations (Seagle et al., 2009):

- Consumption of a low-carbohydrate diet is associated with increased weight and fat loss compared to low-fat diets in the first six months, but these differences are not sustained at one year. Individuals with osteoporosis, kidney disease, or increased LDL should avoid diets with <35% of kilocalories from carbohydrate.
- A low–**glycemic index (GI)** diet is not recommended for weight loss or weight maintenance since evidence is insufficient to demonstrate its effectiveness. However, in order to maintain a healthy weight, one should consume complex carbohydrates, many of which are categorized as low-GI foods, such as oatmeal, pumpernickel bread, grapefruits, strawberries, oranges, and plain yogurt.
- Attention to portion control results in decreased energy intake and enhanced weight loss.
- Total caloric intake should be distributed throughout the day, such that greater consumption occurs during the day compared with the evening.
- For individuals who have difficulty with selection and/or portion control, substituting one to two meals or snacks with meal replacement bars or drinks is a successful weight-loss and weight-maintenance strategy.

Since publication of these recommendations, it also has become clear that a change such as reducing or eliminating consumption of sugar-sweetened beverages such as sodas, sports drinks, and juices will reduce the prevalence of obesity and T2DM (Hu, 2013).

Popular Diets

The best diet for weight loss is a source of contentious debate. From extremely low-fat diets and diets that severely limit carbohydrate intake to meal replacements and strict calorie counting, each method has its followers. Every diet also has people who have failed to achieve their weight-loss goals.

A randomized trial, the gold standard in research design, compared the Atkins (a very low-carbohydrate diet), LEARN (Lifestyle, Exercise, Attitudes, Relationships, and Nutrition; low-fat, high-carbohydrate diet based on national recommendations), Ornish (very high-carbohydrate diet) and Zone diets (low-carbohydrate diet) in 300+ premenopausal women who had overweight or obesity. At 12 months, the Atkins dieters recorded the most significant weight loss (10 pounds; 4.5 kg) (Gardner et al., 2007). The unimpressive amount of weight loss reflects how people struggle to stick to rigid dietary restrictions, though it is worth noting that even a 3 to 5% weight loss confers significant health benefits (Jensen et al., 2013).

A study of 60,000 male and female participants of Jenny Craig, a commercial weight-loss program, found that those who followed the program for one year lost 16% of their body weight. But only 6.6% of the original dieters continued with the program for that long (Finley et al., 2007). Another study found that people who replaced a meal each day with a 100- to 300-calorie substitute, such as a nutrition bar or formulated milkshake meal, maintained a substantial (8.4%) weight loss at four years (Flechthner-Mors et al., 2000).

As Dansinger et al. (2005) concluded after a one-year randomized trial to assess the adherence rate and effectiveness of Atkins, Ornish, Weight Watchers, and the Zone diets, it does not matter what diet a person chooses as long as they can stick to it. This finding is also apparent in the AHA/ACC/TOS obesity guideline, which notes that there is high strength of evidence that all of the following dietary patterns, among others noted in the report, can contribute to weight loss in the context of decreased caloric intake: high-protein, lacto-ovo vegetarian, low-calorie, low-carbohydrate, low-fat plus or minus high dairy plus or minus high fiber plus or minus low–**glycemic load (GL)**, low-GL, Mediterranean, moderate-protein, high-GL, and AHA-style Step I diet (Jensen et al., 2013). Whatever plan is followed, adherence is a lot more difficult than it sounds.

The CMES can guide a client considering a new diet plan to critically evaluate whether or not a particular diet is a good choice. The client should be able to answer the following questions:

- How does the diet cut calories? In order for any diet to work, calories consumed need to be less than calories expended. Remember, it requires approximately a 3,500-calorie deficit to lose close to 1 pound of fat. That is, if a client wants to lose about 1 pound per week (and generally less over time, as described above), they need to eat less and exercise more so that the net calorie balance is about 500 calories less per day than it is currently.
- What is the nutrient density of the diet? The best diets will advocate up to nine servings daily of a variety of fruits and vegetables—low-calorie foods that provide most of the body's needed vitamins, minerals, and phytochemicals (a broad term for a variety of compounds produced by such plants as fruits, vegetables, beans, and grains). Phytochemicals have been linked to decreasing the risk of infection and chronic diseases such as hypertension, stroke, and certain cancers (Boeing et al., 2012; Liu, 2003). Fiber-containing whole grains and calcium-rich low-fat dairy products should also be encouraged. If the diet relies primarily on a supplement to assure sufficient vitamins and minerals, it probably is not the healthiest choice.
- Does the diet advocate exercise? Nutrition is only one component in making a long-term lifestyle change. Exercise not only speeds weight loss by increasing caloric deficit, but it also is essential in keeping the weight off.
- Does it make sense? Some diet plans make claims that oftentimes are based primarily on personal testimony. From promises to lose 10 or more pounds (4.5+ kg) in the first two weeks of a diet to the promotion of supplements that supposedly speed weight loss, diets are marketed as being so easy and effective that they are irresistible—at first. However, weight that is lost quickly is often regained quickly.
- Where is the evidence? Research studies can be a rich source of information on the effectiveness and safety of different diets. When assessing research results, it is important to note the study limitations in addition to the results. For example, most of the diet research has been on middle-aged men and women who have obesity. Thus, the results may not apply to younger people or those who are simply trying to lose 5 or 10 pounds (2.3 to 4.5 kg) but who do not have obesity. Also, most diet studies were conducted over the course of one year or less. Therefore, the differences between the diets or the apparent benefits may not hold true for the long term.
- Does it meet individual needs? The client's health status and other individual factors must be considered when choosing a diet plan. Clients who have a history of significant medical illness, such as (but not limited to) diabetes or heart disease, should talk with their physician before starting a diet or exercise regimen.
- How much does it cost? While clients may initially be able to afford an expensive weight-loss program, they may not be able to sustain the cost for an extended period of time. Help them plan ahead and assess their readiness to change and commit to a program before making huge lifestyle adjustments and financial sacrifices.
- What kind of social support does the client have? Social support is key to successful weight loss. If a diet requires that a client eat different foods than the rest of the family, it is unlikely that they will be successful on the diet. If a client's family is not supportive and committed to helping them make the healthy change, the client will probably struggle.
- How easy is it to adhere to the diet? Long-term adherence to a program (i.e., lifestyle change) is the most important factor for lifelong weight-loss success. It is not necessary to select a specific diet to achieve long-term weight loss. Rather, individuals need to consume fewer calories, while

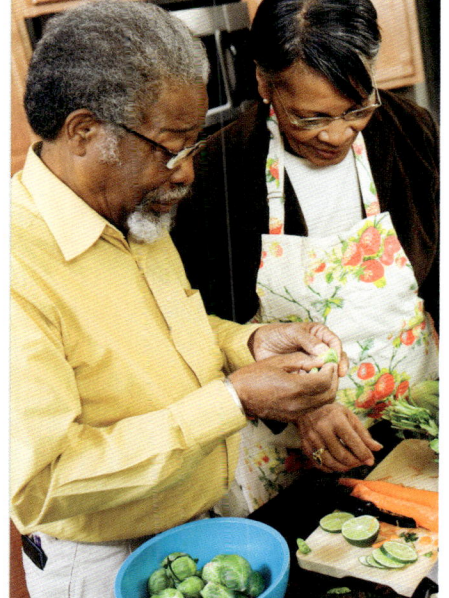

making healthy food choices they like and are likely able to maintain. Regardless of the weight-loss plan, most diets modestly reduce body weight and cardiovascular risk factors, but people who adhere to the diet over the long term have greater weight loss and risk factor reductions (Dansinger et al., 2005). The problem is that most dieters struggle to adhere to restrictive eating plans. A landmark study conducted by the National Institutes of Health (1992) found that most dieters had regained one-third to two-thirds of the weight lost within one year, and within five years dieters had regained almost all of the lost weight. In addition, about one-third to two-thirds of dieters regain more weight than they initially lose (Mann et al., 2007). This reinforces the point that permanent lifestyle change is essential for successful weight loss and subsequent improved health.

Nutritional Considerations for Clients Before and After Bariatric Surgery

Any client who undergoes evaluation for bariatric surgery at a recognized bariatric center will receive an intensive nutritional intervention under the direction of a RD or other appropriately qualified physician or multidisciplinary team. The following is an overview of nutrition for bariatric surgery based on the American Society for Metabolic and Bariatric Surgery's "ASMBS Allied Health Nutritional Guidelines for the Surgical Weight Loss Patient" (Aills et al., 2008).

Preoperative Nutrition Evaluation

The preoperative nutrition evaluation will include **anthropometrics,** weight history including previous weight-loss attempts, medical history, and psychological history, as well as an assessment of current nutrition patterns, physical activity, and psychosocial factors such as readiness to change and extent of social support. Preoperative nutrition education will include behavioral coaching in addition to skill development in self-monitoring nutrition intake and preparation for post-operative nutrition considerations such as meal planning and spacing and tips to maximize food and fluid tolerance; common complaints after surgery like low appetite, nausea, and diarrhea; and strategies for long-term maintenance such as cooking skills and meal-preparation strategies. Typically, prior to surgery the client will also undergo an intensive nutrition and activity intervention, often with the support of obesity medication(s).

Postoperative Nutrition Follow-up

Following bariatric surgery, the nutrition status and habits of post-operative clients will be closely monitored, including current weight and BMI; lab levels of the B vitamins, fat-soluble vitamins (A, D, E, and K), iron, zinc, and protein; medication review; adherence to recommended vitamin and mineral supplementation (which typically includes a multivitamin, B12, calcium, iron, fat soluble vitamins, and an optional B complex); and dietary intake.

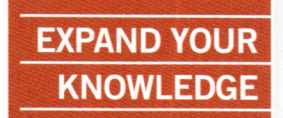

EXPAND YOUR KNOWLEDGE

CONSIDERATIONS FOR OBESITY-RELATED DISORDERS AND DISEASES

A wide range of diseases and health problems are associated with obesity. The CMES should be familiar with the diverse ways that overweight and obesity may be linked with the health and wellness of clients. It is important to note that the research on obesity-related disorders and diseases is very frequently correlational, as opposed to prospective, randomized research. Correlational research explores the statistical association of two or more variables to each other, and this type of study design makes it hard to prove cause and effect. Readers of research results should bear in mind the limitations imposed by the study design. Serious diseases associated with overweight and obesity include CHD, **congestive heart failure,** stroke, **emphysema,** chronic **bronchitis, chronic obstructive pulmonary disease (COPD), deep vein thrombosis,** and some cancers (endometrial, breast, and colon) (NIH, 2012; Patterson et al., 2004). The cardiovascular risk factors related to obesity are hypertension, **hypercholesterolemia** (or elevated cholesterol levels), and T2DM. Patterson and colleagues (2004) note that the numerous medical conditions linked to obesity include **depression,** migraine headaches, asthma, **gastroesophageal reflux disease,** ulcers, diabetes, bladder infections, **osteoarthritis,** yeast infections, and gallbladder disease. A number of other health concerns associated with obesity include osteoporotic fractures (wrist, hip, and forearm), joint pain (neck, back, and knee), stress, fatigue, chronic insomnia, **anxiety,** indigestion, heartburn, constipation, skin problems, and allergies (to plants, trees, molds, dust, or animals) (Patterson et al., 2004). This information clearly depicts the health burden of obesity-related disorders and diseases and the challenges faced by fitness, public health, and medical professionals. It is important for a CMES to realize that a determination of the absolute risk of morbidity and mortality of a client with obesity requires a comprehensive evaluation, including a complete medical history, physical examination, and appropriate laboratory tests.

EXERCISE RECOMMENDATIONS FOR CLIENTS WITH OBESITY

Regular physical activity and exercise have significant benefits in terms of risk reduction for overweight and obesity, insulin resistance, T2DM, blood lipid and lipoprotein abnormalities, hypertension, **peripheral vascular disease,** cerebrovascular disease, and CHD. Not everyone who is physically active on a regular basis will remain free from these vascular and metabolic diseases, but the protective effects and the reduction in risk levels are substantial enough to justify the promotion of a physically active lifestyle in all segments of the population, especially those with overweight or obesity. Continued study of persons with overweight and obesity is needed to better understand the physiological responses to exercise training for this population. Further epidemiological research (the branch of medicine that deals with the incidence, distribution, and possible control of diseases related to health) may uncover new relationships between obesity and health, and extend the understanding of the health benefits of exercise training. Table 11-6 summarizes the physiological effects of cardiovascular and resistance training.

TABLE 11-6
PHYSIOLOGICAL EFFECTS OF CARDIOVASCULAR AND RESISTANCE TRAINING

	Cardiovascular Training	**Resistance Training**
Bone mineral density	Increase	Increase

Hypertension
  Systolic
  Diastolic
	
	Decrease
	Decrease
		
		Possible decrease
		Possible decrease

Resting heart rate	Decrease	Decrease

Blood lipids
  Triglycerides
  Total cholesterol
  LDL cholesterol
  HDL cholesterol
	
	Decrease*
	Decrease*
	Decrease*
	Increase
		
		Possible decrease
		Possible decrease
		Possible decrease
		Possible increase

Glucose metabolism
  Basal insulin levels
  Insulin sensitivity
	
	Decrease
	Increase
		
		Decrease
		Increase

Cardiovascular endurance	Increase	No change

Body composition
  Fat mass
  Fat-free mass
	
	Decrease
	Increase (mild)
		
		Decrease
		Increase

Resting metabolic rate	No change	Increase (mild)
Musculoskeletal health	Increase (mild)	Increase
Functional capabilities	Increase	Increase
Longevity	Increase	Unknown

*A decrease in triglycerides, total cholesterol, and LDL cholesterol from cardiovascular exercise occurs if there is a concurrent loss of body weight.
Note: LDL = Low-density lipoprotein; HDL = High-density lipoprotein
Source: Kravitz, L. (2007). The 25 most significant health benefits of physical activity and exercise. *IDEA Fitness Journal,* 4, 9, 54–63.

The Role of Exercise in Weight Loss and Weight-gain Prevention

Although it is possible to lose weight with physical activity alone, the combination of exercise with a moderate restricted dietary intake is a more meaningful strategy (Donnelly et al., 2009). Exercise positively alters the composition of weight loss so that a greater percentage of weight loss comes from fat, rather than from muscle. Research suggests that for individuals with obesity, logging in more than the consensus public health recommendations of at least 30 minutes per day (150 minutes per week) of moderate-intensity physical activity may be necessary for weight loss and maintenance (ACSM, 2022). Persons expending high volumes of weekly exercise (one hour or more each day) have high success rates in long-term weight-loss maintenance. Performing more than 250 minutes per week (moderate- to vigorous-intensity endurance exercise on five to seven days per week) has been shown to be effective for weight-loss maintenance in adults who have overweight or obesity. In summary, the results of several epidemiological studies consistently reveal that persons who are physically active are much less likely to gain weight over time than those who are not (Donnelly et al., 2009).

Programming and Progressive Exercise Guidelines for Overweight and Obesity

The foundational objectives for exercise guidelines for persons with overweight or obesity include maximizing caloric expenditure to boost weight loss and incorporating exercise into daily life (ACSM, 2022). Exercise guidelines for clients with overweight and obesity include performing cardiorespiratory exercise on at least five days per week and using an exercise mode that involves prolonged, rhythmic activities involving large muscle groups. ACSM (2022) recommends an intensity of exercise of 40 to 59% of $\dot{V}O_2R$ or HRR (progressing to ≥60% of $\dot{V}O_2R$ or HRR) initially, progressing to at least 30 minutes per day. Inherent in these guidelines is the concept of individualizing the program for each person's fitness level, health, age, personal goals, medications, behavioral characteristics, and individual preferences.

ACSM (2022) has published the following guidelines for clients who have overweight or obesity:

- Target a minimal reduction in body weight of at least 3 to 10% of initial body weight over a three- to six-month period.
- Incorporate opportunities to enhance communication between healthcare professionals, dietitians, and exercise professionals and people with overweight and obesity following the initial weight-loss period.
- Target changing eating and exercise behaviors, as sustained changes in both behaviors result in significant long-term weight loss and maintenance.
- Target reducing current energy intake by 500 to 1,000 kcal/day to achieve weight loss. This reduced energy intake should be combined with a reduction in dietary fat.
- Target progressively increasing to a minimum of 150 minutes/week of moderate-intensity physical activity to optimize health/fitness benefits. Physical activity may be accumulated in bouts of at least 10 minutes.
- Progress to higher amounts of exercise and physical activity (i.e., ≥250 minutes/week) to promote long-term weight control.
- Include resistance exercise as a supplement to the combination of aerobic exercise and moderate reductions in energy intake to enhance muscular strength and physical function while also improving CVD, diabetes, and other chronic disease risk factors.
- Incorporate behavioral modification strategies, including goal setting to target short- and long-term weight loss, to facilitate the adoption and maintenance of the desired changes in behavior.

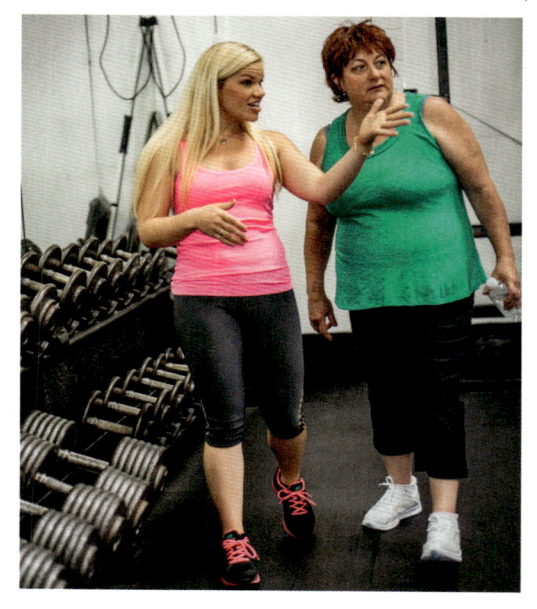

AEROBIC PROGRAM VARIATIONS FOR CLIENTELE WITH OBESITY

Varying aerobic-training programs is encouraged for adults who have overweight or obesity, such that there is an inverse relationship between intensity and volume of training. With aerobic exercise, intensity can be individualized using percent of maximal heart rate, percent of $\dot{V}O_2max$, or RPE, where volume is differentiated by the duration of the session, as well as the frequency of sessions.

The following suggestions can be used to individualize an exercise program to optimize weight loss during aerobic exercise:

- Incorporate frequent cardiorespiratory workouts that are lower in intensity and longer in duration.
- Include some cardiorespiratory workouts that are of higher intensity for a shorter period of time. This objective may best be realized with high-intensity continuous training or with interval training. To avoid physiological and orthopedic stress and injury, it would be prudent to complete only one higher-intensity workout per week.
- Incorporate multimode training. The theory of multimode training (i.e., employing two or more modes of cardiorespiratory exercise) implies that by doing so the body is protected from getting overly fatigued from overuse of the same muscles in the same movement patterns. This technique helps to thwart the occurrence of musculoskeletal system stress, and aids in the prevention of muscle soreness and injuries. Therefore, theoretically, a person will be able to safely do more work more frequently, which equates to higher total energy expenditure and fat utilization.
- Vary the workout designs regularly. Endeavor to find a satisfactory method for each client by which cardiorespiratory workouts vary within each week, weekly, or bi-weekly using the three ideas just listed. Varying the workouts provides a new stimulus to the body's cardiorespiratory system in an effort to avoid the consequences of overuse exercise fatigue.

Cardiorespiratory Exercise Considerations

The preferred type of cardiorespiratory exercise for individuals who have overweight or obesity is a combination of weight-bearing (such as walking and elliptical exercise) and non-weight-bearing (such as cycling and swimming) modes. Exercise choices should be based on an individual's preferences and exercise history. Help each client find modes of exercise where they have a perceived comfort level with few (if any) negative barriers. The majority of the time spent exercising should be at a low-to-moderate intensity level to avoid joint stress and injury. Therefore, running, jumping, and high-impact movements are not recommended. These physical activities may lead to some musculoskeletal problems associated with body weight and impact forces from the repeated (and forceful) foot strikes on the ground surface. The emphasis of the cardiorespiratory exercise programs should be on performing longer and/or more frequent bouts of exercise. It is important to monitor muscle soreness from the exercise and always ask the client if they are experiencing any orthopedic problems or discomfort. Stationary cycling is preferable to road cycling, as it eliminates any balance-related challenges, while also avoiding the hazards of traffic.

OBESITY AND GAIT MECHANICS

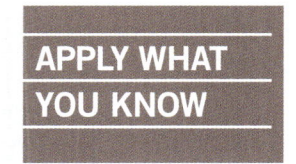

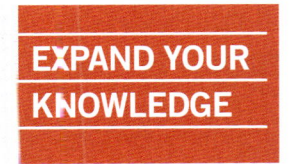

Walking is considered a very good initial exercise because it requires no extra skill. When beginning a walking or weight-bearing exercise regimen with a client, it is important to keep a few things in mind. Obesity has been associated with low walking speed and predicts the development of mobility disability. It has been suggested that excess body weight causes a biomechanical burden to lower-extremity joints, that in turn leads to degenerative joint disease and, eventually, to walking impairment (Houston et al., 2009; Stenholm et al., 2007). Researchers have reported associations between obesity and slower gait speed, wider step width, higher hip medial-lateral rotation, and lower ankle anterior-posterior joint moment. It has been proposed that these walking-pattern characteristics develop as adaptations to excess weight loading on the knee joints while walking (Ko, Stenholm, & Ferrucci, 2010). Further, walking in individuals with obesity can result in a different metabolic cost compared to that seen with normal-weight people. An earlier study by Mattsson, Larsson, and Rossner (1996) presented some very useful data about walking with a female population with obesity. The most interesting finding was that level walking was much harder work for women with obesity when compared to normal-weight women. On average, women with obesity used as much as 56% $\dot{V}O_2$max during walking, as compared to 36% $\dot{V}O_2$max for normal-weight women. The authors noted that even though women with obesity do not necessarily walk with a waddle or straddled legs, they do walk with an abnormal gait pattern that increases their relative oxygen cost. The authors conclude that walking may be too exhausting (and sometimes painful) for some individuals with obesity due to these biomechanical differences in gait and recommend incorporating alternative training modes in the workout design. Swimming and aquatic exercise programs provide total-body exercise with little to no weight-bearing due to the buoyancy of water. Buoyancy is also a benefit for people who have overweight or obesity, who may have joint problems (such as arthritis of the knee, hip, or ankle, or structural problems of these three joints), as well as problems with chafing or thermoregulation.

Fitness facilities have a variety of exercise equipment. The CMES is encouraged to help clients find exercise devices that are easy to use and that do not cause any back, hip, knee, or ankle discomfort. For example, recumbent bikes are great cycling options for individuals with obesity, as compared to stationary or road cycling. However, the CMES must make sure the bike seat is comfortable for the client with overweight or obesity. For walking activities, make sure the person has quality fitness shoes with good shock-absorbing qualities. For some clients with obesity, balance will be an additional challenge with some modes of exercise. If this is the case, the CMES should select exercise devices that have handrails to provide balance support and help prevent falling.

Resistance-training Considerations

There are a few biomechanical concerns to note regarding resistance exercise by persons who have overweight or obesity. For some people with overweight and obesity with mobility and/or balance challenges, seated exercises are good initial options. These types of exercises can be useful in building basic muscle strength. While seated in a chair, individuals are able to do a variety of arm raises, leg lifts, and stretches. Please note that the seats on some exercise machines were not developed for large persons, which may limit the feasibility of using some strength-training equipment. Moreover, weight benches are often quite narrow, which could result in the loss of balance for some clients. In addition, getting into and out of some resistance-training devices may be difficult. It is sometimes preferable not to use exercise devices (such as some abdominal equipment) that are built at floor level, because the person with overweight may have great difficulty getting down to, and up from, the floor. Note that some supine exercises may cause breathing difficulty for some clients with obesity. The CMES must always check to make sure that the client's breathing is regular and uninterrupted during all exercises. Prudence should be taken to avoid doing too much lunge and squat work with persons with overweight, due to possible knee and back discomfort and injury.

EXPAND YOUR KNOWLEDGE

PSYCHOLOGICAL ISSUES ASSOCIATED WITH OBESITY AND RELATED DIETARY PATTERNS

The relationship between obesity and psychological distress is somewhat mixed in the research. Some research does not show statistically significant differences between individuals with obesity and their non-obese counterparts in psychological health and personality profiles (Huang et al., 2007), while other research shows clear associations between obesity and major depressive disorder (Pi-Sunyer, 2009; Gavin, Simon, & Ludman, 2010). Odds of ever having met criteria for major depressive disorder are 20 to 50% higher among individuals with obesity than their normal-weight counterparts (Fabricatore et al., 2011). Some clients with obesity and overweight tend to have a higher prevalence of distress than their non-obese counterparts. These clients often experience adverse feelings of body satisfaction and self-esteem. However, there is a growing body of knowledge that substantiates that physical activity improves psychological well-being in most adults (with and without obesity). Several studies have demonstrated that exercise can positively affect mental health, and a meta-analysis reported that exercise interventions lasting three to 12 weeks can reduce anxiety measures, especially in sedentary subjects with a chronic illness (Hopkins et al., 2012). In addition, the effects of exercise on depression seem equivalent in both sexes and not affected by age or health status. Although no research guidelines exist for actual exercise programming, the evidence suggests that the accepted guidelines for the recommended quantity and quality of exercise for developing and maintaining cardiorespiratory and muscular fitness and flexibility in healthy adults should be followed (ACSM, 2022).

Body image is a complex construct that includes feelings, thoughts, and perceptions about one's physique. Body-image problems are common in people who have overweight or obesity, especially among those seeking treatment, and can undermine successful weight management, increasing chances of relapse. Evidence indicates that there are associations between a range of body-image disturbances and problematic eating behaviors and attitudes. Longitudinal investigations also point to poor body image as a precursor of the adoption of dysfunctional eating behaviors among other unhealthy weight-control strategies (Carraça et al., 2011). For example, Neumark-Sztainer and colleagues (2006) observed that lower levels of body satisfaction were associated with more health-compromising behaviors, such as unhealthy weight-control behaviors and binge eating.

To help improve body-image dissatisfaction, the CMES should be very attentive to the design of fitness facilities to help clients who have overweight or obesity feel more comfortable with their body image. For example, having access to private changing facilities is recommended to help reduce feelings of body-image dissatisfaction. In addition, the CMES needs to be aware that exercise participation may accentuate a person's body-image dissatisfaction and enhance a person's drive for leanness. Therefore, the suggestion or implication that everyone can attain a "model's body" may perpetuate psychological disorders in some clients. Caution is necessary for all exercise professionals when guiding clients, especially clients who have overweight or obesity, toward healthy physical activity, as opposed to leading them to a path obsessed with thinness and the development of eating disorders.

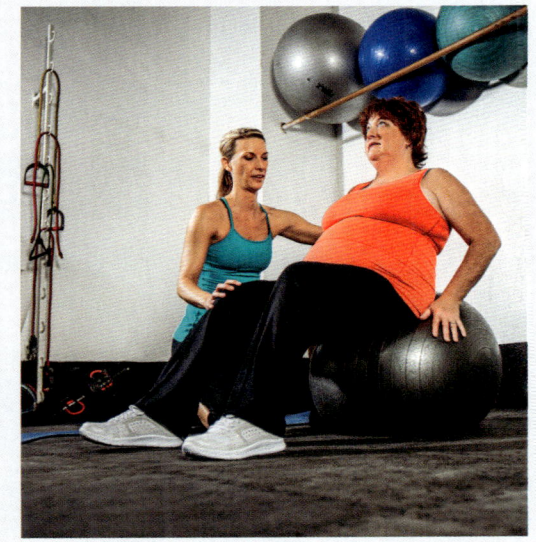

Exercise has a positive connection to improved self-esteem. This link also appears to be more potent among individuals who have lower self-esteem. At this time, available studies indicate that aerobic exercise may have a more pronounced effect, perhaps only because there is so little research available regarding resistance training and self-esteem. However, self-esteem is quite complex and studies suggest that certain subcomponents contribute to a person's self-esteem, including perceived sport competence, physical condition, an "attractive" body, and strength (Elavsky, 2010). Because of the many variables that influence self-esteem, it is important to note that a person may highly value their physical condition and yet have a negative evaluation of their body. The meaningful evidence suggests that aerobic exercise has the most consequential influence on individuals who initially have low self-esteem. An optimal exercise design is uncertain at this time based on published research.

EXERCISE GUIDELINES SUMMARY FOR CLIENTS WITH OBESITY

CARDIORESPIRATORY TRAINING	
Frequency	• ≥5 days per week to maximize caloric expenditure
Intensity	• Intensity may be determined through the following methods: ✓ 40 to 59% HRR or $\dot{V}O_2R$ ✓ RPE of 12–13 on a scale of 6–20 • Eventual progression to a more vigorous intensity (≥60% HRR or $\dot{V}O_2R$) is encouraged to produce greater health/fitness benefits
Time	• Initial goal of 30 minutes per day • Progress to 60 minutes or more per day. • Clients with limited exercise capacity can perform 10-minute bouts accumulated to a total of 30–60 minutes.
Type	• Emphasis should be placed on rhythmic, large muscle group activities, such as: ✓ Walking ✓ Jogging ✓ Cycling ✓ Swimming
Progression	• Progress following the ACE Integrated Fitness Training® Model based on client goals and availability.

MUSCULAR TRAINING	
Frequency	• Perform muscular training two to three days per week, with a day of rest between sessions.
Intensity	• 60–70% 1-RM to begin • Gradually increase to enhance strength and muscle mass
Time	• 2–4 sets of 8–12 repetitions for each major muscle group
Type	• Free weights and/or machines. The decision regarding what form of resistance to use is largely a function of personal preference, training experience, and a client's goals.

Note: $\dot{V}O_2R$ = Oxygen uptake reserve; RPE = Rating of perceived exertion; 1-RM = One-repetition maximum

CMES FOCUS

With the understanding that weight management depends on the relative intake of energy and energy expenditure, the CMES should encourage clients with obesity to reduce current energy intake by 500 to 1,000 calories per day and progressively increase to a minimum of 150 minutes per week of moderate-intensity physical activity. To optimize health/fitness benefits and promote long-term weight control, clients with obesity should be encouraged to progress to greater amounts of exercise (i.e., 250 to 300 minutes per week).

Source: American College of Sports Medicine (2022). ACSM's Guidelines for Exercise Testing and Prescription (11th ed.). Philadelphia: Wolters Kluwer.

CASE STUDIES

Case Study 1

Client Information

Clare is a 52-year-old client who is 5'6" (1.7 m) and weighs 160 pounds (73 kg). Her blood pressure is 110/70 mmHg, her total cholesterol is 200 mg/dL, and she has 33% body fat. She was very athletic in the past and even competed as a middle-distance runner in high school. Clare takes an indoor cycling class lasting 40 minutes three or four days a week and walks leisurely whenever she can. She currently performs no resistance training.

Clare drinks 1.5 liters (0.4 gallons) of water and eats between 2,300 and 2,500 calories each day, including a small breakfast, light snacking in the morning, a light lunch that sometimes includes protein but usually consists of a salad or just vegetables, an afternoon snack, and a dinner of fish or chicken with vegetables and some fat-free ice cream. She also drinks two cups of decaffeinated coffee during the day and has a glass of wine in the evening approximately five days a week.

Clare reports no health conditions and does not take any medications or vitamins. She has a history of yo-yo dieting and did some fasting in her 20s and 30s. She sleeps 5.5 hours each night and has a high-stress job. Her goals are to lose weight (fat) and "firm up."

CMES Approach

Workout and Lifestyle Plan:
- Cardiorespiratory exercise is progressed to the following:
  - ✓ 40 minutes of cardiorespiratory exercise (cycle ergometer or stair stepping) two days a week
  - ✓ Walking for 45 continuous minutes at a self-selected moderate intensity one day a week
  - ✓ Elliptical training for 45 minutes at a self-selected moderate intensity one day a week
  - ✓ Walking moderately for a total accumulated time of at least 90 minutes during the week
- Resistance training
  - ✓ Once Clare demonstrates adequate kinetic-chain mobility and postural stability, and can perform the five primary movement patterns relatively well, the CMES introduces a circuit-training program performed initially two times a week. The circuit-training program includes 10 different exercises targeting the major muscle groups (chest, back, biceps, triceps, deltoids, quadriceps, hamstrings, abdominals, buttocks, lower back) (one circuit).

Dietary Pattern:
- Clare met with a dietitian, who gave her a Mediterranean-type dietary pattern of approximately 1,700 calories a day to follow.

Lifestyle:
- Attempts to sleep 7 hours a night when possible
- Completes extra stretching exercises on high-stress days

Three-month Outcomes:
- Weight = 148 lb (67 kg)
- Blood pressure = 110/70 mmHg
- Total cholesterol = 184 mg/dL
- Body fat = 28%

Six-month Outcomes:
- Weight = 136 lb (62 kg)
- Blood pressure = 101/70 mmHg
- Total cholesterol = 177 mg/dL
- Body fat = 24%

ACE IFT® MODEL AT A GLANCE

Cardiorespiratory Training

This client is performing Fitness Training prior to working with the CMES. As such, her initial program was designed by the CMES to build on her current level of fitness with enhanced programming for Fitness Training.

Muscular Training

Initially, the CMES would help this client to establish adequate postural stability and kinetic-chain mobility with Functional Training exercises to improve muscular endurance, joint function, core function, flexibility, and balance, and progress to Movement Training to help the client develop proficient movement patterns. Once established, the CMES introduces a low-resistance, high-repetition circuit that progresses the client into Load/Speed Training, focused primarily on developing muscular endurance.

Case Study 2

Client Information

Jen is a 19-year-old client who is 5'4" (1.6 m) and weighs 220 pounds (100 kg). Her blood pressure is 124/78 mmHg, her total cholesterol is 210 mg/dL, and she has approximately 40% body fat. Jen walks leisurely twice a week for 25 minutes each time. She currently performs no resistance training.

Jen drinks more than 1.5 liters (0.4 gallons) of water and eats more than 2,800 calories of food each day. Her diet is very high in fats (particularly saturated fat) and **simple carbohydrates** and low in protein. She eats three big meals a day and enjoys a lot of fried and baked foods. She also snacks on sweets (e.g., cookies and cake) during the day. Jen drinks two cups of caffeinated coffee and three or four colas each day. In addition, she drinks three or four alcoholic beverages each weekend.

Jen has elevated blood pressure and hypercholesterolemia and is currently taking no medications or vitamins. She leads what she calls an "inactive lifestyle," sleeps seven hours a night, and has a stress level typical of a college student. Her goal is to lose weight (fat) and get in shape.

ACE IFT® MODEL AT A GLANCE

Cardiorespiratory Training

This client is performing Base Training prior to working with the CMES. As such, her initial program is designed to progress Base Training through positive exercise experiences until the client is able to exercise for 20 to 30 minutes on most days of the week.

Muscular Training

Initially, the Muscular Training program is focused on establishing postural stability and kinetic-chain mobility with Functional Training exercises that will enhance muscular endurance, joint and core function, and flexibility and balance. Next, the program will progress to Movement Training to focus on proficient movement patterns without compromising postural or joint stability before adding external resistance and moving into Load/Speed Training with a focus on muscular strength and endurance, while also boosting caloric expenditure.

CMES Approach

Workout and Lifestyle Plan:

- Cardiorespiratory exercise is progressed to the following:
  ✓ Begin with 20 to 30 minutes of cardiorespiratory exercise (stair stepping, elliptical training, or treadmill walking) performed three days a week. The goal is to progress duration to 60 minutes and frequency to four days a week.
  ✓ Walking at a moderate intensity two times a week for 30 minutes each time
- Resistance training
  ✓ Program would eventually progress to four days a week using an upper- and lower-body split program; each day she does 5 different exercises, 1 to 5 sets of each (never doing more than 20 sets in a workout) consisting of 8 to 12 repetitions per set

Dietary Pattern:

- Met with a dietitian who gave her a heart-healthy diet that meets the recommendations of the Academy of Nutrition and Dietetics (lowering the fats and simple sugars and replacing them with healthy fats and more fruits and vegetables and complex carbohydrates)
- Caloric intake gradually decreased to 1,500 calories per day

Lifestyle:

- Practice meditation 3 or 4 times a week (20 minutes each time) to help manage stress

Three-month Outcomes:

- Weight = 185 lb (84 kg)
- Blood pressure = 110/76 mmHg
- Total cholesterol = 200 mg/dL
- Body fat = 40%

Six-month Outcomes:

- Weight = 150 lb (68 kg)
- Blood pressure = 101/74 mmHg
- Total cholesterol = 185 mg/dL
- Body fat = 32%

SUMMARY

Client education is the framework of successful weight-loss interventions. The CMES is encouraged to inform clients of the health risks of overweight and obesity and the benefits that accompany exercise, weight loss, and lifestyle modifications. The CMES can help clients establish realistic weight-management goals and strategies, and provide the ongoing support for them to keep up these new behaviors. It is important to regularly remind clients that successful energy balance is a life-long process that starts with a commitment to improve the quality of their lives.

REFERENCES

Aills, L. et al. (2008). ASMBS allied health nutritional guidelines for the surgical weight loss patient. *Surgery for Obesity and Related Diseases*, 4, S73–S108.

American College of Sports Medicine (2022). *ACSM's Guidelines for Exercise Testing and Prescription* (11th ed.). Philadelphia: Wolters Kluwer.

Arnardottir, E.S. et al. (2009). Molecular signatures of obstructive sleep apnea in adults: A review and perspective. *Sleep*, 32, 4, 447–470.

Boeing, H. et al. (2012). Critical review: Vegetables and fruit in the prevention of chronic diseases. *European Journal of Nutrition*, 51, 637–663.

Borg, G. (1998). *Borg's Perceived Exertion and Pain Scales*. Champaign, Ill.: Human Kinetics.

Bray, G.A. & Gray, D.S. (1988). Obesity: Part I: Pathogenesis. *Western Journal of Medicine*, 149, 429–441.

Butryn, M.L., Webb, V., & Wadden, T.A. (2011). Behavioral treatment of obesity. *Psychiatric Clinics of North America*, 34, 4, 841–859.

Carraça, E.V. et al. (2011). Body image change and improved eating self-regulation in a weight management intervention in women. *International Journal of Behavioral Nutrition and Physical Activity*, 8, 75.

Casazza, K. et al. (2013). Myths, presumptions, and facts about obesity. *New England Journal of Medicine*, 368, 446–454.

Chapman, C.D. et al. (2012). Lifestyle determinants of the drive to eat: A meta-analysis. *American Journal of Clinical Nutrition*, 96, 3, 492–497.

Dansinger, M.L. et al. (2005). Comparison of the Atkins, Ornish, Weight Watchers, and Zone diets for weight loss and heart disease risk reduction: A randomized trial. *Journal of the American Medical Assocation*, 293, 1, 43–53.

Dempsey, J.A. et al. (2010). Pathophysiology of sleep apnea. *Physiology Reviews*, 90, 1, 47–112. DOI: 10.1152/physrev.00043.2008

Donnelly, J.E. et al. (2009). Position Stand: Appropriate physical activity intervention strategies for weight loss and prevention of weight regain for adults. *Medicine & Science in Sports & Exercise*, 41, 2, 459–471. DOI: 10.1249/MSS.0b013e3181949333

Dreifus, C. (2012). "A Mathematical Challenge to Obesity." *The New York Times*. http://www.nytimes.com/2012/05/15/science/a-mathematical-challenge-to-obesity.html

Elavsky, S. (2010). Longitudinal examination of the exercise and self-esteem model in middle-aged women. *Journal of Sport and Exercise Psychology*, 32, 6, 862–880.

Fabricatore, A.N. et al. (2011). Intentional weight loss and changes in symptoms of depression: A systematic review and meta-analysis. *International Journal of Obesity (London)*, 35, 11, 1363–1376.

Federico, A. et al. (2010). Fat: A matter of disturbance for the immune system. *World Journal of Gastroenterology*, 16, 38, 4762–4772.

Finley, C.E. et al. (2007). Retention rates and weight loss in a commercial weight loss program. *International Journal of Obesity*, 31, 2, 292–298.

Flechtner-Mors, M. et al. (2000). Metabolic and weight loss effects of long-term dietary intervention in obese patients: Four-year results. *Obesity Research*, 8, 5, 399–402.

Gardner, C.D. et al. (2007). Comparison of the Atkins, Zone, Ornish, and LEARN diets for change in weight and related risk factors among overweight premenopausal women: The A to Z Weight Loss Study: A randomized trial. *Journal of the American Medical Association*, 297, 9, 969–977.

Garland, T.G. et al. (2011). The biological control of voluntary exercise, spontaneous physical activity and daily energy expenditure in relation to obesity: Human and rodent perspectives. *Journal of Experimental Biology*, 214, 2, 206–229.

Gavin, A.R., Simon, G.E., & Ludman, E.J. (2010). The association between obesity, depression, and educational attainment in women: The mediating role of body image dissatisfaction. *Journal of Psychosomatic Research*, 69, 6, 573–581.

Gibson, A.L., Wagner, D.R., & Hayward, V.H. (2019). *Advanced Fitness Assessment and Exercise Prescription* (8th ed.). Champaign, Ill.: Human Kinetics.

Gloy, V.L. et al. (2013). Bariatric surgery versus non-surgical treatment for obesity: A systematic review and meta-analysis of randomised controlled trials. *British Medical Journal,* 347, f5934.

Hall, K.D. et al. (2011). Quantification of the effect of energy imbalance on bodyweight. *Lancet,* 378, 9793, 826–837.

Hickey, M.S. & Israel, R.G. (2007). Obesity drugs and drugs in the pipeline. *ACSM's Health & Fitness Journal,* 11, 4, 20–25.

Hopkins, M.E. et al. (2012). Differential effects of acute and regular physical exercise on cognition and affect. *Neuroscience,* 215, 59–68.

Houston, D.K. et al. (2009). Overweight and obesity over the adult life course and incident mobility limitation in older adults: The health, aging and body composition study. *American Journal of Epidemiology,* 169, 927–936.

Hu, F.B. (2013). Resolved: There is sufficient scientific evidence that decreasing sugar-sweetened beverage consumption with reduce the prevalence of obesity and obesity-related diseases. *Obesity Reviews,* 14, 8, 606–619.

Huang, J.S. et al. (2007). Body image and self-esteem among adolescents undergoing an intervention targeting dietary and physical activity behaviors. *Journal of Adolescent Health,* 40, 3, 245–251.

Hui, X. et al. (2012). Adiponectin and cardiovascular health: An update. *British Journal of Pharmacology,* 165, 3, 574–590.

Jakicic, J.M. et al. (2009). ACSM position stand on the appropriate intervention strategies for weight loss and prevention of weight regain for adults. *Medicine & Science in Sports & Exercise,* 33, 2145–2156.

Jensen, M.D. et al. (2013). 2013 AHA/ACC/TOS guidelines for the management of overweight and obesity in adults: A report of the American College of Cardiology/American Heart Association Task Force on Practice Guidelines and The Obesity Society. *Circulation,* DOI:10.1016/j.jacc.2013.11.004

Kaptoge, S. et al. (2010). C-reactive protein concentration and risk of coronary heart disease, stroke, and mortality: An individual participant meta-analysis. *Lancet,* 9, 375, 9709, 132–140. DOI: 10.1016/S0140-6736(09)61717-7

Karra, E., Chandarana, K., & Batterham, R.L. (2009). The role of peptide YY in appetite regulation and obesity. *Journal of Physiology,* 587, Pt 1, 19–25.

Ko, S., Stenholm, S., & Ferrucci, L. (2011). Characteristic gait patterns in older adults with obesity: Results from the Baltimore Longitudinal Study of Aging. *Journal of Biomechanics,* 43, 6, 1104–1110.

Koliaki, C. et al. (2010). The effect of ingested macronutrients on postprandial ghrelin response: A critical review of existing literature data. *International Journal of Peptides,* pii: 710852. DOI: 10.1155/2010/710852

Kravitz, L. (2007). The 25 most significant health benefits of physical activity and exercise. *IDEA Fitness Journal,* 4, 9, 54–63.

Levine, J.A. (2007). Nonexercise activity thermogenesis: Liberating the life-force. *Journal of Internal Medicine,* 262, 3, 273–287.

Levine, J.A. et al. (2005). Interindividual variation in posture allocation: Possible role in human obesity. *Science,* 307, 584–586.

Liu, R.H. (2003). Health benefits of fruit and vegetables are from additive and synergistic combinations of phytochemicals. *American Journal of Clinical Nutrition,* 78, Suppl., 517S–520S.

Lucassen, E.A., Rother, K.I., & Cizza, G. (2012). Interacting epidemics? Sleep curtailment, insulin resistance, and obesity. *Annals of the New York Academy of Science,* 1264, 1, 110–134.

Magee, L. & Hale, L. (2012). Longitudinal associations between sleep duration and subsequent weight gain: A systematic review. *Sleep Medicine Reviews,* 16, 3, 231–241.

Mann, T. et al. (2007). Medicare's search for effective obesity treatments: Diets are not the answer. *American Psychologist,* 62, 3, 220–233.

Mantzoros, C.S. et al. (2011). Leptin in human physiology and pathophysiology. *American Journal of Physiology – Endocrinology & Metabolism,* 301, 4, E567–E584.

Mattsson, E., Larsson, U.E., & Rossner, S. (1996). Is walking for exercise too exhausting for obese women? *International Journal of Obesity and Metabolic Disorders,* 21, 5, 380–386.

Mazza, A.D., Pratley, R.E., & Smith, S.R. (2011. Beta-cell preservation… Is weight loss the answer? *The Review of Diabetic Studies,* 8, 4, 446–453.

Muth, N.D. (2014). *Nutrition for Health Professionals.* Philadelphia: F.A. Davis.

National Heart, Lung, and Blood Institute (2019). *Classification of Overweight and Obesity by BMI, Waist Circumference, and Associated Disease Risks.* www.nhlbi.nih.gov/health/educational/lose_wt/BMI/bmi_dis.htm

National Institutes of Health (2012). *Overweight and Obesity.* www.nhlbi.nih.gov/health/dci/Diseases/obe/obe_whatare.html

National Institutes of Health Technology Assessment Conference Panel (1992). Methods for voluntary weight loss and control. *Annals of Internal Medicine,* 116, 11, 942–949.

Neumark-Sztainer, D. et al. (2006). Does body satisfaction matter? Five-year longitudinal associations between body satisfaction and health behaviors in adolescent females and males. *Journal of Adolescent Health,* 39, 244–251.

Ouellet, V. et al. (2011). Outdoor temperature, age, sex, body mass index, and diabetic status determine the prevalence, mass, and glucose-uptake activity of 18F-FDG-detected BAT in humans. *Journal of Clinical Endocrinology & Metabolism,* 96, 192–199.

Patel, S.R. & Hu, F.B. (2008). Short sleep duration and weight gain: A systematic review. *Obesity (Silver Spring),* 16, 3, 643–653.

Patterson, R.E. et al. (2004). A comprehensive examination of health conditions associated with obesity in older adults. *American Journal of Preventive Medicine,* 97, 5, 385–390.

Pfannenberg, C. et al. (2010). Impact of age on the relationships of brown adipose tissue with sex and adiposity in humans. *Diabetes,* 59, 1789–1793.

Pi-Sunyer, X. (2009). The medical risks of obesity. *Postgraduate Medicine,* 121, 6, 21–33.

Poirier, P. et al. (2011). Bariatric surgery and cardiovascular risk factors: A scientific statement from the American Heart Association. *Circulation,* 123, 1683–1701.

Rasmussen, A.T. (1923). The so-called hibernating gland. *Journal of Morphology,* 38, 147–205.

Scheen, A.J. (2011). Sibutramine on cardiovascular outcome. *Diabetes Care,* 34, Suppl. 2, S114–S119.

Seagle, H.M. et al. (2009). Position of the American Dietetic Association: Weight management. *Journal of the American Dietetic Associatin,* 109, 2, 330–346.

Stanford, K.I. et al. (2013). Brown adipose tissue regulates glucose homeostasis and insulin sensitivity. *Journal of Clinical Investigation,* 123, 1, 215–223. DOI: 10.1172/JCI62308

Stenholm, S. et al. (2007). Effect of comorbidity on the association of high body mass index with walking limitation among men and women aged 55 years and older. *Aging Clinical and Experimental Research,* 19, 277–283.

St-Onge, M-P. (2013). The role of sleep duration in the regulation of energy balance: Effects on energy intakes and expenditure. *Journal of Clinical Sleep Medicine,* 9, 1, 73–80.

Swanson, M. et al. (2011). Intergenerational energy balance interventions: A systematic literature review. *Health Education & Behavior,* 38, 2, 171–197.

Townsend, K. & Tseng, Y-H. (2012), Brown adipose tissue: Recent insights into development, metabolic function and therapeutic potential. *Adipocyte,* 1, 1, 13–24.

Veerman, J.L. et al. (2011). Cost-effectiveness of pharmacotherapy to reduce obesity. *PLoS One,* 6, 10, e26051.

Vijgen, G.H. et al. (2012). Increase in brown adipose tissue activity after weight loss in morbidly obese subjects. *Journal of Clinical Endocrinology & Metabolism,* 97, E1229–E1233.

Vijgen, G.H. et al. (2011). Brown adipose tissue in morbidly obese subjects. *PLoS ONE,* 6, e17247.

Wang, X. et al. (2013). Inflammatory markers and risk of type 2 diabetes: A systematic review and meta-analysis. *Diabetes Care,* 36, 1, 166–175.

Wing, R.R. & Phelan, S. (2005). Long-term weight loss maintenance. *American Journal of Clinical Nutrition,* 82, Suppl., 222S–225S.

Wing, R.R. et al. (2011). Benefits of modest weight loss in improving cardiovascular risk factors in overweight and obese individuals with type 2 diabetes. *Diabetes Care,* 34, 7, 1481–1486.

World Health Organization (2020). *Obesity and Overweight.* www.who.int/news-room/fact-sheets/detail/obesity-and-overweight

Wu, J., Cohen, P., & Spiegelman, B.M. (2013). Adaptive thermogenesis in adipocytes: Is beige the new brown? *Genes & Development,* 27, 3, 234–250.

Xia, Q. & Grant, S.F.A. (2013). The genetics of human obesity. *Annals of the New York Academy of Science,* 1281, 1, 178–190.

Yoneshiro, T. et al. (2011). Age-related decrease in cold-activated brown adipose tissue and accumulation of body fat in healthy humans. *Obesity (Silver Spring),* 19, 1755–1760. DOI: 10.1038/oby.2011.125

Zhou, Y.H. et al. (2012). Effect of anti-obesity drug on cardiovascular risk factors: A systematic review and meta-analysis of randomized controlled trials. *PLoS ONE,* 7, 6, e39062.

SUGGESTED READING

Casazza, K. et al. (2013). Myths, presumptions, and facts about obesity. *New England Journal of Medicine,* 368, 446–454

Chapman, C.D. et al. (2012). Lifestyle determinants of the drive to eat: A meta-analysis. *American Journal of Clinical Nutrition,* 96, 3, 492–497.

Jensen, M.D. et al. (2013). 2013 AHA/AC/TOS guidelines for the management of overweight and obesity in adults: A report of the American College of Cardiology/American Heart Association Task Force on Practice Guidelines and The Obesity Society. *Circulation,* DOI:10.1016/j.jacc.2013.11.004

St-Onge, M-P. (2013). The role of sleep duration in the regulation of energy balance: Effects on energy intakes and expenditure. *Journal of Clinical Sleep Medicine,* 9, 1, 73–80.

Xia, Q. & Grant, S.F.A. (2013). The genetics of human obesity. *Annals of the New York Academy of Science,* 1281, 1, 178–190.

World Health Organization (2020). *Obesity and Overweight.* www.who.int/news-room/fact-sheets/detail/obesity-and-overweight

12 THE METABOLIC SYNDROME

IN THIS CHAPTER

EPIDEMIOLOGY

OVERVIEW

DIAGNOSTIC CRITERIA

TREATMENT OPTIONS
- NON-PHARMACOLOGICAL TREATMENT
- PHARMACOLOGICAL TREATMENT
- SURGICAL TREATMENT
- EXERCISE TREATMENT

NUTRITIONAL CONSIDERATIONS

EXERCISE RECOMMENDATIONS
- TYPE OF EXERCISE
- INTENSITY AND DURATION
- FREQUENCY

EXERCISE GUIDELINES SUMMARY FOR CLIENTS WITH METABOLIC SYNDROME

CASE STUDY

SUMMARY

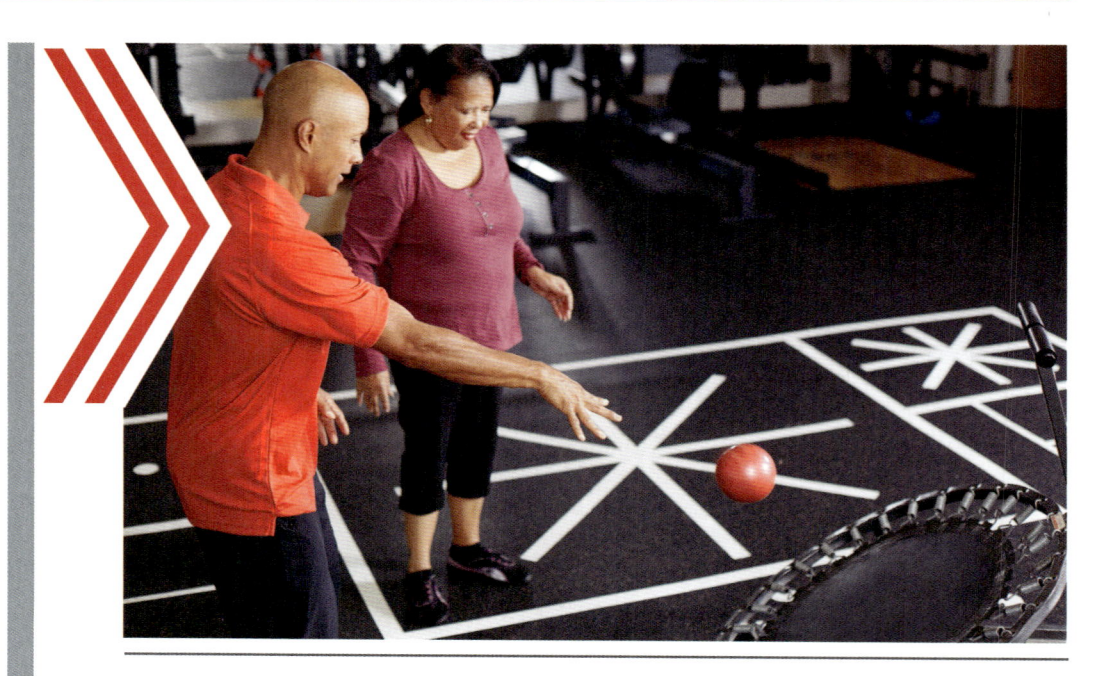

ABOUT THE AUTHORS

Barry A. Franklin, Ph.D., is director of Preventive Cardiology and Cardiac Rehabilitation at William Beaumont Hospital in Royal Oak, Michigan, and professor of Internal Medicine at Oakland University William Beaumont School of Medicine, Rochester, Michigan. Dr. Franklin served as president of the American Association of Cardiovascular and Pulmonary Rehabilitation in 1988 and president of the American College of Sports Medicine in 1999. Currently, he holds editorial positions with numerous scientific and clinical journals, including the *American Journal of Cardiology, The Physician and Sportsmedicine,* and the *Journal of Cardiovascular and Pulmonary Rehabilitation and Prevention.* Dr. Franklin has written or edited more than 600 publications, including 80 book chapters and 25 books.

Wendy M. Miller, M.D., is section head of Nutrition and Preventive Medicine at William Beaumont Hospitals, Royal Oak and Troy, Mich., and professor of Internal Medicine at Oakland University William Beaumont School of Medicine, Rochester, Mich. Dr. Miller is Board Certified in Internal Medicine and Obesity Medicine, and is also certified as a Physician Nutrition Specialist. She serves as director of two comprehensive multidisciplinary weight-control centers, which provide medically supervised weight loss, perioperative, and long-term care of bariatric surgery patients, and a lifestyle-change program for children with obesity. Dr. Miller has published extensively on obesity and its association with diabetes, inflammation, metabolic syndrome, dyslipidemia, and cardiovascular disease.

Peter A. McCullough, M.D., M.P.H., FACC, FACP, FCCP, FAHA, FNKF, oversees cardiovascular education and research at the Baylor Health Care System in Dallas, Tex. He is an internationally recognized authority on the role of chronic kidney disease in cardiometabolic risk state, with more than 1,000 publications, including the "Interface between Renal Disease and Cardiovascular Illness" in *Braunwald's Heart Disease.* In 2013, Dr. McCullough was honored with the International Vicenza Award for Critical Care Nephrology for his outstanding contribution and dedication to the emerging problem of cardiorenal syndromes.

By Barry A. Franklin, Wendy M. Miller, Peter A. McCullough

A SYNDROME IS DEFINED AS A CLUSTERING OF FACTORS that occur together more often than by chance alone, often with uncertain causes. The **metabolic syndrome (MetS)** matches these criteria and is characterized by a constellation of disorders, including **insulin resistance, obesity, visceral adiposity**, glucose intolerance, **dyslipidemia**, and increased blood pressure. Individuals with MetS are at twice the risk of developing **cardiovascular disease (CVD)** over the next decade as those without the syndrome. The risk over a lifetime is even higher. Furthermore, MetS sufferers have a fivefold increase in risk for **type 2 diabetes mellitus (T2DM)** (Alberti et al., 2009).

Complex, mutually reinforcing interactions between obesity and insulin resistance largely account for the pathogenesis of MetS (Figure 12-1). Excess visceral adiposity is both necessary and sufficient for the development of this multifaceted disease state (Batsis, Nieto-Martinez, & Lopez-Jimenez, 2007). Genetically predisposed groups, including Hispanics and Asian Indians, have demonstrated a greater intolerance to excess visceral adiposity, and are known to develop MetS at relatively lesser degrees of adiposity (Caballero, 2005; Misra & Vikram, 2004). More than 95% of individuals with MetS have a **body mass index (BMI)** that is ≥25 kg/m^2; thus, the BMI as a crude measure identifies the majority of individuals at risk for this medical condition.

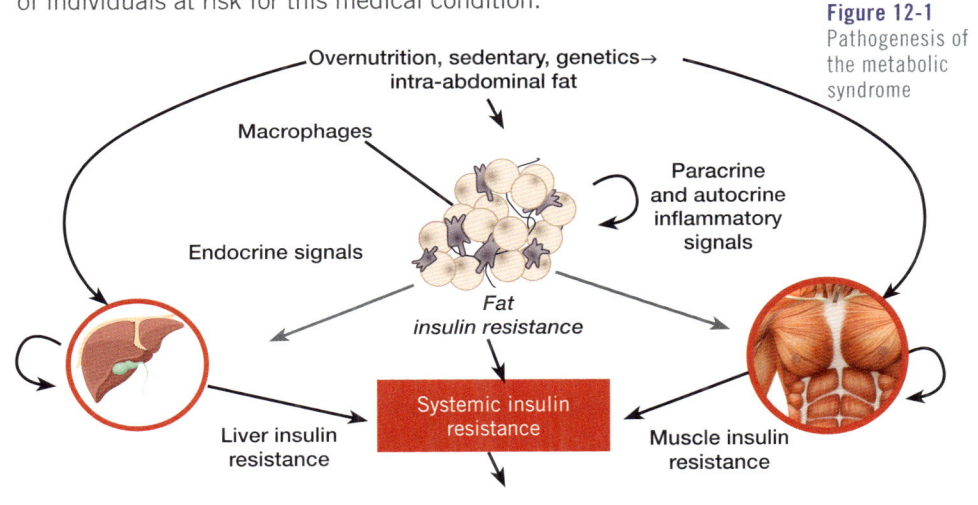

Figure 12-1
Pathogenesis of the metabolic syndrome

Metabolic syndrome: hyperinsulinemia, increased blood pressure, dyslipidemia, hyperglycemia, pro-inflammatory, and hypercoagulable changes

LEARNING OBJECTIVES:

» List the cluster of risk factors that together make up the metabolic syndrome.

» Explain the association between the metabolic syndrome and the risk for cardiovascular disease and diabetes mellitus.

» Describe the treatment options for metabolic syndrome with a specific focus on appropriate lifestyle intervention strategies, including strategies to enhance weight loss, increase physical activity, and eat a non-atherogenic diet.

» Design and implement safe and effective physical-activity programs for clients with the metabolic syndrome who have received medical clearance for exercise participation.

EPIDEMIOLOGY

The epidemiology of MetS directly parallels the obesity epidemic in terms of incidence and prevalence (Ford, Giles, & Dietz, 2002). The many causes for the rise in obesity are complex (see Chapter 11). Follow-up data from the Coronary Artery Risk Development in Young Adults Study (CARDIA) (Figure 12-2) indicate that young adults are at considerable risk to develop MetS if, over time, there has been a consistent increase in body weight (Lloyd-Jones et al., 2007). Further, evidence shows a graded increase in the risk of MetS with an increase in BMI, even with various levels of physical activity (Cheriyath et al., 2010). Although overall body weight and relative adiposity, as reflected in the BMI, identify the greater than two-thirds of Western populations at risk for MetS, those with excessive intra-abdominal adiposity are particularly susceptible. This android or male pattern of fat deposition in the abdomen is easily recognized and can be accurately quantified. If the abdomen is not scaphoid (concave)

Figure 12-2
Incidence of metabolic syndrome at year 15 by sex and change in body mass index. Probability values refer to the comparison with the stable/decreased body mass index group for the same sex.

Reprinted with permission from Lloyd-Jones D.M. et al. (2007). Consistently stable or decreased body mass index in young adulthood and longitudinal changes in metabolic syndrome components: The Coronary Artery Risk Development in Young Adults Study. *Circulation,* 115, 8, 1004.

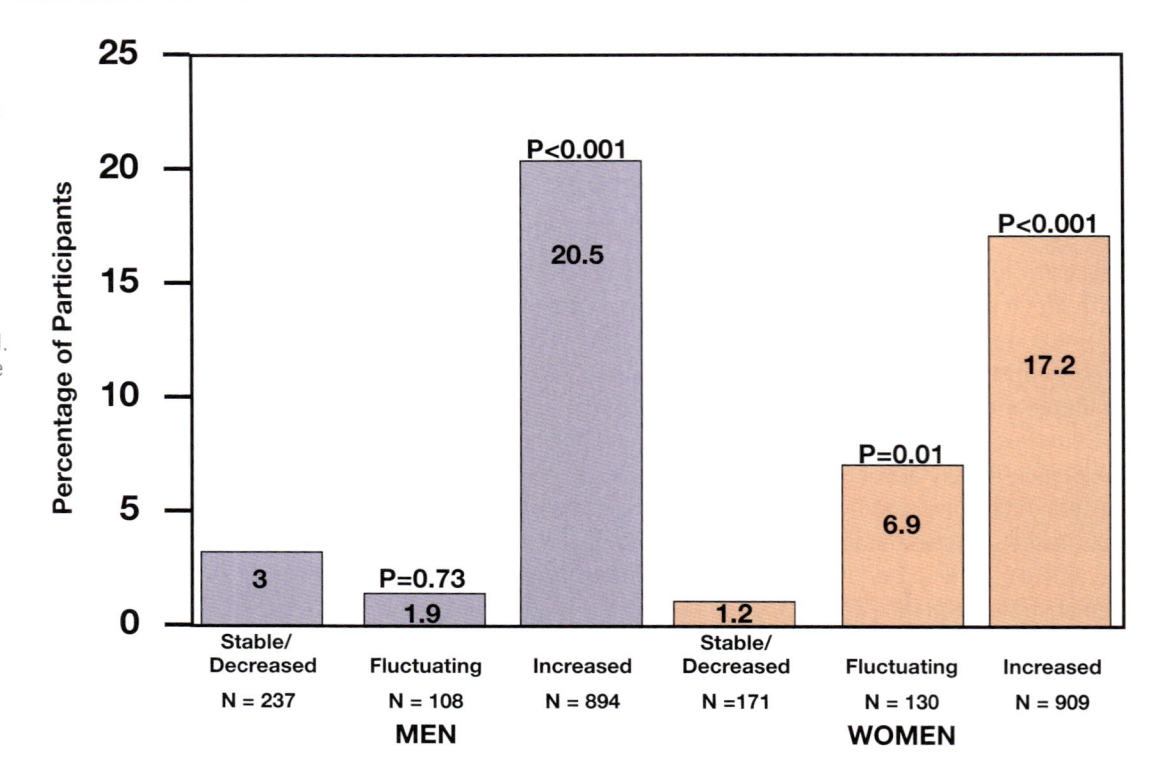

on examination, excess visceral adiposity should be considered. Conversely, a predominantly gynoid pattern of fat deposition in the buttocks and legs with a scaphoid abdomen does not indicate risk for MetS. One practical consideration, however, is that virtually all individuals with a BMI ≥30 kg/m² have excess visceral adiposity irrespective of body shape, with the exception of extremely muscular individuals.

MetS is present in approximately 34% of all adults in the United States. Men who have **overweight** are about six times as likely and men with obesity are about 32 times as likely as normal-weight males to meet the criteria. Women who have overweight are more than five times as likely and women with obesity are more than 17 times as likely as normal-weight females to meet the criteria (Ervin, 2009). Each component of MetS is associated with a heightened risk for developing CVD and **diabetes.** Individuals with MetS have a one-and-a-half- to threefold increased risk for developing **coronary heart disease (CHD)** or **stroke** (Isomaa et al., 2001). In the primary prevention arm of the San Antonio Heart Study, MetS was associated with a twofold higher risk for developing CVD over a mean follow-up of 12.7 years (Hunt et al., 2004). This distinguishes MetS as a unique marker for increased cardiovascular risk, highlighting the need for aggressive risk-factor reduction and treatment.

OVERVIEW

Central pathophysiologic features of MetS as a consequence of excess visceral adiposity include the following (Rader, 2007):
- Insulin resistance at the liver and skeletal muscles
- **Atherogenic dyslipidemia,** chiefly manifested as a triad of low **high-density lipoprotein (HDL)** cholesterol together with increases in **triglycerides** and small, dense **low-density lipoprotein (LDL)** cholesterol particles
- Increased blood pressure or **hypertension**
- A proinflammatory state, with increases in inflammatory markers [e.g., high-sensitivity C-reactive protein (hs-CRP)]
- A prothrombotic state, with increases in plasminogen activator inhibitor (PAI-1) and fibrinogen

The Metabolic Syndrome

Both the proinflammatory and prothrombotic states of MetS derive largely from the secretory activity of intra-abdominal or visceral adipose tissue, which may increase the risk of coronary events. A widely cited report found that increasing BMI was independently associated with prothrombotic factors and impaired fibrinolytic activity in men and women (Rosito et al., 2004). Accordingly, the investigators found greater thrombotic potential in subjects who had overweight or obesity. High-sensitivity C-reactive protein is considered an index of inflammation and is associated with increased cardiovascular risk, particularly the provocation of **angina pectoris** or acute **myocardial infarction (MI).** Values greater than 2 mg/L may serve as a powerful predictor for future cardiovascular events. The American Heart Association/Centers for Disease Control and Prevention (CDC) Scientific Statement on Markers of Intervention and Cardiovascular Disease recommends that in persons with an intermediate Framingham CHD 10-year risk (10 to 20%) and an LDL level that is above average but still below the cutoff for pharmacotherapeutic intervention, it may be appropriate to measure hs-CRP to aid in risk stratification (Pearson et al., 2003).

CLINICAL IMPLICATIONS AND ASSOCIATED DISORDERS OF THE METABOLIC SYNDROME

MetS places an individual at high risk for the development of T2DM and CVD. The transition from MetS to overt T2DM stems from insulin resistance and a decline of pancreatic beta-cell function. Insulin resistance in muscle tissue results in decreased glucose uptake and impaired **glycogen** synthesis. In the liver, insulin resistance results in failure of insulin to suppress hepatic glucose production. Despite these anomalies, individuals are normoglycemic in the early stages of the disease due to a marked increase in pancreatic beta-cell insulin secretion. As the disease progresses, glucotoxicity and lipotoxicity cause beta-cell function to decline, leading to **apoptosis** of pancreatic islet cells (Marchetti et al., 2006). At this point, the lower level of insulin secretion can no longer compensate for the effects of insulin resistance, and serum glucose levels reach the threshold for T2DM.

A variety of pathophysiologic mechanisms initiated by insulin resistance promote CVD. Insulin resistance triggers endothelial dysfunction via glucose intolerance, **hyperglycemia,** and attenuated vascular production of nitric oxide, a factor involved in **vasodilation** and endothelial function (Peppa, Uribarri, & Vlassara, 2003; McFarlane, Banerji, & Sowers, 2001). Additionally, insulin resistance is associated with an atherogenic dyslipidemic profile, including **hypertriglyceridemia;** low HDL; increased proportion of small, dense LDL particles; and increased apolipoprotein B concentrations. Furthermore, insulin resistance contributes to the development of a prothrombotic and proinflammatory state via increased levels of PAI-1 and other inflammatory markers, as well as hypertension.

There are other clinical derangements associated with MetS. Fatty liver disease with **steatosis** can ultimately lead to **fibrosis** and **cirrhosis.** Chronic kidney disease and **microalbuminuria** are more prevalent in those with MetS. There are also relationships between MetS and obstructive sleep apnea, **hyperuricemia,** and **gout.**

EXPAND YOUR KNOWLEDGE

DIAGNOSTIC CRITERIA

The association of visceral obesity and cardiovascular risk stems from the clustering of metabolic conditions, including hypertension, dyslipidemia, and T2DM mediated through insulin resistance, leading to MetS. The purpose of this unique designation was to identify those at higher metabolic risk for CVD and the development of diabetes and to respond with more aggressive strategies for prevention (Alberti et al., 2009; Grundy, 2007). As indicated earlier, MetS should be suspected in all individuals with a BMI ≥25 kg/m^2. Although several different definitions for metabolic syndrome have been proposed, the International Diabetes Federation, NHLBI, AHA, and others have proposed a harmonized definition for MetS (Alberti, 2009). MetS is characterized by a constellation of disorders, and current guidelines suggest that an individual must have three or more of the following to qualify for a diagnosis of MetS:
- Abdominal obesity indicated by a waist circumference ≥40 inches (102 cm) in men and ≥35 inches (88 cm) in women

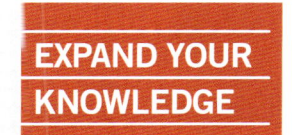

TABLE 12-1	
PATHOPHYSIOLOGIC PROCESSES ASSOCIATED WITH THE METABOLIC SYNDROME	
• Insulin resistance	• Microalbuminuria
• Abnormal fibrinolysis	• Inflammation
• Endothelial dysfunction	• Procoagulation

Source: Grundy S.M. et al. (2004). Implications of recent clinical trials for the National Cholesterol Education Program Adult Treatment Panel III Guidelines. *Circulation,* 110, 2, 227.

- Levels of triglycerides ≥150 mg/dL (1.7 mmol/L) or on drug treament
- HDL levels <40 and <50 mg/dL (1.0 and 1.3 mmol/L) in men and women, respectively, or on drug treatment
- **Blood pressure** levels ≥130/85 mmHg or on drug treament
- Fasting glucose levels ≥100 mg/dL (5.6 mmol/L) or on drug treament

Additional biomarkers that strongly support the diagnosis of MetS include hsCRP >2 mg/L, **hyperinsulinemia** (fasting C-peptide >4.6 ng/mL), and a urinary albumin:creatinine ratio >30 mg/g, which reflects kidney damage due to the vascular consequences of the disease (Table 12-1).

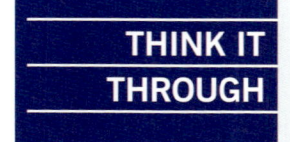

THINK IT THROUGH

The previous section outlines the five diagnostic criteria for MetS. As an ACE® Certified Medical Exercise Specialist (CMES), it is within your scope of practice to measure two of these criteria (i.e., waist circumference and blood pressure). If a new client indicates on their health-history form that they have been diagnosed with one of the other three criteria (i.e., dyslipidemia, elevated fasting glucose levels, or elevated triglycerides) that cannot be measured by an exercise professional, and you ascertain that they also have increased blood pressure and abdominal obesity through your initial assessment, how will you approach the topic of MetS with this client? Respecting your scope of practice, which prohibits you from diagnosing any medical condition, what would you say to the client about their risk factors for disease?

TREATMENT OPTIONS

For management of long-term as well as short-term risk, lifestyle therapies are first-line interventions, as these changes may produce a reduction in all of the metabolic risk factors simultaneously. Ultimately, the greatest benefit for those with MetS will be derived from effective long-term lifestyle intervention.

Non-pharmacological Treatment

The cornerstone treatment of MetS is therapeutic lifestyle modification to reduce body weight and fat stores, increase physical activity, and transition to an anti-**atherogenic** diet—that is, a diet that reduces the risk of developing CVD (Table 12-2). Reduction of abdominal adiposity, the primary underlying cause of MetS, is the main therapeutic target. Although lifestyle intervention is often overlooked in clinical practice (Grundy, 2006), this non-pharmacological approach has been shown to reduce cardiovascular risk and prevent or delay progression to diabetes [Knowler et al., 2002; National Institutes of Health (NIH), 1998].

TABLE 12-2	
EFFECTIVE LIFESTYLE INTERVENTIONS FOR RISK FACTORS OF THE METABOLIC SYNDROME	
Therapeutic Target	**Therapeutic Goal**
Abdominal obesity	Reduced body weight (e.g., 7–10% during first year); continued weight loss thereafter with goal of ultimately achieving desirable weight (BMI <25 kg/m^2)
Physical inactivity	30–60 minutes continuous/intermittent moderate-intensity physical activity; 5 days/week, but preferably daily, complemented by increased lifestyle activity
Atherogenic diet	Reduced intakes of saturated fats (<7% of total fats) and cholesterol (<200 mg/d); avoid trans fat; total fat 25–35% of total calories; most dietary fat should be unsaturated; and simple sugars should be limited

Note: BMI = Body mass index

Source: Grundy, S.M. et al. (2005). Diagnosis and management of the metabolic syndrome: An American Heart Association/National Heart, Lung, and Blood Institute Scientific Statement: Executive summary. *Circulation,* 112, e285–e290.

Pharmacological Treatment

Permanent lifestyle changes are generally considered first-line strategies to address the cardiovascular risk factors that characterize MetS. However, pharmacotherapies may be indicated for individuals unable to adopt healthier lifestyle habits or those failing to reach metabolic goals despite lifestyle change. Agents that can modify the cardiovascular risk may target increased blood pressure (Ruilope, Redón, & Schmieder, 2007; He & Whelton, 1999), insulin resistance (Hu et al., 2002), impaired glucose metabolism (Gerstein et al., 2006; Knowler et al., 2002), dyslipidemia (Grundy et al., 2004; Expert Panel, 2001), obesity, or combinations thereof.

Surgical Treatment

According to the NIH guidelines, bariatric surgery is indicated for those with a BMI of 40 kg/m^2 or greater, or those with a BMI between 35 and 40 kg/m^2 with at least one comorbid condition such as diabetes, hypertension, obstructive sleep apnea, or CHD (NIH, 1998). Bariatric surgery has shown the highest success rates for obesity management, with an average weight loss of 35 to 38% of initial total body weight (Shah, Simha, & Garg, 2006); moreover, it improves all components of MetS. A meta-analysis of bariatric surgery outcomes found that diabetes improved or resolved in 83%, hypercholesterolemia improved in 95%, and hypertension improved or resolved in 87% of patients who underwent gastric bypass surgery (Buchwald et al., 2004).

Exercise Treatment

There is a pathophysiological cascade by which physical inactivity predisposes to a cluster of metabolic diseases, including MetS. With an increasingly hypokinetic lifestyle, skeletal muscle downregulates its capacity to convert nutritional substrates to energy. Inactive skeletal muscle's impaired ability to oxidize glucose and fatty acids is presumably mediated by several mechanisms, including decreased mitochondrial concentration; a reduced ability to remove glucose from blood due to fewer capillaries and diminished glucose transporter; and an attenuated capacity to hydrolyze blood triglycerides to **free fatty acids,** secondary to decreased lipoprotein lipase activity (Chakravarthy & Booth, 2003). Collectively, these metabolic perturbations serve to reduce the capacity to burn fuel, resulting in hyperinsulinemia, hypertriglyceridemia, and ultimately increased cardiovascular risk. On the other hand, moderate-to-vigorous leisure-time physical activity diminishes the magnitude of all five risk factors that are associated with MetS (Rennie et al., 2003) (Table 12-3). An increase in physical activity also improves insulin action in obesity, with or without a concomitant reduction in body weight and fat stores (Kelley & Goodpaster, 1999). This is an important (and often overlooked) salutary effect, suggesting that physical activity is as efficacious in preventing insulin resistance as losing body weight.

TABLE 12-3
INFLUENCE OF PHYSICAL ACTIVITY (AND INACTIVITY) ON THE CHARACTERISTICS OF THE METABOLIC SYNDROME

Characteristics of the Metabolic Syndrome	Impact of Physical Activity	Impact of Physical Inactivity
Large abdominal circumference: Women ≥35 inches (88 cm) Men ≥40 inches (102 cm)	Decreases	Increases
Hypertriglyceridemia: ≥150 mg/dL	Decreases	Increases
Low HDL: Women <50 mg/dL Men <40 mg/dL	Increases	Decreases
Increased blood pressure: ≥130/85 mmHg	Decreases	Increases
High fasting blood glucose: ≥100 mg/dL	Decreases	Increases

Source: The Expert Panel on Detection, Evaluation, and Treatment of High Blood Cholesterol in Adults (2001). Executive Summary of the Third Report of the National Cholesterol Education Program (NCEP) Expert Panel on Detection, Evaluation, and Treatment of High Blood Cholesterol in Adults (Adult Treatment Panel III). *Journal of the American Medical Association,* 285, 19, 2486.

Researchers in Finland examined the effects of moderate and vigorous physical activity over a four-year period in 612 middle-aged men without evidence of MetS (Laaksonen et al., 2002). Subjects who engaged in more than three hours per week of moderate-intensity leisure-time physical activity (LTPA) were half as likely as **sedentary** control subjects to develop MetS. Moreover, vigorous LTPA had an even stronger inverse association, particularly in unfit men. Men in the upper third of $\dot{V}O_2$max were 75% less likely than unfit men to develop MetS. This was the first prospective study to show that low levels of LTPA and aerobic fitness predict the development of MetS, even after adjustments for potential confounding variables (e.g., age, BMI, smoking habit, alcohol intake, socioeconomic status, and other coronary risk factors).

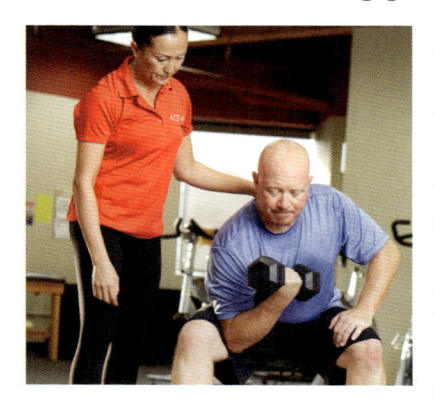

In a more recent investigation, researchers conducted a meta-analysis on prospective cohort studies to assess the effect of LTPA on the risk of MetS (Huang & Liu, 2014). The subjects consisted of healthy adults between the ages of 20 and 70 years who performed either moderate-level physical activity or high-level physical activity. The control group was comprised of subjects with a low level of physical activity. The results indicated that performing moderate-level and high-level physical activity could decrease the risk of MetS. The authors concluded that overall, regular physical activity should be performed on most days of the week and for a longer duration (up to 60 to 90 minutes) at a moderate intensity initially [approximately 40 to 59% **$\dot{V}O_2$ reserve ($\dot{V}O_2R$)** or **heart-rate reserve (HRR)**] and progressing to a more vigorous intensity [≥60% $\dot{V}O_2R$ or HRR] when appropriate over time for optimal metabolic benefits. These results are consistent with the general consensus public health recommendations for adults with overweight or obesity [American College of Sports Medicine (ACSM), 2022].

Several investigators have also examined the relationships among habitual physical activity, cardiorespiratory fitness, MetS, and all-cause and cardiovascular **mortality.** Overall, these studies suggest that higher levels of daily physical activity and/or aerobic fitness are associated with a decreased clustering of risk factors that delineate MetS (LaMonte et al., 2005; Farrell, Cheng, & Blair, 2004; Kullo, Hensrud, & Allison, 2002; Carroll, Cooke, & Butterly, 2000). In one widely cited report (Whaley et al., 1999), the age-adjusted cumulative odds ratio for abnormal markers of MetS was 3.0 for the least-fit men compared with moderately fit ones, and 10.1 when compared with the most-fit men (Figure 12-3). Among women, the age-adjusted cumulative odds ratio was 2.7 for the least-fit women when compared with moderately fit ones, and 4.9 when compared with the most-fit women (see Figure 12-3). Others have reported that higher levels of cardiorespiratory fitness are associated with a substantial reduction in health risk for a given level of visceral and

Figure 12-3
Prevalence of metabolic syndrome increases as cardiovascular fitness decreases

Source: Whaley, M.H. et al. (1999). Physical fitness and clustering of risk factors associated with the metabolic syndrome. *Medicine & Science in Sports & Exercise*, 31, 2, 287.

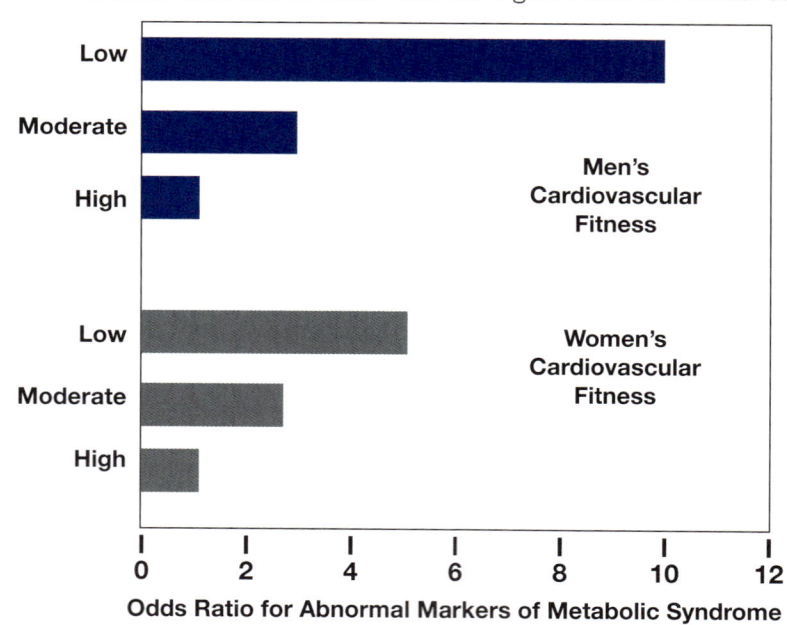

The Metabolic Syndrome

subcutaneous fat (Lee et al., 2005), and that fitness provides a strong protective effect against all-cause and cardiovascular mortality in men with MetS (Katzmarzyk et al., 2005; Katzmarzyk, Church, & Blair, 2004). Accordingly, these data strongly support the role of structured exercise, regular physical activity, or both, in interventions designed to prevent and treat MetS (Janiszewski, Saunders, & Ross, 2008).

PHYSIOLOGIC RESPONSES TO EXERCISE

Numerous studies have clearly demonstrated that the pathogenesis of MetS is largely attributable to a lack of fitness and physical activity (Roberts, Hevener, & Barnard, 2013). Further, MetS is associated with an impaired exercise tolerance, especially among individuals with overweight or obesity and those destined to develop T2DM (Alexander, 1964). Most studies have reported a decreased aerobic power (10 to 20% or more), expressed as milliliters of oxygen per kilogram of body weight per minute (mL O_2/kg/min) or as **metabolic equivalents (METs)** (1 MET = 3.5 mL/kg/min), among individuals with insulin resistance syndrome, as compared with age- and activity-matched controls (Shahid & Schneider, 2000). Moreover, there is an inverse graded relationship between BMI and cardiorespiratory fitness (Gallagher et al., 2005). Common characteristics of individuals with overweight or obesity that may contribute to their reduced functional capacity include heat intolerance; **hyperpnea/dyspnea;** movement restriction; orthopedic pain or discomfort; localized muscular weakness; agility problems; and anxiety about loss of balance during moderate-to-vigorous physical activity.

MetS may also serve as a respiratory stress, especially in individuals with concomitant abdominal obesity (deJong et al., 2008; Buskirk, 1971). As adiposity develops, breathing requires increased effort, owing to the expanded mass of the chest wall, elevation of the diaphragm, and compression by a protruding abdomen. Dyspnea on exertion may result because the depth of breathing (i.e., **tidal volume**) is compromised, and the only way increased ventilation can occur is by increasing the individual's breathing frequency. Varied indices of breathing economy may be adversely affected, such as the relationship between minute ventilation and oxygen uptake or the relationship between minute ventilation and carbon dioxide production (Gallagher et al., 2005). Conversely, related pulmonary abnormalities may exacerbate the obesity because the breathlessness on exertion stimulates the afflicted individuals to avoid moderate-to-vigorous physical activity (Buskirk, 1971).

Individuals with MetS may also be susceptible to altered cardiovascular, hemodynamic, and thermoregulatory responses to exercise. During a progressive treadmill walk, individuals with obesity demonstrate a higher heart rate and **systolic blood pressure (SBP)** at any given work rate as compared with their leaner counterparts (Alexander, 1964). Because subcutaneous fat provides thermal insulation against cold, performance of a given submaximal workload in the cold is accomplished by the person with obesity with a lower body surface temperature but a higher core temperature than a lean person. On the other hand, performance of a fixed work rate involving transport of body weight in a warm environment causes greater thermal strain on individuals with obesity (Buskirk, 1971). The added heat stress results in a higher heart rate and core temperature and a greater sweat rate than in the lean individual.

EXPAND YOUR KNOWLEDGE

NUTRITIONAL CONSIDERATIONS

Several dietary approaches have been advocated for cardiovascular risk reduction in individuals who have overweight or obesity. The Third Report of the National Cholesterol Education Program Adult Treatment Panel recommends a therapeutic lifestyle change (TLC) diet. Table 12-4 shows the overall composition of the TLC diet.

A modified Mediterranean-style diet, which has a similar **macronutrient** composition to the TLC diet, may have particular benefit for individuals with MetS. This diet is high in fruits, vegetables, nuts, whole grains, and olive oil. A two-year randomized, controlled trial of subjects with MetS found superior weight loss with a Mediterranean-style diet as compared to a control prudent diet; moreover, the Mediterranean-style diet group experienced a concomitant reduction in markers of vascular inflammation and insulin (Esposito et al., 2004). Additionally, endothelial function improved in those on the Mediterranean-style diet, but not in the controls.

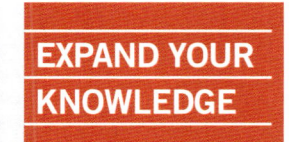

Table 12-4	
NUTRIENT COMPOSITION OF THE THERAPEUTIC LIFESTYLE CHANGES (TLC) DIET	
Nutrient	**Recommended Intake**
Saturated fat*	<7% of total calories
Polyunsaturated fat	Up to 10% of total calories
Monounsaturated fat	Up to 20% of total calories
Total fat	25–35% of total calories
Carbohydrate†	50–60% of total calories
Fiber	20–30 grams/day
Protein	Approximately 15% of total calories
Cholesterol	<200 mg/day
Total calories	Balance energy intake and expenditure to maintain a desirable body weight/prevent weight gain

*Trans fatty acids are another low-density lipoprotein–raising fat that should be severely restricted.

†Carbohydrates should be derived predominantly from foods rich in complex carbohydrates, including grains, especially whole grains, fruits, and vegetables, with an avoidance of simple carbohydrates, which include sugar, and most baked goods and snack foods.

To achieve weight loss in individuals who have overweight or obesity, a reduction in daily calorie intake of 500 to 1,000 kcal is commonly recommended. This degree of caloric deficit should produce a weight loss of 1 pound (0.45 kg) or more per week. Comparisons of popular dietary approaches with unusually high restrictions of various macronutrients, such as very-low-carbohydrate diets, have generally failed to show significant differences in weight loss or cardiovascular risk reduction at one year (Dansinger et al., 2005). Additionally, diets advocating excessive restriction of certain macronutrients are likely to be associated with some nutritional inadequacies and typically are not adhered to over the long term. Therefore, such diet programs should not be recommended. Prevention of weight regain will ultimately depend on the maintenance of substantive lifestyle changes, including healthy dietary modifications and regular physical activity.

Because the nutrition recommendations for individuals with MetS are in alignment with overall recommendations to enhance cardiovascular health and improve the **lipid** profile, refer to the nutrition sections in Chapters 7 and 8 for further details and suggested recommendations to clients.

EXERCISE RECOMMENDATIONS

Because obesity is at the core of MetS, the exercise program should generally follow the guidelines published by ACSM for the treatment of clients who have overweight or obesity (BMI ≥25 kg/m^2 and ≥30 kg/m^2, respectively) (Jakicic et al., 2009), but other components of the cluster of risk factors associated with the condition (i.e., dyslipidemia, hypertension, and if applicable, diabetes) also should be considered. Overall, individuals with MetS have an increased risk of mortality and **morbidity** from CVD and developing diabetes as compared to their age- and gender-matched counterparts without this syndrome. Accordingly, a careful cardiovascular assessment including peak or symptom-limited exercise testing should be considered before beginning a vigorous (≥60% $\dot{V}O_2R$) exercise-training program.

$$\dot{V}O_2 \text{ reserve} = \text{Percent intensity} \times (\dot{V}O_2 \text{ peak} - \dot{V}O_2 \text{ rest}) + \dot{V}O_2 \text{ rest}$$

Both the American College of Cardiology/American Heart Association guidelines on exercise testing and the ACSM guidelines recommend medical clearance for clients with diabetes who are not currently participating in regular exercise, as well as for those who are already participating in regular moderate-intensity exercise and plan to engage in vigorous-intensity exercise or are currently experiencing signs or symptoms suggestive of a metabolic disease (ACSM, 2022; Thompson et al., 2007).

Type of Exercise

Aerobic (or endurance) exercise has been the most frequently studied mode of exercise, and has consistently resulted in improvements in the components of MetS (Shahid & Schneider, 2000). The most effective exercises for the endurance phase employ large muscle groups, are maintained continuously, and are rhythmic in nature, such as walking, jogging, elliptical training, stationary or outdoor cycling, swimming, rowing, stair climbing, and combined arm-leg ergometry. Clearly, it is difficult to achieve an adequate volume of exercising muscle (and caloric expenditure) if the lower extremities are excluded. Other exercise modalities commonly used in physical-conditioning programs for clients with MetS include calisthenics, particularly those involving sustained total-body movement; recreational games; and resistance training. The latter is a particularly important option, since traditional aerobic-conditioning regimens often fail to accommodate participants who have an interest in improving muscular strength and endurance. Moreover, studies have shown that muscular strength is inversely associated with all-cause mortality (FitzGerald et al., 2004) and the prevalence of MetS (Jurca et al., 2005), independent of cardiorespiratory fitness levels.

Walking has several advantages over other forms of exercise during the initial phase of a physical-conditioning program. Brisk walking programs can result in a substantial increase in aerobic power and a reduction in body weight and fat stores, particularly when the walking duration exceeds 30 minutes (Pollock et al., 1971). Walking offers an easily tolerable exercise intensity and causes fewer musculoskeletal and orthopedic problems of the legs, knees, and feet than jogging or running. Moreover, it is a "companionable" activity that requires no special equipment other than a pair of well-fitted athletic shoes. Walking in water, with a backpack, or with a weighted vest are additional options for those who seek to lose body weight and fatness and improve cardiorespiratory fitness.

THE ENERGY COST OF WALKING

APPLY WHAT YOU KNOW

Because most clients with overweight or obesity prefer to walk at moderate intensities, it is helpful to recognize that walking on level ground at 2 and 3 mph (3.2 and 4.8 km/h) approximates 2 and 3 METs, respectively. For clients who prefer the slower walking pace (2 mph; 3.2 km/h), each 3.5% increase in treadmill grade adds approximately 1 MET to the gross energy cost. For example, if a client desires to walk at a 2 mph (3.2 km/h) pace, but requires a 4-MET workload for training, they would be advised to add 7% grade to this speed. For clients who can negotiate the faster walking speed (3 mph; 4.8 km/h), each 2.5% increase in treadmill grade adds an additional MET to the gross energy expenditure. Accordingly, a workload of 3.0 mph (4.8 km/h) at a 5.0% grade would approximate an aerobic requirement of 5 METs. Using this practical rule can be helpful when advising clients regarding walking workloads for training.

Although resistance exercise has generally been considered to be less effective in treating individuals with MetS, some reviews suggest that high-volume resistance training has independent and additive effects to an aerobic exercise program for virtually the entire cluster of associated cardiovascular risk factors (Williams et al., 2007; Braith & Stewart, 2006). For example, numerous studies show that resistance training improves insulin action, significantly decreases **glycosylated hemoglobin (A1c)** and blood pressure in diabetic and hypertensive adults, respectively, and reduces total body-fat mass and visceral adipose tissue in both men and women. In addition, the maintained or enhanced muscle mass resulting from chronic resistance training is associated with a modest increase in **basal metabolic rate (BMR),** which, over time, may facilitate greater success at weight reduction than can be achieved with aerobic exercise alone. Weight training has been shown to attenuate the **rate-pressure product** (Heart rate x Systolic blood pressure) when any given load is lifted (McCartney et al., 1993), which may reduce cardiac demands during daily activities such as carrying packages or lifting moderate-to-heavy objects. There are also intriguing data to suggest that strength training can increase muscular endurance capacity without an accompanying increase in cardiorespiratory fitness (Hickson, Rosenkoetter, & Brown, 1980).

Despite the widely cited *Physical Activity Guidelines for Americans* encouraging people to be more physically active, nearly 80% of adults in the U.S. are not meeting key guidelines for both aerobic and muscle-strengthening activities (U.S. Department of Health & Human Services, 2018). The skyrocketing prevalence of MetS (approximately 34% of U.S. adults) suggests the need for "real world" interventions designed to circumvent and attenuate barriers to achieving an adequate daily energy expenditure (Ervin, 2009). Accordingly, the CMES should encourage clients to integrate multiple short bouts of physical activity into their daily lives.

Intensity and Duration

Structured exercise training sessions should include a preliminary aerobic warm-up (approximately 10 minutes), followed by stretching activities, a conditioning phase (30 minutes or more), a cool-down (five to 10 minutes), and ideally, an optional recreational game. The warm-up facilitates the transition from rest to the conditioning phase by stretching postural muscles and increasing blood flow. A walking cool-down enhances venous return during recovery, reducing the possibility of post-exercise hypotension. In addition, it facilitates more rapid removal of **lactic acid** than stationary recovery and ameliorates the potential deleterious effects of the post-exercise rise in plasma catecholamines (Dimsdale et al., 1984).

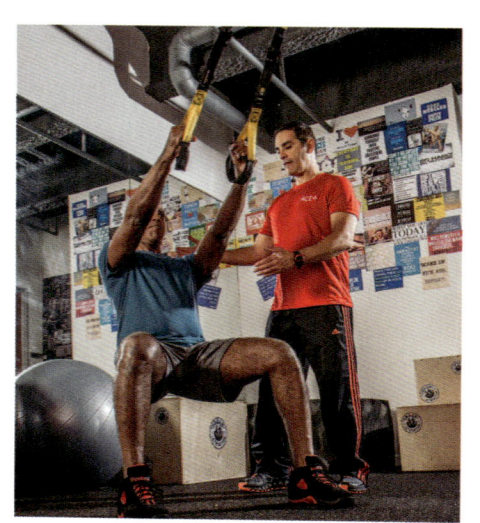

There is some controversy regarding the most appropriate exercise intensity and duration that are needed to optimally train individuals with MetS (Shahid & Schneider, 2000). Different risk factors associated with this condition may optimally respond to different exercise dosages. For example, a randomized, controlled trial of men and women who were sedentary and had overweight and mild-to-moderate dyslipidemia compared the effectiveness of three different exercise regimens versus controls: high-amount, high-intensity exercise; low-amount, high-intensity exercise; and low-amount, moderate-intensity exercise (Kraus et al., 2002). Although all exercise groups had better responses on a variety of lipid and **lipoprotein** variables than the control group, the most beneficial effect of exercise was seen most clearly with the high amount of high-intensity exercise. Because MetS has been associated with a sedentary lifestyle, low cardiorespiratory fitness, and CVD risk factors, the initial exercise program should be at an intensity of approximately 40 to 59% of the $\dot{V}O_2R$ or HRR for a minimum accumulated duration of 30 minutes. Over time, the exercise intensity should be increased to ≥60% $\dot{V}O_2R$ or HRR to provide the stimulus to improve cardiorespiratory fitness and facilitate a progressive overload (i.e., attainment of goal energy expenditure) (ACSM, 2022).

Frequency

The frequency of exercise is an important consideration when structured exercise and/or increased lifestyle activity are used to treat the abnormalities associated with MetS, especially insulin sensitivity and glucose utilization. Because much of the benefit of exercise is related to the cumulative effects of individual bouts of exercise, exercising five or more times a week is ultimately necessary to maximize benefits. In the available research, there are increased insulin sensitivity effects of a single bout of exercise, as well as accumulated bouts, for individuals with MetS, but they are difficult to separate. Nonetheless, it is likely that insulin sensitivity is increased for up to 48 hours after an exercise bout (Roberts, Hevener, & Barnard, 2013). Hence, exercising on most days of the week is appropriate for this population.

EXERCISE GUIDELINES SUMMARY FOR CLIENTS WITH METABOLIC SYNDROME

CARDIORESPIRATORY TRAINING	
Frequency	• At least 3–5 days per week
Intensity	• 40–59% HRR or $\dot{V}O_2R$
	• Below VT1 HR; can talk comfortably
	• RPE 12–13 (6–20 scale)
	• May progress to intensities 60–89% HRR
Time	• 30–60 minutes per day
	• However, 50–60 minutes per day is recommended for weight loss or weight-loss maintenance. Some individuals may need to progress to 60–90 minutes per day to promote or maintain weight loss.
	• 150–450 minutes of physical activity per week
	• Intermittent exercise can be accumulated throughout the day as an alternative to continuous exercise.
Type	• A variety of rhythmic large-muscle-group exercises
Progression	• Progress following the ACE Integrated Fitness Training® Model based on client goals and availability.

MUSCULAR TRAINING	
Frequency	• A minimum of 2 nonconsecutive days per week
Intensity	• 60–70% 1-RM for beginners
	• Experienced exercisers can use more specific repetitions and intensities based on muscular-fitness goals.
Time	• 1–3 sets of 8–10 repetitions (10–15 repetitions to start)
Type	• All major muscle groups
	• Multijoint exercises targeting more than one muscle group and agonist and antagonist muscles
	• Single-joint exercises may also be included after performing multijoint exercises.
	• A variety of equipment can be used, including resistance machines, free weights, and body weight.
Progression	• Progress following the ACE Integrated Fitness Training Model based on client goals and availability.

Note: $\dot{V}O_2R$ = Oxygen uptake reserve; HRR = Heart-rate reserve; RPE = Rating of perceived exertion; 1-RM = One-repetition maximum

CMES FOCUS

The prevalence of MetS is increasing and many individuals who are diagnosed with the condition also have overweight or obesity. It is important to guide clients with MetS toward healthy lifestyle practices that lead to reduced body weight and fat stores, increased physical activity, and a transition to an anti-atherogenic diet, as these therapeutic interventions are essential in reducing the risk for developing CVD and diabetes. Because individuals with MetS will likely present with multiple CVD and diabetes risk factors (e.g., dyslipidemia, hypertension, obesity, and hyperglycemia), the CMES should carefully consider the exercise recommendations based on the presence of these associated factors and the goals of the client and their healthcare provider.

Source: American College of Sports Medicine (2022). *ACSM's Guidelines for Exercise Testing and Prescription* (11th ed.). Philadelphia: Wolters Kluwer.

CHAPTER 12

CASE STUDY

Client Information

Juan, a 57-year-old male, is interested in starting a weight-reduction program, including exercise. His medical history reveals that he has obesity, prediabetes, hypertension, and hyperlipidemia, is currently sedentary, does not smoke cigarettes, and has a family history of premature atherosclerotic CVD (i.e., his father suffered his first acute MI at 53 years of age). Juan is currently taking Toprol XL (metoprolol SR) 50 mg once daily for hypertension, Lipitor (atorvastatin) 40 mg once daily for hyperlipidemia, Niaspan (niacin extended-release tablets) 500 mg twice daily for a reduced HDL level, and aspirin 162 mg once daily for prophylaxis of acute MI. Because he has three or more components of MetS, or takes medications to control them, he is considered to have MetS, even though he is currently asymptomatic.

At his most recent physical examination, his height and weight are 5'7" (1.7 m) and 255 pounds (115 kg), corresponding to a BMI of 40 kg/m^2. He has a waist circumference of 46 inches (117 cm); seated resting blood pressure of 146/94 mmHg; resting heart rate of 64 beats per minute (bpm); and a fasting plasma glucose of 122 mg/dL. With the exception of a low HDL (37 mg/dL), his serum lipids and lipoproteins are at the goal level. The remainder of the physical examination was unremarkable from an exercise programming perspective (e.g., no limiting orthopedic or musculoskeletal problems).

Juan performed a peak or symptom-limited exercise stress test to volitional fatigue using the conventional Bruce treadmill protocol. He intends to exercise at a health club after work and the exercise test was performed in the late afternoon. Juan typically takes his metoprolol SR after breakfast and was instructed to do so on the morning of the exercise test. Immediately prior to the exercise test, in the standing position, his heart rate was 76 bpm and blood pressure was 152/94 mmHg. During the exercise test, Juan demonstrated infrequent unifocal **premature ventricular contractions (PVCs)** and occasional **premature atrial contractions (PACs)** but did not develop chest discomfort, lightheadedness, or significant ST-segment depression. The test was terminated after five minutes because of volitional fatigue [**rating of perceived exertion (RPE)** of 18/20, signifying "very hard" work] and increasing dyspnea (3/4, corresponding to "moderately severe" shortness of breath), indicating an estimated functional capacity of 6.6 METs. He achieved a peak heart rate and blood pressure of 136 bpm (83% of his estimated maximal heart rate) and 186/92 mmHg, respectively. His blunted peak heart rate was most likely attributed, at least in part, to his beta-blocker therapy for hypertension.

ACE IFT® MODEL AT A GLANCE

Cardiorespiratory Training

This client is starting with Base Training, as he needs to develop an aerobic base before progressing. The exercise program includes progressions that should be able to safely allow this client to move to Fitness Training and increase exercise duration and frequency to improve fitness.

Muscular Training

The initial Muscular Training program for Juan is focused on Functional Training to improve posture and joint mobility. Movement Training is introduced after four to eight weeks, depending on his progress, with a focus on good form during the primary movements. From there, external loads can be added to advance the program to focus on muscular endurance and strength during Load/Speed Training.

CMES Approach

Based on Juan's medical history, physical examination, and graded exercise test results, the following exercise program was formulated.

Cardiorespiratory Training Program

- Type: Treadmill walking and combined arm-leg ergometry
- Frequency: Initially three days/week; increase gradually to five to seven days/week
- Duration: Initially 15 to 20 minutes/session, which may be accumulated in two 10-minute exercise bouts; to build up gradually to 45 to 60 or more minutes/session by adding approximately five minutes each week as tolerated
- Intensity: Target heart rate set at 40 to 59% heart-rate reserve = 100 to <120 bpm and target

RPE (6–20 scale) set at 12–13; target MET range initially set at 40 to 59% $\dot{V}O_2R =$ 3–5.9 METs). Estimated treadmill workloads at the lower end of this intensity range (approximately 3.2 METs) might be 2.0 mph, 3.5% grade or, for clients who prefer a faster walking pace, 3.0 mph, 0% grade.

Juan was informed that the time interval between his taking metoprolol SR and exercise training could modify his heart-rate response to exercise, since the effects of beta-blocker therapy are not necessarily uniform over time. Moreover, he was educated about the importance of warming up and cooling down, as well as the significance of warning signs and symptoms (e.g., heart rhythm irregularities, exertional chest pain or pressure, lightheadedness, and unusual shortness of breath) that require the cessation of exercise and immediate medical review.

Muscular Training Program

The CMES designs a Muscular Training program for Juan to complement his cardiorespiratory exercise. The program focuses first on Functional Training to increase strength and endurance of the postural muscles and establishing adequate joint mobility through primarily body-weight exercises performed two to three days/week. Once he can perform one to two sets of 10 to 15 repetitions of each exercise, after approximately four to eight weeks, exercises will be introduced to train the primary movement patterns (i.e., bend-and-lift, single-leg, pushing, pulling, and rotation) to focus on developing good movement patterns without compromising postural or joint stability. A total of eight to 10 exercises will be performed, with a focus on training all major movements of the body. He was advised regarding appropriate lifting and breathing techniques (e.g., avoid the **Valsalva maneuver**). Once Juan displays adequate primary movement patterns, external resistance can be introduced and progressed [approximately 2 to 5 pounds/week (0.9 to 2.25 kg/week) for arms and 5 to 10 pounds/week (2.25 to 4.5 kg/week) for legs] as tolerated.

Lifestyle Activity

Juan was also advised to integrate multiple short bouts of walking into his daily routine. To this end, he purchased a quality pedometer to enhance his awareness of daily physical activity by progressively increasing step totals. Baseline ambulatory studies conducted over one week revealed that he took approximately 3,000 steps/day on average. He was advised to add at least an additional 500 steps/day each week, to ultimately increase his daily step totals to 8,000 to 10,000 steps/day. Moreover, he was provided a "log" to document and track his progress in this regard.

SUMMARY

Obesity and insulin resistance largely account for the pathogenesis of MetS. Although overall body weight and relative adiposity (as reflected in the BMI) identify the greater than two-thirds of Western populations at risk for MetS, those with excessive intra-abdominal adiposity are particularly susceptible.

The cornerstone treatment of MetS is therapeutic lifestyle modification to reduce body weight and fat stores, increase physical activity, and transition to an anti-atherogenic diet. Although lifestyle intervention is often overlooked in clinical practice, this non-pharmacological approach has been shown to reduce cardiovascular risk and prevent or delay progression to diabetes. The CMES can play an important role in providing a safe and effective exercise program that corresponds with the lifestyle-intervention component of metabolic syndrome treatment. Because obesity is at the core of MetS, the CMES should generally follow the guidelines published by ACSM for the treatment of clients who have overweight or obesity when designing exercise programs for this population. Aerobic exercise, resistance training, and increased lifestyle activity are recommended for individuals with MetS.

REFERENCES

Alberti, K.G. et al. (2009). Harmonizing the metabolic syndrome: A joint interim statement of the International Diabetes Federation Task Force on Epidemiology and Prevention; National Heart, Lung, and Blood Institute; American Heart Association; World Heart Federation; International Atherosclerosis Society; and International Association for the Study of Obesity. *Circulation,* 120, 16, 1640–1645. DOI: 10.1161/CIRCULATIONAHA.109.192644

Alexander, J.K. (1964). Obesity and cardiac performance. *American Journal of Cardiology,* 14, 860.

American College of Sports Medicine (2022). *ACSM's Guidelines for Exercise Testing and Prescription* (11th ed.). Philadelphia: Wolters Kluwer.

Batsis, J.A., Nieto-Martinez, R.E., & Lopez-Jimenez, F. (2007). Metabolic syndrome: From global epidemiology to individualized medicine. *Clinical Pharmacology & Therapeutics,* 82, 5, 509.

Braith, R.W. & Stewart, K.J. (2006). Resistance exercise training: Its role in the prevention of cardiovascular disease. *Circulation,* 113, 22, 2642.

Buchwald, H. et al. (2004). Bariatric surgery: A systematic review and meta-analysis. *Journal of the American Medical Association,* 292, 14, 1724.

Buskirk, E.R. (1971). Obesity. In: Downey, J.A. & Darling, R.C. (Eds.) *Physiologic Basis of Rehabilitation Medicine.* Philadelphia: W.B. Saunders Co, pp. 229–242.

Caballero, A.E. (2005). Diabetes in the Hispanic or Latino population: Genes, environment, culture, and more. *Current Diabetes Reports,* 5, 3, 217.

Carroll, S., Cooke, C.B., & Butterly, R.J. (2000). Metabolic clustering, physical activity and fitness in nonsmoking, middle-aged men. *Medicine & Science in Sports & Exercise,* 32, 12, 2079.

Chakravarthy, M.V. & Booth, F.W. (2003). *Hot Topics: Exercise.* Philadelphia: Hanley and Belfus (Elsevier).

Cheriyath, P. et al. (2010). Obesity, physical activity and the development of metabolic syndrome: The Atherosclerosis Risk in Communities study. *European Journal of Cardiovascular Prevention and Rehabilitation,* 17, 3, 309–313. DOI: 10.1097/HJR.0b013e32833189b8

Dansinger, M.L. et al. (2005). Comparison of the Atkins, Ornish, Weight Watchers, and Zone diets for weight loss and heart disease risk reduction: A randomized trial. *Journal of the American Medical Association,* 293, 1, 43.

deJong, A.T. et al. (2008). Peak oxygen consumption and the minute ventilation/carbon dioxide production relation slope in morbidly obese men and women: Influence of subject effort and body mass index. *Preventive Cardiology,* 11, 2, 100.

Dimsdale, J.E. et al. (1984). Post exercise peril: Plasma catecholamines and exercise. *Journal of the American Medical Association,* 25, 5, 630.

Ervin, R.B. (2009). Prevalence of metabolic syndrome among adults 20 years of age and over, by sex, age, race and ethnicity, and body mass index: United States, 2003–2006. *National Health Statistics Report,* 5, 13, 1–7.

Esposito, K. et al. (2004). Effect of a Mediterranean-style diet on endothelial dysfunction and markers of vascular inflammation in the metabolic syndrome: A randomized trial. *Journal of the American Medical Association,* 292, 12, 1440.

Expert Panel on Detection, Evaluation, and Treatment of High Blood Cholesterol in Adults (2001). Executive summary of the Third Report of the National Cholesterol Education Program (NCEP) Expert Panel on the detection, evaluation, and treatment of high blood cholesterol in adults (Adult Treatment Panel III). *Journal of the American Medical Association,* 285, 19, 2486.

Farrell, S.W., Cheng, Y.J., & Blair, S.N. (2004). Prevalence of the metabolic syndrome across cardiorespiratory fitness levels in women. *Obesity Research,* 12, 5, 824.

FitzGerald, S.J. et al. (2004). Muscular fitness and all-cause mortality: Prospective observations. *Journal of Physical Activity & Health,* 1, 1, 7.

Ford, E.S., Giles, W.H., & Dietz, W.H. (2002). Prevalence of the metabolic syndrome among U.S. adults: Findings from the third National Health and Nutritional Examination Survey. *Journal of the American Medical Association,* 287, 3, 356.

Gallagher, M.J. et al. (2005). Comparative impact of morbid obesity vs. heart failure on cardiorespiratory fitness. *Chest,* 127, 6, 2197.

Gerstein, H.C. et al. of the DREAM (Diabetes Reduction Assessment with ramipril and rosiglitazone Medication) Trial Investigators (2006). Effect of rosiglitazone on the frequency of diabetes in patients with impaired glucose tolerance or impaired fasting glucose: A randomized controlled trial. *Lancet,* 368, 9541, 1096.

Grundy, S.M. (2007). Cardiovascular and metabolic risk factors: How can we improve outcomes in the high-risk patient? *The American Journal of Medicine*, 120, 9, Suppl. 1, S3.

Grundy, S.M. (2006). Metabolic syndrome: Connecting and reconciling cardiovascular and diabetes worlds. *Journal of the American College of Cardiology*, 47, 6, 1093.

Grundy, S.M. et al. (2005). Diagnosis and management of the metabolic syndrome: An American Heart Association/National Heart, Lung, and Blood Institute Scientific Statement: Executive summary. *Circulation*, 112, e285–e290.

Grundy, S.M. et al. (2004). Implications of recent clinical trials for the National Cholesterol Education Program Adult Treatment Panel III guidelines. *Circulation*, 110, 2, 227.

He, J. & Whelton, P.K. (1999). Elevated systolic blood pressure and risk of cardiovascular and renal disease: Overview of evidence from observational epidemiologic studies and randomized controlled trials. *American Heart Journal*, 138, 3 pt. 2, 211.

Hickson, R.C., Rosenkoetter, M.A., & Brown, M.M. (1980). Strength training effects on aerobic power and short-term endurance. *Medicine & Science in Sports & Exercise*, 12, 5, 336.

Hu, F.B. et al. (2002). Elevated risk of cardiovascular disease prior to clinical diagnosis of type 2 diabetes. *Diabetes Care*, 25, 7, 1129.

Huang, Y. & Liu, X. (2014). Leisure-time physical activity and the risk of metabolic syndrome: Meta-analysis. *European Journal of Medical Research*, 23, 19, 22. DOI: 10.1186/2047-783X-19-22

Hunt, K.J. et al. (2004). National Cholesterol Education Program versus World Health Organization metabolic syndrome in relation to all-cause and cardiovascular mortality in the San Antonio Heart Study. *Circulation*, 110, 10, 1251.

Isomaa, B. et al. (2001). Cardiovascular morbidity and mortality associated with the metabolic syndrome. *Diabetes Care*, 24, 4, 683.

Jakicic, J.M. et al. (2009). American College of Sports Medicine position stand: Appropriate intervention strategies for weight loss and prevention of weight regain for adults. *Medicine & Science in Sports & Exercise*, 33, 12, 2145.

Janiszewski, P.M., Saunders, T.J., & Ross, R. (2008). Lifestyle treatment of the metabolic syndrome. *American Journal of Lifestyle Medicine*, 2, 2, 99.

Jurca, R. et al. (2005). Association of muscular strength with incidence of metabolic syndrome in men. *Medicine & Science in Sports & Exercise*, 37, 11, 1849.

Katzmarzyk, P.T., Church, T.S., & Blair, S.N. (2004). Cardiorespiratory fitness attenuates the effects of the metabolic syndrome on all-cause and cardiovascular disease mortality in men. *Archives of Internal Medicine*, 164, 10, 1092.

Katzmarzyk, P.T. et al. (2005). Metabolic syndrome, obesity, and mortality. *Diabetes Care*, 28, 2, 391.

Kelley, D.E. & Goodpaster, B.H. (1999). Effects of physical activity on insulin action and glucose tolerance in obesity. *Medicine & Science in Sports & Exercise*, 31, Suppl. 6, S619.

Knowler, W.C. et al. for the Diabetes Prevention Program Research Group (2002). Reduction in the incidence of type 2 diabetes with lifestyle intervention or metformin. *New England Journal of Medicine*, 346, 6, 393.

Kraus, W.E. et al. (2002). Effects of the amount and intensity of exercise on plasma lipoproteins. *New England Journal of Medicine*, 347, 19, 1483.

Kullo, I.J., Hensrud, D.D., & Allison, T.G. (2002). Relation of low cardiorespiratory fitness to the metabolic syndrome in middle-aged men. *American Journal of Cardiology*, 90, 7, 795.

Laaksonen, D.E. et al. (2002). Low levels of leisure-time physical activity and cardiorespiratory fitness predict development of the metabolic syndrome. *Diabetes Care*, 25, 9, 1612.

LaMonte, M.J. et al. (2005). Cardiorespiratory fitness is inversely associated with the incidence of metabolic syndrome: A prospective study of men and women. *Circulation*, 112, 4, 505.

Lee, S. et al. (2005). Cardiorespiratory fitness attenuates metabolic risk independent of abdominal subcutaneous and visceral fat in men. *Diabetes Care*, 28, 4, 895.

Lloyd-Jones, D.M. et al. (2007). Consistently stable or decreased body mass index in young adulthood and longitudinal changes in metabolic syndrome components: The Coronary Artery Risk Development in Young Adults Study. *Circulation*, 115, 8, 1004.

Marchetti, P. et al. (2006). The pancreatic beta-cell in human type 2 diabetes. *Nutrition, Metabolism, and Cardiovascular Diseases*, 16, Suppl. 1, S3.

McCartney, N. et al. (1993). Weight-training-induced attenuation of the circulatory response of older males to weight lifting. *Journal of Applied Physiology,* 74, 3, 1056.

McFarlane, S.I., Banerji, M., & Sowers, J.R. (2001). Insulin resistance and cardiovascular disease. *Journal of Clinical Endocrinology and Metabolism,* 86, 2, 713.

Misra, A. & Vikram, N.K. (2004). Insulin resistance syndrome (metabolic syndrome) and obesity in Asian Indians: Evidence and implications. *Nutrition,* 20, 5, 482.

National Institutes of Health (1998). Clinical guidelines on the identification, evaluation, and treatment of overweight and obesity in adults: The Evidence Report. *Obesity Research,* 6, Suppl. 2, 51S.

Pearson, T.A. et al. (2003). Markers of inflammation and cardiovascular disease: A statement for healthcare professionals from the Centers for Disease Control and Prevention and the American Heart Association. *Circulation,* 107, 499–511.

Peppa, M., Uribarri, J., & Vlassara, H. (2003). Glucose, advanced glycation end products, and diabetes complications: What is new and what works. *Clinical Diabetes,* 21, 4, 186.

Pollock, M.L. et al. (1971). Effects of walking on body composition and cardiovascular function of middle-aged men. *Journal of Applied Physiology,* 30, 1, 126.

Rader, D.J. (2007). Effect of insulin resistance, dyslipidemia, and intra-abdominal adiposity on the development of cardiovascular disease and diabetes mellitus. *American Journal of Medicine,* 120, 3, Suppl. 1, S12.

Rennie, K.L. et al. (2003). Association of the metabolic syndrome with both vigorous and moderate physical activity. *International Journal of Epidemiology,* 32, 4, 600.

Roberts, C.K., Hevener, A.L., & Barnard, R.J. (2013). Metabolic syndrome and insulin resistance: Underlying causes and modification by exercise training. *Comprehensive Physiology,* 3, 1, 1–58. DOI: 10.1002/cphy.c110062

Rosito, G.A. et al. (2004). Association between obesity and a prothrombotic state: The Framingham Offspring Study. *Thrombosis and Haemostasis,* 91, 4, 683.

Ruilope, L.M., Redón, J., & Schmieder, R. (2007). Cardiovascular risk reduction by reversing endothelial dysfunction: ARBs, ACE inhibitors, or both? Expectations from the ONTARGET Trial Programme. *Vascular Health Risk Management,* 3, 1, 1.

Shah, M., Simha, V., & Garg, A. (2006). Review: Long-term impact of bariatric surgery on body weight, comorbidities, and nutritional status. *Journal of Clinical Endocrinology and Metabolism,* 91, 11, 4223.

Shahid, S.K. & Schneider, S.H. (2000). Effects of exercise on insulin resistance syndrome. *Coronary Artery Disease,* 11, 2, 103.

Thompson, P.D. et al. (2007). AHA Scientific Statement: Exercise and acute cardiovascular events. Placing the risks into perspective. *Circulation,* 115, 17, 2358.

U.S. Department of Health & Human Services (2018). *Physical Activity Guidelines for Americans* (2nd ed.). www.health.gov/paguidelines/

Whaley, M.H. et al. (1999). Physical fitness and clustering of risk factors associated with the metabolic syndrome. *Medicine & Science in Sports & Exercise,* 31, 2, 287.

Williams, MA. et al. (2007). AHA Scientific Statement: Resistance exercise in individuals with and without cardiovascular disease: 2007 update. *Circulation,* 116, 5, 572.

SUGGESTED READING

Franklin, B. & Sweetgall, R. (2013). *One Heart, Two Feet.* Clayton, Mo.: Creative Walking.

Grundy, S.M. et al. (2005). Diagnosis and management of the metabolic syndrome: An American Heart Association/National Heart, Lung, and Blood Institute Scientific Statement. *Circulation,* 112, 17, 2735.

Huang, Y. & Liu, X. (2014). Leisure-time physical activity and the risk of metabolic syndrome: Meta-analysis. *European Journal of Medical Research,* 23, 19, 22. DOI: 10.1186/2047-783X-19-22

Piscatella, J.C. & Franklin, B.A. (2011). *Prevent, Halt, and Reverse Heart Disease.* New York: Workman Publishing.

Roberts, C.K., Hevener, A.L., & Barnard, R.J. (2013). Metabolic syndrome and insulin resistance: Underlying causes and modification by exercise training. *Comprehensive Physiology,* 3, 1, 1–58. DOI: 10.1002/cphy.c110062

13 DIABETES MELLITUS

IN THIS CHAPTER

EPIDEMIOLOGY

OVERVIEW
TYPE 1 DIABETES MELLITUS
TYPE 2 DIABETES MELLITUS
GESTATIONAL DIABETES MELLITUS

DIAGNOSTIC CRITERIA
THE METABOLIC SYNDROME

PATHOLOGICAL CONSEQUENCES OF DIABETES MELLITUS
MACROVASCULAR DISEASE
MICROVASCULAR AND NEURAL COMPLICATIONS

TREATMENT OPTIONS
NON-PHARMACOLOGICAL TREATMENT
PHARMACOLOGICAL TREATMENT
SURGICAL TREATMENT
EXERCISE TREATMENT

NUTRITIONAL CONSIDERATIONS
NUTRITIONAL CONSIDERATIONS FOR PREDIABETES
NUTRITIONAL CONSIDERATIONS FOR T1DM AND T2DM
NUTRITIONAL CONSIDERATIONS FOR GESTATIONAL DIABETES MELLITUS

EXERCISE RECOMMENDATIONS
EXERCISE PROGRAMMING IN T1DM
EXERCISE PROGRAMMING IN T2DM
MANAGEMENT OF EXERCISE RISKS IN CLIENTS WITH DIABETES
PROGRESSION OF THE PROGRAM

EXERCISE GUIDELINES SUMMARY FOR CLIENTS WITH DIABETES

CASE STUDIES

SUMMARY

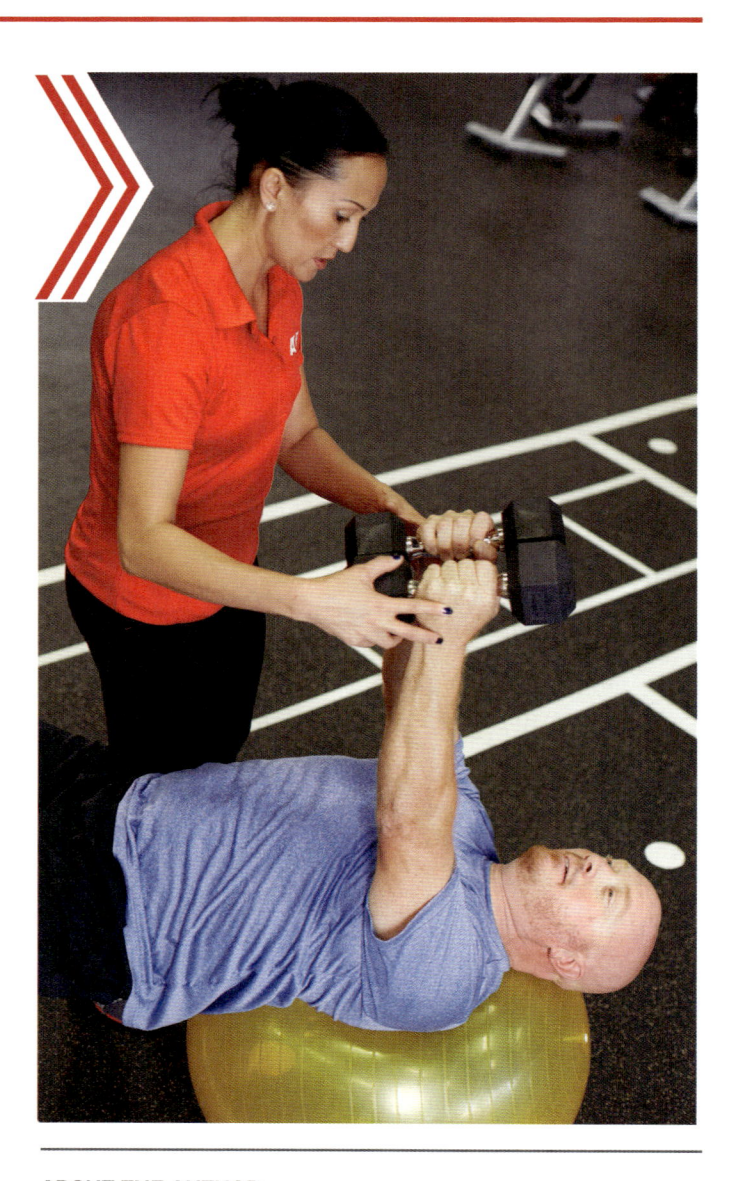

ABOUT THE AUTHOR

Larry S. Verity, Ph.D., FACSM, is Associate Dean of Academic Affairs in the College of Health and Human Services, and is a professor of exercise physiology in the School of Exercise and Nutritional Sciences at San Diego State University. He is a fellow of the American College of Sports Medicine (ACSM) and is certified as an Exercise Specialist. Dr. Verity served on ACSM's CCRB Publications Subcommittee, was co-editor of ACSM's *Certified News*, has written manual chapters for the American Council on Exercise, and has published reviews and original manuscripts on diabetes and exercise in many refereed publications. He has managed type 1 diabetes mellitus for more than 38 years and is without complications.

By Larry S. Verity

ONLY THREE DECADES AGO, PHYSICAL EXERCISE for persons with **diabetes**—also called **diabetes mellitus**—was frowned upon. In fact, diabetes was seen as an excuse to avoid exercise. Questions continue to be asked regarding whether a person with diabetes can safely participate in exercise or physical activity.

Questions that an ACE® Certified Medical Exercise Specialist (CMES) may be asked include the following:
- Does exercise actually help a person with diabetes or does it hamper their condition?
- Can exercise actually control diabetes?
- Is it safe for persons with diabetes to exercise at any time?
- Do diabetes complications affect the ability to regularly and safely participate in exercise?

To answer these questions, the CMES must have a solid understanding of the different types of diabetes to recommended exercise interventions for individuals with this disease, identify practical aspects of physical activity for diabetics, and design and modify exercise programs to improve disease management and health outcomes. This chapter provides a thorough overview of the different types of diabetes, the benefits and risks of exercise for this disease, and assessments that may be performed by the CMES that could aid in the design of a safe and effective exercise program.

EPIDEMIOLOGY

According to the Centers for Disease Control and Prevention (CDC, 2014), an estimated 29 million people in the United States have diabetes, with more than 8 million undiagnosed cases, while prevalence is approximately 9.3% of the population. **Type 2 diabetes mellitus (T2DM)** accounts for 90 to 95% of all cases of diabetes mellitus, and there is a slightly greater prevalence in men (13.6%) versus women (11.2%) (CDC, 2014). The burden of diabetes disproportionately affects minorities. The prevalence rates are about twofold greater in Hispanic Americans, African Americans, Native Americans, Asians, and Pacific Islanders when compared with non-Hispanic whites. **Type 1 diabetes mellitus (T1DM)** accounts for 5 to 10% of all cases of diabetes [American College of Sports Medicine (ACSM), 2022; ACSM, 2014]. Although T1DM is one of the most commonly diagnosed chronic diseases in children, diagnosis of T2DM in youth has risen dramatically over the past two decades. While **obesity** in children and adolescents is not increasing any more in the United States and some countries in Europe, the prevalence of T2DM has increased threefold since the mid-1990s. This has been attributed to the fact that the prevalence of obesity is not increasing, but rather the degree of obesity in affected children and adolescents (Reinehr, 2013).

The CMES should realize that diabetes mellitus is a heterogeneous disease composed of three primary categories: T1DM, T2DM, and **gestational diabetes mellitus (GDM)**. Diagnostic and classification criteria of diabetes focus on cause and pathogenesis. The two major etiopathogenetic categories of diabetes are T1DM and T2DM, each of which has distinguishing characteristics (Table 13-1). All persons with diabetes have elevated blood **glucose** levels, or **hyperglycemia**, caused by either an absolute or relative lack of **insulin,** along with abnormal **protein** and **fat** metabolism. Low blood glucose, or **hypoglycemia**, occurs most often in T1DM, but persons with T2DM and GDM can also experience episodes, although these are infrequent [American Diabetes Association (ADA), 2014]. Acute complications can occur when hypoglycemia or hyperglycemia are present for relatively short periods of time.

LEARNING OBJECTIVES:

» Describe the differences between the major forms of diabetes mellitus (i.e., type 1, type 2, and gestational).

» Identify the diagnostic criteria for the major types of diabetes mellitus.

» Describe how daily nutritional intake and physical activity influence a diabetic's strategies for controlling blood glucose.

» Identify treatment strategies for diabetes, including common medications for glycemic control.

» Explain how each major type of diabetes affects a client's ability to perform physical activity and exercise.

» Design and implement an appropriate exercise program for the major types of diabetes mellitus, taking into account the myriad diabetes-related complications that may occur in clients with this condition.

TABLE 13-1

DISTINGUISHING CHARACTERISTICS OF TYPE 1 (T1DM) AND TYPE 2 DIABETES MELLITUS (T2DM)

	T1DM	T2DM
Synonyms	Insulin requiring (formerly: juvenile onset)	Non–insulin requiring (formerly: adult onset)
Former Abbreviation	IDDM	NIDDM
Age of Onset	Often <30 years, but can occur at any age	Usually >30 years, but can occur at any age
Cases of Diabetes in U.S.	5–10%	90–95%
Pathological Factor	Auto-immune deficiency	Family history and lifestyle factors
Insulin Use	100%	~40%
Body Weight History	Recent weight loss	Weight gain
Obese at Diagnosis	Uncommon	Common (~80% obese)
Insulin Production	None	Deficient
Ketoacidotic Episodes	Common	Uncommon
Response to Diet Alone	Absent	In some mild forms
Insulin Resistance	Uncommon; may be present	Common

Source: American College Sports Medicine (2014). *ACSM's Resource Manual for Guidelines for Exercise Testing and Prescription* (7th ed.). Philadelphia: Wolters Kluwer/Lippincott Williams & Wilkins.

Diabetes mellitus increases the risk for **cardiovascular disease (CVD),** along with other complications. Most notably, macrovascular, microvascular, and nerve disease complications are commonly linked to hyperglycemia and diabetes. A CMES should know whether a client has complications, which reflect the severity and duration of the disease and may contribute to accelerated **morbidity** and excessive **mortality.**

Diabetes mellitus afflicts 26.9 million Americans of all ages, or 8.2% of the population. Overall, diabetes contributes to more than 270,000 deaths in the U.S. each year, making diabetes the seventh leading cause of death in the United States (CDC, 2020a). The presence of diabetes-related complications (DRCs) exacerbates morbidity and increases the likelihood of physical limitation or disability (ADA, 2014). Hyperglycemia for extended periods is linked with chronic abnormalities that worsen macrovascular, microvascular, and neural disease processes. As shown in Table 13-2, DRCs can be quite serious. Because of the daily fluctuations in blood glucose that occur in diabetes, therapeutic interventions are focused on the effective management and control of blood glucose and heart disease risk factors, along with prevention of DRCs to improve health and longevity.

OVERVIEW

Type 1 Diabetes Mellitus

T1DM is the most common form of diabetes in childhood and adolescence, but can occur at any age, even in the elderly (ADA, 2020). It is an immune-mediated disease that selectively destroys the pancreatic **beta cells,** leading to a "central defect" in insulin release upon

TABLE 13-2
DIABETES-RELATED COMPLICATIONS
• Individuals with diabetes are twice as likely to have heart disease or a stroke.
• Hypertension is present in approximately 80% of adults with diabetes.
• Diabetes is the leading cause of blindness among adults 18 to 64 years old.
• 37% of U.S. adults aged 18 and older have chronic kidney disease.
• Half of all people with diabetes have nerve damage.
• in 2016, 130,000 patients with diabetes were discharged from the hospital with a lower-extremity amputation (5.6 per 1,000 adults with diabetes).

Sources: American Diabetes Association (2020). Classification and diagnosis of diabetes: Standards of medical care in diabetes—2020. *Diabetes Care,* 43 (Suppl. 1), S14–S32; Centers for Disease Control and Prevention (2020a) *2020 National Diabetes Statistics Report: Estimated of Diabetes and Its Burden in the United States.* www.cdc.gov/diabetes. pdfs/data/statistics/national-diabetes-statistics-report.pdf; Centers for Disease Control and Prevention (2020b). *Diabetes and Nerve Damage.* www.cdc.gov/diabetes/library/features/diabetes-nerve-damage.html; Whelton, P.K. et al. (2017). 2017 ACC/AHA/AAPA/ABC/ACPM/AGS/APhA/ASH/ASPC/NMA/PCNA guideline for the prevention, detection, evaluation, and management of high blood pressure in adults: A report of the American College of Cardiology/American Heart Association Task Force on Clinical Practice Guidelines. *Journal of the American College of Cardiology,* Nov 7. pii: S0735-1097 (17) 41519-1.

stimulation, or **hypoinsulinemia** (waning of the insulin dose), and resultant hyperglycemia (ADA, 2014). Serologic markers of pancreatic beta-cell destruction (e.g., islet cell autoantibodies, insulin autoantibodies, glutamic acid decarboxylase, and human leukocyte antigens) are common at diagnosis and provide evidence for its autoimmune nature (ADA, 2014).

Onset of T1DM is usually abrupt and accompanied by "classic" signs of diabetes, including frequent urination **(polyuria),** constant hunger **(polyphagia),** excessive thirst **(polydipsia),** and unexplained weight loss (ADA, 2020). An absolute lack of insulin production in T1DM requires exogenous insulin administration (e.g., injections, pump, or inhalation) to maintain normal glucose levels, minimize complications, and prevent excessive use of **fatty acids** for energy, resulting in **ketoacidosis.**

Ketoacidosis occurs when a high level of **ketones** (beta hydroxybutyrate, acetoacetate) are produced as a by-product of fatty-acid metabolism. In T1DM, the combination of deficient insulin and increased counter-regulatory hormones (e.g., **catecholamines, cortisol,** and **glucagon**) results in excessive ketone production and metabolic acidosis. **Diabetic ketoacidosis (DKA)** can result from an infection, acute medical illness, such as heart attack and stroke, diseases of the endocrine axis (acromegaly, Cushing's syndrome), and stress of recent surgical procedures, but is more commonly linked to a lack of insulin, dehydration, and failure to manage glucose levels. Signs and symptoms of DKA include confusion, gastrointestinal (GI) upset, extreme thirst, lethargy, and a fruity breath odor (Gosmanov, Gosmanova, & Dillard-Cannon, 2014). DKA is a serious health issue for individuals with T1DM and, if left untreated, can result in coma or death.

Type 2 Diabetes Mellitus

T2DM usually afflicts persons older than 30 years of age—but it can affect children and adolescents—and is directly related to **insulin resistance.** For those with T2DM, insulin resistance creates a health burden that worsens the ability to manage blood glucose, and significantly increases morbidity and mortality associated with vascular complications of diabetes (ADA, 2014). The pathology and natural history of T2DM onset is illustrated in Figure 13-1. Interestingly, onset of T2DM may actually be present approximately 10 years prior to diagnosis.

Figure 13-1
Pathology and history of onset of T2DM

Reprinted with permission from Peters, A. (2000). The clinical implications of insulin resistance. *American Journal of Managed Care*, 6, 13 Suppl., S668–S674.

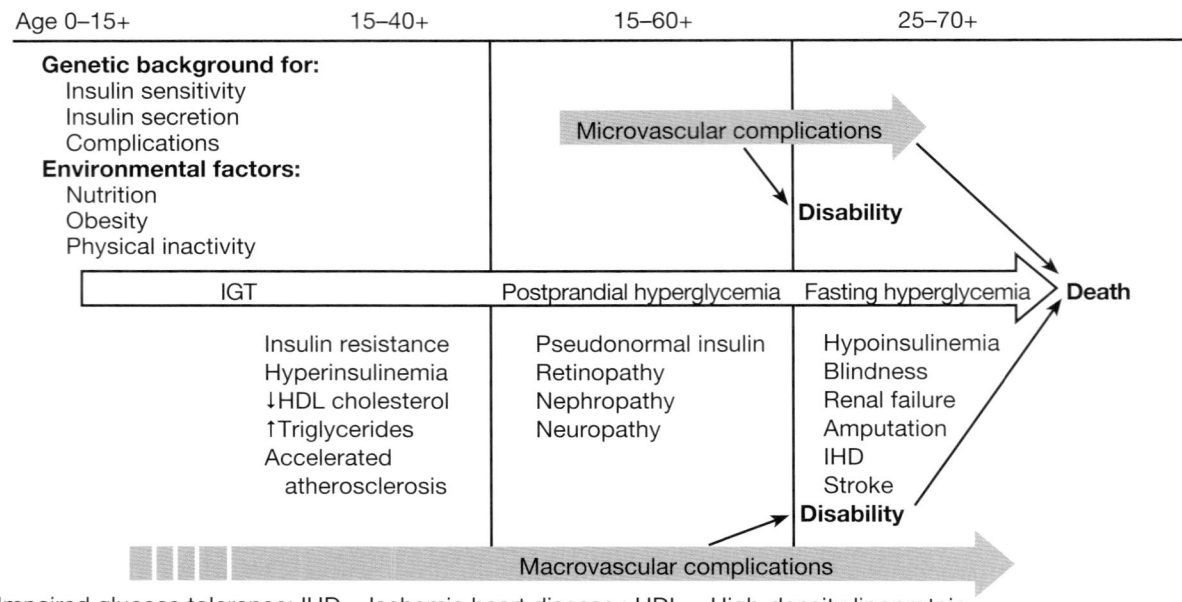

Age 0–15+	15–40+	15–60+	25–70+
Genetic background for: Insulin sensitivity, Insulin secretion, Complications **Environmental factors:** Nutrition, Obesity, Physical inactivity		Microvascular complications → Disability	
IGT	Postprandial hyperglycemia	Fasting hyperglycemia	Death
	Insulin resistance, Hyperinsulinemia, ↓HDL cholesterol, ↑Triglycerides, Accelerated atherosclerosis	Pseudonormal insulin, Retinopathy, Nephropathy, Neuropathy	Hypoinsulinemia, Blindness, Renal failure, Amputation, IHD, Stroke, Disability
Macrovascular complications →			

Note: IGT = Impaired glucose tolerance; IHD = Ischemic heart disease ; HDL = High-density lipoprotein

The role of diabetes and insulin resistance in advancing heart disease and DRCs, or disorders of the eyes, kidneys, heart, blood vessels, and nerves, is well established. T2DM is highly linked with typical CVD risk factors, such as obesity, **hypertension,** and **dyslipidemia** (ADA, 2020). Alarmingly, the incidence of T2DM in children and adolescents has increased in recent years, to the point where approximately 80% of children diagnosed with T2DM in the U.S. have obesity at diagnosis, presumably related to increased levels of obesity secondary to excess caloric intake and too little caloric expenditure (Liu et al., 2010). To this end, the CMES must have a solid understanding of T2DM onset to develop an effective exercise program that can aid in managing T2DM and countering the common coexisting conditions of this disease.

Varying degrees of endogenous insulin production (e.g., normal or elevated) are present in T2DM, which is characterized by insulin resistance or a relative lack of activity in insulin-sensitive tissues to maintain **normoglycemia** (i.e., normal glucose levels) (ADA, 2014). Insulin resistance is considered a "peripheral defect" because of a decrease in insulin-mediated uptake and storage of glucose in the liver and skeletal muscle. Reduced insulin receptor binding at target tissues and impaired postreceptor activities related to insulin function manifest as insulin resistance. Central to postreceptor deficiencies are abnormal translocation of muscle glucose transporters (GLUT-4) and insulin receptor substrates that perform important intermediary phosphorylation processes (ACSM, 2014). Interestingly, these abnormalities may be reversible through weight loss, proper diet, and physical activity. In the prospective Nurses' Health Study II, risk of subsequent diabetes after a history of GDM was significantly lower in women who followed healthy eating patterns. Adjusting for **body mass index (BMI)** moderately, but not completely, attenuated this association (Tobias et al., 2012).

The hyperglycemia present in T2DM suggests that insulin release is inadequate to compensate for the insulin resistance. Over time, the pancreas loses its ability to produce insulin, and the need for exogenous insulin to control blood glucose increases (ADA, 2014).

Control of glucose levels in T2DM is essential to prevent **hyperosmolar hyperglycemic nonketotic syndrome (HHNS),** an emergency condition in which elevated glucose levels are accompanied by dehydration without ketones in the blood or urine (ADA, 2014). Usually, HHNS affects individuals with T2DM and, if not treated over several days to weeks, can lead to coma or death.

Onset of T2DM is associated with insulin secretory defects related to metabolic stress and inflammation and other contributing factors such as genetics (ADA, 2020). The risk of T2DM rises with family history, age, obesity, and inactivity. About 89% of adults with T2DM have overweight or obesity and 38% are physically inactive (participating less than 10 minutes of moderate or vigorous physical activity per week), both of which are related to increased insulin resistance (CDC, 2020a). Lifestyle interventions focusing on weight loss and physical activity are essential strategies to manage diabetes, lessen the onset of DRCs, prevent the onset of T2DM, and prevent the onset of CVD (ADA, 2020).

Gestational Diabetes Mellitus

The CMES should have a sound understanding of all types of diabetes, including the type that occurs during pregnancy. In essence, GDM is an inability to maintain normal glucose or any degree of glucose intolerance during pregnancy, despite being treated with either diet (**class A1GDM**) or medication (**class A2GDM**). According to the American College of Obstetricians (ACOG, 2017), 6 to 9% of pregnancies are complicated by diabetes and approximately 90% of these cases are the result of GDM. High-risk factors for developing GDM include obesity, personal or family history of GDM, and **glycosuria** (an excretion of glucose in the urine). The prevalence of this condition is increasing as obesity and older age at pregnancy become more common. Other risk factors include having a family history of T2DM or belonging to an ethnic group at increased risk for the condition (such as Hispanic, Native American, South or East Asian, African American, or Pacific Islands descent). Women with GDM are at higher risk for **preeclampsia** (9.8 to 18%), and Cesarean delivery (17 to 25%), and have a greater risk of developing diabetes later in life, with 70% of women with GDM developing diabetes within 22 to 28 years after pregnancy (ACOG, 2017).

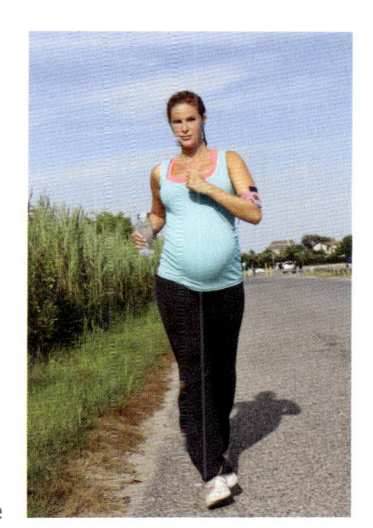

GDM is usually diagnosed by an oral glucose tolerance test between 24 and 28 weeks of gestation. If GDM is diagnosed, therapeutic strategies are used to monitor and manage maternal blood glucose to prevent fetal **macrosomia** (i.e., abnormally high birth weight) and maternal complications (ADA, 2014). GDM resolves postpartum, yet, as noted above, many women who experience GDM eventually develop T2DM. Although not identical in pathophysiology, GDM resembles etiologic features of T2DM, including obesity, insulin resistance, family history, and physical inactivity. As in T2DM, GDM onset is related to genetic predisposition, insulin resistance, and subsequent deficient insulin release (ACSM, 2014). Management of GDM focuses on interventions similar to those that are commonly recommended in T2DM. However, insulin therapy, not oral agent therapy, is usually initiated when glucose control is not achieved (ADA, 2020). Referring women with GDM to an exercise setting that can provide heart-rate monitoring of both mother and fetus is the most appropriate action for the CMES, as women with GDM typically require close medical supervision during exercise.

DIAGNOSTIC CRITERIA

The diagnosis of diabetes mellitus is based on established criteria (Table 13-3). After diagnosis, clinical emphasis is placed on frequent blood glucose monitoring (i.e., three to six glucose checks per day) in conjunction with diet and physical activity to control glucose levels and reduce the risk of complications (ADA, 2020). Glycemic control is assessed using **glycosylated hemoglobin (A1c)**, which reflects a time-averaged blood glucose concentration over the previous two to three months. The recommended A1c goal is set at less than 7.0%, which is approximately 1% above the nor-diabetic range (A1c <6.0%), and it is recommended that it be assessed approximately every three months. Some individuals with stable glycemia may do well with testing only twice per year, while unstable or highly intensively managed patients (e.g., pregnant women with T1DM) may be tested more frequently than every three months (ADA, 2020).

TABLE 13-3
CRITERIA FOR THE DIAGNOSIS OF DIABETES

FPG ≥126 mg/dL (7.0 mmol/L). Fasting is defined as no caloric intake for at least 8 hours.*
OR
2-hour PG ≥200 mg/dL (11.1 mmol/L) during OGTT. The test should be performed as described by the WHO, using a glucose load containing the equivalent of 75 g anhydrous glucose dissolved in water.*
OR
A1C ≥6.5% (48 mmol/mol). The test should be performed in a laboratory using a method that is NGSP certified and standardized to the DCCT assay.*
OR
In a patient with classic symptoms of hyperglycemia or hyperglycemic crisis, a random plasma glucose ≥200 mg/dL (11.1 mmol/L).

Note: DCCT = Diabetes Control and Complications Trial; FPG = Fasting blood glucose; OGTT = Oral glucose tolerance test; WHO = World Health Organization; 2-h PG = 2-hour plasma glucose

*In the absence of unequivocal hyperglycemia, diagnosis requires two abnormal test results from the same sample or in two separate test samples.

Reprinted with permission from American Diabetes Association (2020). Classification and diagnosis of diabetes: Standards of medical care in diabetes—2020. *Diabetes Care,* 43 (Suppl. 1), S14–S32.

Assessment of overall health, especially identification of coexisting CVD risk factors and DRCs, is an essential component of effective diabetes care. A relatively new term has been used to address the complex relationship between diabetes and cardiac risk—**cardiometabolic risk.** The existence of multiple risk factors for CVD, along with metabolic- and diabetes-specific factors, creates an unusually increased likelihood for those with diabetes to develop CVD (Figure 13-2). Recommendations focus on aggressive management of CVD risk factors (ADA, 2020; Buse et al., 2007). Glucose-lowering agents are the primary medications used in diabetes management, supplemented by drugs to prevent CVD, such as antihypertensive drugs, lipid-lowering agents, and antiplatelet medications (ADA, 2020; CDC, 2014).

Figure 13-2
Factors contributing to cardiometabolic risk

Reprinted with permission from Brunzell, J.D. et al. (2008). Lipoprotein management in patients with cardiometabolic risk. *Journal of the American College of Cardiology,* 51, 15, 1512–1524.

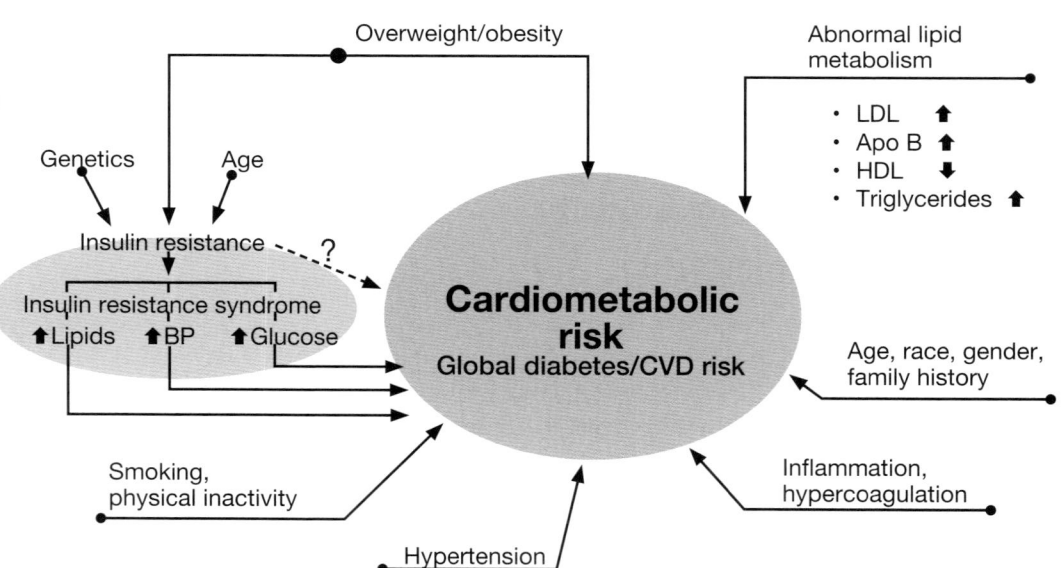

Note: BP = Blood pressure; LDL = Low-density lipoprotein; Apo B = Apolipoprotein B; HDL = High-density lipoprotein; CVD = Cardiovascular disease

Diabetes Mellitus
CHAPTER 13

Whereas body weight is usually normal in T1DM, obesity prevails in T2DM and GDM. BMI often exceeds 30 kg/m^2 and abdominal girth is often large [men ≥40 inches (102 cm); women ≥35 inches (88 cm)] in those with T2DM, placing many patients at high risk for CVD and cancer. Therefore, weight loss is a primary treatment goal to improve insulin action in persons with T2DM (ADA, 2014).

The Metabolic Syndrome

The **metabolic syndrome (MetS)** is commonly seen in T2DM and is linked to physical inactivity, diet, and genetic factors (Alberti et al., 2009) (see Chapter 12). Compared to individuals without the MetS, those with the diagnostic criteria have about a fivefold increased risk of developing T2DM and a one-and-a-half- to threefold relative risk of developing CVD (Alberti et al., 2009; Grundy, 2007). The MetS is characterized by a constellation of disorders, including insulin resistance, obesity, central adiposity, glucose intolerance, dyslipidemia, and hypertension:
- Abdominal obesity indicated by a waist circumference ≥40 inches (102 cm) in men and ≥35 inches (88 cm) in women
- Levels of **triglycerides** ≥150 mg/dL (1.7 mmol/L) or on drug treatment
- **High-density lipoprotein (HDL)** levels <40 and <50 mg/dL (1.0 and 1.3 mmol/L) in men and women, respectively or on drug treatment
- **Blood pressure (BP)** levels ≥130/85 mmHg or on drug treatment
- Fasting glucose levels ≥100 mg/dL (5.6 mmol/L) or on drug treatment

PATHOLOGICAL CONSEQUENCES OF DIABETES MELLITUS

Diabetes leads to a variety of metabolic, physiologic, vascular, and neural problems. The pathology of this disease results in DRCs that primarily affect the macrovascular (e.g., CVD, peripheral vasculature, and cerebral vasculature), microvascular (e.g. small vessels of the retina and kidney), and neural (e.g., peripheral motor and sensory nerves, and autonomic nerves) systems. It is important to note that these DRCs are not always present in clients with diabetes. Diabetes self-management principles suggest maintaining near-normal glucose levels and managing CVD risk factors to reduce the risk for complications. In essence, good metabolic control is associated with a significant reduction in vascular and neural diabetes complications.

Macrovascular, microvascular, and nerve disease complications are commonly linked to hyperglycemia and diabetes [ADA, 2020; American Heart Association (AHA), 2007; Buse et al., 2007]. DRCs reflect the severity and duration of the disease and contribute to accelerated morbidity and excessive mortality in diabetics. Diabetes increases mortality risk from CVD. Thus, the CMES must know the health profile of any client with diabetes to ensure safe and effective exercise participation, while also minimizing risks for untoward outcomes.

Macrovascular Disease

Large-vessel disease, or **macrovascular disease**, is common in persons with diabetes. One type of macrovascular disease, **coronary heart disease (CHD)**, is accelerated in people with diabetes and leads to premature morbidity and mortality. Additionally, diabetes contributes to an accelerated **atherogenic** process in other large vessels, including those in the lower extremities (peripheral vasculature) and in the brain (cerebral vasculature). Lower-extremity complications usually limit the weight-bearing tolerance of afflicted individuals and contribute to a greater risk of non-traumatic amputations. **Cerebral vascular disease** is another serious complication worsened by high BP that increases the risk of stroke in people with diabetes. Consequently, knowing whether a client with diabetes has macrovascular disease is a crucial part of the pre-activity screening process. If macrovascular disease is present, obtaining physician approval of exercise and modifying the assessment, programming, and leadership accordingly is prudent.

Multiple, coexisting risk factors for macrovascular disease are commonly present in T1DM and T2DM, as indicated by the cardiometabolic risk profile (ADA, 2020). As in non-diabetic populations, modification of CVD risk factors (e.g., smoking, elevated lipid levels, high BP, and physical inactivity) aid in minimizing the risk of macrovascular disease. Additionally, T2DM is the most common form of diabetes among individuals of older age or with obesity, visceral fat, insulin resistance, hypertension, dyslipidemia, and inactivity, which commonly coexist, and thus, increase the risk for macrovascular disease (ADA, 2020; AHA, 2007).

Physiological and metabolic abnormalities of diabetes that are believed to exacerbate the macrovascular atherogenic process are glucose intolerance, hyperglycemia, and insulin resistance (Garcia-Touza & Sowers, 2012). Though there may be different mechanisms responsible for the pathogenesis of atherosclerosis in T1DM and T2DM, modification of CVD risk factors and improvement of glucose control and insulin sensitivity are keys to lessening the risk of atherosclerotic vascular disease (ADA, 2020).

Microvascular and Neural Complications

Small-vessel diseases, or microvascular complications, and nerve diseases are common outcomes of long-standing diabetes. Usually, the onset of **microvascular disease** progressively contributes to failure of the target tissue involved. The three different types of microvascular and neural complications are **retinopathy** (eye disease), **nephropathy** (kidney disease), and **neuropathy** (nerve disease) (see page 393). These complications of diabetes are the leading causes of new blindness, end-stage renal disease and kidney failure in adults, and nervous system damage leading to numerous amputations, respectively (see Table 13-2). Moreover, these complications affect work performance and tolerance, as well as the mode and intensity of work performed. The CMES must know whether microvascular complications exist to safely and effectively devise an exercise program for a client with diabetes.

Compelling data link diabetes complications with poor blood glucose control, and provide diabetes healthcare professionals with persuasive evidence about the importance of vigilant management of metabolic factors through **self–blood glucose monitoring [SBGM]** to prevent or delay the progression of complications (ADA, 2020). Thus, a CMES can help in diabetes management by encouraging clients to maximize glucose control and regulation, while lessening the progression of small-vessel complications in these clients.

TREATMENT OPTIONS

The cornerstones of therapy for self-management of diabetes include insulin (or oral drugs), diet, and exercise, as well as a focus on blood glucose regulation. The primary goal is not only to normalize glucose metabolism, but also to delay or prevent disease complications common to diabetes. Therapeutic strategies for treatment encompass various allied health professionals in conjunction with the physician to enhance self-care management of the disease (Figure 13-3). The CMES is part of the management team and can help in motivating clients to safely and regularly participate in physical activity. Also, proactive communication with other members of the treatment team (e.g., personal physician and nurse educator) to ensure the safety and effectiveness of a physical-activity program is an essential responsibility of the CMES.

Precise hormonal and metabolic events that normally regulate glucose **homeostasis** are disrupted in diabetes because of defects in insulin release, action, or both, and result in an excess release of counter-regulatory hormones. Glucose control requires near-normal balance between hepatic glucose production and peripheral glucose uptake, combined with effective insulin responses. An inability to precisely match glucose production with glucose use results in daily glucose excursions that require regular glucose monitoring and adjustments in the dosage of exogenous insulin or oral agent, combined with adjustments in dietary intake, particularly when anticipating exercise or physical activity.

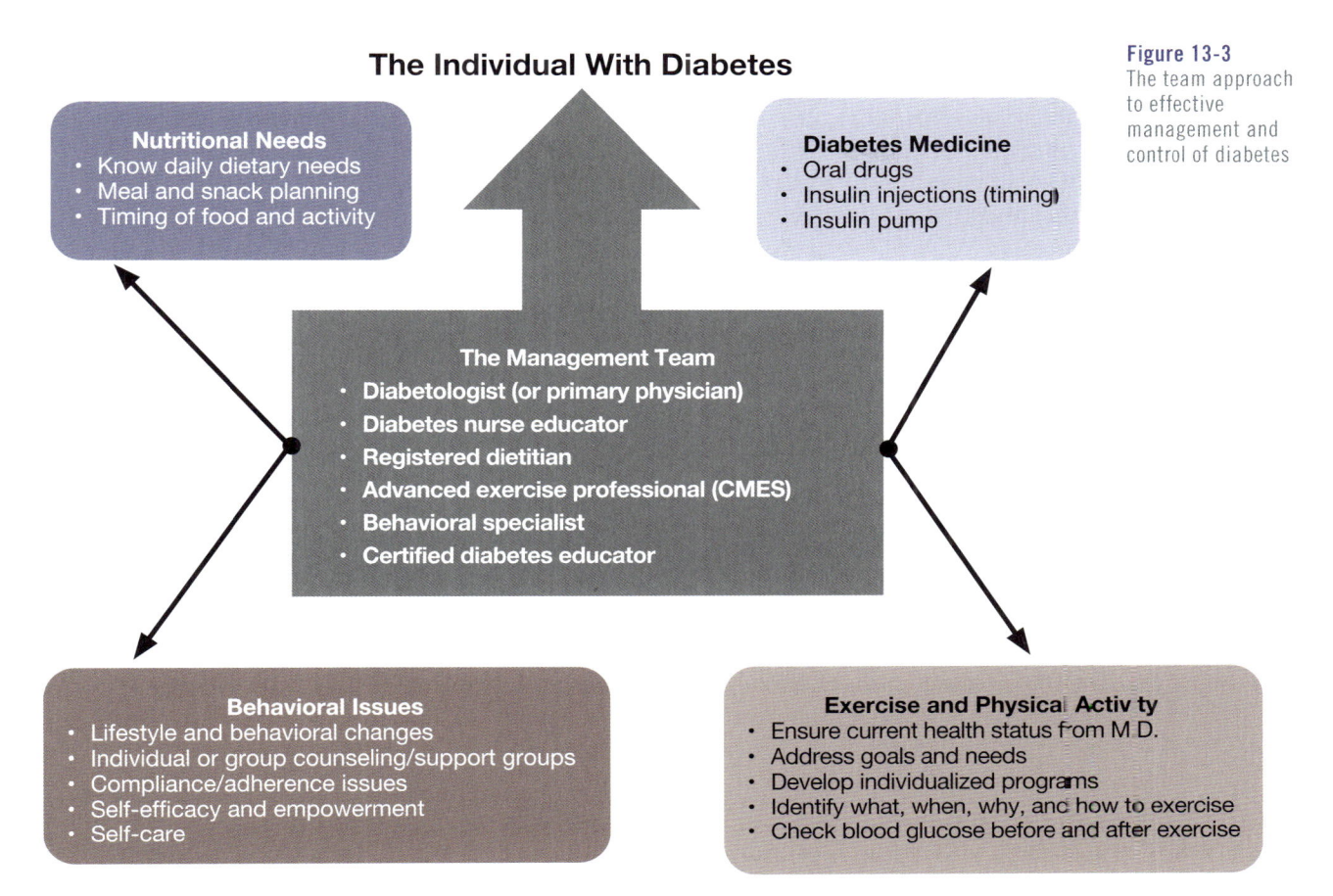

Diabetes Mellitus   CHAPTER 13

The Individual With Diabetes

Nutritional Needs
- Know daily dietary needs
- Meal and snack planning
- Timing of food and activity

Diabetes Medicine
- Oral drugs
- Insulin injections (timing)
- Insulin pump

The Management Team
- Diabetologist (or primary physician)
- Diabetes nurse educator
- Registered dietitian
- Advanced exercise professional (CMES)
- Behavioral specialist
- Certified diabetes educator

Behavioral Issues
- Lifestyle and behavioral changes
- Individual or group counseling/support groups
- Compliance/adherence issues
- Self-efficacy and empowerment
- Self-care

Exercise and Physical Activity
- Ensure current health status from M.D.
- Address goals and needs
- Develop individualized programs
- Identify what, when, why, and how to exercise
- Check blood glucose before and after exercise

Figure 13-3
The team approach to effective management and control of diabetes

Non-pharmacological Treatment

Therapeutic intervention involves a multidisciplinary team of specialists that includes the diabetes physician, diabetes nurse educator, **registered dietitian (RD),** and exercise specialist to facilitate patient education and necessary lifestyle changes to manage this disease (ADA, 2020). Intensive SBGM, combined with balancing diet, oral drugs or exogenous insulin (or both), and exercise are the established cornerstones of therapy to facilitate near-normal to normal metabolic function (ADA, 2020). In general, management of blood glucose level involves a planned regimen of insulin or oral medication (or both), frequent SBGM, an individualized **medical nutrition therapy (MNT)** plan, and participation in a regular physical-activity program. Self-management skills are essential to the successful management of diabetes. The use of diabetes self-management education (DSME) is also an important tool to improve control (ADA, 2020). The use of a continuous glucose monitoring system has been shown to improve the management of diabetes, but remains a limited therapeutic intervention due to third-party reimbursement issues.

The primary goal of therapy for all diabetics focuses on SBGM to achieve acceptable blood glucose control (A1c <7.0%), thereby limiting the development and progression of DRCs (ADA, 2020). Both T1DM and T2DM show reduced risk for retinopathy, nephropathy, and neuropathy with intensive therapy and the potential for a reduction of CVD with improved glycemic control (ADA, 2020). Glycemic control is best achieved through SBGM combined with nutrition, adjustment of medications, and physical activity.

The CMES should address the ABCs of diabetes with respect to clients' health (NIH, 2013):
- A1c% (glycosylated hemoglobin): <7%; checked at least twice a year
- Blood pressure: Work with your doctor to set a goal that is right for you
- Cholesterol: **Low-density lipoprotein (LDL)** <100 mg/dL; checked at least once a year

Managing the ABCs of diabetes aids in reducing cardiometabolic risk and managing risk for CVD onset. Cardiovascular risk factors, along with symptomatic and asymptomatic CVD, are common in diabetes (ADA, 2014; Buse et al., 2007). Identification of macrovascular disease and comorbidities and aggressive intervention are crucial in minimizing their progression, particularly factors linked with the MetS (ADA, 2014; Buse et al., 2007). CVD morbidity and mortality in diabetes can be favorably affected through lifestyle interventions. Prudent lifestyle interventions focus on minimizing progression of CVD through the management of CVD risk factors. Lifestyle strategies lower CVD risk factors by favorably modifying BP, blood lipids, glucose tolerance, and body weight. Lifestyle strategies for managing CVD risk include the following (ADA, 2020):

- Dietary intervention where calories and fat intake are restricted
- Weight management and/or weight loss
- Regular physical activity
- Smoking cessation
- DSME

The coexistence of multiple CVD risk factors and hyperglycemia requires a vigilant lifestyle intervention to lessen risk and prevent CVD (ADA, 2020; Buse et al., 2007).

Pharmacological Treatment

The CMES should have a general understanding of common medications that are prescribed, their action(s), and the impact of exercise with respect to the medication. Classically, there are different medications that aid in controlling blood glucose. The CMES should recognize that medication is taken by injection/infusion or orally.

Insulin Injections or Continuous Subcutaneous Insulin Infusion

Individuals with T1DM require multiple daily insulin injections or must use an insulin pump—also called continuous subcutaneous insulin infusion (CSII)—to facilitate glucose uptake and control glucose levels (ADA, 2020). An insulin pump can be used by some individuals to manage T2DM and GDM. Insulin administered by syringe is injected into subcutaneous tissue using a rotation of sites, including the abdomen (fastest absorption rate), upper arms, lateral thigh, and buttocks (Berger, 2002). CSII is subcutaneously delivered only in the abdominal area.

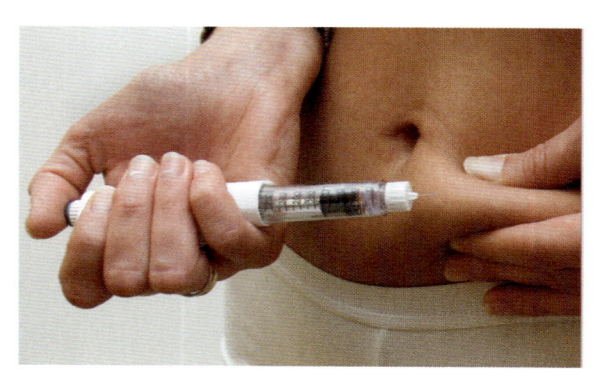

Insulin administered by syringe can be rapid-acting (peak action: 30 minutes to one hour) (Humalog), short-acting (peak action: two to three hours) (Regular), intermediate-acting (peak action: four to 10 hours) (Humulin L or N), or long-acting (peak action: sustained for 20 to 24 hours) (Humulin U). A mixed dose of different types of insulin produces a more normal glucose response and is used most commonly in T1DM. Usually, rapid-acting insulin is used with CSII. Exercise can accelerate the mobilization of insulin if the injection site is in the exercising muscle. Therefore, it is essential that the CMES understands the importance of avoiding injection of insulin into working muscle. Also, insulin dosage (pump or injection) can be reduced prior to exercise to avoid hypoglycemia. Frequent adjustments in insulin administration are generally needed to effectively manage diabetes. These insulin adjustments involve a trial-and-error process that requires an understanding of insulin action and the impact of exercise, food intake, and medication on glucose excursions, combined with frequent routine SBGM (Toni et al., 2006; Berger, 2002).

There are also two injectable medications that aid in glucose management. Byetta (exenatide or extendin-4) is used for T2DM and Symlin (pramlintide), a synthetic form of amylin, which is a hormone co-released from pancreatic beta cells with insulin, is used for T1DM (Joy, Rodgers, & Scates, 2005; Ryan, Jobe, & Martin, 2005). For the CMES, the main exercise-related concern with these medications is that they both delay the emptying of food from the gut after a meal and could slow the release of ingested **carbohydrates** taken to prevent or treat low blood glucose levels during a bout of exercise. Consequently, to err on the side of safety, neither Byetta nor Symlin should be injected within two hours prior to scheduled physical activity.

Oral Hypoglycemic Agents

Oral agents are widely prescribed for individuals with T2DM when onset is recent and little or no insulin is taken (e.g., <20 units) (ACSM, 2014). As with insulin injections, oral agents are prescribed individually or in combination to optimize glucose control in T2DM. Four major groups of oral agents are used to control glucose: beta-cell stimulants for insulin release, drugs to improve insulin sensitivity, drugs to abate intestinal absorption of carbohydrates and drugs to extend the action of insulin. Their mechanisms of action and effects on exercise are discussed in the following sections.

Beta-cell Stimulants for Insulin Release

Sulfonylurea and meglitinide drugs are taken at mealtime to stimulate insulin release and manage **postprandial glycemia.** Because of insulin stimulation, these oral agents can lead to hypoglycemia with or without exercise. The prolonged length of action in these oral agents increases the risk for low blood glucose and requires more frequent monitoring during exercise (ACSM, 2014). Sulfonylureas include the following:
- Chlorpropamide (Diabinese)
- Glipizide (Glucotrol and Glucotrol XL)
- Glyburide (Micronase, Glynase, and Diabeta)
- Glimepiride (Amaryl)

The CMES should recognize that individuals taking these types of longer-lasting oral hypoglycemic medications will need to check their blood glucose levels more often when exercising (and afterward). When exercise becomes a habit, it is a good idea to encourage these clients to check with their healthcare providers about lowering their medication doses, particularly if they are experiencing more frequent low glucose readings with exercise.

Drugs to Improve Insulin Sensitivity

The thiazolidinediones [rosiglitazone (Avandia) and pioglitazone (Actos)] improve insulin sensitivity at muscle and adipose tissue, and the biguanides [e.g., metformin (Glucophage and Glucophage XR)] promote muscle glucose uptake and inhibit hepatic glucose output overnight. Consequently, these types of medications have little effect on exercise responses. Insulin sensitizers mainly improve the action of insulin at rest, not during exercise, so the risk of them causing exercise-associated hypoglycemia is very low (ACSM, 2014).

Drugs to Abate Intestinal Absorption of Carbohydrates

Alpha-glucosidase inhibitors [acarbose (Precose) and miglitol (Glyset)] decrease the carbohydrate absorption rate and slow the increase in postprandial (i.e., after-meal) blood glucose level. These medications do not directly affect exercise, but can delay effective treatment of hypoglycemia during activities by slowing the absorption of carbohydrates ingested to treat this condition (ACSM, 2014).

Drugs to Extend the Action of Insulin

Dipeptidyl peptidase-4 inhibitors (DDP-4 inhibitors) are the newest class of oral diabetic drugs. The primary action of these drugs is to extend the action of insulin, but they may not increase the risk of exercise-induced hypoglycemia in individuals with T2DM who are already being treated with metformin (Charbonnel et al., 2006).

THINK IT THROUGH

If you work with clients who have diabetes, you should be prepared to handle situations wherein a client's blood sugar drops excessively. In fact, low blood sugar events most commonly happen in the beginning of the program or after about four weeks, as a new participant is able to increase exercise intensity, has been able to increase muscle strength, and has increased blood sugar uptake. Spend some time thinking about how you will handle this situation with clients, should it occur. What will you say to reassure the client if they appear anxious? Will you have a high-carbohydrate snack on hand, or will you ask that the client always carry a snack to the exercise sessions? Being prepared for hypoglycemic occurrences will help you handle them with confidence and professionalism.

Surgical Treatment

Although lifestyle modifications and medical therapy are the mainstays of management for T2DM, adequate glycemic control remains a challenge for most individuals with obesity and T2DM. Only 52% of diabetics in the U.S. are achieving the ADA's recommended glycosylated hemoglobin (A1c) goal of 7.0%. Furthermore, many patients with obesity and T2DM also have hypertension and dyslipidemia (specifically, high LDL) and only 18.2% of patients in the U.S. are currently achieving the targeted goals of therapy for all three conditions (Stark et al., 2013). Hence, there has been an increased interest in strategies to better these clinical results. As such, an emergence of evidence supporting surgical treatment of diabetes has led the International Diabetes Federation (Dixon et al., 2011) and ADA (ADA, 2020) to recognize bariatric surgery as an effective treatment option for patients with obesity and T2DM. In their study on the long-term metabolic effects of bariatric surgery in patients with obesity and T2DM, Brethauer and colleagues (2013) found that bariatric surgery can induce a significant and sustainable remission and improvement of T2DM and other metabolic risk factors in patients with severe obesity. Further, the researchers found that surgical intervention within five years of diagnosis was met with a high rate of long-term remission (Brethauer et al., 2013).

In cases where diabetes is poorly controlled, surgery may have to be performed on the lower extremity to remove necrotic tissue. To avoid surgery, one of the most valuable strategies is to prevent the development of foot complications, since neuropathic foot ulceration can often lead to loss of a limb due to a major amputation (Nather & Wong, 2013). Thus, patients diagnosed with diabetes must be subjected to early annual foot screening programs. A CMES can help in this regard by regularly asking diabetic clients about their routine foot care (e.g., taking time at the beginning/end of each exercise session to check the feet). Once a diabetic foot complication has developed, the next best strategy is to treat this complication early in a hospital setting by a multidisciplinary diabetic foot team in hopes of salvaging the foot in order to avoid the loss of a limb from a major amputation (Nather et al., 2010).

Exercise Treatment

Regular physical activity and exercise offer multiple well-known health benefits for both T1DM and T2DM (Table 13-4). Mild-to-moderate intensity exercise may assist with daily glucose regulation on a short-term basis for both T1DM and T2DM, which may explain the role of regular exercise to favorably alter metabolic functions related to glucose metabolism. Regular exercise helps lessen CVD and cardiometabolic risk factors, such as mild to moderate hypertension, insulin action and resistance, glucose metabolism, vascular inflammation and altered vascular reactivity, impaired **fibrinolysis,** and abnormal lipid profiles. Also, regular exercise favorably affects not only cardiovascular and metabolic health, but also the psychological and cognitive health of individuals with T1DM and T2DM. Clearly, the CMES should understand the benefits of chronic exercise and its adaptations in clients with diabetes.

Long-term Benefits of Exercise in T1DM

Current knowledge about the long-term benefits of regular exercise on various health aspects offers a persuasive rationale for persons with T1DM to participate in physical activities. While effective exercise programming is based upon an understanding of short-term benefits, it is the benefits of chronic exercise that help to maximize health and manage risks for CVD and DRCs.

A single session of exercise acutely lowers blood glucose in individuals with T1DM for a variable amount of time, as long as the pre-exercise blood glucose level is approximately 250 mg/dL or less. The synergistic effect of exercise and insulin on lowering blood glucose is well established, and is the typical focus regarding the role of exercise as part of diabetes management. As the pre-exercise blood glucose increases beyond 250 to 300 mg/dL (with or without ketones), exercise causes skeletal muscle to increase blood glucose utilization; however, the relative amount of glucose use is countered with an excessive amount of glucose production from the liver. Thus, the CMES should understand that the pre-exercise blood glucose has an effect on the exercise-related blood glucose response. Requiring blood glucose checks for all individuals with T1DM before and after exercise is a safe and effective strategy to minimize untoward outcomes of exercise.

Evidence suggests that physical-activity levels are suboptimal in people with T1DM because of a fear of hypoglycemia or due to low levels of cardiorespiratory fitness (Valletta et al., 2014). Additionally, people with T1DM may struggle with how best to ensure good glucose control in the presence of varying levels of food intake and insulin doses throughout the day. Nonetheless, physical training through aerobic workouts and/or resistance training is commonly recommended for individuals with T1DM who are without complications. Such individuals tend to exhibit chronic exercise benefits similar to those observed in non-diabetics (ADA, 2020). However, regular exercise is not effective for improving blood glucose control of T1DM and should not be the sole means of doing so (ACSM, 2014; Verity, 2010). Adjusting therapeutic medication and nutritional regimens is an important management strategy for individuals with T1DM, along with SBGM (ADA, 2020). Although regular exercise improves metabolism in individuals with T1DM, it does not facilitate the desired level of metabolic control. The CMES should help educate clients on daily use of SBGM, insulin adjustment, and nutritional needs combined with regular exercise to facilitate the management of glucose.

The CMES should recommend regular physical exercise for cardiovascular conditioning and modification of cardiovascular risk factors in individuals with T1DM, rather than only as a means for better glucose control. Research suggests that cardiovascular training in T1DM favorably alters common CVD risk factors, including blood lipids, BP, insulin resistance, and glucose control (ADA, 2020; Valletta et al., 2014). Therefore, improving aerobic fitness and muscular fitness in individuals with T1DM is central to improving cardiovascular health and lessening CVD risk.

The CMES must understand that physical training (e.g., cardiorespiratory or resistance exercise) enhances the sensitivity of peripheral tissue to insulin action in T1DM, as is commonly reflected by reduced daily insulin dosage (Giannini, Mohn, & Chiarelli, 2006; Riddell & Iscoe, 2006; Berger, 2002). While physical activity augments insulin-mediated glucose disposal into skeletal muscle and improves insulin action after a single exercise session, regular exercise (e.g., aerobic training for 12 weeks) dramatically improves glucose uptake through important glucose transport activities (e.g.,

TABLE 13-4
THE BENEFITS OF REGULAR EXERCISE IN T1DM AND T2DM

	Relative Change
Cardiovascular Aspects • Aerobic power, or fitness level • Resting heart rate • Blood pressure—chronic outcome	↑ ↓ ↓
Lipid/Lipoprotein Alterations • HDL • LDL • VLDL/triglycerides • Total cholesterol • Risk ratio (total cholesterol/HDL)	↑ ↔ ↓ ↓ ↔ ↓ ↓
Body Composition • Body fat, especially in obese • Fat-free mass • Visceral body fat	↓ ↑ ↓
Metabolic Aspects • Insulin sensitivity • Glucose metabolism • Intracellular insulin action—insulin signaling • Basal and postprandial insulin needs	↑ ↑ ↑ ↓
Psychological Aspects • Self-concept/self-esteem • Depression • Stressor response to psychologic stimuli	↑ ↓ ↓

Note: T1DM = Type 1 diabetes mellitus; T2DM = Type 2 diabetes mellitus; ↑ = increase; ↓ = decrease; ↔ = no change; HDL = High-density lipoprotein; LDL = Low-density lipoprotein; VLDL = Very-low-density lipoprotein

GLUT-4) (Stehno-Bittel, 2014). Physical activity has a transient, or short-term, effect on glucose transport because insulin sensitivity begins to decline within days after physical activity ceases. To minimize insulin needs and maximize insulin action, regular exercise participation is strongly recommended for individuals with T1DM. Further, consistency is a key factor in managing blood glucose. That is, keeping the same daily routine (e.g., exercising at noon and eating essentially the same types of foods at the same times), can help an individual better control the amount of insulin needed. For this reason, the CMES should stress consistency.

Beyond the physiological and metabolic benefits of chronic exercise, the psychological benefits of regular exercise for those with T1DM are beginning to receive attention. The rigors of diabetes management are emotionally stressful, particularly for young children and adolescents. **Depression** is common in people with T1DM and can adversely influence adherence to diabetes self-management regimens and result in poor glycemic control (Huang et al., 2013). Because of poor glycemic control, T1DM can also increase the risk for diabetes complications. Given that regular exercise may help lessen physiological reactivity to mental stressors, it may help reduce stress, thereby enhancing psychological well-being, lessening depressed feelings, and improving the quality of life for individuals with T1DM (ACSM, 2014). Chronic exercise is a powerful tool for those with T1DM to empower themselves to keep control of their lives. The CMES must continually promote the mind-body value of exercise for individuals with T1DM.

Long-term Benefits of Exercise in T2DM

Of the many coexisting conditions presented in T2DM, insulin resistance is central to muscle glucose metabolism and numerous health-related problems that only worsen the health profile. Consequently, the strategic focus of therapeutic interventions in waging war against these combined health risks is to manage glucose levels and reverse insulin resistance, or improve insulin sensitivity, which favorably affects glucose metabolism, glucose control, lipid metabolism, inflammatory reactions, and vascular wall functions—all while focusing on the reduction of cardiometabolic risk. Individuals with T2DM may also suffer from abnormal insulin secretion and hepatic and peripheral insulin resistance. Obesity, hyperglycemia, **hyperinsulinemia,** dyslipidemia, and physical inactivity also contribute to insulin resistance. Presently, diabetes management includes strategies to not only control blood glucose levels, but also to lessen morbidity and mortality in T2DM via aggressive lifestyle interventions.

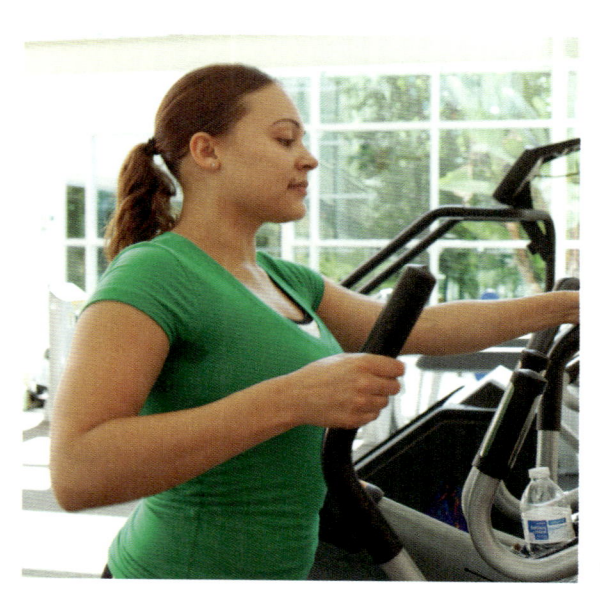

In addition to glucose control through self-management skills, T2DM interventions include nutritional changes, weight loss, CVD risk-factor management, and physical activity. These strategies are recommended based on results of the Diabetes Prevention Program Research Group (2005), where modest lifestyle changes—including dietary changes in line with current recommendations, weight loss between 5 and 7%, and increased physical activity—reduced the risk of T2DM onset by 58% in those with impaired glucose tolerance. Just as these lifestyle strategies are used to prevent the onset of T2DM, the same strategies can be implemented secondarily to lessen the progression of cardiometabolic risks associated with T2DM (Buse et al., 2007).

The favorable effects of regular exercise have been reported for insulin signaling, insulin resistance, and T2DM (Aguiar et al., 2014). It can be stated that the more that individuals with T2DM engage in physical activity throughout each week, the lower the insulin levels and the greater the insulin sensitivity or the lower the insulin resistance. To maximize health benefits, regular aerobic and resistance exercise, combined with individualized nutrition therapy, are the key weapons used to combat T2DM and insulin resistance (Aguiar et al., 2014; Buse et al., 2007).

Diabetes Mellitus

CHAPTER 13

The combined therapeutic interventions promote myriad beneficial health outcomes, including improved cardiovascular and metabolic functions, reduced risk of cardiac morbidity and mortality, and favorable changes in lipids and lipoproteins (increased HDL and decreased triglycerides and LDL), BP, body weight, fat-free mass (maintained or decreased), fat mass, body-fat distribution and morphology, insulin sensitivity and insulin concentrations, and glucose metabolism (ADA, 2020). Also, strength training has been shown to improve muscle function and quality, while increasing insulin sensitivity in individuals with T2DM (Aguiar et al., 2014). Most importantly, the glucose metabolic defects found in previously sedentary individuals with T2DM are reversed with exercise, while both insulin signaling and exercise signaling of glucose transport are markedly improved with moderate-intensity exercise performed consistently over time (Zierath, 2002). Consequently, regular exercise training improves glucose control (e.g., A1c) in T2DM, primarily through improved insulin signaling and insulin sensitivity. These combined physiological changes can actually lower daily medication dose (e.g., insulin and/or oral agent) for individuals with T2DM.

Interestingly, increased energy expenditure through aerobic exercise and/or strength training is independently linked with reducing insulin resistance, while improving insulin sensitivity. Both physical activity/aerobic exercise and muscle-strengthening activities have been shown to improve insulin-mediated glucose uptake, GLUT-4 transporters, insulin-signaling capabilities, and insulin sensitivity—all of which are essential in glucose metabolism and management. In general, exercise training appears to reverse inflammatory markers and postreceptor insulin-signaling defects, and encourage intramuscular and abdominal fat use, while simultaneously lowering the metabolic and atherosclerotic risks associated with T2DM (ACSM, 2014; ADA, 2020).

Additionally, regular exercise may favorably alter stress-related psychological factors and cognitive function in diabetes. Depression is common in people with diabetes (Huang et al., 2013; Renoir, Hasebe, & Gray, 2013). Unfortunately, depression can interfere with the management of diabetes and worsen glucose control in T2DM. Because glucose control plays a pivotal role in minimizing the risk for complications, individuals with T2DM are at increased risk for diabetes complications. Thus regular exercise may assist in countering depression and **anxiety,** while improving glucose control and lessening the risk for complications. Moreover, nontraditional exercise modalities in which mind-body interventions are the focus have become more popular and have been integrated into the overall programs of clients with diabetes (Alexander et al., 2008). For example, **tai chi, yoga,** and **Pilates** are becoming more common as alternative exercises for clients with T2DM. These types of exercise not only improve functional fitness and flexibility, but also aid in glucose management. Because the mind-body interventions aid in self-care and self-knowledge, there is a psychological outcome that has important outcomes for those with T2DM (Kinser, Goehler, & Taylor, 2012). Furthermore, regular exercise may enhance psychological well-being and quality of life for individuals with T2DM (Colberg et al., 2010). The CMES must recognize the value of traditional and nontraditional exercise to facilitate improved diabetes management and health outcomes in individuals with T2DM.

NUTRITIONAL CONSIDERATIONS

Nutrition plays an important role in the management of diabetes. The nutrition section of this chapter describes general nutrition recommendations for **prediabetes**—the precursor to T2DM—as well as T2DM, T1DM, and GDM. In general, the primary goal of nutrition therapy is to help improve overall health and quality of life for those with or at high risk of diabetes through three mechanisms (Evert et al., 2013):
- Optimize cardiometabolic risk profile through attainment of a hemoglobin A1c <7%, BP <130/80 mmHg, LDL cholesterol <100 mg/dL, triglycerides <150 mg/dL, and HDL cholesterol >40 mg/dL for men and >50 mg/dL for women.
- Achieve and maintain a healthy weight, or a 7% reduction in body weight for those who have overweight or obesity.
- Delay or prevent complications associated with diabetes.

Strategies to achieve these objectives while also preserving the pleasure of eating, enhancing **self-efficacy** to effectively manage the disease, and respecting cultural preferences and traditions are provided here. These suggestions are based on the best scientific evidence to date.

Nutritional Considerations for Prediabetes

Prediabetes is characterized by insulin resistance. Thus, the main objective of a nutritional plan for prediabetes is to reverse insulin resistance. A groundbreaking study published in 2002 in the New England Journal of Medicine found that certain lifestyle changes are highly effective in preventing the progression of prediabetes to T2DM and undoing insulin resistance (Knowler et al., 2002). This program, known as the Diabetes Prevention Program (DPP), serves as a useful model for providing nutrition and physical-activity recommendations for individuals with prediabetes. The study found that losing about 5 to 7% of body weight and maintaining that weight loss in combination with 150 minutes per week of physical activity decreases the risk of progression from prediabetes to T2DM by 58% (Knowler et al., 2002). Thus, the main nutritional objective for an individual with prediabetes is to decrease caloric consumption to facilitate weight loss. The DPP helps participants obtain this objective as well as increase physical activity through 16 weekly core sessions and up to 15 monthly post-core sessions. The downloadable DPP curriculum and further information is available at www.cdc.gov/diabetes.

Nutritional Considerations for T1DM and T2DM

In 2013, the ADA published a comprehensive position statement on nutrition recommendations for adults with T1DM and T2DM (Evert et al., 2013). Highlights of that report are included here, though readers are strongly encouraged to view the full report for further information. (The report is available free of charge at www.diabetes.org).

- Medical nutrition therapy: Individuals with diabetes should receive MNT provided by an RD with knowledge of diabetes management as well as diabetes self-management education (DSME) and diabetes self-management support (DSMS). ADA standards for DSME and DSMS are detailed in Haas et al., 2012.
- Energy balance: For those who have overweight, modest weight loss is best achieved through energy balance and maintenance of a healthy eating pattern. Evidence suggests the most effective strategies to do this include weekly self-weighing, eating breakfast, decreasing fast-food intake, increasing physical activity, reducing portion sizes, using meal replacements when appropriate, and eating healthful foods. Weight loss appears to provide most benefit early in the disease process. Evidence suggests a 5 to 7% weight loss combined with regular physical activity and frequent contact with an RD provides the most health benefit. Healthcare providers should focus coaching efforts on nutrition, physical activity, and behavior change.
- Eating patterns and macronutrient composition: There is no ideal "diabetes eating plan" or preferred percentage of calories from carbohydrates, fats, and proteins for individuals with diabetes. In fact, many eating patterns have shown benefit, including the **Healthy Mediterranean-Style Dietary Pattern,** the **Dietary Approaches to Stop Hypertension (DASH) eating plan,** and vegetarian, low-fat, and low-carbohydrate diets. Eating plans should be based on personal preferences and cardiometabolic goals, ideally in consultation with an RD. Older adults and those with lower literacy levels who have T2DM may benefit most from a simple meal planning approach like portion control or learning to make more healthful food choices.
- Carbohydrates: There is no established ideal carbohydrate intake for people with diabetes. Monitoring carbohydrate intake in relation to insulin availability is a key nutritional strategy and those with T1DM benefit from training in carbohydrate counting as well as consistent timing and amount of carbohydrate on a day-to-day basis if fixed insulin amounts are used. The best sources of carbohydrate include vegetables, fruits, whole grains, legumes, and dairy products.

Fiber intake recommendations mirror those for the general public (i.e., 25 grams per day for women and 38 grams per day for men).
- Glycemic load: Substituting low–**glycemic load** foods for high–glycemic load foods may improve blood sugar control, though the evidence is inconclusive.
- Sucrose (sugar) intake: While sugar intake has the same effect on blood glucose as other carbohydrates, sugar intake is best minimized so as not to replace nutrient-dense foods. Sugar-sweetened beverages are best avoided or limited due to risk of weight gain and disruption of cardiometabolic profile.
- Fructose: Free fructose (such as that found in fruit) is not more harmful than other sugars, as long as it does not comprise more than 12% of total calories.
- Sugar substitutes (non-nutritive sweeteners): Non-nutritive sweeteners may help decrease caloric intake from caloric sweeteners as long as individuals do not compensate by increased intake of other calorie-containing foods.
- Protein: Specific protein recommendations do not exist, so overall intake should be individualized. Protein does not need to be limited below usual intake in individuals with diabetes, even those with kidney disease. For individuals with T2DM, a high-protein carbohydrate snack should not be given when treating hypoglycemia, as ingested protein appears to increase insulin response with no effect on blood sugar.
- Fat: Fat quality is more important than fat quantity, as long as caloric balance is maintained. **Monounsaturated** and **polyunsaturated fats** provide health benefits. While **omega-3 fatty acid** supplementation probably does not decrease risk of cardiovascular events, consumption of fish at least two times per week does. Recommended intakes of **saturated fat,** cholesterol, and **trans fat** is the same as those for the general population.
- Plant stanols and sterols: Consumption of 1.6 to 3.0 grams/day of plant **stanols** or **sterols** can reduce total and LDL cholesterol.
- Micronutrients: Vitamin and mineral supplementation is not necessary. Supplementation with vitamins A, C, or E or carotene may be harmful. Despite purported benefits, chromium, magnesium, vitamin D, and cinnamon supplementation does not provide benefit beyond what is attained from a healthy, balanced eating plan.
- Alcohol: Alcohol should be consumed in moderation, if at all. Alcohol intake may cause delayed hypoglycemia, which is of particular concern for those with T1DM.
- Sodium: Sodium should be limited to 2,300 mg/day, in alignment with recommendations for the general population. Intake should be lower for those with hypertension.

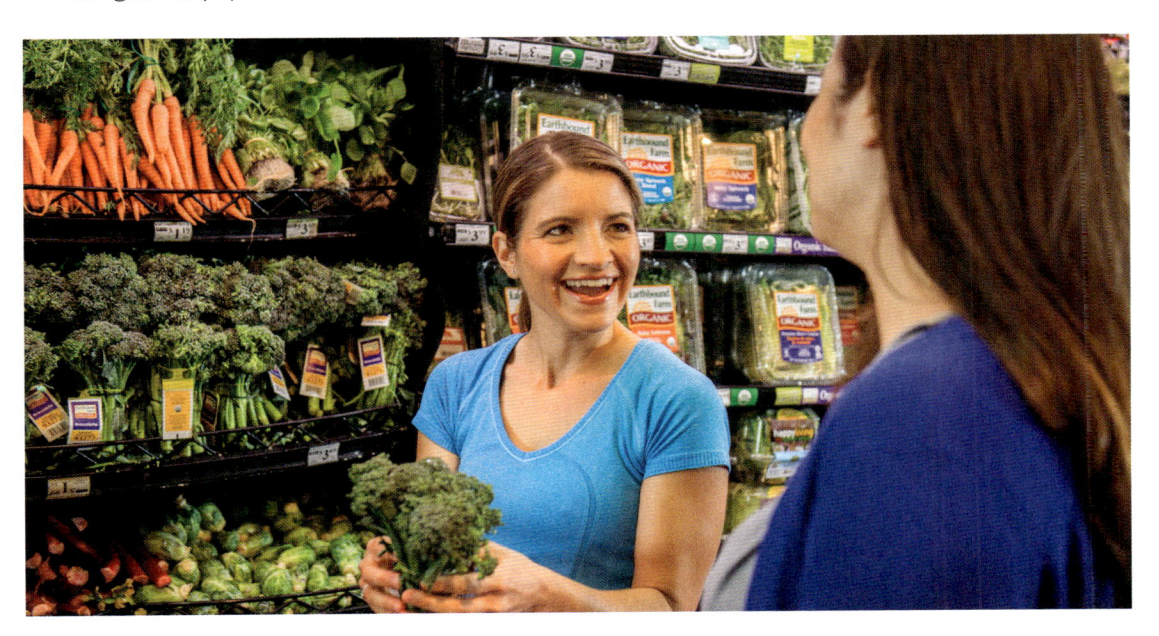

- Medication management: Medication and food intake should be coordinated. Nutritional recommendations vary based on the type of medication used, per the following:
  - ✓ Insulin secretagogues (promote increased insulin secretion) such as glyburide and glipizide: Moderate carbohydrate intake through scheduled and consistent meals and snacks. Have a source of carbohydrate on hand when doing physical activity in case of hypoglycemia.
  - ✓ Biguanides (decrease sugar release from the liver) such as Metformin: The physician should titrate the dose to minimize GI side effects. Take with food or 15 minutes after a meal to minimize GI symptoms.
  - ✓ Alpha-glucosidase inhibitors (delay digestion and absorption of carbohydrates) such as acarbose: The physician should titrate the dose to minimize GI side effects. For optimal efficacy, take at the start of a meal.
  - ✓ Incretin mimetics (control post-meal glucagon so as to help reduce post-meal blood sugar) such as GLP-1 analogs (injection) and DPP-4 inhibitors (oral medication): The physician should titrate the dose to minimize side effects. For the GLP-1 analogs, if given once or twice per day as an injection, should be provided pre-meal. If given as a weekly injection, it may be taken at any time. DPP-4 inhibitors can be taken at any time, but may be most effective if taken at the start of a meal.
  - ✓ Insulin: If taken via a pump or multiple injections per day, insulin should be taken at mealtimes before eating. If physical activity is performed within one or two hours of meal time, the dose may need to be lowered. If on a premixed insulin plan, insulin should be given and meals should be consumed at consistent times each day. Physical activity may decrease blood glucose so individuals should also have a rapid-acting source of carbohydrate on hand. If on a fixed insulin plan, the individual should eat similar amounts of carbohydrate each day to match set doses of insulin.

Of note, while the report advises that individuals with diabetes see an RD for nutrition intervention, as suggested by the Academy of Nutrition and Dietetics (A.N.D.) Evidence Analysis Library, the authors acknowledge that few individuals with diabetes ever see a dietitian and that the need to provide nutrition guidance spans the continuum of health professionals who work with individuals with diabetes. For that reason, the report and its recommendations are written for the non-RD health professional.

APPLY WHAT YOU KNOW

A PRIMER ON CARBOHYDRATE COUNTING

Carbohydrate counting is a method in which a meal plan is broken down by the number of carbohydrates to consume at each meal and snack. This method is used most often in individuals with T1DM who need to match insulin dosing with carbohydrate intake. An RD typically works closely with the individuals in developing and explaining the meal plan and carbohydrate counting method. The process typically includes three steps:

- Determine the meal plan in terms of the number of servings of each food group for breakfast, lunch, dinner, and snacks.
- Calculate carbohydrates. Grains/starch/sugars, vegetables, fruits, and dairy contain carbohydrates, while pure fats and proteins do not. As a general rule, the number of carbohydrates per serving in each food group can be estimated as presented in Table 13-5.
- Match food intake with allotted number of carbohydrates per meal and snack.

TABLE 13-5

CARBOHYDRATES PER SERVING

Food Group	Grams of Carbohydrates per Standard Serving Size
Grains/starch/sugars	15
Fruit	15
Vegetables	5
Dairy	12
Protein	0
Fats	0

Note: Table 13-5 is included for informational purposes only. Client meal planning and carbohydrate counting should be developed and overseen by an RD or certified diabetes educator.

> **EXPAND YOUR KNOWLEDGE**
>
> **MEDICAL NUTRITION THERAPY AND THE IMPROVEMENT OF DIABETES OUTCOMES**
>
> The A.N.D. Evidence Analysis Library suggests—and the American Diabetes Association endorses (Evert et al., 2013)—that individuals with both T1DM and T2DM receive at least three or four encounters with a diabetes educator lasting 45 to 90 minutes each within the first three to six months after diagnosis (A.N.D., 2008a). Additionally, the individuals should receive at least one follow-up visit annually. This level of intervention is associated with a 0.25 to 2.9% reduction in hemoglobin A1c after three to six months (A.N.D., 2008a), as well as 5 to 8% reduction in daily fat intake, 2 to 4% reduction in saturated fat consumption, 200 to 700 reduction in daily caloric intake, 11 to 31% decrease in triglycerides, 7 to 22% reduction in LDL cholesterol, and 7 to 21% reduction in total cholesterol (Evert et al., 2013). Despite these recommendations, about half of people with diabetes report receiving no structured diabetes education; a small minority have seen an RD—even though the service is covered by most insurance companies for people with diabetes (Evert et al., 2013).

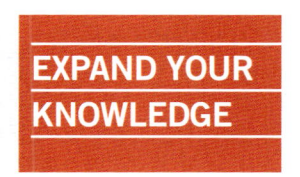

Nutritional Considerations for Gestational Diabetes Mellitus

All pregnant women are assessed for GDM, with screening generally occurring between 24 and 28 weeks gestation. If the woman tests positive for GDM, treatment is imperative. If left untreated, GDM increases the risk of poor maternal and neonatal outcomes.

Typically, an obstetrician will refer a woman with GDM to an RD who will implement MNT, ideally within the first week after diagnosis. Nutrition assessment includes dietary intake, level of physical activity, food preferences, weight gain, and any special concerns or considerations. The nutrition plan will help the woman achieve weight gain within the Institute of Medicine recommendations (see Chapter 21), and slow weight gain if it has occurred too rapidly, typically with a nutrition prescription of caloric intake of about 70% of the **Dietary Reference Intake (DRI)** for pregnant women. A typical recommendation would be to include about 45% of calories from carbohydrate, but no fewer than 175 grams of carbohydrate per day to provide sufficient glucose to the fetal brain and to prevent ketosis. Protein and fat recommendations generally align with the DRIs. Women with GDM should monitor blood glucose while fasting and after mealtimes; if numbers are consistently elevated, the obstetrician may initiate medication management (A.N.D., 2008b). All pregnant women are advised to eat a healthy, balanced diet and ensure adequate intake of key nutrients including folic acid, iron, and calcium.

EXERCISE RECOMMENDATIONS

Developing an exercise plan by using the FITT acronym (frequency, intensity, time, and type) is commonplace. Using **rating of perceived exertion (RPE)** and ventilatory thresholds to identify exercise intensity is prudent, as disease progression and complications (e.g., autonomic and **peripheral neuropathy**) can limit the ability to accurately assess **heart rate (HR).** Additionally, the FITT program for healthy adults typically applies to individuals with diabetes, as well. Participating in regular exercise brings about important benefits for individuals with T1DM and T2DM, with improved CVD risk factors, improved overall quality of life, reduced all-cause mortality, and improved psychological profile being key outcomes for both types (ACSM, 2022). Also, individuals with diabetes are encouraged to engage in at least 150 minutes of moderate-intensity exercise each week (or 75 minutes of vigorous exercise each week for those with T1DM), primarily focusing on caloric expenditure and weight-management issues. The CMES must consider the risk for muscular injury whenever they recommend higher-intensity exercise, especially for clients with T2DM. For long-term weight-loss maintenance, larger volumes of exercise (seven hours/week of moderate or vigorous activity, with an expenditure of more than 2,000 kcal/week) are recommended for clients with T2DM. Consideration of personal interests, past and/or present activity habits, and the goals and needs of a physical-activity program is critical for successful participation, especially in those with T2DM. Individuals who use insulin should engage in daily physical activity to improve the balance between insulin dose and caloric needs (ACSM, 2014; Colberg et al., 2010).

Resistance training is recommended for persons with diabetes who have no contraindications (ADA, 2020) and follows apparently healthy guidelines, with age and experience as prime considerations in program development. Interestingly, evidence suggests that there is no difference between resistance training and aerobic exercise when it comes to impact on cardiovascular risk markers and safety in those with T2DM. Also, for those with T1DM, performing muscular training before cardiorespiratory training on combined training days or performing **high-intensity interval training (HIIT)** combining both anaerobic and aerobic exercise may lower the risk of post-exercise hypoglycemia (ACSM, 2022). When working with clients who have diabetes complications, the CMES must either obtain specific instructions from the physician for safe and effective participation, or refer the client to an appropriately monitored setting. Strength or resistance training appears to offer specific improvements in insulin sensitivity (Cheng et al., 2007) and glucose control in those with T2DM (Sigal et al., 2007; Castenada et al., 2002; Dunstan et al., 2002). Therefore, the CMES is strongly encouraged to have all appropriate diabetes clients engage in resistance training to accrue its many potential benefits. Appropriate attention to modifying the intensity of the resistance-training session may lessen the risk for elevations in BP and glucose, and for the onset of musculoskeletal injury. Research suggests that higher-intensity resistance exercise is safe and effective in lowering A1c (ACSM, 2014; ADA, 2020). Caution should be reserved when recommending higher-intensity resistance exercise for those with diabetes. For safe and effective exercise participation, it is imperative that glucose levels be carefully managed. Moreover, initiation of a resistance-exercise program requires that clients do not have complications that might prevent safe and effective outcomes. To lessen exercise-induced BP elevations, modifications may need to be made, including lowering the intensity of each lift, requiring higher repetitions, foregoing lifting to exhaustion, and limiting **isometric** contractions. Further, clients should be directed to avoid the **Valsalva maneuver** and breathe during effort in order to avoid increased BP that may lead to retinal damage (ACSM, 2014).

Flexibility exercises are appropriate for clients with diabetes, but should not be performed in place of other training (ACSM, 2014). Balancing the selection of exercises between the upper and lower body, as well as for the core area, is important. Essentially, the flexibility-exercise recommendations are very similar between T1DM and T2DM (Table 13-6). The CMES must ensure that clients do not hold their breath for the entire range of motion of any movement, even when statically holding a given stretch. Proper breathing will limit the Valsalva maneuver, which causes increased **systolic blood pressure (SBP)** and may be detrimental to individuals with CVD or to those who have DRCs.

TABLE 13-6

RECOMMENDED FITT PROGRAM FOR FLEXIBILITY AND BALANCE TRAINING IN INDIVIDUALS WITH DIABETES

Variable	Recommendation
Frequency	At least 2–3 days/week
Intensity	Stretch to the point of tightness or slight discomfort. Perform balance exercises at a light to moderate intensity.
Time	10–30 seconds/stretch 2–4 repetitions/stretch Balance for any duration
Type of stretching exercise	Static, dynamic, other stretching, and yoga

Source: American College of Sports Medicine (2022). *ACSM's Guidelines for Exercise Testing and Prescription* (11th ed.). Philadelphia: Wolters Kluwer.

Diabetes Mellitus   CHAPTER 13

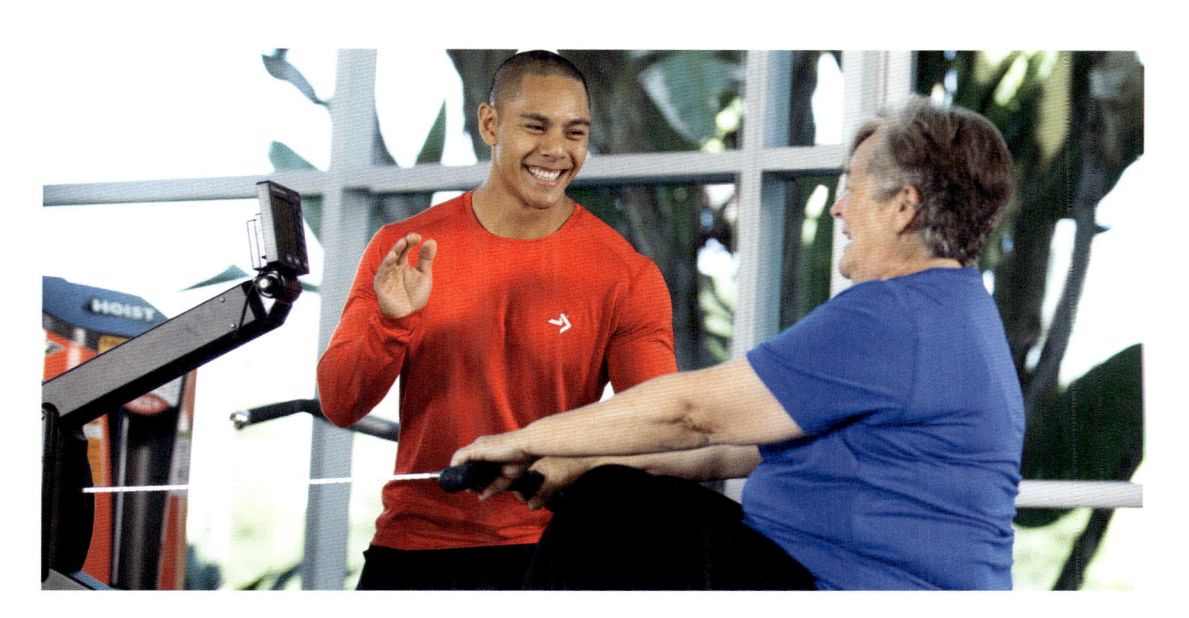

PREPARTICIPATION HEALTH SCREENING AND CLIENT ASSESSMENT

The diabetes management team must encourage clients to participate in physical activity and reduce sedentary behavior. While regular exercise carries significant benefits, there may also be risks for individuals with underlying CVD who perform unaccustomed vigorous physical activity. It is best to proceed cautiously. Before initiating exercise with clients who have diabetes, the CMES must acquire information about their client to ensure safe and effective participation in physical activity. By implementing a preparticipation health screening (e.g., PAR-Q+), the CMES will have crucial information about the client's current health and risk factors; current level of physical activity; the presence of signs or symptoms and/or known cardiovascular, renal, or metabolic disease; evidence of any DRCs and physical limitations; and exercise recommendations from the physician. Thus, the preparticipation health screening provides an excellent opportunity for the CMES to obtain important health information about a client with diabetes. Assessment of clients with diabetes includes the following key areas related to diabetes:

- Medical information
- Medical clearance when needed
- Lifestyle and habits questionnaire
- PAR-Q+ (see Figure 3-3, pages 74–77)
- Pre-test screening
- Health-related fitness assessment

APPLY WHAT YOU KNOW

Medical Information and Physician Approval

For clients with diabetes, medical clearance may be the first step to safely beginning or increasing the intensity of an exercise program. The CMES should know the health of their client and whether vascular and/or neural complications exist. Therefore, learning about a client's health and clinical status is essential for the CMES to effectively engage a client in an exercise program. Additionally, identifying questions that reflect the potential needs of the client is encouraged, including the following:

- How long has the client suffered from diabetes?
- How long have they taken medication?
- Are other coexisting conditions present (e.g., hypertension, elevated lipids, smoking habits, or obesity)?

Because diabetes is a disease that increases the risk for coexisting conditions, the CMES should develop a continuing-care plan that requires clients to have periodic medical evaluations (e.g., at least one physician visit per year). These follow-up visits may identify the onset or progression of complications.

When initiating an exercise program of light-to-moderate intensity, exercise testing is typically not necessary for individuals with diabetes who may be asymptomatic for CVD (ACSM, 2022). Stress tests may be advisable for persons with diabetes who have been sedentary and desire to participate in vigorous-intensity activities (ACSM, 2022). CVD risk is increased with both T1DM and T2DM, and an exercise test may aid in identifying safe exercise heart-rate limits for persons with or without neural complications (e.g., **autonomic neuropathy**), and/or hypertensive response(s) to exercise. From this physician-derived information, the CMES can then design a safe program for this type of higher-risk client.

The CMES must understand the nature of each client's health- and diabetes-management plan. Given this perspective, the CMES should ask their clients about current medication(s) for diabetes and any other coexisting conditions (e.g., high BP and abnormal lipids). All individuals with T1DM and some with T2DM use insulin to aid in lowering blood glucose, while many, but not all, people with T2DM use oral medications to manage blood glucose levels. Thus, prior to initiating any exercise program, it is important for the CMES to pinpoint the daily dose(s) of insulin and the location of the insulin injection. They must also keep a ready supply of simple sugar (e.g., candy bars and snacks) to counter the likelihood of hypoglycemia. In some clients who require insulin injections, physical activity combined with close monitoring of blood glucose may contribute to a lowering of the daily insulin requirement. However, any adjustment of insulin dosage must be carefully balanced with nutritional needs and close glucose monitoring. Any change must also be thoroughly discussed with the client's physician, diabetes educator, or nurse practitioner. Under no circumstances should a CMES recommend an unusual lowering of daily insulin dosage.

Oral medications are commonly prescribed for those with T2DM, while fewer than 20% of individuals with T2DM are prescribed insulin alone or in combination with oral medications (CDC, 2014). The purpose of oral drugs is to lower blood glucose by augmenting insulin release and insulin action or sensitivity. Once again, the CMES should ask clients to identify the daily dosage of oral medications. Oral agents to lower blood glucose for T2DM include:

- Glucotrol XL (glipizide extended release)
- Prandin (repaglinide)
- Amaryl (glimepiride)
- Glucophage (metformin)
- Micronase (glyburide)

Medication dosage can be reduced following a period of weight loss and/or physical activity. However, only the client's physician should make changes in oral medications. The CMES should encourage clients who are taking oral medications to regularly monitor and record their blood glucose and then provide this information to a physician, which may help the physician in determining dosage.

About 73% of all persons with diabetes develop hypertension (CDC, 2014). Hypertensive medications are outlined in Chapter 8. Drugs commonly prescribed to treat high BP can adversely elevate blood glucose. These include **diuretics,** beta blockers, and calcium channel blockers. Furthermore, beta blockers are known to mask the symptoms related to low blood glucose. Other hypertensive medications may actually lower blood glucose, including angiotensin-converting enzyme (ACE) inhibitors and alpha-adrenergic antagonists (Rizos & Elisaf, 2014). The varying effect of hypertensive medications is further reason to monitor blood glucose.

Using a questionnaire (e.g., health history or PAR-Q+) is appropriate. If the client responds positively to a question, its significance must be ascertained through a follow-up with the client's physician. Whenever a client with diabetes presents a history of heart disease, the CMES should refer the client to a clinical setting for supervised exercise.

Lifestyle and Habits Questionnaire

The CMES should consider a number of factors before developing an exercise program for clients with diabetes. Based on current health profile, fitness assessment outcomes, and limitations identified by the physician, a safe and effective individualized exercise program can be devised. Central to the safety of an exercise program is ensuring that a client with diabetes monitor and manage their blood glucose to minimize risks of exercise and onset of complications. To motivate the client, the CMES should devise an exercise program that considers personal interests, past and/or present exercise habits, and short- and long-term goals that are achievable, as doing so is central to the client's successful adherence to the exercise program.

Because most people with diabetes do not engage in regular physical activity (Valletta et al., 2014; Colberg et al., 2010), developing an activity program that is motivational, develops long-term habits, and addresses each client's personal goals is key to a successful program.

Identifying the personal goals and needs in a physical-activity program is crucial to maintain the interest and focus of a client with T2DM. Additionally, past exercise habits can provide important insight regarding present exercise interests, commitments, and/or habits. Previous habits and interests can also provide information about the client's awareness and knowledge of their disease, and about their effort in trying to control blood glucose. Glucose control is a life-long habit and helps ensure that exercise is safe and effective.

Education about the role of SBGM before and after each exercise session is usually presented in diabetes education classes. If a client with diabetes has not participated in a series of diabetes education classes, the CMES should encourage them to do so. These classes will increase the client's understanding of the disease and reemphasize the importance of regular glucose monitoring. Also, the CMES may provide the client with a list of diabetes educators and other resources.

Screening

The CMES should administer the PAR-Q+, informed consent, and possibly release forms, and then measure **resting heart rate (RHR)** and BP. From their most recent physician visit, the client with diabetes should know their A1c (%) and inform the CMES of this value for baseline information. Also, the client with diabetes should bring their glucose meter on the day of the health-related fitness assessment and or subsequent exercise days for glucose monitoring before and after each exercise session.

RHR and BP assessment are commonly used as screening aids for apparently healthy persons who wish to partake in physical activity. More than 60% of persons with T2DM have hypertension (Colberg et al., 2010). Some medications used to treat hypertension may actually lower the RHR; however, resting BP may remain elevated. Consequently, a client with diabetes may have a normal RHR but elevated BP.

A RHR above 120 bpm and resting BP exceeding 180/105 mmHg are contraindications to exercise (Gordon, 2002). Other contraindications to exercise follow previously established guidelines (ACSM, 2022).

Health-related Fitness Assessment

Fitness assessments are integral to effective exercise programming. The CMES can chart client progression and set goals to motivate clients. Fitness evaluations may include body morphology and/or composition, cardiorespiratory fitness, and musculoskeletal fitness tests. Although fitness assessments can be administered, the CMES may have to adapt the procedure for some clients with diabetes. Whenever testing procedures are changed, the CMES should record the modifications of the client's initial test so that subsequent evaluations are consistent.

Body Morphology and/or Composition

Excessive body weight and/or body fat is common in individuals with T2DM, while those with T1DM are commonly normal weight. Most persons with T2DM have overweight or obesity (ADA, 2020), while the distribution of body fat is predominantly in the abdominal region. This type of body morphology, or body-fat distribution, increases the risk for CVD, insulin resistance, and abnormal lipids. One method to determine body composition is by using skinfold thickness measures. The use of circumferential measures aids the CMES in understanding the distribution of body fat, or the client's morphology. Normally, it is acceptable to use the same generalized equations that have established norms for age and gender of apparently healthy persons for those with T1DM. When working with individuals with T2DM, the determination of body fat is difficult and may not be very useful, as most of these individuals have obesity. However, the CMES can measure and record skinfold thickness to observe subtle changes over time. Also, circumference measures (e.g., abdominal, waist, and hip) can be obtained and recorded for clients with T2DM to derive a baseline from which program goals may be targeted. Overall, these types of morphologic measures have far greater practical outcomes and can be easily compared with previous assessments.

Cardiorespiratory Fitness

Clients with diabetes tend to participate less frequently in regular physical activity than non-diabetics (Valletta et al., 2014; Colberg et al., 2010). Low cardiorespiratory fitness is strongly linked with cardiac mortality in individuals with diabetes (Boulé et al., 2003). Moreover, research suggests that people with T2DM consume a lower amount of oxygen than non-diabetics across different intensity levels of work; this suggests that the delivery of oxygen to the muscles is impaired and is in agreement with the finding that diabetics also have a lower **cardiac output** (Regensteiner et al., 1995). Therefore, improving cardiorespiratory fitness is an important health outcome that can be accomplished through regular exercise (Buse et al., 2007; Boulé et al., 2003; Stewart, 2002). The CMES is encouraged to use standard submaximal testing protocols to assess cardiorespiratory fitness in persons with diabetes. Also, heart-rate data and RPE should be obtained during cardiorespiratory assessments.

A valid submaximal test can be difficult with diabetics. Many persons with diabetes are hypertensive and take heart rate–altering medications, which make a submaximal test to assess cardiorespiratory fitness invalid. In some clients, a bicycle protocol may be appropriate (e.g., YMCA protocol). To ensure the validity of submaximal outcomes, the CMES must know whether a client has a neural condition called **cardiac autonomic neuropathy (CAN)**, because this DRC slows the HR and limits the validity of submaximal protocols that assess heart-rate responses to submaximal work.

The CMES may find field tests (e.g., 12-minute walk/run test) to be suitable for clients with T1DM, but not for those with T2DM. Performance in this type of test requires motivation to achieve a near-maximal effort and knowledge of pacing oneself. The use of a field test of this type may be useful only for those who have a recent history of regular exercise.

For those clients who undergo a stress test with their physicians, it is always a good idea to obtain a copy of this report through client consent. In cases where the cardiorespiratory fitness assessment cannot be administered, the information from a stress test can be used to aid in developing an aerobic program for a client.

Musculoskeletal Fitness

Administration of tests to assess muscle endurance, muscle strength, and joint flexibility in clients with diabetes is appropriate only in those who are not limited by diagnosed complications, especially microvascular complications, and have been cleared for physical activity by their physician (Aiello et al., 2002; Albright et al., 2000). Prior to initiating any portion of the muscular-strength and/or endurance assessments, the CMES should ensure an appropriate medical health status, especially the absence of microvascular complications. The CMES is encouraged to use standard testing protocols that do not use **one-repetition maximum (1-RM)** to assess musculoskeletal fitness.

Exercise Programming in T1DM

Daily aerobic exercise has been recommended for individuals with T1DM to better regulate insulin dosage and diet needs for glucose control. Improving glucose control for individuals with T1DM is best achieved through intensive insulin therapy combined with SBGM (ADA, 2020). The CMES should know that exercise is not recommended for glucose control in T1DM, and that daily exercise may be unrealistic. Moreover, high-intensity activity can increase the risk of elevating blood glucose and suffering musculoskeletal injuries (Hornsby & Albright, 2009; Gordon, 2002). Clients with T1DM who do not have complications can safely exercise at a moderate to vigorous intensity between 40 and 89% of $\dot{V}O_2R$ or at an RPE of 12 to 17 (using the 6 to 20 scale) depending on their current level of conditioning. Each activity session should last about 20 to 30 minutes to spur improved aerobic fitness and health-related benefits.

Finally, strength training for clients with T1DM may increase muscle mass and improve glucose control by increasing insulin sensitivity (Riddell & Iscoe, 2006). Clients with T1DM who do not have complications can participate in a moderate-intensity strength-training program that mimics a program nondiabetics would use.

Diabetes Mellitus   CHAPTER 13

Exercise Programming in T2DM

Exercise programming for individuals with T2DM follows the FITT principle (see page 394). The focus of such programming is to burn calories and lose weight (ADA, 2020; Colberg et al. 2010). Physical activity of 30 to 60 minutes per day at an intensity of 40 to 60% or greater of $\dot{V}C_2R$ is appropriate for persons who have overweight or obesity to burn an adequate number of calories (ACSM, 2022). Overall, the therapeutic effects of regular exercise have health benefits for those with T2DM. Because obesity is a problem, more moderate exercise reduces the likelihood of foot irritation and/or musculoskeletal injury (Verity, 2010; Gordon, 2002).

Exercising three to seven days per week maximizes the caloric expenditure necessary for weight management. Although walking is the most convenient activity, persons with **claudication** pain may have to perform low- or non-weight-bearing activity (e.g., swimming, aquatic exercise, or stationary cycling), or alternate between weight-bearing and non-weight-bearing activities. Moreover, peripheral neuropathy, which may lead to foot irritation, may preclude weight-bearing activities due to the possibility of foot irritation.

Finally, it may also benefit individuals with T2DM to engage in moderate-intensity resistance training, which increases muscle mass, lowers basal insulin levels, improves insulin action and sensitivity, and aids in glucose control. Resistance training is a safe, effective, and highly recommended component of a comprehensive exercise program that provides cardiovascular and metabolic benefits for those with T2DM (Hornsby & Albright, 2009). However, it is important for clients with T2DM to participate regularly in an aerobic-training program before the start of a resistance-training program, as most of these clients are severely deconditioned. Dynamic, whole-body activity in the aerobic exercise program will enhance their abilities to accommodate the muscular strength, endurance, and flexibility requirements.

GUIDELINES FOR EXERCISE LEADERSHIP

APPLY WHAT YOU KNOW

Clients with diabetes should consider numerous factors before starting an exercise program. Safety before, during, and after exercise is of paramount importance. Ensuring that clients learn certain practical information before exercising is central to safe and effective exercise participation, and providing practical exercise advice is a strong asset for a CMES.

Documenting each exercise session helps when communicating with a client's physician about cardiovascular adaptations and metabolic changes resulting from regular exercise. A daily log may be a particularly efficient way to record vital information—both quantitative and qualitative.

In fact, a qualitative assessment of the client's ability and performance is essential. Additionally, evaluating the client's self-concept, self-esteem, motivation to exercise regularly, and other quality-of-life issues is important for the CMES. Any noticeable dysfunctional changes should immediately be reported to the client's physician. These changes may include:
- An inability to accurately palpate and obtain the HR
- A loss of sensation in the feet or toes during weight-bearing activities
- Increasing pain in the legs during weight-bearing activities
- Difficulty reading the RPE chart
- Unusual forgetfulness or memory problems
- Persistent fatigue

The CMES must evaluate the client each time they come to exercise and report both quantitative and qualitative information regarding the exercise session. Barring more immediate problems, written documentation can be submitted to the client's physician on an annual basis. This documentation may compare various fitness assessments to those from the previous year. They may include the frequency and amount of daily submaximal work and HR, medication doses, glucose levels before and after sessions (averaged weekly or monthly), and any qualitative assessments previously described.

TABLE 13-7
PRACTICAL TIPS FOR CLIENTS WITH T1DM AND T2DM WHEN ENGAGING IN EXERCISE

Check with your physician.
- Clients may need to limit the intensity of physical activity, especially if disease complications are present.
- Clients may need to join a supervised program for guidance and assistance, especially if they have not been physically active for a long period of time.

Utilize self–blood glucose monitoring (SBGM).
- Clients should perform SBGM before and after each physical-activity session. SBGM is excellent cognitive training for diabetics to understand individual glucose response to physical activity. It is important to ensure that blood glucose is in relatively good control before engaging in purposeful exercise. If blood glucose is:
  - ✓ ≥300 mg/dL but the person feels good and has no ketones present (blood or urine), they may continue to exercise up to a moderate intensity
  - ✓ ≤100 mg/dL, the client should eat a snack consisting of carbohydrates and recheck blood glucose before exercising
  - ✓ Between 100 and 250 mg/dL, physical activity can be safely performed
- Postpone exercise when ketones and hyperglycemia are present.
  - ✓ Individuals with T1DM should test for urine ketones when blood glucose levels are ≥250 mg/dL.

Keep a daily log.
- Clients should record the value and the time of day the SBGM is performed and the amount/timing of any pharmacological agent (e.g., oral drugs or insulin). Also, they should include approximate time (minutes), intensity (heart rate), and distance (miles or meters) of each activity session. This information will aid the diabetic in understanding the type of response to possibly expect from specific physical-activity bouts.

Plan for an exercise session.
- How much activity is anticipated (e.g., time and intensity)?
- If needed, clients should carry extra carbohydrate snacks (~20–30 g of carbohydrate per 30 minutes of exercise).

Exercise with a partner.
- Exercising with a partner affords a "support system" for the physical-activity habit. Initially, diabetics should exercise with a partner until glucose response is known. Ideally, a partner who accompanies the physically active diabetic will be a source of social support and encourage continued participation in this healthy lifestyle.

Wear a diabetes I.D.
- Never leave home without it. Hypoglycemia or other problems can arise that require an understanding of the condition.

Wear good shoes.
- Proper-fitting and comfortable footwear can minimize foot irritations and sores, and reduce the occurrence of orthopedic injuries to the foot and lower leg.

Practice good hygiene.
- Clients should always take extra care to inspect their feet for any irritation spots to prevent possible infection. They should tend to all sores immediately and report hard-to-heal sores to a physician. Clients can prevent irritations when physically active by using Vaseline on the feet and wearing socks inside-out.

Modify caloric intake accordingly.
- Through frequent SBGM, caloric intake can be regulated more carefully on days of, and following, physical activity. For those clients requiring insulin, blood glucose can drop significantly after physical activity and latent post-exercise hypoglycemia can be prevented via SBGM. Also, in consultation with the client's physician, a decrease in insulin dosage may be necessary.

Note: T1DM = Type 1 diabetes mellitus; T2DM = Type 2 diabetes mellitus

Diabetes Mellitus CHAPTER 13

RISKS OF EXERCISE IN CLIENTS WITH T1DM AND CLIENTS WITH T2DM WHO REQUIRE INSULIN

Although individuals with T1DM and some individuals with T2DM require exogenous insulin derived from an injection site, or through a continuous infusion pump, exogenous insulin absorption does not mimic the normal insulin secretory pattern, especially during physical exercise. Consequently, insulin administration poses a potential problem for these individuals as they work to sustain near-normal glucose levels while exercising (Toni et al., 2006). In non-diabetics, metabolic responses to most exercise are balanced between adequate insulin release and an intricately matched glucose utilization and glucose production (Figure 13-4a). The maintenance of a normal glucose response, or **euglycemia,** during exercise is always achieved in normal clientele. Because of the need for exogenous insulin, it is important for the CMES to identify the risks for individuals with T1DM and T2DM who wish to safely participate in exercise.

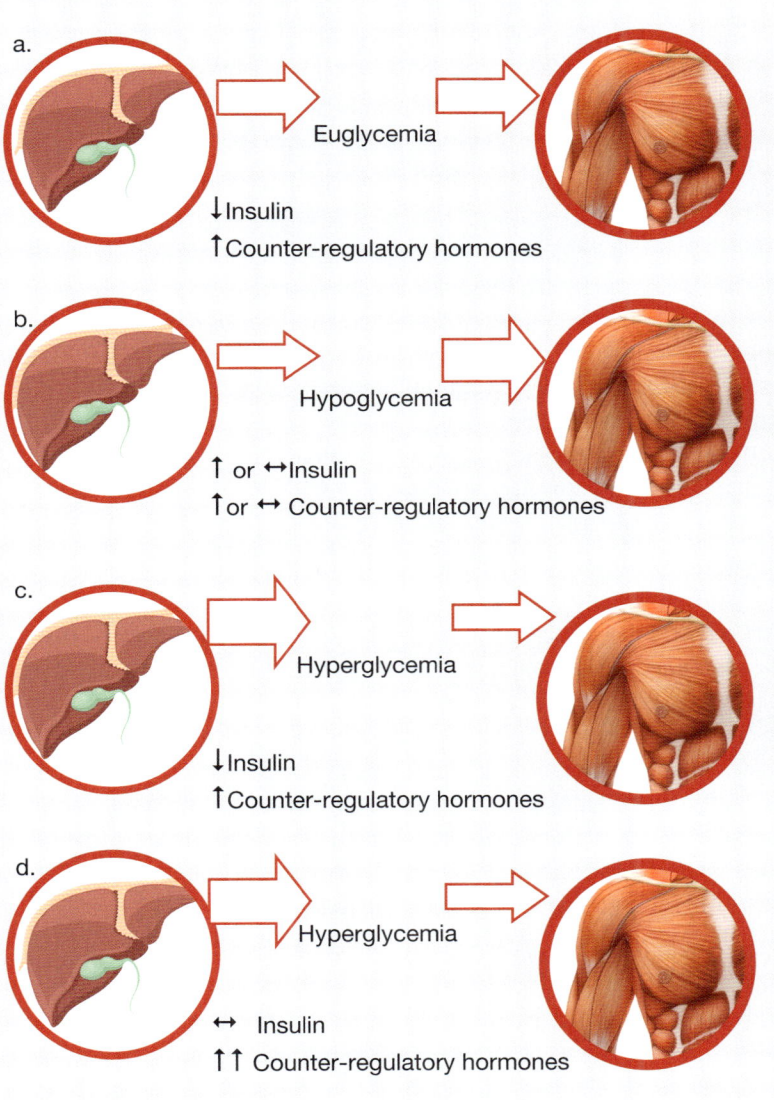

EXPAND YOUR KNOWLEDGE

a. → Euglycemia
↓ Insulin
↑ Counter-regulatory hormones

b. → Hypoglycemia
↑ or ↔ Insulin
↑ or ↔ Counter-regulatory hormones

c. → Hyperglycemia
↓ Insulin
↑ Counter-regulatory hormones

d. → Hyperglycemia
↔ Insulin
↑↑ Counter-regulatory hormones

Figure 13-4
Schematic illustration of the blood glucose response to exercise. (a) Non-diabetic response or ideally controlled T1DM where hepatic glucose production matches skeletal muscle glucose utilization and blood glucose does not change. (b) Hyperinsulinemia, or excessive insulin, results in low hepatic glucose production and enhanced skeletal muscle glucose uptake, yielding a low blood glucose, or hypoglycemia. (c) Hypoinsulinemia, or insulin deficiency, results in elevated counter-regulatory hormones, causing an imbalance between excessive hepatic blood glucose production and an inadequate skeletal muscle glucose uptake, thereby yielding an increase in blood glucose. (d) The stress of high-intensity exercise, competition, or heat can dramatically increase counter-regulatory hormones that increase hepatic glucose output with diminished skeletal muscle glucose uptake resulting in hyperglycemia.

Note: ↑ = Increase; ↓ = Decrease; ↔ = No change; ↑↑ = Large increase

Reprinted with permission from Riddell, M.C. & Iscoe, K.E. (2006). Physical activity, sport, and pediatric diabetes. *Pediatric Diabetes, 7,* 60–70.

Insulin injection therapy for most individuals with T1DM typically consists of multiple-dose insulin injections, while those who use CSII infuse a single type of fast-acting insulin (Toni et al., 2006). In some clients with T2DM, insulin is commonly introduced into an existing treatment regimen of oral medications as a single evening or bedtime dose of basal insulin. Because of this regimen, those with T2DM are less likely to experience the common risks of insulin injections/infusions observed in those with T1DM.

Exogenous insulin absorption is not well regulated and results in varying degrees of insulin excess or deficiency in the peripheral blood. Insulin levels are very important during the increased metabolic demands of physical exercise. In T1DM, several factors influence the blood glucose response to exercise, including the time of the insulin injection; the location of insulin injection (e.g., active vs. non-active muscle); pre-exercise glucose; pre-exercise nutrition; intensity and duration of the exercise session; and the novelty of the exercise performed (Toni et al., 2006).

Given so many factors to regulate, it is not surprising that physical exercise brings about unpredictable blood glucose responses in individuals with T1DM. Because of the dependency on exogenous insulin and an inability to regulate the absorption of insulin, people with T1DM commonly oscillate between insulin excess and insulin deficiency. Hence, the degree of "insulinization" and the level of blood glucose before the start of exercise determine the blood glucose response during and after exercise for those with T1DM. In well-controlled or well-insulinized T1DM clients, a single session of moderate exercise brings about normal metabolic responses. Under certain conditions, blood glucose may increase or decrease, depending on insulin levels (see Figure 13-4).

Hyperinsulinemia

Hyperinsulinemia, or high insulin levels, usually occurs when the clearance of exogenous insulin from the injection site is accelerated by increased muscle contraction and blood flow (Figure 13-4b). This situation can cause exercise-induced hypoglycemia. Insulin injection into non-active muscle is recommended on exercising days, although the strict use of non-active muscle as an injection site may not prevent hypoglycemia during exercise in those with T1DM (Toni et al., 2006).

Elevated insulin levels suppress hepatic glucose production, which causes an imbalance between the rate of peripheral glucose use and production, and results in the lowering of blood glucose. Although a decrease in blood glucose is a beneficial short-term effect of exercise, prolonged exercise can bring about hypoglycemia. Consequently, blood glucose lowering is dependent upon such factors as pre-exercise levels of blood glucose and insulin, antecedent nutrition, and exercise duration and intensity. Regular SBGM and modifying food intake and insulin dose on exercise days are useful strategies to prevent hypoglycemia in clients with T1DM.

Hypoinsulinemia

Hypoinsulinemia, or insulin deficiency, results in elevated blood glucose and ketone bodies before exercise (Figure 13-4c). Insulin-deficient diabetics rely heavily upon **free fatty acids (FFA)** as a primary energy source, which may lead to elevated ketones in the blood and urine.

What happens when an insulin-deficient client exercises? As work increases, there is an increase in metabolic functions to provide adequate fuel for the body. Unfortunately, a person with inadequate insulin is not able to effectively regulate blood glucose levels, and therefore experiences an increase in blood glucose, along with an increase in FFA use and ketone production. Exercise seems to worsen hyperglycemia in an insulin-deficient state because insulin action does not promote normal metabolic functions. Clients with diabetes should use SBGM before exercise, as this is the safest way to determine whether exercise will help improve insulin action and lower glucose levels.

Exercise-induced Hyperglycemia

During heavy, or high-intensity, exercise in clients with T1DM, glucose levels increase because of stress responses to the intensity of work that result in excessive release of glucose from the liver and limit skeletal muscle glucose use (Figure 13-4d). Typically, the T1DM is in good control prior to exercise and the elevation of blood glucose is singularly due to the stressors of high-intensity exercise. Therefore, the CMES should always have their T1DM clients check their blood glucose to enhance effective management of their exercise-induced responses.

Post-exercise Hypoglycemia

Although hypoglycemia can occur during exercise, low blood glucose can develop many hours after an acute exercise bout in those with T1DM. Although short-lived, post-exercise metabolic adjustments increase the risk for hypoglycemia in the first few hours following an exercise bout. To prevent acute and late-onset hypoglycemia, strategies should combine aggressive post-exercise SBGM with the adjustment of pre- and post-exercise insulin and caloric intake, as changes in insulin dose and caloric intake are not totally effective.

Postprandial Exercise Responses

The majority of individuals with T1DM exercise after a meal, rather than in a postabsorptive, or fasted, state. Usually, persons with T1DM have glucose fluctuations with each meal, due to the relative timing of insulin injection or infusion and the rate of insulin absorption from the injection/infusion site. Mild exercise after breakfast blunts glucose elevations throughout the course of a day in those with T1DM. Exercise performed after breakfast may also prove valuable because of a reduced risk for hypoglycemia during and following exercise. However, the postprandial response to exercise in those with T1DM is quite variable, and is dependent upon the pre-exercise glucose level, the timing of the insulin injection and food consumption before activity, and exercise intensity and duration.

Management of Exercise Risks in Clients With Diabetes

As a client with diabetes engages in regular physical activity, are there risks associated with participation? Will they develop problems? If so, what are the signs and symptoms of these problems?

The CMES should know that the most common problem encountered by exercising clients with T1DM (and some T2DM) is low blood glucose. Hypoglycemia can occur at any time (i.e., before, during, or after exercise) and is defined as blood glucose less than 70 mg/dL. Clients may be experiencing hypoglycemia or an insulin reaction when they exhibit:

- Abnormal sweating
- Nervousness and anxiety
- Shakiness
- Tingling of the mouth and fingers
- Hunger
- Weakness
- Lightheadedness or pass out

It is important for clients to consult with their healthcare provider to discuss a plan for appropriate dietary and/or medication changes to maintain euglycemia. Clients should keep glucose tablets or other rapid carbohydrate treatment with them (ACSM, 2022). Following an insulin reaction, the client may not feel comfortable exercising. At this point, the exercise session should be terminated.

Hypoglycemia is not totally preventable. Exercise-induced hypoglycemia most commonly occurs in insulin-requiring diabetics. To minimize the occurrence of low blood glucose, the CMES should link each exercise session to the timing and site of insulin injection or the use of CSII, the antecedent and post-exercise nutrition, the time of day, and the pre- and post-exercise blood glucose monitoring.

For those who use insulin injections, the insulin injection should occur at least one hour before exercising, and preferably in a non-exercising area. Some insulin-requiring clients can reduce the dosage of intermediate insulin by 30 to 50%, whether using injections or CSII (Toni et al., 2006). For persons on insulin pumps, a reduction in basal insulin dosage is recommended during and after mild to moderate exercise to minimize the risk of acute and late-onset hypoglycemia (Verity, 2010).

Consumption of carbohydrates is critical for individuals with T1DM to avoid low blood glucose levels. Between 15 and 30 grams of carbohydrates should be consumed for every 30 minutes of moderate exercise (Verity, 2010). A complex carbohydrate snack helps lessen post-exercise reductions in blood glucose and late-onset hypoglycemia.

The timing of exercise for those with T1DM may be a key in avoiding hypoglycemia. Depending on insulin administration and nutrient intake, the best time for some clients with T1DM to exercise is one to two hours after breakfast, or at least in the morning hours. For some with T1DM, postprandial exercise aids in mitigating glucose excursions throughout the day, and leaves them less susceptible to dramatic decrements in blood glucose (Toni et al., 2006). It is also important to individualize an exercise regimen. A program must fit into a client's schedule.

SBGM is essential for clients with T1DM and is strongly recommended for those with T2DM. Glucose monitoring is appropriate before and after exercising. Given the understanding of glucose levels, those with diabetes can minimize severe glucose shifts, especially after exercise.

Elevated blood glucose occurs in clients with diabetes who are not well insulinized because of excessive caloric intake and/or not enough insulin. Exercise will only worsen the hyperglycemia and ketone levels when pre-exercise glucose levels are elevated. Pre-exercise glucose levels ≥250 mg/dL with ketones indicate poor control and necessitate postponement of exercise. A log enables a management team to evaluate glucose excursions and prevent a reoccurrence. When blood glucose is high, clients with T1DM need an appropriate dosage of insulin, while those with T2DM may be able to engage in low-intensity physical activity without medication adjustment. For those with T1DM, exercise is not recommended until blood glucose is below 250 mg/dL.

High-intensity exercise has been found to elevate blood glucose from a normal to hyperglycemic level. It is believed that the role of counter-regulatory hormones on glucose production plays a major part in this type of glycemic excursion. Moderate-intensity exercise is recommended to facilitate more normal glucose levels and lessen the likelihood of musculoskeletal injury.

Progression of the Program

The progression of the aerobic and musculoskeletal programs is determined by several factors, including age, functional capacity, medical and disease complications, and personal preferences and goals. Initial changes in FITT programming for clients with diabetes should focus on the duration of the exercise session rather than the intensity, particularly for those with T2DM. This programming adjustment can prevent blood glucose increases, provide a safe and effective workout that is not unduly taxing, and increase the likelihood that the program will be sustained.

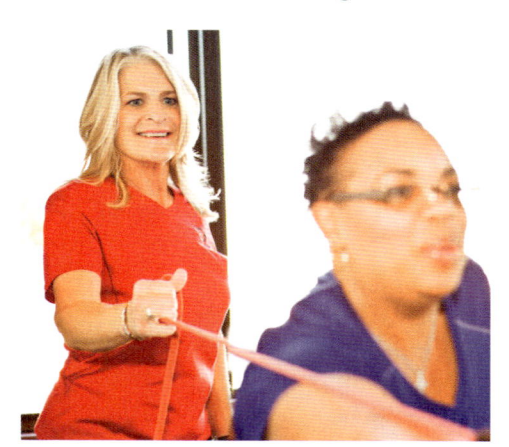

For clients without complications, initial ability levels are quite different between types of diabetes. For example, individuals with T1DM follow a similar FITT program to that of apparently healthy persons. They can initially engage in continuous, moderate-intensity physical activity for 20 minutes, while those with T2DM may only be able to engage in low-intensity physical activity for five to 10 minutes before fatiguing. The initial phase of FITT programming for clients with T2DM requires low-intensity and short-duration (e.g., less than 15 minutes) activity at least three times per week, and preferably seven times per week (ACSM, 2014). Individuals with T1DM may not require significant modifications in the initial phase of FITT programming. By closely observing client response to a program and modifying it to prevent fatigue, the CMES will enhance the client's enjoyment and commitment to such a lifestyle change.

Progression of the program after the initial phase should be approached with caution, especially when working with clients with T2DM. For both types of diabetes, the duration of an activity should be increased before the intensity. The duration should be gradually increased to accommodate the ability and clinical status of each client. Because clients with T2DM are more likely to have obesity and be older, they may require a longer period of time to adapt to program changes. Once the client is able to exercise for a desired amount of time, programmatic changes should be small and be approached with caution to lessen the risk of undue fatigue, musculoskeletal injuries, and/or relapse.

Some clients with well-controlled T1DM may set a goal to participate in competitive athletics (e.g., 10Ks, marathons, triathlons, and biathlons). A small number of these clients may require

Diabetes Mellitus — CHAPTER 13

higher-intensity, longer-duration workouts. Successful participation in competitive athletics by an individual with T1DM is dependent upon rigorous SBGM, appropriate insulinization, proper nutrient intake, and regular medical visits. Still, most diabetics will not strive to compete in athletics. Instead, they will need to improve functional aspects that relate to quality of life. Because T2DM onset is related to older age, obesity, and dysfunction of physiologic and neurologic processes, the most valuable aspect of any program should relate to functional outcomes specific to each client and their abilities and limitations.

MEDICAL CONCERNS AND DISEASE COMPLICATIONS

Although complications are common in diabetes, their existence does not preclude physical activity. Rather, there are physical-activity precautions and limitations for clients with diabetes who have one or more types of microvascular and/or neural complications. The options for diabetics with disease complications are discussed in the following sections. The CMES should familiarize themself with the many diabetic complications. Clients with those complications should often be referred to a clinical setting where close supervision and monitoring of exercise can safely occur.

Retinopathy

Although exercise increases systemic and retinal BP, studies suggest that low-intensity training in individuals with T1DM and T2DM can improve cardiovascular function without adverse retinal outcomes (ACSM, 2014). However, SBP should be monitored during each exercise session and limited to 20 to 30 mmHg above resting. Clients with retinopathy may exercise safely when they are properly supervised.

Clients with retinopathy have a higher risk for retinal detachment and vitreous hemorrhage associated with vigorous-intensity exercise. Thus, high-intensity aerobic or resistance exercise should be avoided, as these activities may cause SBP to rise dramatically. Under such circumstances, increased BP may increase the likelihood of retinal hemorrhaging when proliferative retinopathy is present. Also, inverted (i.e., head-down) activities and jumping or jarring movements should be excluded from the exercise program because of the increased hemorrhage risk (ACSM, 2014).

Nephropathy

Approximately 30% of individuals with diabetes develop nephropathy (Coccheri, 2007; Bo et al., 2005). Increased BP is a common precursor to worsening of this microvascular disease. It is prudent to avoid activities that cause SBP to rise to 180 to 200 mmHg (e.g., Valsalva maneuver, or high-intensity aerobic or strength exercises), as systemic pressure increases could potentially exacerbate the progression of this disease. Persons with progressive nephropathy or end-stage renal disease may benefit from lower-intensity physical activities. Most clients with nephropathy should be referred to a clinical setting where their fragile metabolic condition may be carefully monitored. In many cases, clients with this disease participate in physical-activity sessions while undergoing renal dialysis.

Neuropathy

Neuropathy is a nerve disorder. The two main nerve diseases related to diabetes are autonomic neuropathy (AN), and peripheral neuropathy (PN). Persons with AN have impaired sweating and thermoregulatory abilities and impaired hypoglycemia awareness. When this disease affects the autonomic nerves to the heart, it is called cardiac autonomic neuropathy (CAN). The HR is altered and the maximal HR is blunted, while RHR increases (e.g., RHR >100 bpm). CAN causes hypertension and **hypotension** and increases the risk for exercise-induced hypotension after strenuous activity. Approximately 22% of those with T2DM have CAN, the presence of which doubles the risk of mortality (Colberg et al., 2010). Persons with CAN exhibit a lower fitness level and fatigue at relatively low workloads due to the disruption in nerve innervation to the heart, which indicates the use of RPE as a method to monitor intensity. Consequently, physical activity for these persons should focus on low-level daily activities, where mild changes in HR and BP can be accommodated. Before beginning any exercise program for persons with AN or CAN, the CMES should gain physician approval and proceed cautiously.

Peripheral nerve disease affects the extremities, especially the lower legs and feet. Up to 40% of diabetic individuals may experience PN, and 60% of lower-extremity amputations in Americans are related to diabetes

EXPAND YOUR KNOWLEDGE

(Colberg et al., 2010). Repeated weight-bearing activities on insensitive feet can lead to chronic irritation, open sores, and musculoskeletal injuries, especially fractures. Persons with PN are susceptible to overstretching due to loss of sensation, as well as infection, particularly when daily hygiene is lacking. Proper footwear for any weight-bearing activity is important to prevent undetectable sores, which may turn into infections. However, people with PN should also participate in non-weight-bearing activities. Such interventions may include aquatic exercise, recumbent cycling, chair exercises, and upper-extremity exercises. Additionally, activities requiring a full range of joint motion are highly effective in reducing stiffness due to muscle contractures. Some mindful forms of exercise (e.g., yoga, Pilates, and tai chi) may be prudent for the client who has PN.

EXERCISE GUIDELINES SUMMARY FOR CLIENTS WITH DIABETES

CARDIORESPIRATORY TRAINING	
Frequency	• 3–7 days per week with no more than 2 consecutive days without activity to prevent excessive decline in insulin action/sensitivity in T2DM • 3 days of vigorous or 5 days of moderate intensity (greater regularity may facilitate diabetes management)

Intensity	• Moderate intensity
	  ✓ Below VT1 HR; can talk comfortably
	  ✓ 40–59% HRR or $\dot{V}O_2R$
	  ✓ RPE 12–13 (6–20 scale)
	• Vigorous intensity
	  ✓ HR from VT1 to just below VT2
	  ✓ 60–89% HRR or $\dot{V}O_2R$
	  ✓ RPE 14–17 (6–20 scale)

Time	• 150 minutes per week at moderate to vigorous intensity
Type	• A variety of prolonged rhythmic large-muscle-group exercises
Progression	• Progress following the ACE Integrated Fitness Training® Model based on client goals and availability.
MUSCULAR TRAINING	
Frequency	• A minimum of 2 nonconsecutive days per week, preferably 3
Intensity	• 50–85% 1-RM (lower intensity to start)
Time	• At least 8–10 exercises • 1–3 sets of 10–15 repetitions to near fatigue per set initially
Type	• All major muscle groups • Resistance machines, free weights, resistance bands, and/or body weight
Progression	• Progress following the ACE Integrated Fitness Training Model based on client goals and availability.

Note: VT1 = First ventilatory threshold; HR = Heart rate; HRR = Heart-rate reserve; $\dot{V}O_2R$ = Oxygen uptake reserve; RPE = Rating of perceived exertion; VT2 = Second ventilatory threshold; 1-RM = One-repetition maximum

Diabetes Mellitus   CHAPTER 13

CMES FOCUS

The recommendations for exercise for healthy individuals generally apply to those with diabetes. However, a CMES who works with clients who have been diagnosed with diabetes must be aware of the myriad comorbidities that can occur with this condition. Accordingly, the exercise programming for clients with T1DM and T2DM must be tailored to accommodate any DRCs (e.g., macrovascular and microvascular conditions) and should be undertaken at the recommendations of the client's healthcare provider. Further, understanding the implications of impaired glucose control and insulin administration surrounding exercise is a must for working with clients who present with diabetes.

Sources: American College of Sports Medicine (2022). *ACSM's Guidelines for Exercise Testing and Prescription* (11th ed.). Philadelphia: Wolters Kluwer; American College Sports Medicine (2014). *ACSM's Resource Manual for Guidelines for Exercise Testing and Prescription* (7th ed.). Philadelphia: Wolters Kluwer/Lippincott Williams & Wilkins.

CASE STUDIES

Case Study 1

Client Information

Jim is 35 years old and has had T1DM since the age of 13. He is 5'10" (1.8 m) and weighs 165 pounds (75 kg). Jim was highly involved in high school and college sports, but has not been regularly active for about 12 years. He currently uses an insulin pump and monitors his blood glucose once or twice each day. He visits his doctor each year and his self-reported health is good. He reports no diabetes-related complications and believes his A1c was 8.5% when it was measured about eight months ago. Jim's goal is to begin an exercise program so that he can run a 10K with his son, who is 12. He has come to a CMES for professional assistance.

CMES Approach

As a general rule, a CMES must obtain more information about Jim's health before developing an exercise program. According to established guidelines (ACSM, 2022), it is prudent for the CMES to obtain medical clearance before working with Jim. Also, it is essential that Jim completes a health-history appraisal to ascertain any known CVD, DRCs, and potential limitations with exercise. Additionally, the CMES should assess Jim's exercise history and obtain information about his usual meal times and insulin pump routine before developing an exercise plan.

From this screening, Jim should either plan to visit his diabetes educator or enroll in a diabetes education class to improve his diabetes self-management skills and education. Although Jim uses an insulin pump, his one or two daily blood glucose checks may not be adequate to effectively manage his blood glucose levels. Also, his A1c is high. He should strive to get his A1c below 7.0%. More frequent A1c assessments are strongly encouraged, as A1c is highly linked with risk for CVD, as well as onset/progression of DRCs. With more rigorous monitoring and visits with his diabetes educator, Jim may see his A1c gradually decline. SBGM before and after each exercise session is a requirement for him.

To develop an appropriate exercise regimen, the CMES can ask Jim about his preferences (e.g., walking or cycling) to focus on enjoyment and moving more consistently while establishing basic cardiorespiratory endurance. Results from his initial fitness assessment reveal that his percent body fat as determined from skinfold assessment was 17%, while his musculoskeletal fitness was good. Results from the fitness and exercise habits assessments suggest that Jim can immediately

ACE IFT® MODEL AT A GLANCE

Cardiorespiratory Training

Jim will start with Base Training until he establishes basic cardiorespiratory endurance and can exercise continuously for 20 minutes or more on at least three days per week. He will then transition to Fitness Training, where he will focus first on increasing exercise duration while incorporating jogging intervals that improve fitness and his ability to run for longer periods of time and increased frequency of sessions.

Muscular Training

Jim's initial Muscular Training program is focused on Functional Training to establish postural stability and kinetic-chain mobility before progressing to Movement Training. Once he can perform the movements correctly, external loads will be added to increase the intensity to build muscular endurance and strength in Load/Speed Training.

participate in moderate-intensity cardiorespiratory activities. His initial Cardiorespiratory Training program can focus primarily on walking at a moderate intensity below the talk-test threshold to build his fitness for consistent running during a 10K. The initial session should be 10 to 20 minutes in duration, based on Jim's tolerance, eventually progressing to a walk/jog workout that builds to a maximal distance of six or more miles (approximately 10 km). As endurance increases, jogging intervals can be introduced until Jim can eventually run all or most of the 10K continuously. His desire to participate in a 10K does not preclude alternate activities (e.g., recumbent cycle ergometer, upright cycle ergometer, or stair stepping). Blood glucose readings should be recorded, and if his pre-exercise blood glucose is ≥250 mg/dL with ketones present, the CMES should postpone the session until his glucose is below 250 mg/dL. If Jim's pre-exercise blood glucose is 100 mg/dL or lower, he should consume about 15 to 30 grams of carbohydrates for every 30 minutes of anticipated exercise to limit hypoglycemia onset.

When initiating a resistance-training program, the CMES should begin at the lower end of the range of each FITT element. It is essential that Jim learns proper lifting techniques and breathing cues (e.g., breathe on effort) before adding external resistance. The goal will be to perform one to three sets of eight to 10 exercises, making sure to focus on all major movements of the body (e.g., squat, lunge, push, pull, and rotation). If Jim performs resistance-training exercises following his cardiorespiratory exercise, he should check his blood glucose after each exercise session. If there is a long delay (e.g., several hours) between the cardiorespiratory and resistance-training exercise, then Jim should do the SBGM before and after each respective regimen.

Case Study 2

Client Information

Nandita is 55 years old and was diagnosed with T2DM about three years ago. Nandita is 5'3" (1.6 m) and weighs 180 pounds (82 kg). She is currently taking an oral medication (metformin) for her diabetes and antihypertensive medications for her high BP (ACE inhibitor: lisinopril, 40 mg; beta blocker: atenolol, 25 mg), and she does not regularly monitor her blood glucose. She reports SBGM about twice per week and her A1c is about 9%. Nandita reports that her health is good. She does not suffer from diabetes complications, but gets easily fatigued doing housework and cleaning. Furthermore, she reports that taking a 15- to 25-minute stroll with her husband at the local mall creates discomfort in her knees and hips. She has not seen her doctor in more than a year; however, her diabetes educator has encouraged her to participate in regular physical activity. She has asked the CMES for assistance in the development of an exercise program. Her goals are to improve her endurance and lose about 45 pounds (20 kg).

CMES Approach

Nandita requires an annual check-up on the clinical status of her diabetes (e.g., the evaluation of the presence/absence/progression of disease complications). She must receive her physician's approval to begin an exercise program with the CMES, who should encourage this client to improve management of her diabetes by getting routine physician check-ups and blood work. Also, the CMES should recommend that Nandita work with an RD who specializes in working with clients who have diabetes to determine the most appropriate plan for her to safely and effectively lose the desired weight.

Nandita should complete a thorough health-risk appraisal and PAR-Q+ questionnaires to seek medical clearance and identify possible limits in her exercise program. Her discomfort while walking requires further evaluation. The lack of regular blood glucose monitoring must be addressed, along with her elevated A1c%.

Once medical clearance is received with disease status and limitations, an individualized exercise program can be created. Of greatest importance are the client's personal interests and goals. Because Nandita has difficulty with short-term weight-bearing activity, the CMES can help her choose activities that are less wearing on her joints and identify enjoyable activities that she would more likely engage in on a regular basis.

Nandita should exercise in a comfortable environment where weight bias is limited or nonexistent. This is an important issue because the wrong exercise environment could adversely affect her motivation to maintain her physical-activity program.

An initial cardiorespiratory exercise program for Nandita can focus on the lower end of the range for each FITT element. The program must be safe, effective, reasonable, and prudent for this type of client. The FITT should look as follows:
- F = 3–7 days per week
- I = RPE approximately 3–4 (on the 0–10 scale)
- T = 15–30 minutes
- T = alternate between weight-bearing (e.g., walking) and non-weight-bearing (e.g., aquatic exercise; recumbent ergometer; chair exercises) activities

Body-composition assessment is not necessary when someone is already known to have obesity, but an anthropometric assessment can be administered. Initial measures should include body weight, as well as hip and waist circumferences. These measurements provide a good baseline for serial assessments. Nandita's measurements were as follows:
- Body weight: 180 lb (82 kg)
- Waist circumference: 42 in (107 cm)
- Hip circumference: 48 in (123 cm)

Weight loss will have a favorable impact on Nandita's anthropometric measurements. The measurements may also be motivating for Nandita as she strives to improve her fitness and lose weight.

Musculoskeletal fitness should not be assessed in the initial phase of the program. Nandita has enough to do at this point. Incorporating an additional routine into Nandita's activity regimen is not appropriate at the outset. As previously indicated, the CMES should start with Cardiorespiratory Training to engage Nandita in an exercise routine before initiating a Muscular Training program.

The CMES must recommend that Nandita perform SBGM before and after each exercise session as a prerequisite to safe exercise programming. Nandita may be able to engage in low-intensity exercise if her pre-exercise blood glucose is ≥300 mg/dL if no ketones are present and she feels good. If Nandita's pre-exercise blood glucose is below 100 mg/dL, then she should consume about 15 to 30 grams of carbohydrates for every 30 minutes of anticipated exercise. Nandita's beta blocker for hypertension can mimic the symptoms of hypoglycemia, so the CMES should periodically have Nandita check her blood glucose, especially at the start of a program.

Nandita is willing to come to a fitness facility two days each week. For Nandita to succeed in her exercise program, she should exercise on at least two additional days, especially at the beginning. As she progresses and wants to lose more weight, then she should do something every day, if possible. She should be instructed on the correct use of RPE and the talk test to ensure a safe and effective exercise environment when she is not supervised.

During the first activity session, Nandita should be closely supervised and should be comfortable when exercising. The intensity level should be appropriate. She should expend as much energy as she can comfortably do during each bout of exercise so that she can accumulate more calories used each day. Also, she must accurately monitor her blood glucose. For Nandita to exercise for the recommended 30- to 60-minute exercise period, she may need to alternate between a circuit of five-minute cardiorespiratory activities with 10-minute rest intervals or initiate a low-intensity

ACE IFT® MODEL AT A GLANCE

Cardiorespiratory Training

Nandita will start her Cardiorespiratory Training program at a low intensity, with a primary goal of establishing a cardiorespiratory base through Base Training. Once her endurance improves to where she can perform 20 minutes or more of continuous, moderate-intensity exercise, she can progress to Fitness Training, where the goal will be to increase exercise duration and session frequency, plus the introduction of aerobic intervals.

Muscular Training

Nandita's initial program includes Functional Training exercises incorporated into her warm-up and cool-down to improve core and postural stability and joint function. Once she improves her cardiorespiratory fitness and develops foundational core and postural stability, basic exercises to improve the performance of the primary movement patterns without compromising postural or joint stability (Movement Training) can be introduced as a preliminary step toward future Load/Speed Training.

aerobic interval program of similar work and rest intervals. Keep in mind that a client with T2DM must be closely monitored and given prompt feedback about accomplishments and progress. Also, the CMES must ensure that blood glucose levels are normal when the client leaves the facility to minimize the risk of low glucose or hypoglycemia problems.

SUMMARY

The CMES must realize that physical activity and/or exercise is an essential part of the therapeutic regimen in diabetes management and care. Diabetes presents challenges for exercise that requires the CMES to perform careful assessment of client status, determine client ability, and individualize the exercise program to meet the needs and goals of those with either T1DM or T2DM. Careful attention to the client and their diabetes-related comorbidities is a must for safe and effective exercise-training administration. The CMES should also maintain close communication with each client's physician to update progress or address any issues/concerns of the exercise program and/or responses that may need attention.

REFERENCES

Academy of Nutrition and Dietetics (2008a). Diabetes type 1 and 2 evidence-based nutrition practice guideline for adults. *Evidence Analysis Library.* www.andevidencelibrary.com

Academy of Nutrition and Dietetics (2008b). Gestational diabetes mellitus evidence-based nutrition practice guidelines. *Evidence Analysis Library.* www.andevidencelibrary.com

Aguiar, E.J. et al. (2014). Efficacy of interventions that include diet, aerobic and resistance training components for type 2 diabetes prevention: A systematic review with meta-analysis. *International Journal of Behavioral Nutrition and Physical Activity,* 11, 2. DOI: 10.1186/1479-5868-11-2

Aiello L.P. et al. (2002). Retinopathy. In: Ruderman, N. et al. (Eds). *Handbook of Exercise in Diabetes* (2nd ed.) pp. 401–413. Alexandria, Va: American Diabetes Association.

Alberti, K.G. et al. (2009). Harmonizing the metabolic syndrome: A joint interim statement of the International Diabetes Federation Task Force on Epidemiology and Prevention; National Heart, Lung, and Blood Institute; American Heart Association; World Heart Federation; International Atherosclerosis Society; and International Association for the Study of Obesity. *Circulation,* 120, 16, 1640–1645. DOI: 10.1161/CIRCULATIONAHA.109.192644

Albright, A. et al. (2000). Exercise and type 2 diabetes: Position stand. *Medicine & Science in Sports & Exercise,* 32, 1345–1360.

Alexander, G.K. et al. (2008). Contextualizing the effects of yoga therapy on diabetes management: A review of the social determinants of physical activity. *Family and Community Health,* 31, 3, 228–239. DOI: 10.1097/01.FCH.0000324480.40459.20

American College of Obstetricians and Gynecologists (2017). Practice Bulletin No. 180: Gestational diabetes mellitus. *Obstetrics & Gynecology,* 130, 1, e17–e31.

American College of Sports Medicine (2022). *ACSM's Guidelines for Exercise Testing and Prescription* (11th ed.). Philadelphia: Wolters Kluwer.

American College Sports Medicine (2014). *ACSM's Resource Manual for Guidelines for Exercise Testing and Prescription* (7th ed.). Philadelphia: Wolters Kluwer/Lippincott Williams & Wilkins.

American Diabetes Association (2020). Classification and diagnosis of diabetes: Standards of medical care in diabetes--2020. *Diabetes Care,* 43 (Suppl. 1), S14–S32.

American Diabetes Association (2014). Diagnosis and classification of diabetes mellitus. *Diabetes Care,* 37, Suppl., S81–S90. DOI: 10.2337/dc14-S081

American Heart Association (2007). *The Heart of Diabetes:*℠ *Understanding Insulin Resistance.* www.heart.org/HEARTORG/Conditions/Diabetes/Diabetes_UCM_001091_SubHomePage.jsp

Berger M. (2002). Adjustment of insulin and oral agent therapy. In: Ruderman, N. et al. (Eds.). *Handbook of Exercise in Diabetes* (2nd ed.) pp. 365–381. Alexandria, Va: American Diabetes Association.

Bo, S. et al. (2005). Renal damage in patients with type 2 diabetes: A strong predictor of mortality. *Diabetic Medicine,* 22, 3, 258–265.

Boulé, N.G. et al. (2003). Meta-analysis of the effect of structures exercise training on cardiorespiratory fitness in type 2 diabetes. *Diabetologia,* 46, 1071–1081.

Brethauer, S.A. et al. (2013). Can diabetes be surgically cured? Long-term metabolic effects of bariatric surgery in obese patients with type 2 diabetes mellitus. *Annals of Surgery,* 258, 4, 628–636; discussion 636–637. DOI: 10.1097/SLA.0b013e3182a5034b

Brunzell, J.D. et al. (2008). Lipoprotein management in patients with cardiometabolic risk. *Journal of the American College of Cardiology,* 51, 15, 1512–1524.

Buse, J.B. et al. (2007). Primary prevention of cardiovascular diseases in people with diabetes mellitus: A scientific statement from the American Heart Association and the American Diabetes Association. *Circulation,* 115, 114–126.

Castenada, C. et al. (2002). A randomized controlled trial of resistance exercise training to improve glycemic control in older adults with type 2 diabetes. *Diabetes Care,* 25, 2335–2341.

Centers for Disease Control and Prevention (2020a). *2020 National Diabetes Statistics Report: Estimated of Diabetes and Its Burden in the United States.* www.cdc.gov/diabetes/pdfs/data/statistics/national-diabetes-statistics-report.pdf

Centers for Disease Control and Prevention (2020b). *Diabetes and Nerve Damage.* www.cdc.gov/diabetes/library/features/diabetes-nerve-damage.html

Centers for Disease Control and Prevention (2014). *National Diabetes Statistics Report: Estimates of Diabetes and Its Burden in the United States.* Atlanta: U.S. Department of Health and Human Services.

Charbonnel, B. et al. (2006). Efficacy and safety of the dipeptidyl peptidase-4 inhibitor sitagliptin added to ongoing metformin therapy in patients with type 2 diabetes inadequately controlled with metformin alone. *Diabetes Care,* 29, 12, 2638–2643.

Cheng, Y.J. et al. (2007). Muscle-strengthening activity and its association with insulin sensitivity. *Diabetes Care,* 30, 9, 2264–2270.

Coccheri, S. (2007). Approaches to prevention of cardiovascular complications and events in diabetes mellitus. *Drugs,* 67, 7, 997–1026.

Colberg, S.R. et al. (2010). Exercise and type 2 diabetes: The American College of Sports Medicine and the American Diabetes Association: Joint position statement. *Diabetes Care,* 33, 12, e147–e167. DOI: 10.2337/dc10-9990

Diabetes Prevention Program Research Group (2005). Impact of intensive lifestyle and metformin therapy on cardiovascular disease risk factors in the diabetes prevention program. *Diabetes Care,* 28, 4, 888–894.

Dixon, J.B. et al. (2011). Bariatric surgery for diabetes: The International Diabetes Federation takes a position. *Journal of Diabetes,* 3, 261–264.

Dunstan, D.W. et al. (2002). High-intensity resistance training improves glycemic control in older patients with type 2 diabetes. *Diabetes Care,* 25, 1729–1736.

Evert, A.B. et al. (2013). Nutrition therapy recommendations for the management of adults with diabetes. *Diabetes Care,* 36, 3821–3842.

Garcia-Touza, M. & Sowers, J.R. (2012). Evidence-based hypertension treatment in patients with diabetes. *Journal of Clinical Hypertension,* 14, 2, 97–102. DOI: 10.1111/j.1751-7176.2011.00570.x

Giannini, C., Mohn, A., & Chiarelli, F. (2006). Physical exercise and diabetes during childhood. *ACTA Biomedica,* 77 (Suppl. 1), 18–25.

Gosmanov, A.R., Gosmanova, E.O., & Dillard-Cannon, E. (2014). Management of adult diabetic ketoacidosis. *Journal of Diabetes, Metabolic Syndrome and Obesity,* 7, 255–264. DOI: 10.2147/DMSO.S50516

Gordon, N. (2002). The exercise prescription. In: Ruderman, N. et al. (Eds.). *Handbook of Exercise in Diabetes* (2nd ed.) pp. 269–288. Alexandria, Va: American Diabetes Association.

Grundy, S.M. (2007). Cardiovascular and metabolic risk factors: How can we improve outcomes in the high-risk patient? *The American Journal of Medicine,* 120, 9, Suppl. 1, S3.

Haas L. et al. (2012). 2012 Standards Revision Task Force: National standards for diabetes self-management education and support. *Diabetes Care,* 35, 2393–2401.

Hornsby, W.G. & Albright, A.L. (2009). Diabetes. In: Durstine, L. et al. (Eds.). *ACSM's Exercise Management for Persons with Chronic Disease and Disabilities* (3rd ed.). pp. 182–191. Champaign, Ill.: Human Kinetics.

Huang, Y. et al. (2013). Collaborative care for patients with depression and diabetes mellitus: A systematic review and meta-analysis. *BMC Psychiatry,* 13, 260. DOI: 10.1186/1471-244X-13-260

Joy, S., Rodgers, P., & Scates, A. (2005). Incretin mimetics as emerging treatment for type 2 diabetes. *Annals of Pharmacotherapy,* 39, 1, 110–118.

Kinser, P.A., Goehler, L., & Taylor, A.G. (2012). How might yoga help depression? A neurobiological perspective. *Explore,* 8, 2, 118–126. DOI: 10.1016/j.explore.2011.12.005

Knowler, W.C. et al. (2002). Reduction in the incidence of type 2 diabetes with lifestyle intervention or metformin. *New England Journal of Medicine,* 346, 6, 393–403.

Liu, L.L. et al. (2010). Prevalence of overweight and obesity in youth with diabetes in USA: The SEARCH for Diabetes in Youth study. *Pediatric Diabetes,* 11, 1, 4–11. DOI: 10.1111/j.1399-5448.2009.00519.x

Nather, A. & Wong, K.L. (2013). Distal amputations for the diabetic foot. *Diabetic Foot and Ankle,* 4. DOI: 10.3402/dfa.v4i0.21288

Nather A. et al. (2010). Value of team approach combined with clinical pathway for diabetic foot problems: A clinical evaluation. *Diabetic Foot and Ankle,* 1, 5731.

National Institutes of Health (2013). *Control the ABCs of Diabetes.* https://www.nhlbi.nih.gov/health/educational/healthdisp/pdf/tipsheets/Control-the-ABCs-of-Diabetes.pdf

Peters, A. (2000). The clinical implications of insulin resistance. *American Journal of Managed Care,* 6, 13, Suppl., S668–S674.

Regensteiner, J. et al. (1995). Effects of non-insulin dependent diabetes on oxygen consumption during treadmill exercise. *Medicine & Science in Sports & Exercise,* 27, 875–881.

Reinehr, T. (2013). Type 2 diabetes mellitus in children and adolescents. *World Journal of Diabetes,* 15, 4, 6, 270–281. DOI: 10.4239/wjd.v4.i6.270

Renoir, T., Hasebe, K., & Gray, L. (2013). Mind and body: How the health of the body impacts on neuropsychiatry. *Frontiers in Pharmacology,* 4, 158. DOI: 10.3389/fphar.2013.00158

Riddell, M.C. & Iscoe, K.C. (2006). Review article: Physical activity, sport, and pediatric diabetes. *Pediatric Diabetes,* 7, 60–70.

Rizos, C.V. & Elisaf, M.S. (2014). Antihypertensive drugs and glucose metabolism. *World Journal of Cardiology,* 6, 7, 517–530.

Ryan, G., Jobe, L., & Martin, R. (2005). Pramlintide in the treatment of type 1 and type 2 diabetes mellitus. *Clinical Therapeutics,* 27, 10, 1500–1512.

Sigal, R.J. et al. (2007). Effect of aerobic training, resistance training, or both on glycemic control in type 2 diabetes: A randomized control. *Annals of Internal Medicine,* 147, 357–369.

Stark, S. et al. (2013). The prevalence of meeting A1C, blood pressure, and LDL goals among people with diabetes, 1988–2010. *Diabetes Care,* 36, 8, 2271–2279.

Stehno-Bittel, L. (2012). Organ-based response to exercise in type 1 diabetes. *ISRN Endocrinology,* 318194. DOI: 10.5402/2012/318194

Stewart, K.J. (2002). Exercise training and the cardiovascular consequences of type 2 diabetes and hypertension: Plausible mechanisms for improving cardiovascular health. *Journal of the American Medical Association,* 288, 13, 1622–1631.

Tobias, D.K. et al. (2012). Healthful dietary patterns and type 2 diabetes mellitus risk among women with a history of gestational diabetes mellitus. *Archives of Internal Medicine,* 172, 1566–1572.

Toni, S. et al. (2006). Managing insulin therapy during exercise in type 1 diabetes mellitus. *ACTA Biomedica,* 77 (Suppl. 1), 34–40.

Valletta, J.J. et al. (2014). Daily energy expenditure, cardiorespiratory fitness and glycaemic control in people with type 1 diabetes. *PloS One,* 9, 5, e97534. DOI: 10.1371/journal.pone.0097534

Verity, L. (2010). Exercise prescription in patients with diabetes. In: *ACSM's Resource Manual for Guidelines for Exercise Testing and Prescription* (6th ed.). Philadelphia: Wolters Kluwer/Lippincott Williams & Wilkins.

Whelton, P.K. et al. (2017). 2017 ACC/AHA/AAPA/ABC/ACPM/AGS/APhA/ASH/ASPC/NMA/PCNA guideline for the prevention, detection, evaluation, and management of high blood pressure in adults: A report of the American College of Cardiology/American Heart Association Task Force on Clinical Practice Guidelines. *Journal of the American College of Cardiology,* Nov 7. pii: S0735-1097 (17) 41519–1.

Zierath, J.R. (2002). Exercise effects of muscle insulin signaling and action—Invited review: Exercise training-induced changes in insulin signaling in skeletal muscle. *Journal of Applied Physiology,* 93, 773–781.

SUGGESTED READING

Aguiar, E.J. et al. (2014). Efficacy of interventions that include diet, aerobic and resistance training components for type 2 diabetes prevention: A systematic review with meta-analysis. *International Journal of Behavioral Nutrition and Physical Activity,* 11, 2. DOI: 10.1186/1479-5868-11-2

American College of Sports Medicine (2009). *ACSM's Exercise Management for Persons with Chronic Disease and Disabilities* (3rd ed.). Champaign, Ill.: Human Kinetics.

American Diabetes Association (2014). Clinical practice recommendations. *Diabetes Care,* 30 (Suppl. 1), S1–S155.

Evert, A.B. et al. (2013). Nutrition therapy recommendations for the management of adults with diabetes. *Diabetes Care,* 36, 3821–3842

Leroux, C. et al. (2014). Lifestyle and cardiometabolic risk in adults with type 1 diabetes: A review. *Canadian Journal of Diabetes,* 38, 1, 62–69. DOI: 10.1016/j.jcjd.2013.08.268

Umpierre, D. et al. (2011). Physical activity advice only or structured exercise training and association with HbA1c levels in type 2 diabetes: A systematic review and meta-analysis. *Journal of the American Medical Association,* 305, 17, 1790–1799. DOI: 10.1001/jama.2011.576

Verity, L. (2010). Exercise prescription in patients with diabetes. In: *ACSM's Resource Manual for Guidelines for Exercise Testing and Prescription* (6th ed.). Philadelphia: Wolters Kluwer/Lippincott Williams & Wilkins.

PART V
MUSCULOSKELETAL DISORDERS

CHAPTER 14
POSTURE AND MOVEMENT

CHAPTER 15
BALANCE AND GAIT

CHAPTER 16
ARTHRITIS

CHAPTER 17
OSTEOPOROSIS AND OSTEOPENIA

CHAPTER 18
MUSCULOSKELETAL INJURIES OF THE LOWER EXTREMITY

CHAPTER 19
MUSCULOSKELETAL INJURIES OF THE UPPER EXTREMITY

CHAPTER 20
LOW-BACK PAIN

14 POSTURE AND MOVEMENT

IN THIS CHAPTER

MOVEMENT
LENGTH-TENSION RELATIONSHIP
FORCE-COUPLE RELATIONSHIPS
NEURAL CONTROL

OVERVIEW OF POSTURAL ASSESSMENT

STATIC POSTURAL ASSESSMENT
PLUMB LINE INSTRUCTIONS
PLUMB LINE POSITIONS
DEVIATION 1: FOOT PRONATION/SUPINATION AND THE EFFECT ON TIBIAL AND FEMORAL ROTATION
DEVIATION 2: HIP ADDUCTION
DEVIATION 3: PELVIC TILTING (ANTERIOR OR POSTERIOR)
DEVIATION 4: SHOULDER POSITION AND THE THORACIC SPINE
DEVIATION 5: HEAD POSITION
POSTURAL ASSESSMENT CHECKLIST AND WORKSHEETS

MOVEMENT SCREENS
BEND-AND-LIFT SCREEN
HURDLE-STEP SCREEN
SHOULDER-PUSH STABILIZATION SCREEN
THORACIC-SPINE MOBILITY SCREEN

FLEXIBILITY AND MUSCLE-LENGTH TESTING
THOMAS TEST FOR HIP FLEXION/QUADRICEPS LENGTH
PASSIVE STRAIGHT-LEG (PSL) RAISE
SHOULDER FLEXION AND EXTENSION
APLEY'S SCRATCH TEXT FOR SHOULDER MOBILITY

RESTORATIVE EXERCISE FOR POSTURAL COMPENSATION

EXERCISE EXAMPLES FOR STABILITY AND MOBILITY
PROXIMAL STABILITY: CORE FUNCTION
PROXIMAL MOBILITY: HIPS AND THORACIC SPINE
PROXIMAL STABILITY OF THE SCAPULOTHORACIC REGION AND PROXIMAL MOBILITY OF THE GLENOHUMERAL JOINT

PRACTICAL APPROACHES FOR DESIGNING AND IMPLEMENTING RESTORATIVE EXERCISE PROGRAMS
USING INFORMATION FROM SCREENS AND ASSESSMENTS
PRIORITIZING SOURCE VS. SYMPTOM
THE PROCESS

OTHER CONSIDERATIONS
BODY MECHANICS IN THE GYM SETTING
PHYSIOLOGICAL CONSIDERATIONS

CASE STUDY

SUMMARY

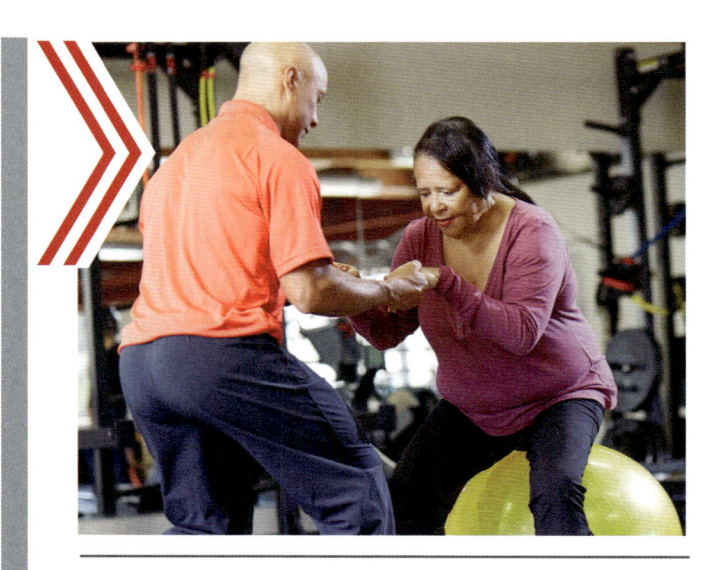

ABOUT THE AUTHORS

Fabio Comana, M.A., M.S., is a faculty instructor at San Diego State University, UC San Diego, and the National Academy of Sports Medicine. Previously, Comana was an exercise physiologist and certification manager for the American Council on Exercise, where he was a significant contributor to the development of the ACE Integrated Fitness Training® Model and live personal training educational workshops. His previous experiences include collegiate head coaching, strength and conditioning coaching, and opening and managing health clubs for Club One. As a national and international presenter, he is frequently featured on television, radio, internet, and in print publications. Comana has authored chapters in various textbooks and publications, and is presently authoring upcoming academic and consumer books.

Chris McGrath, M.S., is the founder of Movement First, a New York City–based health and fitness education, consulting, and training organization. Drawing on more than 20 years of fitness and coaching experience, Chris specializes in a variety of training modalities, including sports performance, injury prevention, post-rehabilitation, and lifestyle and wellness coaching. He has successfully established himself as an international fitness expert and has presented and consulted for some of the most successful fitness organizations in the world, including ACE, Functional Movement Systems, TRX, Reebok, EA Sports Active, and numerous others. Chris holds a master's degree in exercise science, a bachelor's degree in health education, and he currently serves as an adjunct professor at Long Island University in Brooklyn, N.Y.

By Fabio Comana & Chris McGrath

THE HUMAN BODY IS DESIGNED TO MOVE AND develop in response to the stresses placed upon the joints, bones, muscles, and tissues. Efficient movement often originates from good posture, defined as that state of musculoskeletal alignment and balance that allows muscles, joints, and nerves to function efficiently (Kendall et al., 2005). Correct posture contributes to the well-being of the individual by placing less stress on muscles, bones, and joints. Poor posture, on the other hand, is the faulty alignment of various body parts, producing increased stress and strain on supporting structures, ultimately compromising **balance** and movement efficiency and leading to degenerative changes and possibly pain (Kendall et al., 2005).

"Stand tall… stop slouching… pull your shoulders back…" These familiar comments, which most people heard repeatedly throughout childhood and adolescence, are equally important in adulthood to cue better posture. Occupational and lifestyle positions (e.g., driving a car, working at a computer, repetitive movements, wearing high heels, holding static positions for long periods, and improper weight-training techniques) and poor movement technique often create postural challenges that, over time, can result in poor posture and muscle imbalance. Muscle imbalance and postural deviations can be attributed to many factors, such as repetitive movement (pattern overload) and habitual poor posture (positions and movements).

Muscle imbalance generally alters physiological properties and function within muscle by changing the muscle's length-tension curve and force-coupling relationship. This often alters movement at the joint (**arthrokinetics**) and beyond the joint of **origin** (e.g., an **anterior** pelvic tilt may change the static position, and movement, of the cervical vertebrae). As joints bear weight and move abnormally, the body strives to discover paths of lesser resistance (law of facilitation), potentially overloading the musculoskeletal system (VanGelder, Hoogenboom, & Vaughn, 2013; Page, 2011). This could increase the likelihood of discomfort, injury, and pain. When there is associated pain, the ACE® Certified Medical Exercise Specialist (CMES) should refer the client to a qualified medical professional.

LEARNING OBJECTIVES:

» Explain the relationship between posture and movement, including how each can influence the other.

» Describe the fundamentals of movement, including the contributions of the musculoskeletal and nervous systems.

» Differentiate between the various approaches to working with clients who have postural deviations and pain.

» Identify important postural deviations from three different observational views.

» Identify and administer appropriate movement screens and flexibility tests to clients.

» Design and implement safe and effective restorative exercise programs for improving clients' posture, stability, and mobility.

» Consider body mechanics and other important physiological issues when working with clients who have postural and movement problems.

DOES EVIDENCE SUPPORT THE USE OF SPECIFIC INTERVENTIONS FOR CORRECTING POSTURE AND PAIN?

Despite a common assumption that posture is related to back pain, studies of interventions that include measurement of changes to posture are scarce, and a relationship between postural modification and improvements to pain or activity limitation has not been established. Further, the ability to change movement patterns with specific interventions is not well supported by the research currently available (Laird, Kent, & Keating, 2012). Part of the difficulty of finding research that supports specific interventions for improving posture and pain lies in the heterogeneity among studies conducted to date. More research with better designs is required to advance the understanding of movement modification and pain reduction through exercise. The exercise strategies presented in this chapter may be helpful for clients who present with poor posture by improving core function and movement awareness. However, the CMES should be diligent about reviewing the scientific literature as it becomes available to stay current on best practices for exercise and posture.

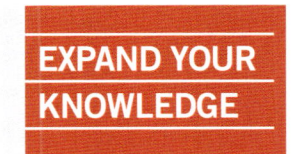

EXPAND YOUR KNOWLEDGE

MOVEMENT

One fundamental objective that all exercise professionals should share is to improve clients' movement efficiency and ability to perform daily activities. This is one of many possible definitions of functional training. Movement is the result of muscle force, where actions at one body segment affect successive body segments along the kinetic chain. While an individual produces forces to move, the body must also tolerate the imposed forces of any external load, gravity pulling down on the body, and **ground reaction forces** pushing upward through the body, if it is to remain stable.

Consequently, the ability of an individual to move efficiently requires that their body possesses appropriate levels of both **stability** and **mobility.**

- Joint stability is defined as the ability to maintain or control joint movement or position. It is achieved by the synergistic actions of the components of the joint (e.g., muscles, **ligaments,** and **joint capsule**) and the neuromuscular system, and must never compromise joint mobility (Houglum, 2010).
- Joint mobility is defined as the range of uninhibited movement around a joint or body segment. It is achieved by the synergistic actions of the components of the joint and the neuromuscular system, and must never compromise joint stability (Houglum, 2010).

Individuals who exhibit optimal levels of stability and mobility receive and interpret sensory information efficiently regarding movement (i.e., anticipate movement and stabilization needs), and then elicit the necessary motor responses. Sensory input and motor output are contingent on collaborative contributions from the neurological and physiological systems, as well as proper joint mechanics (**arthrokinematics**) (Figure 14-1).

Figure 14-1
The movement efficiency model

Source: Sahrmann, S.A. (2002). *Diagnosis and Treatment of Movement Impairment Syndromes.* St. Louis, Mo.: Mosby.

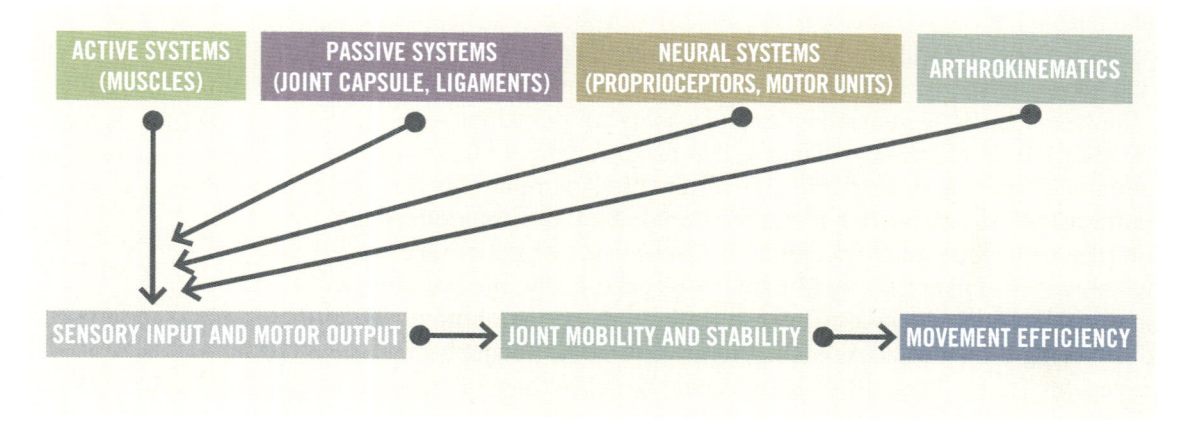

Movement efficiency involves a synergistic approach between stability and mobility where "**proximal** stability promotes **distal** mobility." For example, if the hips, trunk, and shoulder girdle are stable, it facilitates greater mobility of the legs and arms. While this is fundamentally true, the relationship between stability and mobility throughout the kinetic chain is slightly more complex. The CMES should understand this relationship, as it serves as the foundation from which all **flexibility** and resistance programming originates.

It is important to remember that while all joints demonstrate varying levels of stability and mobility, they tend to favor one over the other, depending on their function within the body (Figure 14-2) (Cook & Jones, 2007a; Cook & Jones, 2007b). For example, while the lumbar spine demonstrates some mobility (approximately 15 degrees of **rotation**), it is generally stable, protecting the low back from injury. On the other hand, the thoracic spine is designed to be more mobile to facilitate a variety of movements in the upper extremity. The scapulothoracic joint is a more stable joint formed by collective muscle attachments between the scapulae and rib cage that provide a solid platform for pulling and pushing movements at the glenohumeral joint and must tolerate the reactive forces transferred into the body during

Posture and Movement

CHAPTER 14

GLENOHUMERAL = MOBILITY
SCAPULOTHORACIC = STABILITY
THORACIC SPINE = MOBILITY
LUMBAR SPINE = STABILITY
HIP = MOBILITY
KNEE = STABILITY
ANKLE = MOBILITY
FOOT = STABILITY

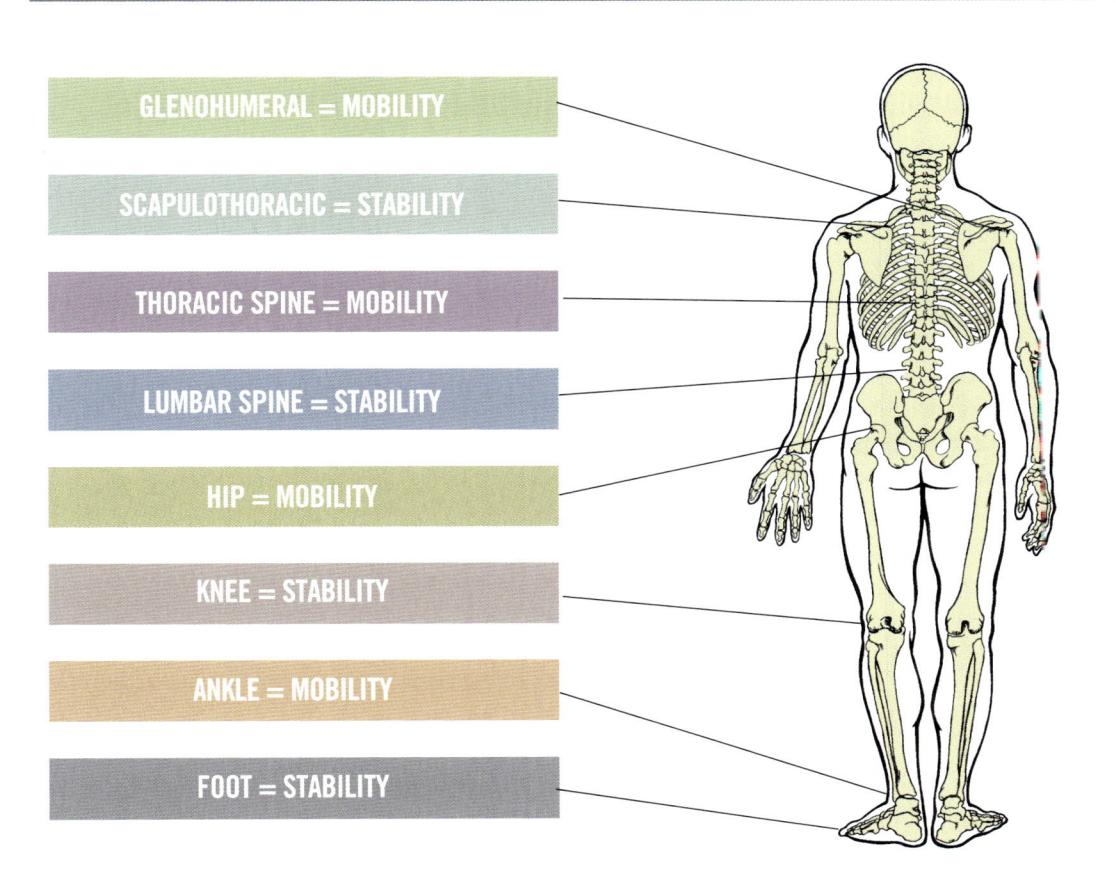

Figure 14-2
Mobility and stability of the kinetic chain

these movements. The foot is unique, as its level of stability varies during the **gait** cycle. Given its need to provide a solid platform for force production against the ground during push-off (heel-off and toe-off **instants**), it is stable. However, as the foot transitions from the heel strike to accepting body weight on one leg (load-response instant), the ankle moves into **pronation** (with accompanying calcaneal **eversion** that increases the space between the tarsal and metatarsal bones), and the foot forfeits some stability in exchange for increased mobility to help absorb the impact forces. As the foot prepares to push off, the ankle moves back into **supination** (with accompanying calcaneal **inversion** that decreases the space between the tarsal and metatarsal bones), becoming more rigid and stable again to increase force transfer into motion.

Individuals who exhibit good posture generally demonstrate an improved relationship between stability and mobility throughout the kinetic chain, but concern arises when an individual exhibits bad posture. What happens when a joint lacks the appropriate level of mobility needed for movement? When mobility is compromised, the following movement compensations typically occur:

- The joint will seek to achieve the desired **range of motion (ROM)** by incorporating movement into another plane. For example, if a client performs a bird dog exercise with hip **extension** (**sagittal plane** movement) (see Figure 15-42, page 517) and lacks flexibility in the hip flexors, it is common to see the extended leg and hips externally rotate in the **transverse plane,** thereby producing a compensated movement pattern.
- Adjacent, more stable joints may need to compromise some degree of stability to facilitate the level of mobility needed. For example, if a client exhibits **kyphosis** and attempts to extend the thoracic spine, an increase in lumbar **lordosis** often occurs as a compensation for the lack of thoracic mobility.

EXPAND YOUR KNOWLEDGE

APPLICATION OF THE JOINT-BY-JOINT APPROACH TO MOBILITY AND STABILITY

It should be noted that mobility and stability are used as relative terms. Stable joints are not to be thought of as "stiff and rigid," but instead of as providing greater stability over mobility. Naturally, mobile joints can become hypermobile, resulting in other movement- and posture-related issues. Stable joints should rarely have much in the way of multiplanar mobility relative to mobile joints (consider the knee, which has a lot of ROM in the sagittal plane but very little in the **frontal plane** and transverse plane). Conversely, a significant amount of stability is required in mobile joints for certain activities and functions. For example, the hip is a ball-and-socket joint and requires ROM in all three planes (**flexion/extension, internal/external rotation, abduction/adduction,** and **circumduction**), but is required to stabilize greatly in functional movements with little to no ROM (e.g., walking or single-leg stand). Figure 14-3 provides an example of how a compromised and/or injured joint can influence the entire chain.

Dysfunction in the lower extremity can influence movement up the chain. However, dysfunction higher up the chain can also influence movement down the chain. In other words, issues can originate down and influence upward, originate upward and influence downward, or originate in the middle and influence upward and downward. Determining where the issue started on the chain can present a conundrum for the CMES. Determining how a compromised joint will influence the rest of the chain can be equally perplexing. There are endless combinations of movements, making it virtually impossible to know precisely how each part will influence, or be influenced by, other parts in every given set of circumstances. It is important for the CMES to appreciate and respect these potential influences of compensatory behavior and patterns. A greater level of awareness can, at the very least, help eliminate risky movements, exercises, and activities and prevent perpetuating issues.

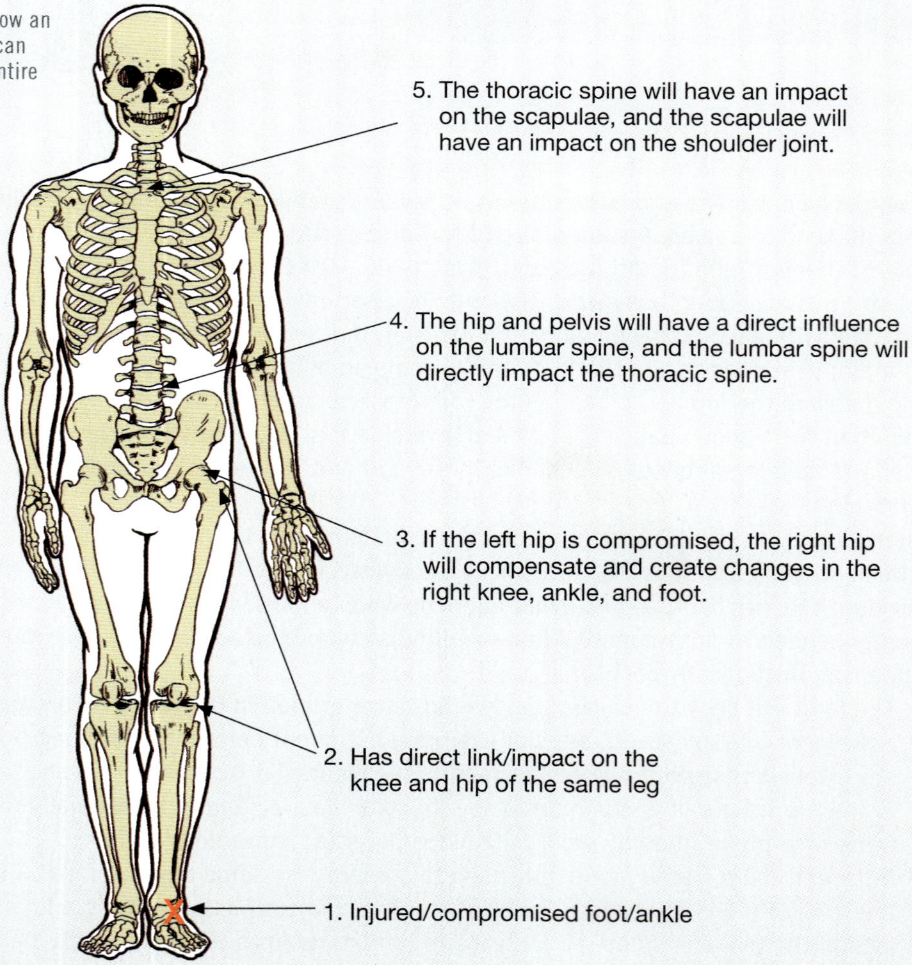

Figure 14-3
Example of how an ankle injury can impact the entire kinetic chain

5. The thoracic spine will have an impact on the scapulae, and the scapulae will have an impact on the shoulder joint.

4. The hip and pelvis will have a direct influence on the lumbar spine, and the lumbar spine will directly impact the thoracic spine.

3. If the left hip is compromised, the right hip will compensate and create changes in the right knee, ankle, and foot.

2. Has direct link/impact on the knee and hip of the same leg

1. Injured/compromised foot/ankle

Posture and Movement CHAPTER 14

A lack of mobility can be attributed to numerous factors, including reduced levels of activity and actions and conditions that promote muscle imbalance (e.g., repetitive movements, habitually poor posture, side-dominance, poor exercise technique, and imbalanced strength-training programs) (Kendall et al., 2005). This loss of mobility leads to compensations in movement and potential losses to stability at subsequent joints. Muscle imbalances alter the physiological and neurological properties of muscles in a way that ultimately contributes to dysfunctional movement (Figure 14-4).

Figure 14-4
Dysfunctional movement

MUSCLE IMBALANCE ATTRIBUTED TO:
- Repetitive motion
- Awkward positions/postures
- Work environment
- Side-dominance
- Poor exercise technique
- Imbalanced resistance-training programs
- Congenital conditions (e.g., scoliosis)
- Pathologies (e.g., arthritis)
- Structural deviations (e.g., tibial torsion and femoral anteversion)
- Trauma (e.g., surgery, injury, and amputations)

→ **ALTERS MUSCLE PHYSIOLOGICAL AND NEUROLOGICAL PROPERTIES**

↓

COMPROMISES THE MOBILITY-STABILITY RELATIONSHIP
- Compromises are largest at subsequent joints (proximal and distal)
- Demonstrates continued effects along the kinetic chain

↓

THE BODY SUBSCRIBES TO THE LAW OF FACILITATION
- Achieves the desired movement following the path of least resistance

↓

DYSFUNCTIONAL MOVEMENT
- Develops faulty neural pathways and strategies

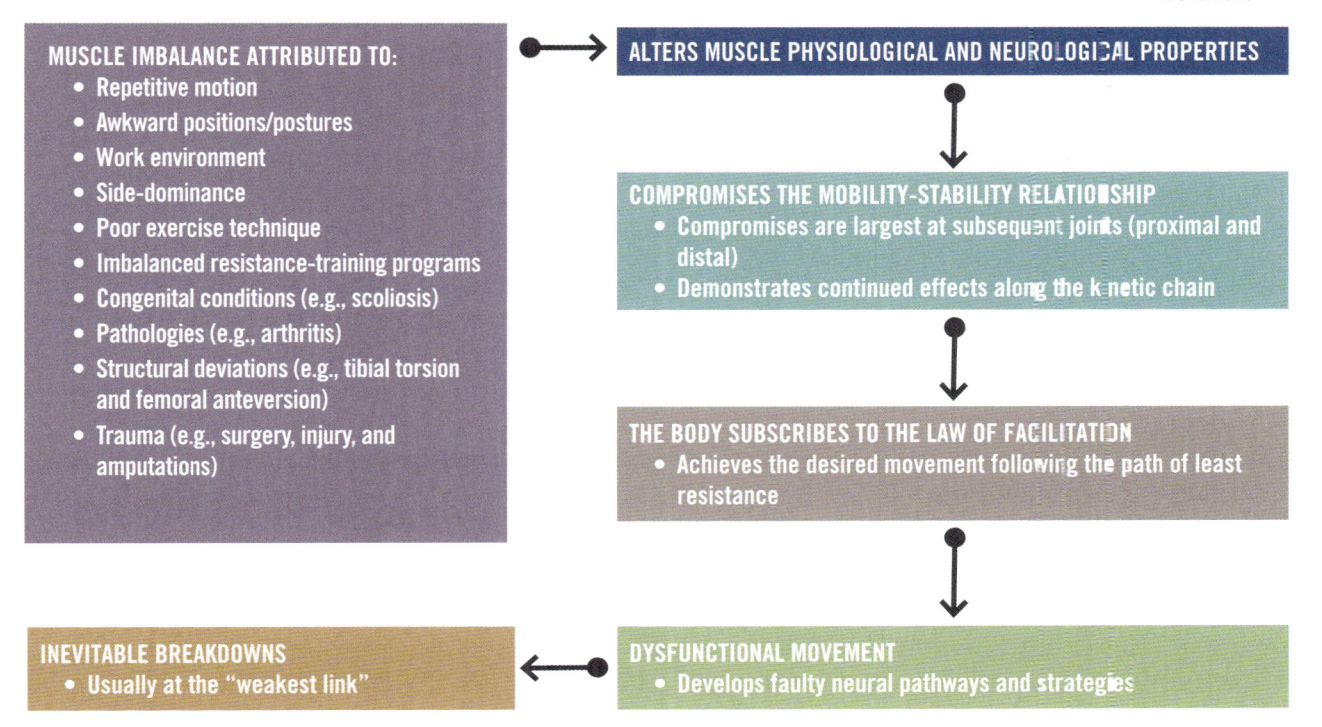

← **INEVITABLE BREAKDOWNS**
- Usually at the "weakest link"

Technology is another contributing factor that promotes dysfunctional movement. As technology continues to advance the complexity of exercise equipment, many exercises and drills have become equally technical. For example, with the introduction of the free-standing, dual-stack, low-high pulley cable systems that move in multiple directions, advanced exercises like the high-to-low cable chop (see Figure 15-40, page 516) are now common practice in most fitness settings. Individuals who exhibit limited mobility and stability will often resort to compensated movement when performing complex exercises or using advanced equipment. This raises the potential concern of whether exercise without regard for an individual's levels of stability and mobility throughout the kinetic chain is actually doing more harm than good, advancing the concept of "dysfunctional fitness."

Movement compensations generally represent an inability to maintain muscle balance and neutrality at the joint (Kendall et al., 2005). Periods of inactivity when joints are held passively in shortened positions result in muscle shortening (e.g., prolonged periods of sitting without hip extension shortens the hip flexors). As one muscle (the **agonist**) shortens, the opposing muscle (the **antagonist**) at the joint tends to lengthen. Muscle shortening and lengthening alter both the physiological and neural properties within the muscle (i.e., length-tension and force-coupling relationships).

Length-tension Relationship

The length-tension relationship is the relationship between the **contractile proteins** (e.g., **actin** and **myosin**) of a **sarcomere** and their force-generating capacity. A slight stretching of the sarcomere beyond its normal resting length increases the spatial arrangement between the muscle's contractile proteins and increases its force-generating capacity (Figure 14-5). Further stretching of the sarcomere beyond optimal length, however, reduces the potential for contractile protein binding and decreases the muscle's force-generating capacity (Kenney, Wilmore, & Costill, 2012; Krans, 2010). Similarly, shortening the sarcomere beyond resting length results in an overlap of contractile proteins, which also reduces the muscle's force-generating potential.

Muscle immobilization, passive shortening, trauma, and aging all shorten muscles, thereby shifting the length-tension curve to the left (Figure 14-6) (Lieber, 2009; MacIntosh, Gardiner, & McComas, 2006; Williams & Goldspink, 1978). This represents a loss in the number of sarcomeres within the **myofibril** of the muscle fiber (a typical muscle myofibril may have approximately 500,000 sacromeres arranged in series). While the muscle may demonstrate good force-generating capacity in the shortened position, it demonstrates reduced force-generating capacity in both the normal-resting-length (good posture) and lengthened positions. Muscles can shorten in as little as two to four weeks when held in passively shortened positions without being stretched or used through a full or functional ROM (e.g., continuous bouts of sitting hunched over a desk without extension activity within the upper thorax can shorten the pectoralis major). Simply stretching a tight muscle does not immediately restore its normal force-generating capacity due to the reduced number of sarcomeres present within the myofibril. Passive stretching or elongation of a tightened muscle will gradually add sarcomeres back in line and help restore the muscle's normal resting length and its length-tension relationship (Williams, 1990).

Figure 14-5
Length-tension relationship of a sarcomere

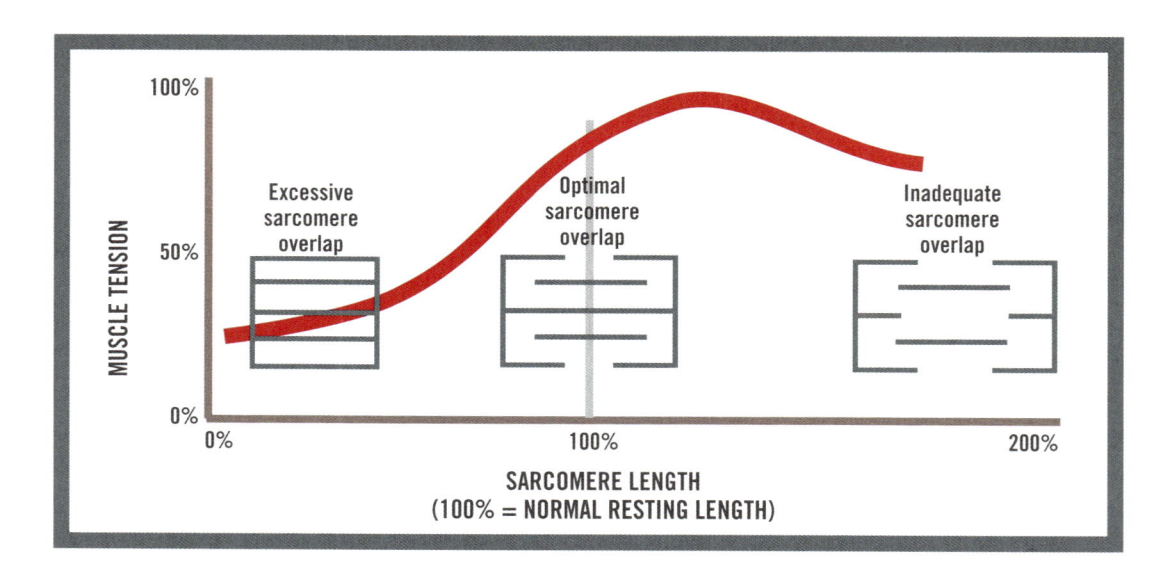

Figure 14-6
Alterations to the length-tension relationship of a sarcomere

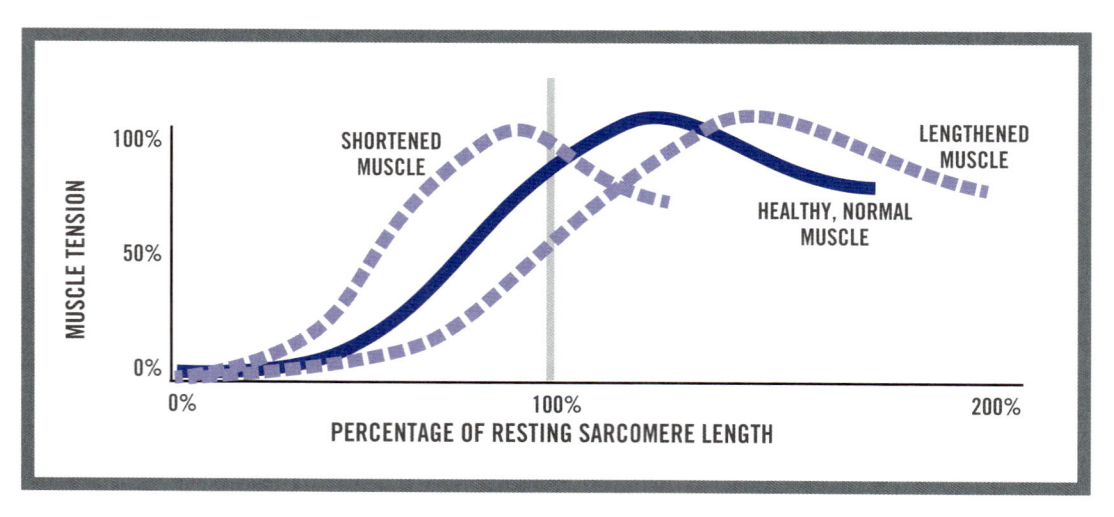

Posture and Movement   CHAPTER 14

Also illustrated in Figure 14-6 is what happens to the lengthened muscles on the opposing side of the joint. These muscles undergo an adaptive change and add sarcomeres in series, shifting the length-tension curve to the right (Lieber, 2009; MacIntosh, Gardiner, & McComas, 2006; Williams & Goldspink, 1978). They demonstrate greater force-generating capacities in lengthened positions, but demonstrate reduced force-generating capacity in the normal-resting-length (good posture) or shortened positions. Restoring the normal resting length and the muscle's force-generating capacity requires a physiological adaptation best achieved by strengthening a muscle in normal-resting-length positions, but not in lengthened positions. For example, when a client exhibits protracted shoulders, performing high-back rows using a full ROM to strengthen the rhomboids and **posterior** deltoids is not recommended initially. As the rhomboids demonstrate good strength in the lengthened position, the momentum generated during a full-ROM row will carry the movement through the weaker region, essentially decreasing the ability to strengthen the muscle where it needs strengthening. A more appropriate approach is to perform this same exercise initially with either an **isometric** contraction in a good postural position or through a limited ROM.

Force-couple Relationships

Muscles rarely ever work in isolation, but instead function as integrated groups. Many function by providing opposing, directional, or **contralateral** pulls at joints (termed force-couples) to achieve efficient movement (Houglum, 2010; Sahrmann, 2002). For example, maintenance of a neutral pelvic position is achieved via opposing force-couples between four major muscle groups that all have attachments on the pelvis. The rectus abdominis pulls upward on the anterior, **inferior** pelvis, while the hip flexors pull downward on the anterior, **superior** pelvis (Figure 14-7). On the posterior surface, the hamstrings pull downward on the posterior, inferior pelvis, while the erector spinae pull upward on the posterior, superior pelvis. When these muscles demonstrate good balance, the pelvis holds an optimal position. However, when one muscle becomes tight, it alters this relationship and changes the pelvic position. Changes to pelvic position will affect the position of the spine above and the femur below, thereby altering posture and the loading on the joints along the kinetic chain (Panjabi, 1992).

Another example of a force-couple occurs at the glenohumeral joint between the deltoids and rotator cuff muscles during arm abduction (Figure 14-8). While the deltoid acts as the

Figure 14-7
Pelvic force-couples

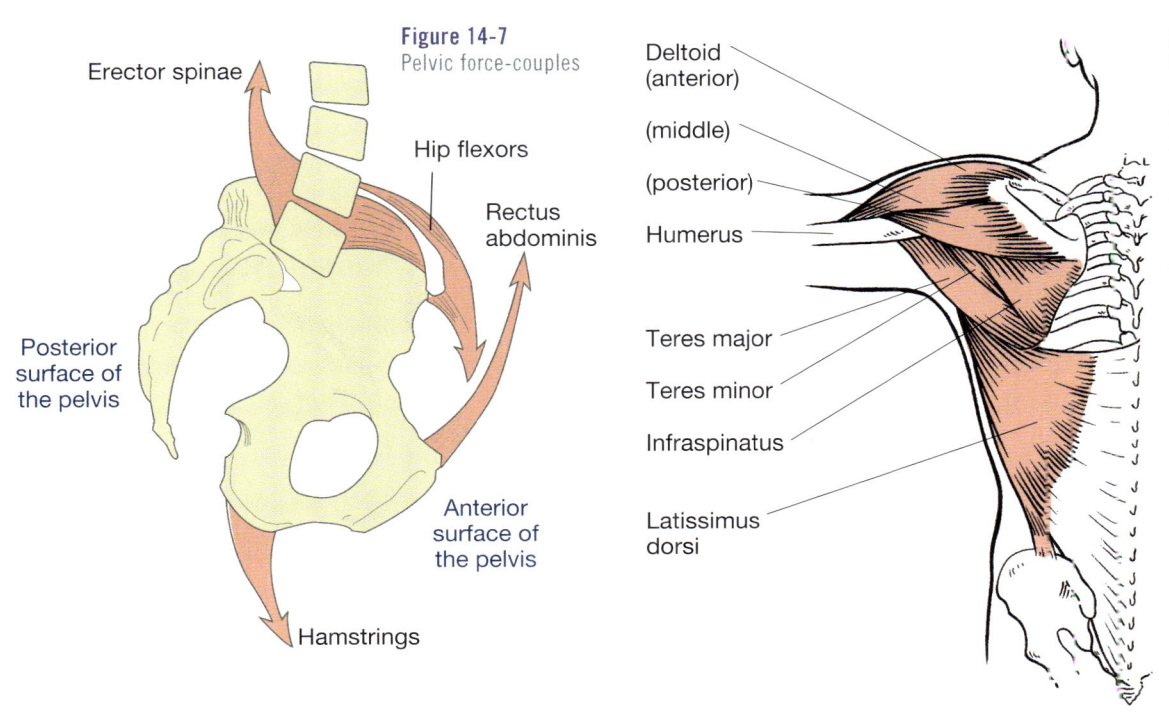

Figure 14-8
Superficial musculature of the superior and inferior shoulder joint, prime movers for shoulder abduction (deltoid) and adduction (latissimus dorsi and teres major)

prime mover in arm abduction, it is the collaborative action of the rotator cuff muscles, with respect to magnitude and timing of contraction, that counters the direct upward pull of the deltoid to produce rotation. Without the action of the rotator cuff muscles that allows the humeral head to glide inferiorly during rotation, the isolated, upward pull of the deltoid would impinge the humeral head upward against the coracoacromial arch (Houglum, 2010; Cook & Jones, 2007a).

Neural Control

Joint movement is dependent on nerve activity, in that impulses are transmitted to the intended muscles. To help stabilize and control movement within the joint, some degree of simultaneous **co-contraction** of the antagonist also occurs. However, when a muscle becomes shortened, this increases **tonicity** within that muscle (i.e., **hypertonicity**), implying that the muscle now requires only a smaller or weaker nerve impulse to activate a contraction (i.e., lowered irritability threshold) (Levine, Richards, & Whittle, 2012). Thus, when an individual tries to activate the antagonist at a joint, the reduced irritability threshold of the agonist may prematurely activate the muscle and in turn inhibit the action of the antagonist (e.g., tight hip flexors will fire prematurely and may inhibit gluteus activation during hip extension). Consequently, hypertonic muscles decrease the neural drive to the opposing muscle via **reciprocal inhibition.** While both muscles on either side of the joint demonstrate weakness due to their altered length-tension relationship, the reciprocal inhibition of the opposing muscles contributes to further weakening of the antagonist, thereby reducing its ability to generate adequate levels of force to move the joint. When this occurs, the body has to call on other muscles at the joint (i.e., the synergists) that will assume the responsibility of becoming the prime mover, a process called **synergistic dominance** (Sahrmann, 2002). For example, a tight hip flexor may inhibit and weaken the gluteus maximus, forcing the hamstrings (a synergist) to assume a greater role in hip extension (Figure 14-9). Unfortunately, the hamstrings are not designed for this function and may suffer from overuse or overload, increasing the likelihood for tightness and injury. Additionally, as the hamstrings do not offer the same degree of movement control of the femoral head during hip extension as the gluteus maximus does, this also increases the likelihood for dysfunctional movement and injury to the hip over time.

Figure 14-9
Posterior musculature of the hip and knee, prime movers for hip extension (gluteus maximus and hamstrings) and knee flexion (hamstrings and gastrocnemius)

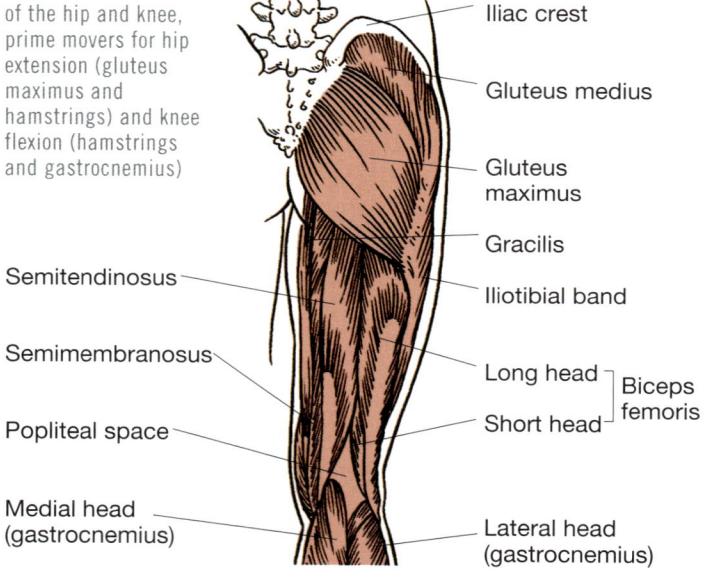

Compromised joint movement alters neuromuscular control and function, prompting additional postural misalignments and faulty loading at the joints that inevitably increases overload and the likelihood for further injury and pain (Figure 14-10). It is therefore imperative that the CMES works to restore and maintain normal joint alignment, joint movement, muscle balance, and muscle function, all of which are critical for optimal health and longevity. Effective programming and attention to exercise technique will help the CMES achieve this goal.

OVERVIEW OF POSTURAL ASSESSMENT

Initial assessments of posture are conducted to estimate the position of the skeletal structures by observing the contours and alignment of the body in comparison to "ideal posture" (Figure 14-11). This evaluation provides a baseline with which to measure a client's starting point and ultimate progress. According to Kendall et al. (2005), ideal posture

Figure 14-10
Pain-compensation cycle

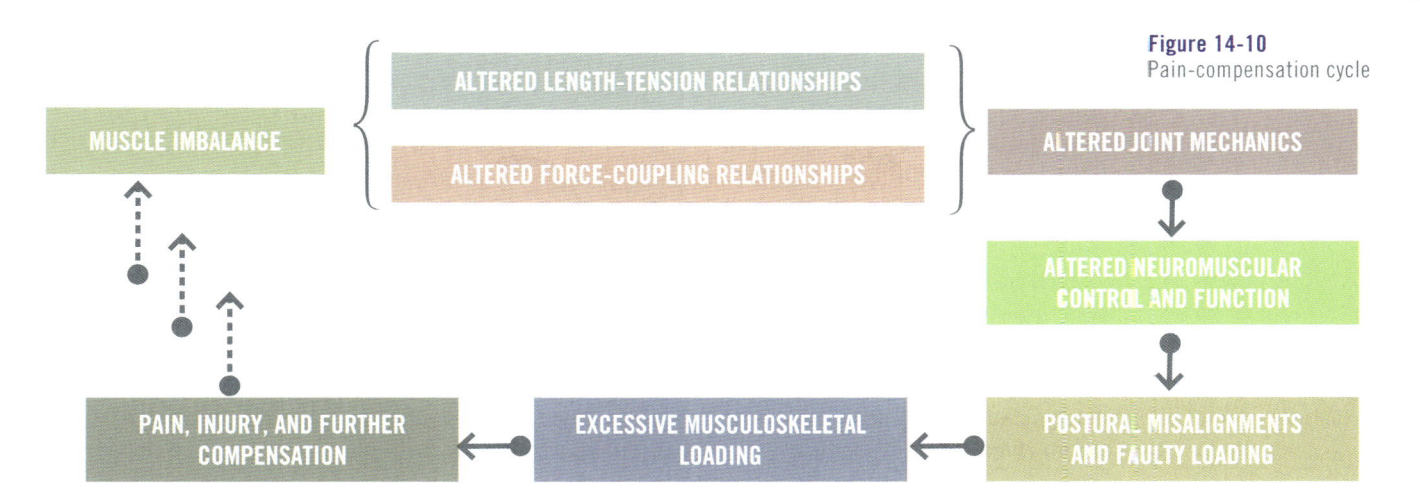

Figure 14-11
Frontal and sagittal views of the spine

represents normal spinal curves, with the bones of the lower extremities in ideal alignment for weight bearing. The "neutral" position of the pelvis allows for a good alignment of the abdomen and trunk and of the extremities below. Optimal functioning of the respiratory organs occurs when the chest and upper back are properly aligned. Lastly, when the head is erect and in a well-balanced position, it minimizes stress on the neck musculature (Kendall et al., 2005).

Postural assessments can provide information that guides exercise programming and helps the CMES achieve an important objective of "straightening the body before strengthening it." This may potentially avoid exacerbating existing postural and movement compensations and muscle–joint imbalances. It is important to remember, however, that while postural assessments provide valuable information, they are only one piece (a starting point) of the movement-efficiency puzzle, and therefore should not be overemphasized. The CMES is encouraged to focus on the obvious, gross imbalances, and avoid getting caught up on minor postural asymmetries. Regardless, the CMES must always respect the **scope of practice,** particularly in the presence of pain or injury, and understand the need for referral to more qualified professionals.

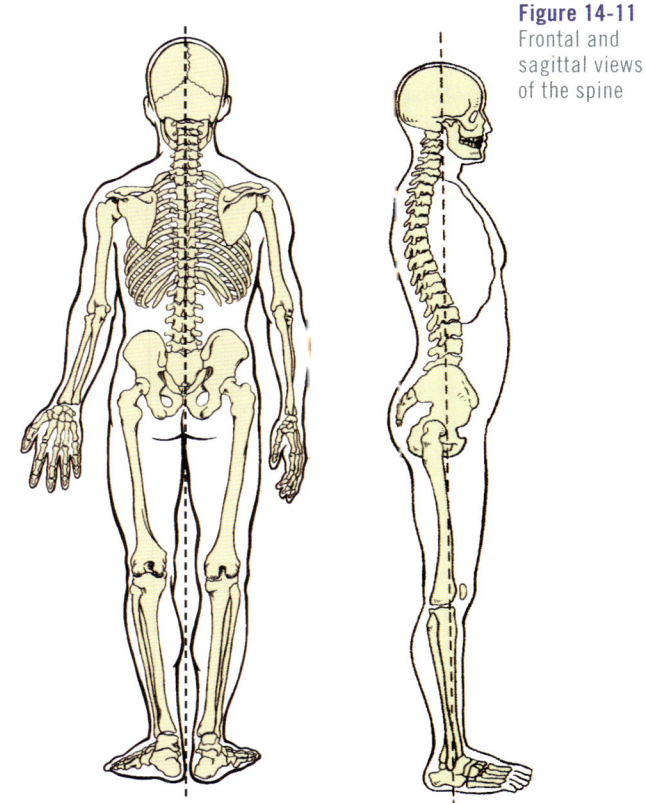

PRACTICAL APPROACHES TO WORKING WITH CLIENTS WHO HAVE PAIN

It is beyond the scope of practice for the CMES to work with clients who currently experience pain from posture or during movement unless cleared by an appropriate orthopedic specialist. In some instances (such as arthritic conditions), the client may be unlikely to be completely pain-free. If a client is cleared with pain conditions, the pain symptoms must be respected and strategies should be implemented to avoid exacerbating painful conditions. In these circumstances, the role of the CMES is to help manage painful conditions. This can be accomplished through integrated approaches designed to prevent excessive stresses to susceptible areas.

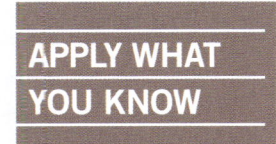

APPLY WHAT YOU KNOW

There are essentially four categories within which clients will fall. A comprehensive screening process should identify and classify a client in one of the following categories:
1. The client has no existing postural/movement faults and experiences no pain.
2. The client has existing postural/movement faults but experiences no pain.
3. The client has no existing postural/movement faults but experiences pain.
4. The client has existing postural/movement faults and experiences pain.

Clients who fall in categories 1 and 2 experience no pain under normal postural or movement conditions and therefore would not necessarily require medical/orthopedic clearance. Category 1 is obviously the best-case scenario, as a client in this category is cleared to begin or continue a fitness-related program that matches their goals and current physiological fitness level (assuming no other risk factors are present). When a client is identified as being in category 2, they would be unlikely to see a doctor or a rehabilitation specialist, as these practitioners are traditionally designated to work with individuals who are injured and/or experiencing pain. In other words, clients do not typically see a doctor, nor do doctors typically refer to rehabilitation experts, if pain and/or injury are not present. It is in these situations that the CMES acts as a preventive expert.

Clients in categories 3 and 4 experience pain and must therefore be referred to an appropriate orthopedic specialist for further diagnosis. Even though category 3 identifies a client who appears to have normal posture and apparently good movement strategies, pain is present and therefore may be a sign that a more serious abnormality or structural issue exists that is impossible to identify through screens and movement/fitness-related analysis. In other words, just because a client moves well does not ensure that they are free of musculoskeletal-related conditions that are beyond the scope for the CMES. Therefore, it is imperative that a CMES never assume a client who moves well, yet experiences pain, is appropriate for an exercise program.

Category 4 identifies clients who experience pain and demonstrate poor posture and movement. In such cases, an evaluation by an orthopedic expert is warranted. However, the CMES does not need to be completely removed from the process. If possible, attempt to communicate with the client's physicians. In most cases, orthopedic experts focus primarily on rehabilitation. With effective communication between practitioners, the CMES can help supervise home-exercise programs prescribed by a rehabilitation expert, as well as identify exercise strategies that are safe to perform with the client.

Client Example

If a client presents with knee pain, for example, it could be determined through clinical evaluations that no structural damage or abnormalities exist in the knee and, therefore, the client could be cleared for exercise. The pain may be a result of postural/movement dysfunction in surrounding areas that are leading to knee discomfort or pain. The CMES may use this opportunity to explore the functionality of movement as a whole. Improvements to knee symptoms in a structurally sound knee may be achieved by exploring a client's movement patterns. Inefficient movement patterns distribute forces unevenly to other parts of the body and may result in discomfort or pain. By improving movement patterns, stresses may be properly redistributed to other areas of the body, alleviating excessive stress to the symptomatic area.

Exploring the functionality of the surrounding areas can also be beneficial. Special considerations for foot/ankle and hip function should be explored. When considering the chain reactions throughout the body, dysfunction at the foot/ankle and/or the hip can have a direct impact on knee mechanics. Therefore, if the knee experiences discomfort or pain and the client is not cleared for standard exercises involving the knee, strategies may be applied that address the areas that are pain-free, but inefficient or dysfunctional. Foot and ankle stability and mobility exercises, as well as hip-dominant exercises designed to identify and improve mobility and stability, will avoid stressing the knee and may aid in improving the functionality of the lower extremity as a whole.

The same can be true of other common problematic areas such as the low back and shoulders. For example, a client may have an arthritic lumbar region. Poor rotational hip mobility and/or poor thoracic rotation mobility may result in the lumbar spine taking on excessive rotational forces, irritating arthritic conditions. If the hips and thoracic spine are pain-free, strategies to improve mobility in these areas can create opportunities to re-educate movement patterns that can reduce stresses on the lumbar region. With regards to the shoulder, thoracic mobility and scapular stability can have an impact on the glenohumeral joint.

STATIC POSTURE IS ONLY ONE PIECE OF THE ASSESSMENT PUZZLE

The purpose of postural assessments is to observe the joint positions relative to one another. When postural alignment is altered, joint positions provide information regarding which muscles elongated and which muscles shortened (Kendall et al., 2005). For example, an anterior pelvic tilt means the pelvis is rotated anteriorly relative to the femur and the lumbar spine. This places the hip into relative flexion, holding the origin and **insertion** points of the hip flexor muscles closer together. This would indicate, at rest, that the hip flexors are in a shortened position relative to ideal posture and alignment. Conversely, the hip extensor muscles would then have greater separation from their origin and insertion points, indicating a relative lengthening of these muscles.

If misalignment is identified, the positioning of the joints and muscles are difficult to dispute. However, while associations are found, such as short muscles being "tight" and elongated muscles being "weak," these results cannot be assumed. Some clients may demonstrate altered positions, yet the "shortened" muscles may in fact be flexible and the position of the body may change readily, indicating that other factors may be contributing to the altered position (Kendall et al., 2005). Therefore, while it is important for the CMES to identify postural misalignments and be familiar with common associations for the misalignment, it is equally important not to jump to conclusions about the possible cause.

Static postural assessments provide an opportunity to explore abnormalities more quickly, resulting in identifying effective solutions more efficiently. Additional assessments can help determine and/or confirm the functionality of the muscles associated with joint misalignment. A static postural assessment is best used as a baseline for unconscious postural control and to help identify areas that may need further evaluation. By combining postural assessments with movement assessments, a larger picture can be developed, equipping the CMES with more comprehensive information for program strategies.

EXPAND YOUR KNOWLEDGE

STATIC POSTURAL ASSESSMENT

Static posture represents the alignment of the body's segments, or how the person holds themselves "statically" or "isometrically" in space (Figure 14-12). Holding a proper postural position involves the actions of multiple postural muscles, which are generally the deeper muscles that contain greater concentrations of **type I muscle fibers** and function to hold static positions or low-grade isometric contractions for extended periods. Good posture or structural integrity is defined as that state of musculoskeletal alignment and balance that allows muscles, joints, and nerves to function efficiently (Kendall et al., 2005). However, if a client exhibits deviations in their static position from good posture, this may reflect muscle-endurance issues in the postural muscles and/or potential imbalance at the joints (Tables 14-1 through 14-4 and Figure 14-13). Movement begins from a position of static posture. Therefore, the presence of poor posture is a good indicator that movement may be dysfunctional. Although movement screens offer valuable information related to neuromuscular efficiency, a static postural assessment is considered very useful and serves as a starting point from which a CMES can identify muscle imbalances and potential movement compensations associated with poor posture (Kendall et al., 2005; Sahrmann, 2002). A static posture assessment may offer valuable insight into:

- Muscle imbalance at a joint and the working relationships of muscles around a joint
  - ✓ Muscle imbalance often contributes to dysfunctional movement.
- Altered neural action of the muscles moving and controlling the joint
  - ✓ For example, tight or shortened muscles are often overactive and dominate movement at the joint, potentially disrupting healthy joint mechanics.

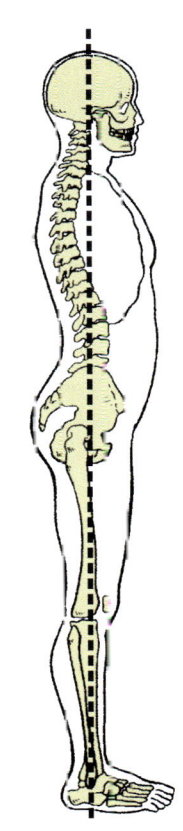

Figure 14-12
Neutral spine alignment with slight anterior (lordotic) curves at the neck and low back and a posterior (kyphotic) curve in the thoracic region

CHAPTER 14
Posture and Movement

TABLE 14-1	
MUSCLE IMBALANCES ASSOCIATED WITH LORDOSIS POSTURE	
Facilitated/Hypertonic (Shortened)	Inhibited (Lengthened)
Hip flexors	Hip extensors
Lumbar extensors	External obliques
	Rectus abdominis

TABLE 14-2	
MUSCLE IMBALANCES ASSOCIATED WITH KYPHOSIS POSTURE	
Facilitated/Hypertonic (Shortened)	Inhibited (Lengthened)
Anterior chest/shoulders	Upper-back extensors
Latissimus dorsi	Scapular stabilizers
Neck extensors	Neck flexors

TABLE 14-3	
MUSCLE IMBALANCES ASSOCIATED WITH FLAT-BACK POSTURE	
Facilitated/Hypertonic (Shortened)	Inhibited (Lengthened)
Rectus abdominis	Iliacus/psoas major
Upper-back extensors	Internal obliques
Neck extensors	Lumbar extensors
Ankle plantar flexors	Neck flexors

TABLE 14-4	
MUSCLE IMBALANCES ASSOCIATED WITH SWAY-BACK POSTURE	
Facilitated/Hypertonic (Shortened)	Inhibited (Lengthened)
Hamstrings	Iliacus/psoas major
Upper fibers of posterior obliques	Rectus femoris
Lumbar extensors	External obliques
Neck extensors	Upper-back extensors
	Neck flexors

Figure 14-13
Postural deviations

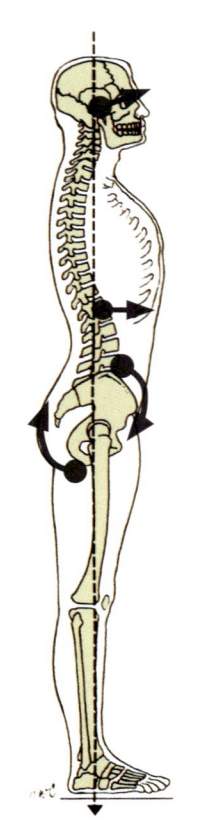

a. Lordosis: increased anterior lumbar curve from neutral

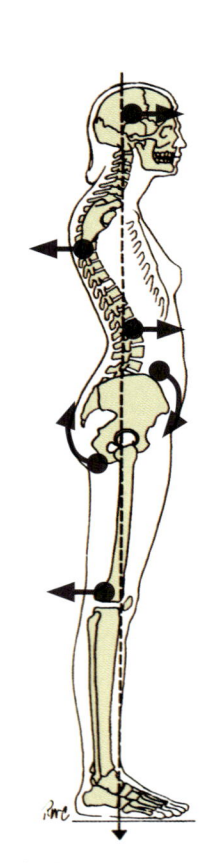

b. Kyphosis: increased posterior thoracic curve from neutral

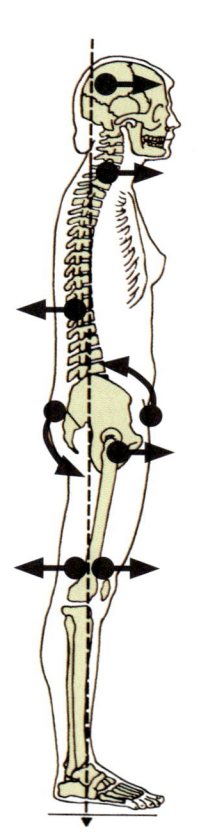

c. Flat back: decreased anterior lumbar curve

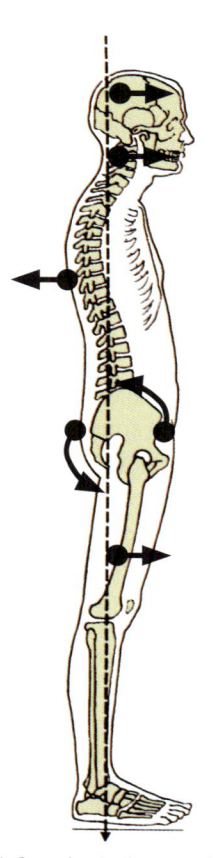

d. Sway back: decreased anterior lumbar curve and increased posterior thoracic curve from neutral

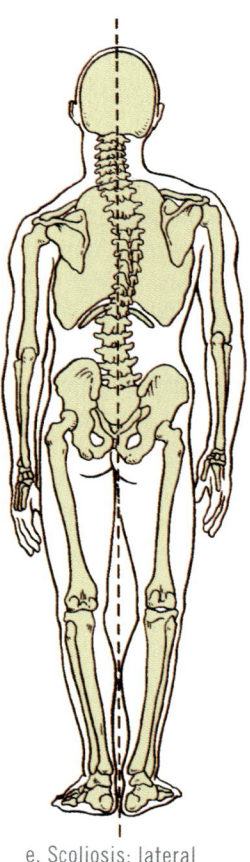

e. Scoliosis: lateral spinal curvature often accompanied by vertebral rotation

Posture and Movement   CHAPTER 14

> **THINK IT THROUGH**
>
> Carefully read through the information presented in Tables 14-1 through 14-4. Because the postures depicted are common deviations, you are likely to observe clients with one or more of these variants. Think about methods you would employ to help clients with these muscle imbalances. Can you come up with at least one stretch for each tight muscle group and one strengthening exercise for each inhibited muscle group?

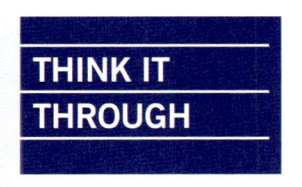

Muscle imbalance and postural deviations can be attributed to many factors that are both correctable and non-correctable, including the following:
- Correctable factors:
  - ✓ Repetitive movements (muscular pattern overload)
  - ✓ Awkward positions and movements (habitually poor posture)
  - ✓ Side dominance
  - ✓ Lack of joint stability
  - ✓ Lack of joint mobility
  - ✓ Imbalanced strength-training programs
- Non-correctable factors:
  - ✓ Congenital conditions (e.g., **scoliosis**)
  - ✓ Some pathologies (e.g., **rheumatoid arthritis**)
  - ✓ Structural deviations (e.g., tibial or femoral **torsion,** or femoral **anteversion**)
  - ✓ Certain types of trauma (e.g., surgery, injury, or amputation)

Proper postural alignment promotes optimal neural activity of the muscles controlling and moving the joint. When joints are correctly aligned, the length-tension relationships and force-coupling relationships function efficiently. This facilitates proper joint mechanics, allowing the body to generate and accept forces throughout the kinetic chain, and promotes joint stability and mobility and movement efficiency. Figure 14-14 illustrates the importance of muscle balance and its contribution to movement efficiency. Given how an individual's static posture reflects potential muscle imbalance, it stands to reason that a CMES should consider conducting a static postural assessment on their clients as an initial assessment.

Given the propensity many individuals have toward poor posture, an initial focus of the CMES should be to restore stability and mobility within the body and attempt to "straighten the body before strengthening it." The CMES can therefore start by looking at a client's static posture following the right-angle rule of the body (Kendall et al., 2005). This model demonstrates how the human body represents itself in vertical alignment across the major joints—the ankle (and subtalar joint), knee, hip, and shoulder, as well as the head. This model allows the observer to look at the individual in all three planes to note specific "static" asymmetries at the joints (e.g., front to back and left to right). As illustrated in Figure 14-15,

Figure 14-14
Movement efficiency pattern

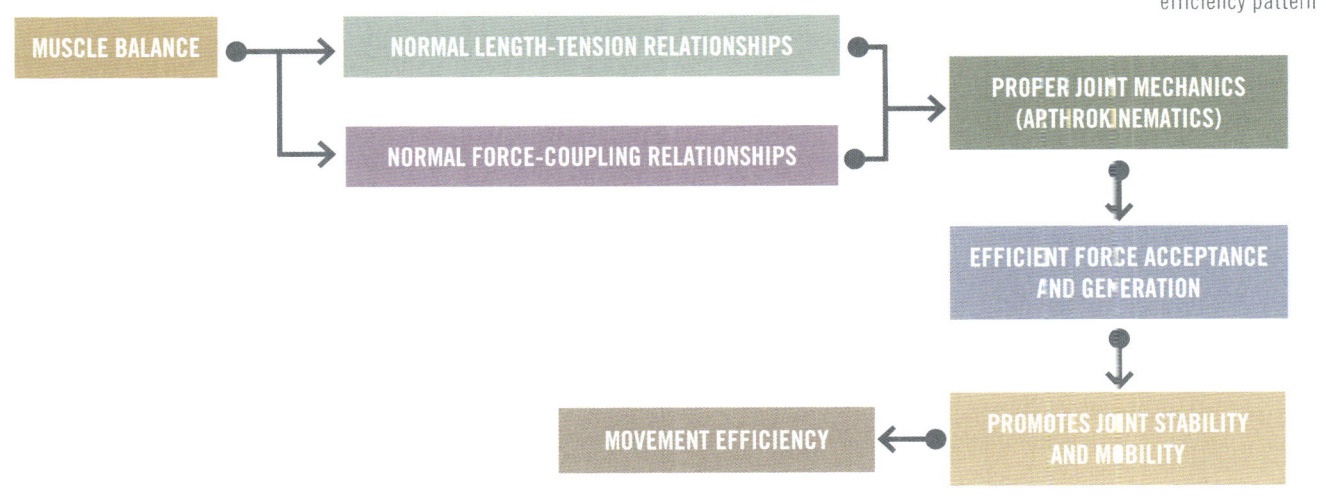

Figure 14-15
The right-angle rule (frontal and sagittal views)

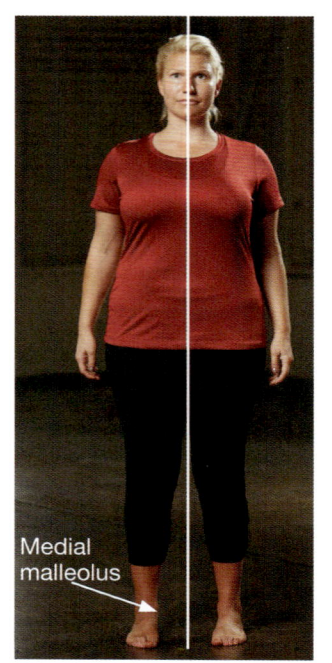

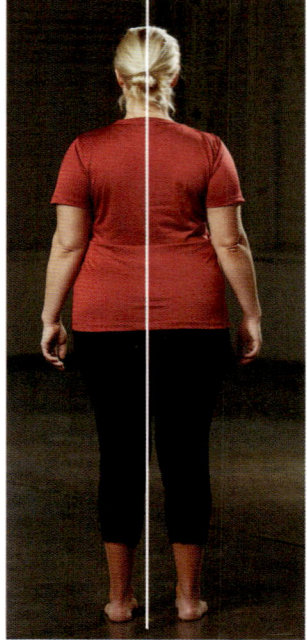

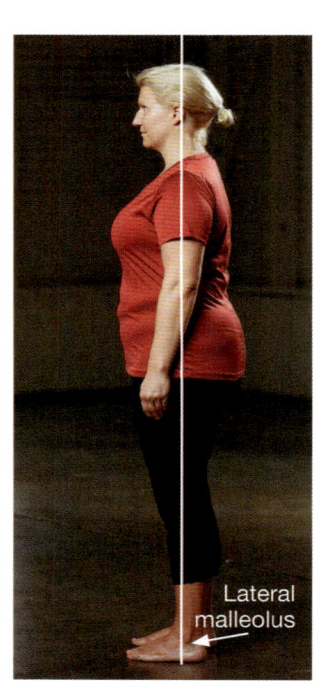

a. Frontal view (anterior)   b. Frontal view (posterior)   c. Sagittal view

the right-angle model implies a state from a frontal view wherein the two hemispheres are equally divided, and wherein the anterior and posterior surfaces appear in balance from a sagittal view. The body is in good postural position when the body parts are symmetrically balanced around the body's **line of gravity,** which is the intersection of the mid-frontal and mid-sagittal planes and is represented by a plumb line hanging from a fixed point overhead.

While this model helps the CMES identify postural compensations and potential muscle imbalances, it is important to recognize that limitations exist in using this model.

Plumb Line Instructions

Using a length of string and an inexpensive weight (e.g., a washer), a CMES can create a plumb line that suspends from a ceiling or fixed point to a height 0.5 to 1 inch (1.3 to 2.5 cm) above the floor. It is important to select a location that offers a solid, plain backdrop or a grid pattern with vertical and horizontal lines that offer contrast against the client. When conducting these assessments, the CMES should instruct the client to wear form-fitting athletic-style clothing to expose as many joints and bony landmarks as possible, and have the client remove their shoes and socks. The use of adhesive dots placed upon the bony landmarks may assist the CMES in identifying postural deviations.

The objective of this assessment is to observe the client's symmetry against the plumb line and the right angles that the weight-bearing joints make relative to the line of gravity. Individuals will consciously or subconsciously attempt to correct posture when they are aware they are being observed. The CMES should encourage clients to assume a normal, relaxed posture, and utilize distractions such as casual conversation to encourage this relaxed posture. It is important to remember that while postural assessments provide valuable information, they are only one piece to the movement-efficiency puzzle, and thus should not be overemphasized.

The CMES should focus on the obvious, gross imbalances and avoid getting caught up in minor postural asymmetries. Bear in mind that the body is rarely perfectly symmetrical (such as the slight imbalance in weight-bearing between the right and left feet of the subject in Figure 14-15) and that overanalyzing asymmetries is time-consuming, potentially intimidating to clients, and may induce muscle fatigue in the client that can alter their posture even further. Therefore, when looking for gross deviations, the CMES should select an acceptable margin of asymmetry that they will allow and focus on larger, more obvious discrepancies. For example, start by focusing on gross deviations that differ by a quarter-inch (0.6 cm) or more between the compartments of the body.

Plumb Line Positions

Frontal Views (Anterior and Posterior)
Source: Kendall et al., 2005
- For the anterior view, position the client between the plumb line and a wall, facing the plumb line with the feet equidistant from the suspended line (using the inside of the heels or medial malleoli as a reference) (see Figure 14-15a).
- With good posture, the plumb line will pass equidistant between the feet and ankles, and intersect the pubis, umbilicus, sternum, mandible (chin), maxilla (face), and frontal bone (forehead).
- For the posterior view, position the individual between the plumb line and a wall, facing away from the plumb line with the insides of the heels equidistant from the suspended line (see Figure 14-15b).
- With good posture, the plumb line should ideally bisect the sacrum and overlap the spinous processes of the spine.

Sagittal View
Source: Kendall et al., 2005
- Position the individual between the plumb line and the wall, facing sideways with the plumb line aligned immediately anterior to the lateral malleolus (anklebone) (see Figure 14-15c).
- With good posture, the plumb line should ideally pass through the anterior third of the knee, the greater trochanter of the femur, and the acromioclavicular (AC) joint, and slightly anterior to the mastoid process of the temporal bone of the skull (in line with, or just behind, the ear lobe) (see Figure 14-12).

Transverse View
Source: Kendall et al., 2005
- All transverse views of the limbs and torso are performed from frontal- and sagittal-plane positions.
- The CMES should look for an obvious misalignment in rotation at the limbs and the torso For example, a patella that faces any direction other than forward, or a hip or rib that protrudes more prominently than the other could indicate transverse plane faults.

The CMES must respect scope of practice when performing a postural assessment on clients, particularly in the presence of pain or injury. It is important to understand the need for referral to more qualified healthcare professionals when pain or underlying pathologies are present (e.g., scoliosis).

When conducting assessments of posture and movement, the following key components should be included (Figure 14-16).
- Client history—written and verbal
    - ✓ Collect information on musculoskeletal issues, congenital issues (e.g., scoliosis), trauma, injuries, pain and discomfort, the site of pain or discomfort, and what aggravates and relieves pain or discomfort (e.g., with discomfort in the upper back, the client may feel temporary relief by hunching forward and rounding the shoulders).
    - ✓ Collect lifestyle information, including occupation, side-dominance, and habitual patterns (information regarding these patterns may take time to gather).
- Visual and manual observation
    - ✓ Identify observable postural deviations.
    - ✓ Verify muscle imbalance as determined by muscle-length testing.
    - ✓ Determine the impact on movement ability or efficiency by performing movement screens.
    - ✓ Facilitate movement to distinguish correctable from non-correctable compensations.

While postural assessments can be performed in great detail, the following sections address five key postural deviations that occur frequently in individuals.

Figure 14-16
A chronological plan for conducting postural assessments and movement screens

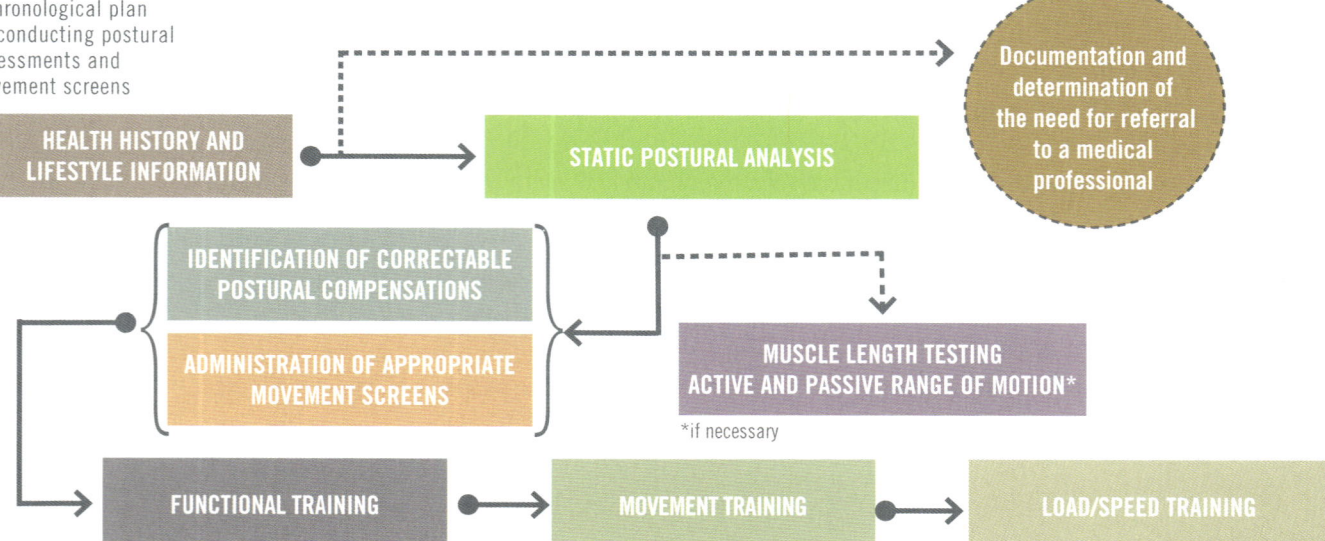

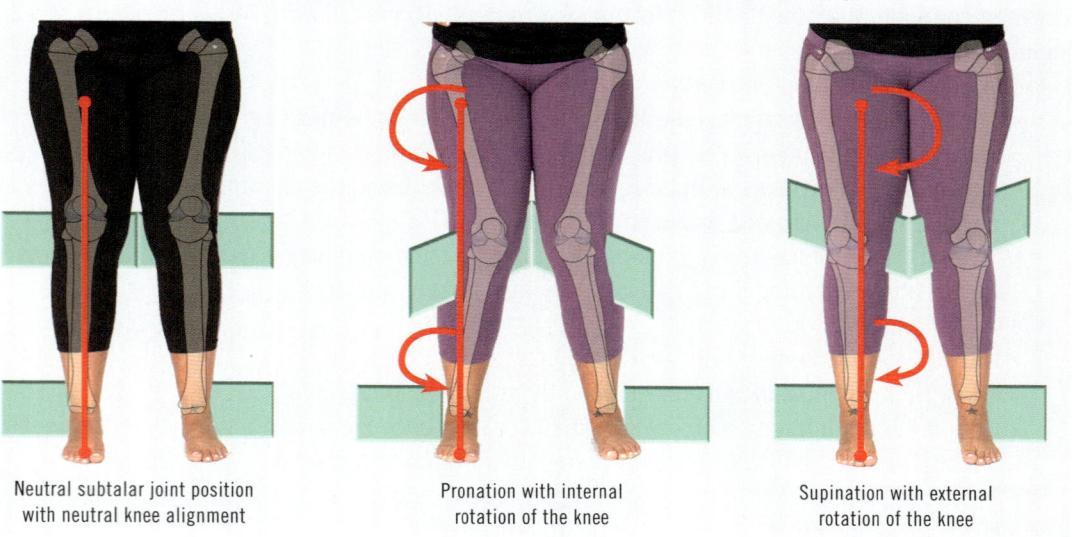

Deviation 1: Foot Pronation/Supination and the Effect on Tibial and Femoral Rotation

Both feet should face forward in parallel or with slight (8 to 10 degrees) external rotation (toes pointing outward from the midline, as the ankle joint lies in an oblique plane with the medial malleolus slightly anterior to the lateral malleolus) (see Figure 14-15). The toes should be aligned in the same direction as the feet and any excessive pronation (arch flattening) or supination (high arches) at the subtalar joint should be noted.

APPLY WHAT YOU KNOW

KINETIC CHAIN: SUBTALAR POSITION AND TIBIAL AND FEMORAL ROTATION

Because the body is one continuous kinetic chain, the position of the subtalar joint will impact the position of the tibia and femur. Barring structural differences in the skeletal system (e.g., tibial torsion or femoral anteversion), a pronated subtalar joint position typically forces internal rotation of the tibia and slightly less internal rotation of the femur (Figure 14-17 and Table 14-5). To demonstrate this point, stand with shoes off and place the hands firmly on the fronts of the thighs. Notice what happens to the orientation of the knees and thighs when moving between pronation and supination. Additionally, notice how the calcaneus everts as the subtalar joint is pronated.

Figure 14-17
Foot pronation and supination and the effects up the kinetic chain

Neutral subtalar joint position with neutral knee alignment

Pronation with internal rotation of the knee

Supination with external rotation of the knee

Posture and Movement

CHAPTER 14

TABLE 14-5
SUBTALAR JOINT PRONATION/SUPINATION AND THE EFFECT ON THE FEET, TIBIA, AND FEMUR

Subtalar Joint Movement	Foot Movement	Tibial (Knee) Movement	Femoral Movement	Frontal Plane
Pronation	Eversion	Internal rotation	Internal rotation	Anterior view
Supination	Inversion	External rotation	External rotation	Anterior view

Subtalar joint pronation forces internal rotation at the tibia, flexion at the knee, and hip flexion and internal rotation when weight bearing. Additional stresses on some knee ligaments and the integrity of the joint itself may lead to injury during ambulation if the joint remains in pronation (Houglum, 2010). Additionally, closed-chain pronation tends to move the calcaneus into eversion, which may actually lift the outside of the heel slightly off the ground (moving the ankle into **plantar flexion**). In turn, this may tighten the calf muscles and potentially limit ankle **dorsiflexion,** but the CMES should keep in mind that the opposite is also true: A tight gastrocnemius and soleus complex (triceps surae) may force calcaneal eversion in an otherwise neutral subtalar joint position (Gray & Tiberio, 2006) (Figure 14-18).

To illustrate this point, stand barefoot facing a wall with the feet 36 inches (0.9 m) away. Extend both arms in front of the body, placing the hands on the wall for support. Slowly lean forward, flexing the elbows and dorsiflexing the ankles while keeping both heels firmly pressed into the floor. Observe for any movement in the feet (e.g., appearance of the arch collapsing with calcaneal eversion). As a tight gastrocnemius and soleus complex reach the limit of their extensibility, the body may need to evert the calcaneus to allow further movement. This scenario may occur repeatedly in gait immediately prior to the push-off phase if the gastrocnemius and soleus complex are tight, forcing calcaneal eversion and subtalar joint pronation.

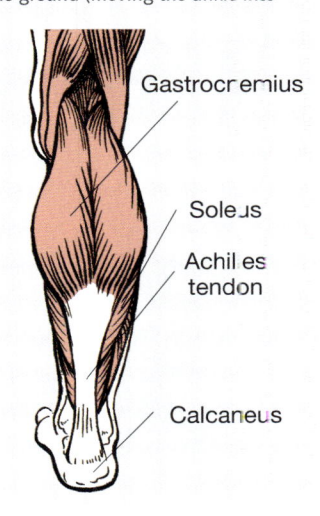

Figure 14-18
Triceps surae (i.e., gastrocnemius and soleus) are the posterior tibial compartment muscles primarily responsible for plantar flexion of the ankle

Deviation 2: Hip Adduction

In standing and in gait, hip adduction is a lateral tilt of the pelvis that elevates one hip higher than the other (also called "hip hiking"), which may be evident in individuals who have a limb-length discrepancy (Sahrmann, 2002). If a person raises the right hip as illustrated in Figure 14-19, the line of gravity following the spine tilts over toward the left, moving the right thigh closer to this line of gravity. Consequently, the right hip is identified as moving into adduction. This position progressively lengthens and weakens the right hip abductors, which are unable to hold the hip level (Table 14-6). Sleeping on one's side can produce a similar effect, as the hip abductors of the upper hip fail to hold the hip level.

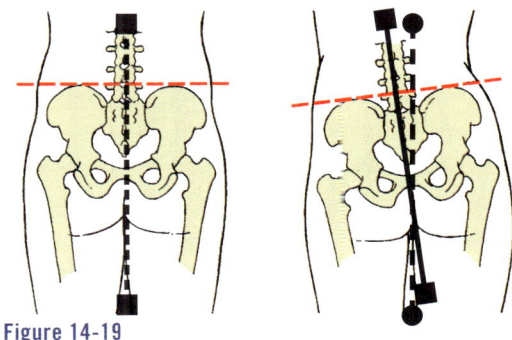

Figure 14-19
Normal hip position versus right hip adduction (posterior view)

Source: LifeART image copyright 2008 Wolters Kluwer Health, Inc., Lippincott Williams & Wilkins. All rights reserved.

TABLE 14-6
HIP ADDUCTION

Observation	Position	Alignment	Frontal Plane
Right hip adduction	Elevated (vs. left side)	Hips usually shifted right	Posterior view
Left hip adduction	Elevated (vs. right side)	Hips usually shifted left	Posterior view

Figure 14-20
Anterior musculature of the hip and knee, prime movers for hip flexion (iliacus, psoas major and minor) and knee extension

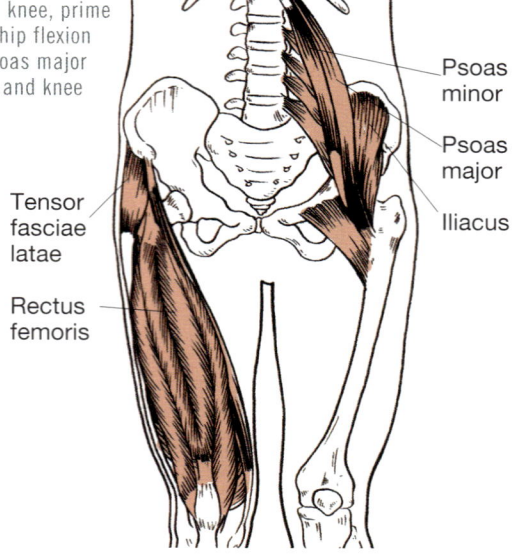

Deviation 3: Pelvic Tilting (Anterior or Posterior)

Anterior tilting of the pelvis frequently occurs in individuals with tight hip flexors, which is generally associated with **sedentary** lifestyles where individuals spend countless hours in seated (i.e., shortened hip flexor) positions (Kendall et al., 2005) (Figure 14-20). With standing, this shortened hip flexor pulls the pelvis into an anterior tilt (i.e., the superior, anterior portion of the pelvis rotates downward and forward) (see Figure 14-7). As illustrated in Figure 14-21, an anterior pelvic tilt rotates the superior, anterior portion of the pelvis forward and downward, spilling water out of the front of the bucket, whereas a posterior tilt rotates the superior, posterior portion of the pelvis backward and downward, spilling water out of the back of the bucket. Figure 14-22 illustrates the alignment of the anterior superior iliac spine and posterior superior iliac spine in neutral alignment, as well in anterior and posterior pelvic tilts.

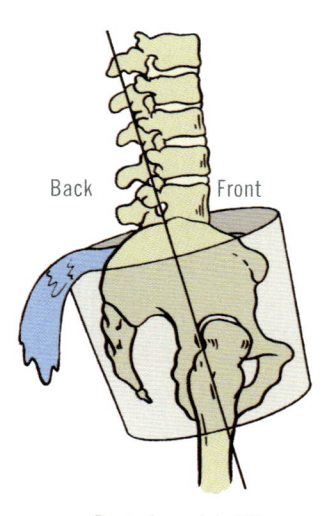

Figure 14-21
Anterior and posterior tilting of the pelvis—sagittal (side) view

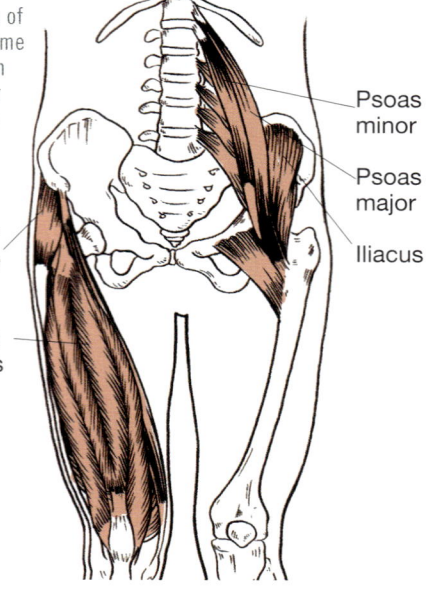

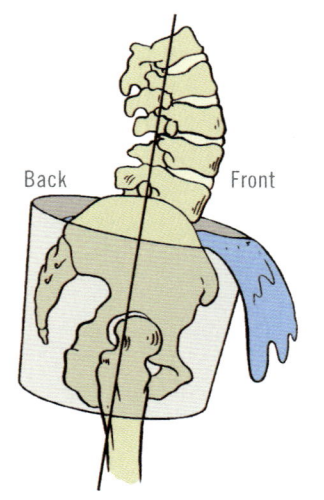

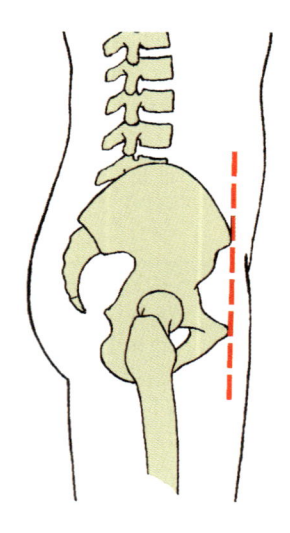

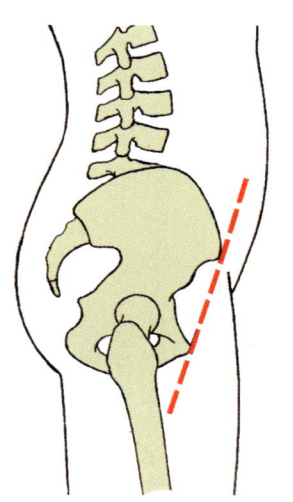

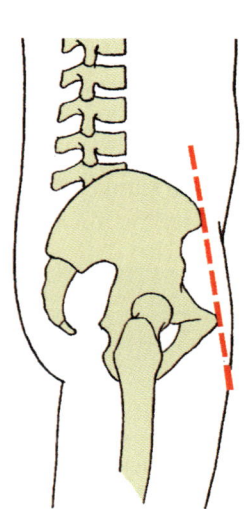

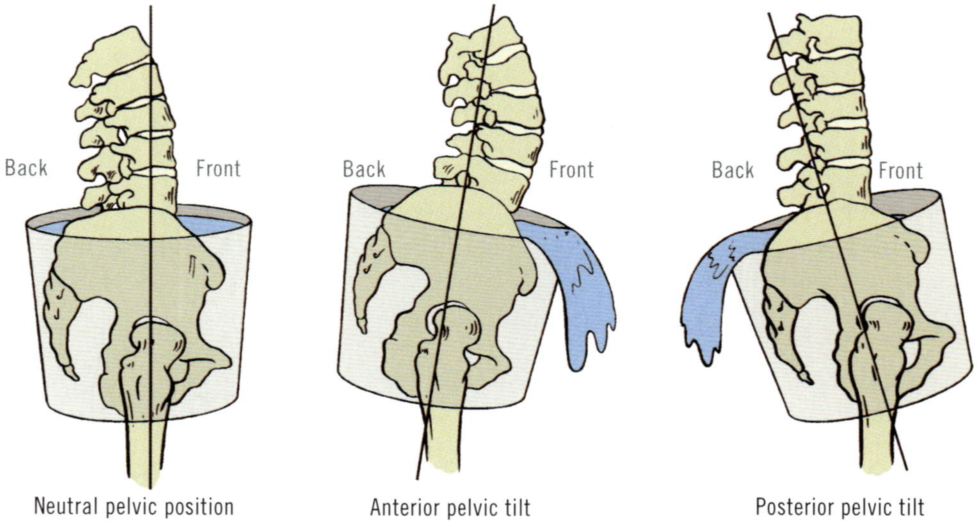

Figure 14-22
Alignment of the anterior superior iliac spine (ASIS) and pubic bone

Source: LifeART image copyright 2008 Wolters Kluwer Health, Inc., Lippincott Williams & Wilkins. All rights reserved.

Posture and Movement

CHAPTER 14

PELVIC TILT

An anterior pelvic tilt will increase lordosis in the lumbar spine, whereas a posterior pelvic tilt will reduce the amount of lordosis in the lumbar spine. To demonstrate this point, a CMES can stand with hands placed on the hips and gently tilt their pelvis anteriorly, noticing the change in position and increase in muscle tension in the lumbar region. Likewise, the CMES can tilt the pelvis posteriorly and notice how the lumbar spine flattens and reduces tension in the lumbar extensors.

APPLY WHAT YOU KNOW

Tight or overdominant hip flexors are generally coupled with tight erector spinae muscles (Figure 14-23), producing an anterior pelvic tilt, while tight or overdominant rectus abdominis muscles are generally coupled with tight hamstrings, producing a posterior pelvic tilt (Table 14-7). This coupling relationship between tight hip flexors and erector spinae is defined by Vladimir Janda as lower-cross syndrome (Morris et al., 2006). With foot pronation and accompanying internal femoral rotation, the pelvis may tilt anteriorly to better accommodate the head of the femur, demonstrating the point of an integrated kinetic chain whereby foot pronation can increase lumbar lordosis due to an anterior pelvic tilt (Sahrmann, 2002).

Figure 14-23
The erector spinae muscles and hamstrings (posterior view)

- Longissimus
- Spinalis
- Iliocostalis
- Biceps Femoris
- Semitendinosus
- Semimembranosus

TABLE 14-7
PELVIC TILT

	Anterior Tilt	Posterior Tilt
Rotation	ASIS tilts downward and forward	ASIS tilts upward and backward
Muscles suspected to be tight	Hip flexors, erector spinae	Rectus abdominis, hamstrings
Muscles suspected to be lengthened	Hamstrings, rectus abdominis	Hip flexors, erector spinae
Plane of view	View from the side	View from the side

Note: ASIS = Anterior superior iliac spine

Deviation 4: Shoulder Position and the Thoracic Spine

Limitations and compensations to movement at the shoulder occur frequently due to the complex nature of the shoulder-girdle design and the varied movements performed at the shoulder. It is important that the CMES understand the collaborative function of the scapulothoracic region (the scapulae and associated muscles attaching them to the thorax) and glenohumeral joint to produce shoulder movements. While the glenohumeral joint is highly mobile and perhaps a less stable joint, the scapulothoracic joint is designed to offer greater stability with less mobility. However, it is important to remember that it still contributes approximately 60 degrees of movement in raising the arms overhead, with the glenohumeral joint contributing the remaining 120 degrees (Figure 14-24). The scapulothoracic joint also promotes many important movements of the scapulae (Figure 14-25). Collectively, however, they allow for a diverse range of movements in the

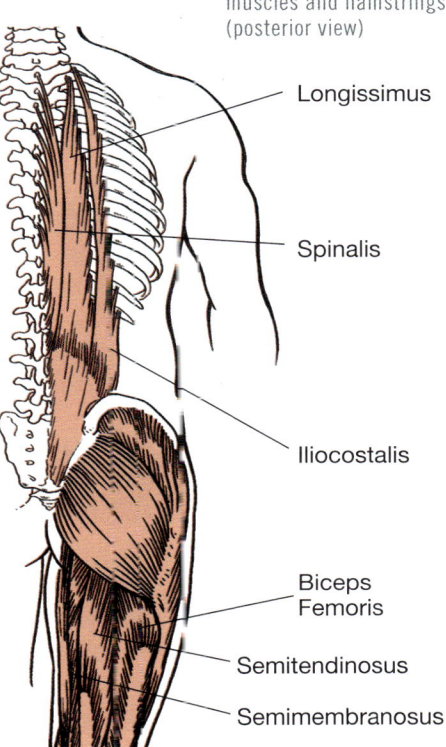

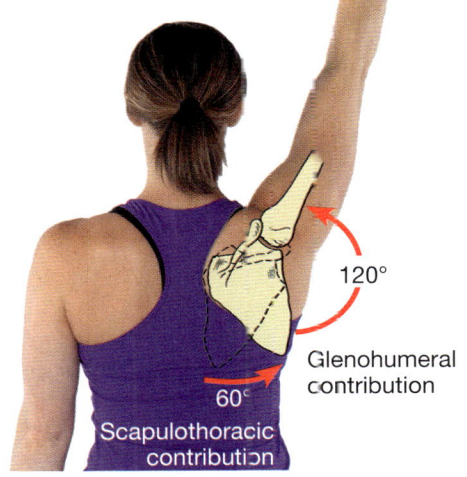

Figure 14-24
Scapulohumeral rhythm

The movement of the arm is accompanied by movement of the scapula—a ratio of approximately 2° of arm movement for every 1° of scapular movement occurs during shoulder abduction and flexion.

Figure 14-25
Scapular movements

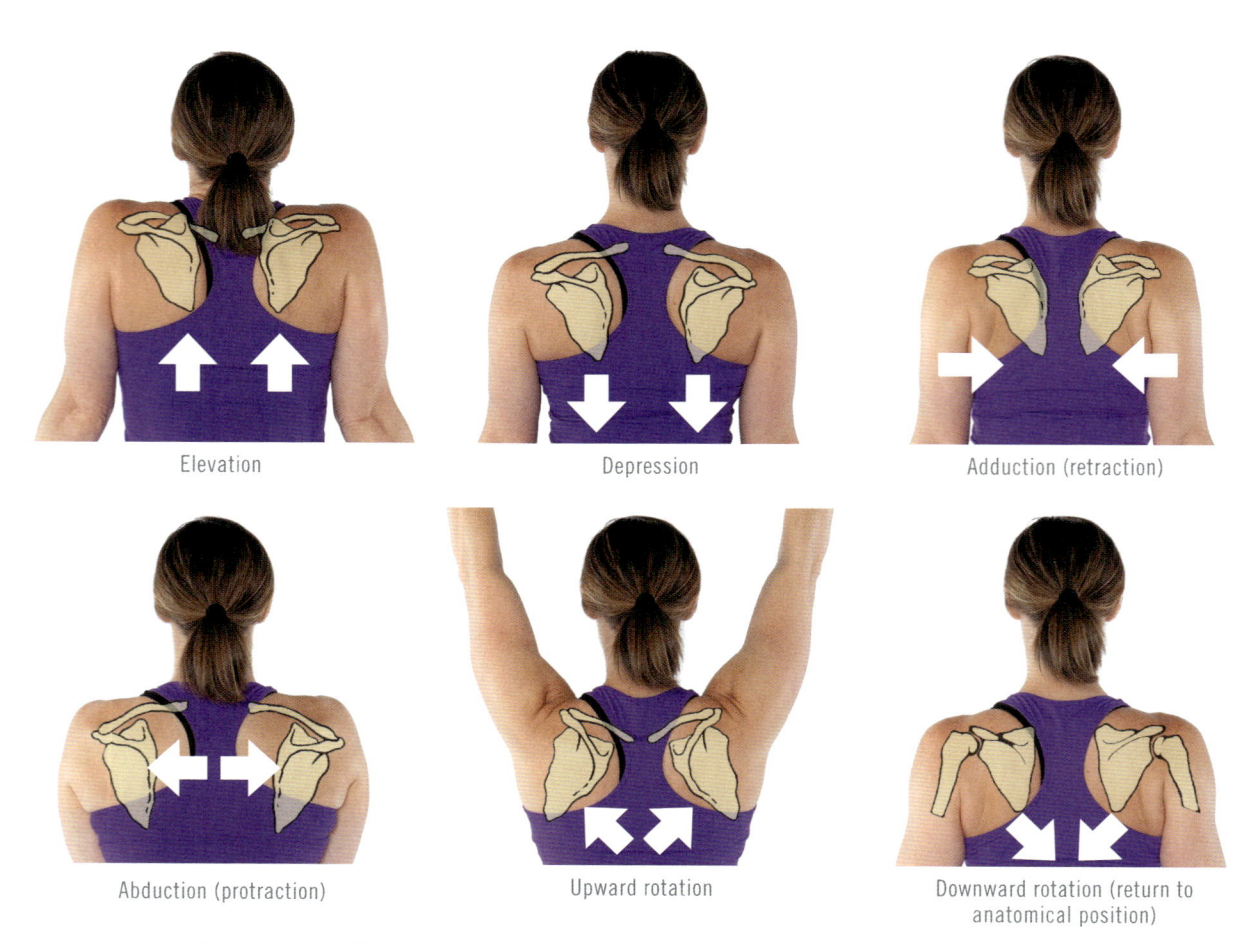

Elevation

Depression

Adduction (retraction)

Abduction (protraction)

Upward rotation

Downward rotation (return to anatomical position)

shoulder complex. Observation of the position of the scapulae in all three planes provides good insight into a client's quality of movement at the shoulders.

Figure 14-26 illustrates the "resting" position of the scapulae, which can vary considerably from person to person. The vertebral (**medial**) border of the scapula is typically positioned between the second and seventh ribs and vertically about 2 inches (5.1 cm) from the spinous processes (Houglum, 2010; Kendall et al., 2005). While the glenoid fossa is tilted upward 5 degrees and anteriorly 30 degrees to optimally articulate with the head of the humerus, the scapulae usually lie flat against the rib cage (Kendall et al., 2005). While the scapulae should appear flat against the rib cage, their orientation depends on the size and shape of the person and the rib cage.

Figure 14-26
The normal position of the scapulae

- Medial border of the scapula
- Head of the humerus
- Glenoid fossa
- Inferior angle of the scapula

SCAPULAR WINGING AND SCAPULAR PROTRACTION

The CMES can perform a quick observational assessment to identify scapular winging and scapular protraction. While looking at the client from the posterior view, if the vertebral (medial) and/or inferior angle of the scapulae protrude outward, this indicates an inability of the scapular stabilizers (primarily the rhomboids and serratus anterior) to hold the scapulae in place. Noticeable protrusion of the vertebral (medial) border outward is termed "scapular protraction" (Figure 14-27a), while protrusion of the inferior angle and vertebral (medial) border outward is termed "winged scapulae" (Figure 14-27b).

Scapular protraction can also be identified from the anterior view. If the palms face backward instead of to the sides, this generally indicates internal (medial) rotation of the humerus and/or scapular protraction (Figure 14-28).

Table 14-8 lists key deviations of the thoracic spine and shoulders in various planes of view.

Note: There is often a natural amount of "shrugging" inward with scapular protraction.

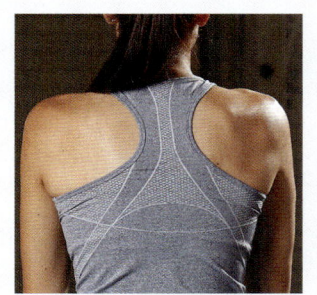

APPLY WHAT YOU KNOW

a. Scapular protraction

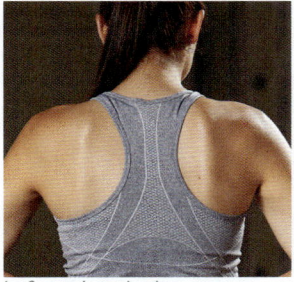

b. Scapular winging

Figure 14-27
Scapular protraction and winging: Posterior view

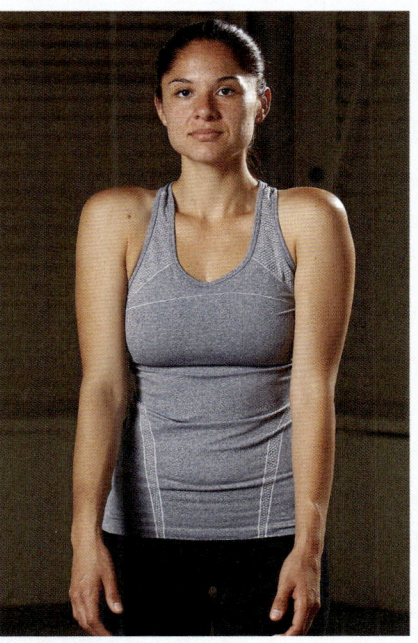

Figure 14-28
Scapular protraction: Anterior view

TABLE 14-8
SHOULDER POSITION

Observation	Muscles Suspected to Be Tight	Plane of View
Shoulders not level	Upper trapezius, levator scapula, rhomboids on the elevated side	Frontal
Asymmetry to midline	Lateral trunk flexors (flexed side)	Frontal
Protracted (forward, rounded)	Serratus anterior*, anterior scapulo-humeral muscles, upper trapezius	Sagittal
Medially rotated humerus	Pectoralis major and latissimus dorsi (shoulder adductors), subscapularis	Frontal
Kyphosis and depressed chest	Shoulder adductors, pectoralis minor, rectus abdominis, internal oblique	Sagittal

*Serratus anterior is usually tight with scapular protraction and is usually lengthened with scapular winging.

Deviation 5: Head Position

With good posture, the earlobe should align approximately over the acromion process, but given the many awkward postures and repetitive motions of daily life, a forward-head position is very common (Table 14-9) (Kendall et al., 2005). This altered position does not tilt the head downward, but simply shifts it forward so that the earlobe appears significantly forward of the acromioclavicular joint. To observe the presence of this imbalance, use the sagittal view, aligning the plumb line with the acromioclavicular joint, and observe its position relative to the ear (Figure 14-29) (Price, 2010). A forward-head position represents tightness in the cervical extensors and lengthening of the cervical flexors. To demonstrate this point, a CMES can place one thumb on their manubrium (top of the sternum) and the index finger of the same hand on the chin. Slowly slide the head forward and observe how the spacing between the fingers increases, representing the change in muscle length. An alternative option for observing forward-head position is via the alignment of the cheek bone and the collarbone. With good posture, they should almost be in vertical alignment with each other. To demonstrate this point, have a client place one finger on their collar bone (aligned under the cheek) and place another finger on the cheek bone (aligned under the eye) as illustrated in Figure 14-30 (Price, 2010). From the sagittal plane, the CMES can observe the vertical alignment of the two fingers.

TABLE 14-9
HEAD POSITION

Observation	Muscles Suspected to Be Tight	Plane of View
Forward-head position	Cervical spine extensors, upper trapezius, levator scapulae	Sagittal

Figure 14-29
Alignment of the acromioclavicular joint with the ear

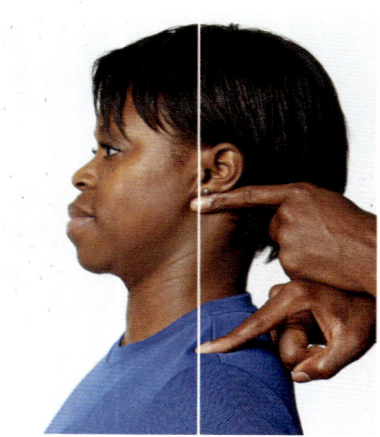

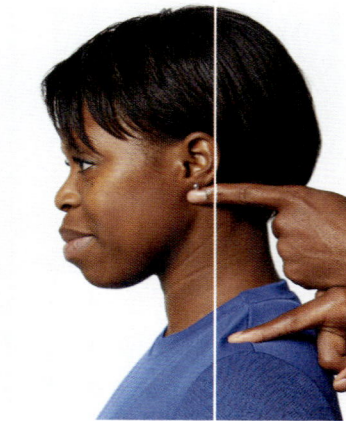

Good posture | Forward-head position

Figure 14-30
Alignment of the collar bone and cheek bone

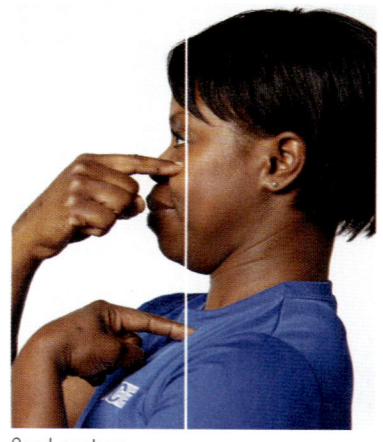

Good posture | Forward-head position

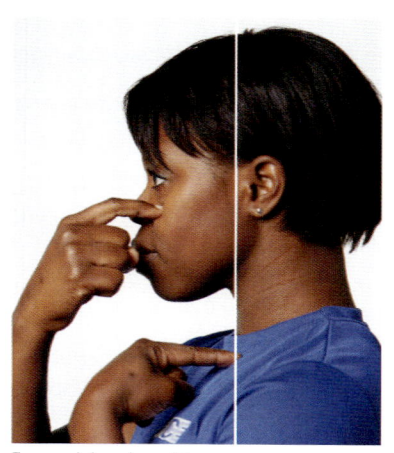

Postural Assessment Checklist and Worksheets

When performing basic postural assessments, the CMES can use the checklist provided in Figure 14-31 to guide themself through the observations, and complete the worksheets provided in Figures 14-32 and 14-33 to mark any postural compensations identified.

	ANTERIOR VIEW
☐	Overall body symmetry: symmetrical alignment of the left and right hemispheres
☐	Ankle position: observe for pronation and supination
☐	Foot position: observe for inversion and eversion
☐	Knees: rotation and height discrepancies
☐	Hip adduction and shifting: observe for shifting to a side as witnessed by the position of the pubis in relation to the line of gravity
☐	Alignment of the iliac crests
☐	Alignment of the torso: position of the umbilicus and sternum in relation to the line of gravity
☐	Alignment of the shoulders
☐	Arm spacing: observe the space to the sides of the torso
☐	Hand position: observe the position relative to the torso
☐	Head position: alignment of the ears, nose, eyes, and chin

	POSTERIOR VIEW
☐	Overall body symmetry: symmetrical alignment of the left and right hemispheres
☐	Alignment of the spine: vertical alignment of the spinous processes (may require forward bending)
☐	Alignment of the scapulae: inferior angle of scapulae and presence of winged scapulae
☐	Alignment of the shoulders
☐	Head: alignment of the ears

	SIDE VIEW
☐	Overall body symmetry: symmetrical alignment of load-bearing joint landmarks with the line of gravity
☐	Knees: flexion or extension
☐	Pelvic alignment for tilting: relationship of ASIS to PSIS
☐	Spinal curves: observe for thoracic kyphosis, lumbar lordosis, or flat-back position
☐	Shoulder position: forward rounding (protraction) of the scapulae
☐	Head position: neutral cervical curvature (versus forward position) and level (position above the clavicle)

Note: ASIS = Anterior superior iliac spine; PSIS = Posterior superior iliac spine

Figure 14-31
Postural assessment checklist

Visit www.ACEfitness.org/CMESresources to download a free PDF of the postural assessment checklist and worksheets, as well as other forms and tools that you can use throughout your career as a CMES.

CHAPTER 14

Posture and Movement

ANTERIOR VIEW:			POSTERIOR VIEW:		
L	R	DEVIATION	L	R	DEVIATION
☐	☐	1.	☐	☐	1.
☐	☐	2.	☐	☐	2.
☐	☐	3.	☐	☐	3.
☐	☐	4.	☐	☐	4.
☐	☐	5.	☐	☐	5.
☐	☐	6.	☐	☐	6.
☐	☐	7.	☐	☐	7.
CIRCLE OR MARK OBSERVED DEVIATIONS			**CIRCLE OR MARK OBSERVED DEVIATIONS**		

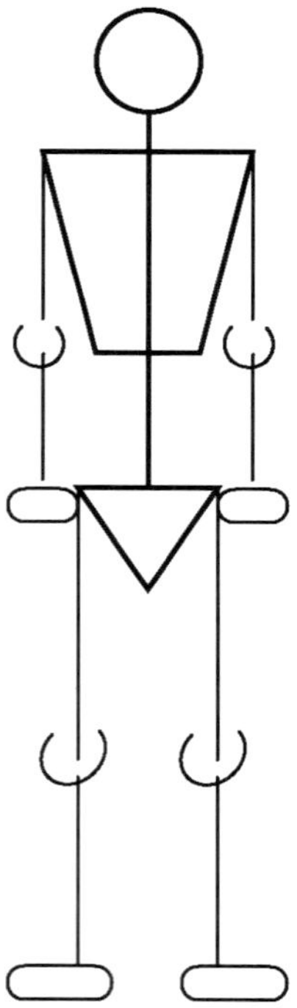

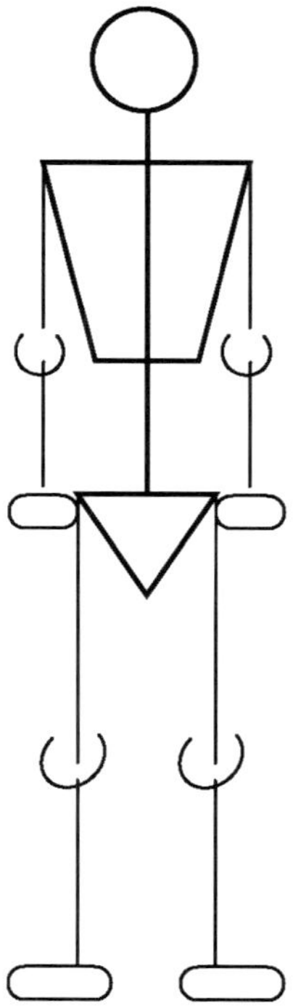

Figure 14-32
Anterior/posterior worksheet

Posture and Movement

CHAPTER 14

L	SAGITTAL: LEFT SIDE DEVIATION	R	SAGITTAL: RIGHT SIDE DEVIATION
☐	1.	☐	1.
☐	2.	☐	2.
☐	3.	☐	3.
☐	4.	☐	4.
☐	5.	☐	5.
☐	6.	☐	6.
☐	7.	☐	7.

CIRCLE OR MARK OBSERVED DEVIATIONS	CIRCLE OR MARK OBSERVED DEVIATIONS

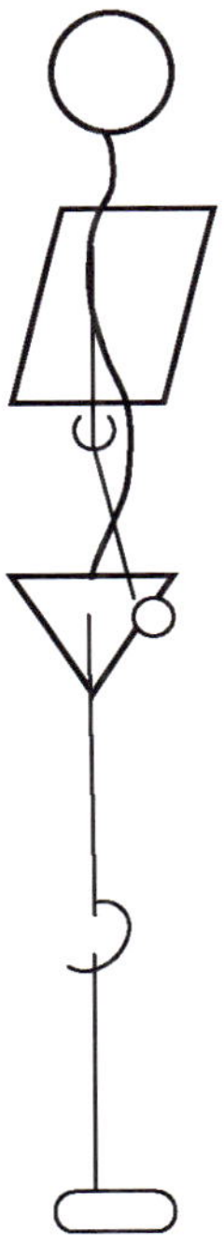

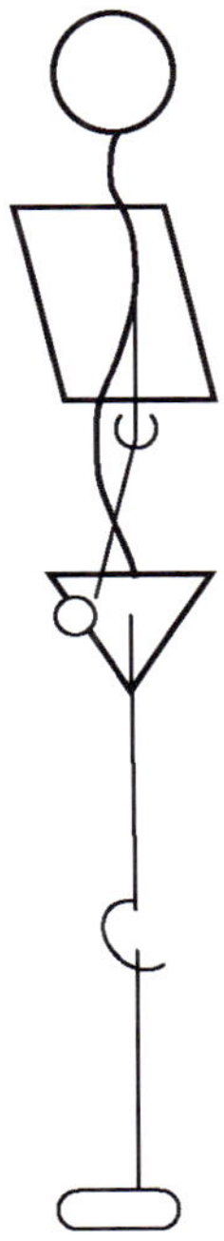

Figure 14-33
Sagittal worksheet

MOVEMENT SCREENS

Observing movement is an effective method to determine the contribution that muscle imbalances and poor posture have on neural control, and also helps identify movement compensations (Whiting & Rugg, 2012; Sahrmann, 2002). When compensations occur during movement, they are usually indicative of some form of altered neural action, commonly referred to as "faulty neural control," which normally manifests due to muscle tightness or an imbalance between muscles acting at the joint.

Movement can essentially be broken down and described by five primary movements that people perform during many daily activities (Cook, 2003):
- Bending/raising and lifting/lowering movements (e.g., squatting)
- Single-leg movements
- Pushing movements (in vertical/horizontal planes) and resultant movement
- Pulling movements (in vertical/horizontal planes) and resultant movement
- Rotational movements

Activities of daily living (ADL) are essentially the integration of one or more of these primary movements. For example, the action of picking up a child and turning to place the child in a car seat involves a squatting movement, a rotational movement, a possible single-leg movement if stepping is involved, a pushing movement, and finally a pulling movement to resist the effects of gravity as the child is lowered into the seat.

Movement screens help the CMES observe the ability and efficiency with which a client performs many ADL. The movement screens, however, must be skill- and conditioning-level appropriate, and be specific to the client's needs. It is important to remember that almost any screen can evaluate **functional capacity,** as long as it is relevant to client needs and challenges, and provides useful feedback on movement efficiency (Sahrmann, 2002). Screens generally challenge clients with no recognized pathologies to perform basic movements and evaluate their ability to demonstrate appropriate levels of stability and mobility throughout the entire kinetic chain—namely, at the feet, knees, lumbo-pelvic-hip complex, shoulders, and head. If the client experiences pain during a movement screen, the test should be stopped and the client should be referred to their healthcare provider to have the painful area evaluated before performing that type of movement in a future exercise session.

Bend-And-Lift Assessment: Squat Pattern

Objective: To assess symmetrical lower-extremity mobility and stability and trunk mobility and stability during a bend-and-lift movement

Equipment:
- None

Instructions:
- Briefly discuss the protocol so the client understands what is required.
- Ask the client to stand with the feet shoulder-width apart with the arms hanging freely to the sides.
- Ask the client to perform five to 10 bend-and-lift movements (i.e., squats), lowering as deep as is comfortable. It is important not to cue the client to use good technique, but instead observe their natural movement.

Observations (Table 14-10):
- Anterior view (Figure 14-34):
  - ✓ Feet: Is there evidence of pronation, supination, eversion, or inversion?
  - ✓ Knees: Do they move inward or outward?
  - ✓ Torso: How is the overall symmetry of the entire body over the **base of support**? Is there evidence of a lateral shift or rotation?
- Side view (Figure 14-35):
  - ✓ Feet: Do the heels remain in contact with the floor throughout the movement?

Posture and Movement — CHAPTER 14

TABLE 14-10
BEND-AND-LIFT ASSESSMENT: SQUAT PATTERN

View	Location	Compensation	Key Suspected Compensations: Overactive (Tight)	Key Suspected Compensations: Underactive (Lengthened)
☐ Anterior	Feet	Lack of foot stability: Ankles collapse inward/feet turn outward	Soleus, lateral gastrocnemius, peroneals	Medial gastrocnemius, gracilis, sartorius, tibialis group
☐ Anterior	Knees	Move inward	Hip adductors, tensor fascia latae	Gluteus medius and maximus
☐ Anterior	Torso	Lateral shift to a side	Side dominance and muscle imbalance due to potential lack of stability in the lower extremity during joint loading	
☐ Side	Feet	Unable to keep heels in contact with the floor	Plantar flexors	None
☐ Side	Hip and knee	Initiation of movement	Movement initiated at knees may indicate quadriceps and hip flexor dominance, as well as insufficient activation of the gluteus group	
☐ Side	Hip and knee	Unable to achieve tops of thighs parallel to the floor	Poor mechanics, lack of dorsiflexion due to tight plantar flexors (which normally allow the tibia to move forward)	
	Contact behind knee	Hamstrings contact back of calves	Muscle weakness and poor mechanics, resulting in an inability to stabilize and control the lowering phase	
☐ Side	Lumbar and thoracic spine	Back excessively arches (i.e., lumbar dominance)	Hip flexors, back extensors, latissimus dorsi	Core, rectus abdominis, gluteal group, hamstrings
		Back rounds forward	Latissimus dorsi, teres major, pectoralis major and minor	Upper back extensors
☐ Side	Head	Downward	Increased hip and trunk flexion	
		Upward	Compression and tightness in the cervical extensor region	

Sources: Kendall, F.P. et al. (2005). *Muscles Testing and Function with Posture and Pain* (5th ed.). Baltimore, Md.: Lippincott Williams & Wilkins; Cook, G. (2003). *Athletic Body in Balance*. Champaign, Ill.: Human Kinetics; Donnelly, D.V. et al. (2006). The effect of directional gaze on kinematics during the squat exercise. *Journal of Strength and Conditioning Research*, 20, 145–150; Fry, A.C., Smith J.C., & Schilling, B.K. (2003). Effect of knee position on hip and knees torques during the barbell squat. *Journal of Strength and Conditioning Research*, 17, 629–633; Abelbeck, K.G. (2002). Biomechanical model and evaluation of a linear motion squat type exercise. *Journal of Strength and Conditioning Research*, 16, 516–524; Sahrmann, S.A. (2002). *Diagnosis and Treatment of Movement Impairment Syndromes*. St. Louis, Mo.: Mosby.

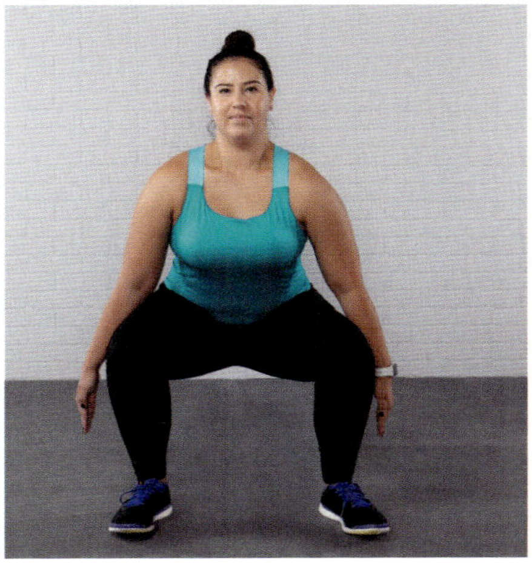

Figure 14-34
Bend-and-lift assessment (squat pattern): Anterior view

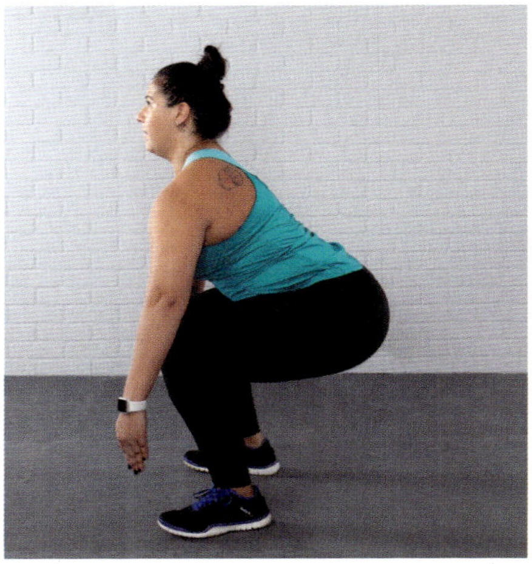

Figure 14-35
Bend-and-lift assessment (squat pattern): Side view

Visit www.ACEfitness.org/CMESresources to download a free PDF of the bend-and-lift screen observations table, as well as other forms and tools that you can use throughout your career as a CMES.

✓ Hip and knee: Does the client exhibit "glute" or "quadriceps dominance" (i.e., is the descent initiated by driving the knees forward or by pushing the hips backward)?
✓ Hip and knee: Does the client achieve a parallel position between the top of the thighs and the floor?
✓ Knee: Does the client control the descent to avoid resting the hamstrings against the calves at the bottom of the squat?
✓ Lumbar and thoracic spine: Does the client exhibit an exaggerated curve in the lumbar (i.e., "lumbar dominance") or thoracic spine during the descent?
✓ Head: Are any changes in the position of the head observed during the movement?

Interpretation:
- Identify origin(s) of movement limitation or compensation.
- Evaluate the impact on the entire kinetic chain.

EXPAND YOUR KNOWLEDGE

MOVEMENT PATTERNS DURING A SQUAT

The gluteals and core musculature play an important role in the squat movement, during which individuals can exhibit "lumbar dominance," "quadriceps dominance," or "glute dominance."

- *Lumbar dominance:* This implies a lack of core and gluteal muscle strength to counteract the force of the hip flexors and erector spinae as they pull the pelvis forward during a squat movement. In this scenario, the individual experiences excessive loads within the lumbar spine as it moves into extension during the squat. The muscles of the abdominal wall and gluteal complex do not contribute enough in this situation to spare the back and foster proper execution of the squat (McGill, 2017). Chronically tight hip flexors, such as those experienced by individuals who sit for prolonged periods throughout the day, may also contribute to the problem.

- *Quadriceps dominance:* This implies reliance on loading the quadriceps group during a squat movement. The first 10 to 15 degrees of the downward phase are initiated by driving the tibia forward, creating shearing forces across the knee as the femur slides over the tibia. In this lowered position, the gluteus maximus does not eccentrically load and cannot generate much force during the upward phase. Quadriceps-dominant squatting transfers more pressure into the knees, placing greater loads on the **anterior cruciate ligament (ACL)** (Wilthrow et al., 2005).

Figure 14-36
Hip hinge

- *Glute dominance:* This implies reliance on eccentrically loading the gluteus maximus during a squat movement. The first 10 to 15 degrees of the downward phase are initiated by pushing the hips backward, creating a hip hinge (Figure 14-36). In the lowered position, this maximizes the eccentric loading on the gluteus maximus to generate significant force during the upward, concentric phase. The glute-dominant squat pattern is the preferred method of squatting, as it spares the lumbar spine and relieves undue stress on the knees. Glute dominance also helps activate the hamstrings, which pull on the posterior surface of the tibia and help unload the ACL to protect it from potential injury (Hauschildt, 2008).

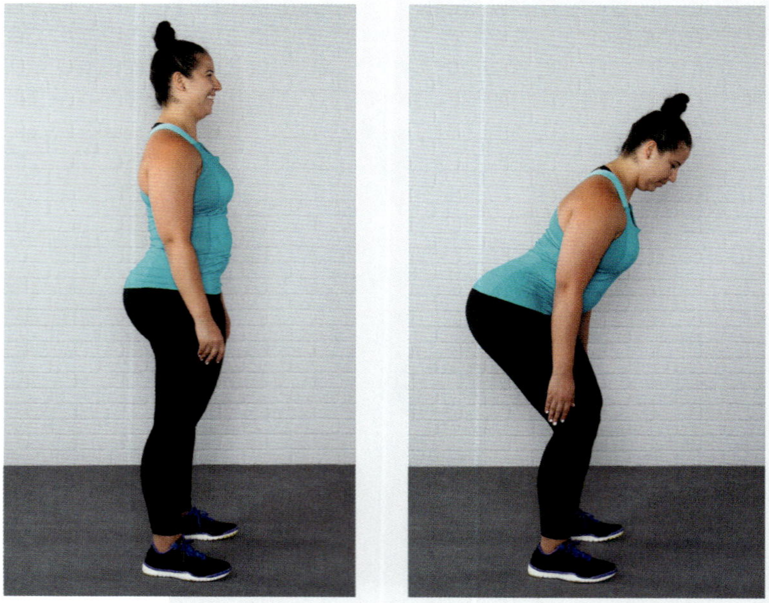

SQUATS AND LUNGES: IS "NEVER LET THE KNEES GO PAST THE TOES" AN APPROPRIATE MOVEMENT CUE?

EXPAND YOUR KNOWLEDGE

While it is appropriate to avoid excessive forward movement of the knee during squatting and lunging movements, it is a myth that exercisers should "never let the knees go past the toes" while doing a squat or lunge. This common movement cue originated from a 1978 study that found that keeping the lower leg as vertical as possible reduced shearing forces on the knees during a squat (McLaughlin, Lardner, & Dillman, 1978). In truth, leaning the trunk too far forward is more likely the cause of any injury.

In 2003, researchers confirmed that knee stress increased by 28% when the knees were allowed to move past the toes while performing a squat (Fry, Smith, & Schilling, 2003). However, hip stress increased by nearly 1,000% when forward movement of the knee was restricted. In addition, in group exercise, the cue "don't let your knees go over your toes" has long been an effective general rule when trying to teach an exercise to a room full of people with different skill levels, abilities, and goals. When a class has a large number of participants, it is difficult to help each individual participant with their specific ROM, so providing this general cue is an effective way of erring on the side of caution for the group fitness instructor.

The general pointer while performing a lunge is to try to keep the knees aligned over the second toe so that the knee is moving in the same direction as the ankle joint. However, in reality, clients often find the knee translating forward to the toes or beyond in a squat or lunge movement, so there are other things that must be considered, specifically limb length.

During lunge or squat movements, personal trainers should always emphasize beginning the movement by pushing the hips backward before lowering toward the floor (an action referred to as "hip hinging"; see Figure 14-36). This technique prevents premature forward movement of the knee by shifting the hips backward. As the exerciser continues to lower their body downward, this creates a healthy hinge effect at the knee, but there comes a time where the knee (tibia) will begin to move forward in order to maintain balance (keeping the **center of mass** within the base of support). If an exerciser happens to have long limbs, then it is realistic to expect the knees to move forward over or beyond the toes. Any attempt to prevent this motion will result in either the client falling backward or bad squat or lunge technique that places increased loads on the low back. As long as personal trainers teach the lunge/squat movement correctly by first initiating the movement at the hips and avoid premature forward movement of the knees, then the fact that the knees are moving forward is quite safe.

Single-Leg Assessment: Step-Up

Objective: To assess symmetrical lower-extremity mobility and stability and trunk mobility and stability during a single-leg (step-up) movement

Equipment:
- Bench; select a bench height that allows the client to start with the hip and knee at approximately a 90-degree angle.

Instructions:
- Briefly discuss the protocol so the client understands what is required.
- Ask the client to stand with the feet shoulder-width apart with the arms hanging freely to the sides.
- Instruct the client to place one leg up squarely on the bench while maintaining an upright posture.
- Instruct the client to push off with the heel of the foot on the bench while simultaneously bringing the opposite leg up to a 90-degree angle.
- Instruct the client to return slowly to the starting position in a one-two-three rhythm.
- Ask the client to perform five to 10 single-leg (step-up) movements.
- Switch the leg positioned on the bench and repeat the above steps.
- It is important not to cue the client to use good technique, but instead observe their natural movement.

Observations (Table 14-11):
- Anterior view (Figure 14-37):
  - ✓ First repetition: Observe the stability of the foot (i.e., evidence of pronation, supination, eversion, or inversion).
  - ✓ Second repetition: Observe the alignment of the stance-leg knee over the foot (i.e., evidence of knee movement in any plane).
  - ✓ Third repetition: Watch for excessive hip adduction greater than 2 inches (5.1 cm) as measured by excessive stance-leg adduction or downward hip-tilting toward the opposite side.
  - ✓ Fourth repetition: Observe the stability of the torso.
  - ✓ Fifth repetition: Observe the alignment of the moving leg (i.e., lack of dorsiflexion at the ankle, deviation from the sagittal plane at the knee or ankle, or hiking of the moving hip).
- Side view (Figure 14-38):
  - ✓ First repetition: Observe the stability of the torso and stance leg.
  - ✓ Second repetition: Observe the mobility of the hip (i.e., allowing 70 degrees of hip flexion without compensation—anterior tilting) of the moving leg.

Interpretation:
- Identify origin(s) of movement limitation or compensation.
- Evaluate the impact on the entire kinetic chain.

TABLE 14-11

SINGLE-LEG ASSESSMENT: STEP-UP

	View	Location	Compensation	Key Suspected Compensations: Overactive (Tight)	Key Suspected Compensations: Underactive (Lengthened)
☐	Anterior	Feet	Lack of foot stability: Ankles collapse inward/feet turn outward	Soleus, lateral gastrocnemius, peroneals	Medial gastrocnemius, gracilis, sartorius, tibialis group, gluteus medius and maximus—inability to control internal rotation
☐	Anterior	Knees	Move inward	Hip adductors, tensor fascia latae	Gluteus medius and maximus
☐	Anterior	Hips	Hip adduction* >2 inches (5.1 cm)	Hip adductors, tensor fascia latae	Gluteus medius and maximus
			Stance-leg hip rotation (inward)	Stance-leg or raised-leg internal rotators	Stance-leg or raised-leg external rotators
☐	Anterior	Torso	Lateral tilt, forward lean, rotation	Lack of core stability	
☐	Anterior	Raised-leg	Limb deviates from sagittal plane Hiking the raised hip	Ankle plantar flexors Raised-leg hip extensors Stance-leg hip flexors—limiting posterior hip rotation during raise	Ankle dorsiflexors Raised-leg hip flexors

Posture and Movement
CHAPTER 14

TABLE 14-11 (continued)

	Side	Pelvis and low back	Lack of ankle dorsiflexion	Stance-leg hip flexors	Rectus abdominis and hip extensors
			Anterior tilt with forward torso lean	Rectus abdominis and hip extensors	Stance-leg hip flexors
			Posterior tilt with hunched-over torso		

*Hip adduction involves weight transference over the stance leg while preserving hip, knee, and foot alignment. This weight transference requires a 1- to 2-inch (2.5- to 5-cm) lateral shift over the stance-leg, with a small hike in the stance-hip of 4 to 5 degrees or less.

Sources: Kendall, F.P. et al. (2005). *Muscles Testing and Function with Posture and Pain* (5th ed.). Baltimore, Md.: Lippincott Williams & Wilkins; Cook, G. (2003). *Athletic Body in Balance.* Champaign, Ill.: Human Kinetics; Sahrmann, S.A. (2002). *Diagnosis and Treatment of Movement Impairment Syndromes.* St. Louis, Mo.: Mosby.

Figure 14-37
Step-up: Anterior view

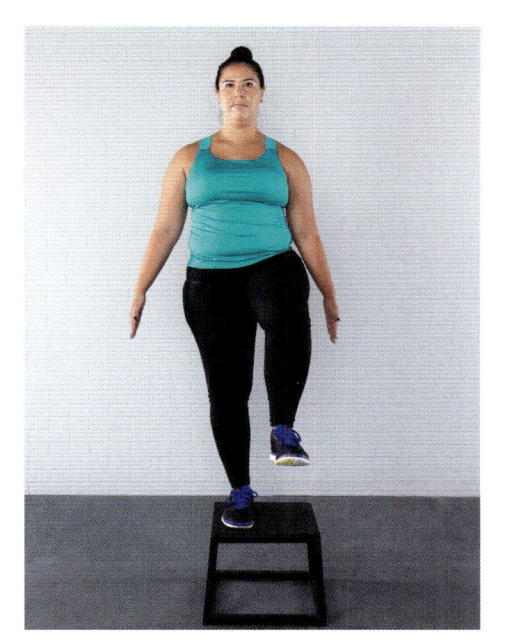

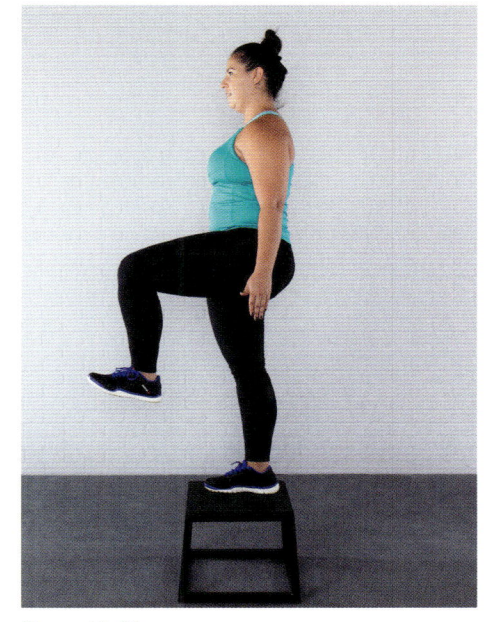

Figure 14-38
Step-up: Side view

Visit www.ACEfitness.org/CMESresources to download a free PDF of the step-up screen observations table, as well as other forms and tools that you can use throughout your career as a CMES.

Push Assessment: Shoulder Push Stabilization

Objective: To assess stabilization of the scapulothoracic joint and core control during closed-kinetic-chain pushing movements

Instructions:
- Briefly discuss the protocol so the client understands what is required.
  - ✓ The client presses their body off the ground as the personal trainer evaluates the ability to stabilize the scapulae against the thorax (rib cage) during pushing-type movements (Figure 14-39).
- Instruct the client to lie prone on the floor with arms abducted in the push-up position or bent-knee push-up position.
- Ask the client to perform several push-ups to full arm extension.
  - ✓ Subjects should perform full push-ups; modify to bent-knee push-ups if necessary.
  - ✓ It is important to remember not to cue the client to use good technique, but instead observe their natural movement.
  - ✓ Repetitions need to be performed slowly and with control.

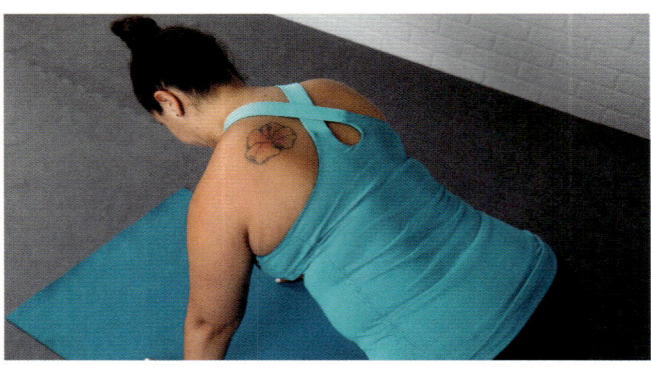

Figure 14-39
Push assessment: Shoulder push stabilization

Visit www.ACEfitness.org/CMESresources to download a free PDF of the shoulder-push stabilization screen observations table, as well as other forms and tools that you can use throughout your career as a CMES.

Observations (Table 14-12):
- Observe any notable changes in the position of the scapulae relative to the rib cage at both end-ranges of motion (i.e., the appearance of scapular "winging") (see Figure 14-27b).
- Observe for lumbar hyperextension in the press position.

General interpretations:
- Identify the origin(s) of movement limitation or compensation.
- Evaluate the impact on the entire kinetic chain.

TABLE 14-12
PUSH ASSESSMENT: SHOULDER PUSH STABILIZATION

View	Joint Location	Compensation	Key Suspected Compensations
☐ Side	Scapulothoracic	Exhibits "winging" during the push-up movement	Inability of the parascapular muscles (i.e., serratus anterior, trapezius, levator scapula, rhomboids) to stabilize the scapulae against the rib cage. Can also be due to a flat thoracic spine.
☐ Side	Trunk	Hyperextension or "collapsing" of the low back	Lack of core, abdominal, and low-back strength, resulting in instability

Sources: Kendall, F.P. et al. (2005). *Muscles Testing and Function with Posture and Pain* (5th ed.). Baltimore, Md.: Lippincott Williams & Wilkins; Sahrmann, S.A. (2002). *Diagnosis and Treatment of Movement Impairment Syndromes.* St. Louis, Mo.: Mosby.

Pull Assessment: Standing Row

Objective: To assess movement efficiency and potential muscle imbalances during pulling movements

Equipment:
- Selectorized cable machine with handle attachments or resistance band with handles

Instructions:
- Briefly discuss the protocol so the client understands what is required.
- A light resistance appropriate for the client should be selected.
- Ask the client to stand with feet shoulder-width apart and knees slightly bent.
- Position the anchor point at a height that aligns with the client's xiphoid process.
- Instruct the client to grab the handles.
- Instruct the client to pull the bar or handle toward their pectoral muscles/torso while keeping the chest forward and back straight (Figure 14-40). The client should briefly pause and then return to the starting position.
- Ask the client to perform several repetitions slowly and with control.
- It is important to remember not to cue the client to use good technique, but instead observe their natural movement.

Observations (Table 14-13):
- Observe for shoulder elevation or head migrating forward.
- Observe for lumbar hyperextension in the pull position.

General interpretations:
- Identify the origin(s) of movement limitation or compensation.
- Evaluate the impact on the entire kinetic chain.

Posture and Movement

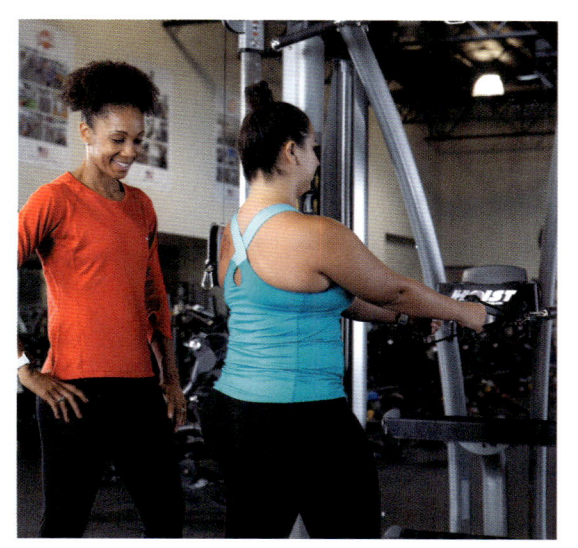

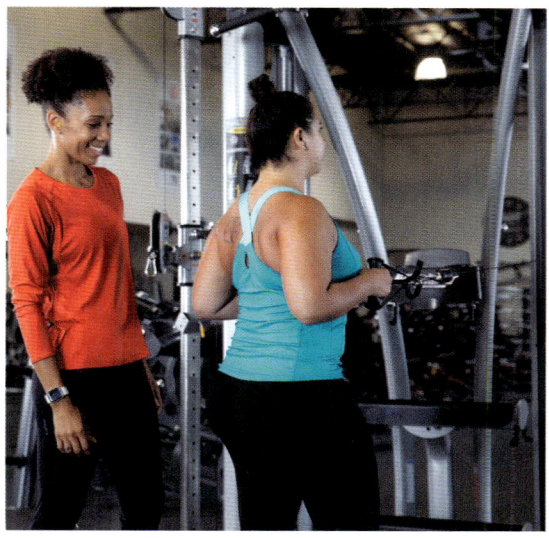

CHAPTER 14

Figure 14-40
Pull assessment:
Standing row

TABLE 14-13
PULL ASSESSMENT: STANDING ROW

View	Location	Compensation	Key Suspected Compensations: Overactive (Tight)	Key Suspected Compensations Underactive (Lengthened)
☐ Side	Lumbar spine	Hyperextension	Hip flexors, back extensors	Core, rectus abdominis, gluteal group, hamstrings
☐ Posterior	Scapulothoracic	Elevation	Upper trapezius, levator scapulae, rhomboid major and minor	Mid and lower trapezius
☐ Side	Head	Migrates forward (protraction)	Cervical spine extensors, upper trapezius, levator scapulae	Cervical spine flexors
☐ Posterior	Scapulothoracic	Abduction (protraction)	Serratus anterior, anterior scapulohumeral muscles, upper trapezius	Rhomboid major and minor, middle trapezius

Rotation Assessment: Thoracic Spine Mobility

Objective: To assess bilateral mobility of the thoracic spine. Lumbar spine rotation is considered insignificant, as it only offers approximately 15 degrees of rotation.

Equipment:
- Chair
- Squeezable ball or block
- 48-inch (1.2-m) dowel

Instructions:
- Briefly discuss the protocol so the client understands what is required.
- Instruct the client to sit upright toward the front edge of the seat with the feet together and firmly placed on the floor. The client's back should not touch the backrest. Place a squeezable ball or block between the knees and a dowel across the front of the shoulders, instructing the client to hold the bar in the hands (i.e., front barbell squat grip) (Figure 14-41a).

- While maintaining an upright and straight posture, the client squeezes the block to immobilize the hips and gently rotates left and right to an end-ROM without any bouncing (Figure 14-41b).
    ✓ It is important to remember not to cue the client to use good technique, but instead observe their natural movement.
    ✓ Ask the client to perform a few repetitions in each direction, slowly and with control.

Observation (Table 14-14):
- Observe any bilateral discrepancies between the rotations in each direction.

General interpretations:
- Identify the origin(s) of movement limitation or compensation. As an individual rotates, the facet joints of each vertebra experience shearing forces against each other. One way to reduce this force and promote greater movement is to laterally flex the trunk during the movement or at the end-range of movement. This assessment evaluates trunk rotation in the transverse plane. Therefore, any lateral flexion of the trunk (dowel tilting up or down) must be avoided.
- Evaluate the impact on the entire kinetic chain. Remember that the lumbar spine generally exhibits limited rotation of approximately 15 degrees (Sahrmann, 2002), with the balance of trunk rotation occurring through the thoracic spine. If thoracic spine mobility is limited, the body strives to gain movement in alternative planes within the lumbar spine (e.g., increase in lordosis to promote greater rotation).

Figure 14-41
Rotation assessment: Thoracic spine mobility

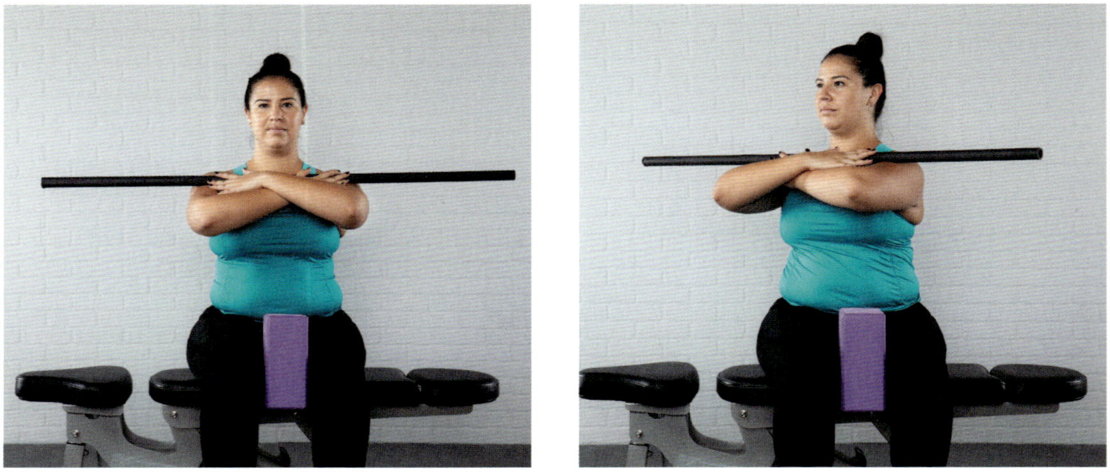

a. Starting position

b. Assessment position

Visit www.ACEfitness.org/CMESresources to download a free PDF of the thoracic-spine mobility screen observations table, as well as other forms and tools that you can use throughout your career as a CMES.

TABLE 14-14

ROTATION ASSESSMENT: THORACIC SPINE MOBILITY

View	Location	Compensation	Possible Biomechanical Problems
☐ Anterior or posterior	Trunk	None if trunk rotation achieves 45 degrees in each direction	
☐ Anterior or posterior	Trunk	Bilateral discrepancy (assuming no existing congenital issues in the spine)	Side-dominance Differences in paraspinal development Torso rotation, perhaps associated with some hip rotation *Note:* Lack of thoracic mobility will negatively impact glenohumeral mobility

Source: Sahrmann, S.A. (2002). *Diagnosis and Treatment of Movement Impairment Syndromes.* St. Louis, Mo.: Mosby.

Posture and Movement CHAPTER 14

FLEXIBILITY AND MUSCLE-LENGTH TESTING

During the initial assessments of posture and movement, a CMES may opt to assess the flexibility of specific muscle groups that they suspect demonstrate tightness or limitations to movement. While Figures 14-42 through 14-44 illustrate normal ranges of motion for healthy adults at each major joint, specific muscle groups that frequently demonstrate tightness or limitations to movement are discussed in this section. In addition, Table 14-15 presents the average ROM at various joints for healthy adults. Figure 14-45 can be used to keep records when conducting the flexibility assessments presented in this section.

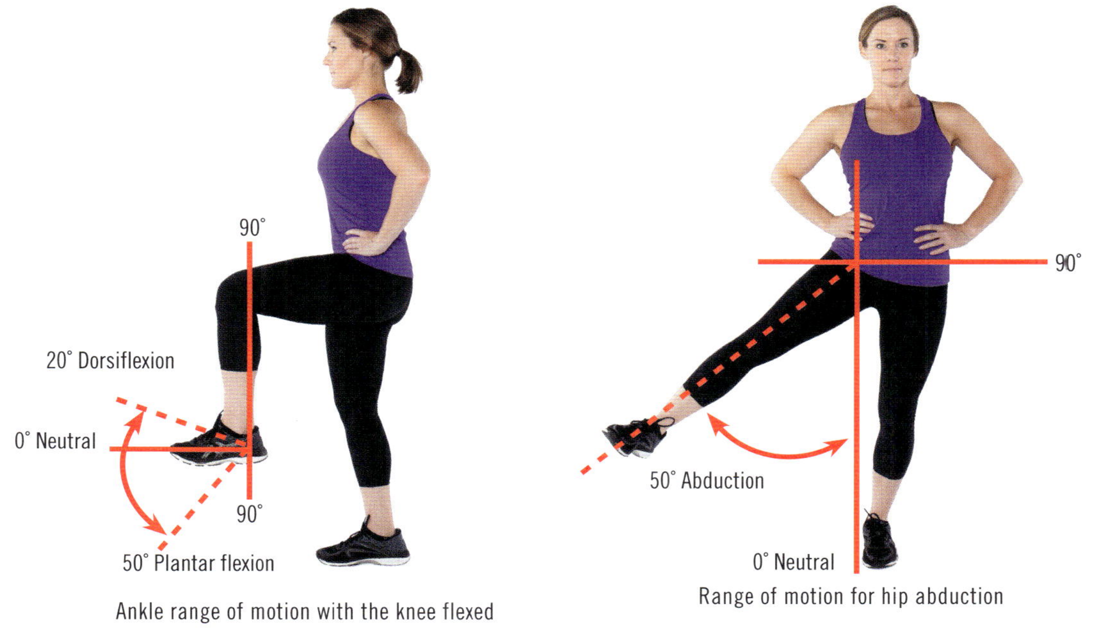

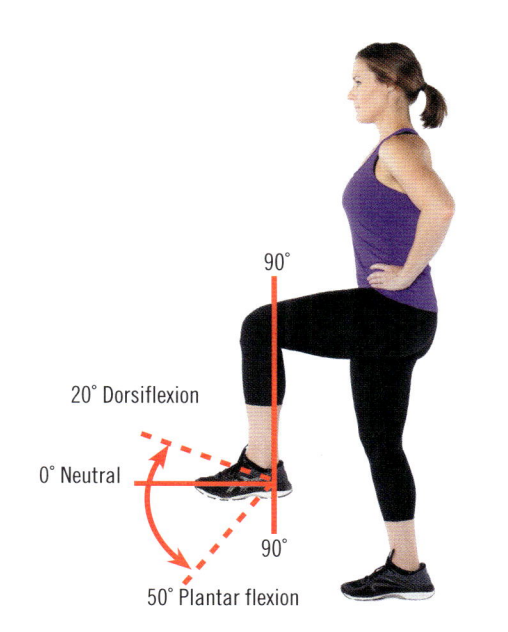

Figure 14-42
Lower-extremity movements and active ranges of motion

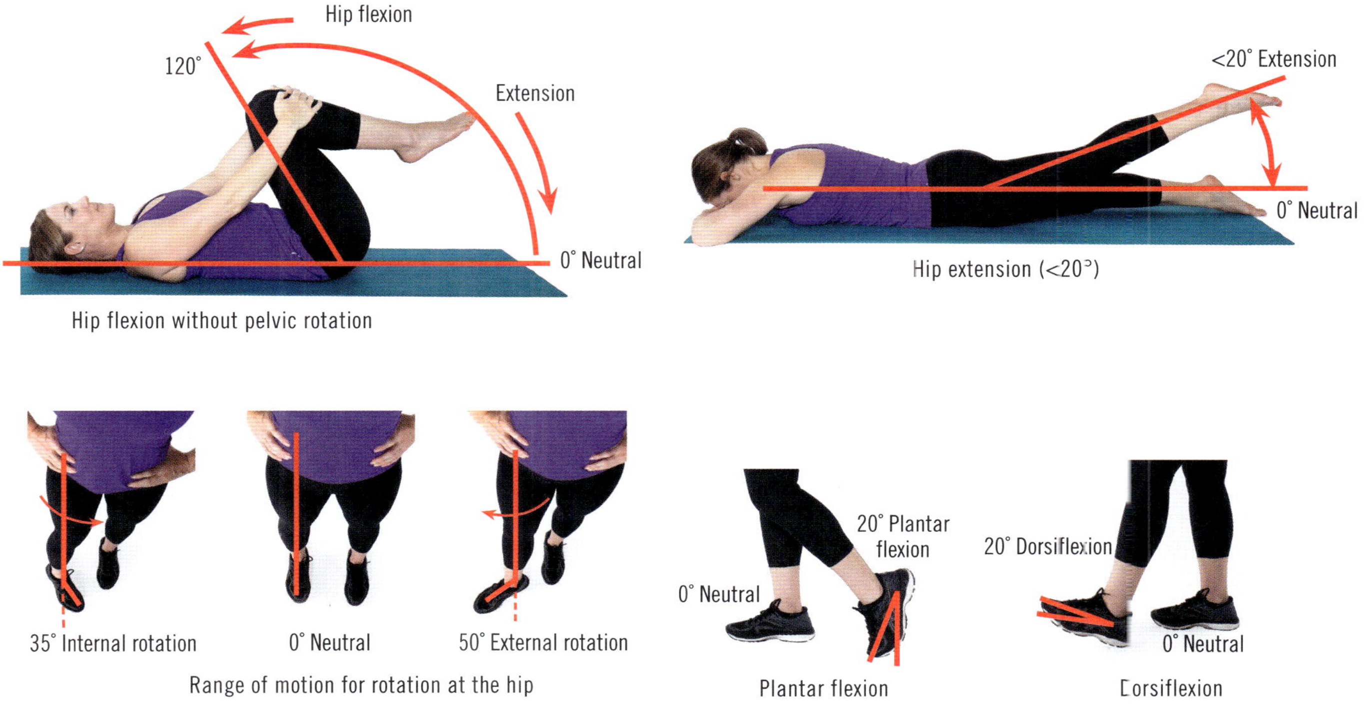

Ankle range of motion with the knee flexed — 20° Dorsiflexion, 0° Neutral, 50° Plantar flexion, 90°

Range of motion for hip abduction — 50° Abduction, 0° Neutral, 90°

Hip flexion without pelvic rotation — 120° Hip flexion, Extension, 0° Neutral

Hip extension (<20°) — <20° Extension, 0° Neutral

Range of motion for rotation at the hip — 35° Internal rotation, 0° Neutral, 50° External rotation

Plantar flexion — 0° Neutral, 20° Plantar flexion

Dorsiflexion — 20° Dorsiflexion, 0° Neutral

CHAPTER 14 — Posture and Movement

Figure 14-43
Shoulder joint range of motion

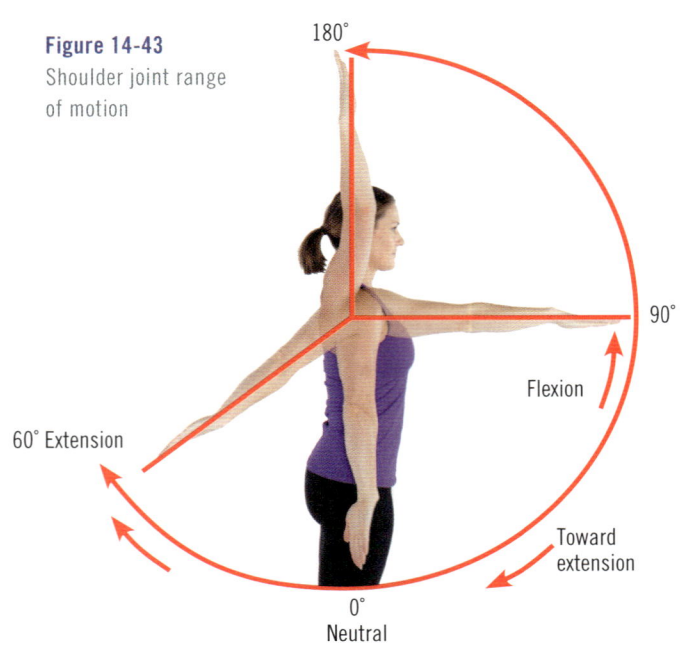

Shoulder range of motion in the sagittal plane: Flexion 180°, extension to 0°, hyperextension 60°

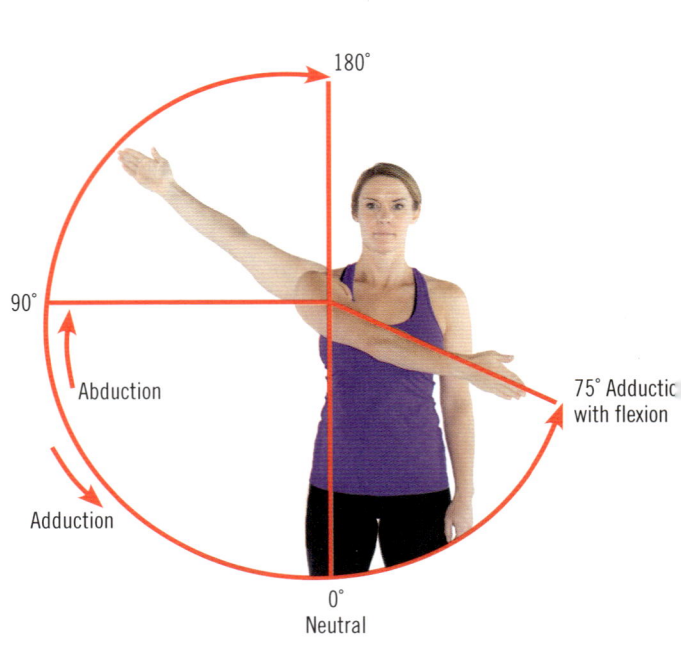

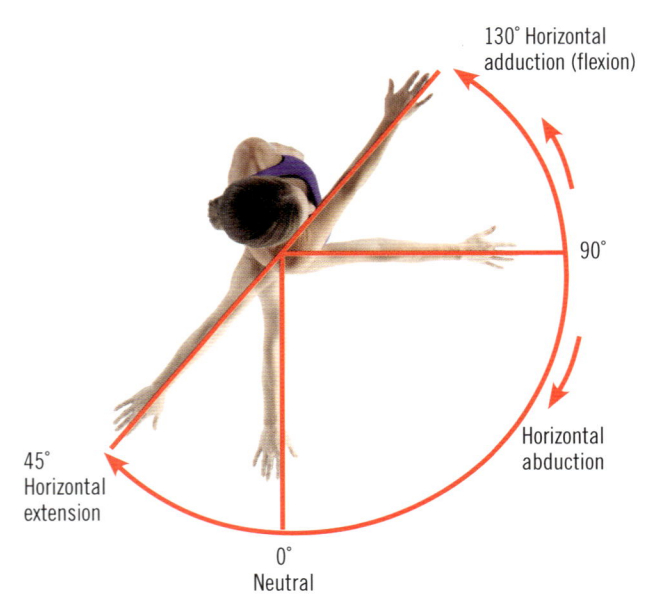

Shoulder range of motion in the transverse plane: Horizontal adduction (flexion) 130°, horizontal abduction to 0°, horizontal extension 45° past neutral

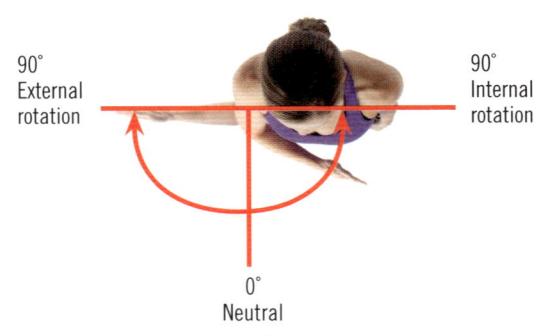

Shoulder rotation range of motion in the transverse plane (shoulder is adducted to 0°): External rotation 90°, internal rotation 90°

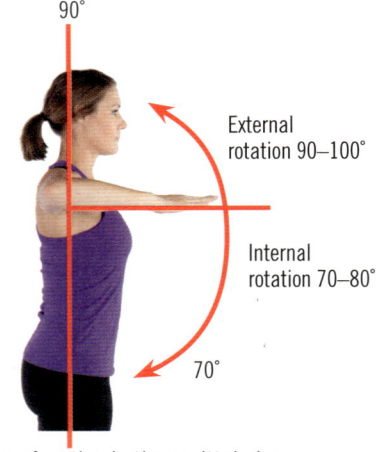

Shoulder rotation range of motion in the sagittal plane: External rotation 90–100°, internal rotation 70–80°

Posture and Movement

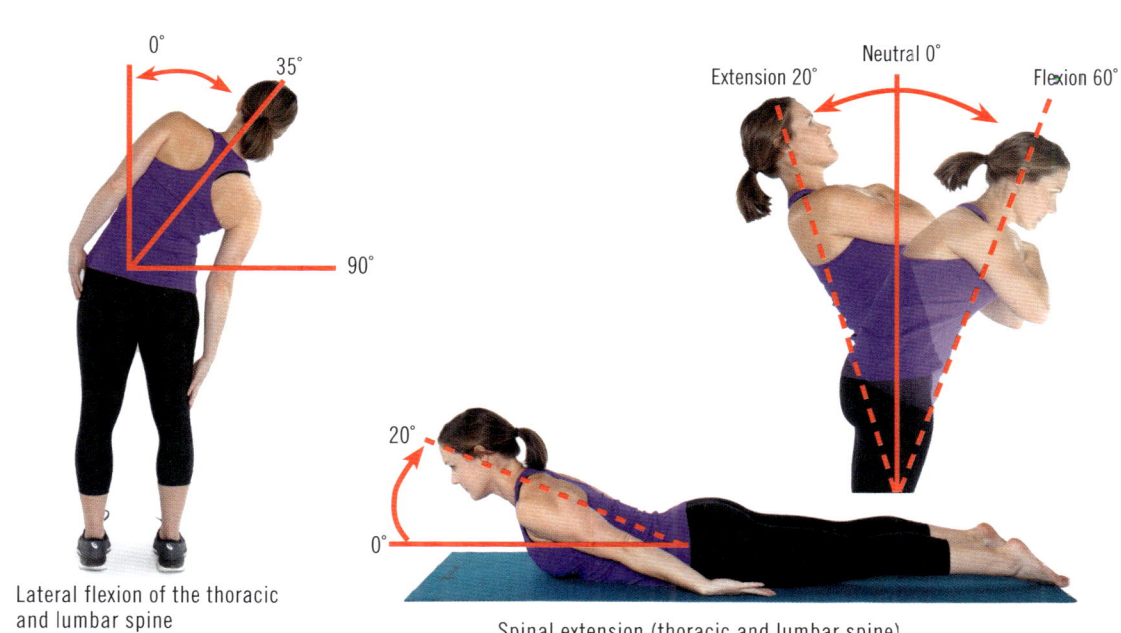

CHAPTER 14

Figure 14-44
Active range of motion of the thoracic and lumbar spine

Lateral flexion of the thoracic and lumbar spine

Spinal extension (thoracic and lumbar spine)

TABLE 14-15
AVERAGE RANGE OF MOTION (ROM) OR HEALTHY ADULTS

JOINT AND MOVEMENT	ROM (°)	JOINT AND MOVEMENT	ROM (°)
Shoulder/Scapulae		*Thoraco-lumbar Spine*	
Flexion	150–180	Lumbar flexion	40–45
Extension	50–60	Thoracic flexion	30–40
Abduction	180	Lumbar extension	30–40
Internal/medial rotation	70–80	Thoracic extension	20–30
External/lateral rotation	90	Lumbar rotation	10–15
Shoulder horizontal adduction	90*	Thoracic rotation	35
Shoulder horizontal abduction	30–40*	Lumbar lateral flexion	20
		Thoracic lateral flexion	20–25
Elbow		*Hip*	
Flexion	145	Flexion	100–120
Extension	0	Extension	10–30
		Abduction	40–45
		Adduction	20–30
		Internal/medial rotation	35–45
		External/lateral rotation	45–60
Radio-ulnar		*Knee*	
Pronation	90	Flexion	125–145
Supination	90	Extension	0–10
Wrist		*Ankle*	
Flexion	80	Dorsiflexion	20
Extension	70	Plantar flexion	45–50
Radial deviation	20		
Ulnar deviation	45		
Cervical Spine		*Subtalar*	
Flexion	45–50	Inversion	30–35
Extension	45–75	Eversion	15–20
Lateral flexion	45		
Rotation	65–75		

*Zero point (0 degrees) is with the arms positioned in frontal-plane abduction at shoulder height.
Source: Kendall, F.P. et al. (2005). *Muscles Testing and Function with Posture and Pain* (5th ed.). Baltimore, Md.: Lippincott Williams & Wilkins.

THOMAS TEST							
Left hip:	Normal ☐	Tight ☐		Right hip:	Normal ☐	Tight ☐
Additional notes:_____				Additional notes:_____		
PASSIVE STRAIGHT-LEG RAISE							
Left hamstrings:	Normal ☐	Tight ☐		Right hamstrings:	Normal ☐	Tight ☐
Additional notes:_____				Additional notes:_____		
SHOULDER FLEXION							
Left shoulder:	Normal ☐	Tight ☐		Right shoulder:	Normal ☐	Tight ☐
Additional notes:_____				Additional notes:_____		
SHOULDER EXTENSION							
Left shoulder:	Normal ☐	Tight ☐		Right shoulder:	Normal ☐	Tight ☐
Additional notes:_____				Additional notes:_____		
INTERNAL ROTATION							
Left shoulder:	Normal ☐	Tight ☐		Right shoulder:	Normal ☐	Tight ☐
Additional notes:_____				Additional notes:_____		
EXTERNAL ROTATION							
Left shoulder:	Normal ☐	Tight ☐		Right shoulder:	Normal ☐	Tight ☐
Additional notes:_____				Additional notes:_____		
APLEY'S SCRATCH TEST							
Left reach-under:	Normal ☐	Tight ☐		Right reach-under:	Normal ☐	Tight ☐
Additional notes:_____				Additional notes:_____		
Left reach-over:	Normal ☐	Tight ☐		Right reach-over:	Normal ☐	Tight ☐
Additional notes:_____				Additional notes:_____		

Figure 14-45
Worksheet for conducting flexibility assessments

Visit www.ACEfitness.org/CMESresources to download a free PDF of a worksheet for conducting flexibility assessments, as well as other forms and tools that you can use throughout your career as a CMES.

Posture and Movement CHAPTER 14

Thomas Test for Hip Flexor Length

Objective: To evaluate the length of the muscles involved in hip flexion (i.e., hip flexors and rectus femoris). This test assesses the length of the primary hip flexors. It should not be conducted on clients suffering from low-back pain, unless cleared by their physician.

Equipment:
- Stable table

Instructions:
- Given the nature of the movement associated with this test, personal trainers may want to consider draping a towel over the client's groin area.
- Explain the objective of the test and allow a warm-up.
- Instruct the client to sit at the end of a table with the mid-thigh aligned with the table edge (Figure 14-46a).
- While supporting the client, instruct them to flex one thigh toward the chest and gradually assist as they roll to the table top with back and shoulders flat.
- Instruct the client to continue to pull one knee toward the chest only until the low back is flat (Figure 14-46b).

Observations:
- Observe whether the back of the lowered thigh touches the table (hips positioned in 10 degrees of extension).
- Observe whether the knee of the lowered leg achieves 80 degrees of flexion.
- Observe whether the knee remains aligned straight or falls into internal or external rotation.

Interpretation:
- Use the information provided in Table 14-16 to determine the location and identity of the tight or limiting muscles

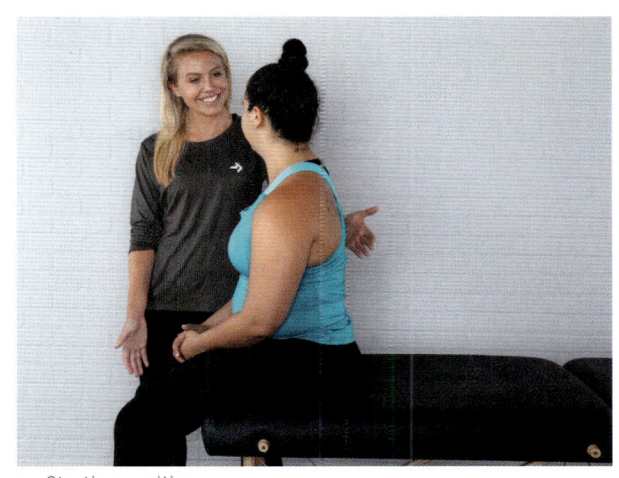

a. Starting position

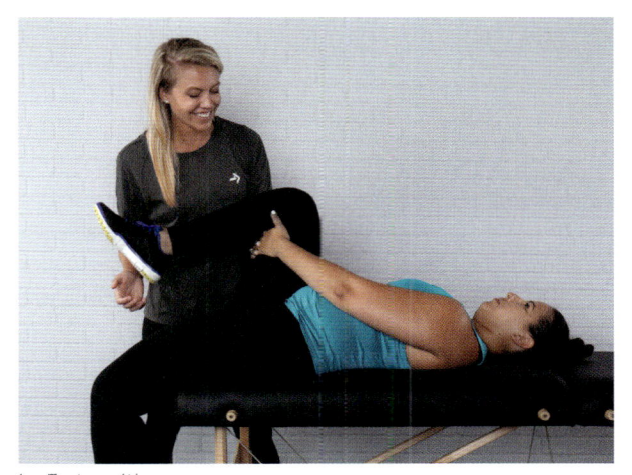

b. Test position
Figure 14-46
Thomas test for hip flexor length

TABLE 14-16	
INTERPRETATION OF THE THOMAS TEST	
Movement/Limitation	**Suspected Muscle Tightness**
With the back and sacrum flat: • The back of the lowered thigh does not touch the table • The knee *does not* flex to 80 degrees	Primary hip flexor muscles
With the back and sacrum flat: • The back of the lowered thigh does not touch the table • The knee *does* flex to 80 degrees	The iliopsoas, which is preventing the hip from rotating posteriorly and inhibiting the thigh from being able to touch the table
With the back and sacrum flat: • The back of the lowered thigh does touch the table • The knee *does not* flex to 80 degrees	The rectus femoris, which does not allow the knee to bend

Source: Kendall, F.P. et al. (2005). *Muscles Testing and Function with Posture and Pain* (5th ed.). Baltimore, Md.: Lippincott Williams & Wilkins.

Passive Straight-leg Raise

Objective: To assess the length of the hamstrings

Equipment:
- Stable table or exercise mat

Instructions:
- Explain the objective of the assessment and allow a warm-up.
- Instruct the client to lie supine on a mat or table with the legs extended and the low back and sacrum flat against the surface.
- Place one hand under the calf of the leg that will be raised while instructing the client to keep the opposite leg extended on the mat or table. Restrain that leg from moving or rising during the assessment.
- Slide the other hand under the lumbar spine into the space between the client's back and the mat or table (Figure 14-47).
- Advise the client to gently plantar flex their ankles to point the toes away from the body. This position avoids an assessment limitation due to a tight gastrocnemius muscle (which would limit knee extension with the ankle in dorsiflexion). Additionally, a straight-leg raise with dorsiflexion may increase tension within the sciatic nerve and create some discomfort.
- Slowly raise the one leg, asking the client to keep that knee loosely extended throughout the movement.
- Continue to raise the leg until firm pressure can be felt from the low back pressing down against the hand (Figure 14-48).
- This indicates an end-ROM of the hamstrings, with movement now occurring as the pelvis rotates posteriorly.
- Throughout the movement, the client needs to maintain extension in the opposite leg and keep the sacrum and low back flat against the mat or table.
  - ✓ If the assessment is performed with the opposite hip in slight flexion, this allows the pelvis more freedom to move into a posterior tilt, allowing a greater ROM and falsely increasing the length of the hamstrings.

Observation:
- Note the degree of movement attained from the table or mat that is achieved before the spine compresses the hand under the low back or the opposite leg begins to show visible signs of lifting off the table or mat.
  - ✓ The mat or table represents 0 degrees.
  - ✓ The leg perpendicular to the mat or table represents 90 degrees.

Interpretation:
- Use the information provided in Table 14-17 to determine the limitation(s).

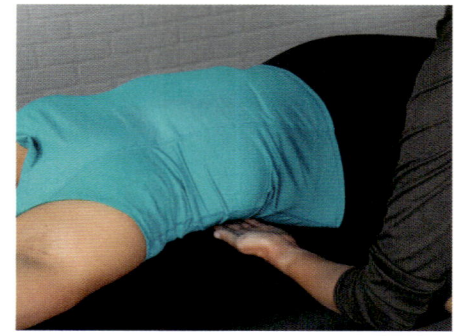

Figure 14-47
Passive straight-leg raise: Personal trainer's hand position

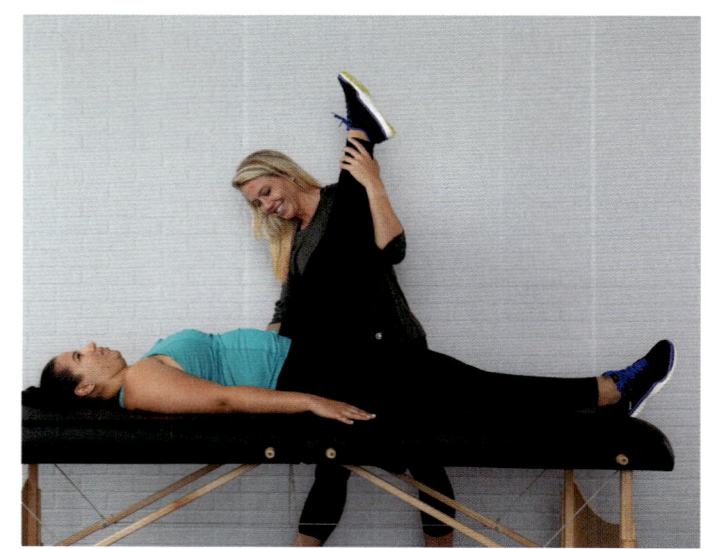

Figure 14-48
Passive straight-leg raise: Assessment position

TABLE 14-17	
INTERPRETATION OF THE PASSIVE STRAIGHT-LEG RAISE	
Movement/Limitation	**Hamstrings Length**
The raised leg achieves ≥80 degrees of movement before the pelvis rotates posteriorly.	Normal hamstrings length
The raised leg achieves <80 degrees of movement before the pelvis rotates posteriorly or there are any visible signs in the opposite leg lifting off the mat or table.	Tight hamstrings

Source: Kendall, F.P. et al. (2005). *Muscles Testing and Function with Posture and Pain* (5th ed.). Baltimore, Md.: Lippincott Williams & Wilkins.

Shoulder Flexion and Extension

Objective: To assess the degree of shoulder flexion and extension
Equipment:
- Exercise mat
- Pillow (optional)

Instructions:
- Explain the purpose of the assessment.
- Shoulder flexion:
  ✓ Instruct the client to lie supine on a mat, with the back flat and a bent-knee position (knees and second toe aligned with the hips), and with the arms at the sides.
  ✓ Have the client engage the abdominal muscles to hold a neutral spine without raising the hips from the mat.
  ✓ Instruct the client to raise both arms simultaneously into shoulder flexion, moving them overhead, keeping them close to the sides of the head, and bringing them down to touch the floor or as close to the floor as possible (Figure 14-49).
    - The client must maintain extended elbows and neutral wrist position (the arms will naturally rotate internally during this movement).
    - Have the client avoid any arching in the low back during the movement.
    - Have the client avoid any **depression** of the rib cage, which may pull the shoulders off the mat.
- Shoulder extension:
  ✓ Instruct the client to lie prone, extending both legs, with arms at the sides, and resting the forehead gently on a pillow or the mat.
  ✓ Ask the client to slowly raise both arms simultaneously into extension, lifting them off the mat while keeping the arms close to the sides (Figure 14-50) (the arms will naturally rotate internally during this movement).
    - A small amount of extension in the thoracic spine is acceptable during the movement.
    - The client should avoid any arching in the low back or any rotation of the torso during the movement.
    - The client should avoid any attempts to lift the chest or head off the mat during the movement.

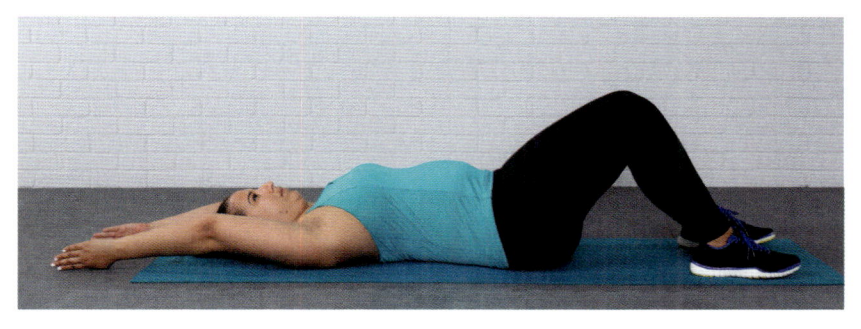

Figure 14-49
Shoulder flexion assessment

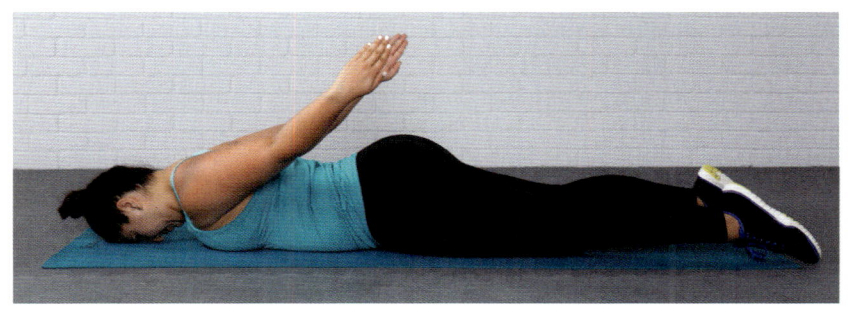

Figure 14-50
Shoulder extension assessment

Observations:
- Measure the degree of movement in each direction.
- Note any bilateral differences between the left and right arms in performing both movements.

Interpretation:
- Use the information provided in Table 14-18 to determine the limitation(s) in these shoulder flexibility assessments.

TABLE 14-18
INTERPRETATION OF THE SHOULDER FLEXION AND EXTENSION ASSESSMENTS

Movement/Limitation—Flexion	Shoulder Mobility
Ability to flex the shoulders to 170–180 degrees (hands touching/nearly touching floor)	Good shoulder mobility
Inability to flex the shoulders to 170 degrees or discrepancies between the limbs	• Potential tightness in the pectoralis major and minor, latissimus dorsi, teres major, rhomboids, and subscapularis • Tightness in the latissimus dorsi will force the low back to arch. • Tightness of the pectoralis minor may tilt the scapulae forward (anterior tilt) and prevent the arms from touching the floor. • Tight abdominals may depress the rib cage, tilting the scapulae forward (anterior tilt), and prevent the arms from touching the floor. • Thoracic kyphosis may round the thoracic spine and prevent the arms from touching the floor.
Movement/Limitation—Extension	Shoulder Mobility
Ability to extend the shoulders to 50–60 degrees off the floor	Good shoulder mobility
Inability to extend the shoulders to 50 degrees or discrepancies between the limbs	• Potential tightness in pectoralis major, abdominals, subscapularis, certain shoulder flexors (anterior deltoid), coracobrachialis, and biceps brachii • Tightness in the abdominals may prevent normal extension of the thoracic spine and rib cage. • Tightness in the biceps brachii may prevent adequate shoulder extension with an extended elbow (but may permit extension with a bent elbow).

Source: Houglum, P.A. (2010) *Therapeutic Exercise for Musculoskeletal Injuries* (3rd ed.). Champaign, Ill.: Human Kinetics.

Apley's Scratch Test for Shoulder Mobility

Objective: To assess simultaneous movements of the shoulder girdle (primarily the scapulothoracic and glenohumeral joints)

Movements include:
- Shoulder extension and flexion
- Internal and external rotation of the humerus at the shoulder
- Scapular abduction and adduction

Instructions:
- Explain the purpose of the test and allow a warm-up (e.g., forward and rearward arm circles).
- Shoulder flexion, external rotation, and scapular abduction
    ✓ From a sitting or standing position, the client raises one arm overhead, bending the elbow and rotating the arm outward while reaching behind the head with the palm facing inward to touch the medial border of the contralateral scapula or to reach down the spine (touching vertebrae) as far as possible (Figure 14-51).
    ✓ The client should avoid any excessive arching in the low back or rotation of the torso during the movement.
    ✓ Have the client repeat the test with the opposite arm.

Posture and Movement   CHAPTER 14

- Shoulder extension, internal rotation, and scapular adduction
  - ✓ From a sitting or standing position, the client reaches one arm behind the back, bending the elbow and rotating the arm inward with the palm facing outward to touch the inferior angle of the contralateral scapula or to reach up the spine (touching vertebrae) as far as possible (Figure 14-52).
  - ✓ The client should avoid any excessive arching in the low back or rotation of the torso during the movement.
  - ✓ Have the client repeat the test with the opposite arm.

Observations:
- Note the client's ability to touch the medial border of the contralateral scapula or how far down the spine they can reach with shoulder flexion and external rotation.
- Note the client's ability to touch the opposite inferior angle of the scapula or how far up the spine they can reach with shoulder extension and internal rotation.
- Observe any bilateral differences between the left and right arms in performing both movements.

General interpretations:
- Use the information provided in Table 14-19 to determine the limitation(s) in this flexibility test.

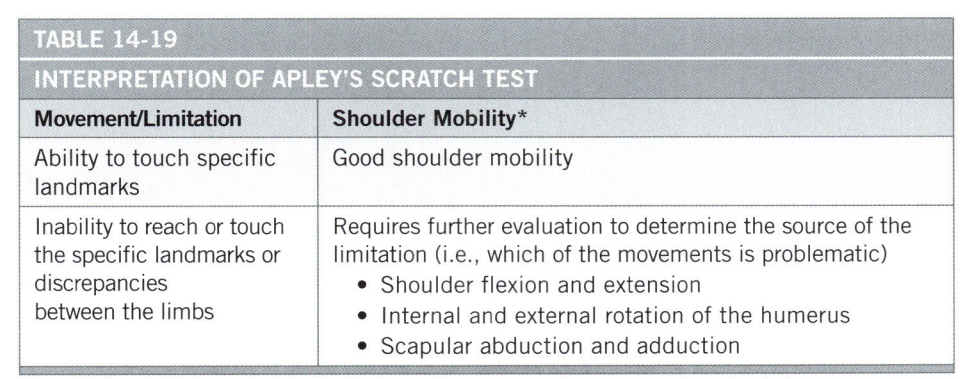

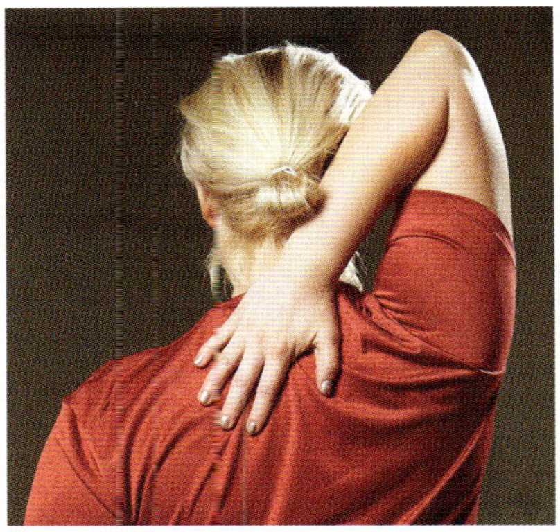

Figure 14-51
Apley's scratch test: Shoulder flexion, external rotation, and scapular abduction

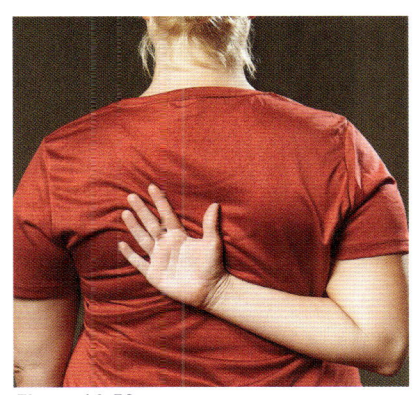

Figure 14-52
Apley's scratch test: Shoulder extension, internal rotation, and scapular adduction

TABLE 14-19

INTERPRETATION OF APLEY'S SCRATCH TEST

Movement/Limitation	Shoulder Mobility*
Ability to touch specific landmarks	Good shoulder mobility
Inability to reach or touch the specific landmarks or discrepancies between the limbs	Requires further evaluation to determine the source of the limitation (i.e., which of the movements is problematic) • Shoulder flexion and extension • Internal and external rotation of the humerus • Scapular abduction and adduction

*Tightness of the joint capsules and ligaments may also contribute to limitations. It is common to see greater restriction on the dominant side due to increased muscle mass.

Source: Kendall, F.P. et al. (2005). *Muscles Testing and Function with Posture and Pain* (5th ed.). Baltimore, Md.: Lippincott Williams & Wilkins.

RESTORATIVE EXERCISE FOR POSTURAL COMPENSATION

The overall goal with programming is to restore muscle balance, enhance muscle's physiological properties, and improve neuromuscular control of movement by re-educating faulty neural pathways. However, unless *awareness* of poor posture and *intention* to improve are key objectives of the program, individuals are not likely to attain great success. Table 14-20 presents the basic programming principles surrounding:

- Stretching hypertonic (tight and overactive) muscles through passive elongation to increase ROM
- Strengthening latent (weak and inactive) muscles with isometric or limited-ROM exercises in normal resting-length positions

The initial emphasis placed on passive elongation (static stretching) to reduce muscle tightness may not be considered functional by some, but its objective is to reset muscle tone (in the hypertonic muscle), correct side asymmetry, and introduce normal ROM and muscle length prior to integrating movement patterns. This is especially important if muscle length or tone restricts efficient movement. McGill (2016), however, claims that static stretching deadens the muscle from a neural perspective, diminishing the stretch reflex and reducing peak strength and power. Consequently, the

TABLE 14-20
KEY STEPS OF RESTORATIVE EXERCISE PROGRAMMING

Restorative Progression Steps	Modality
Inhibit hypertonic muscles	Myofascial release, static stretching, PNF, isometric contractions, active isolated stretches
Lengthen hypertonic muscles	Static stretching, PNF
Activation of latent muscles	Isometric contractions, active isolated stretches, muscle activation techniques, dynamic contractions
Integration into functional movement*	Part-to-whole progression of movement patterns

*An example of integrated movement is the progression from a shoulder-bridge knee-tuck to stretch tight hip flexors and activate a weak gluteus maximus to more functional walking lunges with overhead triplanar arm reaches that engage more of the entire body.

Note: PNF = Proprioceptive neuromuscular facilitation

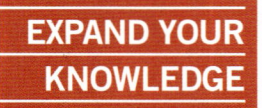

EXPAND YOUR KNOWLEDGE

KEEPING THE TERMS (AND CONCEPTS) STRAIGHT

Muscles that are found to be shortened or lengthened through postural observations have terms that are commonly associated with each. These terms are sometimes defined incorrectly and are often mistakenly used interchangeably. It is important for the CMES to appropriately use this terminology when addressing postural issues.

Shortened Muscles and Associated Terms

- *Tight:* The association between "short" and "tight" appears logical and at times they will coincide. However, these terms are not synonymous. Consider, for instance, a male gymnast who has heavily developed upper-body muscles. It is not uncommon to observe a slight rounding of the shoulder girdle and internal rotation at the glenohumeral joint in these individuals. This passive position would indicate that the internal rotators of the shoulder (including the pectoralis major, latissimus dorsi, and anterior deltoid) are in a shortened position at rest, but do these muscles actually lack flexibility? Considering that gymnasts are required to maintain tremendous levels of flexibility throughout the shoulder joint, it is very unlikely that these muscles would lack ROM.
- *Strong:* A muscle that is "shortened" can also be misrepresented as a "strong" muscle. When a "strong" muscle causes muscle imbalances, it is typically from overdevelopment either from training or from repetitive physical activities without balancing the strength with counter movements. For example, some exercisers participate in workouts wherein pectoralis major and latissimus dorsi exercises dominate. This can influence rounded shoulders and internal rotation—sometimes referred to as "bench press shoulders." However, similar postural imbalances may be found in a non-exerciser, but not from overdevelopment or "strength" in the associated muscles. Based on the principles associated with the length-tension relationship, muscles in a shortened position may actually test weak (Sahrmann, 2002). Therefore, it is important to avoid assumptions that a shortened muscle is short due to higher levels of strength and overdevelopment.
- *Overactive:* Shortened muscles are often believed to be "overactive," indicating they carry excessive tension at rest. Over-activity (also referred to as hypertonicity) can be just as common as tightness and overdeveloped muscles, but once again, not necessarily at the same time. Short muscles can be tight, overdeveloped, and overactive. However, a muscle can be short and not overactive, just as overactive muscles are not necessarily short. Overactive muscles can be found just as readily in ideal posture, as well as in those with lengthened muscles.

Lengthened Muscles and Associated Terms

- *Weak:* Muscles that are lengthened at rest are often assumed to be "weak." This is very common, but it should be noted that this is in relation to their functional antagonists—at rest. Another way to look at a "weak" muscle is to observe whether it is allowing the opposite action to happen. In other words, it is not necessarily active at holding a position deemed desirable. This can be misleading, especially when considering the example of the male gymnast who has rounded and internally rotated shoulders. The scapular retractors and external rotators appear to

"allow" protraction and internal rotation. However, once again, you would not necessarily find weak retractors or external rotators on a gymnast. Caution should be used when assuming a lengthened muscle is weak. The term "underactive" is a more appropriate term in most cases, as it refers once again to "allowing" a position to take place, rather than balancing a joint in a neutral position.
- *Flexible:* Lengthened muscles may not be flexible at all. The term lengthened refers to a resting position. Consider, for example, the hamstrings, which are a commonly tight muscle group. A client may have an anterior pelvic tilt, indicating that the hamstrings are in a lengthened position. However, it is common to find people who present with an anterior pelvic tilt and yet have very inflexible hamstrings. At the same time, the hamstrings at rest are not near their lengthened capacity, which means that some extra room to extend exists. Therefore, it should not be assumed that a lengthened muscle is flexible.

The significance of terminology distinction and clarification is that it can have a profound impact on programming strategies. For example, if a shortened muscle is presumed tight, flexibility strategies would likely be implemented. This may be appropriate if the muscle in fact lacks extensibility. However, a short muscle may not lack flexibility and, therefore, implementing a stretching program may have little impact on corrective strategies and could even be inappropriate. Another scenario could present where a muscle is hyperactive, but not tight. Stretching the muscle may not help change the over-activity. In fact, it may perpetuate it (McGill, 2016). In such cases, self-**myofascial release** techniques (see page 45) may be more appropriate for reducing the tension.

dominance of static-type stretching should be limited to the initial part of the program until the client is capable of integrating movement patterns. As the client progresses through the program, the static-type stretches will be replaced with more dynamic-type movement patterns.

A common issue of debate is whether hypertonic agonists should first be stretched or the weakened antagonists should first be strengthened. Several approaches exist, but a basic approach of stretch-then-strengthen delivers effective results. This approach involves inhibiting and reducing tension in the hypertonic (tight) muscles, and stretching the tight muscles before strengthening the latent (weakened) muscles to facilitate their full activation. Janda studied electromyography (EMG) activity on hypertonic erector spinae and normotensive rectus abdominis muscles during trunk flexion exercises (Arokoski et al., 2001). Test subjects demonstrated reduced rectus abdominis activity with tight erector spinae during normal trunk flexion, yet when the erector spinae were first stretched, they exhibited increased rectus abdominis activity and reduced erector spinae activity. It therefore appears that the neurological principles of **autogenic inhibition** serve an important role in restorative exercise.

Low-force, longer-duration static stretches evoke low-grade muscle spindle activity and a temporary increase in muscle tension due to muscle lengthening. This low-grade muscle response progressively decreases due to a gradual desensitization of the muscle spindle activity as the duration of the stretch progresses. After approximately seven to 10 seconds of a low-force stretch, the increase in muscle tension activates a **Golgi tendon organ (GTO)** response. Under GTO activation, muscle spindle activity within the stretched muscle is temporarily inhibited, allowing further muscle stretching. This concept defines autogenic inhibition (Whittle, 2007). For example, passively holding a hamstrings stretch to the point of resistance for the appropriate timeframe will elicit this neurological response. After the removal of the stretch stimulus, however, the muscle spindle quickly reestablishes its stretch threshold to approximately 70% of full recovery within the first five seconds (MacIntosh, Gardiner, & McComas, 2006).

Increasing ROM is best accomplished through prolonged passive elongation at lower intensities (Sahrmann, 2002). While passively positioning shortened muscles in elongated positions for 10-minute-plus intervals effectively stimulates increases in sarcomere number, these timeframes prove unrealistic and unmanageable for most. Consequently, the CMES must encourage clients to follow their stretching programs as frequently as possible, as stretching adaptations are dose-dependent on volume (repetitions x duration x frequency) and the quality of the repetitions completed.

Active agonist contraction and reciprocal inhibition are alternative approaches to restorative exercise. Active agonist contractions involve a series of repeated, low-grade isometric or dynamic contractions of the hypertonic agonist to reduce its irritability threshold via GTO activation (MacIntosh, Gardiner, & McComas, 2006). This facilitates stretching of the agonist, which is followed by strengthening of the antagonist. For example, a sequence at the pelvis would include low-grade concentric or isometric contractions of the hip flexors preceding hip flexor stretching, followed by gluteus maximus strengthening.

Reciprocal inhibition involves first performing isometric or dynamic contraction with the weakened antagonist to reciprocally inhibit the hypertonic agonist, which can then be stretched. Low-grade muscle contractions at approximately 50% of maximal force in the antagonist for a total duration of six to 15 seconds inhibit or reduce muscle spindle activity within the agonist muscle (Whittle, 2007). For example, a low-grade isometric contraction of the gluteus maximus reciprocally inhibits the hip flexors, which can then be stretched, followed again by gluteus maximus strengthening.

Table 14-21 provides general guidelines for the CMES to follow when designing a restorative exercise program for a client.

TABLE 14-21
RESTORATIVE EXERCISE PROGRAMMING GUIDELINES (F.I.R.S.T.)

Program Modality	Tightened Muscles—Stretching	Lengthened Muscles—Strengthening
Frequency	Best accomplished with prolonged passive elongations (10-minute-plus intervals), but unrealistic/unmanageable for most As adaptations are dose-dependent, aim for 1–2 times/day	Perform 1–2 times/day with the stretching program
Intensity	**Static stretching:** To the point of tension Always control joint movements in bi-articulate (two-joint) muscles **Dynamic patterns:** Controlled tempos to the point of resistance Maintain full neuromuscular control of movement—higher intensities may call upon existing faulty strategies	Provide small overload in controlled positions Generally need only around 50% of MVC Focus on strengthening with the joint position near neutral position Use the body's resistance or fixed surfaces (e.g., the floor) Higher intensities may call upon existing faulty strategies Lower intensities also allow faster muscle recovery and more frequent training
Repetitions and sets	**Static stretching:** 2–4 repetitions x 30–60 seconds each **Dynamic movements:** 1–2 sets x 5–10 repetitions progressing to 3 sets x 15–20 repetitions	**Isometric contractions:** 2–4 repetitions x 5–10 seconds each Emphasize uniplanar action **Dynamic contractions:** 1–2 sets x 12–20 repetitions with slow, controlled tempos Progress to 2–3 sets x 10–15 repetitions Introduce triplanar action
Timeframe	Plan sessions between 30–45 minutes (depending on the amount of muscle imbalance noted) Plan for 1–3 months of participation, depending on the degree of imbalance and volume of exercise performed, or until noticeable body alignment and movement efficiency are restored After 2 weeks of overload, small strength gains are evident, but they are 20% morphological and 80% neural 4–6 weeks may be required to demonstrate more significant morphological changes in muscle	

Note: MVC = Maximal voluntary contraction

LOMBARD'S PARADOX

The concept of reciprocal inhibition during single-joint movements has its own limitations when addressing functional, dynamic movements. The agonist/antagonist relationship during some of the most fundamental movements, to some degree, contradicts the mechanism of reciprocal inhibition. For example, when looking at knee flexion and extension, the hamstrings and the quadriceps are clearly antagonists. More precisely, the rectus femoris, (which extends the knee and flexes the hip) is the antagonist to the semitendinosus, semimembranosus, and the long head of biceps femoris (during flexion of the knee and extension of the hip). However, when palpating the quadriceps and the hamstrings during a sit-to-stand, the quadriceps and the hamstrings all engage to perform this multijoint movement. This is referred to as Lombard's paradox (Cook, 2010).

An argument can be made that the more dynamic the movement, the harder it is to find true agonist/antagonist relationships. This does not eliminate the possibility of altered neural drive from faulty postural positions. However, when creating programs for clients, this paradox must be considered.

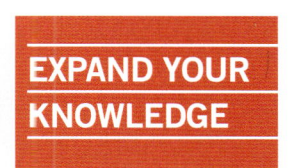

EXPAND YOUR KNOWLEDGE

EXERCISE EXAMPLES FOR STABILITY AND MOBILITY

This section provides basic examples of stretches and exercises to improve mobility and stability of the lumbo-pelvic and scapulothoracic regions.

Proximal Stability: Core Function

Exercise 1: Supine Drawing-in (Centering)

- Ask the client to assume a supine, bent-knee position, align the knees and second toe with the ASIS, and hold this position throughout the exercise (Figure 14-53).
  - ✓ Instruct the client to place the hands immediately medial to the ASIS, in line with the umbilicus (belly button), and rest the fingers over the transverse abdominis (TVA).
- All muscle contractions should be of a moderate intensity (≤50% of maximal effort).
  - ✓ Throughout these exercises, there should be no movement of the pelvis, low back, or rib cage.
  - ✓ Movement of these joints indicates activation of the rectus abdominis and an inability to activate the TVA in an isolated manner.
- Have the client follow the exercise progression outlined in Table 14-22.

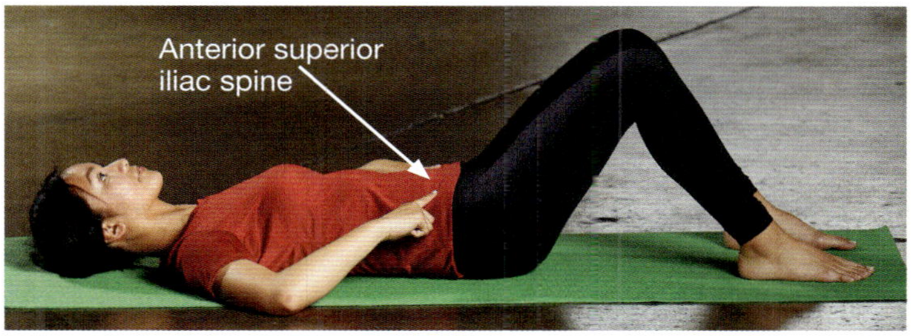

Figure 14-53
Supine drawing-in body position

TABLE 14-22	
EXERCISE PROGRESSION FOR CORE ACTIVATION	
Pelvic floor contractions ("Kegels," or the contraction to interrupt the flow of urine)	Perform 1–2 sets x 10 repetitions with a 2-second tempo, 10–15 second rest intervals between sets
TVA contractions (drawing the belly button toward the spine)	Perform 1–2 sets x 10 repetitions with a 2-second tempo, 10–15 second rest intervals between sets
Combination of both contractions	Perform 1–2 sets x 10 repetitions with a 2-second tempo, 10–15 second rest intervals between sets
Contractions with normal breathing	Perform 1–2 sets x 5–6 repetitions with slow, 10-second counts while breathing independently, 10–15 second rest intervals between sets
	Progress to 3–4 sets x 10–12 repetitions, each with a 10-second count, 10–15 second rest intervals between sets

Note: TVA = Transverse abdominis

✓ During the TVA contractions, the client should feel some tension develop under the fingers. This may not be possible with heavier individuals.
✓ The purpose of these exercises is to re-educate faulty neural pathways. Thus, the appropriate exercise volume conducted via perfect exercise technique will help regain the reflexive function of the core musculature.
✓ Teach the client how to perform these exercises by providing a demonstration of the progressions and instructing them to perform them as frequently as possible for one to two weeks.

Exercise 2: Quadruped Drawing-in (Centering) With Extremity Movement

Once the client effectively demonstrates their ability to activate the core and pelvic floor muscles independent of the diaphragm (during breathing), the CMES can have them follow the exercise progression for core stabilization. These exercises train clients to stabilize the lumbar spine with minimal loading on the spine during movements of the hips and shoulders.

The purpose of this exercise sequence is to activate the core muscles by working against gravity while placing small loads on the spine by moving the hips and shoulders. Clients should activate the core muscles, as demonstrated in the core-activation exercises (see Table 14-21), and continue to breathe independently.

- Have the client adopt the quadruped position with the knees under the hips and the hands under the shoulders. The client must maintain a neutral spine (Figure 14-54a).
  ✓ Due to limb-length discrepancies between the arms and legs, the slope of the spine may range from parallel with the floor to a slight incline or decline.
  ✓ The goal of this exercise is to elevate one arm and/or leg 0.5 to 1 inch (1.25 to 2.5 cm) off the floor and perform slow, controlled extremity movements through a short distance without losing control of the lumbar spine (Figure 14-54b). Extending the limbs too far may result in a loss of lumbar stability (increased lordosis) or force hip and shoulder rotation due to a lack of mobility within those joints, and therefore should be avoided.
  ✓ Encourage clients to perform this exercise adjacent to a mirror and use visual feedback to monitor and control changes in spinal position (e.g., increased lordosis), which indicate a loss of core control.
- Have clients follow the exercise progression outlined in Table 14-23.
- The purpose of these exercises is to reestablish core control with minimal loading on the spine during hip and shoulder movements. Thus, appropriate exercise volume conducted via perfect exercise technique will help clients regain reflexive control of loading along the lumbar spine.
  ✓ Teach the client how to perform these exercises by providing a demonstration of the progressions and instructing them to perform them as frequently as possible for one to two weeks.

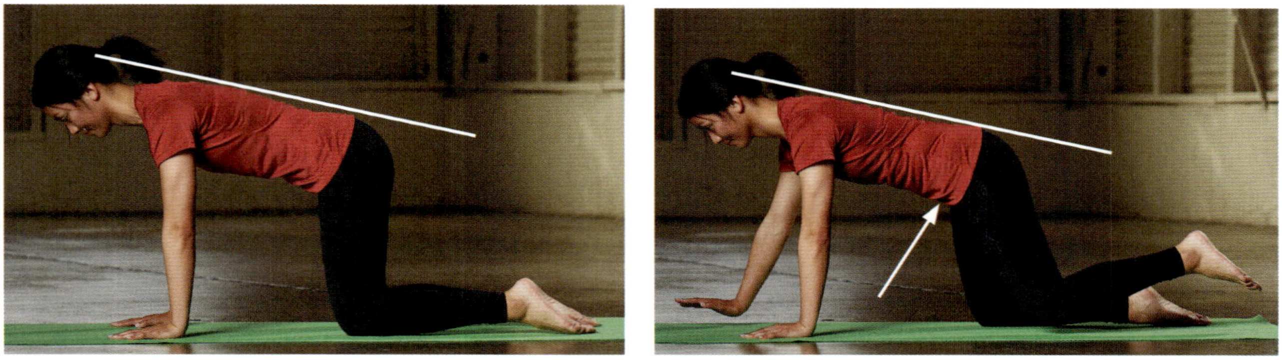

Figure 14-54
Quadruped drawing-in with extremity movement

Posture and Movement   CHAPTER 14

TABLE 14-23
EXERCISE PROGRESSION FOR CORE STABILIZATION

1. Raise one arm 0.5 to 1 inch (1.25 to 2.5 cm) off the floor and perform the sequence of controlled shoulder movements: • 6–12 inch (15–30 cm) sagittal plane shoulder movements (flexion/extension) • 6–12 inch (15–30 cm) frontal plane shoulder movements (abduction/adduction) • 6–12 inch (15–30 cm) transverse plane shoulder movements (circles or circumduction)	Perform 1–2 sets x 10 repetitions with a 2-second tempo, use 10–15 second rest intervals between sets
2. Raise one knee 0.5 to 1 inch (1.25 to 2.5 cm) off the floor and perform the sequence of controlled hip movements: • 6–12 inch (15–30 cm) sagittal plane hip movements (flexion/extension) • 6–12 inch (15–30 cm) frontal plane hip movements (abduction/adduction) • 6–12 inch (15–30 cm) transverse plane hip movements (circles)	Perform 1–2 sets x 10 repetitions with a 2-second tempo, use 10–15 second rest intervals between sets
3. Raise contralateral limbs (i.e., one arm and the opposite knee) 0.5 to 1 inch (1.25 to 2.5 cm) off the floor and perform the sequence of movements: • Repeat the above movements in matching planes (i.e., simultaneous movement in the same plane with both limbs) or alternating planes (i.e., mixing the planes between the two limbs). • This contralateral movement pattern mimics the muscle-activation patterns used during the push-off phase portion of walking and is an effective exercise to train this pattern.	Perform 1–2 sets x 10 repetitions with a 2-second tempo, use 10–15 second rest intervals between sets

Proximal Mobility: Hips and Thoracic Spine

The goal of this stage is to improve mobility of the two joints immediately adjacent to the lumbar spine. Based on observations made during the postural assessments and movement screens, limitations in mobility within these two areas in any of the three planes should become the focus. The CMES should follow some fundamental principles when programming to improve mobility in these body regions:

- Although these two regions should exhibit good mobility in all three planes, they are typically prone to poor mobility. Consequently, some static stretching to improve muscle flexibility (or extensibility) should precede dynamic mobilization exercises.
- When attempting to improve muscle flexibility or joint mobility, clients must avoid undesirable or compensated movements at successive joints (e.g., avoid any increases in lumbar lordosis associated with a tight latissimus dorsi muscle during an overhead stretch).
- The CMES should be familiar with muscle anatomy and differentiate between mono- or uniarticulate muscles and biarticulate muscles.
  - ✓ A monoarticulate muscle crosses one joint (e.g., soleus muscle), whereas a biarticulate muscle crosses two joints (e.g., hamstrings).
  - ✓ When stretching a biarticulate muscle, joint movement must be controlled at both ends

of the muscle to avoid any compromise to stability at adjacent joints. For example, when performing a passive straight-leg raise to stretch the hamstrings, posterior tilting of the pelvis must be avoided when the hamstrings reach their limit of flexibility, because further stretching forces pelvic rotation and a flattening of the low back, which compromises the stability of the lumbar spine.

- Because the body still lacks the ability to effectively stabilize the entire kinetic chain, supportive surfaces should be utilized while promoting mobility (e.g., floor, benches, or backrests).
    - ✓ Once an individual effectively demonstrates the ability to stabilize the more proximal regions of the body (i.e., the lumbar spine and scapulothoracic region), exercises can become more unsupported in nature. This transition should coincide with a shift from more isolated exercises to more integrated multijoint and multiplanar movements.
- Because muscles contribute to movement in all three planes, the CMES should incorporate flexibility exercises that lengthen the muscles in all three planes. It is important, however, to focus on the muscle's primary plane of movement before adding complexity by introducing movement in other planes. For example, when stretching the hip flexors using a half-kneeling lunge stretch, the client should stretch the muscle in the sagittal plane before incorporating any frontal or transverse plane movements into the stretch (e.g., a lateral trunk lean or trunk rotation).

Exercises and Stretches

The exercises presented in Figures 14-55 through 14-65 promote mobility of the hips and thoracic spine.

Figure 14-55
Cat-cow

Objective: To improve extensibility within the lumbar extensor muscles

Note: The cat-cow exercise is intended as a motion exercise—not a stretch—so the emphasis is on motion rather than "pushing" at the end ranges of flexion and extension.

Preparation and position:
- Assume the quadruped position with the hands positioned directly under the shoulders (shoulder-width apart) and the knees positioned directly under the hips (shoulder-width apart).
- Engage the core muscles to create a neutral spine in this starting position.
- The elbows should remain extended throughout the exercise.

Exercise:
- From this starting position, exhale slowly while contracting the abdominals [draw the belly button toward the spine (i.e., "hollowing")], gently pushing and rounding the entire back upward. Drop the head, bringing the chin toward the chest (a).
- Slowly inhale, relax, and return to the starting position, but allow the stomach and spine to sag toward the floor. Allow the shoulders to collapse (adduct) toward the spine, and tilt the head upward (b).
- Perform two to four repetitions.

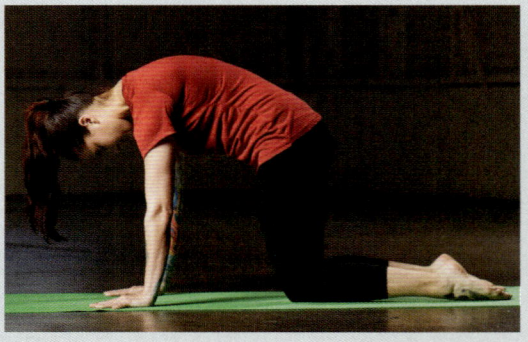

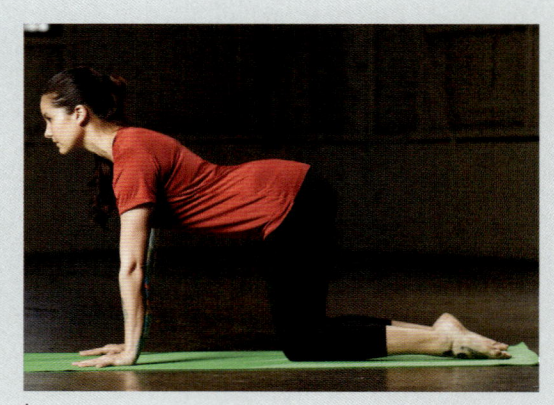

Posture and Movement
CHAPTER 14

Figure 14-56
Pelvic tilts

Objective: To improve hip mobility in the sagittal plane

Preparation and position:
- Lie supine with the knees bent and the feet placed flat on the floor, aligning the anterior superior iliac spine (ASIS) with the knee and second toe. Place a rolled-up towel under the low back, which can be used by the client to monitor any changes in the low-back position kinesthetically during this exercise. An alternative option is to place one hand in the natural curve under the low back to control changes in the low-back position.
- Abduct the arms to shoulder height, resting them on the floor with the arms externally rotated (palms facing upward) (a).

Exercise:
- Slowly contract the abdominals to tilt the pelvis posteriorly, hold briefly, relax, and then contract the erector spinae muscles and hip flexors to tilt the pelvis anteriorly (b).
- Perform one or two sets of five to 10 controlled repetitions, holding the end position for one or two seconds, with 30-second rest intervals between sets.

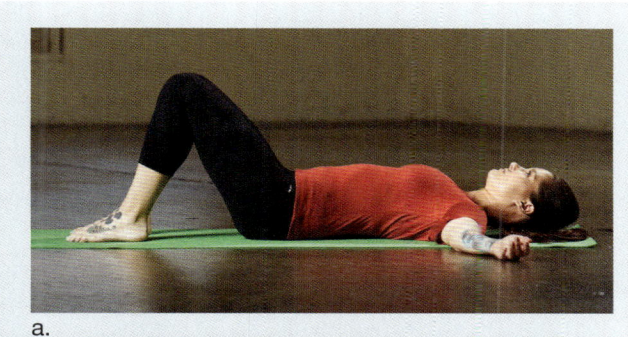

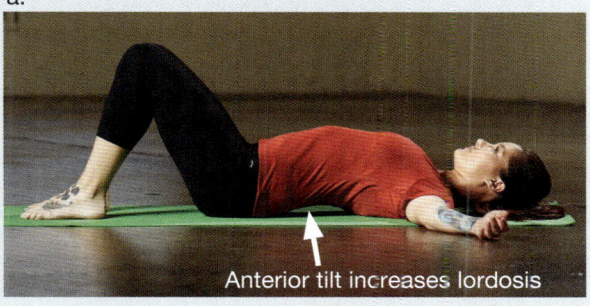

a.

b. Anterior tilt increases lordosis

Figure 14-57
Pelvic-tilt progressions: Supine bent-knee marches

Objective: To improve hip mobility in the sagittal plane without compromising lumbar stability during lower-extremity movement

Preparation and position:
- Lie supine with the knees bent and the feet placed flat on the floor, aligning the anterior superior iliac spine (ASIS) with the knee and second toe. Place a rolled-up towel under the low back, which can be used by the client to monitor any changes in the low-back position kinesthetically during this exercise. An alternative option is to place one hand in the natural curve under the low back to control changes in the low-back position.
- Abduct the arms to shoulder height, resting them on the floor with the arms externally rotated (palms facing upward).
- Engage the core muscles to stabilize the lumbar spine in the neutral position (a).

Exercise:
- Slowly raise one leg, maintaining a bent-knee position, and drive the knee toward the chest, stopping when the thigh is perpendicular to the ground (b).
- Hold this position briefly before returning to the starting position.
- Repeat this same movement with the opposite leg.
- Perform one or two sets of five to 10 controlled repetitions per leg, holding the end range of motion for one or two seconds, with 30-second rest intervals between sets.

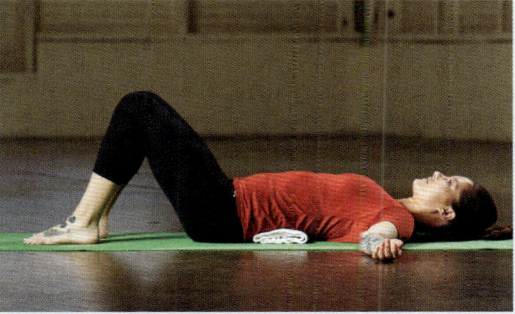

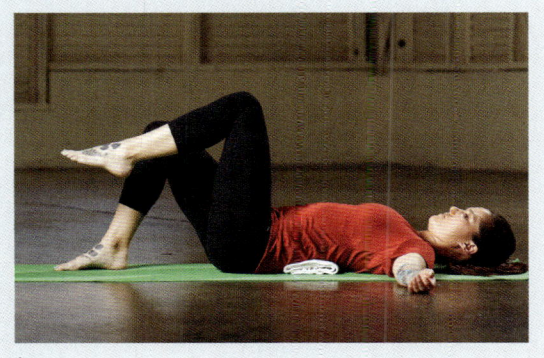

Figure 14-58
Pelvic-tilt progressions: Modified dead bug with reverse bent-knee marches

Objective: To improve hip mobility in the sagittal plane without compromising lumbar stability during lower-extremity movement

Note: Introduce this exercise as a progression to the exercise presented in Figure 14-62.

Preparation and position:
- Lie supine and place a rolled-up towel under the low back, which can be used by the client to monitor any changes in the low-back position kinesthetically during this exercise (a). An alternative option is to place one hand in the natural curve under the low back to control changes in the low-back position.
- Engage the core muscles to stabilize the lumbar spine in the neutral position.
- Raise both legs until the hips and knees are flexed to approximately 90 degrees (feet in the air), aligning the anterior superior iliac spine (ASIS) with the knee and second toe (b).

Exercise:
- Exhale while slowly lowering one leg toward the floor and maintaining a bent-knee position (c). Avoid any loss of lumbar stability throughout the movement.
- Hold this position briefly before returning to the starting position.
- Repeat this same movement with the opposite leg.
- Perform one or two sets of five to 10 controlled repetitions per leg, holding the end range of motion for one or two seconds, with 30-second rest intervals between sets.

Progression—Dead bug with reverse bent-knee and arm movements: Assume the same starting position, but flex both shoulders to raise the arms perpendicular to the floor in line with the shoulders (d). Exhale while simultaneously lowering one leg and the same-side (ipsilateral) arm toward the floor and maintaining a bent-knee position (e). Avoid any loss of lumbar stability throughout the movement. Hold this position briefly before returning to the starting position. Additional progressions include moving contralaterally (opposite arm and leg) or bilaterally (both arms and legs simultaneously).

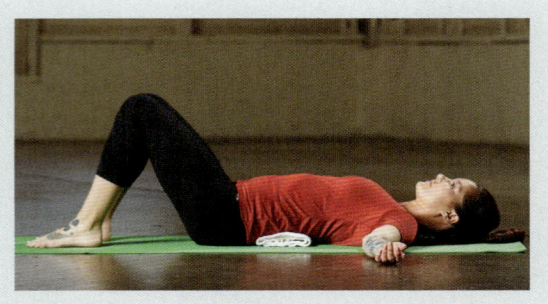

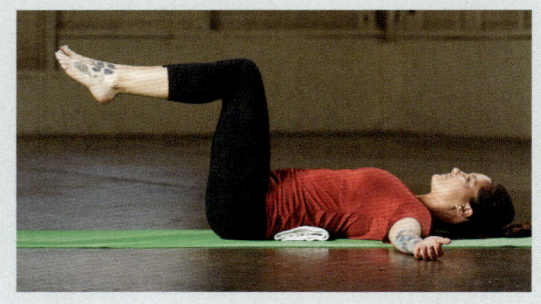

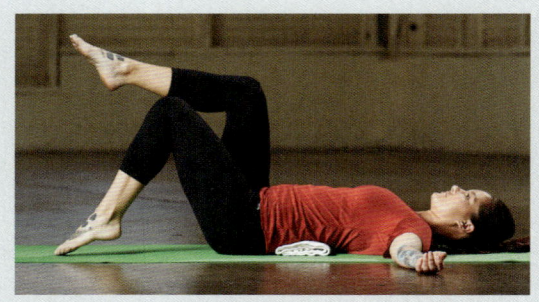

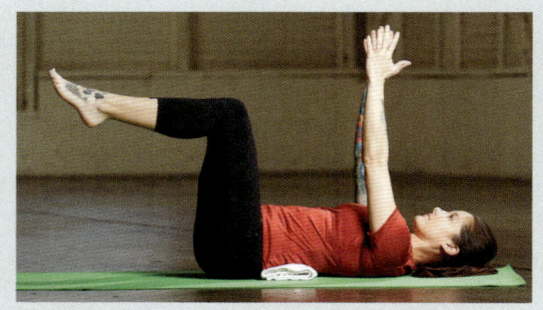

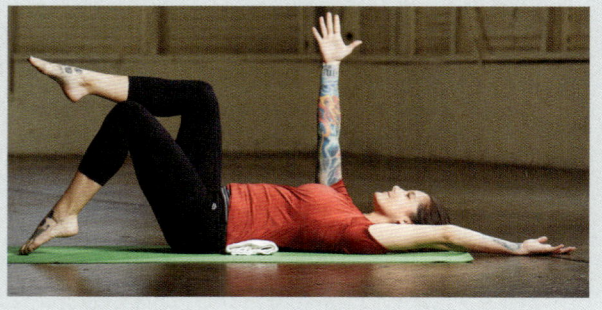

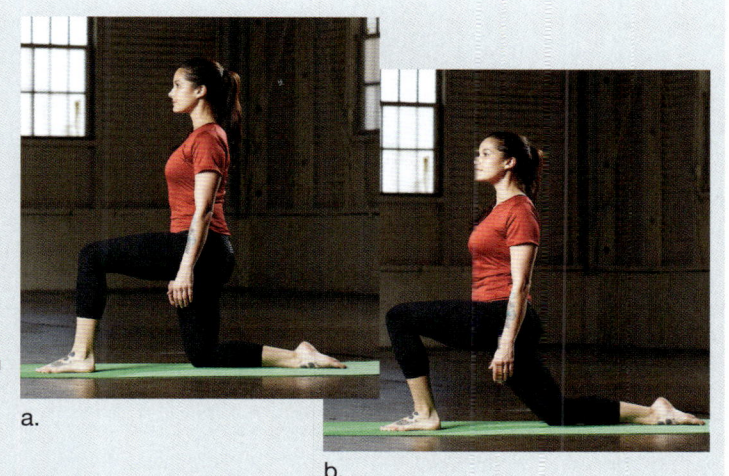

Posture and Movement **CHAPTER 14**   457

Figure 14-59
Hip-flexor mobility: Lying hip-flexor stretch

Objective: To improve mobility of the hip flexors in the sagittal plane without compromising lumbar stability

Preparation and position:
- Lie supine with the knees bent and the feet placed flat on the floor, aligning the anterior superior iliac spine (ASIS) with the knee and second toe.
- Engage the core muscles to stabilize the lumbar spine in the neutral position and maintain this position throughout the exercise.

Exercise:
- Reach both hands behind one knee and gently pull the knee toward the chest (a).
- Slowly extend the opposite leg until it is either fully extended or lumbar stability is compromised (b).
- Perform two to four repetitions per side, each for a minimum of 15 seconds.

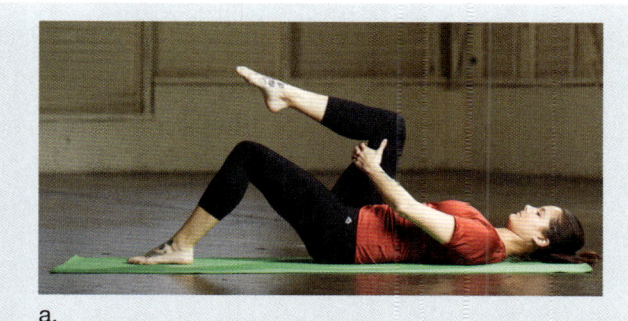

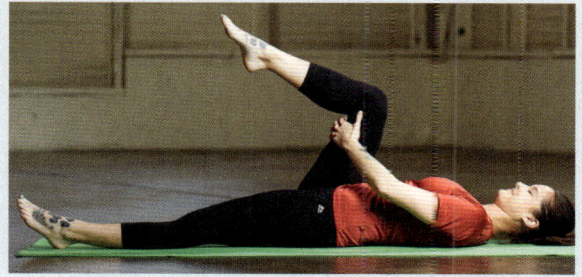

Figure 14-60
Hip-flexor mobility progression: Half-kneeling triplanar stretch

Objective: To improve mobility of the hip flexors in all three planes without compromising lumbar stability

Preparation and position:
- Assume a half-kneeling lunge position, placing the rear leg directly under the hips and torso (a).
- Engage the core muscles to stabilize the lumbar spine in the neutral position. Maintain this position throughout the exercise.

Exercise:
- Exhale and slowly lunge forward to stretch the hip flexors (b). Avoid any forward tilt of the pelvis that increases lordosis in the low back.
- Perform two to four repetitions per side.
- Hold each stretch for a minimum of 15 seconds.

Progression—sagittal plane: While maintaining a neutral lumbar spine, extend the arm opposite the forward leg overhead (c). Slowly reach the arm behind the head while slowly lunging forward, avoiding any increase in lumbar lordosis. Perform two to four repetitions per side and hold each stretch for a minimum of 15 seconds.

Progression—frontal plane: While maintaining a neutral lumbar spine, extend the arm opposite the forward leg overhead. Laterally flex the torso over the leading leg while slowly lunging forward, avoiding any increase in lumbar lordosis (d).

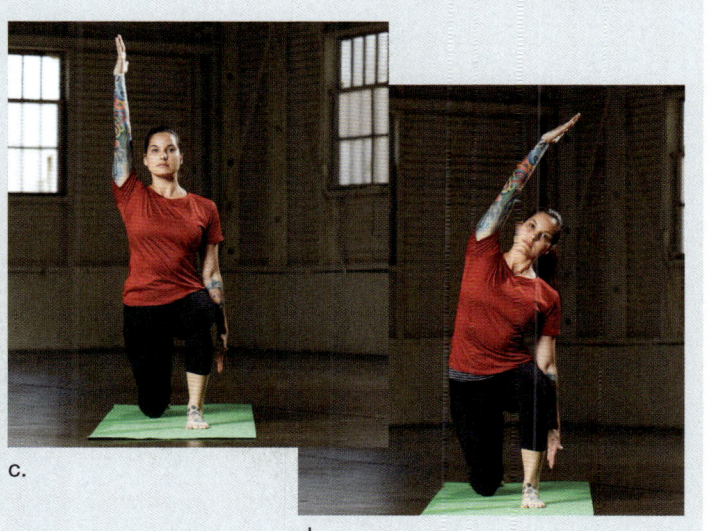

Perform two to four repetitions per side and hold each stretch for a minimum of 15 seconds.

Progression—transverse plane: While maintaining a neutral lumbar spine, place the arm opposite the leading leg behind the head (prisoner position). Rotate the torso over the leading leg while slowly lunging forward, avoiding any increase in lumbar lordosis (e). Perform two to four repetitions per side and hold each stretch for a minimum of 15 seconds.

Progression—spiral pattern: Assume a staggered-stance position, elevating the front leg and placing the foot on a riser or chair. Slowly lunge forward, avoiding any increase in lumbar lordosis, while simultaneously reaching both arms upward toward the side of the trailing leg as if preparing to swing a club or axe (f). Return to the starting, upright position as the arms swing down and across the front of the body (g). Perform one or two sets of five to 10 controlled repetitions per side, holding the end range of motion for one or two seconds, with 30-second rest intervals between sets.

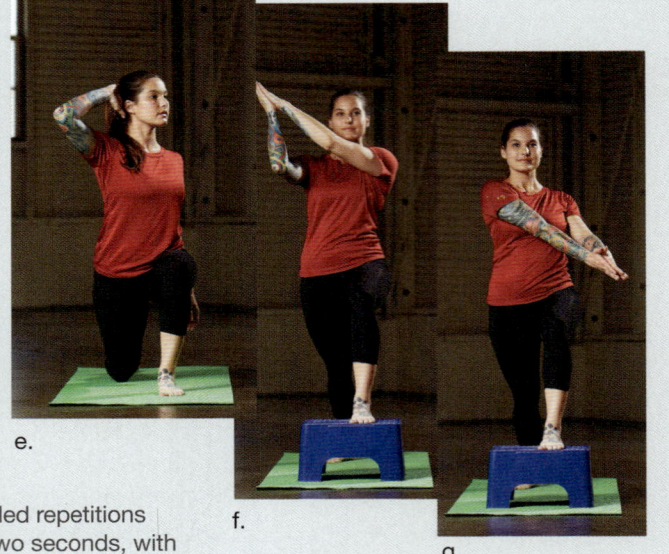

Figure 14-61
Hamstrings mobility: Lying hamstrings stretch

Objective: To improve mobility of the hamstrings in the sagittal plane without compromising lumbar stability

Preparation and position:
- Lie supine inside a door jamb with one knee bent and the foot placed flat on the floor, aligning the anterior superior iliac spine (ASIS) with the knee and second toe.
- Engage the core muscles to stabilize the lumbar spine in the neutral position, and maintain this position throughout the exercise.
- Raise the opposite leg to rest it on the door jamb with slight flexion in the knee and plantar flexion at the ankle (to remove any limitation from the gastrocnemius during the stretch) (a).

Exercise:
- Exhale and slowly extend the raised leg, stretching the hamstrings.
- The objective is to promote hamstrings flexibility with the extended leg positioned at an 80- to 90-degree angle with the floor.
- Perform two to four repetitions per side, each for a minimum of 15 seconds.

Progression: Perform a series of pelvic tilts, holding the anterior pelvic tilt to increase the magnitude of the stretch (b).

Progression: Extend the lower leg for the duration of the stretch without compromising lumbar stability (c).

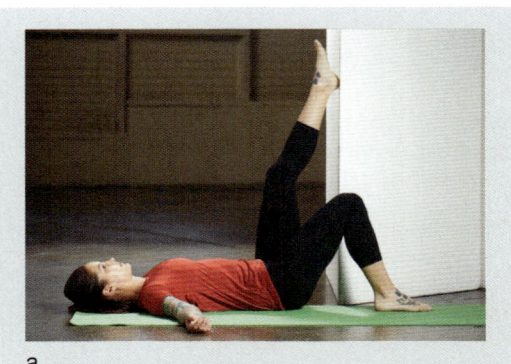

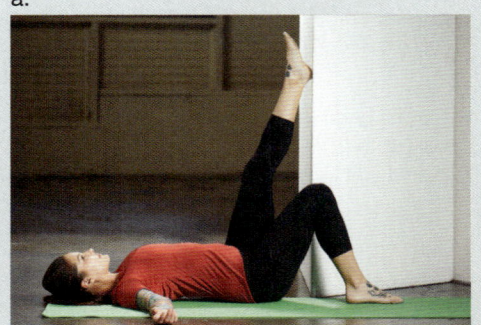

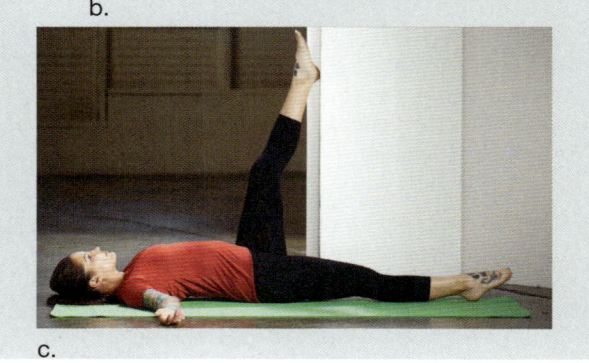

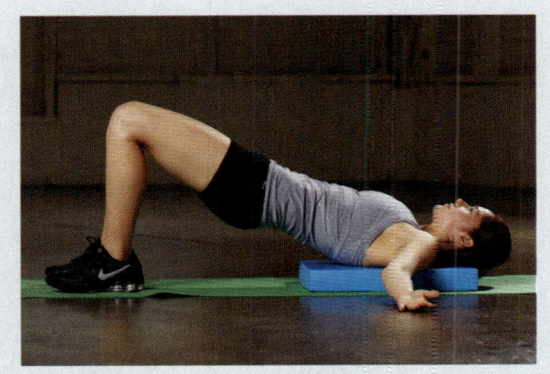

Posture and Movement

CHAPTER 14

Figure 14-62
Hip mobilization with glute activation: Shoulder bridge (glute bridge)

Objective: To improve hip mobility and stability and core stability by activating the gluteal muscle groups

Preparation and position:
- Lie supine with knees bent and the feet placed flat on the floor, aligning the anterior superior iliac spine (ASIS) with the knee and second toe (a).
- Engage the core muscles to stabilize the lumbar spine in the neutral position and maintain this position throughout the exercise. A common mistake made during this exercise is an increased lordosis in the up or "bridge" position due to a lack of lumbar stability. Recognizing the frequency of this compensation, full activation of the abdominals to tilt the pelvis posteriorly may be needed initially to prevent any increase in lordosis.

Exercise:
- Exhale and activate the gluteal muscles to elevate the hips off the floor into hip extension without increasing lordosis (b).
- Perform one or two sets of five to 10 controlled repetitions per side, holding the end range of motion for one or two seconds, with 30-second rest intervals between sets.

Progression: From the starting position, gently pull one knee toward the chest, tilting the pelvis posteriorly, and hold this knee to the chest while raising the body into the bridge position (c).

Progression: Place a riser or pad under the thoracic spine. This permits additional thoracic extension and increases the core challenge (d).

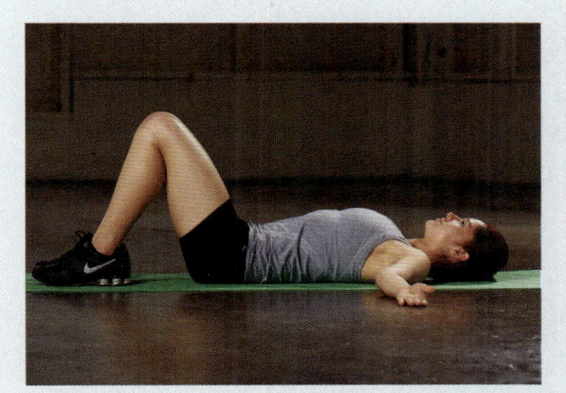

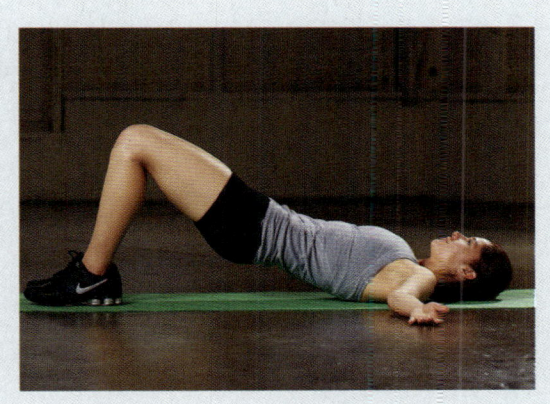

a.

b.

c.

d.

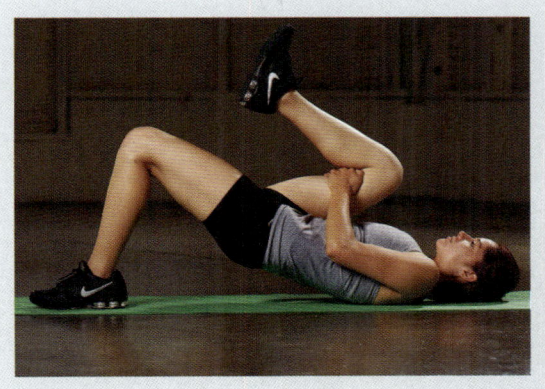

Figure 14-63
Hip mobilization: Supine 90-90 hip rotator stretch

Objective: To improve hip mobility in the transverse plane

Preparation and position:
- Lie supine with both feet placed against a wall, with an approximately 90-degree bend at the knees and 60 to 80 degrees of flexion at the hips (a).
- Cross one leg over the opposite knee, resting that ankle on the knee.
- Engage the core muscles to stabilize the lumbar spine in the neutral position and maintain this position throughout the exercise.
- Place one hand on the crossed knee.

Exercise:
- Exhale and gently push the crossed knee away from the body while simultaneously lifting the opposite foot off the wall, increasing the degree of hip flexion (b).
- Perform two to four repetitions per side.
- Hold each stretch for a minimum of 15 seconds.

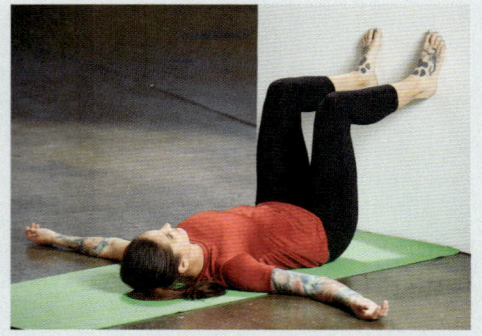

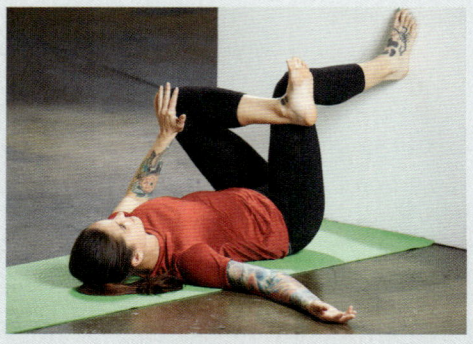

a.

b.

Figure 14-64
Thoracic-spine (T-spine) mobilization exercises: Spinal extensions and spinal twists

Spinal Extensions
Objective: To promote thoracic extension

Preparation and position:
- Lie supine with the knees bent and feet placed flat on the floor, aligning the anterior superior iliac spine (ASIS) with the knee and second toe.
- Position the arms at the sides with elbows extended.
- Engage the core muscles to stabilize the lumbar spine (avoiding increased lordosis during the exercise) and maintain this contraction throughout the exercise.
- Depress and retract the scapulae while stabilizing the low back (a).

Exercise:
- Exhale and slowly flex the shoulders, raise both arms overhead, and attempt to bring both hands to touch the floor overhead ("I" position) (b). Since the arms tend to internally rotate during shoulder flexion, and shrugging of the shoulders often occurs, attempt to depress the scapulae and keep the arms in a neutral or externally rotated position.
- Slowly return to the starting position.
- Perform one or two sets of five to 10 controlled repetitions, holding the end range of motion for one to two seconds, with 30-second rest intervals between sets.
- Repeat the entire movement from the starting position, but move into a "Y" formation, abducting the arms to 135 degrees (c).

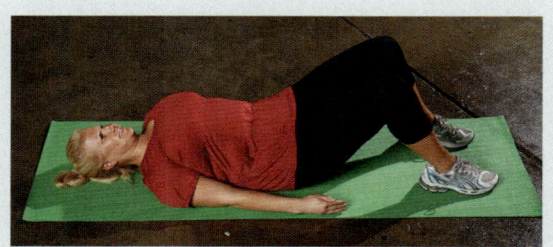

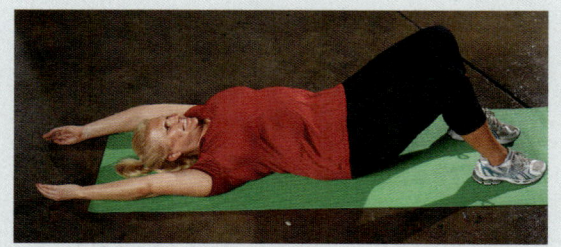

a.

b.

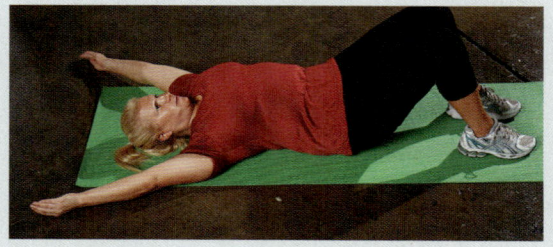

c.

Continued on next page

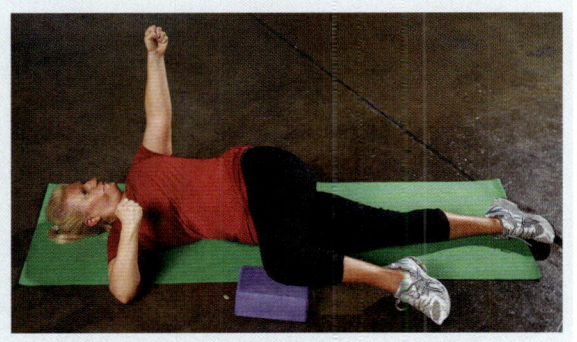

Posture and Movement

CHAPTER 14

- Repeat the entire movement from the starting position, but move in a "T" formation, sliding the arms along the floor and abducting them to 90 degrees (d).
- Repeat the entire movement from the starting position, but, with the elbows bent, move in a "wiper formation," sliding the arms along the floor from the sides to an overhead position.

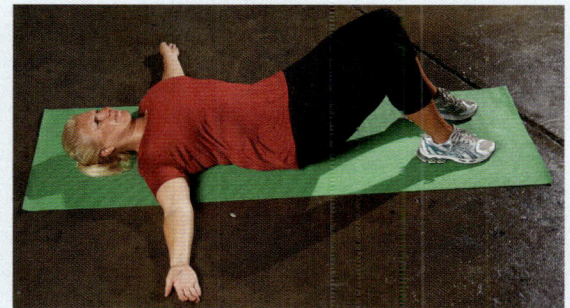

Spinal Twists

Objective: To promote trunk rotation, primarily through the thoracic spine with some lateral hip mobility

Preparation and position:
- Lie on one side, bending both knees to 90 degrees, flexing the hips to 90 to 100 degrees, and aligning both knees together, resting them on a ball or riser. Keep the lower knee on the ball or riser throughout this first exercise progression and keep both knees aligned. Engage the core muscles to stabilize the lumbar spine (avoiding increased lordosis) and maintain this contraction throughout the exercise.
- Reach the upper arm across and in front of the body, grasping the rib cage on the opposite side of the trunk (e).

Exercise:
- Exhale and slowly rotate the torso by pulling on the rib cage. Attempt to avoid any rotational movement of the hips and knees.
- Perform two to four repetitions to each side.
- Hold each pull for 15 to 30 seconds.

Progression: Repeat the same stretch, but place a squeezable object (e.g., a soft ball or yoga block) between the knees, positioning the lower knee on the floor.

Progression: Repeat the same stretch, but extend the lower leg and rest the inside of the upper knee on a squeezable object.

Progression: Repeat the same stretch, but change the upper arm from the rib-grab position to abducting the arm to 90 degrees with an extended elbow, and attempt to bring the upper arm down to touch the floor (f).

Progression—push-pull: Assume any of the starting positions for the lower extremity on one side. Depress and retract both scapulae, then move the upper arm to the start position of a press movement (e.g., bench press), while the lower arm moves into the start position of a pull movement (without protracting the scapula) (g & h). Simultaneously perform an upward press with the upper arm and a high-back row with the lower arm. Perform one or two sets of five to 10 controlled repetitions per side, holding the end range of motion for one or two seconds, with 30-second rest intervals between sets.

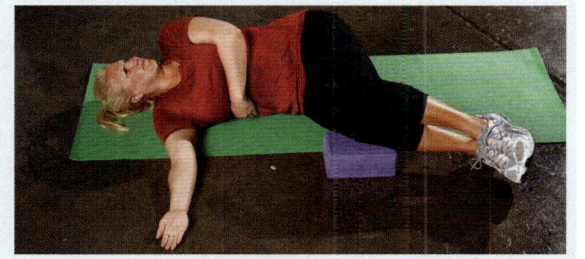

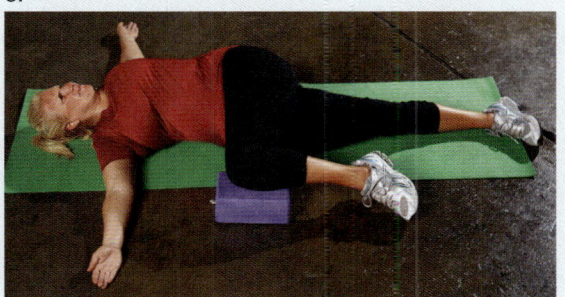

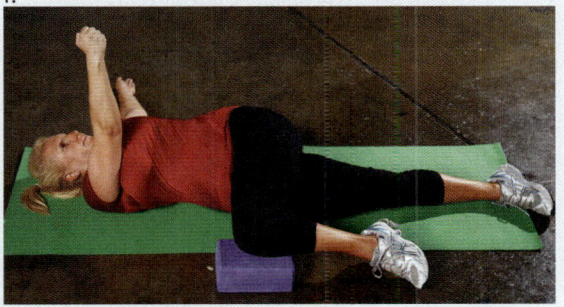

Figure 14-65
Posterior mobilization: Rocking quadrupeds

Objective: To promote hip and thoracic mobility while simultaneously maintaining lumbar stability

Preparation and position:
- Assume the quadruped position adjacent to a mirror, placing both hands directly under the shoulders (shoulder-width apart) and knees directly under the hips (hip-width apart) (a).
- Engage the core muscles to create a neutral spine. Maintain this flat or neutral spine throughout the exercise.

Exercise:
- While focusing on the spine, slowly rock backward and forward using visual feedback to control the range of movement, as dictated by a changing position of the spine (rounding during the backward roll and arching into lordosis during the forward rock) (b & c).
- Perform one or two sets of five to 10 controlled repetitions, holding the end range of motion for one or two seconds, with 30-second rest intervals between sets.

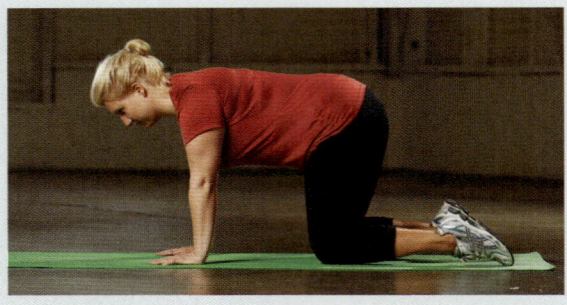

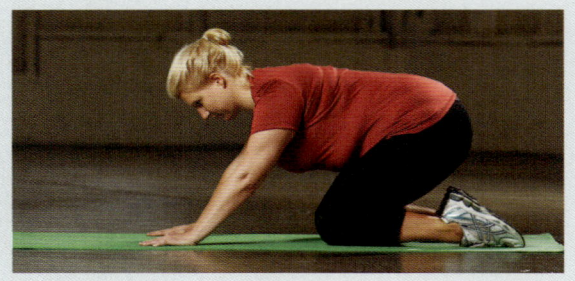

a.

b.

c.

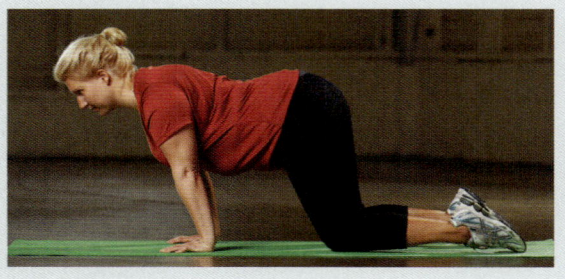

Proximal Stability of the Scapulothoracic Region and Proximal Mobility of the Glenohumeral Joint

This stage is designed to improve stability within the scapulothoracic region during upper-extremity movements (e.g., push- and pull-type motions). The glenohumeral joint is a highly mobile joint and its ability to achieve this degree of movement is contingent upon the stability of the scapulothoracic region (i.e., the ability of the scapulae to maintain appropriate proximity against the rib cage during movement) (Houglum, 2010; Sahrmann, 2002). It is the synergistic actions of muscle groups working through force-couples in this region that help achieve this stability, considering that the scapulae attach only to the axial skeleton via the clavicles. Promoting stability within this joint, therefore, requires muscle balance within the force-couples of the joint. Additionally, as many of these muscles also cross the glenohumeral joint, they require substantial levels of mobility. This implies that a program promoting scapulothoracic stability may need to include stretches to promote extensibility of both the muscle and joint structures. Therefore, static stretches to improve tissue extensibility should precede dynamic movement patterns and strengthening exercises.

A normally positioned scapula promotes muscle balance and effective force-coupling relationships. However, given the design of the shoulder girdle (favoring mobility at a cost of stability) and the propensity toward bad posture in the upper extremity due to a myriad of lifestyle-related positions and activities, compensated movement and shoulder injuries occur very frequently. Perhaps the most problematic movements are associated with arm abduction and a lack of scapular stability during horizontal push-and-pull movements.

Posture and Movement

CHAPTER 14

During abduction, the rotator cuff muscles play an important role in initiating movement and facilitating an inferior glide of the humeral head (Houglum, 2010). This glide is critical, as the articular surface of the humeral head is almost twice the size of the glenoid fossa, and therefore cannot operate as a true ball-and-socket joint. The rotator cuff muscles contract in anticipation of deltoid action. It is the collaborative action of the supraspinatus acting as the primary abductor for the first 15 degrees of abduction and the infraspinatus, subscapularis, and teres minor depressing the head of the humerus inferiorly within the glenoid fossa that permit rotation to occur (in this case, abduction of the shoulder) (Figure 14-66) (Cook & Jones, 2007a; Kendall et al., 2005). After approximately 15 degrees of abduction, the deltoid takes over as the primary abductor, while the rotator cuff muscles continue to depress and stabilize the humeral head, along with the anterior and posterior deltoid. If the deltoid acted alone, pure superior glide would occur, which would impinge the humeral head against the coracoacromial arch at approximately 22 degrees of abduction.

During pushing and pulling movements, key parascapular muscles (i.e., serratus anterior, rhomboids, and lower trapezius) co-contract to permit movement of the scapulae, yet help it maintain proximity against the rib cage. When the thoracic spine lacks appropriate mobility, what often results is compensation to stability within the scapulothoracic region, which in turn affects mobility within the glenohumeral joint and muscle action within that joint. However, with good thoracic mobility and muscle balance in the scapulothoracic region to effectively stabilize the scapula and control its movement, the more distal mobilizers (e.g., deltoid) can generate larger amounts of force. It therefore appears that promoting stability within the scapulothoracic region requires thoracic mobility in addition to other key factors:

- Tissue extensibility (both active and passive structures)
- Healthy rotator cuff muscle function
- Muscle balance within the parascapular muscles
- The ability to resist upward glide and impingement against the coracoacromial arch during deltoid action

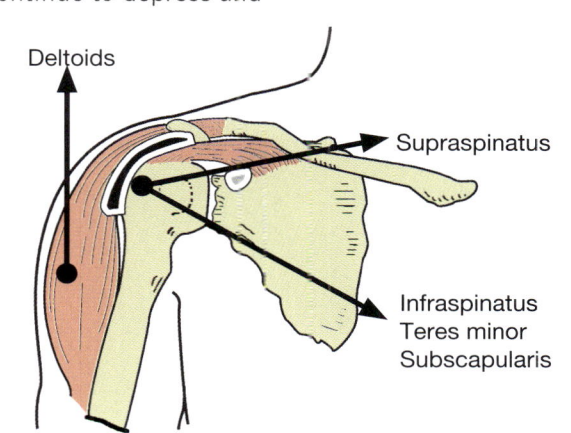

Figure 14-66
Muscle action involved in abducting (raising) the arm

To enhance tissue extensibility, the CMES can employ several different stretching modalities. Self–myofascial release using a stick or foam roller—moving across the tender spots—may help increase ROM and reduce hypertonicity. This should precede static stretching of the shoulder capsule and of specific muscles of the scapulae. When stretching the shoulder capsule with a client, the CMES must address the inferior, posterior, anterior, and superior components.

- Stretch the inferior capsule using an overhead triceps stretch (Figure 14-67).
- Stretch the posterior capsule by bringing the arm across and in front of the body (Figure 14-68a). An alternative position for this stretch is to stand adjacent to a wall flexing the arm in front of the body to 90 degrees and resting the full length of the arm against the wall, then slowly rotate the trunk inward toward the wall (Figure 14-68b & c). Since this movement also produces scapular abduction, and since it is common for clients to have abducted scapulae as a postural deviation, it should be a minimal focus during shoulder stretching.
- Stretch the anterior capsule using a pectoralis stretch (Figure 14-69).
- Stretch the superior capsule by placing a rolled-up towel 2 inches (5.1 cm) above the elbow against the trunk (bent-elbow position at the side of the body), grasping the base of the elbow and pulling it downward and inward (Figure 14-70).

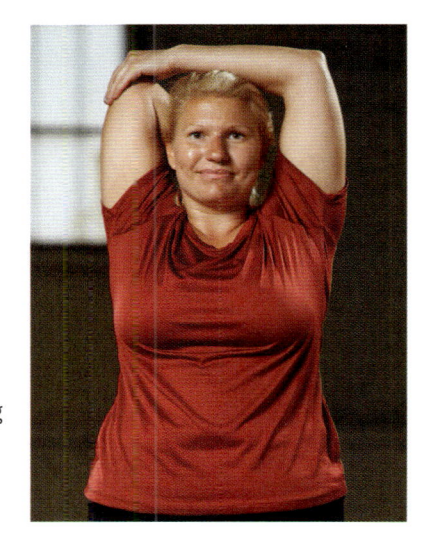

Figure 14-67
Inferior capsule stretch

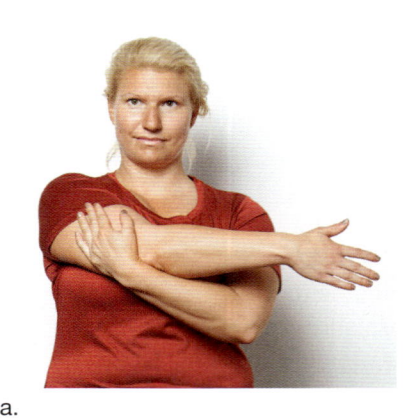

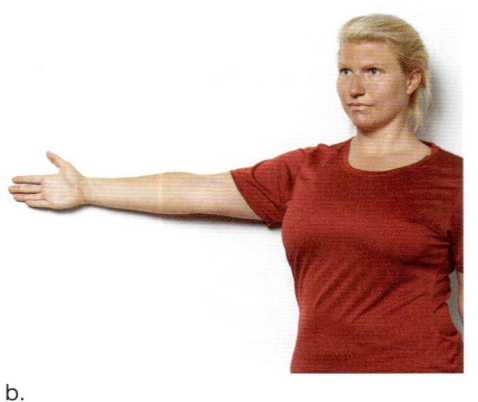

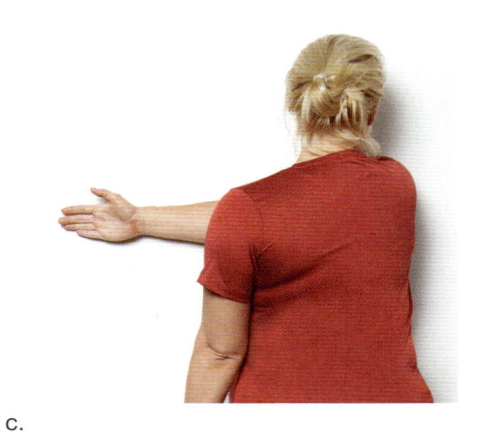

Figure 14-68
Posterior capsule stretches

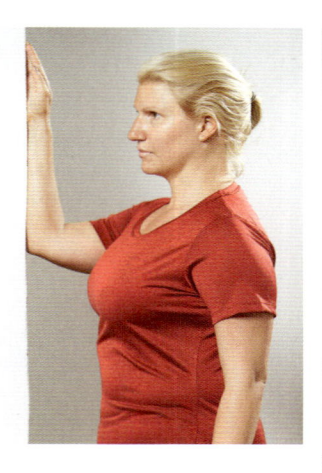

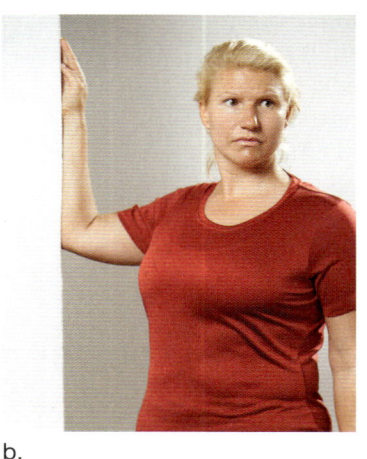

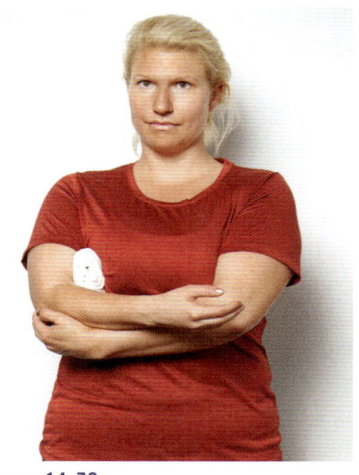

Figure 14-69
Anterior capsule (pectoralis) stretch

Figure 14-70
Superior capsule stretch

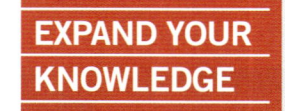

EXPAND YOUR KNOWLEDGE

OPEN- AND CLOSED-KINETIC-CHAIN MOVEMENTS

One important consideration for promoting scapulothoracic stability revolves around the type of exercises selected (i.e., closed-chain or open-chain exercises). During closed-kinetic-chain (CKC) movements where the distal segment is more fixed (e.g., pull-ups and push-ups), a key role of the serratus anterior is to move the thorax toward a more fixed, stable scapulae (Houglum, 2010; Cook & Jones, 2007a). During open-kinetic-chain (OKC) movements, however, a key role of the serratus anterior is to control movement of the scapulae against a more fixed rib cage (Houglum, 2010; Cook & Jones, 2007a).

CKC movements are generally considered more functional, as they closely mimic daily activities. CKC exercises load and compress joints, increasing kinesthetic awareness and proprioception, which translates into improved parascapular and shoulder stability (Cook & Jones, 2007a). Isolated OKC exercises, on the other hand, are not as effective in restoring coordinated parascapular control. One challenge with CKC exercises is that many are too challenging for deconditioned individuals. Thus, it is important to initially use the floor to provide kinesthetic feedback and OKC movements to improve control and movement efficiency and increase kinesthetic awareness of shoulder position. The CMES can start by first helping the individual recognize the normal resting position of the scapulae kinesthetically (i.e., feel the correct scapular position against the floor). The exercise presented in Figure 14-71 helps achieve this awareness by instructing the client on how to "pack" the scapulae.

Posture and Movement

CHAPTER 14

Figure 14-71
Shoulder packing

Objective: To kinesthetically improve awareness of good scapular position, improving flexibility and strength of key parascapular muscles

Preparation and position:
- Lie supine on a mat with knees bent to 90 degrees and the feet placed flat on the floor, aligning the anterior superior iliac spine (ASIS) with the knee and second toe.
- Position the arms at the sides of the trunk with the palms facing upward.
- Engage the core muscles to stabilize the lumbar spine in the neutral position. Maintain this position throughout the exercise (a).

Exercise:
- Exhale and perform two to four repetitions of each of the following, holding each contraction for five to 10 seconds (b):
    ✓ Scapular depression
    ✓ Scapular retraction
- Using passive assistance from the opposite arm, gently push down on the shoulder (posterior tilt on scapula) without losing lumbar stability. Hold this position for 15 to 60 seconds.
- Relax and repeat two to four times on each shoulder.

Note: These exercises can be performed standing against a wall in a quarter-squat position for people who cannot tolerate getting down onto the floor or lying on their back (e.g., those who have obesity or are pregnant, or have orthopedic problems) (c & d).

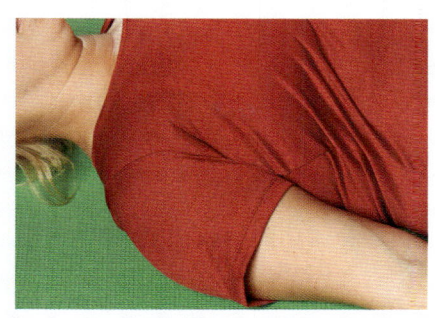

a.

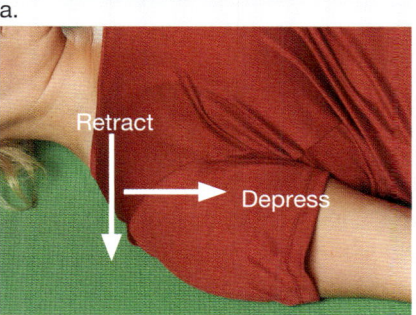

b.

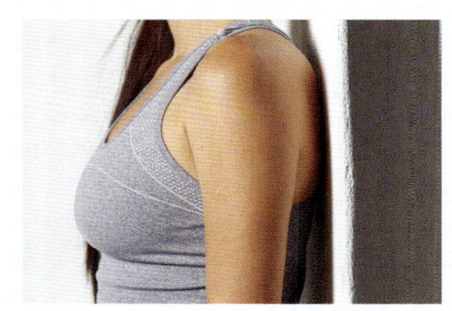

c.

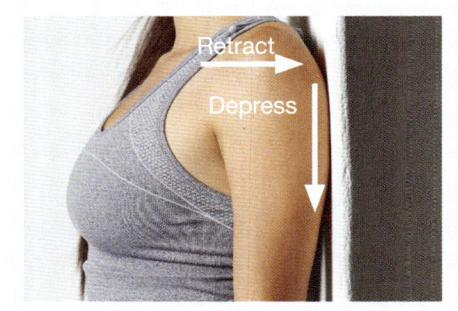

d.

A variety of exercises can be used to condition the rotator cuff muscles, but whichever exercises the CMES and client select, the client must perform them from the packed shoulder position. Figures 14-72 through 14-76 provide examples of OKC and CKC rotator-cuff exercises that promote scapulothoracic stability.

Figure 14-72
External and internal humeral rotation

Objective: To improve rotator cuff function while maintaining good scapular position

Preparation and position:
- Lie supine on a mat with knees bent and feet placed flat on the floor, aligning the anterior superior iliac spine (ASIS) with the knee and second toe.
- Engage the core muscles to stabilize the lumbar spine in the neutral position and maintain this position throughout the exercise.
- Pack both scapulae and maintain this position throughout the exercise.
- Abduct the arms to 90 degrees (shoulder height), resting the backs of the upper arms on the mat, and bend the elbows 90 degrees so that the forearms are perpendicular to the floor (a).

Exercise:
- External rotation: Slowly externally rotate the arms backward, bringing the forearms toward the floor. The ultimate goal is to achieve movement so that the back of the forearm rests on the floor (90 degrees of movement) (b).
- Hold this position for 15 to 60 seconds and repeat two to four times.
- Internal rotation: From the starting position, internally rotate the arms forward, bringing the forearms toward the floor. The ultimate goal is to achieve movement so that the forearms reach an angle of 20 to 30 degrees above the floor (60 to 70 degrees of movement) (c).
- Hold this position for 15 to 60 seconds, and repeat two to four times.

Progression: Once the end ranges can be reached, add resistance to condition these muscles (d & e). Remember, these are small muscles with higher concentrations of type I fibers, so they respond best to volume training. Add no more than 5 pounds (2.3 kg) of external resistance (cable or dumbbell) and build volume toward three sets of 12 to 15 repetitions, with 30-second rest intervals between sets.

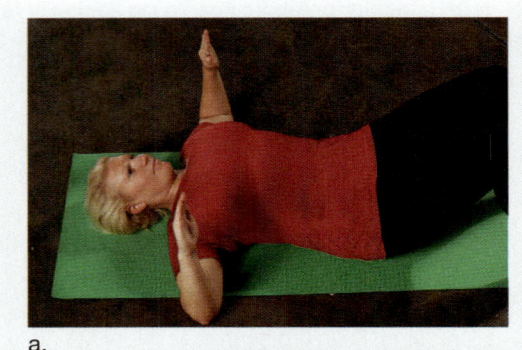

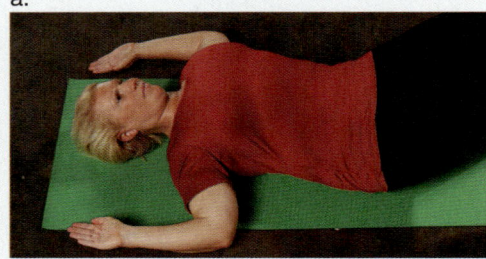

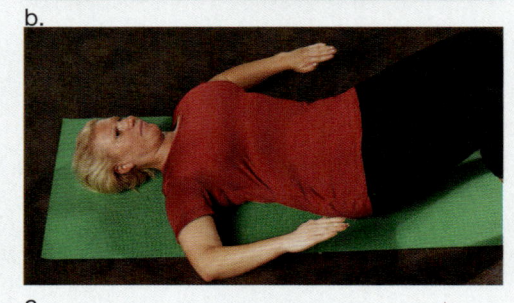

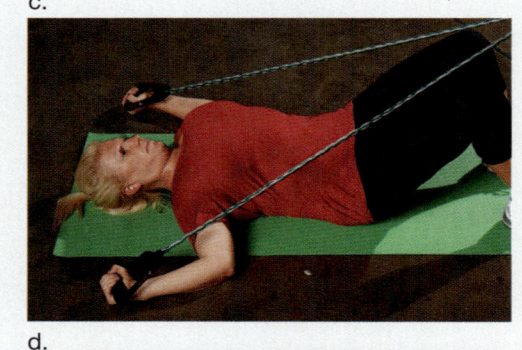

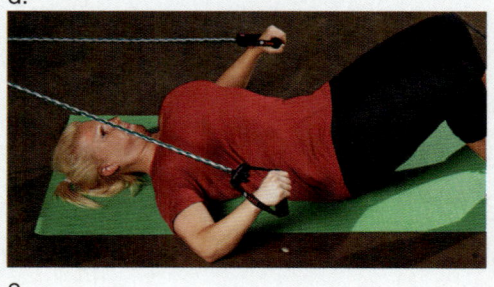

Posture and Movement CHAPTER 14

Figure 14-73
Diagonals

Objective: To improve rotator cuff function with four integrated movements (in two diagonal patterns) at the glenohumeral and scapulothoracic joints

Preparation and position:
- Lie supine on a mat with knees bent and feet placed flat on the floor, aligning the anterior superior iliac spine (ASIS) with the knee and second toe.
- Engage the core muscles to stabilize the lumbar spine in the neutral position and maintain this position throughout the exercise.
- Pack both scapulae and maintain this position throughout the exercise.

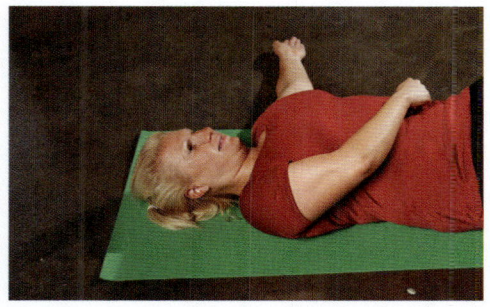

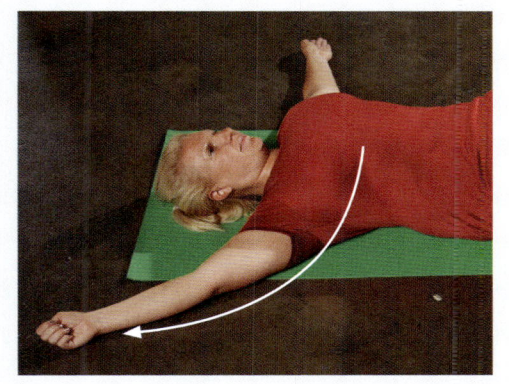

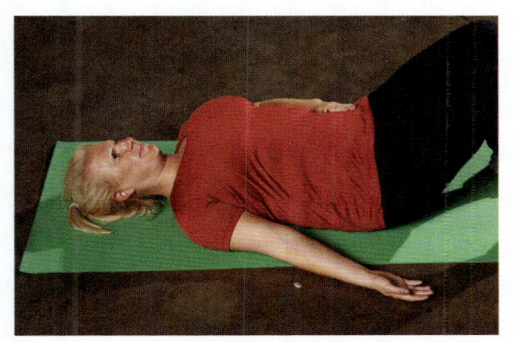

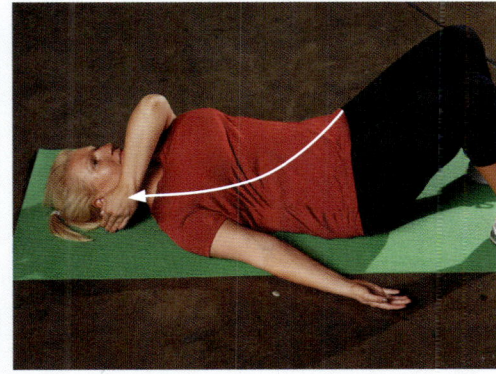

Exercises:
- *Diagonal 1:* Start with one arm extended and placed across the body in an internally rotated position (as if reaching across to withdraw a sword from its sheath) (a). Pull the arm back across the body, externally rotating and abducting the arm to 90 degrees (b). This movement combines elevation, adduction, and upward rotation of the scapulae with extension, abduction, and external rotation of the glenohumeral joint. Perform the opposite movement to return to the starting position. Perform one or two sets of five to 10 controlled repetitions per arm, holding the end range of motion for one or two seconds, with 30-second rest intervals between sets.

- *Diagonal 2:* Start with one arm extended and placed at the side of the body in an internally rotated position (c). Pull the arm across the body, toward the opposite shoulder, externally rotating and adducting the arm as it moves toward that shoulder (with the palm toward the face) (d). This movement combines elevation, abduction, and upward rotation of the scapulae with flexion, adduction, and external rotation of the glenohumeral joint. Perform the opposite movement to return to the starting position. Perform one or two sets of five to 10 controlled repetitions per arm, holding the end range of motion for one or two seconds, with 30-second rest intervals between sets.

a.

b.

c.

d.

Progression: Repeat the four diagonal movements, but add light cable resistance. Remember, these are small muscles with higher concentrations of type I fibers, so they respond best to volume training. Add no more than 5 pounds (2.3 kg) of external resistance (cable or dumbbell) and build volume toward three sets of 12 to 15 repetitions, with 30-second rest intervals between sets.

Figure 14-74
Reverse flys with supine 90-90

Objective: To strengthen the posterior muscles of the shoulder complex

Preparation and position:
- Lie supine on the floor with both legs draped over a chair or riser. The height of the chair or riser should allow the knees and hips to flex to 90 degrees without elevating the hips off the floor.
- Align the anterior superior iliac spine (ASIS) with the knee and second toe and use supports to hold the feet in this position (e.g., pillows), preventing any external or internal rotation of the feet and lower legs, which would alter pelvic and low-back position.
- Abduct the arms to 90 degrees (shoulder height), resting the backs of the upper arms on the mat and bending the elbows 90 degrees so that the forearms are perpendicular to the floor.
- Engage the core muscles to stabilize the lumbar spine in the neutral position and maintain this position throughout the exercise (a).
- Pack both scapulae and maintain this position throughout the exercise.

Exercise:
- Exhale and press the back of the arms into the floor with less than 50% of maximal voluntary contraction, without altering the position of the lumbar spine.
- Perform two to four repetitions, holding each isometric contraction for five to 10 seconds.

Progression: Lying supine, build exercise volume toward three sets of 12 to 15 repetitions, with 30-second rest intervals between sets.

Progression: Seated with the back flat against a wall and knees bent, perform three sets of 12 to 15 repetitions, with 30-second rest intervals between sets. Maintain contact between the sacrum, low back, scapulae, and back of the head and the wall (b).

Figure 14-75
Prone arm lifts

Objective: To strengthen the parascapular muscles

Preparation and position:
- Lie prone on a mat with both legs extended and arms positioned overhead with bent elbows, resting the forearms on a mat.
- Engage the core muscles to stabilize the lumbar spine in the neutral position and maintain this position throughout the exercise.
- Pack both scapulae and maintain this position throughout the exercise (a).

Exercise:
- "I" formation: Exhale and lift both arms 2 to 4 inches (5 to 10 cm) off the floor (keeping the elbows bent), while maintaining a depressed scapular position (avoiding scapular elevation) (b).

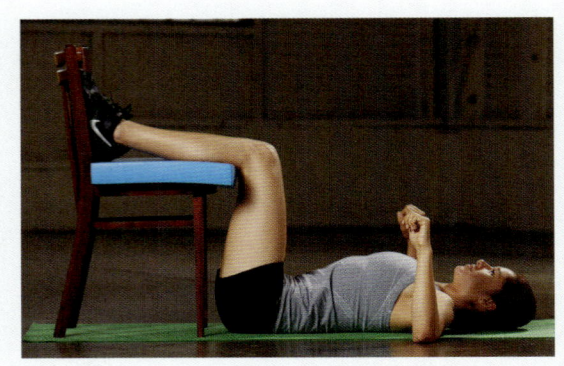

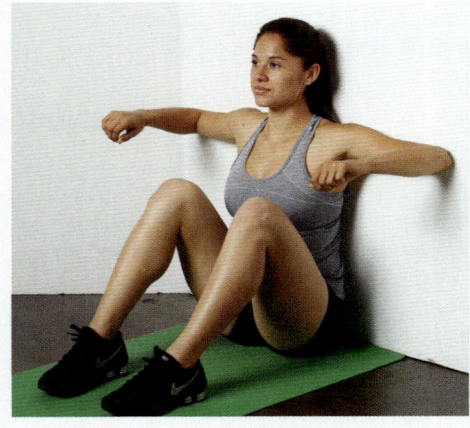

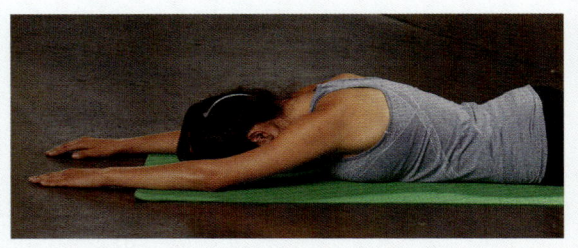

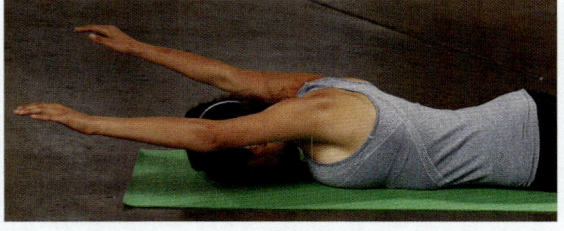

Posture and Movement
CHAPTER 14

- Perform two to four repetitions, holding each repetition for five to 10 seconds.
- *"Y" formation:* Slide both arms out to a 135-degree position, keeping the elbows bent, but resting the arms on the mat (forming the letter "Y"). Exhale and lift both arms 2 to 4 inches (5 to 10 cm) off the floor while maintaining a depressed scapular position (avoiding scapular elevation) (c).
- Perform two to four repetitions, holding each repetition for five to 10 seconds.
- *"W" formation:* Slide both arms out to 90 degrees (shoulder height), resting the arms on the mat (forming the letter "W"). Exhale and lift both arms 2 to 4 inches (5 to 10 cm) off the floor while maintaining a depressed scapular position (avoiding scapular elevation) (d).
- Perform two to four repetitions, holding each repetition for five to 10 seconds.
- *"O" formation:* Reach behind the back and interlock the fingers, forming a giant letter "O" on the back, resting both forearms on the back. Exhale and lift both arms 2 to 4 inches (5 to 10 cm) off the back, while maintaining a depressed scapular position (avoiding scapular elevation) (e).
- Perform two to four repetitions, holding each repetition for five to 10 seconds.

Progression: Repeat the "I", "Y," and "W" formations with fully extended arms (note that the "W" formation becomes a "T" formation with the arms fully extended). Build the exercise volume toward three sets of 12 to 15 repetitions with 30-second rest intervals between sets. These exercises can ultimately be progressed to an incline position on a stability ball, standing, or in a hip-hinge or forward-bending position (hips flexed 90 degrees).

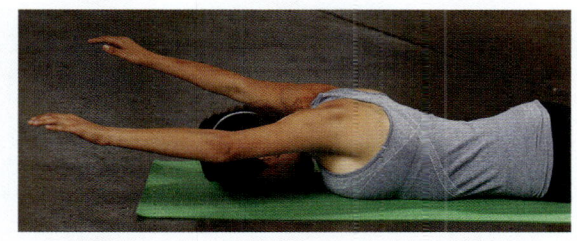

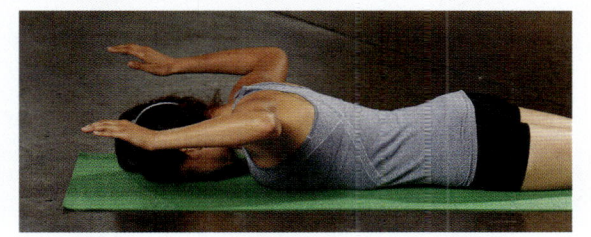

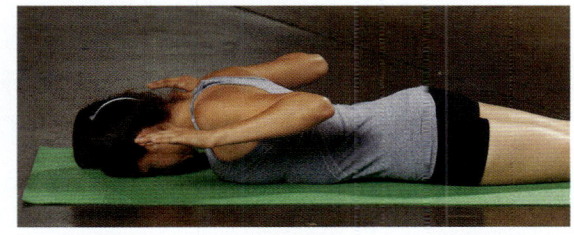

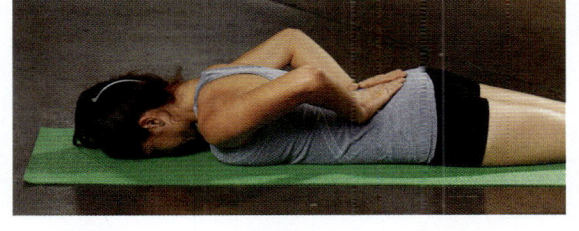

b.

c.

d.

e.

Figure 14-76
Closed-kinetic-chain weight shifts

Objective: To stabilize the scapulothoracic joint and lumbar spine in a closed-kinetic-chain (CKC) position

Preparation and position:

- Lie prone on a mat, placing the hands directly under the shoulders and extending both legs.
- Engage the core muscles to stabilize the lumbar spine in the neutral position. Maintain this position throughout the exercise.
- Pack the shoulders (see Figure 14-71) and maintain this position throughout the exercise (a).
- Press the body upward to assume a full or bent-knee push-up position (b).

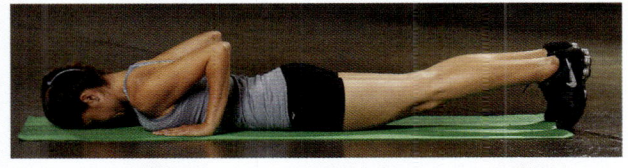

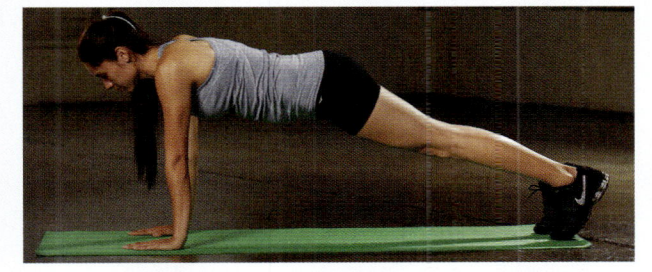

a.

b.

Figure 14-76
Closed-kinetic-chain weight shifts *(continued)*

Exercise:

- Slowly shift the body weight 3 to 6 inches (8 to 15 cm) forward, backward, left, and right without moving the hands (c).

- Perform two to four repetitions, holding each for five to 10 seconds.

Progression: Offset one hand into a staggered position by moving it 6 to 12 inches (15 to 30 cm) forward of the shoulder and repeat the movement (d). Perform two to four repetitions, holding each for five to 10 seconds. Repeat to the opposite side.

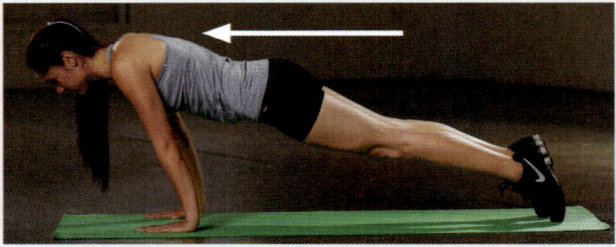

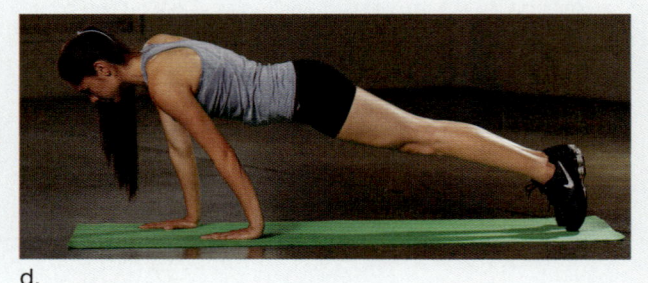

PRACTICAL APPROACHES FOR DESIGNING AND IMPLEMENTING RESTORATIVE EXERCISE PROGRAMS

Posture and movement analysis is a relatively direct process with generally accepted standards for identifying abnormalities. While developing an expert eye for deviations takes time and practice, all practitioners essentially work from the same baseline—ideal posture. However, identifying the cause of faulty posture and movement, as well as generating strategies for improving them, are not quite so direct or clear-cut. Given the many variables that can influence posture and movement, it is difficult to create a standard set of procedures for improvement. The CMES must respect that no one clear solution is guaranteed to solve even the most common issues and should remain open to a trial-and-error process. Trial and error is not only relevant, it allows practitioners to remain objective and scrutinize the effectiveness of each strategy implemented.

It should be noted that trial and error is not an arbitrary selection of techniques. On the contrary, it can be driven by a systematic approach that will help identify priorities and narrow strategic options more efficiently. To develop a systematic approach, it will be beneficial to draw distinctions between two commonly used evaluation terms—screens and assessments. Along with other terms (e.g., tests, evaluations, and analysis), "screens" and "assessments" are often used interchangeably. However, drawing on the subtle distinctions between them can help the CMES develop an efficient and effective process that will streamline efforts and benefit individual clients.

Using Information from Assessments and Screens

Initial observations should be comprehensive, yet remain broad. In general, gross deviations should be sought out first and can be done so through sweeping observations. This is the "postural assessment" process. Screens take a global look at movement and simply identify if faults exist, not why they exist.

For example, if it is observed that a client's knees present with a **valgus** movement (collapse inward) during a postural assessment, it is simply noted in the initial phase. Provided a client is pain-free, they should be able to safely perform fundamental movements for further evaluation. If squatting and lunging movements, for example, demonstrate further knee valgus, it too should be noted and can be recognized as a pattern. The initial observations, or screening, may not shed any light on possible causes, and therefore developing corrective strategies at this stage is premature. A more thorough exploration of the possible cause of the knee valgus will help determine appropriate initial strategies, as well as help identify exercises that may need to be excluded from a program. In this example, the posture, squat, and lunge observations are part of the screening process and help pinpoint what requires further assessment. If no deviations are observed, standard strategies for exercise programming can be explored.

Posture Assessment = Identify possible cause
Movement Screens = Identify possible risks

Prioritizing

In the event that a client has only one obvious postural alignment fault, priorities would naturally focus on the area where the fault is found. However, in the unfortunate event that a client has multiple postural and movement-control issues, prioritizing can be perplexing. Attempting to address all issues may be unrealistic and can also be overwhelming for the client. In the case of multiple postural issues, it is important to develop a prioritization system. While this is another aspect left to discretion of the CMES, there are considerations that can help identify the highest-priority needs for each individual:

- *Severity of faults:* If one area (postural) or one movement appears to have more significant faults than other areas that would place the client at risk and/or interfere with normal exercise programming, this would indicate a higher priority.
- *ADL assessment:* Understanding the individual's ADL—recreational, vocational, or other regular physical requirements—can help identify higher priorities.
- *History of injury:* The CMES would not work with a client during acute stages of injury. However, the likelihood of working with clients who have an injury history and/or have undergone musculoskeletal surgical procedures is very plausible. This can help identify areas of highest priority.

If there appears to be no specific threat to ADL and no history of injury or musculoskeletal-related surgery, the CMES should address the most obvious faults first. This does not mean that other faults should be ignored, but to ensure the client is not overwhelmed, it may be important to apply corrections in relatively small doses.

Source vs. Symptom

Given the interconnectedness of the body, dysfunctional alignment in one area may be the cause of alignment or pain-related issues in other areas of the body. Drawing a distinction, whenever possible, between a symptom and a source can also help ensure strategies are not misdirected. For example, a history of minor knee issues may be a result of poor foot/ankle movement and/or hip movement. Recognizing these dynamics can help the CMES address movement-correction strategies from a more comprehensive and integrated perspective.

The Process

- Posture assessment
- Movement screens and flexibility tests
- Implement restorative exercise
- Re-screen

The ultimate objective for the CMES is to identify the most appropriate solutions that fall within scope of practice. The process of assess → screen/test → implement → re-screen illustrates a systematic trial-and-error approach. Over time, it is easy for practitioners to develop biases toward certain methods. Even if specific methods have a tendency to work in *most* situations, it is the professional and ethical responsibility of the CMES to avoid assuming that a method will work in *all* situations. Therefore, by following this process, the CMES can essentially grade the strategies that are implemented. Applying strategies without evaluating their effectiveness can waste time and limit progress. It is important for the CMES to understand the principles and purpose behind methods rather than memorize the details of a specific method. This allows for an objective approach and will help increase efficiency of efforts.

Posture Assessment

The posture assessment process will explore how a client's joints align in relation to one another during restful standing. Generally speaking, posture- and movement-related limitations are caused by either mobility issues or stability issues. Mobility refers to the ability of a joint to move freely, while stability refers to the relative control of a joint or joints under load and through movement. In other words, a mobility issue is a movement limitation due to some form of "tightness," while stability is a limitation due to poor control or inefficient recruitment strategies.

Mobility issues are most often a result of soft-tissue restrictions from tight muscles, myofascial restrictions, and/or joint restrictions. In a postural assessment, mobility problems could appear as joints that are held in a constant state of flexion, extension, or rotation rather than in ideal neutral or centered position. If mobility restrictions are found, implementing flexibility strategies to increase the extensibility of the soft tissue and increase mobility within the joint may be necessary to enhance the range of a movement and improve the movement pattern. Applying any number of strategies may be helpful. These could include static, active, and dynamic stretching methods; myofascial work (e.g., foam rolling); relaxation techniques; and modification of behaviors and activities that may perpetuate stiffness.

It should be noted that some muscles may appear "tight," but may carry only excessive tension, or hypertonicity. In other words, they may not lack necessary ranges of motion needed for fundamental movements. This can be a result of repetitive movements, physical strain, poor posture, mental stress, poor sleep habits, and/or other incomplete recovery habits. In some of these cases, lifestyle habits may need to be addressed to prevent further exacerbation of tension-related issues. However, simply changing a lifestyle stimulus does not address the cumulative tension that may have developed. Therefore, appropriate mobility strategies should be explored to help alleviate muscular tension.

Movement Screens and Flexibility Tests

As already mentioned, screens are not designed to identify cause. They simply act as a filter to determine if an issue is present. Movement screenings observe alignment, as well as the overall ability to efficiently move through a pattern. Each movement can be labeled as either efficient (sufficient movement strategies) or inefficient (insufficient movement strategies). Because movement screens are not a measurement of volume (fitness capacity or strength), an individual's fitness and strength levels are not typically factors. In fact, it is possible for an untrained individual to move and screen well, while an extremely fit individual may move poorly and therefore screen poorly for movement.

In general, screens search for restrictions and movement inabilities. Some movements in a screening process may appear restricted. For example, a client may have a limited ROM when attempting to perform a full body-weight squat. It would appear that that a mobility issue is present. However, this cannot be conclusively determined simply by observing the movement. A limited-ROM squat would be categorized as inefficient and would need to be assessed further. Some movements may demonstrate appropriate ROM, but could demonstrate poor alignment and control of the desired path or plane of motion. These too would be labeled as inefficient. If further investigation is deemed necessary by the CMES, another option is to perform muscle length tests (also called flexibility tests) on the areas in question. Determining a client's passive ROM through a static flexibility test on joints that appear inflexible is an additional process exercise professionals can use to confirm findings from a posture assessment and/or movement screen.

Implement Restorative Exercise

The CMES must be able to implement effective and progressive exercise strategies for clients. While this is an integral part of the CMES's professional responsibility, the ability to regress exercises and identify exercises that may need to be excluded from a program, especially when it pertains to clients with postural and movement faults, may be even more important. Regressions require an intimate understanding of the various components involved in a movement, including

Posture and Movement   CHAPTER 14

> **APPLY WHAT YOU KNOW**
>
> ## AN EXAMPLE OF REPETITIVE MOVEMENT NEGATIVELY INFLUENCING MOBILITY
>
> Consider a client who wears high-heeled shoes every day. This places the calf muscles in a shortened position with near-constant activation when walking. This client may develop short, tight calf muscles, causing a restriction in dorsiflexion due to poor extensibility of the gastrocnemius and soleus, which can be observed in the posture screen as ankle joints that appear more open, or extended beyond neutral. Evaluating her ankle ROM through the squat movement screen can help identify whether or not it is limited in dorsiflexion. For example, if her calf muscles carry excessive tension, this could be evidenced by her heels lifting off of the floor during the descent of the squat.
>
> Determining whether a muscle(s) lacks ROM or simply carries excessive tension can influence corrective strategies. A tight muscle may require extensive stretching and flexibility work, while a hypertonic muscle may need less stretching but may benefit more from tension-releasing techniques, such as myofascial release. Following the assess → screen/test → implement → re-screen process will help determine if strategies are improving the conditions to move.

mobility and stability requirements, coordination, and timing. Understanding developmental patterns can help guide the CMES "backward" to the most fundamental needs that connect to effective functional movement patterns.

Exercise exclusion requires a thorough understanding of a movement, but perhaps more importantly, how a client responds to that movement. For example, a client may demonstrate an effective lunge with no pain or obvious deviations, yet may be unable to squat well and/or may feel discomfort during squatting motions. Provided the client is cleared to exercise, lunges may safely be included in an exercise program, while squats may be excluded. Since squatting is a fundamental and necessary part of the performance of ADL, regression strategies should be explored to help improve the squat.

Re-screen

In fitness, it is common to perform fitness evaluations routinely and at designated times—quite often every two to four months. Formal and comprehensive re-screening can be instituted during this time as well. However, during the earliest stages of training, constant monitoring of movement progress is imperative, especially when applying corrective strategies. When addressing posture and movement-related faults, re-screening should be frequent and can actually be used after each strategy has been applied, as some strategies may be more effective than others. At the same time, other strategies may be completely ineffective or may even exacerbate a movement fault. If several exercises that are designed to improve posture or movement-related issues are applied before re-screening, it will be difficult to determine which exercises or strategies had a positive influence and which ones may have had little to no influence. This can slow down progress and may increase time spent performing unnecessary strategies. This is part of the trial-and-error process and can help develop the most efficient and effective approach for the individual

In the case of significant mobility restrictions (tightness), the process will likely take time. Re-screening can still be frequently performed. However, mobility strategies for significant restrictions may produce only minor and temporary changes. Nevertheless, minor improvements to mobility are still a positive sign and indicate opportunities for consistent improvement if frequent application is administered.

In the case of stability-related issues, it is possible to see immediate results after applying strategies designed to improve stability. Because stability is about control, modifying the environment for the client can produce marked improvements. Making a movement less challenging may provide an opportunity to retrain and build. In other words, if a regression strategy improves the stability of a movement, it creates a positive and manageable environment.

For example, a client may be able to complete one full push-up, but with poor scapular stabilization. This is not only inefficient, but it can also place heavy stresses on the glenohumeral joint, thereby increasing the risk of wear and tear and possible injury. By implementing, for example, an assisted technique (modifying the conditions by reducing the load), the client may be able to effectively recruit their scapular stabilizers and perform a push-up with efficient form. With time and practice, the stabilizers can develop greater strength and stability during the push-up movement. Over time, as success dictates, the assistance can be lessened and eventually removed. The end result should be a retrained movement with better overall stability. From there, traditional, progressive fitness and strength strategies can be explored.

EXPAND YOUR KNOWLEDGE

STABILITY VS. BALANCE

Stability and balance are sometimes mistaken as being the same. For the purposes of programming, the CMES should consider these concepts as being uniquely separate. Balance is essentially about maintaining equilibrium, whereas stability is about timing and control of the separate parts throughout the kinetic chain. Balance, or equilibrium, can be accomplished in the absence of adequate kinetic-chain stability. This indicates a level of effectiveness (i.e., not falling), but does not necessarily denote maximized efficiency. In other words, it is feasible to observe individuals who have poor stability throughout the kinetic chain, yet find ways to maintain balance throughout their ADL. This likely indicates compensatory patterns to prevent falling, indicating inefficient strategies, but balance is nonetheless maintained. Therefore, it can be argued that stability is required for efficient balance.

The importance of this distinction significantly affects programming. If balance is compromised due to instability in the chain, an individual will develop strategies to maintain balance that may further perpetuate the instability. Addressing and improving instability issues can restore balance through more effective patterns, thereby minimizing risks associated with long-term inefficient strategies.

For example, a client can learn to perform a single-leg balance exercise with instability in the standing foot and/or leg. However, they will likely do so through compensations up the chain to prevent falling. Therefore, asking clients to simply perform a single-leg standing exercise may not result in beneficial strategies regardless of the time spent balancing on one leg. In other words, the client is balancing in spite of instability. To restore balance through kinetic-chain stability, the areas of instability should be identified. Additionally, the CMES can explore in which plane(s) the instability seems to break down the most. For example, if the femur tends to valgus (adduct) during single-leg standing, it could indicate an inability to stabilize in the frontal plane. Therefore, applying exercises to address hip abduction strength and stability may have a positive influence on regaining efficient balancing strategies.

In the case of an alignment condition that is deemed irreversible, similar approaches can be still be implemented. If, for example, a senior-aged client has had flat feet their whole life, nothing can be done to change the actual structure of the feet. However, strategies can still address the areas where the greatest lack of control/stability exists. Reactive exercises can help enhance multiplanar control. This can have a profound impact on proprioception and reaction abilities for the client. The client may continue to exist with limitations, but they can develop greater control within their limitations.

OTHER CONSIDERATIONS

In situations where there are imbalances between the strength of muscles on each side of the body, unilateral machines will reveal the differences in strength. For example, the muscles surrounding the right scapula may be stronger than the muscles surrounding the left scapula. Keep in mind that the exercises may progress from the seated, stationary position to standing, unbalanced positions, and then to multijoint exercises.

Body Mechanics in the Gym Setting

Many fitness/health facilities have standard resistance equipment that is adaptable to individuals of various sizes. The CMES can assist guests or visitors as they "fit" the equipment to

Posture and Movement

their particular needs. Just because one individual is 5'9" (1.8 m), this does not mean that the equipment will be optimally set for another person of the same height, as some individuals have longer legs and others have longer torsos.

Fitness equipment often has joint "cam" markers on the equipment for the knees, shoulders, or hips. These markers should assist with the placement of seat heights, backrests, or leg lengths on the equipment. Individuals new to the fitness facility should begin on the equipment that requires settings and not perform multijoint exercises until they have adequate body awareness and strength.

Once the fixed equipment is mastered and muscle memory is created with correct postural movement, the client can advance to the cable machines. After the cable equipment is mastered, multijoint functional movement patterns can be implemented with resistance bands, stability balls, and unstable surfaces. For a CMES, having a varied program design allows for creativity, as long as the joint alignments are correct and not placed in faulty torque positions.

Physiological Considerations

Several issues need to be considered when discussing posture and movement. It is essential to have a physician's authorization when postural compensation has been detected and the client is experiencing sharp pain or pain that has become chronic. A great rule of thumb is to initially decrease the ROM and progress as muscle memory and strength are accrued. For compensation of the upper scapulothoracic region, it is often necessary to perform three or four rhomboid/scapula **retraction** exercises for every chest (pectoralis major) exercise. The corrective exercises can thereby prevail as dominant, while still working the opposite muscle group. Keep in mind that when retracting the scapula, the client is also stretching the tight pectoral muscles. It is important not to forget the coupling effect that the agonist and antagonist have on one another.

CASE STUDY

Client Information

Elizabeth is a 59-year-old female who works as a professional realtor. She signs up to work with a CMES to start an exercise program. The CMES conducts a postural assessment with Elizabeth during the initial session and makes the following observations:

- The backs of her hands are visible from the anterior view.
- From the side view, both shoulders are rounded forward.
- Also from the side view, a tendency toward a stooped posture (forward flexion of the upper spine with forward lean of the torso) is present.

In addition, when performing Apley's back scratch test, Elizabeth reports pain in her shoulders and cannot place either hand at the middle of her back. During the shoulder flexion test, she could reach only 120 degrees. Lastly, the shoulder rotation test revealed that she could achieve only 45 degrees of external rotation. What can be determined from this information? The rounded shoulders, stooped posture, inability to perform the back scratch, and the poor ROM on the shoulder flexion could mean that she has an exaggerated kyphotic posture. In addition, the muscles responsible for shoulder internal rotation could be tight due to the position of her arms during the postural assessment and the poor ROM on the external shoulder rotation test.

CMES Approach

Due to her shoulder pain during the Apley's back scratch test and her exaggerated kyphotic posture, Elizabeth must receive medical clearance before the CMES can perform additional assessments or begin a restorative exercise program. The medical clearance should address any concerns about shoulder issues that would limit participation in a medical exercise program or and any spinal injuries or diseases. Once given medical clearance and physician guidance, the CMES should also keep in mind that there are many approaches to address this client's postural issues and various options may need to be considered. Thoracic-spine mobility may need to be addressed, which

ACE IFT® MODEL AT A GLANCE

Cardiorespiratory Training

This case study does not provide a specific cardiorespiratory program for Elizabeth, as the primary concern during her initial visit with the CMES is her stooped posture and need for further medical screening. The scenario does state that she is looking to start an exercise program. Initial exercise programs for clients who are not regularly physically active should start with Base Training to establish basic cardiorespiratory endurance for improved health and as the foundation for improved fitness, with progression to Fitness Training as appropriate based on the client's goals and response to the initial program.

Muscular Training

Following medical clearance for her exaggerated kyphosis and shoulder pain, the CMES would design a program for Elizabeth that focuses first on improved thoracic mobility and shoulder stability, and would also include complementary exercises for improved lumbar stability for postural balance. This is a Functional Training program, focused first on proximal stability and mobility and addressing the pain-compensation cycle. The CMES would progress the program as appropriate by first including exercises to improve stability and mobility of the distal joints, and then introducing exercises to improve primary movement patterns. Any progressions to Load/Speed Training would be focused on muscular endurance after Elizabeth demonstrates success with maintaining postural and joint stability while performing the five primary movement patterns.

could be done through ROM exercises paired with deep breathing. If the scapulae appear to be elevated and protracted, the CMES may need to coach Elizabeth to work on positioning the scapula in depression and retraction (i.e., shoulder packing). The CMES may need to instruct her on how to perform these movements, cueing with mirrors and kinesthetic touch. The scapulae may initially move with difficulty, but once the movement is achieved and she has awareness and feels the muscle action, the stretching and strengthening program can begin. This may include the use of a foam roller along with the stretching and strengthening exercises to promote better posture.

SUMMARY

Efficient movement often originates from good posture. Therefore, an assessment of static posture should be considered a prerequisite screening for all programming. Postural restorative exercises strive to "straighten the body before strengthening it" and potentially avoid exacerbating existing postural and movement compensations, muscle-joint imbalances caused by numerous factors including occupational and lifestyle positions, and poor movement technique. These factors alter key physiological properties and functions within muscle, changing arthokinetics at and beyond the joint of origin.

Postural assessments follow the right-angle rule, identifying how the body aligns across four joints. This model divides the body into two hemispheres while observing symmetry between the joints in all three planes of motion. Following a postural assessment, the CMES may want to validate their observations by measuring the length of specific muscles and conduct movement screens to evaluate the impact of muscle imbalance on movement. When muscle tightness is a primary limitation, limitations are evident with passive muscle stretching. However, when compensatory movements occur during active muscle contraction or movement, it is usually indicative of faulty neural control. Consequently, active movement is an effective method of determining the effect that muscle imbalance and poor posture have on neural control, and to identify limitations to movement. The active movements selected as screens, however, must be skill- and conditioning-level appropriate, allow practice trials, and be specific to the client's needs. It is important to remember that almost any screen can evaluate functional capacity, as long as it is relevant to client needs and challenges and provides useful feedback on movement efficiency. It is also imperative to distinguish correctable from non-correctable postural compensations. While a client's health history may provide valuable information to determine this, the objective is to coach the client to move the joint in question toward neutral and evaluate their ability to do so without compromise or pain.

The overall goal with exercise programming is to restore muscle balance and muscle's physiological properties, and improve neuromuscular control of movement by re-educating faulty neural pathways. However, unless awareness of poor posture and intention to improve are key objectives of this program, individuals are not likely to achieve great success. Restorative exercise programs focus upon stretching hypertonic muscles through passive elongation to increase ROM and then strengthen latent muscles with isometric or limited-ROM exercises in normal resting-length positions.

REFERENCES

Abelbeck, K.G. (2002). Biomechanical model and evaluation of a linear motion squat type exercise. *Journal of Strength and Conditioning Research,* 16, 516–524.

Arokoski, J.P. et al. (2001). Back and abdominal muscle function during stabilization exercises. *Archives Physical Medicine and Rehabilitation,* 82, 1089–1098.

Cook, G. (2010). *Movement: Functional Movement Systems—Screening, Assessment, Corrective Strategies.* Aptos, Calif.: On Target Publications.

Cook, G. (2003). *Athletic Body in Balance.* Champaign, Ill.: Human Kinetics.

Cook, G. & Jones, B. (2007a). *Secrets of the Shoulder.* www.functionalmovement.com

Cook, G. & Jones, B. (2007b). *Secrets of the Hip and Knee.* www.functionalmovement.com

Donnelly, D.V. et al. (2006). The effect of directional gaze on kinematics during the squat exercise. *Journal of Strength and Conditioning Research,* 20, 145–150.

Fry, A.C., Smith J.C., & Schilling, B.K. (2003). Effect of knee position on hip and knees torques during the barbell squat. *Journal of Strength and Conditioning Research,* 17, 629–633.

Gray, G. & Tiberio, D. (2006). *Chain Reaction Function.* Adrian, Mich.: Wynn Marketing.

Hauschildt, M. (2008). Landing mechanics: What, why and when? *NSCA's Performance Training Journal,* 7, 1, 13–16.

Houglum, P.A. (2010) *Therapeutic Exercise for Musculoskeletal Injuries* (3rd ed.). Champaign, Ill.: Human Kinetics.

Kendall, F.P. et al. (2005), *Muscles: Testing and Function With Posture and Pain* (5th ed.). Philadelphia: Lippincott Williams & Wilkins.

Kenney, W.L., Wilmore, J.H., & Costill, D.L. (2012). *Physiology of Sport and Exercise* (5th ed.). Champaign, Ill.: Human Kinetics.

Krans, J.L. (2010). The sliding filament theory of muscle contraction. *Nature Education,* 3, 9, 66–70.

Laird, R.A., Kent, P., & Keating, J.L. (2012). Modifying patterns of movement in people with low back pain – Does it help? A systematic review. *BMC Musculoskeletal Disorders,* 13, 169, DOI: 10.1186/1471-2474-13-169

Levine, D., Richards, J., & Whittle, M. (2012). *Whittle's Gait Analysis* (5th ed.). London: Churchill Livingstone.

Lieber, R.L. (2009). *Skeletal Muscle Structure, Function, and Plasticity: The Physiological Basis of Rehabilitation.* Baltimore, Md.: Lippincott Williams & Wilkins.

MacIntosh, B.R., Gardiner, P., & McComas, A.J. (2006). *Skeletal Muscle* (2nd ed.). Champaign, Ill.: Human Kinetics.

McGill, S.M. (2017). *Ultimate Back Fitness and Performance* (6th ed.). Waterloo, Canada: www.Backfitpro.com

McGill, S.M. (2016). *Low Back Disorders: Evidence Based Prevention and Rehabilitation* (3rd ed.). Champaign, Ill.: Human Kinetics.

McLaughlin, T., Lardner, T., & Dillman, C. (1978). Kinetics of the parallel squat. *Research Quarterly,* 49, 2, 175–189.

Morris, C.E. et al. (2006). Vladimir Janda: Tribute to a master of rehabilitation. *Spine,* 31, 9, 1060–1064.

Page, P. (2011). Shoulder muscle imbalance and subacromial impingement syndrome in overhead athletes. *International Journal of Sports and Physical Therapy,* 6, 1, 51–58.

Panjabi, M.M. (1992). The stabilizing system of the spine. Part I: Function, dysfunction, adaptation and enhancement. *Journal of Spinal Disorders,* 5, 380–389.

Price, J. (2010). The fundamentals of structural assessment. In: *The BioMechanics Method Corrective Exercise Program.* San Diego: The BioMechanics. www.thebiomechanicsmethod.com

Sahrmann, S.A. (2002). *Diagnosis and Treatment of Movement Impairment Syndromes.* St. Louis, Mo.: Mosby.

VanGelder, L.H., Hoogenboom, B.J., & Vaughn, D.W. (2013). A phased rehabilitation protocol for athletes with lumbar intervertebral disc herniation. *International Journal of Sports Physical Therapy,* 8, 4, 482–516.

Whiting, W.C. & Rugg, S. (2012). *Dynatomy: Dynamic Human Anatomy.* Champaign, Ill.: Human Kinetics.

Whittle, M. W. (2007). *Gait Analysis: An Introduction* (4th ed.). Edinburgh: Butterworth Heineman Elsevier.

Williams, P.E. (1990). Use of intermittent stretch in the prevention of serial sarcomere loss in immobilised muscle. *Annals of Rheumatic Disease,* 49, 5, 316–317.

Williams, P. & Goldspink, G. (1978). Changes in sarcomere length and physiologic properties in immobilized muscle. *Journal of Anatomy,* 127, 459.

Wilthrow, T.J. et al. (2005). The relationship between quadriceps muscle force, knee flexion and anterior cruciate ligament strain in an in vitro simulated jump landing. *American Journal of Sports Medicine,* 34, 2, 269–274.

SUGGESTED READING

Cook, G. (2010). *Movement: Functional Movement Systems—Screening, Assessment, Corrective Strategies.* Aptos, Calif.: On Target Publications.

McGill, S.M. (2017). *Ultimate Back Fitness and Performance* (6th ed.). Waterloo, Canada: www.Backfitpro.com

Page, P. (2011). Shoulder muscle imbalance and subacromial impingement syndrome in overhead athlete. *Internal Journal of Sports and Physical Therapy,* 6, 1, 51–58.

Price, J. (2010). The fundamentals of structural assessment. In: *The BioMechanics Method Corrective Exercise Program.* San Diego: The BioMechanics. www.thebiomechanicsmethod.com

15 BALANCE AND GAIT

IN THIS CHAPTER

THE CORE IN BALANCE

CORE ANATOMY

MOVEMENT

GAIT: THE FUNDAMENTAL PATTERN OF HUMAN MOVEMENT

MYOFASCIAL SLINGS

CORE FUNCTION ASSESSMENTS

MCGILL'S TORSO MUSCULAR ENDURANCE TEST BATTERY

OTHER ASSESSMENTS

ASSESSMENT OF BALANCE AND GAIT

GAIT ANALYSIS

GAIT EXERCISES

EXERCISES FOR THE MYOFASCIAL SLINGS

ANTERIOR OBLIQUE SLING

POSTERIOR OBLIQUE SLING

LATERAL SLING

DEEP LONGITUDINAL SLING

CASE STUDY

SUMMARY

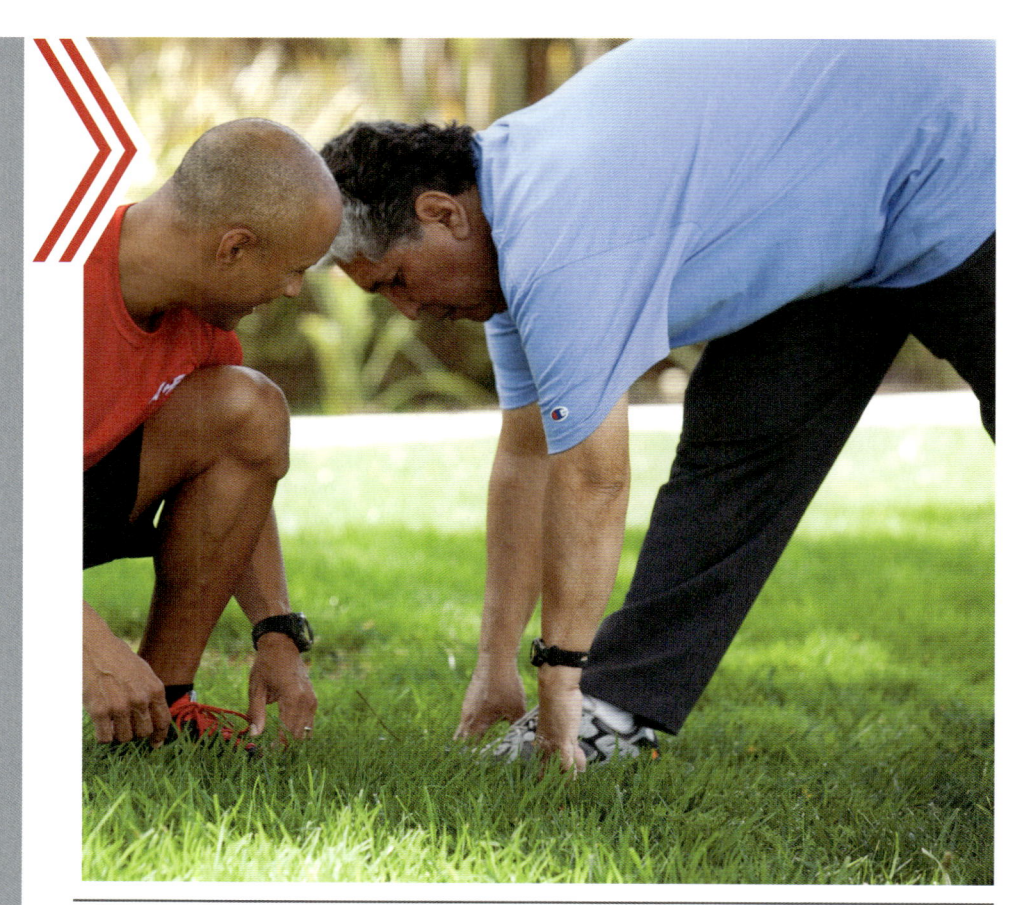

ABOUT THE AUTHORS

Michol Dalcourt is an internationally recognized expert in human movement and performance. He is the founder of the Institute of Motion, inventor of ViPR, and co-founder of PTA Global. As an international lecturer and educator, Dalcourt has authored numerous articles on human design and function. He has served as adjunct faculty at the University of San Francisco in the Department of Sports Science and also as faculty at the NAIT College School of Health Sciences in Canada. Dalcourt received his education from the University of Alberta in the area of Exercise Science (Faculty of Physical Education).

Fabio Comana, M.A., M.S., is a faculty instructor at San Diego State University, UC San Diego, and the National Academy of Sports Medicine. Previously, Comana was an exercise physiologist and certification manager for the American Council on Exercise, where he was a significant contributor to the development of the ACE Integrated Fitness Training® Model and live personal training educational workshops. His previous experiences include collegiate head coaching, strength and conditioning coaching, and opening and managing health clubs for Club One. As a national and international presenter, he is frequently featured on television, radio, internet, and in print publications. Comana has authored chapters in various textbooks and publications, and is presently authoring upcoming academic and consumer books.

By Michol Dalcourt and Fabio Comana

MOVEMENT IS ESSENTIAL TO COMPLETE ALL activities of daily living (ADL), and a person's ability to move efficiently requires control of the body's postural alignment. Control of postural stability is termed **balance.** More specifically, balance is subdivided into static balance—referring to the ability to maintain the body's **center of gravity (COG)** within its **base of support (BOS)**—and **dynamic balance**—referring to the ability to move outside of the body's BOS, yet maintain postural control (Shumway-Cook & Woollacott, 2012).

A body's COG, also called the **center of mass (COM),** is that point around which all weight is evenly distributed. It is generally located 2 inches (5 cm) anterior to the spine in the S2 (second sacral vertebra) location (Figure 15-1), but the location varies by gender, body shape, body size, and even age (Rose, 2010; Kendall et al., 2005). The COG in males tends to be slightly higher than in females because of the greater quantity of upper-body musculature. Additionally, the body's COG continually shifts by changing position, moving, or adding external resistance.

The BOS can be described as the two-dimensional distance between and including a body's points of contact with a surface (Houglum, 2010). For example, when standing with the feet 12 inches (30 cm) apart, the BOS represents the areas that the feet contact and the area between the feet. Moving the feet to 6 inches (15 cm) apart reduces this area and the BOS, thereby reducing balance.

A body is stable when its **line of gravity** falls within its BOS. The line of gravity is a theoretical vertical line passing through the COG, dissecting the body into two hemispheres. When this line of gravity or the COG falls outside of the BOS, or when the body's **limits of stability (LOS)** are challenged, maintaining balance becomes more difficult. The LOS is the degree of allowable sway from the line of gravity without a need to change the BOS. Healthy adults normally tolerate about 12 degrees in anterior-posterior sway and about 16 degrees laterally (Rose, 2010). Muscle weakness, a deconditioned core, reduced **joint mobility,** and neurological and proprioceptive losses reduce the LOS.

Good balance generally exists because multiple systems provide accurate and precise information and commands. Sensory input from the visual, vestibular, and kinesthetic receptors provide important sensory information to the **peripheral nervous system (PNS)** and **central nervous system (CNS),** while motor responses result in reflexive or voluntary muscle action. Voluntary motor commands are relatively slow in comparison to automated or reflexive movements. Therefore, balance efficiency is dependent, in part, on the effectiveness of automated or reflexive systems.

Three measurable dimensions of balance exist and merit consideration when evaluating postural control and designing programs for improving balance and mobility: anticipatory, reactive, and adaptive postural control (Rose, 2010).

Anticipatory postural control involves stabilization of the body in anticipation of voluntary disruptive events that may require postural changes and potential losses in balance.

Reactive postural control occurs in response to unexpected threats to balance that cause the line of gravity to move away from the BOS. This control is necessary to restore balance and prevent a fall. If the disturbance does not exceed the LOS, the righting response may not require a change to the BOS, but if the disturbance is significantly large, it does require a change in BOS (e.g., taking a step or multiple steps to avoid a fall).

LEARNING OBJECTIVES:

» Explain the importance of the core in balance and gait, including anatomical structure and function.

» Describe the fundamentals of the human gait pattern, including the contribution of various myofascial slings.

» Differentiate the myofascial slings and the anatomical structures associated with each.

» Identify and implement important assessments for core, balance, and gait.

» Design and implement safe and effective exercise programs for improving clients' core function, balance, and gait.

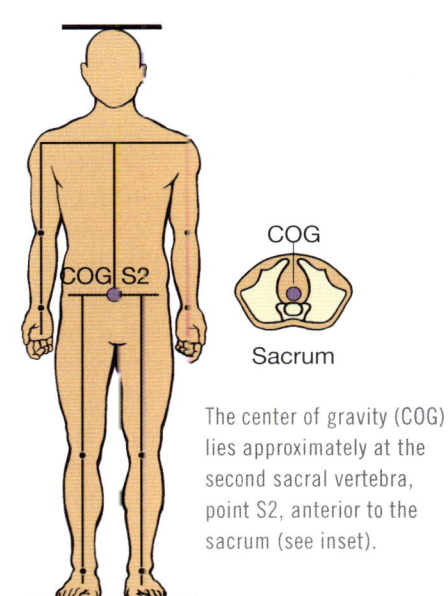

Figure 15-1
Center of gravity

The center of gravity (COG) lies approximately at the second sacral vertebra, point S2, anterior to the sacrum (see inset).

Adaptive postural control is the control of posture through the integration of afferent information from all three sensory systems and efferent (neuromuscular) commands. This allows the body to modify the sensory and motor systems in response to the environment and situational changes.

Maintaining balance relies on three distinct strategies utilized consciously or subconsciously. They involve the ankle, hip, and knee (Rose, 2010). These strategies normally function in sequence and along a continuum, depending on the magnitude and speed of the balance disturbance (Figure 15-2). While these strategies are discussed relative to the **sagittal plane,** they also apply to balance disturbances in the **frontal** and **transverse planes** as an individual exceeds the LOS.

Figure 15-2
Three postural control strategies used to control balance

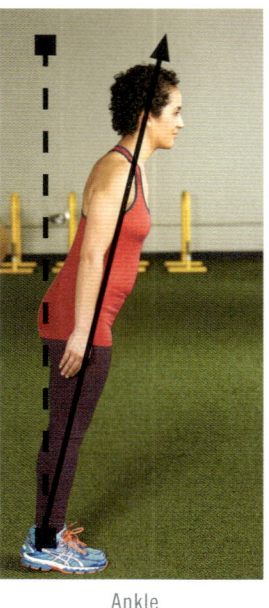

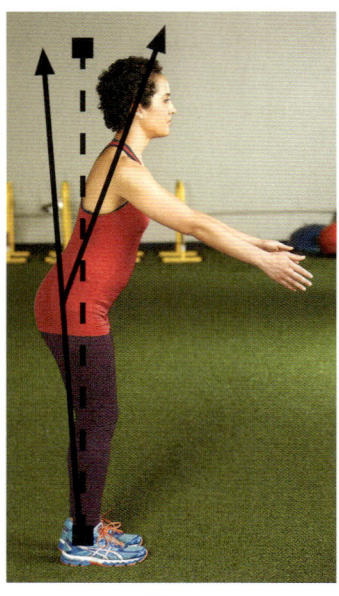

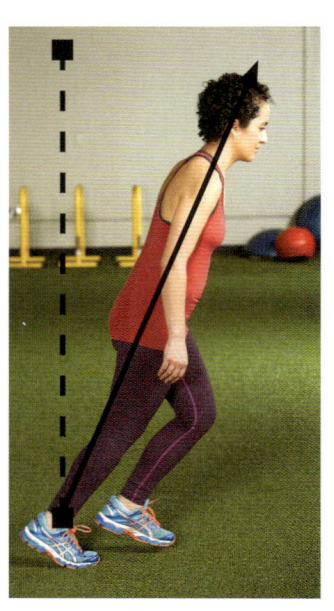

Ankle   Hip   Knee

Ankle strategies occur in response to small disturbances in balance to restore the COG within the BOS by action at the ankle joint. This strategy primarily involves activation of either the plantar flexors or dorsiflexors, resulting in simultaneous sway, or movement of the upper and lower body in the same direction to restore balance. Given the relative weakness of the musculature of the ankle, this strategy generates small amounts of force and responds to minimal balance disturbances, such as normal postural sway.

Hip strategies occur in response to larger and/or faster disturbances in balance necessitating faster restorations of the COG within the BOS. Given the larger magnitude of correction required, the larger hip muscles are recruited to move the lower and upper extremities in opposite directions to restore balance.

Knee or step strategies respond when ankle and hip strategies are ineffective in restoring balance, given that the balance disturbance has exceeded the body's static LOS. Movement is required in the direction of the disturbance by taking a step to restore balance under a new BOS without losing postural control. Knee and hip strategies are vital to maintaining dynamic balance during movement.

These strategies require adequate flexibility at the involved joints, along with strength, power, reactivity, and normal neuromuscular input and responses. Three peripheral systems—visual, somatosensory, and vestibular—provide sensory input:

- The **visual system** provides visual layouts; spatial location relative to objects; a reference of verticality and head motion; navigation, anticipation, and avoidance; and generally accounts for 75% of human sensory input.
- The **somatosensory system** provides spatial position and movement relative to support surfaces, position and movement of body segments relative to each other, and assists with balance and navigation in the absence of vision.

Balance and Gait
CHAPTER 15

- The **vestibular system** provides internal gravitational, linear, and angular acceleration information in relation to inertial space and head position, and becomes important when visual and somatosensory inputs are absent, distorted, or in conflict (e.g., the sensation of a vehicle rolling at a stoplight when another vehicle pulls alongside).

Any change to these intrinsic systems reduces the ability to accurately and rapidly perceive sensory information, compromising balance and mobility.

THE CORE IN BALANCE

Balance is the foundational skill element to all programming, whether functional or sports-related. Balance not only enhances physical performance, but also contributes to improving the cognitive and affective (emotional) domains and building **self-efficacy** and confidence. Improvements to balance result from increased postural stability, a key function of the core musculature. Core conditioning therefore involves balance and the use of controlled, yet exaggerated, positions of static and dynamic imbalance to generate effective neural feedback and evoke appropriate levels of neuromuscular responses.

The concept of the core refers to the trunk, or more specifically the lumbo-pelvic region. Core stability is the ability to control the position and movement of the central portion of the body (Wang et al., 2012). Panjabi (1992a; 1992b) defines core stability as the capacity of the stabilizing systems to maintain the inter-vertebral neutral zones within physiological limits. The stabilizing system consists of three components (Wang et al., 2012; Panjabi, 1992b):

- The passive joint subsystem (spinal column, **fascia,** joint shape, joint structure, and ligaments)
- The active muscle subsystem (muscle and associated tendon action)
- The neural subsystem [CNS and PNS (feedback and control)]

As the passive subsystem generally allows the lumbar spine to support a limited load of about 22 pounds (10 kg), it is the active muscle subsystem that must contribute significantly to supporting body mass, plus any additional loads associated with external resistance and dynamic movement. The active muscle subsystem therefore plays a critical role in stabilization of the lumbo-pelvic region (Figure 15-3) (McGill et al., 2003; McGill, 2001).

Core Anatomy

The different layers of muscles within this region each have specific roles in movement and stabilization. The larger, more superficial muscles are primarily responsible for movement and force transfer between the pelvis and thoracic cage, while the smaller, deeper muscles are more responsible for intersegmental motion and stabilization of the spine.

Cresswell and Thorstensson (1994) demonstrated that the key muscle that works with the neural subsystem is the transverse abdominis. It functions primarily to increase intra-abdominal pressure, reducing compressive forces along the spine. In healthy individuals, this muscle fires in anticipation of voluntary or involuntary loading of the spine to reduce compressive forces (Hodges & Richardson, 1996; Hodges et al., 1996). Given the different roles muscles play within this region, it may be easier to review the muscle anatomy by function and location, rather than exclusively by location.

Figure 15-3
Model of core stability

Reprinted with permission from Willardson, J.M. (2007). Core stability training: Applications to sports conditioning programs. *Journal of Strength and Conditioning Research*, 21, 3, 979–985.

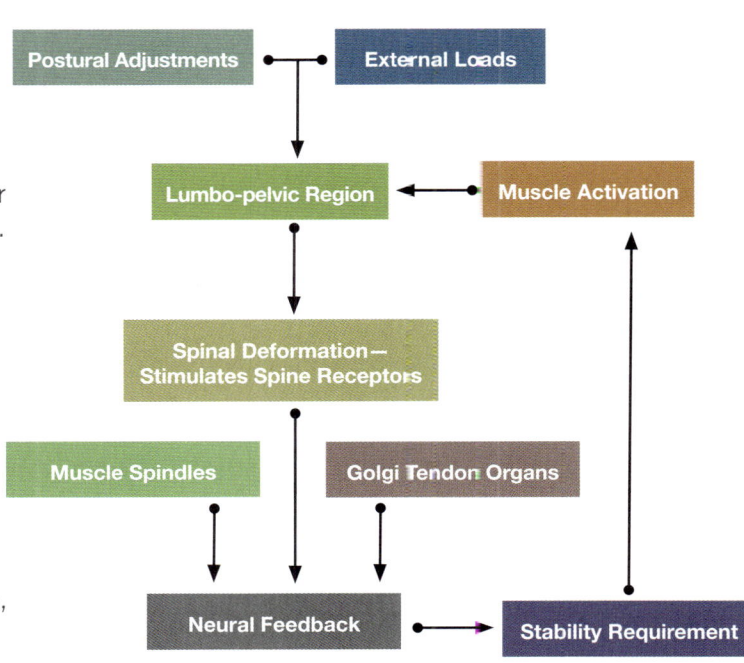

The deep layer, or inner unit, consists of small muscles (rotatores, interspinali, intertransversarii) that span single vertebrae and are generally too small to offer stabilization of the entire spine. They offer segmental stabilization of each vertebra, especially at end ranges of motion, and are rich in sensory nerve endings that provide feedback information to the brain relating to spinal position.

The middle layer forms a box spanning several vertebrae, from the diaphragm to the pelvic floor, with muscles and fascia enclosing the back, front, and sides (Figure 15-4). The group consists of the transverse abdominis, multifidi, quadratus lumborum, posterior fibers of the internal oblique, the diaphragm, the pelvic floor musculature, and the adjoining fascia (i.e., linea alba and thoracolumbar fascia). This box allows the spine and sacroiliac joint to stiffen in anticipation of loading and movement, and provides a working foundation from which the body can operate (Bergmark, 1989).

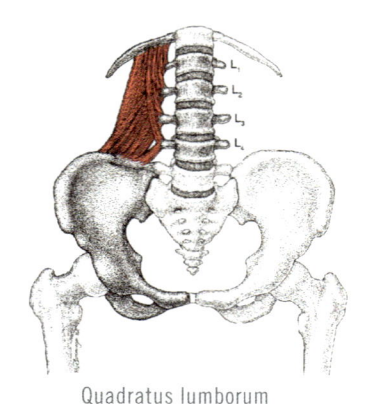

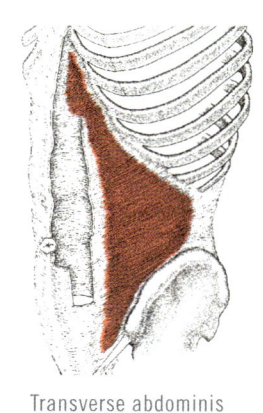

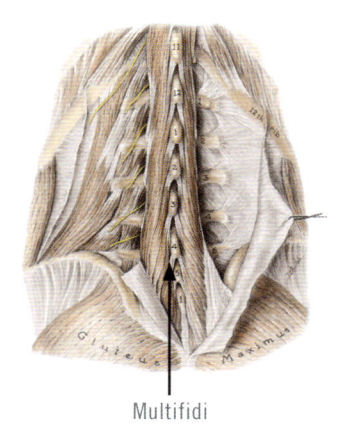

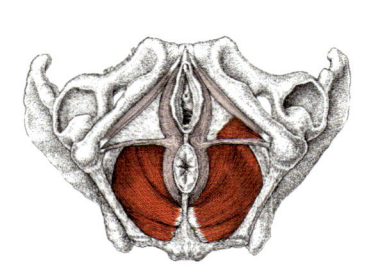

Figure 15-4
Middle layer of core muscles

Source: LifeART image copyright 2008 Wolters Kluwer Health, Inc., Lippincott Williams & Wilkins. All rights reserved.

Quadratus lumborum — Transverse abdominis — Multifidi — Pelvic floor musculature

The relationship between the vertebrae and core musculature (local layer) can be likened to a segmented flagpole with guy wires controlled by the neural subsystem (Figure 15-5) (Bergmark, 1989). The segmented pole represents the vertebra, while the guy wires represent the core muscles. Balanced tension within the guy wires increases tension to stiffen the flagpole or lumbar vertebrae and enhance spinal stability.

The outer layer consists of big powerful muscles that span many vertebrae and are involved in gross movement of the trunk (Figure 15-6) (Bergmark, 1989). These muscles include the rectus abdominis, erector spinae group, external and internal oblique, iliopsoas, and latissimus dorsi.

In healthy individuals without low-back pain, the core musculature functions reflexively to stabilize the spine under voluntary or involuntary loading without the need for conscious muscle control. This anticipatory muscle action minimizes the equilibrium disturbances provoked by the voluntary action. During voluntary or involuntary multiplanar loading and movement, effective core action optimizes force production and transfer through the trunk to the extremities, thereby enabling more efficient control of integrated movement; improving the ability to tolerate loading forces; protecting the spine from potential injury; and improving balance, coordination, dynamic postural strength, and control.

Hodges and Richardson (1996) discovered that delayed activation or minimal activation of the transverse abdominis muscle and limited co-contraction of core muscles in individuals suffering from low-back pain indicated some neural control deficits. Delayed onset of the transverse abdominis may cause inadequate stabilization of the lumbar spine during movements of the upper extremity (Sahrmann, 2002). Deconditioned individuals who spend much of their time in supported devices (e.g., with back rests) may demonstrate similar neural control deficits. Consequently, balance and core training must begin with exercises that emphasize re-education of these faulty motor patterns and is best achieved by activating the core musculature in isolation in stable, supported environments.

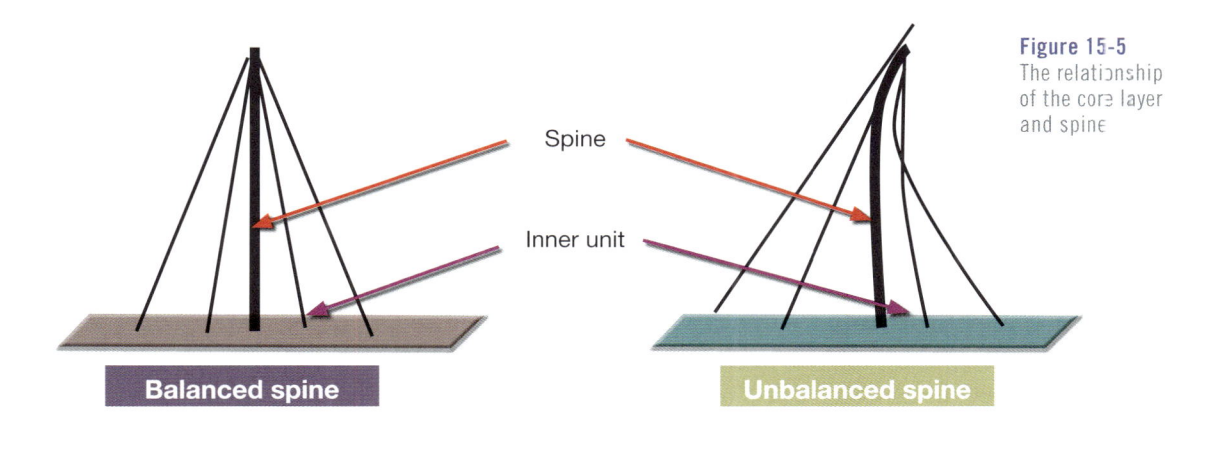

Balance and Gait

CHAPTER 15

Figure 15-5
The relationship of the core layer and spine

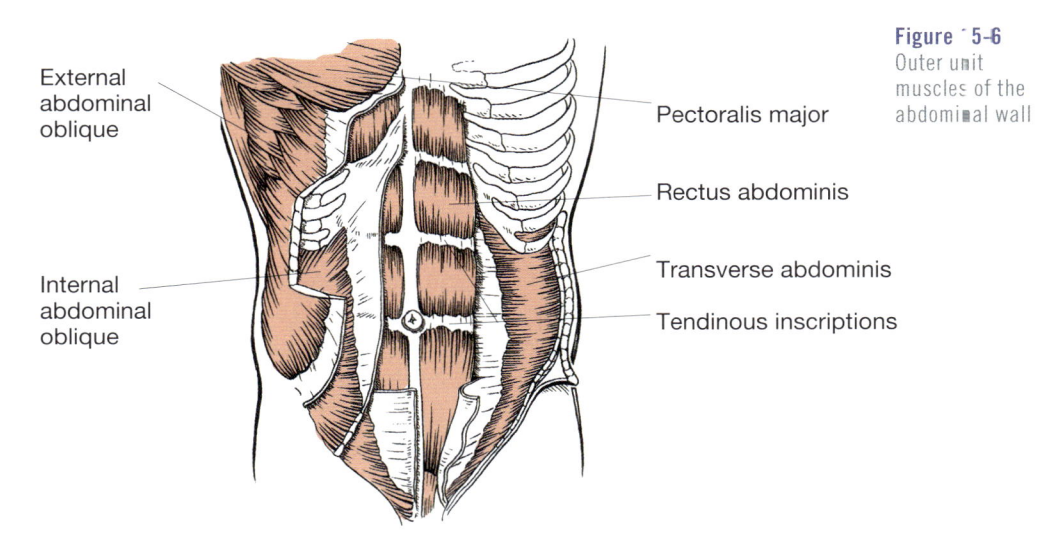

Balanced spine | Unbalanced spine

Figure 15-6
Outer unit muscles of the abdominal wall

External abdominal oblique
Internal abdominal oblique
Pectoralis major
Rectus abdominis
Transverse abdominis
Tendinous inscriptions

McGill (2016) claims that the relative contributions of the core muscles continually change throughout movement to accommodate postural adjustments and spinal loading. Core muscle involvement therefore is dynamic, and effective core training must ultimately simulate the patterns and planes of natural movement. McGill also states that the development of core endurance should take precedence over core strength, as muscular endurance better correlates with spinal stability and a lower risk of injury. Arokoski and colleagues (2001) agree, indicating that the lumbar-stabilizing multifidi muscles are primarily type I fibers, best trained with lighter loads and more repetitions.

McGill (2016) also states that while **abdominal hollowing,** or "centering," the isolated activation of the inner unit that draws the umbilicus inward and upward, serves essential motor re-education purposes, it does not ensure the same degree of stability as "bracing," which involves the co-contraction of both the core and abdominal muscles to create a more rigid and wider BOS for spinal stabilization. Ultimately, clients should implement bracing, as it is a more effective method of stabilizing the spine (Gambetta, 2007).

Intra-abdominal Pressure

Contraction of the inner unit produces a "hoop tension" effect similar to the effect of cinching a belt. This contraction, primarily of the transverse abdominis, pulls on the linea alba, thereby pulling the abdominal wall inward and upward. This contraction compresses the internal organs to push upward against the diaphragm and downward against the pelvic floor musculature. According to Cresswell and Thorstensson (1994), this increases intra-abdominal pressure (IAP), creating a lift pressure against the diaphragm. Since the diaphragm has attachments on the second and third lumbar vertebrae, contraction of the inner unit pulls them upward, increasing traction between the lumbar vertebrae. The increased traction reduces joint and disc compression on the lumbar discs by as much as 40% and creates a rigid cylinder (spinal stiffening) to stabilize the spine during loading.

Thoracolumbar Fascia Gain

The synergistic contractions of the transverse abdominis and obliques, and increased IAP, generate lateral tension on the thoracolumbar fascia, creating an **extension** force on the second through fifth lumbar vertebrae (McGill, 2016; Gracovetsky, Farfar, & Lamy, 1992; Gracovetsky, Farfar, & Helleur, 1985). This extension force is termed thoracolumbar fascia gain and is believed to assist with buffering force transfer between the muscular and ligament systems of the spine during trunk **flexion** and extension movements. Only a small amount of muscle activity in the multifidi and transverse abdominis is required to create this effect.

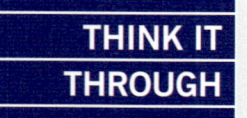

> **THINK IT THROUGH**
>
> The concepts related to core anatomy and function are complex, especially for clients who presumably do not have a background in fitness. Think about how you will explain the importance of a properly functioning core as it contributes to balance and movement to clients who are hearing this information for the first time.

MOVEMENT

Movement involves integrated action along the kinetic chain, where action at one segment affects successive segments within the chain. Efficient movement involves the synergistic contributions of mechanics, and the cohesive actions of the neurological and physiological systems working together to achieve simultaneous stability and mobility at the moving joints. The effective contributions of these systems allows the body to accurately receive and interpret sensory information, anticipate stabilization and movement demands, and allow for the selection and execution of appropriate motor responses to bring about efficient movement (Figure 15-7) (Cook, 2003).

Joint mobility is the range of uninhibited movement around a joint or body segment. **Joint stability** is the ability to maintain or control joint movement or position. Both joint mobility and stability are attained by the interaction of all components surrounding the joints and the neuromuscular system.

Flawed movement patterns, poor posture, improper exercise technique, and poorly designed exercise equipment may force unnatural joint movements and muscle action, thereby overtaxing muscles and increasing the potential for muscle imbalance. These types of misalignments and compensated movements due to faulty mechanics ultimately result in injury.

Locomotion is the act of moving from one location to another. **Gait** defines a particular form of locomotion, most commonly used in the context of describing walking and running (Whiting & Rugg, 2006). Although gait differs among people, there are basic similarities. Major differences result from postural variations, muscle weaknesses and imbalances, structural abnormalities or variances, and soft-tissue length alterations (Houglum, 2010). While walking appears to be a simple movement task, it actually entails a complex set of coordinated neuromuscular and mechanical events. This section provides a comprehensive review of the gait cycle and describes the movements involved.

Although the higher brain centers provide overall control, variation, and adaptability to gait patterns, neuron complexes (central pattern generators) in the spinal cord control rhythmic and

Figure 15-7
The movement efficiency model

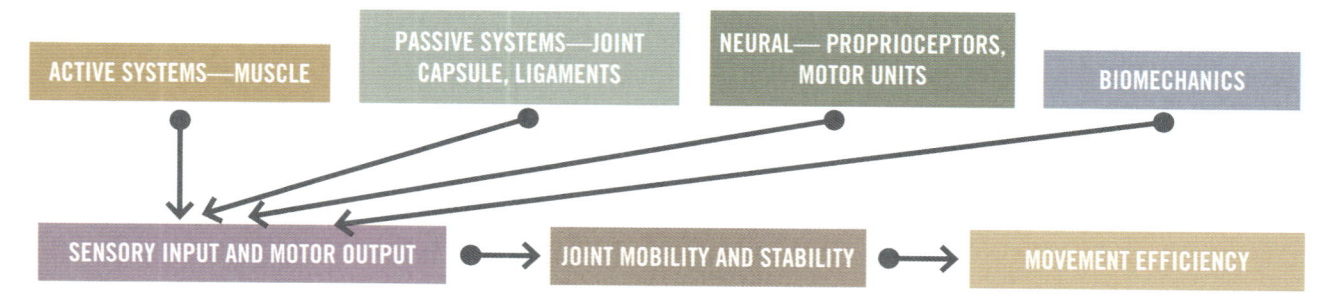

subconscious muscle activation and coordination patterns during walking. These patterns integrate sensory information from the three sensory systems (vision, vestibular, and somatosensory) that control and modify gait in anticipation of, or in reaction to, obstacles (Rose, 2010). Proactive visual control involves avoidance strategies, momentary modifications in gait patterns to avoid obstacles, accommodation strategies, and the adaptation of gait patterns in response to changing surfaces. The vestibular system works together with the visual system to stabilize vision during gait while the head is moving via the vestibulo-occular reflex. Somatosensory feedback provides continual information regarding limb orientation during the gait cycle.

Gait: The Fundamental Pattern of Human Movement

Mobility and balance are discrete inputs of human movement that rely directly on one another to allow an individual to achieve optimal mechanical efficiency and maximize performance during the gait cycle. Due to the forward lean exhibited when walking, gait can be described as a series of losses and recoveries of balance (Myers, 2014; Cook, 2010; Neumann, 2010). Each of the component systems—muscle, fascia, skeletal structures, and the CNS—plays important and essential roles in establishing the mobility and balance required to execute the gait cycle with optimal mechanical efficiency.

From an early age, motor coordination and movement development are based on learning how to execute the gait cycle, making it the foundational pattern of human movement (Abernathy et al., 2005; Schultz & Feitis, 1996). The components of the body discussed in this chapter work in synergy to create the requisite mobility and dynamic balance to help an infant learn how to progress from lying **supine** to upright walking. For an infant, the act of rolling over involves rotating the trunk over a relatively fixed pelvis and is the initial motor skill that ultimately develops into the ability to walk in an upright fashion. The phases of developing gait include lifting the head from a **prone** position, rolling over from front-to-back and back-to-front, belly crawling, crawling with the arms and legs in synchronous motion, standing with support, walking with support, and finally walking without assistance (Abernathy et al., 2005).

When learning to walk, each phase progressively improves the ability of the upper body to work with the pelvis and hips to create movement (Cook, 2010; Abernathy et al., 2005; Schultz & Feitis, 1996). Rolling over is initiated with either the shoulder or hip and the rest of the body follows. Crawling involves coordinated, synergistic actions of the opposite hips and shoulders and is the foundation for the counter-rotation of the trunk and pelvis experienced during upright gait. The initial phases of standing require the upper body to hold onto a stable surface while the hips work to support the trunk and upper extremity. Even though a toddler is holding on for support, this phase is critical for learning how to balance while also developing mobility in the hips.

Only when a child has developed the innate ability to control their COG will they feel comfortable attempting to take the first steps without holding on to any support. From rolling over to standing with support, each of these phases plays an instrumental role in helping a child develop mobility in the hips and shoulders, as well as the balance required to walk successfully (Cook, 2010; Abernathy et al., 2005; Schultz & Feitis, 1996). Throughout childhood, traditional play and athletic activities enhance dynamic balance and mobility, leading to healthy, resilient, and optimally functional muscular, fascial, skeletal, and nervous systems.

As individuals enter adulthood, many will experience a change in behavior that can lead to being **sedentary** for a number of hours a day with only a minimal level of physical activity. Sitting or remaining stationary for extended periods of time can change the function of muscle, fascia, bone, and neural sensory receptors, which can ultimately reduce mobility and disrupt dynamic balance to the point where efficient movement through the gait cycle can become a challenge. If simply walking becomes difficult or physically uncomfortable, this could lead to a series of cascading negative health outcomes such as excessive weight gain.

The Gait Cycle

The gait cycle is the period of time between the initial ground contact by the heel of one foot and the next ground contact with the heel of the same foot; this is called a stride (Figure 15-8). A stride is composed of two steps, with a step being the period of time from initial ground contact of one leg to initial ground contact of the opposite, or **contralateral,** leg (Neumann, 2010).

Gait speed is based on a number of factors, including height (which is related to limb length), injury history, physical disability, fitness level, and age. The two primary components determining the velocity of locomotion, whether walking or running, are stride length and stride frequency.

Stride length is the distance between initial ground contact with the right foot and the point where the right foot makes the next ground contact. Stride frequency, or cadence, is the number of steps per minute. Healthy adult males have a walking speed that averages between 90 and 120 steps per minute, while women are typically capable of maintaining a pace six to nine steps per minute faster than men. Factors that can limit walking speed include reduced step frequency, a longer period of time spent when both feet are on the ground (the double-leg support phase), and cautious load acceptance when transitioning from one leg to the other, all of which can be related to losses of joint mobility and balance (Figure 15-9) (Neumann, 2010; Abernathy et al., 2005).

The gait cycle is made up of periods when one foot is in contact with the ground (stance phase) while the opposite leg is swinging through the air to initiate forward movement (swing phase). During the stance phase, when only one foot is on the ground, that leg and hip are supporting the

Figure 15-8
Step length, stride length, and step width (measured at the center of the heel of each foot)

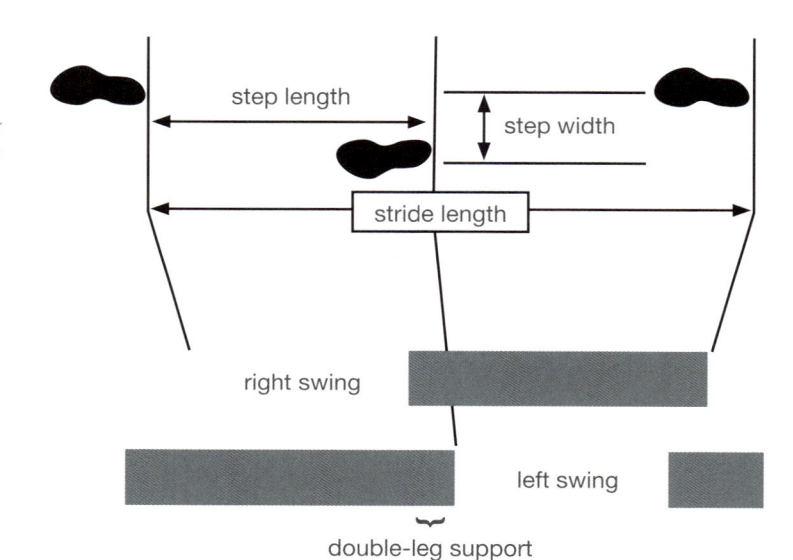

Figure 15-9
The phases and instants of the gait cycle

Source: Adapted from Whiting W.C. & Rugg, S. (2006). *Dynatomy: Dynamic Human Anatomy.* Champaign, Ill.: Human Kinetics.

entire weight of an individual's body; this is referred to as single-leg support. The moment when the heel of the forward foot has made ground contact while the heel of the back foot is still on the ground is known as the double-leg support phase. Each stride includes two moments of single-leg support, each representing 40% of the gait cycle, and two periods of double-leg support, each representing approximately 10% of the gait cycle.

The gait cycle for human locomotion consists of two phases for each lower-body limb. The two phases work together to create alternating motions of hip flexion and extension, which load, store, and release mechanical energy in fascia and elastic **connective tissue.** It is important to note that during the gait cycle, the body will experience upward **ground reaction forces** as the feet make contact with the ground while simultaneously being forced to mitigate the downward acceleration of gravity (Neumann, 2010; Enoka, 2008; Abernathy et al., 2005). A combination of joint mobility and dynamic balance allows the body to experience uninhibited motion through the phases of the gait cycle (Table 15-1).

TABLE 15-1
PHASES OF THE GAIT CYCLE

Phase	Description	Functional Response
Heel strike (initial contact)	When one foot makes contact with the ground and prepares to accept the weight of the body as the other foot prepares to come off the ground for the swing phase. At heel strike, the hip experiences a triplanar motion of flexion, adduction, and internal rotation, requiring mobility to allow elastic connective tissues to load and store mechanical energy in the fascia responsible for creating hip extension, abduction, and external rotation.	When the right foot makes initial contact with the ground, the right hip experiences torque from flexion, adduction, and internal rotation, which lengthens the fascia responsible for extending the right hip during the next phase (mid-stance) of the gait cycle.
Mid-stance	A moment when a single leg is responsible for supporting the body weight as the lower leg (tibia and fibula) translates over a relatively stationary and fixed foot. During mid-stance, the fascia responsible for creating the motion of hip extension, abduction, and external rotation are shortening to help create hip extension. The motion of the opposite leg, which is simultaneously transitioning through its swing phase, also helps to generate momentum for forward movement.	As the right leg is in mid-stance and the right hip is transitioning from flexion to extension, the left leg is experiencing the swing phase, which helps create the forward momentum that moves the right hip into extension.
Heel-off and preswing (terminal stance)	As the body moves forward, the weight is removed from the stance leg and prepares to transition to the opposite leg, which is preparing to repeat the cycle when the heel strikes the ground at initial contact. During heel-off, the fascia and elastic connective tissue responsible for producing hip flexion torque are lengthened with mechanical energy to prepare for the upcoming swing phase.	As the right heel comes off the ground, the hip has moved into extension, which lengthens the fascia responsible for creating hip flexion during the upcoming swing phase for the right leg.
Swing phase	This occurs when a leg transitions from hip extension at heel-off to hip flexion at heel strike; represents approximately 38% of the gait cycle.	The right leg swings forward under the body, causing the pelvis to rotate to the left and the left hip to move into extension. Once the right foot leaves the ground, the fascia of the left hip pulls that joint into extension, abduction, and external rotation while the fascia of the right hip, combined with the pull of gravity, moves the right hip through flexion to prepare for the next heel-strike moment.
Terminal swing phase	The hip has moved into flexion and the knee has transitioned into extension to prepare for the next impact of heel strike.	Early swing occurs during the heel-off phase, when the hip is in extension and the fascia creating hip flexion is lengthened and stored with mechanical energy.

Mobility During the Gait Cycle

Maximal efficiency of the gait cycle requires a high level of mobility from both the hips and the feet while exhibiting sufficient balance to maintain the body's COG as an individual transitions from one leg to the other. The hips require the mobility to allow efficient movement in the sagittal plane to move from flexion at heel-strike to extension at heel-off, the strength and balance to minimize unwanted motion in the frontal plane as the body has to stabilize itself when it is in single-support during mid-stance while the opposite leg is off the ground during swing phase, and triplanar mobility in the transverse plane as the hip moves from internal rotation at heel-strike to external rotation at heel-off (Figure 15-10). The feet require the mobility to pronate, a combination of **dorsiflexion, eversion,** and **abduction,** in order to absorb and dissipate ground reaction forces at heel strike and convert to **supination,** a combination of **plantar flexion, inversion,** and **adduction** (Neumann, 2010). During gait, the thoracic spine and pelvis are counter-rotating as the arms and legs create the momentum for forward movement. As the right leg swings into hip flexion during the swing phase, the left shoulder swings into flexion, creating counter-rotation (Figure 15-11). Any loss of mobility in the feet, hips, spine, or shoulders can change the mechanics of the gait cycle and restrict an individual's ability to walk.

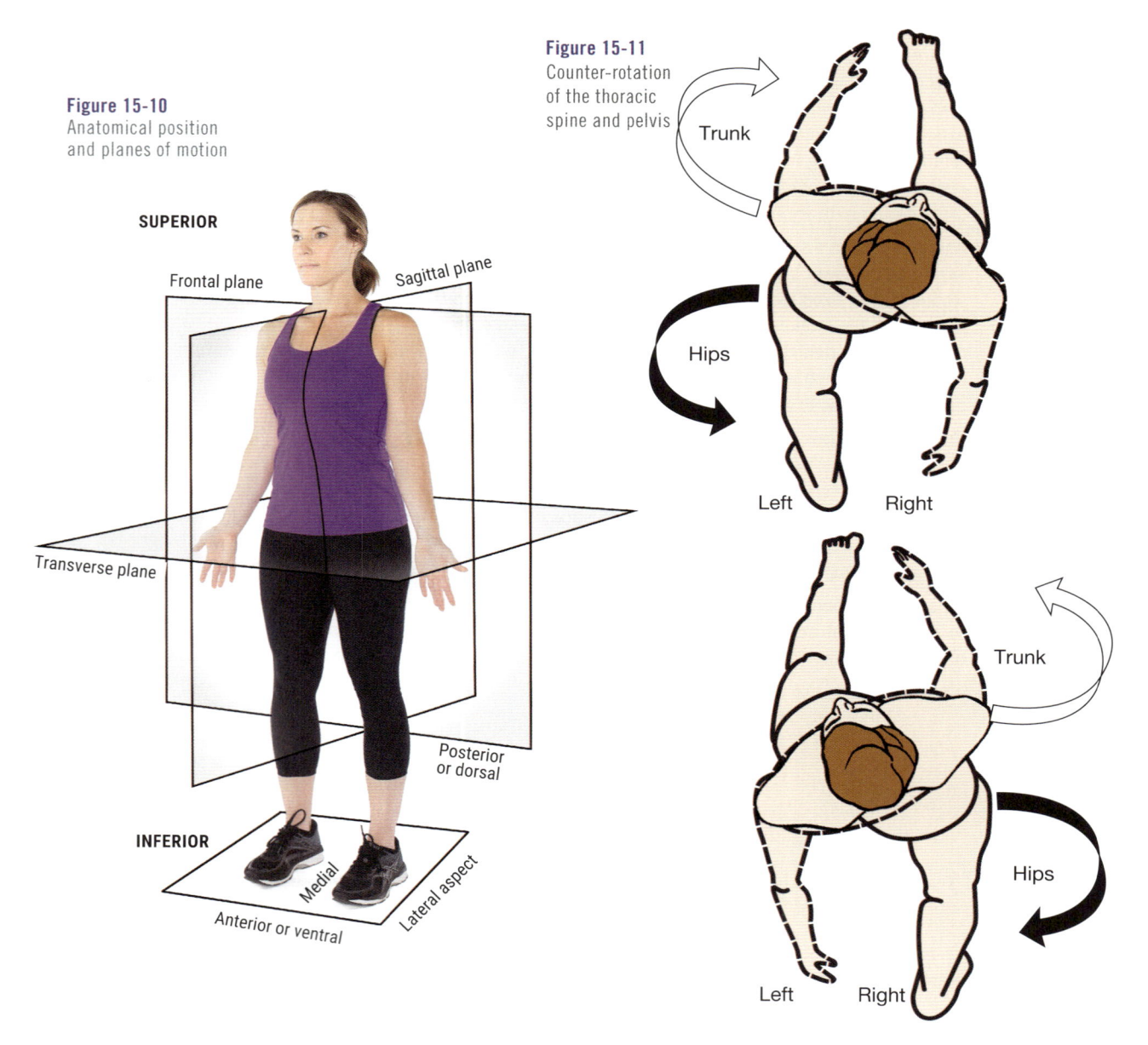

Figure 15-10
Anatomical position and planes of motion

Figure 15-11
Counter-rotation of the thoracic spine and pelvis

Balance and Gait   CHAPTER 15

Muscle is responsible for producing force within the human body, while fascia is responsible for organizing it (Myers, 2014). Following the **biotensegrity** structure of the human body, when it is vertical, upright, and moving across the ground, it must account for the competing bottom-up forces of ground reaction and top-down forces from gravity, with the network of fascia and elastic connective tissue becoming the primary system for controlling these forces (Schleip et al., 2012; Enoka, 2008). Whereas the CNS sends signals via electrical impulses, the structural network of muscle and fascia create a system that communicates by transferring forces from one section of tissue to another (Myers, 2014; Schleip et al., 2012).

UNDERSTANDING BIOTENSEGRITY

Biotensegrity describes how the body has a natural, structural tendency to balance forces (Myers, 2014; Schleip et al., 2012; Levin, 2007). Traditional anatomy teaches that muscles attach to bones via tendons; however, following the model of biotensegrity suggests that skeletal structures float within a three-dimensional matrix of muscle and connective tissue (Myers, 2014; Schultz & Feitis, 1996).

The concept of biotensegrity explains how mechanical behaviors can emerge through multicomponent interactions, making the whole much greater than the sum of its parts (Schleip et al., 2012). If the functions of the skeletal, muscular, and fascial systems are not coordinated by the CNS, then forces such as compression, tension, torsion, or shear can change the architecture and function of the human body, thereby limiting an individual's joint mobility and ultimately their ability to balance and move efficiently through the gait cycle (Neumann, 2010).

As it relates to mobility, balance, and gait, biotensegrity explains how movement, or lack of movement, at one segment of the body can influence the movement and function at other segments of the body. If an individual loses mobility at essential joints or the ability to control balance, they could experience dysfunction through the gait cycle, leading to performance decrements in many essential ADL. An effective way to enhance movement skill to develop dynamic balance and mobility is to train fundamental movement patterns, not isolated muscle actions (Cook, 2010). Understanding the human body as a mechanical structure based on the principle of biotensegrity is helpful for designing exercise programs to improve the skills of mobility and balance that are essential to efficiency through the gait cycle, the fundamental pattern of movement.

A bicycle wheel offers a mechanical model of **tensegrity**. The spokes of the wheel create a tensional balance between the rim and the hub containing the **axis of rotation**. As long as all of the spokes are properly aligned and adjusted, forces are equally distributed throughout the structure, creating balanced equilibrium and allowing the wheel to roll in a straight line. However, if one or more of the spokes become too tight or too loose, then the forces are not equally distributed and can disrupt the function of the entire wheel. Similarly, if muscle and its surrounding fascia are not able to efficiently distribute forces throughout the entire body, this could restrict joint mobility which ultimately changes the structure of the skeletal system and reduces the ability to balance and move efficiently through the gait cycle (Cook, 2010; Neumann, 2010).

EXPAND YOUR KNOWLEDGE

During upright movement, as the network of muscle and fascia has to control forces acting on the body, a single muscle may have some **fascicles** that are lengthening while other fascicles are shortening (Myers, 2014; Schleip et al., 2012; Siff & Verkoshansky, 2009). In reference to the agonist-antagonist model of muscle function, Lombard's paradox describes what occurs when muscles on opposite sides of a joint work synergistically to create motion at that joint (Cook, 2010; Siff & Verkoshansky, 2009; Enoka, 2008). For example, the hamstrings and quadriceps work together to create knee extension when the foot is planted on the ground (during the mid-stance phase of gait) and the gluteus maximus and iliopsoas work together to decelerate hip internal rotation in the transverse plane (during the heel-strike phase of gait) (Figures 15-12 through 15-14). It is important to have clients perform exercises that recreate these actions to improve function during the gait cycle.

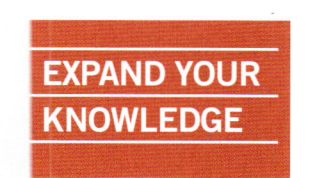

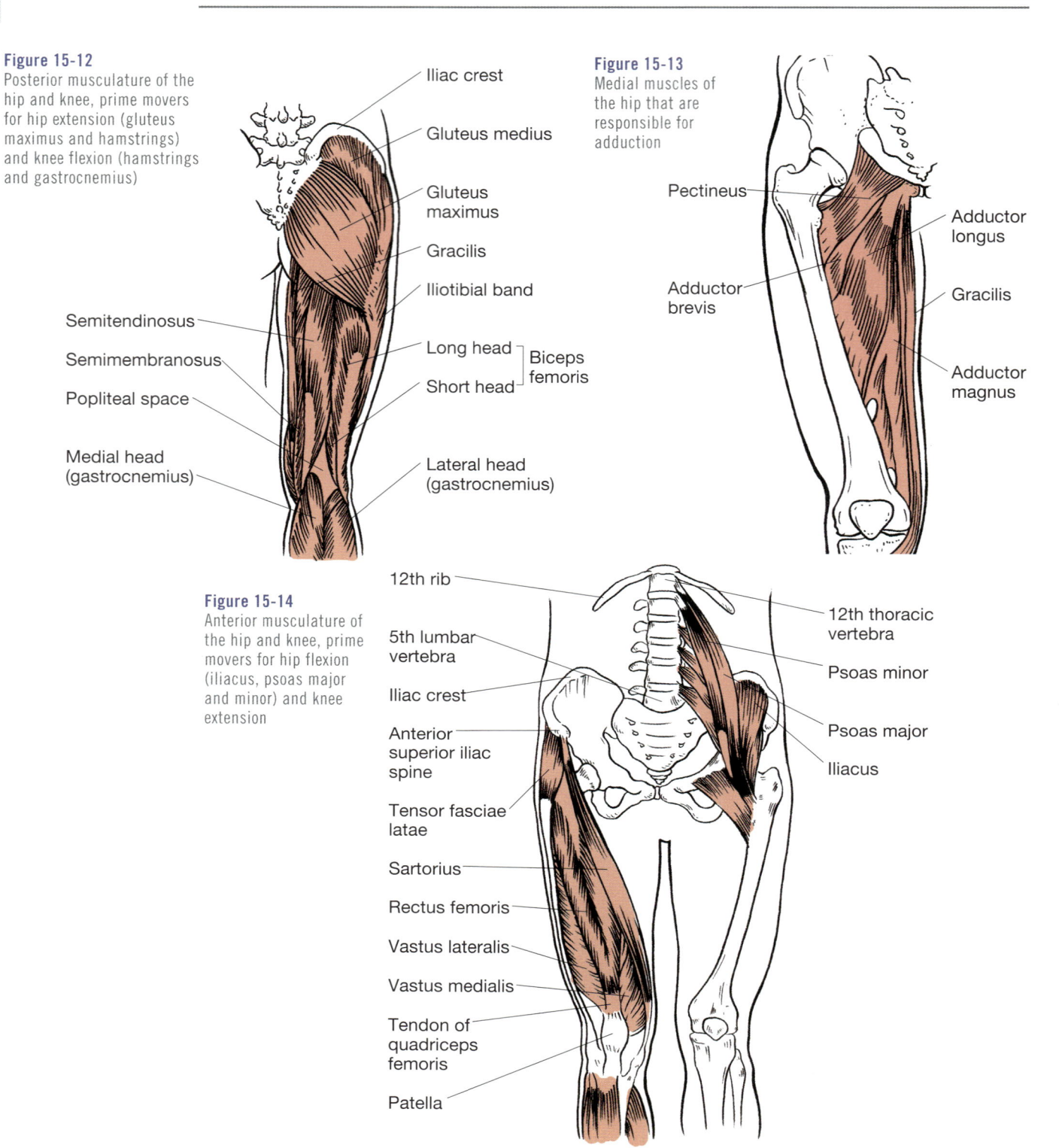

Figure 15-12
Posterior musculature of the hip and knee, prime movers for hip extension (gluteus maximus and hamstrings) and knee flexion (hamstrings and gastrocnemius)

Figure 15-13
Medial muscles of the hip that are responsible for adduction

Figure 15-14
Anterior musculature of the hip and knee, prime movers for hip flexion (iliacus, psoas major and minor) and knee extension

During gait, the trunk and upper body rotate around the longitudinal axis in the transverse plane. This rotational motion is created and driven by the counter-movement of the arms and legs during the gait cycle. This is why the position of the thoracic spine becomes so important related to optimal mobility and balance during gait. If the thoracic spine loses its ability to maintain a neutral extension and flexes into a posture of excessive **kyphosis,** then it will restrict this rotational motion and reduce the ability of the arms and legs to swing and generate momentum to produce mechanical energy (Neumann, 2010).

Balance and Gait

The Role of Muscle in Gait

Customary exercise training focuses on using the contractile element of **actin** and **myosin** myofilaments to generate concentric forces. However, during upright, functional movement like walking through the gait cycle, it is the fibrous component of the fascia responsible for organizing and mitigating the forces that produce and control movement. During dynamic movements, a muscle exhibits patterns of **isometric** contractions where the fibers of the contractile element shorten to create tension in the elastic component as it stores mechanical energy during lengthening, which is then released as mechanical energy when the tissue returns to its normal resting length (Myers, 2014; Schleip et al., 2012; Siff & Verkoshansky, 2009).

The **sliding filament theory** of actin-myosin cross-bridging describes how the contractile element of muscle functions to produce joint mobility (Figure 15-15). As the actin and myosin slide across one another, this shortens the sarcomeres of a particular myofibril; when a number of myofibrils shorten at the same time it causes the **distal** end of a muscle to move closer to the **proximal** attachment, moving the bone it is attached to. The function of the contractile element of muscle is to generate and modulate the internal forces responsible for initiating movement of the skeletal structure (Myers, 2014). In response to afferent sensory input from the PNS, muscle fibers respond by either shortening to create force or allowing rapid lengthening as muscles on the other side of the joint shorten (Cook, 2010; Neumann, 2010; Siff & Verkoshansky, 2009).

Figure 15-15
The sliding filament theory

Myofibril at rest

- Uncoupled cross-bridges
- Myosin myofilament
- Actin myofilament

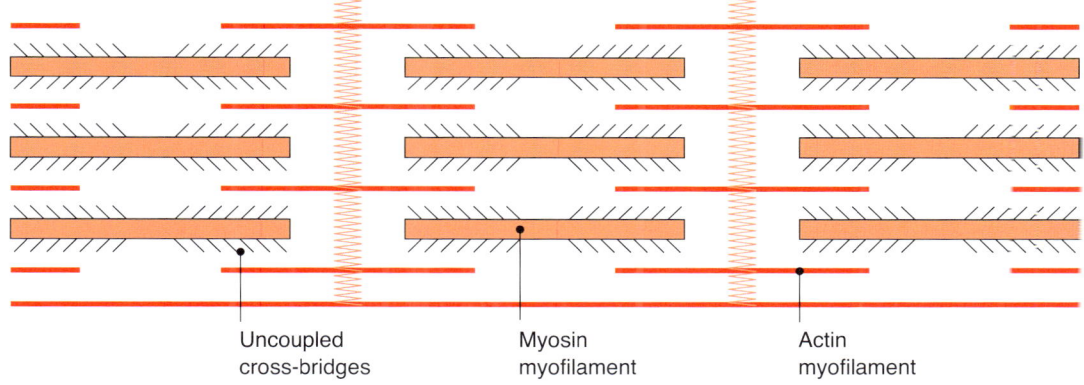

Contracted myofibril

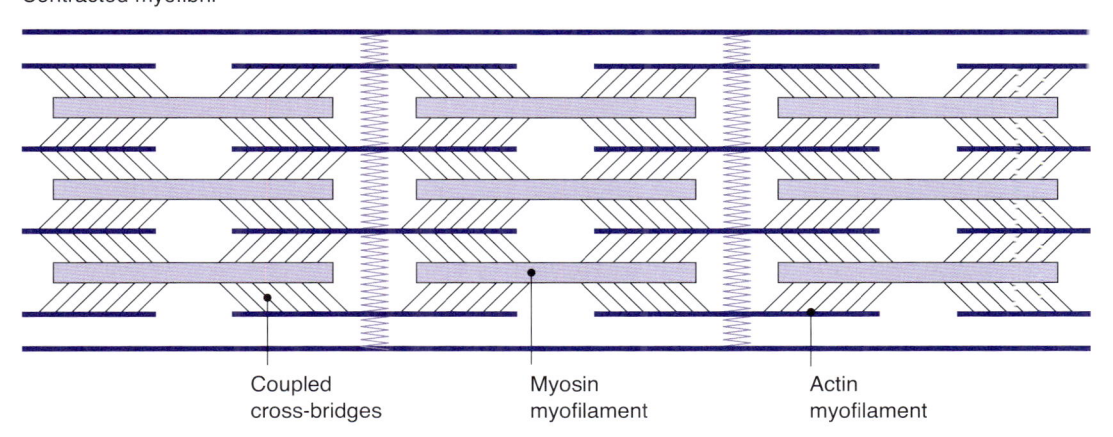

- Coupled cross-bridges
- Myosin myofilament
- Actin myofilament

Much of the work of the muscular system is performed at the subconscious level in reaction to sensory input from **joint capsules,** ligament and tendon endings, and intrafusal fibers that provide constant feedback on the need for tension regulation to control the body's COG over its BOS (Cook, 2010). Changes in COG influence the storage and release of mechanical energy. During mid-stance, the COG is at its highest position relative to the ground, which is the greatest position of storing mechanical energy. As the body transitions to heel-strike with double stance, the COG lowers and kinetic energy is released, moving the body forward (Abernathy et. al, 2005).

When a muscle and its involved connective tissue eccentrically lengthen, the muscle experiences a tensile force that causes it to store elastic mechanical energy. When that same bundle of muscle and connective tissue shortens, it then releases the energy stored during the lengthening phase. During upright human movement like walking through the gait cycle, the network of muscle and fascia functions as a mechanical system balancing the competing tensile and compressive forces responsible for storing and releasing mechanical energy, demonstrating the body's role as a biotensegrity structure. Therefore, it is easy to see how movements or exercises that isolate a specific muscle group or joint can lead to imbalances that then affect the system as a whole.

Traditional anatomy teaches muscle function from the perspective of when the body is in a neutral, anatomical position and does not account for how gravity and ground reaction forces influence movement. Additionally, anatomy teaches that a muscle can only influence motion at a joint that it crosses. However, when the human body is vertical and moving upright across the ground through forces created by gravity and ground reaction, muscles play an important role in generating stiffness through isometric contractions in order to allow the fascia and elastic connective tissue to lengthen and store mechanical energy. When this happens, muscles can actually perform different functions than what is traditionally taught and can actually create motions at joints they do not cross, making it more accurate to describe muscular anatomy as one integrated system with specific lines of pull controlling how forces move and dissipate through the entire body (Myers, 2014; Cook, 2010; Schultz & Feitis, 1996).

For example, it has been traditionally taught that the hamstring muscles flex the knee, which they can do when the foot is off of the ground. However, when the foot is on the ground, specifically during the terminal phase of leg swing and the load-bearing mid-stance phases of the gait cycle, the hamstrings actually function to extend the knee by creating a posterior slide of the proximal tibia on the distal ends of the femur. Another example involves the foot passing under the COG during the transition from the mid-stance to the heel-off phases of the gait cycle. The soleus muscle, which does not cross the knee joint, isometrically contracts to restrict forward motion of the tibia on the calcaneus, helping to extend the knee (Neumann, 2010; Abernathy et. al, 2005).

Muscles play an important role in the mobility of the skeletal structure. By contracting to initiate movement or create tension on the fascia and elastic connective tissue, muscles generate internal forces that dictate the structure and function of the skeletal system. If internal muscle tension becomes too great as the result of either repetitive motions or lack of motion, it can change the alignment of the skeletal structure and reduce the ability of a joint to mobilize through its designed **range of motion (ROM).**

The Role of Fascia in Gait

Movement efficiency and optimal task performance are derived from the design of the human body to be energy-efficient and maximize the use of mechanical energy from the fibrous components of fascia. Forces applied to the human body, whether external from gravity and ground reaction forces, or internal in response to an imbalance in muscle tension, can change the shape and function of fascia, muscle, and bone (Neumann, 2010). During upright, functional movements, mechanical energy is created as the contractile elements sustain shortening during an isometric contraction, which increases the load on elastic tissues.

Increasing elasticity of fascia can improve the ability to store and use mechanical energy during the gait cycle. Enhanced elasticity allows for more efficient storage and release of mechanical energy. A significant amount of energy used when walking emanates from elasticity of involved fascia and connective tissue. The lengthening and shortening of elastic fascia can be responsible for producing the mechanical energy to fuel the cyclic motion of gait (Schleip et al., 2012).

EXPAND YOUR KNOWLEDGE

UNDERSTANDING FASCIA

Fascia is organized to accommodate three-dimensional forces, mitigate stresses, and create equilibrium to establish an efficient structure in the human skeleton. Fascia possesses an ability to adapt and recreate its structure relative to applied forces. Loading patterns create the strain and tensile forces, which ultimately determine whether fascia has a linear or multidirectional structural pattern. Repeated application of strain and tensile forces can increase the density of fascia, enhancing its ability to dissipate these forces. Because they remodel their architecture in response to applied stresses all the way to the microscopic level of individual cells, fascia and elastic connective tissue play an important role in adapting to the applied demands of physical activity (Myers, 2014; Schleip et al., 2012; Neumann, 2010).

Understanding fascia means understanding how the body functions as one unit to create movement. Fascia is a living structure capable of reshaping itself in response to applied forces. This network of fascia and elastic connective tissue that is interwoven throughout all of the tissues in the human body maximizes resiliency while providing protection against injury. All connective tissue differs in form based on density and directional alignment of collagen fibers, creating the structure in which the elasticity of fascia allows multidirectional forces, greatly enhancing the mobility inherent to the human body (Schleip et al., 2012; Schultz & Feitis, 1996).

The fascia contains up to 10 times more afferent nerve endings than the contractile element of muscle and is considered by some researchers to be the richest sensory organ in the human body (Schleip et al., 2012). Bundles of muscle attach to one another via the **epimysium**, which forms the tendons as it tapers to a thicker band or rope-like structure as it continues toward the attachment site on bone. Thus, the epimysium and tendons are responsible for connecting the contractile element to the skeletal structure. The fascia and connective tissue surrounding an individual muscle is responsible for transferring forces between different sections of neighboring muscle. This system repeats itself on every level, from the endomysium between individual muscle fibers to the micro-level where connective tissue forms a lattice-work connecting every single cell in the human body (Schleip et al., 2012).

When one part of the body moves, it can influence motion at all other parts of the body. The tissue optimized to produce such responsiveness is fascia. A well-designed exercise program can enhance the elasticity and structural integrity of fascia, restore the ability of muscle tissue to perform multiplanar movements, and allow optimal joint ROM. An additional benefit of enhancing optimal joint mobility is that multidirectional and multispeed exercises for the entire fascial network can help produce more elastic tissue that is more youthful in architecture and function and reduce the effects of the normal biological aging process (Myers, 2014; Schleip et al., 2012).

One of the more effective ways to enhance a client's mobility and movement skill is to minimize the transition time from muscle lengthening to shortening in a particular movement, known as the **stretch-shortening cycle (SSC)** (Siff & Verkoshansky, 2009). For example, most of the energy for gait is mechanical and generated by the fascia as it lengthens and shortens in response to the anterior and posterior swinging movements of the legs as they transition through the gait cycle. During the swing phase, the mass of the leg acts like a pendulum to create forward momentum.

The muscles will shorten to create tension in the fascia and elastic connective tissue in order to store mechanical energy in the hip flexors as the legs transition from mid-stance to heel-off. Improving the ability of the hip fascia to transition from lengthening to shortening can improve a client's movement efficiency.

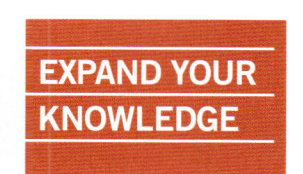

If a constant mechanical stress or tension from repetitive movements or maintaining a poor posture is applied, it can lay down inelastic collagen fibers to mitigate these stresses and protect itself from damage (Myers, 2014; Neumann, 2010). When collagen binds between these layers, it can reduce their ability to slide against one other, which ultimately alters the function of involved joints. If an individual participates in activities requiring multidirectional movements at a variety of speeds, then they can create a more elastic, resilient muscle and fascia system that allows optimal joint mobility (Schleip et al., 2012). Over the course of the natural biological aging process, adults who participate in dynamic activities based on multiplanar movements such as dance or martial arts can experience higher levels of muscle strength and function, which enhances overall quality of life. However, if an individual becomes and remains sedentary and restricts their movement patterns to predictable, repetitive actions, then they can experience a significant loss of elasticity from fascia and elastic connective tissue, which can greatly change the function of a joint and reduce its ROM.

Lack of movement, especially in multiple planes and directions, can create collagen adhesions responsible for limiting joint motion and reducing mobility (Myers, 2014; Cook, 2010). For example, individuals who spend a large portion of their time seated can develop collagen adhesions between the layers of the iliacus and psoas major muscles that contribute to producing hip flexion and reducing the motion of hip extension (see Figure 15-14). The tightness from the hip flexors can limit the ability of the femur to go through the movement of extension and thereby reduce the neural drive to the gluteus maximus (the primary muscle responsible for hip extension), changing the function of the muscle and the mobility of the joint. Many common injuries restricting joint mobility can be related to fascia and connective tissue being loaded beyond its existing capacity (Schleip et al., 2012).

Injuries related to the loss of joint mobility can be prevented. The ability of fascia and elastic connective tissue to lengthen allows a joint to move through a complete ROM that supports optimal joint mobility. If joints designed to be mobile allow unrestricted freedom of movement, this can reduce stress across the entire system and lower the risk of injury (Schleip et al., 2012).

Following the biotensegrity model, when forces are introduced at one point in the human body, they are simultaneously transmitted to other parts of the body. The human body contains specific subsystems of fascia that act to initiate and control movement while dissipating forces between the upper and lower extremities (Table 15-2). During gait, ground reaction forces are transmitted upward, creating a bottom-up force, while gravity simultaneously applies a top-down force (Neumann, 2010). There are different models for how fascia and muscles interact to create lines of pull through the body (Scheip et al., 2012). One model involves **myofascial slings,** or subsystems, that help create specific lines of pull to allow mobility and control balance during the gait cycle (Vleeming et al., 2007). Understanding how these subsystems synergistically produce and reduce force during gait can help exercise professionals develop exercise programs to enhance movement efficiency.

The Role of the Skeletal System in Gait

Bone is responsible for creating structure for the human body and providing attachment points for the contractile element of muscle through the tendons, which are comprised of fibrous connective tissue (Cook, 2010; Neumann, 2010). The structural design and placement of bones within the skeletal system help to dissipate and reduce both internal and external forces experienced by the body. Bone is living tissue and, like fascia and muscle, will develop and grow in response to applied stresses (Neumann, 2010; Enoka, 2008).

The point where two bones come in close proximity to one another, but do not touch, is called a joint. The structural system of the skeleton is designed to allow mobility at certain joints while providing stability at others. Joints that allow movement around a fluid-filled cavity are called **synovial joints.** The articular cartilage at the end of a bone, as well as the connective tissue forming

TABLE 15-2
THE FOUR FASCIAL SUBSYSTEMS

Myofascial Sling	Muscles Involved
Deep longitudinal	Peroneus longus
	Tibialis anterior
	Biceps femoris
	Sacrotuberous ligament (linking the ischium and sacrum)
	Contralateral (opposite) erector spinae
Lateral	Gluteus medius and minimus
	Adductor complex
	Contralateral quadratus lumborum
Anterior oblique	Adductor group
	Internal oblique
	Contralateral external oblique
	Intervening anterior abdominal fascia
Posterior oblique	Gluteus maximus
	Contralateral latissimus dorsi
	Intervening thoracolumbar fascia

the joint capsule, fibrous membranes—such as the menisci in the knees—and the synovial fluid enclosed within the joint capsule ensure that the ends of bones do not touch and provide the lubrication that allows joint mobility (Neumann, 2010). An imbalance of the forces of tension and compression can change the position of a bone in a joint, which ultimately changes the function of that joint. If joint function changes, it will change the length of the fascia and muscle surrounding it, which subsequently changes the sensory inputs to the CNS. A change in structure and function at one joint can change the structure and function of surrounding joints, which can greatly reduce mobility and balance (Cook, 2010).

At any synovial joint allowing motion, one articular surface is concave while the other is convex. This unique function creates curvilinear motion that is actually a combination of three distinct motions: spinning, sliding, and rolling (Table 15-3).

These movements ensure that instead of being associated with one fixed axis of rotation, joint mobility is actually based upon a constantly changing axis of rotation (Neumann, 2010). The muscle and fascia surrounding a joint function will create both the stability responsible for controlling joint position while it is in motion and the force moving the joint along its instantaneous axis of rotation (Cook, 2010). Optimal mobility allows a joint to experience full, unrestricted motion while controlling the constantly moving axis of rotation. Regular exercise and physical activity can ensure that a joint maintains a volume of synovial fluid, as well as the elasticity of the attached connective tissues to ensure functional performance over the course of the lifespan. Lack of movement and articulation through a ROM can actually lead to a loss of fluid and **atrophy** of the structures that provide necessary support and stabilization (Myers, 2014).

TABLE 15-3
THE COMPONENTS OF CURVILINEAR JOINT MOTION

Joint Motion	Definition
Spinning	A single point on one articular surface rotates on a single point of another articular surface.
Sliding	A single point on one articular surface contacts multiple points on another articular surface.
Rolling	Multiple points along one articular surface contact multiple points on another articular surface.

During movement, joint motion can be described as either the proximal segment moving on a distal segment or the distal segment moving on a proximal segment. For example, during the mid-stance phase of the gait cycle, the pelvis of the stance leg is moving on top of the femur, and during the swing phase of the gait cycle the distal tibia is extending on the proximal femur (Neumann, 2010).

The pelvis is constantly moving during the gait cycle. In the sagittal plane, the pelvis experiences anterior and posterior tilting created by the flexion and extension of the femurs at the iliofemoral joints. The pelvis also experiences movement in the frontal and transverse planes as the COG translates laterally in the transverse plane and the pelvis glides over the heads of the femurs during mid-stance. The pelvis also rotates up to 200 degrees around the longitudinal axis in the transverse plane and lists up to 100 degrees side-to-side in the frontal plane as the legs cycle through the phases of gait (Abernathy et al., 2005). If the skeletal structures and tissues of the iliofemoral joint lose mobility in any one of the three planes of motion, it will affect motion in the other two planes and cause the body to seek the movement either up the chain in the lumbar spine or down the chain in the knees or feet in order to create the mobility to allow the COG to shift in response to the storage and release of mechanical energy (Enoka, 2008; Abernathy et al., 2005). In addition, the lateral translation of the pelvis during gait leads to a response in the lower-body fascia where fibroblasts increase the density of the tissue on the medial structures of the thigh (Schleip et al., 2012). If the gait cycle is disrupted, then it could lead to additional accumulation of tissue, which could lead to further performance decrements that significantly impact the ability to engage in physical activity.

The three segments of the body allowing the greatest mobility are the foot and ankle complex (actually a number of joints that will be organized into one structure for the purpose of this discussion), the hip, and the intervertebral segments of the thoracic spine (again, actually a number of separate joints that function together in one unit).

- Foot/ankle complex (Table 15-4)
    - ✓ If the foot/ankle complex loses the ability to convert from pronation to supination during the gait cycle, this could lead to lower-extremity muscle imbalances affecting the knee, hip, and lumbar spine.
    - ✓ Movement efficiency of the foot/ankle complex is observed during single-leg movements such as single-leg balance stances, step-ups, single-leg Romanian deadlifts, lunges, and bounds.
    - ✓ Training for movement efficiency requires adequate stabilization training of the core to improve stability of the lumbo-pelvic hip complex before progressing to dynamic movements.
- Hip (Table 15-5)
    - ✓ Movement efficiency of the hip is observed during both bend-and-lift and single-leg patterns; the key observations are whether the hip can successfully:
        - Transition from flexion to extension without motion from the lumbar spine in the sagittal plane
        - Transition from adduction to abduction and from internal to external rotation without excessive motion from the lumbar spine, **ipsilateral** (i.e., same side) knee, or ipsilateral foot/ankle complex in the frontal plane
- Thoracic spine (Table 15-6)
    - ✓ Movement efficiency of the thoracic spine is observed by viewing a client's posture; if a client has a tall, erect posture with proper thoracic extension, it will allow the thoracic spine to move freely in the transverse plane. Excessive kyphosis and protracted shoulders will limit the ability of the thoracic spine to rotate, directing more torque to the lumbar spine.
    - ✓ Movement efficiency of the thoracic spine can also be viewed during push and pull movements; an individual should be able to maintain a neutral position with adequate thoracic extension while using the upper extremities to manipulate loads.
    - ✓ Training for movement efficiency of the thoracic spine first requires establishing effective stabilization of the pelvis and scapulothoracic joints before progressing to integrated movements. An individual should be able to "set" their scapulothoracic joint before initiating either a push or pull movement with the arms.

TABLE 15-4
MOVEMENTS OF THE FOOT/ANKLE COMPLEX

Primary Joint(s)	Actions During Gait	Influence of Gravity	Influence of Ground Reaction Forces
Transverse tarsal Subtalar Talocrural	Converts from mobility (pronation) at ground contact to stability (supination) at heel-off	The anterior oblique, posterior oblique, and lateral slings work synergistically to control movement of the spine on the pelvis and the pelvis on the femurs. If the pelvis experiences too much adduction on the femur during the mid-stance phase of gait, this increases internal rotation of the femur, which increases pronation of the foot/ankle and limits the ability to convert to a stable lever for toe-off.	Controlled by the deep longitudinal sling, which extends all of the way to the peroneus longus and anterior tibialis The peroneus longus and anterior tibialis attach at the same point (medial cuneiform) on the bottom of the foot to control the transverse tarsal joint as it transitions from mobility to stability.

TABLE 15-5

MOVEMENTS OF THE HIP

Primary Joint(s)	Actions During Gait	Influence of Gravity	Influence of Ground Reaction Forces
Iliofemoral	Converts from flexion, adduction, and internal rotation at ground contact to extension, abduction, and external rotation at heel-off	All four myofascial slings influence motion of the spine on the pelvis and the pelvis on the femurs. The iliopsoas can become hypertonic and restrict the ability of the femur to successfully transition from flexion with internal rotation to extension with external rotation during gait. A hypertonic iliopsoas can inhibit actions of the gluteus maximus, causing the hamstrings to become synergistically dominant during concentric hip extension and deceleration of hip flexion. If the hip loses mobility in all three planes during the gait cycle, this can cause the lumbar spine, knee, or foot/ankle complex to lose mobility, leading to compensations at those joints.	Controlled primarily by the deep longitudinal myofascial sling with synergistic contributions from the lateral, anterior oblique, and posterior oblique slings to control movements of the femur as it transitions from flexion, adduction, and internal rotation to extension, abduction, and external rotation during gait. The motions of hip flexion and extension during the gait cycle are controlled by the adductor complex. When the iliofemoral joint is flexed, the adductors create hip extension; when the iliofemoral joint is extended, the adductors create hip flexion.

TABLE 15-6

MOVEMENT OF THE THORACIC SPINE

Primary Joint(s)	Actions During Gait	Combined Influence of Gravity and Ground Reaction Forces
Facet joints of the 12 thoracic vertebra The scapulothoracic joints	The counter-rotation between the thoracic spine and pelvis is critical for storing and releasing mechanical energy during the gait cycle.	Gravity and ground reaction forces are mitigated by synergistic actions of all four slings, which control movement of the spine, rib cage, and pelvis (via the obliques, quadratus lumborum, latissimus dorsi, and gluteus maximus). The thoracic vertebrae allow the greatest freedom of movement in the transverse plane to accommodate trunk rotation created by the acyclic actions of the arms and legs during the gait cycle. If an individual has excessive kyphosis (thoracic curvature) in the sagittal plane, it will affect the ability of the thoracic spine to rotate in the transverse plane; the scapulothoracic joints, designed to provide a stable platform for the glenohumeral joints, and the lumbar spine will try to increase mobility in the transverse plane to accommodate the loss of motion.

The joints comprising these three segments of the body provide important mobility in all three planes of motion that is essential for optimal movement efficiency of the gait cycle. The loss of mobility at one joint in these segments, even the loss of mobility in a single plane of motion, can affect the structure and function of the entire body. If a joint loses mobility, it could affect joints above or below it, greatly altering their ability to function.

The Function of Lower Limbs During Gait

During the heel strike moment of gait, biomechanical reactions originating from the foot and ankle complex dissipate forces upward to the knee and hip:

- The impact of heel strike causes the calcaneus to move into eversion to absorb ground reaction forces.
- The talus rests on the calcaneus and slides medially, causing pronation in the foot and internal rotation of the tibia.
- Internal rotation of the tibia moves the femur into a greater degree of internal rotation, forcing the knee into abduction (valgus position, with the tibia moving away from the midline of the body), placing stress on the anterior cruciate ligament (ACL) (Figure 15-16).

The body is designed to resist this tendency toward internal rotation and knee abduction:

- The ACL connects from the posterior-lateral femur to the anterior-medial tibia and is a very important stabilizer of the femur on the tibia, preventing it from sliding forward (anterior translation) and rotating inward excessively during dynamic activities.
- The medial collateral ligament (MCL) on the medial surface of the knee resists excessive knee abduction (see Figure 15-16).
- Strong deltoid ligaments at the medial surface of the ankle resist excessive pronation.
- Large posterior-lateral muscles at the hips function to decelerate internal rotation.
  - ✓The internal rotation eccentrically loads the gluteal group (primarily the gluteus maximus), which acts to decelerate this movement and helps protect the knee.
  - ✓Additionally, the gluteus maximus and iliopsoas muscles work synergistically to slow internal rotation, although they are considered antagonists during sagittal plane action.

Figure 15-16
Knee joint anatomy depicting the anterior cruciate ligament (ACL), the medial collateral ligament (MCL), the posterior cruciate ligament (PCL), and the medial and lateral menisci

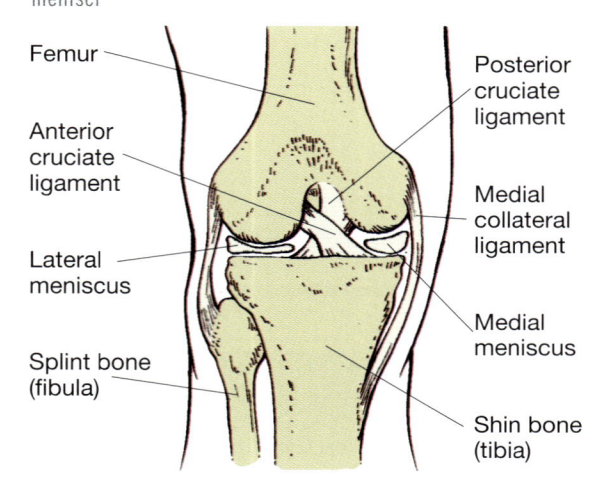

Role of the Central Nervous System in Gait

The CNS plays an essential role in supporting optimal mobility. Sensory nerves detect changes to mechanical loading and positioning of body segments. The CNS has sensory receptors located in the contractile elements of muscle, mechanoreceptors in fascia and joint capsules, and the ability to monitor movement of skeletal structures. For every sensory nerve in muscle, there are up to 10 in fascia and connective tissue (Myers, 2014; Schleip et al., 2012). The high level of sensory nerve endings in fascia makes it a huge influence on the signals the CNS sends to create and organize effective motion.

According to physical therapist Gray Cook (2010), "Movement influences proprioception and proprioception influences movement." The sensory receptors located in ligaments, joint capsules, muscles, and connective tissue provide specific information about the position of a joint and its rate of change as it moves through a ROM. The sensory information is communicated through the spinal cord to the brain to determine the most effective motor output to produce mobility and control a joint through its entire ROM (Neumann, 2010).

Muscle motor units consist of the motor neuron and its attached muscle fibers. Motor neurons respond to signals from the CNS to stimulate contraction in muscles to produce the necessary levels of muscle force to achieve a specific task. As mentioned earlier, muscle and fascia create the balance of tension and compression responsible for supporting the entire skeletal structure. The sensory nerves communicate with the muscle and fascia to detect whether a compressive force is needed or a tensile force should be allowed. Since muscles work in synergies around a joint, as one muscle compresses to initiate movement, a muscle on the opposite side of the joint will experience a tensile force to allow the joint to articulate. Optimal efficiency of the CNS will ensure that a muscle is able to rapidly lengthen to allow a compressive contractile force to create joint movement.

Type I motor units are attached to the **type I muscle fibers** that are generally involved with providing tonic structural support to control posture. Type II motor units stimulate larger muscle fibers involved with generating higher levels of force related to initiating and controlling movement. Mobility at a joint is controlled by the force-producing actions of the type I muscle fibers responsible for stabilizing joint position and the **type II muscle fibers** involved with initiating movement of a bone (Abernathy et al., 2005).

A muscle in a constant state of tension will not be able to shorten effectively to produce a force and will not be able to lengthen to allow motion to occur. More importantly, muscle, fascia, and connective tissue in a constant state of tension will create rigidity and restrict joint mobility.

Exercise programs need to follow an appropriate progression of movement complexity and intensity to allow the CNS to develop efficient motor timing to control compression and tension within the muscle and fascia network.

The CNS plays a number of different functions as it relates to receiving sensory input to determine the proper motor output. The most important roles related to mobility, balance, and gait are the reflexes related to maintaining equilibrium and dynamic balance.

Every client will have different needs for balance. Some clients will need to improve static balance—the ability to maintain a stable COG over a static BOS. Other clients will need to improve dynamic balance—maintaining control of a shifting COG over a moving BOS. Individuals in occupations focused on driving, working in an office, or standing in a relatively static position like a bank teller or check-out clerk will have far different balance requirements than those individuals who spend their days working at construction sites, warehouses, or as restaurant servers. Each activity requires balance specific to the demands placed on the body by gravity and ground reaction forces. The purpose of an exercise program is to improve mobility and balance, which can ultimately lead to greater levels of strength and coordination.

Static balance simply requires holding a position with little-to-no movement. Dynamic balance requires controlling a moving COG and is based on two distinct reflexes:
- *Righting reactions:* Reflexive motor responses for controlling balance when standing on a fixed or stable surface. For example, if an individual stumbles while walking along a sidewalk, the righting reflex is used to regain stability and prevent a fall (Enoka, 2008).
- *Equilibrium reactions:* Equilibrium is a reflexive motor reaction responsible for maintaining or regaining control of the body's COG over its BOS when standing on a moving or unstable surface. When a surface moves under an individual, like a treadmill or moving sidewalk, the equilibrium reflex helps to maintain stability and balance. Examples include wind surfing, working on a boat, riding a horse, driving a motorcycle, riding on a subway train, skiing, snowboarding, and riding a skateboard.

Myofascial Slings

There are four systems within the body that provide dynamic stabilization during movement (see Table 15-2) (Vleeming et al., 2007; Vleeming et al., 1990a; Vleeming et al., 1990b). In particular, Vleeming and colleagues (2007) give attention to the ligaments and muscles spanning the sacroiliac joint, given its capacity for movement and the need for stabilization in controlling force transfer between the trunk and lower limbs. Stabilization or force closure relates to the ability of the muscle system, through its attachments into connective tissue, to compress the joint surfaces of the sacrum and iliac bones together. During gait, ground reactive forces transmit superiorly, while the force of gravity transmits forces inferiorly. While these myofascial slings facilitate efficient movement and help stabilize joints, they buffer forces, distributing them throughout the kinetic chain. These slings are defined as the posterior longitudinal, or deep longitudinal, system; the lateral system; the anterior oblique system; and the posterior oblique system (Myers, 2014; Vleeming et al., 2007). In addition to the four slings identified by Vleeming and colleagues (2007), other slings have been identified, including the **serape effect**, which describes a sling that facilitates rotational movements of the torso.

Deep Longitudinal Sling

The deep longitudinal myofascial sling (Figure 15-17) provides stabilization to the sacroiliac joint during the swing phase of gait as the body prepares for heel strike (when the body receives the greatest bottom-up ground reaction forces).

- As the swing-leg moves forward, it produces hip and torso rotation, generating tension within the contralateral erector spinae group that creates an upward pull on the sacrotuberous ligament.
- Simultaneously, the eccentric lengthening of hip flexion and knee extension by the biceps femoris creates an inferior pull on the sacrotuberous ligament.
- These opposing forces at the sacrotuberous ligament act to stabilize the sacroiliac joint during gait.
- In anticipation of heel strike, the tibialis anterior prepares to decelerate plantar flexion eccentrically while the peroneus longus acts eccentrically to control pronation and stabilize the foot.

Lateral Sling

When the body is on a single leg during the mid-stance phase of the gait cycle, the lateral myofascial sling (Figure 15-18) plays an important role in stabilizing the pelvis to maintain proper alignment of the hip and knee over the foot. This sling decelerates pelvis-on-femur adduction and is very important during single-leg stance positions.

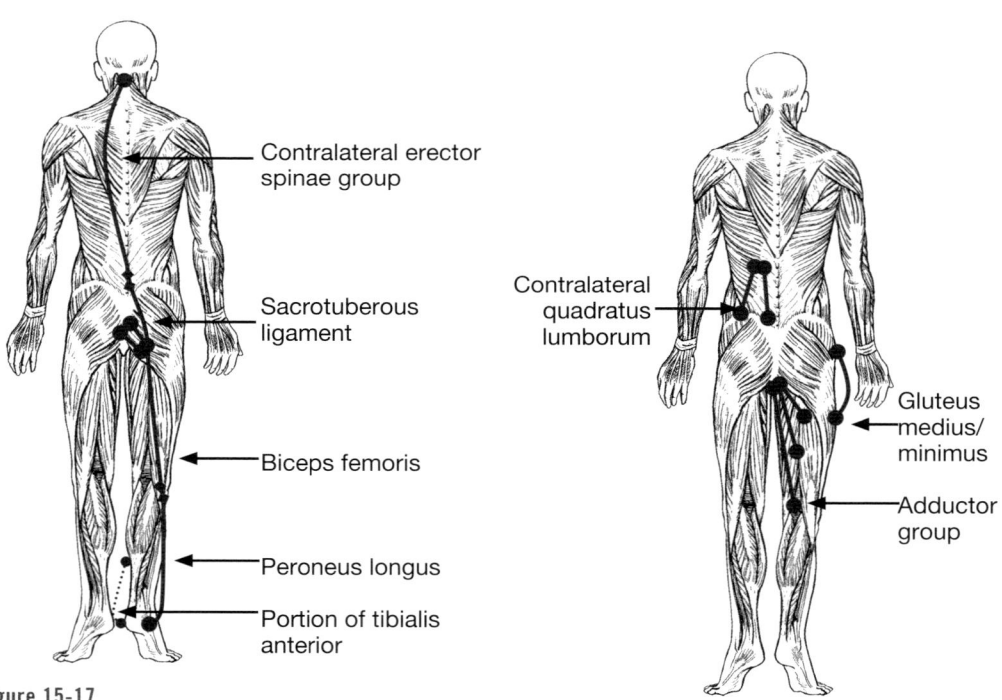

Figure 15-17
The posterior longitudinal, or deep longitudinal, myofascial sling

Source: LifeART image copyright 2008 Wolters Kluwer Health, Inc., Lippincott Williams & Wilkins. All rights reserved.

Figure 15-18
The lateral myofascial sling

Source: LifeART image copyright 2008 Wolters Kluwer Health, Inc., Lippincott Williams & Wilkins. All rights reserved.

The action of the gluteal and adductor groups stabilizes the pelvis to prevent excessive pelvis-on-femur adduction, which can cause internal rotation and abduction of the tibia during the mid-stance phase of the gait cycle.

During the brief moment that the body is in mid-stance, if the lateral sling cannot stabilize the pelvis on the femur while the opposite leg is transitioning through the swing-phase, the pelvis could drop toward the midline of the body, which then changes the position of the hip, knee, and foot of the stance leg. The amount of drop is controlled by the action of the stance-leg abductors (gluteus medius and minimus) and the concentric action of the contralateral quadratus lumborum.

EXPAND YOUR KNOWLEDGE

THE ROLE OF THE LATERAL SUBSYSTEM DURING GAIT

During gait, excessive lateral motion of the hip increases pelvis-on-femur adduction, placing stress on the knee and potentially enhancing the risk of injury. The mid-stance phase of gait requires the lateral subsystem (LSS) (gluteus medius and minimus, hip adductors, and contralateral quadratus lumborum) to create balance and stabilize on the stance leg while the opposite leg is simultaneously moving through the swing phase. The LSS controls and stabilizes the pelvis-on-femur motions during gait, specifically the gluteal complex on the stance-side (working in the frontal plane to control and decelerate pelvis-on-femur hip adduction) and on the contralateral (opposite-side) quadratus lumborum (functioning to prevent excessive hip drop by stabilizing the opposite pelvis side of the pelvis) to help protect the knee during the mid-stance phase.

When the right foot hits the ground in early heel-strike, the body moves to accept weight onto that leg, requiring a weight shift onto the right hip that requires the gluteus medius, gluteus minimus, and contralateral quadratus lumborum to maintain stability at the pelvis and alignment between the hip, knee, and foot. As the right foot transitions into mid-stance, hip adduction occurs as the pelvis glides over a relatively fixed femur; this motion involves the muscles of the LSS to create stability of the pelvis and hip, which protects both the knee and foot as the weight of the body transfers over the stance leg. Any weaknesses in these muscle groups may enhance the probability of a knee injury due to instability in the frontal plane.

Anterior Oblique Sling

During the stance phase, the swing-leg will advance forward of the stance-leg to its new position. While the adductors act to anchor and fix the pelvis, the torso rotates and the opposite arm swings to facilitate forward momentum. The structures of the anterior oblique myofascial sling (Figure 15-19) act to provide anterior stabilization of the sacroiliac joint during forward rotational movements of the stance phase of gait.

- The stance-leg assumes load and allows the opposite leg to prepare for its swing phase.
- The stance-leg adductors work to control and decelerate hip internal rotation.
- Simultaneous ipsilateral internal oblique and contralateral external oblique action rotates the torso.

Posterior Oblique Sling

As the stance-leg hip moves into extension in preparation for toe-off, activation of the gluteus maximus extends the hip and externally rotates the femur. As the right leg swings forward preparing for ground contact, the contralateral (left side) latissimus dorsi is lengthened by the motion of the left arm swinging forward, lengthening the posterior oblique sling (Figure 15-20). This sling provides posterior stabilization of the sacroiliac joint during the hip extension and trunk rotation movements of the gait cycle.

- Concentric contraction of gluteus maximus pulls the hip into extension with a slight external rotation, pulling inferiorly on the thoracolumbar fascia.
- Simultaneously, the contralateral latissimus dorsi contracts, extending and posteriorly rotating the shoulder in the opposite direction of the hips, which pulls superiorly upon the thoracolumbar fascia.

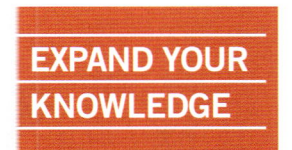

Figure 15-19
The anterior oblique sling

Source: LifeART image copyright 2008 Wolters Kluwer Health, Inc., Lippincott Williams & Wilkins. All rights reserved.

Forward rotation of the left hip and torso with the right leg in stance phase

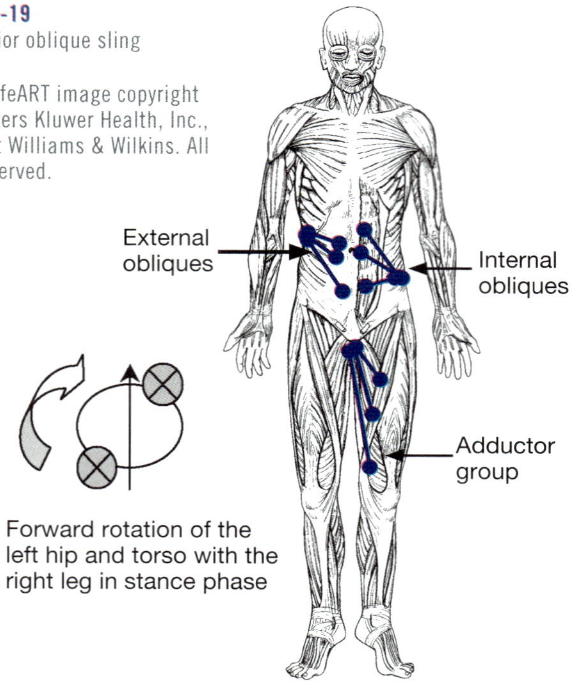

Figure 15-20
The posterior oblique sling

Source: LifeART image copyright 2008 Wolters Kluwer Health, Inc., Lippincott Williams & Wilkins. All rights reserved.

Backward (counterclockwise) rotation of the torso under action of the contralateral latissimus dorsi

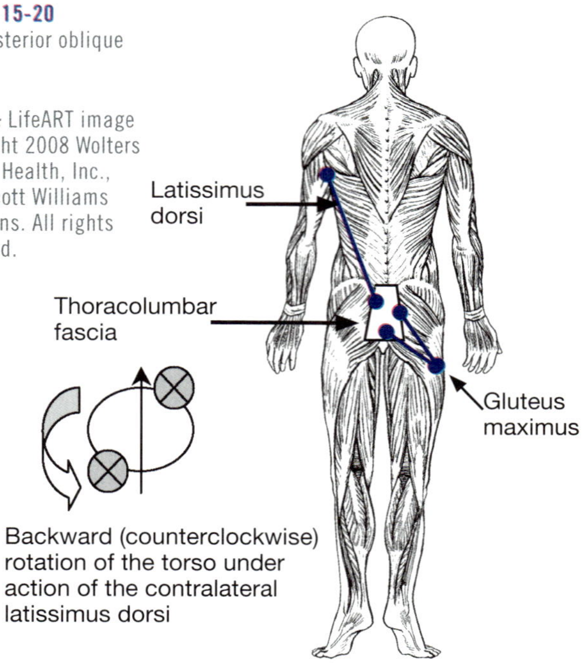

CORE FUNCTION ASSESSMENTS
McGill's Torso Muscular Endurance Test Battery

Optimally functioning core muscles help clients perform ADL like lifting a heavy laundry basket or recreational activities like swinging a golf club. Further, back dysfunction may be reversed by having a conditioned core. To evaluate balanced core endurance and stability, it is important to assess all sides of the torso. Each of the following assessments is performed individually, then evaluated collectively. Poor endurance capacity of the torso muscles or an imbalance among these three muscle groups is believed to contribute to low-back dysfunction and core instability.

Trunk Flexor Endurance Test

The trunk flexor endurance test is the first in the battery of three tests that assesses muscular endurance of the trunk flexors (i.e., rectus abdominis, external and internal obliques, and transverse abdominis). It is a timed test involving a static, isometric contraction of the anterior muscles, stabilizing the spine until the individual exhibits fatigue and can no longer hold the assumed position.

> **Contraindications**
> This test may not be suitable for individuals who suffer from low-back pain, have had recent back surgery, and/or are in the midst of an acute low-back flare-up.

Equipment:
- Stopwatch
- Board (or step)
- Strap (optional)

Pre-assessment procedure:
- After explaining the purpose of the flexor endurance test, describe the proper body position.
    ✓ The starting position requires the client to be seated, with the hips and knees bent to 90 degrees, aligning the hips, knees, and second toe.
    ✓ Instruct the client to fold their arms across the chest, touching each hand to the

Balance and Gait

CHAPTER 15

opposite shoulder, lean against a board positioned at a 50- to 60-degree incline, and keep the head in a neutral position (Figure 15-21).
- ✓ It is important to ask the client to press the shoulders into the board and maintain this "open" position throughout the test after the board is removed.
- ✓ Instruct the client to engage the abdominals to maintain a flat-to-neutral spine. The back should never be allowed to arch during the test.
- ✓ The CMES can anchor the toes under a strap or manually stabilize the feet if necessary.
- The goal of the test is to hold this 50- to 60-degree position for as long as possible without the benefit of the back support.
- Encourage the client to practice this position prior to attempting the test.

Assessment protocol and administration:
- The CMES starts the stopwatch as they move the board about 4 inches (10 cm) back, while the client maintains the 50- to 60-degree, suspended position.
- Terminate the test when there is a noticeable change in the trunk position:
  - ✓ Watch for a deviation from the neutral spine (i.e., the shoulders rounding forward) or an increase in the low-back arch.
  - ✓ No part of the back should touch the back rest.
- Record the client's time on the testing form.

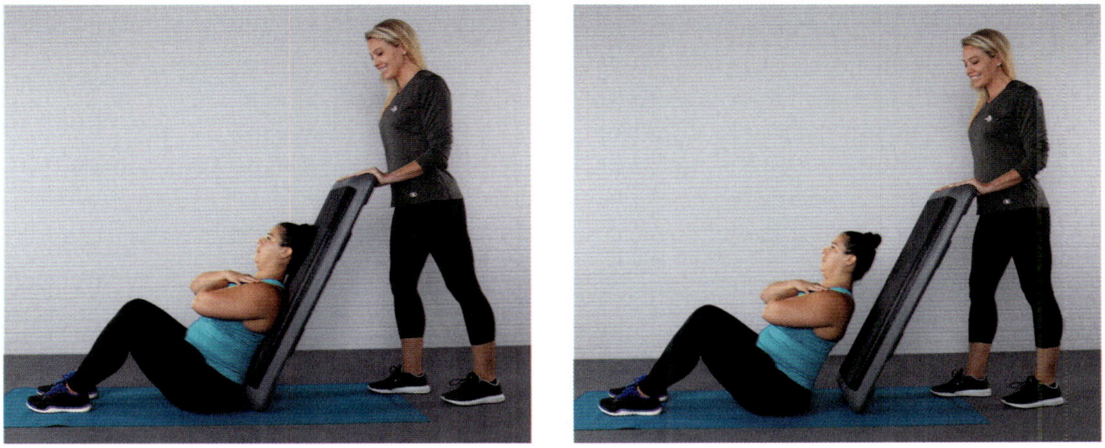

Figure 15-21
Trunk flexor endurance test

Trunk Lateral Endurance Test

The trunk lateral endurance test, also called the side-bridge test, assesses muscular endurance of the lateral core muscles (i.e., transverse abdominis, obliques, quadratus lumborum, and erector spinae). This timed test involves static, isometric contractions of the lateral muscles on each side of the trunk that stabilize the spine.

Contraindications
This test may not be suitable for individuals:
- With shoulder pain or weakness
- Who suffer from low-back pain, have had recent back surgery, and/or are in the midst of an acute low-back flare-up

Equipment:
- Stopwatch
- Mat (optional)

Pre-assessment procedure:
- After explaining the purpose of this test, describe the proper body position.
  - ✓ The starting position requires the client to be on their side with extended legs, aligning the feet on top of each other or in a tandem position (heel-to-toe).

- ✓ Have the client place the lower arm under the body and the upper arm on the side of the body.
- ✓ When the client is ready, instruct them to assume a full side-bridge position, keeping both legs extended and the sides of the feet on the floor. The elbow of the lower arm should be positioned directly under the shoulder with the forearm facing out (the forearm can be placed palm down for balance and support) and the upper arm should be resting along the side of the body or across the chest to the opposite shoulder.
- ✓ The hips should be elevated off the mat and the body should be in straight alignment (i.e., head, neck, torso, hips, and legs). The torso should only be supported by the client's foot/feet and the elbow/forearm of the lower arm (Figure 15-22).
   - *Modification*: If a client is unable to support their body weight while balancing on the feet, an alternative is for the client to rest on the side of the lower leg with both knees bent in the hook-lying position (Figure 15-23), thereby shortening the lever of the legs and increasing the surface area on which to balance. If this modification is used, be sure to perform subsequent assessments in the modified position so that the results are comparable. Because the original test battery was not performed using this modification, the scoring and reliability of results will vary.
- The goal of the test is to hold this position for as long as possible. Once the client breaks the position, the test is terminated.
- Encourage the client to practice this position prior to attempting the test.

Assessment protocol and administration:
- The CMES starts the stopwatch as the client moves into the side-bridge position.
- Terminate the test when there is a noticeable change in the trunk position
   - ✓ A deviation from the neutral spine (i.e., the hips dropping downward)
   - ✓ The hips shifting forward or backward in an effort to maintain balance and stability
- Record the client's time on the testing form.
- Repeat the test on the opposite side and record this value on the testing form.

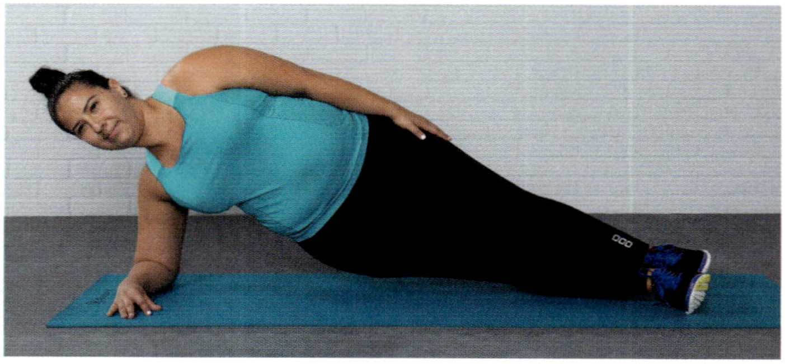

Figure 15-22
Trunk lateral endurance test

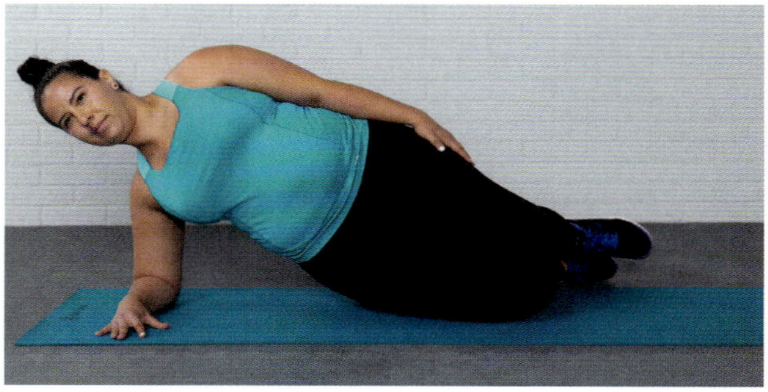

Figure 15-23
Trunk lateral endurance test: Modified hook-lying position

Trunk Extensor Endurance Test

The trunk extensor endurance test is generally used to assess muscular endurance of the torso extensor muscles (i.e., erector spinae and multifidi). This is a timed test involving a static, isometric contraction of the trunk extensor muscles that stabilize the spine.

Contraindications
This test may not be suitable for:
- A client with major strength deficiencies, where the individual cannot even lift the torso from a forward flexed position to a neutral position
- A client with a high body mass, in which case it would be difficult for the CMES to support the client's suspended upper-body weight
- Individuals who suffer from low-back pain, have had recent back surgery, and/or are in the midst of an acute low-back flare-up

Balance and Gait   CHAPTER 15

Equipment:
- Elevated, sturdy exam table
- Nylon strap
- Stopwatch

Pre-assessment procedure:
- After explaining the purpose of the test, explain the proper body position.
    - ✓ The starting position requires the client to be prone, positioning the iliac crests at the table edge while supporting the upper extremity on the arms, which are placed on the floor or on a riser.
    - ✓ While the client is supporting the weight of their upper body, anchor the client's lower legs to the table using a strap. If a strap is not used, the CMES will have to use their own body weight to stabilize the client's legs (Figure 15-24a).
- The goal of the test is to hold a horizontal, prone position for as long as possible. Once the client falls below horizontal, the test is terminated.
- Encourage the client to practice this position prior to attempting the test.

Assessment protocol and administration:
- When ready, the client lifts/extends the torso until it is parallel to the floor with their arms crossed over the chest (Figure 15-24b).
    - ✓ *Modification:* If a client is unable to support their body weight while hanging off the edge of a table, an alternative is for the client to lie prone on the floor and come into spinal extension (Figure 15-25), thereby eliminating the need for a table and strap (or for the CMES to hold the client's legs). The client should be instructed to keep the thighs in contact with the floor throughout the duration of the assessment. If this modification is used, be sure to perform subsequent assessments in the modified position so that the results are comparable. Because the original test battery was not performed using this modification, the scoring and reliability of results will vary.
- Start the stopwatch as soon as the client assumes this position.
- Terminate the test when the client can no longer maintain the position.
- Record the client's time on the testing form.

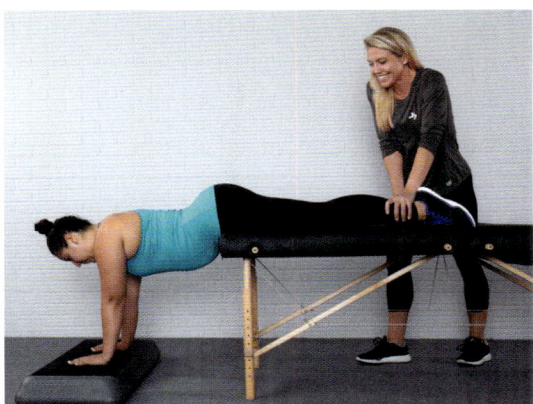

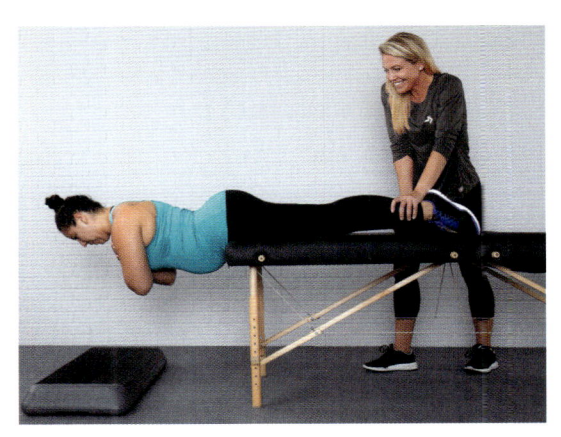

Figure 15-24
Trunk extensor endurance test

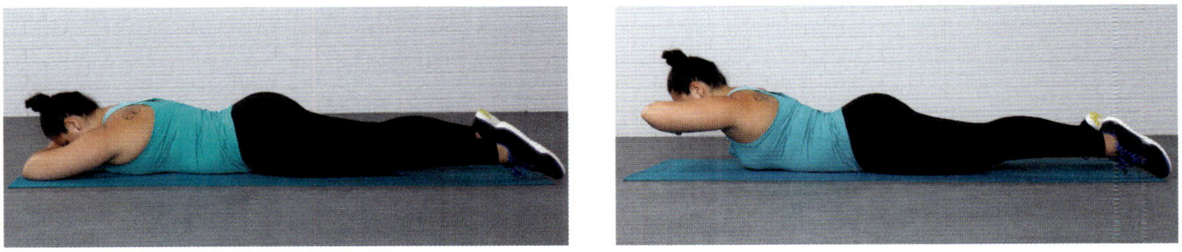

a. Starting position

b. Test position

Figure 15-25
Trunk extensor endurance test: Modified position

a. Starting position

b. Test position

Total Test Battery Interpretation

Each individual test in this testing battery is not a primary indicator of current or future back problems. McGill (2016) has shown that the relationships among the tests are more important indicators of muscle imbalances that can lead to back pain compared to looking at the individual results of each test because the torso extensors, flexors, and lateral musculature are involved in virtually all tasks. In fact, even in a person with little or no back pain, the ratios can still be off, suggesting that low-back pain may eventually occur without diligent attention to a solid core-conditioning program. McGill (2016) suggests the following ratios indicate balanced endurance among the muscle groups:

- Flexion:extension ratio should be less than 1.0
  - ✓ For example, a flexion score of 120 seconds and extension score of 150 seconds generates a ratio score of 0.80
- Right-side bridge (RSB):left-side bridge (LSB) scores should be no greater than 0.05 from a balanced score of 1.0 (i.e., 0.95 to 1.05)
  - ✓ For example, a RSB score of 88 seconds and an LSB score of 92 seconds generates a ratio score of 0.96, which is within the 0.05 range from 1.0
- Side bridge (either side):extension ratio should be less than 0.75
  - ✓ For example, a RSB score of 88 seconds and an extension score of 150 seconds generates a ratio score of 0.59

Demonstrated deficiencies in these core functional assessments should be addressed during exercise programming as part of the foundational exercises for a client. The goal is to create ratios consistent with McGill's recommendations. Muscular endurance, more so than muscular strength or even ROM, has been shown to be an accurate predictor of back health (McGill, 2016). Low-back stabilization exercises have the most benefit when performed daily. When working with clients with low-back dysfunction, it is prudent to include daily stabilization exercises in their home exercise plans. After completing all elements of McGill's torso muscular endurance test battery, the CMES can use Figure 15-26 to record the client's data.

Figure 15-26
McGill's torso muscular endurance test battery—record sheet

Visit www.ACEfitness.org/CMESresources for a record sheet for McGill's torso muscular endurance test battery, as well as other forms and tools that you can use throughout your career as a CMES.

Trunk flexor endurance test

Time to completion: _____

Trunk lateral endurance test

Right side time to completion: _____ Left side time to completion: _____

Trunk extensor endurance test

Time to completion: _____

Ratio of Comparison	Criteria for Good Relationship Between Muscles
Flexion:extension	Ratio less than 1.0
Right-side bridge:left-side bridge	Scores should be no greater than 0.05 from a balanced score of 1.0
Side bridge (each side):extension	Ratio less than 0.75

Flexion:extension ratio: _____ Rating: ❏ Good ❏ Poor

Right-side bridge:left-side bridge ratio: _____ Rating: ❏ Good ❏ Poor

Side-bridge (each side):extension ratio: _____ Rating: ❏ Good ❏ Poor

Balance and Gait CHAPTER 15

> **EXPAND YOUR KNOWLEDGE**
>
> **EVALUATION AND APPLICATION OF PERFORMANCE FOR MCGILL'S TORSO MUSCULAR ENDURANCE TEST BATTERY**
>
> Each individual test in this testing battery is not a primary indicator of current or future back problems. McGill (2016) has shown that the relationships among the tests are more important indicators of muscle imbalances that can lead to back pain. In fact, even in a person with little or no back pain, the ratios can still be off, suggesting that low-back pain may eventually occur without diligent attention to a solid core-conditioning program. McGill (2016) suggests the following ratios indicate balanced endurance among the muscle groups:
> - Flexion:extension ratio should be less than 1.0
>   - ✓ For example, a flexion score of 120 seconds and extension score of 150 seconds generates a ratio score of 0.80
> - Right-side bridge (RSB):left-side bridge (LSB) scores should be no greater than 0.05 from a balanced score of 1.0 (i.e., 0.95 to 1.05)
>   - ✓ For example, a RSB score of 88 seconds and an LSB score of 92 seconds generates a ratio score of 0.96, which is within the 0.05 range from 1.0
> - Side bridge (either side):extension ratio should be less than 0.75
>   - ✓ For example, a RSB score of 88 seconds and an extension score of 150 seconds generates a ratio score of 0.59
>
> Demonstrated deficiencies in these core functional assessments should be addressed during exercise programming as part of the foundational exercises for a client. The goal is to create ratios consistent with McGill's recommendations. Muscular endurance, more so than muscular strength or even ROM, has been shown to be an accurate predictor of back health (McGill, 2016). Research shows that low-back stabilization exercises have the most benefit when performed daily. When working with clients with low-back dysfunction, it is prudent to include daily stabilization exercises in their home-exercise plans.
>
> Since most Americans will experience low-back pain at some point in their lives, a comprehensive fitness program should incorporate spinal-stabilization exercises. Even when working with clients who have yet to develop an interest in the health of their back, core stability should still be a key element in any training program. For example, if the core is not strong, the back may be compromised during a dumbbell shoulder press, creating excessive lumbar lordosis.
>
> The same break in position can happen during a squat or a bench press, thus creating excess stress on the lumbar spine. Improper alignment can create a whole host of problems for the lower back, ranging from herniated discs to sciatic pain. Clients' training objectives can vary from rehabilitation or prevention of low-back pain to optimizing health and fitness or maximizing athletic performance. All clients will benefit from exercises targeting core stability.

Other Assessments

Sahrmann (2002) offers screening tools to identify movement impairments within the lumbar spine and hip. While a CMES is not qualified to make any diagnoses or treat movement-impairment syndromes, familiarization with some of the protocols offered in this reference will help the CMES better understand the roles these muscles play across the lumbo-pelvic region in stabilizing the spine and improving balance. Houglum (2010) and Kendall et al. (2005) also offer valuable insight.

ASSESSMENT OF BALANCE AND GAIT

A thorough health history is always a prerequisite to conducting assessments and includes a review of medications and any potential side effects the medications may have on balance (e.g., psychotropic and antihypertensive medications). The CMES should also conduct a needs assessment to determine the appropriateness of testing based upon the client's needs, skill level, and functional capacity. The CMES must then give consideration to prioritizing the assessments and establish timelines for testing, as many clients may find a battery of tests conducted at the onset overwhelming. To further complicate matters, the **scope of practice** for the CMES includes additional evaluations such as posture and movement. Figure 15-27 provides an overview of how a CMES can sequence assessments.

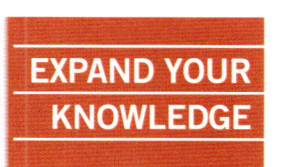

The use of population-specific protocols that are appropriate to functional capacity is recommended when working with older adults, given their propensity for functional limitations and considering the fact that many industry-standardized protocols are not appropriate nor validated for this age group (Rikli & Jones, 2013; Nagi, 1991). Figure 15-28 illustrates the progression of age-related changes in physiological function toward disability.

Several researchers and practitioners have developed and validated population-specific protocols. These protocols generally evaluate a cross-section of the major health- and skill-related fitness components associated with independent living, including balance. Balance tests assess basic static balance (standing or unsupported sitting); static balance challenges (manipulating BOS and COG, challenging LOS, and sensory integration); dynamic balance (rising out of chairs and gait); and anticipatory or adaptive control (movement around and over obstacles). Rose's *Fall Proof* (2010) and Rikli and Jones's *Senior Fitness Test Manual* (2013) are excellent resources for many of these protocols.

Figure 15-27
Sequencing of assessments

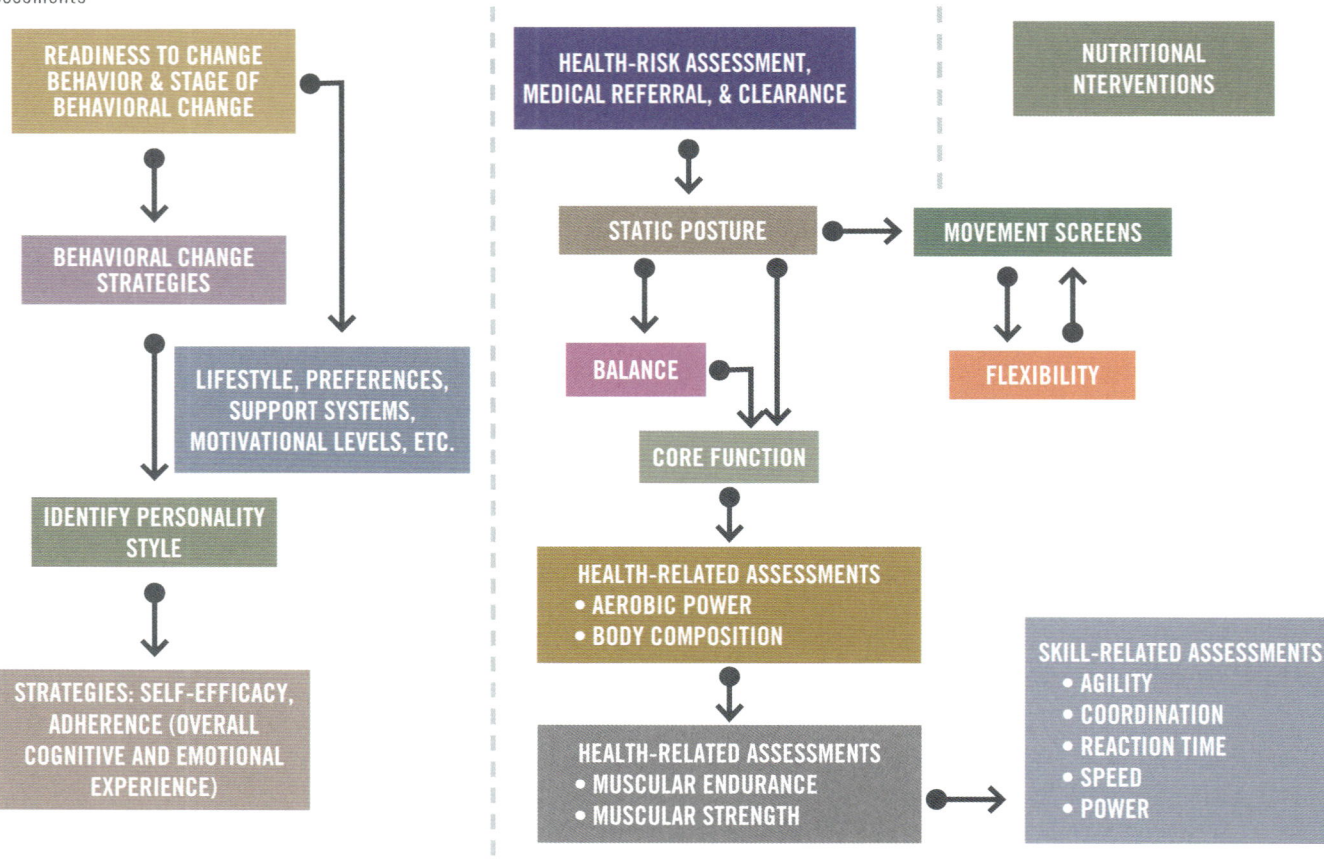

Figure 15-28
The modified disability model

Source: Adapted from Nagi, S.S (1991). Disability concepts revisited: Implication for prevention. In: Pope, A.M. & Tarlov, A.R. (Eds). *Disability in America: Toward a National Agenda for Prevention.* Washington, D.C.: National Academy Press.

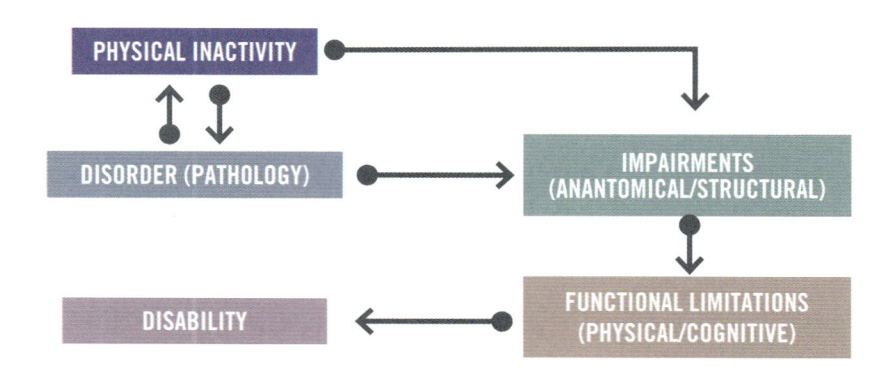

GAIT ANALYSIS

The detailed analysis of gait is a complicated process ideally performed by a qualified professional, although the CMES can perform some basic evaluations of walking patterns, as illustrated in Figure 15-29. A CMES should be able to recognize postural deviations and muscle imbalances, and identify the impact they might potentially have on movement efficiency. A CMES can also identify compensations at the joints and within the kinetic chain, distinguish correctable from non-correctable deviations (see page 417), and then apply their knowledge of neuromuscular physiology and biomechanics to help the client restore anatomical joint neutrality, which in turn might improve balance and gait efficiency. For example, if excessive pronation is identified at the subtalar joint, the CMES can direct the client to find the neutral subtalar position while standing. If the client is able to correct the position without further compensations along the kinetic chain and hold this position free of pain or discomfort, it is likely that a program of stretching **hypertonic** (tight) muscles and strengthening **latent** (weakened) muscles, coupled with neural reeducation and conscious awareness of posture, can help restore neutrality at the joint. However, the CMES must understand the limitations of this approach and respect the scope of practice. Structural deviations or limitations within the skeletal system may limit the client's ability to restore or correct joint position (e.g., anteversion/retroversion due to an abnormal rotational angle of the femoral neck in relation to the femur's long axis alters knee alignment and the forces acting throughout the lower kinetic chain). If a client presents with a structural deviation and/or persistent pain, a referral to the appropriate medical professional is warranted.

Visit www.ACEfitness.org/CMESresources for a walking patterns worksheet, as well as other forms and tools that you can use throughout your career as a CMES.

Figure 15-29
Basic evaluation of walking patterns

Instructions:

The client walks toward the CMES along a 10-to 15-yard (9.1- to 13.6-m) hallway, following a straight line marked on the floor or carpeting, or walks toward a full-length mirror (repeat as needed).

1.	Does the gait follow a straight line?	❏
2.	Do the two hemispheres of the body appear symmetrical?	❏
3.	Does the body appear to maintain extension?	❏
4.	Are the hips and shoulders level?	❏
5.	Do the knees point forward?	❏
6.	Do the arms swing rhythmically and appear to swing symmetrically (observe for rotation)?	❏
7.	Do the step lengths appear equal?	❏
8.	Does the foot appear to make initial contact in supination, then pronate during load response?	❏
9.	After heel strike, do the toes have a controlled eccentric movement toward the floor?	❏

The client walks 10 to 15 yards (9.1 to 13.6 m) from left to right along a line or parallel to a full-length mirror (repeat as needed).

1.	Do the heels make initial contact with the floor after the swing phase?	❏
2.	Does the foot follow from heel-off to toe-off?	❏
3.	Is the knee almost fully extended immediately prior to heel strike?	❏
4.	Does the torso maintain good extension with alignment of the head and torso?	❏
5.	Are the steps of equal length?	❏
6.	Are the arms swings of equal length?	❏

GAIT EXERCISES

Gait is perhaps the most functional movement in humans, yet people face significant challenges in maintaining gait function and mobility as they age and develop disorders, functional limitations, or impairments. As gait function is vital to functional independence, people must continue to train the necessary parameters that contribute to gait, including balance, agility, strength, power, flexibility, coordination, reactivity, and sensorimotor integration. Once good posture is restored, faulty core neural pathways are re-educated, confidence and efficiency with static balance is achieved, and sensory acuity and postural-control strategies are enhanced. Assuming there is no need for prerequisite lower-extremity strengthening and flexibility, the programming focus should turn to improving gait. Basic gait exercises begin with static balance and progress to dynamic balance and include:

- Static weight shifting (weight transference) in anterior-posterior and lateral directions
- Stepping in anterior-posterior and lateral directions
- In-place marching (progress in-place marching to include 90-degree turns)
- The CMES can introduce directional walking, directional changes, and directional changes with abrupt stops and starts as the next progression (Figure 15-30).

Figure 15-30
Directional progression of gait drills

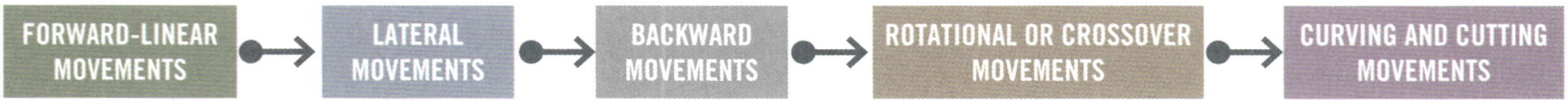

FORWARD-LINEAR MOVEMENTS → LATERAL MOVEMENTS → BACKWARD MOVEMENTS → ROTATIONAL OR CROSSOVER MOVEMENTS → CURVING AND CUTTING MOVEMENTS

Curving movements generally involve stepping into the curve with the inside leg, dropping the inside shoulder and arm toward the marker, and pushing off the outside leg through the curve. Cutting movements generally involve eccentric deceleration and loading on the outside leg while maintaining foot, knee, hip, and shoulder alignment, followed by a push-off of the outside leg while stepping in the new direction with the inside leg.

To lead a client through directional walking drills, the CMES should:
- Create a 10- to 15-foot (3.0- to 4.6-m) walking pathway using cones as markers
- Instruct the client to walk through the drill as quickly as possible while maintaining postural control
- Gradually increase repetitions from two to five per exercise
- Observe efficiency in executing directional changes, offering feedback and correction as needed (Figure 15-31)

The development of agility and coordination are essential skill elements for efficient movement. Traditional exercises and drills for these skill parameters are usually performed at high speeds with athletes, but can be simplified and slowed down with individuals seeking gait improvement. Predetermined agility drills with predesignated foot placements are taught before introducing reactionary drills, a more advanced exercise format in which the client reacts to stimuli and instructions. The CMES can teach drills in a segmented or part-to-whole format to facilitate learning and mastery.

When training for agility, the CMES can use the same exercise equipment used for sports-conditioning drills (e.g., cones, risers, agility ladders, and hurdles). While agility ladders are an effective learning tool for developing agility, these drills need to progress to hurdles and risers that emphasize leg lift and clearance, mimicking true gait patterns, as opposed to the foot shuffles with minimal ground clearance used when working with the ladders. Agility ladder drills for foot patterns can be simple, unidirectional, slow-walking exercises that gradually increase to more advanced, faster, multidirectional, runs, jumps, and hops incorporating obstacles and simultaneous coordination drills often used with more athletic individuals. Examples of agility ladder drills include:

- Forward walks or runs (single-foot step into each square, double-foot step into each square)
- Forward jumps or hops (double hops, single hops, jumping jacks, hopscotch patterns)
- Lateral shuffles (basic, crossovers, **carioca,** grapevines)

Balance and Gait   CHAPTER 15

- Lateral hops (double hops, single hops, split jumps)
- Backpedaling (single-foot step into each square, double-foot step into each square)
- Multidirectional (lateral-forward patterns, zigzags, slaloms or "Ickey shuffles," double slalom, Ws, Ms, machine gunners, multidirectional hops) (Figure 15-32)

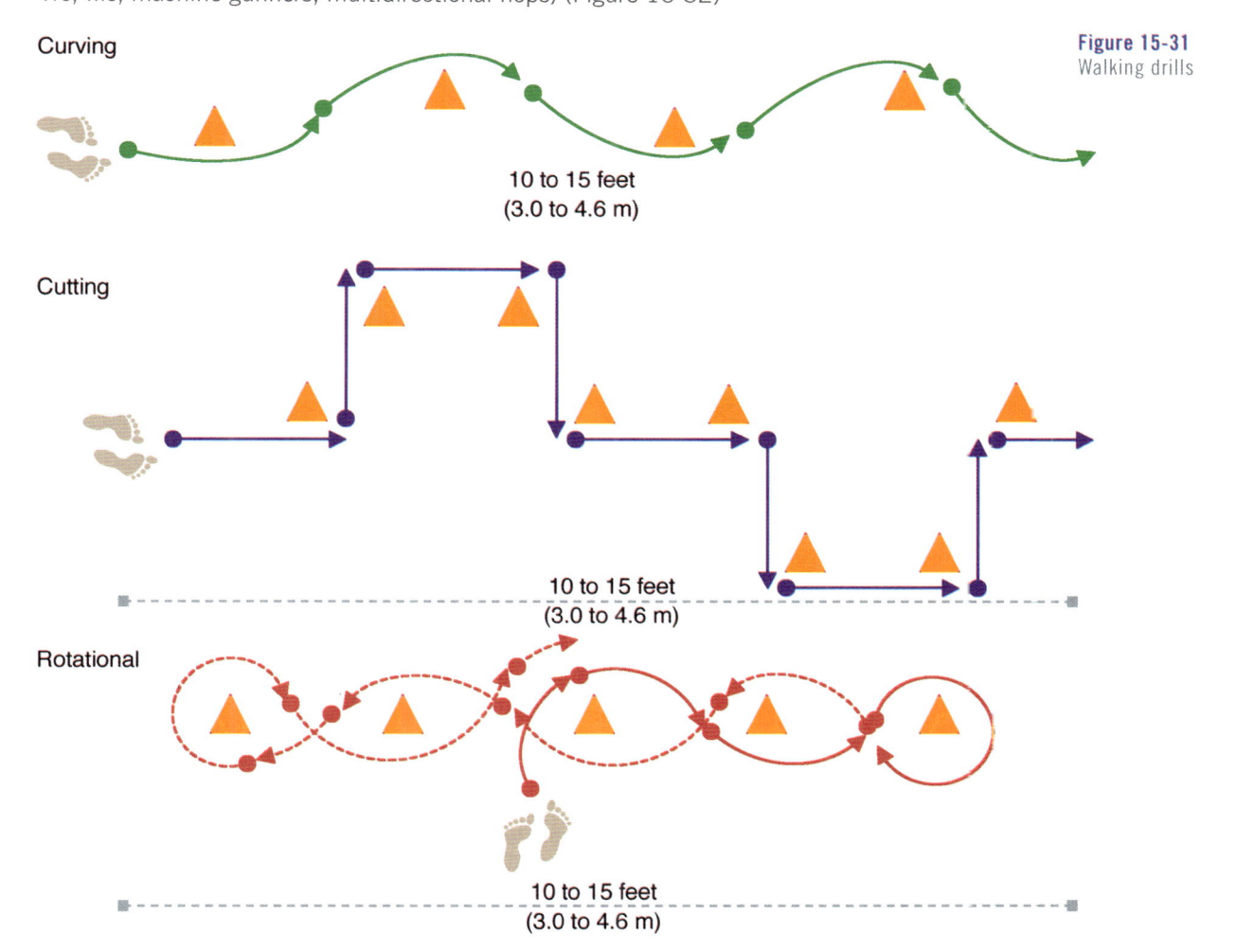

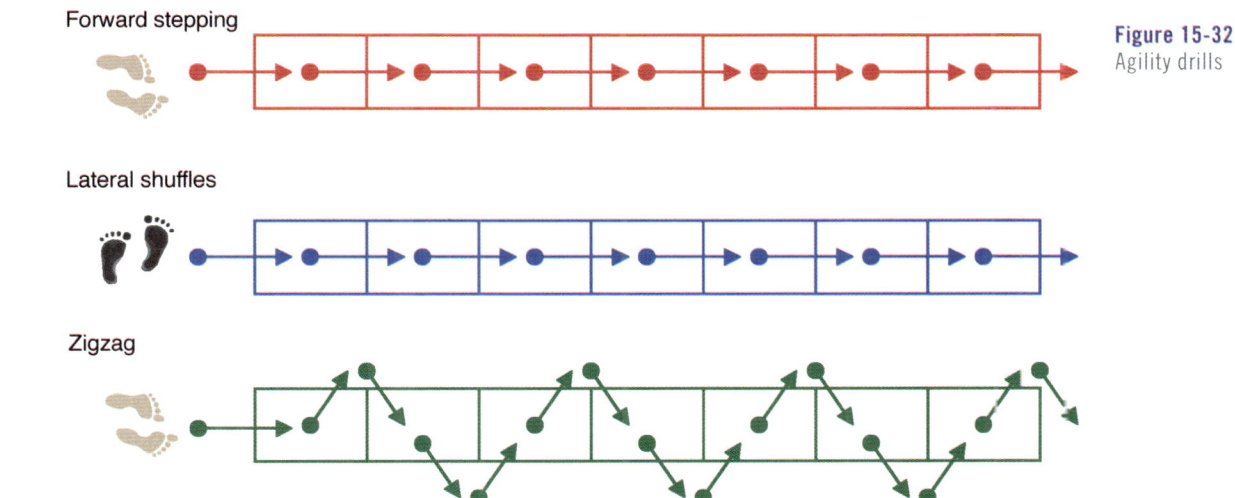

Figure 15-31
Walking drills

Curving

10 to 15 feet
(3.0 to 4.6 m)

Cutting

10 to 15 feet
(3.0 to 4.6 m)

Rotational

10 to 15 feet
(3.0 to 4.6 m)

Figure 15-32
Agility drills

Forward stepping

Lateral shuffles

Zigzag

ACE MEDICAL EXERCISE SPECIALIST MANUAL   AMERICAN COUNCIL ON EXERCISE

Gait exercises can be advanced further with the addition of walking with altered bases of support, and by changing the speed, distance, and complexity of the exercise by introducing the following tasks:
- Narrow, wide, or alternating narrow-wide step widths
- Tandem or heel-to-toe walks
- High-knee, stiff-legged march walks
- Heel-off or toe-off walks
- Crossover walks

They can also be advanced by adding obstacle walks using risers, steps, and even unstable surfaces for more advanced individuals (Figure 15-33). Obstacle walking involves walking along narrow beams or inverted half–foam rollers or performing step-up, step-over, or step-down exercises over the same height or pyramiding heights on similar or different surfaces. The CMES should begin with a forward-linear direction, introducing directional changes as mastery is achieved. The treadmill is also an effective training modality for gait, although clients may experience a little instability at first if unfamiliar with the device. Allow adequate opportunities for each client to develop confidence and balance on a treadmill before using it as a training tool.

Figure 15-33
Obstacle walking using different equipment as props

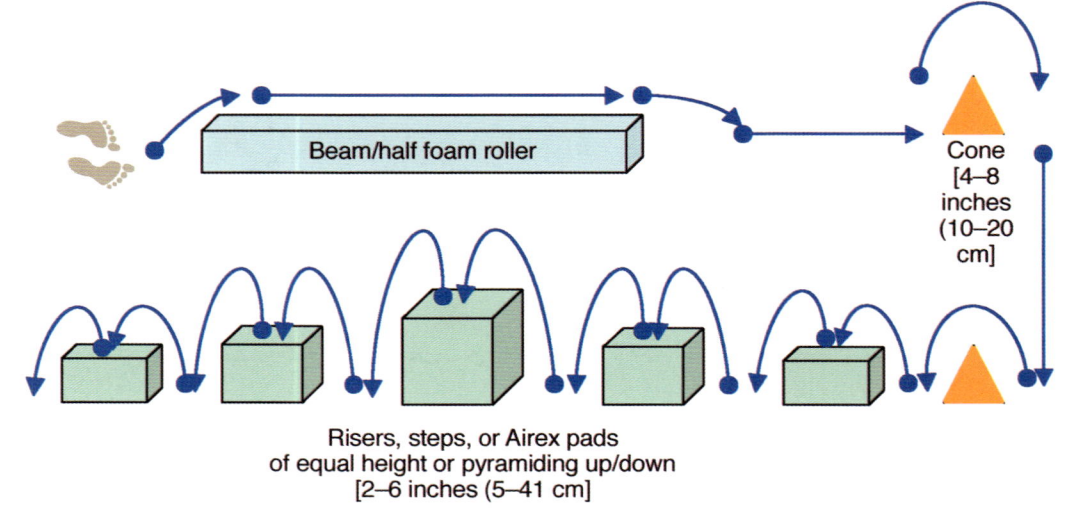

Coordination is the ability to train the body to enable each muscle involved in a movement to provide an accurate response in both timing and intensity. There are specific requirements for coordinated movement:
- Perception of the activity or awareness of volitional muscle activity, joint position, and movement. This element originally stems from visual feedback (a slower process), but with repetition and mastery, it may originate from proprioceptive feedback (a more rapid process).
- Feedback during and following activity, as the cognitive and nervous systems evaluate performance and make any necessary adjustments
- Perfect repetitions with increasing accuracy as mastery increases, potentially decreasing the required effort and overflow from other muscles (overstimulation of muscles compensating for weaker muscles that decrease response accuracy in both timing and intensity)
- The ability to inhibit undesired muscle activity and response is facilitated by precise, slow and controlled movement until motor patterns are developed, after which speed and intensity can be increased.

Training the skill of coordination involves advancing the complexity of the more basic gait and agility drills and/or simultaneously integrating motor and cognitive tasks (e.g., having a client process questions or tasks cognitively while performing motor tasks, such as having them perform simple mathematical calculations while moving through the agility ladders or around cones).

Balance and Gait   CHAPTER 15

Often, when clients who are regularly active develop chronic injuries, they are surprised to learn that potential causes for their problems are related to core imbalances or fundamental movement dysfunctions. Consequently it may be difficult for clients who are skilled in fitness pursuits (e.g., weightlifting and recreational sports) to regress their exercise programs to include basic exercises that are corrective in nature. How would you address the concerns of a client who is worried that performing exercises to develop basic core function and movement skills will set them back in terms of maintaining their achievements in other fitness-related pursuits?

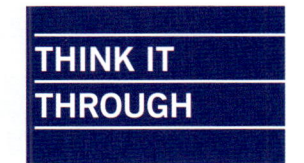

THINK IT THROUGH

APPLY WHAT YOU KNOW

SAMPLE BALANCE AND GAIT EXERCISE PROGRAM

INITIAL PHASE EXERCISES

	Repetitions	Intensity	Sets	Tempo	Rest Interval
Core stabilization					
Pelvic tilts	12–15	Body weight	2–3	Slow	45 seconds
Quadruped bird dog	10–12	Body weight	2–3	Slow	45 seconds
Lateral planks	1	Body weight	2–3	Hold–15 seconds	45 seconds
Glute bridges	12–15	Body weight	2–3	Slow	45 seconds
Mobility					
Rocking quadriceps	10–12	Body weight	2–3	Slow	45 seconds
Spinal twists	8–10	Body weight	2–3	Slow	45 seconds
Lateral lunge with reach for ground	8–10	Body weight	2–3	Moderate	45 seconds
Balance					
Single-leg balance	10–12	Body weight	2–3	Slow	45 seconds
Lateral step-up	10–12	Body weight	2–3	Slow	45 seconds

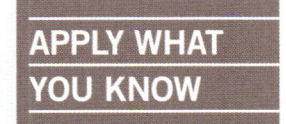

EXERCISE PROGRESSIONS

	Repetitions	Sets	Tempo	Rest Interval
Core stabilization				
Supine bent-knee marches	10–12	2–3	Slow	30 seconds
Single-leg supine glute bridge	10–12	2–3	Slow	30 seconds
Front plank with hip extension	6	2–3	Slow	30 seconds
Standing bilateral cable press	8–10	2–3	Slow	30 seconds
Mobility				
Right lateral lunge with left-hand opposite reach at shoulder height (alternating)	8–10	2–3	Moderate	Circuit format; no rest between exercises; 2 minutes of rest at the end
Half-kneeling triplanar stretch	8–10	2–3	Moderate	
Lateral plane lunge with bilateral rm rotation at shoulder height (alternating sides)	8–10	2–3	Moderate	
Balance				
Prone plank to standing single-leg balance	8–10	2–3	Slow	30 seconds between each leg
Lateral bounds to balance	4–6	2–3	Fast	
Lateral plane lunge to single-leg balance	6–8	2–3	Moderate	

EXERCISES FOR THE MYOFASCIAL SLINGS

Applying the biotensegrity model of structural mechanics, as the body changes positions during the gait cycle, the muscles experience both compressive and tensile forces. To help a client improve mobility and balance to enhance their performance through the gait cycle, the CMES can design exercise programs to integrate and coordinate the actions of the muscle, fascia, skeletal structures, and CNS as they function during upright movement.

Instead of simply having clients do an exercise for a specific muscle, the CMES should use integrated movement patterns based on the lines of pull of the myofascial slings in an effort to help remodel the muscle and fascia into a more efficient structure capable of balancing and controlling the forces of compression and tension. It is recommended to start by teaching clients exercise movements in a stable environment such as lying on the ground before progressing to standing position that requires the ability to control forces created by gravity and ground reaction.

The five foundational patterns of movement: squatting (or bending at the hips), lunging (or stepping on a single leg), pushing (either toward the front of the body or overhead), pulling (either from the front of the body or an overhead position), and rotating (which is the synchronized combination of a push and pull movement) can be seen in the different phases of the gait cycle. Therefore, teaching clients how to perform exercises based on these patterns can enhance mobility and balance to improve performance through gait, as well as many other ADL.

Walking through the gait cycle involves the shoulders counter-rotating with the contralateral hips to create efficient movement. The most effective exercises for training the CNS to coordinate the efforts of muscle and fascia to control movement of the skeletal structures involve the upper and lower limbs moving at the same time, similar to how they function during gait. Clients should first learn how to perform the basic patterns of movement before progressing to integrated patterns involving multiple movements, which can help realign the network of muscle and fascia and enhance the biotensegrity of the human body. For example, clients can begin in a staggered stance and perform arm reaches. Adopting the staggered position facilitates the necessary pelvic rotation and relative foot placement required for gait, and performing the arm reaches induces counter-rotation of the shoulders. Mobility strategies such as this will help provide the required joint ROM to efficiently pattern gait.

Body-weight exercises featuring the basic patterns of movement can be used as a progression of a dynamic warm-up before increasing the intensity and challenge to include multiplanar movements using a variety of traditional and nontraditional resistance-training equipment. To develop optimal coordination and have the greatest training effect on the entire myofascial system, it is important to load specific lines of fascia and muscle tissue.

The exercises presented here are examples of how to engage the muscle and fascia involved in the various slings. Starting with exercises in a supine or prone position takes away the force of gravity and can be effective for improving cognitive action of the involved muscles. As the client demonstrates improvements in strength and body control, they can be progressed to standing exercises that require more input from the reflexes responsible for maintaining upright position and equilibrium. Some exercises will certainly involve the muscles from more than one sling and that is acceptable as long as the client can maintain good posture and control of their COG. Once movement efficiency has been enhanced, the client can progress to either classic resistance training using external loads to improve force output or reactive **plyometrics** with body weight to enhance fascial elasticity. The client's fitness level, movement skill, and training goal will dictate the specific application of variables (intensity, repetitions, sets, and rest interval) for their exercise program.

Anterior Oblique Sling

The anterior oblique myofascial sling is responsible for rotating the trunk over the pelvis during gait and creating dynamic stability of the upper body during upright movements involving pushing motions. This sling can be strengthened with movements that involve an upright stance with split-leg or single-leg positions and trunk rotation. Figures 15-34 through 15-40 present exercises for the anterior oblique sling.

Balance and Gait CHAPTER 15

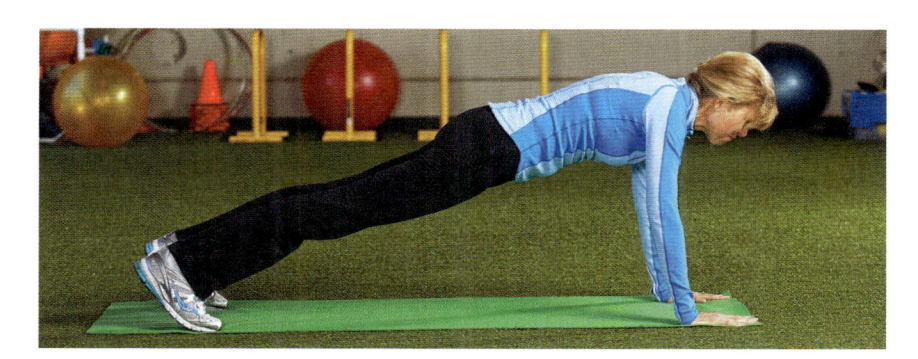

Figure 15-34
Front plank

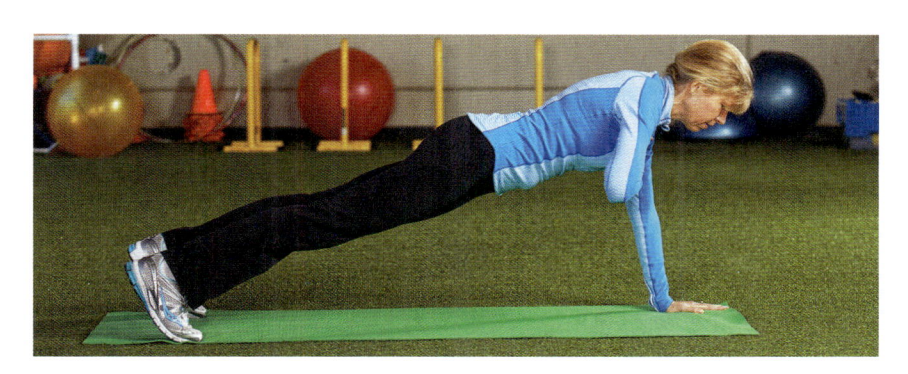

Figure 15-35
Single-arm front plank

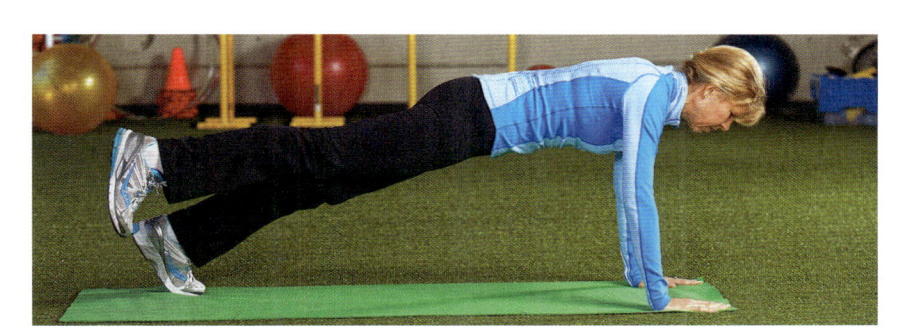

Figure 15-36
Front plank (or push-up) with hip extension

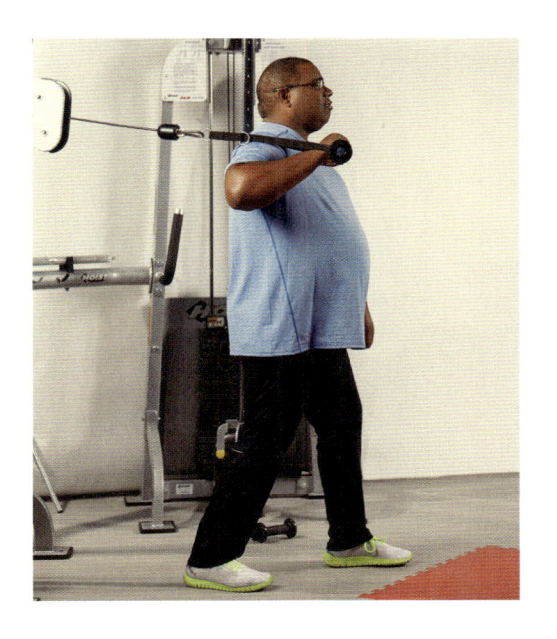

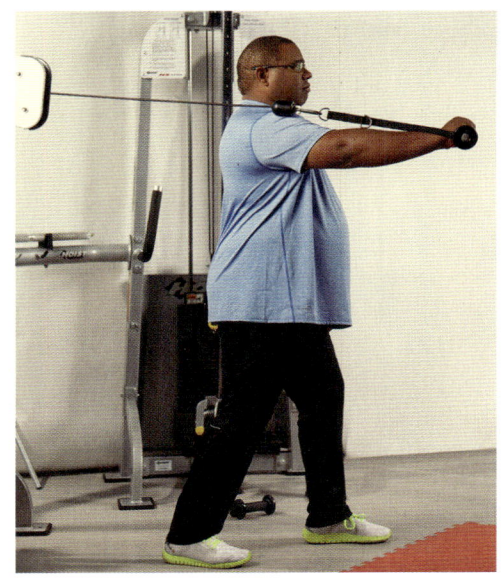

Figure 15-37
Standing single-arm cable press

Figure 15-38
Standing bilateral cable press

Figure 15-39
Anterior lunge with bilateral overhead reach (or shoulder press)

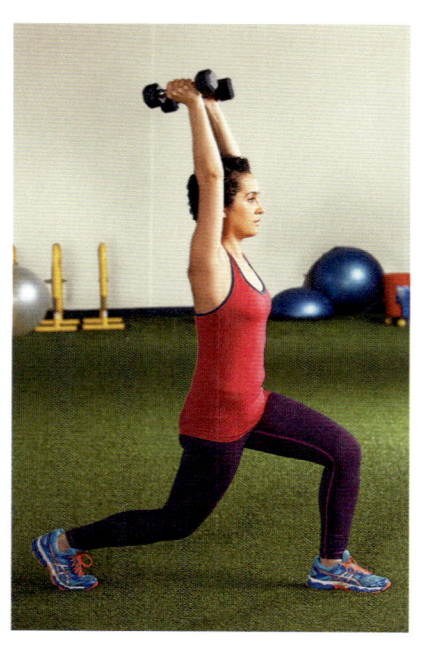

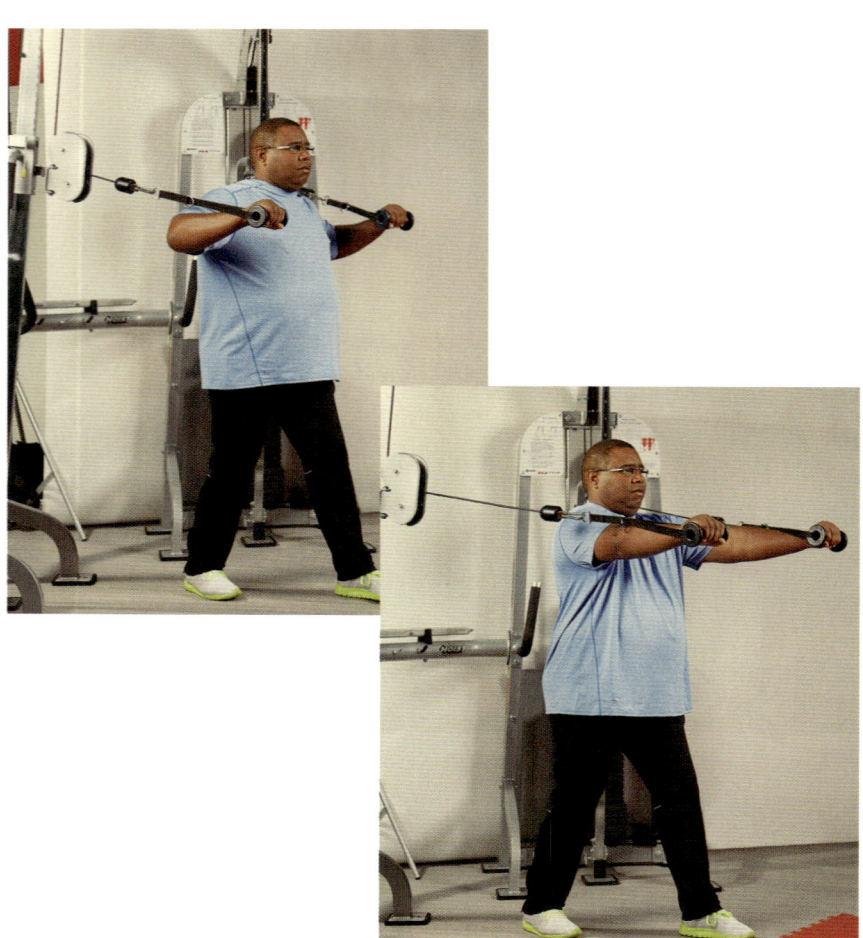

Figure 15-40
High-to-low cable chop

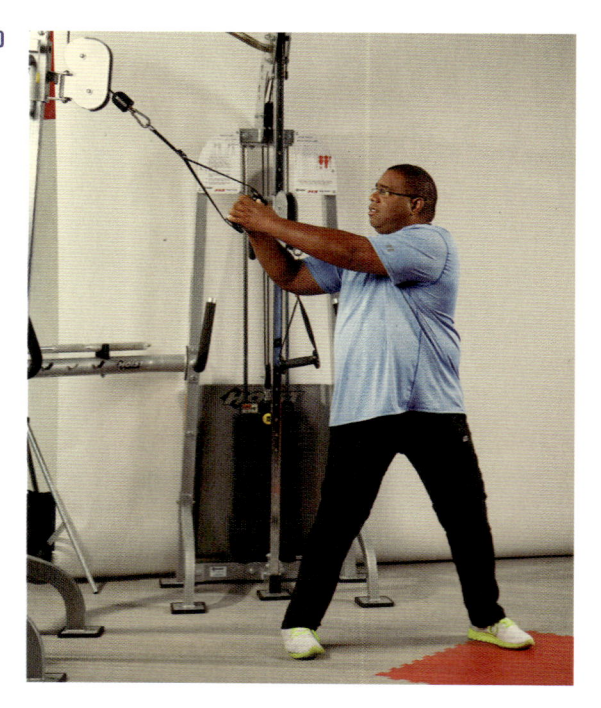

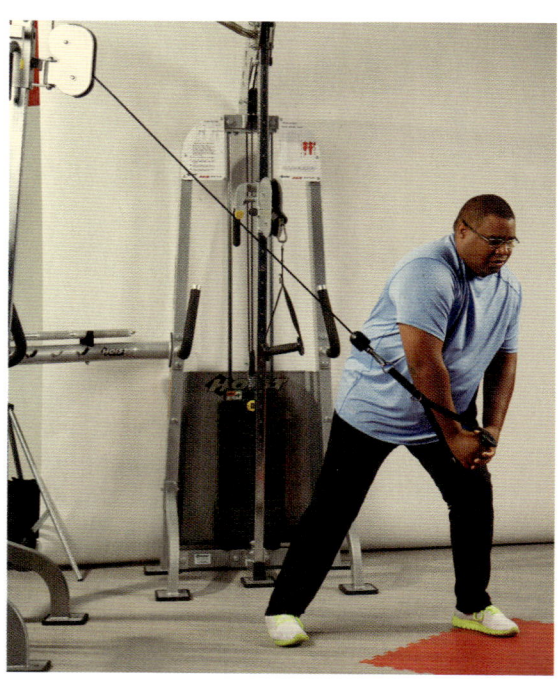

Balance and Gait

CHAPTER 15

Posterior Oblique Sling

The role of the posterior oblique myofascial sling is to help with rotation of the trunk over the pelvis during gait and to create dynamic stability during upright movements featuring pulling motions. Figures 15-41 through 15-46 present exercises for the posterior oblique sling.

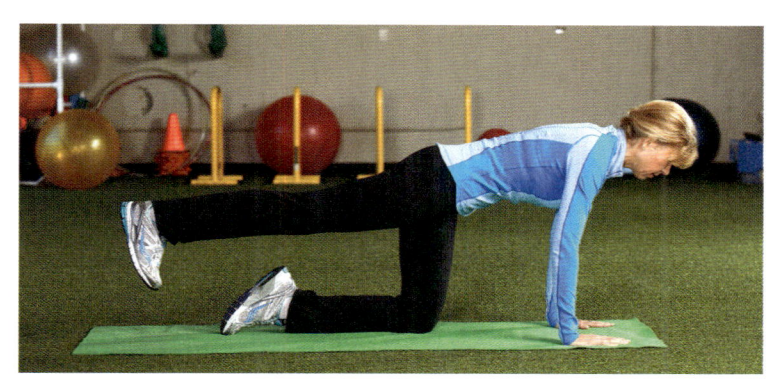

Figure 15-41
Quadruped hip extension

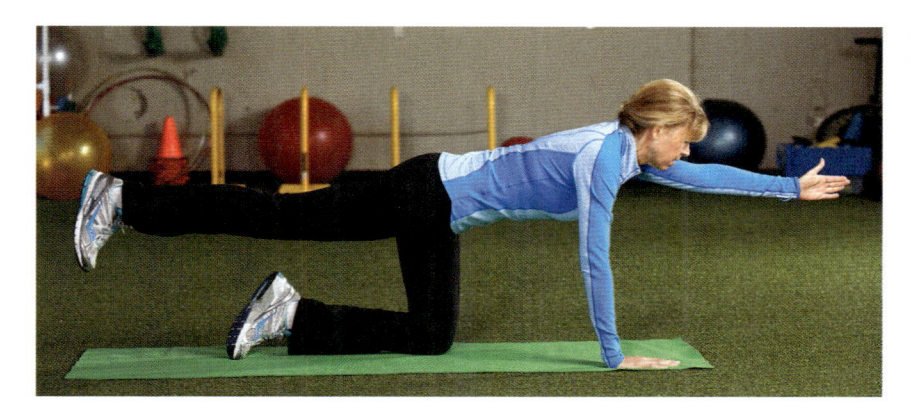

Figure 15-42
Quadruped bird dog

Figure 15-43
Single-leg Romanian deadlift

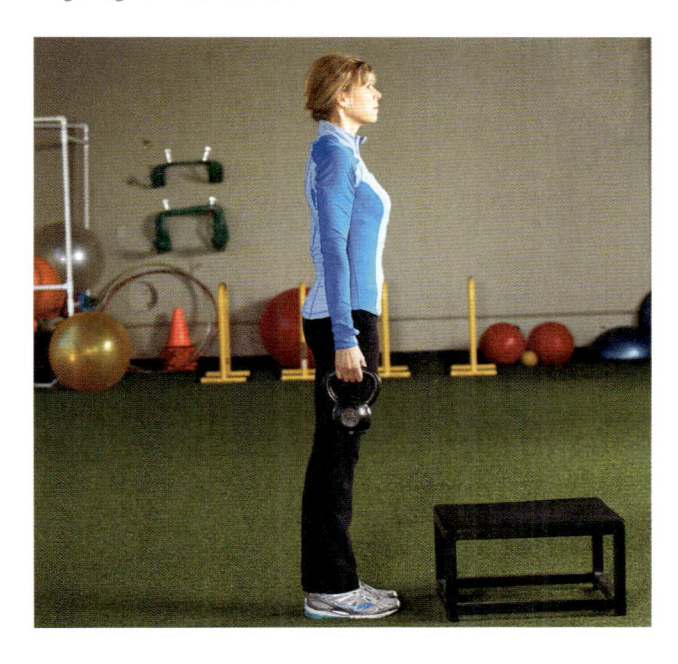

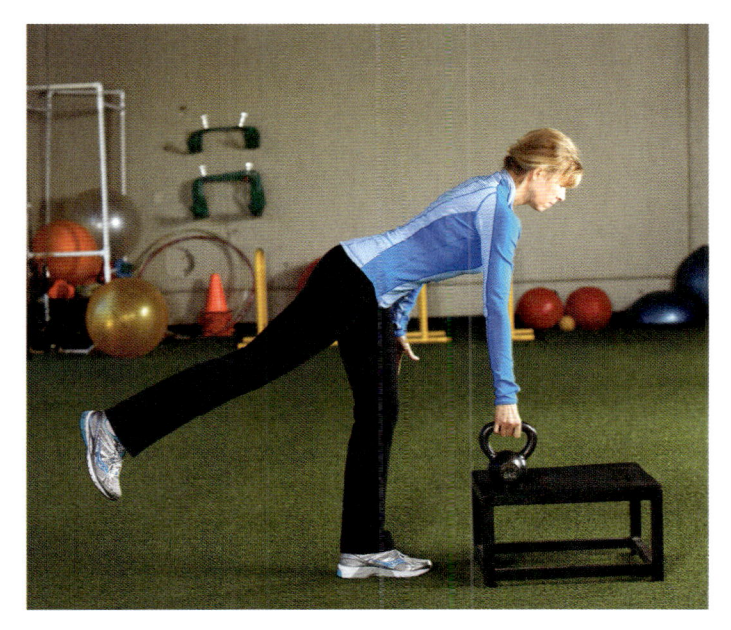

ACE MEDICAL EXERCISE SPECIALIST MANUAL   AMERICAN COUNCIL ON EXERCISE

CHAPTER 15 Balance and Gait

Figure 15-44
Lunge to single-arm cable pull

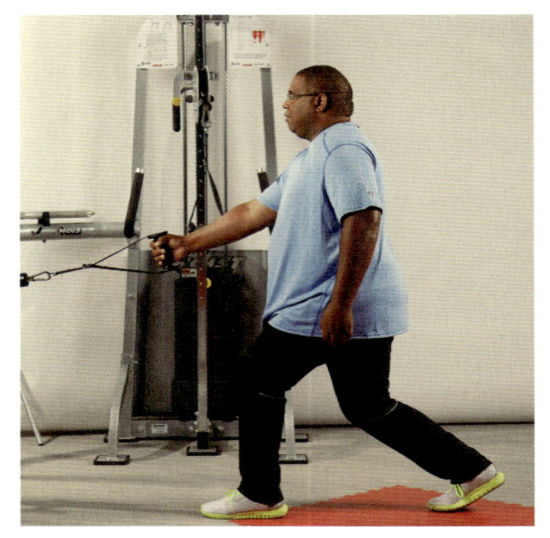

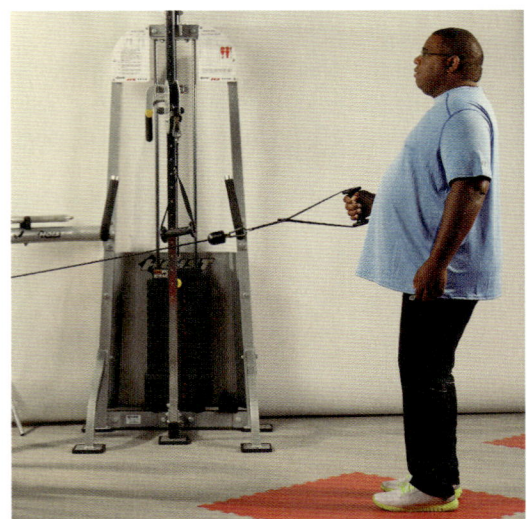

Figure 15-45
Anterior lunge with medicine ball lift

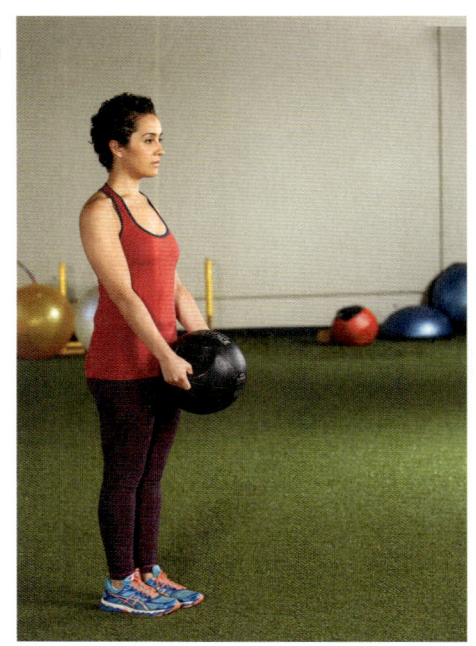

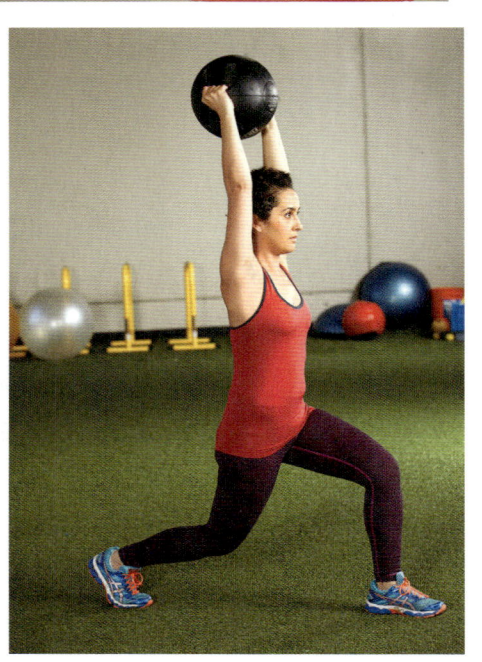

Figure 15-46
Bent-over barbell row

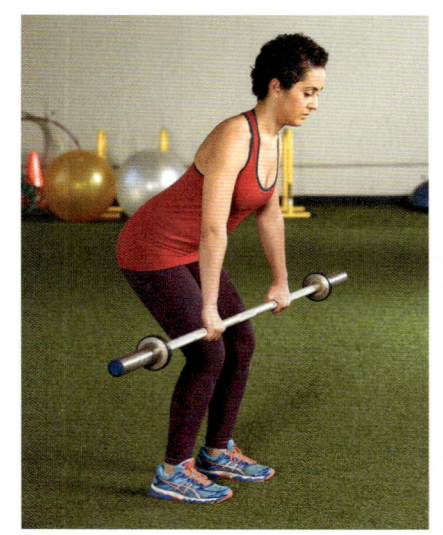

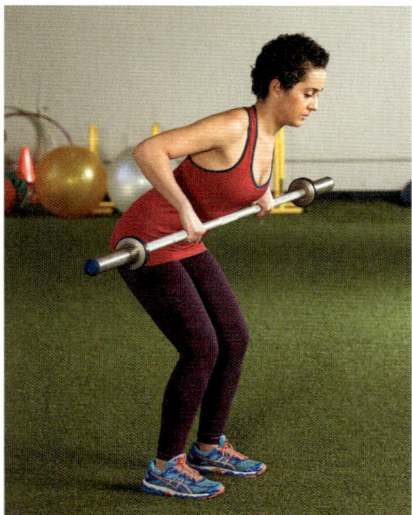

Balance and Gait   CHAPTER 15

Lateral Sling

The role of the lateral myofascial sling is to stabilize the frontal plane mechanics of pelvis-on-femur movement during the gait cycle. This sling can be strengthened with movements that emphasize single-leg balance or moving laterally in the frontal plane. Figures 15-47 through 15-50 present exercises for the lateral sling.

Figure 15-47
Lateral plank

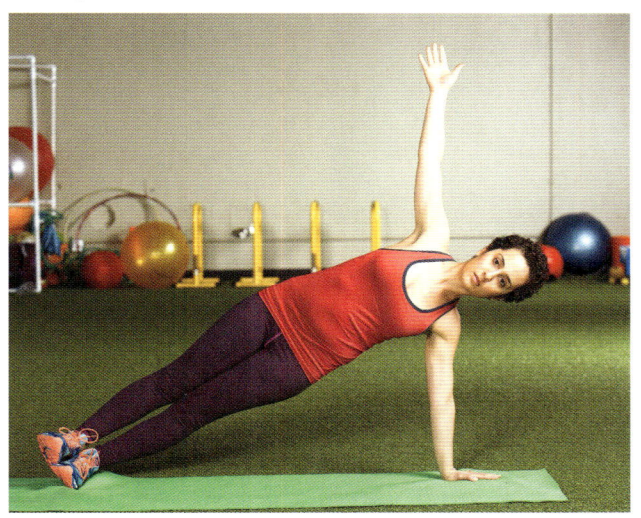

Figure 15-48
Lateral step-up

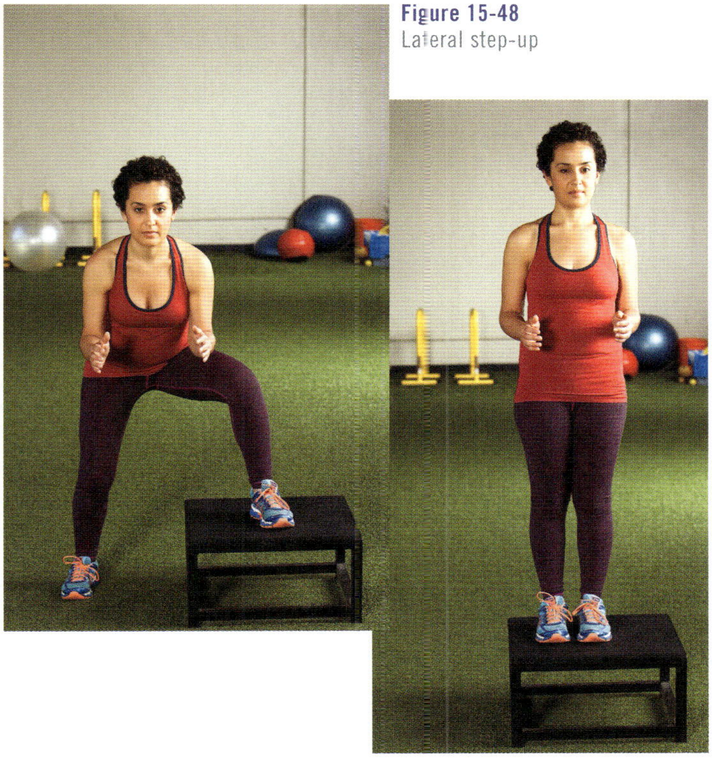

Figure 15-49
Single-leg balance with contralateral shoulder press

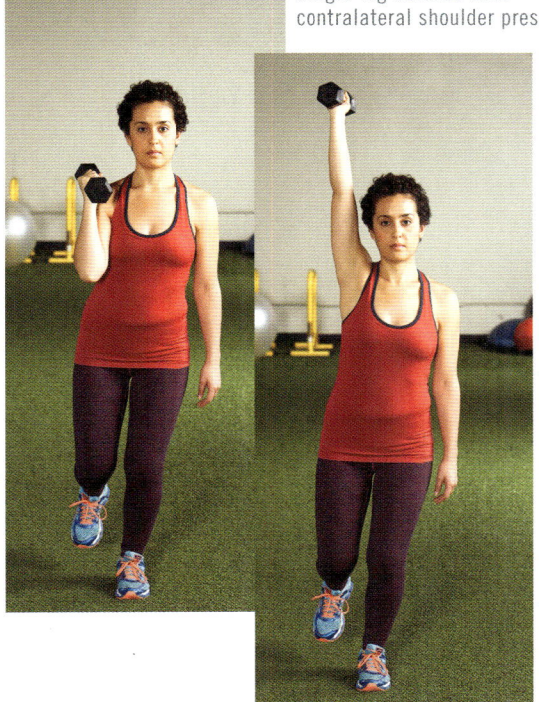

Figure 15-50
Lateral lunge
To advance the progression, reach both hands forward (anterior).

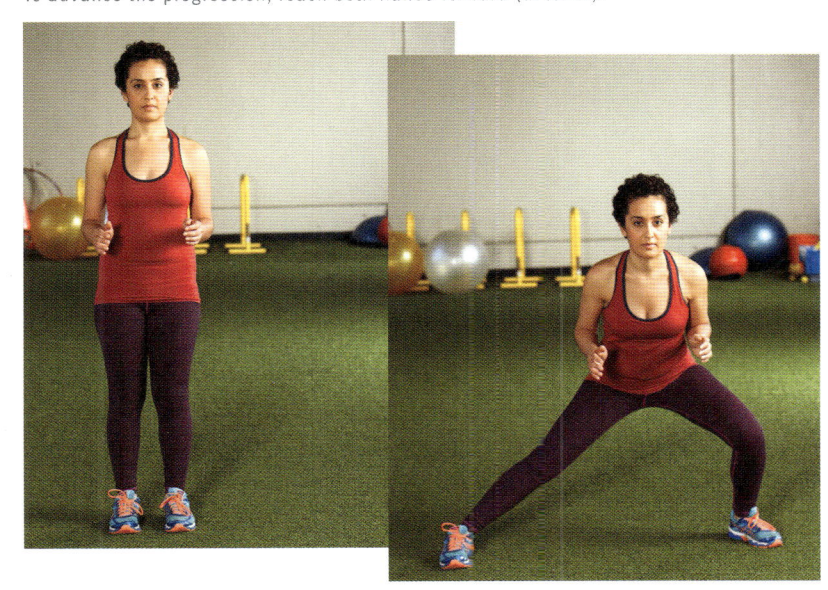

Deep Longitudinal Sling

The role of the deep longitudinal myofascial sling is to decelerate forward flexion of the trunk created by gravity while creating stability along the spinal column, extending the femur and creating stability in the mid-foot during the gait cycle. This sling can be trained with movements (isolated or integrated) that promote spinal stability and extension through the posterior chain. Figures 15-51 through 15-57 present exercises for the deep longitudinal sling.

Figure 15-51
Glute bridge

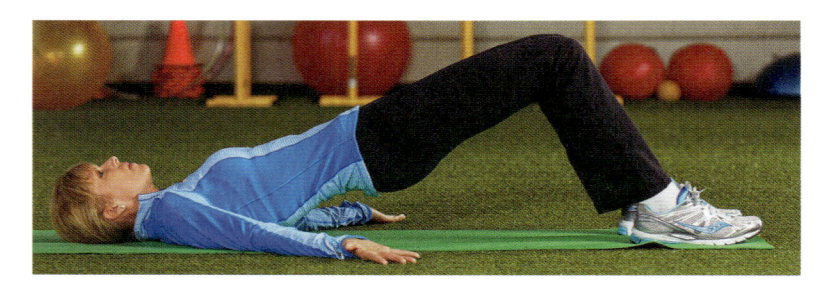

Figure 15-52
Single-leg supine glute bridge

Figure 15-53
Step-up

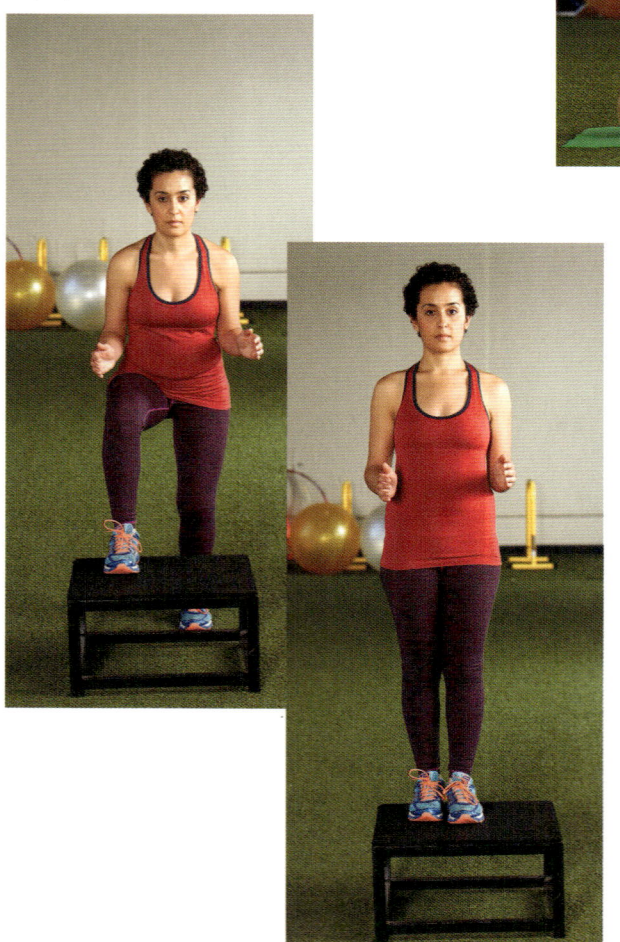

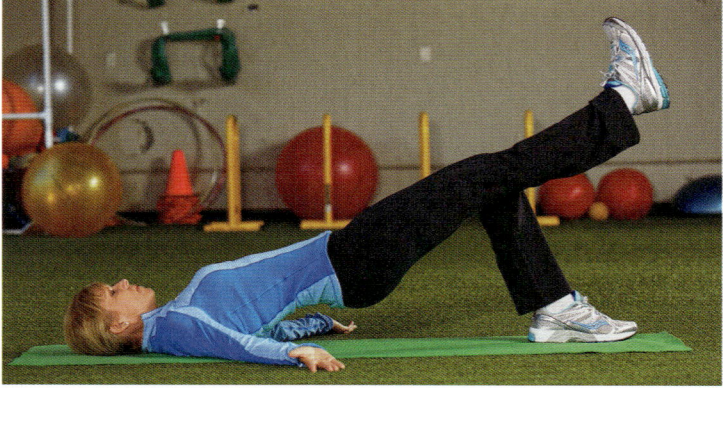

Figure 15-54
Romanian deadlift

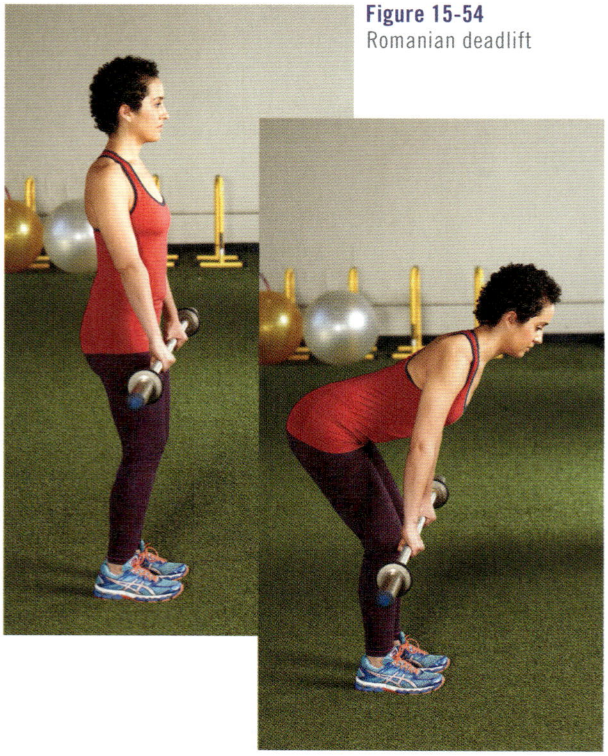

Balance and Gait

CHAPTER 15

Although incorporating kettlebell exercises into a client's functional-training program is an effective approach to enhancing gait, the CMES should complete additional continuing education on the proper instruction and implementation of kettlebell training before teaching these movements to their clients.

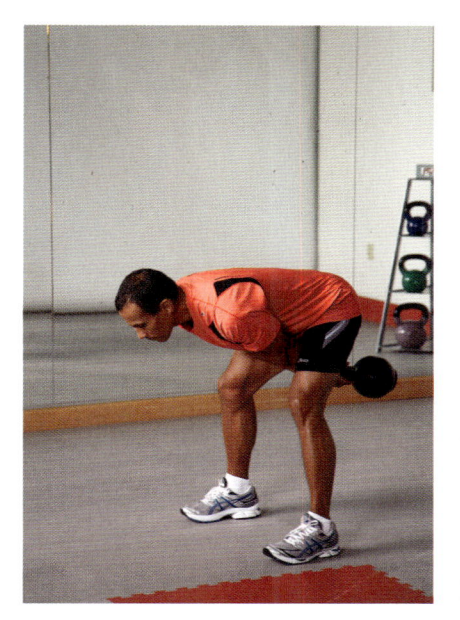

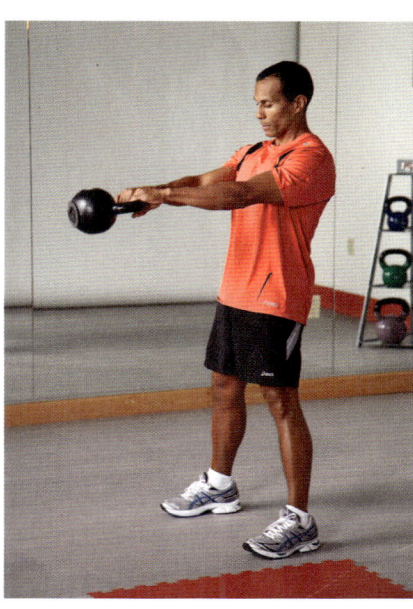

Figure 15-55
Kettlebell swing

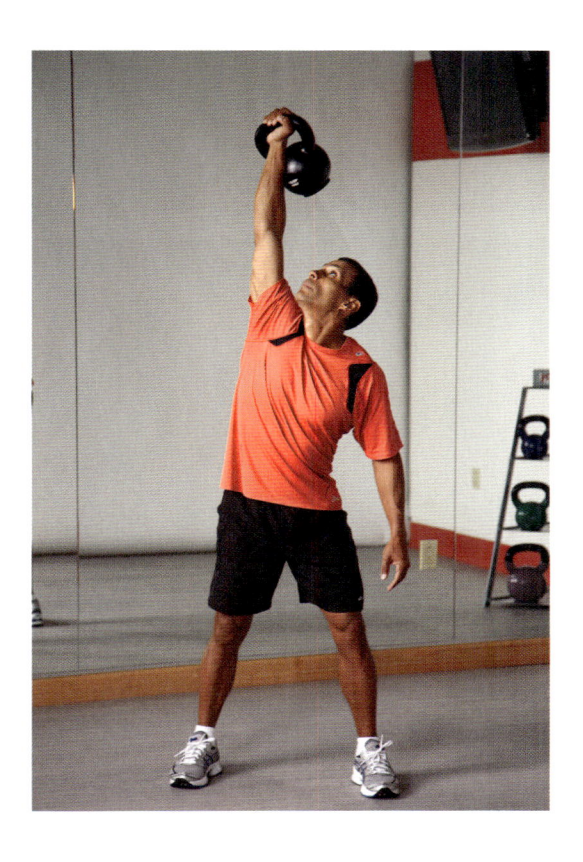

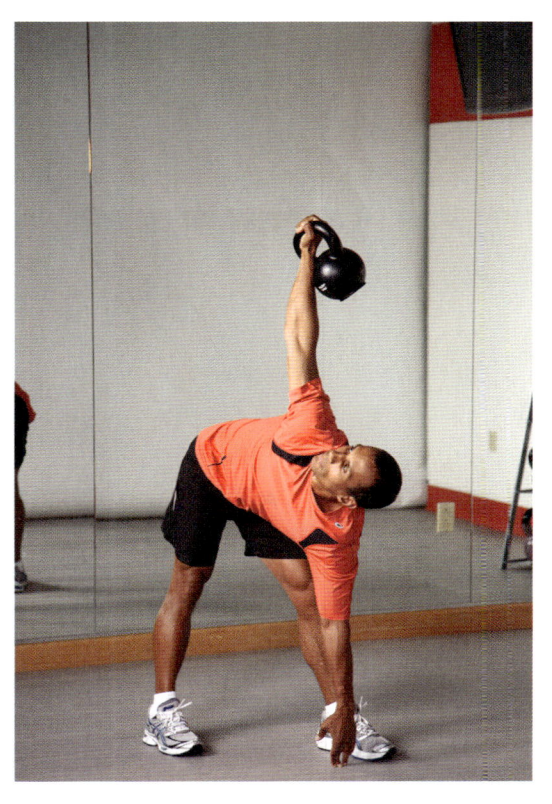

Figure 15-56
Kettlebell windmill

Figure 15-57
Kettlebell Turkish get-up

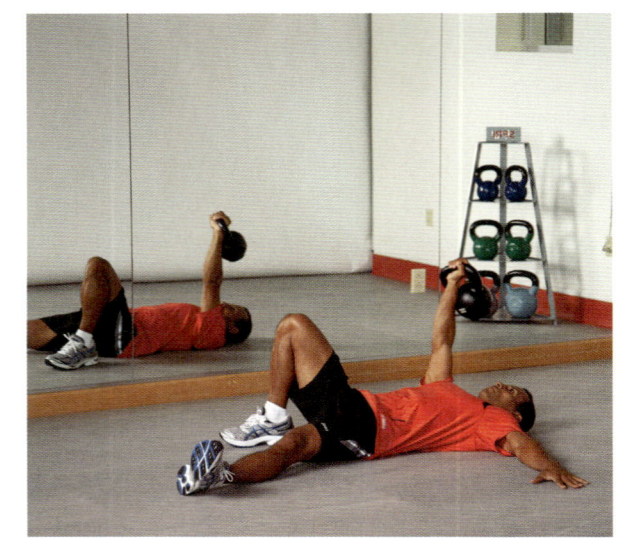

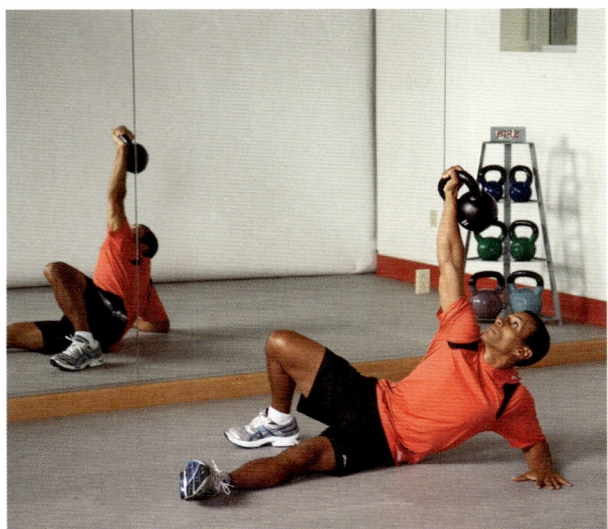

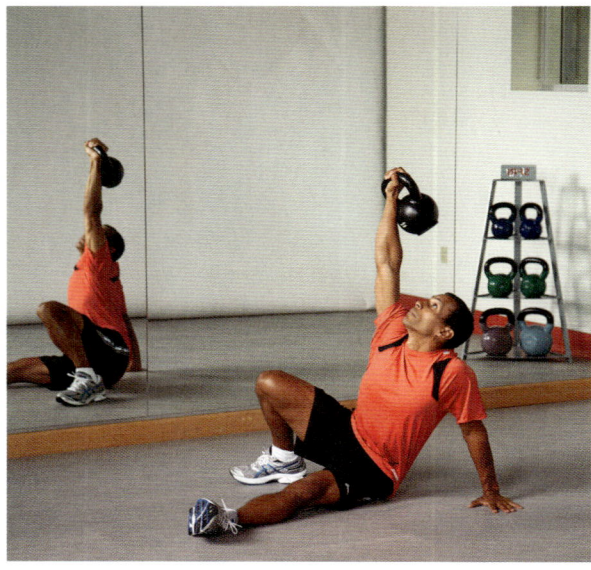

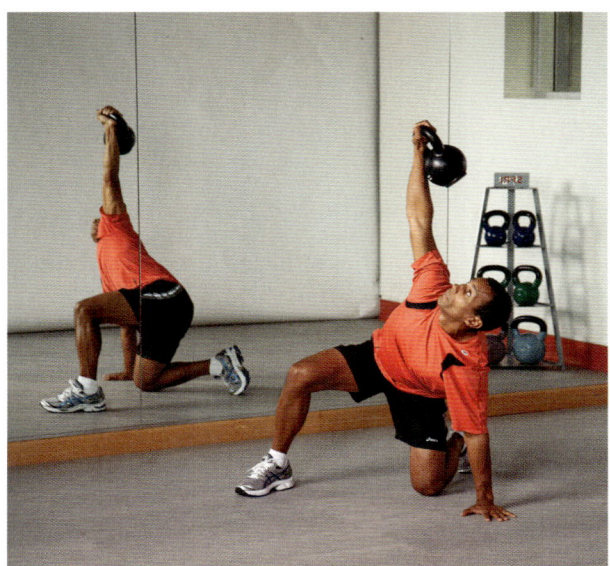

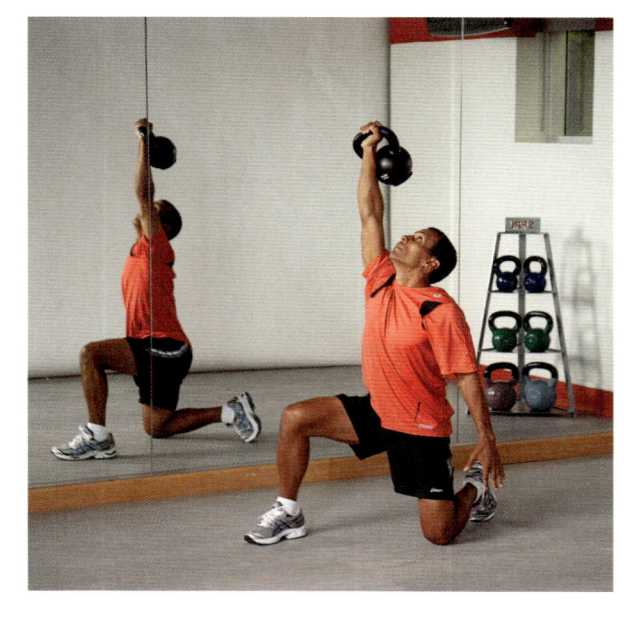

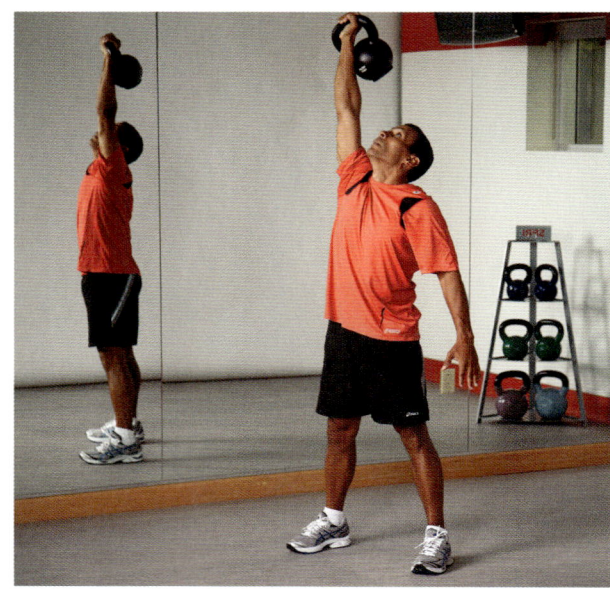

CASE STUDY

Client Information

Joe is a 42-year-old business executive who hires a CMES after he decides that he would like to start participating in a recreational basketball league with some of his coworkers. He was physically active throughout college and has maintained sporadic bouts of activity since he turned 35. He appears to be about 20 pounds (9 kg) overweight. His current activity involves infrequent walks with his wife and golfing two or three times a month with clients. His health history reveals no significant risk factors and he has obtained clearance from his physician to exercise. His current complaints include some mild low-back discomfort, a general lack of conditioning, and a lack of power with his golf drives, which he would like to improve. The CMES completes the initial assessments (static postural assessment, movement screens, core activation, body composition, and balance) that reveal a need to improve Joe's core conditioning, balance, and posture as foundational components. After the CMES briefs Joe on these findings and shares recommendations, Joe agrees to focus on these parameters as his initial goal. He makes a commitment to train with the CMES two times per week in addition to following the programming recommendations when at home and while traveling. The following outlines the core-conditioning portion of Joe's overall program.

CMES Approach

Based on the information gathered during the assessment process, the CMES determines his low-back discomfort could be related to a loss of mobility in the hips and thoracic spine. The CMES designs a total-body exercise program to improve Joe's core strength, dynamic balance, and mobility of his hips and thoracic spine to address the items found during his assessments. In addition, improving thoracic spine and hip mobility can help Joe add power to his golf swing and help him prepare for playing basketball. The program will first use stabilization exercises to improve strength of the deep core muscles and then progress to dynamic movement exercises that can help promote hip and thoracic mobility.

- *Frequency:* During the initial phase of Joe's exercise program, the CMES will meet with him two times a week for 30 minutes at a time.
- *Duration:* The CMES will work with Joe for an initial period of six weeks. During this time, the CMES will encourage Joe to do the exercises on his own at least one other time a week and try to make time for two 30-minute moderate-intensity walks with his wife (**rating of perceived exertion** of 3 to 4 on the 0 to 10 scale).

Joe meets with the CMES consistently two times a week for six weeks. Joe twice skips doing his own workout and notices the difference in the way his back feels and begins to understand the effect the exercise program is having on improving his mobility and movement skill. Because he is feeling better, Joe adds a third walk with his wife each week. At the end of the initial six week program, the CMES performs a few of the movement screens and core activation assessments to show Joe the progress he has achieved. Based on his progress, Joe's program is progressed as follows:

- *Frequency:* Joe continues to work with the CMES and begins to meet him for two one-hour sessions a week. The CMES uses the initial stabilization program for one set of each as a

ACE IFT® MODEL AT A GLANCE

Cardiorespiratory Training

Joe's training program includes 30-minute moderate-intensity walks with his wife, performed two, and then three days per week. These initial sessions meet the criteria for transitioning from Base Training to Fitness Training. His progressions to more frequent and longer-duration exercise sessions, and the addition of recreational basketball to his weekly physical activity, advance his cardiorespiratory training program. He is also ready for the introduction of higher-intensity intervals to improve fitness and health.

Muscular Training

This case study describes a very common scenario. With increased desk work and decreased physical activity, Joe has lost mobility in his hips and thoracic spine, placing additional stress on his low back, which is designed to be more stable. By starting with a Functional Training program, the CMES is able to help Joe improve posture, mobility, core function, and balance. Progressing to Movement Training, the CMES helps Joe to further improve his postural stability and kinetic-chain mobility, which enhances his golf swing and helps him get back into recreational basketball. The end result is decreased low-back discomfort and improved movement, fitness, activities of daily living, and self-efficacy for additional physical activity.

dynamic warm-up before progressing to a more challenging mobility-based workout program. The CMES encourages Joe to do the stabilization program on his own two days a week and increase the distance he walks with his wife.
- *Duration:* The CMES will work with Joe for another six weeks before conducting a re-assessment to determine the amount of improvement during the entire 12-week program.

Over the course of working with the CMES, Joe begins to notice a remarkable difference in his energy levels and a significant reduction in his low-back pain. Because he feels so much better, Joe is able to be more active and enjoys walks with his wife as well as playing basketball with some of his friends and coworkers. Joe becomes more physically active at work and invests in a stand-up desk because he finds that despite the success in his exercise program, sitting too long during a workday may initiate a recurrence of low-back pain.

When Joe first started working with the CMES, he was surprised that they did no resistance-training exercises but is amazed at how much better he feels as a result of his exercise program. By improving core stability and enhancing joint mobility, the CMES was able to help Joe become more physically active, which helped him lose 15 pounds (6.8 kg). In addition, Joe has become a better golfer and begins to prepare for a vacation hiking with his wife in the Grand Canyon. Because the CMES identified a number of issues related to lost joint mobility during the assessment process, Joe was able to follow an exercise program designed to address his specific needs.

SUMMARY

Movement is essential to complete all ADL, and static and dynamic balance are critical to efficient movement. Older adults generally suffer losses to multiple senses that impact balance and, consequently, their movement efficiency. Balance, therefore, is the foundational skill element to all programming, whether functional or sports-related. It enhances physical performance, but also contributes to improving the cognitive and affective (emotional) domains and building self-efficacy and self-confidence. Improvements to balance result from increased postural stability, a key function of the core musculature. Core conditioning is a critical component of balance training and must therefore be considered a prerequisite to effective training. While the science of the core is generally well understood, a sequential approach to programming for the core is not. Balance training improves movement and the most functional of all movement is gait. While gait is briefly reviewed, the myofascial slings involved in gait are discussed to help the CMES understand the involvement of the entire kinetic chain. All movement can essentially be described by the five primary movements, and training programs should aim to initially target these movements prior to mimicking the specific movement patterns.

REFERENCES

Abernathy, B. et al. (2005). *The Biophysical Foundations of Human Movement* (2nd ed.). Champaign, Ill.: Human Kinetics.

Arokoski, J.P. et al. (2001). Back and abdominal muscle function during stabilization exercises. *Archives of Physical Medicine and Rehabilitation,* 82, 1089–1098.

Bergmark, A. (1989) Stability of the lumber spine: A study in mechanical engineering. *Acta Orthopedia Scandinavia*, 230 (Suppl.), 20–24.

Cook, G. (2010). *Movement: Functional Movement Systems.* Santa Cruz, Calif.: On Target Publications.

Cook, G. (2003). *Athletic Body in Balance.* Champaign, Ill.: Human Kinetics.

Cresswell, A.G. & Thorstensson, A. (1994). Changes in intra-abdominal pressure, trunk muscle activation and force during isokinetic lifting and lowering. *European Journal of Applied Physiology,* 68, 315–321.

Enoka, R. (2008). *Neuromechanics of Human Movement* (4th ed.). Champaign, Ill.: Human Kinetics.

Gambetta, V. (2007). *Athletic Development: The Art and Science of Functional Sports Conditioning.* Champaign, Ill.: Human Kinetics.

Gracovetsky, S., Farfan, H.F., & Helleur, C. (1985). The abdominal mechanism. *Spine,* 10, 317–324.

Gracovetsky, S., Farfan, H.F., & Lamy, C. (1992). The mechanisms of the lumbar spine. *Spine,* 6, 1, 249–262.

Hodges, P.W. & Richardson, C.A. (1996). Inefficient muscular stabilization of the lumbar spine associated with LBP: A motor control evaluation of the TVA. *Spine,* 21, 2640–2650.

Hodges, P. et al. (1996). Evaluation of the relationship between laboratory and clinical tests of transversus abdominis function. *Physiotherapy Research International,* 1, 1, 30–40.

Houglum, P.A. (2010) *Therapeutic Exercise for Musculoskeletal Injuries* (3rd ed.). Champaign, Ill.: Human Kinetics.

Kendall, F.P. et al. (2005). *Muscles: Testing and Function with Posture and Pain* (5th ed.). Baltimore, Md.: Lippincott Williams & Wilkins.

Levin, S.M. (1997). A different approach to the mechanics of the human pelvis: Tensegrity. In: Vleeming, A. et al. (Eds.) *Movement, Stability and Low Back Pain.* London, Churchill Livingston.

McGill, S.M. (2016). *Low Back Disorders: Evidence-Based Prevention and Rehabilitation* (3rd ed.). Champaign, Ill.: Human Kinetics.

McGill, S.M. (2001). Low back stability: From formal description to issues for performance and rehabilitation. *Exercise and Sports Science Review,* 29, 1, 26–31.

McGill, S.M. et al. (2003). Coordination of muscle activity to assure stability of the lumbar spine. *Journal or Electromyography and Kinesiology,* 13, 353–359.

Myers, T. (2014). *Anatomy Trains: Myofascial Meridians for Manual and Movement Therapists* (3rd ed.). London: Elsevier.

Nagi, S.S. (1991). Disability concepts revisited: Implication for prevention. In: Pope, A.M. & Tarlov, A.R. (Eds.) *Disability in America: Toward a National Agenda for Prevention.* Washington, D.C.: National Academy Press.

Neumann, D. (2010). *Kinesiology of the Musculoskeletal System: Foundations for Rehabilitation* (2nd ed.). St. Louis, Mo.: Elsevier.

Panjabi. M.M. (1992a). The stabilizing system of the spine. Part I. Function, dysfunction, adaptation and enhancement. *Journal of Spinal Disorders,* 5, 380–389.

Panjabi. M.M. (1992b). The stabilizing system of the spine. Part II. Neutral zone and instability hypothesis. *Journal of Spinal Disorders,* 5, 390–397.

Rikli, R.E. & Jones, J.C. (2013). *Senior Fitness Test Manual* (2nd ed.). Champaign, Ill.: Human Kinetics.

Rose, D.J. (2010). *Fall Proof* (2nd ed.) Champaign, Ill.: Human Kinetics.

Sahrmann, S. (2002). *Diagnosis and Treatment of Movement Impairment Syndromes.* St. Louis, Mo.: Mosby.

Schleip, R. et al. (2012) *Fascia: The Tensional Network of the Human Body.* London: Churchill Livingstone.

Schultz, L. & Feitis, R. (1996). *The Endless Web.* Berkeley, Calif.: North Atlantic Books.

Shumway-Cook, A. & Woollacott, M.H. (2012). *Motor Control: Translating Research into Clinical Practice* (4th ed.). Philadelphia: Wolters Kluwer/Lippincott Williams & Wilkins.

Siff, M. & Verkhoshansky, Y. (2009). *Supertraining* (6th ed.). Denver: Supertraining Institute.

Vleeming, A. et al. (2007). *Movement, Stability & Lumbopelvic Pain: Integration of Research and Therapy* (2nd ed.). London: Churchill Livingstone.

Vleeming A. et al. (1990a). Relation between form and function in the sacroiliac joint. Part 1: Clinical anatomical concepts. *Spine,* 15, 2, 130–132.

Vleeming A. et al. (1990b). Relation between form and function in the sacroiliac joint. Part 2: Biomechanical concepts. *Spine,* 15, 2, 133–136.

Wang, X.Q. et al. (2012). A meta-analysis of core stability exercise versus general exercise for chronic low back pain. *PLoS One,* 7, 12, e52082. DOI: 10.1371/journal.pone.0052082

Whiting W.C. & Rugg, S. (2006). *Dynatomy: Dynamic Human Anatomy.* Champaign, Ill.: Human Kinetics.

Willardson, J.M. (2007). Core stability training: Applications to sports conditioning programs. *Journal of Strength and Conditioning Research,* 21, 3, 979–985.

SUGGESTED READING

McGill, S.M. (2016). *Low Back Disorders: Evidence-Based Prevention and Rehabilitation* (3rd ed.). Champaign, Ill.: Human Kinetics.

Rikli, R.E. & Jones, J.C. (2013). *Senior Fitness Test Manual* (2nd ed.). Champaign, Ill.: Human Kinetics.

Rose, D.J. (2010). *Fall Proof* (2nd ed.). Champaign, Ill.: Human Kinetics.

Schleip, R. et al. (2012) *Fascia: The Tensional Network of the Human Body.* London: Churchill Livingstone.

Wang, X.Q. et al. (2012). A meta-analysis of core stability exercise versus general exercise for chronic low back pain. *PLoS One,* 7, 12, e52082. DOI: 10.1371/journal.pone.0052082

Whittle, M.W. (2007). *Gait Analysis: An Introduction* (4th ed.). Edinburgh, Scotland: Butterworth Heinemann Elsevier.

16 ARTHRITIS

IN THIS CHAPTER

EPIDEMIOLOGY
OSTEOARTHRITIS
RHEUMATOID ARTHRITIS
JUVENILE ARTHRITIS

OVERVIEW
OSTEOARTHRITIS
RHEUMATOID ARTHRITIS
JUVENILE ARTHRITIS

DIAGNOSTIC CRITERIA
OSTEOARTHRITIS
RHEUMATOID ARTHRITIS
JUVENILE ARTHRITIS

TREATMENT OPTIONS
NON-PHARMACOLOGICAL TREATMENT
PHARMACOLOGICAL TREATMENT
SURGICAL TREATMENT
EXERCISE TREATMENT

NUTRITIONAL CONSIDERATIONS
A KEY ROLE FOR FATTY ACIDS
THE HEALTHY MEDITERRANEAN-STYLE DIETARY PATTERN AS DISEASE MODIFIER
NUTRIENTS IN QUESTION
SUPPLEMENTS UNDER INVESTIGATION
ELIMINATION DIETS: HELP OR HYPE?

EXERCISE RECOMMENDATIONS
CONTRAINDICATIONS AND PRECAUTIONS
CARDIORESPIRATORY ENDURANCE EXERCISE
RESISTANCE EXERCISE
FLEXIBILITY EXERCISE

SAMPLE EXERCISES

EXERCISE GUIDELINES SUMMARY FOR CLIENTS WITH ARTHRITIS

CASE STUDY

SUMMARY

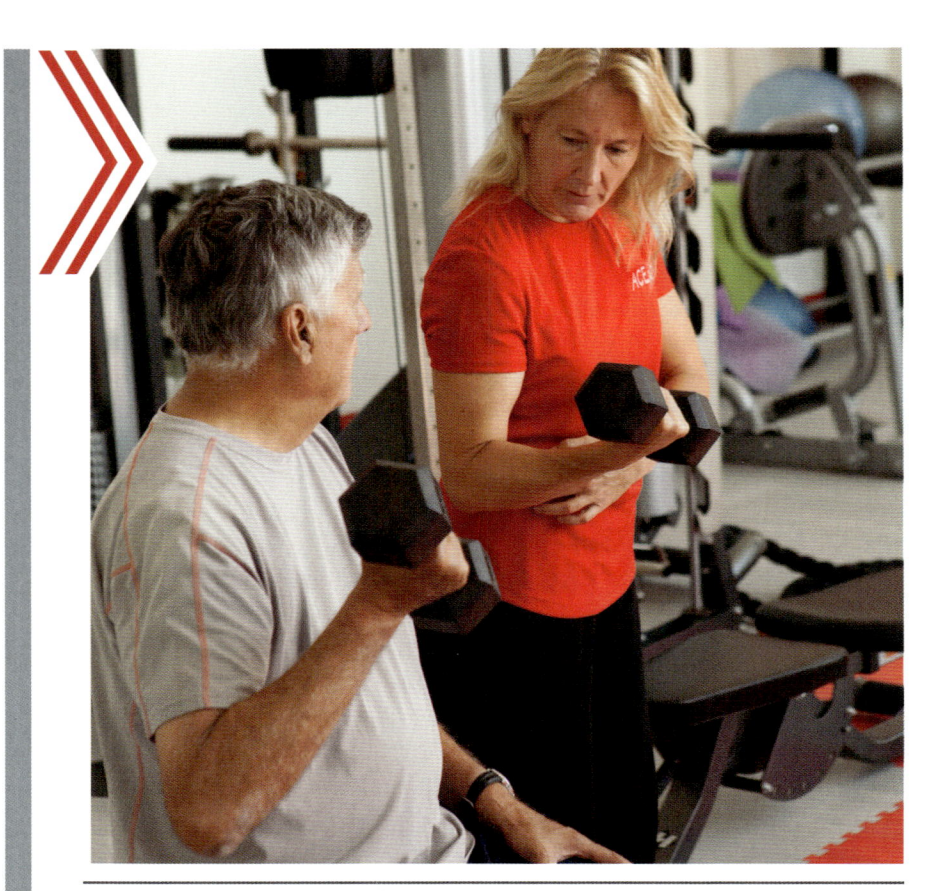

ABOUT THE AUTHORS

The late John G. Aronen, M.D., FACSM, was an orthopedic sports medicine specialist. After retiring from the Navy in 1996, Dr. Aronen was a consultant for the Center for Sports Medicine, Saint Francis Memorial Hospital in San Francisco. Dr. Aronen was a selected member of the American Orthopedic Society for Sports Medicine and the American Medical Society for Sports Medicine, and a fellow of the American College of Sports Medicine. Following two years of specialty training in sports medicine, Dr. Aronen founded and served as the head of the Sports Medicine Division of the Department of Orthopedic Surgery at the United States Naval Academy and head team physician from 1979 to 1987. Dr. Aronen then founded and directed a four-week CME/GME course for primary care providers and second-year physician assistant students in the "Evaluation and Management of Musculoskeletal Injuries Commonly Seen in Military Personnel."

Kent A. Lorenz, Ph.D., CSCS, NSCA-CPT, is an instructor in the Exercise Science and Health Promotion program in the College of Health Solutions at Arizona State University, specializing in physical activity promotion and strength and conditioning. Dr. Lorenz teaches courses in strength and conditioning, health and physical activity promotion, and physical education. His research emphasis is currently centered on creating school environments that are favorable for promoting physical activity and other healthy behaviors for students and staff.

By John G. Aronen and Kent A. Lorenz

THE TERM "ARTHRITIS" LITERALLY REFERS to joint inflammation. However, as a disease, arthritis is actually a complex family of musculoskeletal disorders consisting of more than 100 different diseases or conditions that can affect people of all ages, races, and genders. Three common forms are **osteoarthritis (OA), rheumatoid arthritis (RA),** and **juvenile arthritis (JA)**. While it might be common to associate arthritis with old age, two-thirds of people with the disease are under the age of 65, including 300,000 children (Arthritis Foundation, 2019).

OA results from a degeneration of **synovial fluid** and generally progresses into a loss of **articular cartilage**, which typically presents itself as localized joint pain and a reduction of **range of motion (ROM)**. RA is a systemic autoimmune disease characterized by the inflammation of the membranes lining the joint, which causes pain, stiffness, warmth, swelling, and potential severe joint damage. JA is an umbrella term used to describe the many autoimmune and inflammatory conditions that can develop in children ages 16 and younger (Arthritis Foundation, 2019).

As with all chronic conditions, the ACE® Certified Medical Exercise Specialist (CMES) should communicate with their clients to discuss what types of activities they are able to do—and how much. If a client presents with some of the signs and symptoms of OA, RA, or JA, and has not sought medical advice, the CMES should refer the individual to a medical professional before the exercise program begins. In more severe cases, where the majority of weight-bearing activity is painful or limited, the CMES may want to refer to a physical therapist or occupational therapist.

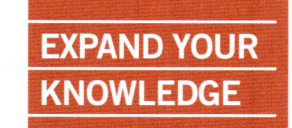

LEARNING OBJECTIVES:

» Describe the differences among the three main types of arthritis: osteoarthritis, rheumatoid arthritis, and juvenile arthritis.

» Explain the basic diagnostic criteria and treatment options associated with the main types of arthritis.

» Briefly explain the different stages of arthritis progression as they relate to joint structure and function.

» Design and implement safe and effective exercise programs for clients in the various stages associated with the main forms of arthritis.

» Explain to clients the latest evidence on nutrition and supplements related to managing arthritis symptoms.

EXPAND YOUR KNOWLEDGE

ETIOLOGY OF JOINT PATHOLOGY

Medical conditions (e.g., illnesses and injuries) are typically placed into one of two categories based on their suspected cause, or **etiology**—primary or secondary. The determination of a condition's category is based on whether the underlying cause for the problem can be identified. If the underlying cause for a problem cannot be identified, the problem falls into the primary category (i.e., the individual has the problem, but physicians cannot determine why or what is causing or contributing to the problem). For primary problems, treatment and management must be directed at the symptoms associated with the condition. Unfortunately, while this approach may provide resolution of the symptoms, the underlying cause will continue to contribute to the natural progression of the problem.

If the underlying cause that contributed to the onset of the condition and/or continues to contribute to the condition can be identified, the condition is categorized as secondary. With a problem that is secondary, the emphasis of the treatment and management program must be directed at eliminating or minimizing the underlying cause. Failure to recognize that proper management of a secondary condition includes management of both the symptoms and, more importantly, the underlying cause(s) of the symptoms, will result in only short-term relief from the presenting symptoms, as the underlying cause is allowed to continue to contribute to the natural progression of the problem.

Injuries to a joint occur either acutely or insidiously (i.e., over a prolonged period of time). Any injury to a joint that causes detrimental changes to its structural integrity becomes the starting point for the onset and progression of osteoarthritic changes. For example, because there are typically detrimental changes to the structural integrity of the knee with an **acute** injury, such as a sprain of the anterior cruciate ligament (ACL), a tear of a meniscus, or patellar dislocation, the starting point for the onset of osteoarthritic changes is the time of the injury. In many acute injuries, due to the severity of the initial changes to the structural integrity of the joint, the starting point for osteoarthritic changes is also the starting point for discomfort and/or swelling, constant reminders to the individual that they no longer have an entirely healthy or normal joint. For others, the initial changes to the structural integrity of the joint are not severe enough to result in the onset of discomfort and/or swelling from the time of the injury. The starting point for changes to the structural integrity with an injury of insidious onset, as may be seen in the knees and hips with a steady regimen of distance running, is ill defined, as it does not come on acutely, but rather over time. Unfortunately, with the normal progression of degenerative changes that occurs in osteoarthritic joints, discomfort and/or swelling will become evident eventually.

Structural integrity of a joint refers primarily to the following:
- Articular cartilage, which consists of hyaline cartilage, is free of pain receptors and covers the portions of bone that articulate with each other within a joint. Articular cartilage is also referred to as chondral cartilage.
- Subchondral bone, which underlies the articular cartilage, must be healthy to provide appropriate structural support to the articular cartilage overlying it.
- Discomfort and/or swelling are the earliest symptoms or physical findings that indicate that changes have occurred to the structural integrity and that the joint is no longer an entirely healthy or normal joint. Typically, the amount of discomfort and/or swelling is an indicator of the severity of changes to the structural integrity of the joint.

EPIDEMIOLOGY

According to a report from the Centers for Disease Control and Prevention (CDC), 54.4 million U.S. adults had arthritis in 2013–2015, an increase from 2007–2009 (50 million) (CDC, 2018). This estimate matches future projected prevalence estimates of 78.4 million by the year 2040. Further, the data revealed that 23.7 million individuals (43.5% of adults with arthritis) have activity limitations because of their arthritis (CDC, 2019a). Arthritis-attributable activity limitations (AAAL) are more common in adults who have arthritis as well as one of three coexisting chronic health conditions—**diabetes,** heart disease, or **obesity.** Accordingly, people with these conditions also have higher than average rates of arthritis, approximately 1.7, 1.9, and 1.5 times more likely, respectively. The data showed that approximately 47% of adults with diabetes, 49% with heart disease, and 31% with obesity also have arthritis, and that more than 49 to 54% of those adults with any of those conditions and arthritis reported AAAL [54.5% (heart disease), 54% (diabetes), and 49% (obesity)] (Barbour et al., 2017).

Osteoarthritis

About 33 million people in the U.S. have OA (CDC, 2020), and OA is the most common cause of disability in adults in the United States (Arthritis Foundation, 2019). It affects millions of individuals aged 55 years and older, often leading to physical disability and reduced quality of life. Symptomatic knee OA occurs in 5.9 to 13.5% of men and 7.2 to 18.7% of women aged 45 years or older (Arthritis Foundation, 2019). These percentages are likely to increase due to the aging of the population and the obesity epidemic. Old age, female gender, **overweight** and obesity, knee injury, repetitive use of joints, bone density, muscle weakness, and joint laxity all contribute to the development of joint OA, particularly in the weight-bearing joints (i.e., the knee, followed by the hip). With the exception of age and gender, modifying these factors may reduce the risk of OA and prevent subsequent pain and disability.

EXPAND YOUR KNOWLEDGE

A BRIEF HISTORY OF OSTEOARTHRITIS

Prior to the 1980s, OA, often referred to as **degenerative joint disease,** was believed to occur only in men who suffered an injury to a joint, most commonly the knee, while involved in a contact sport. Because the onset of OA was thought to be caused by the initial injury to the knee, the OA that occurred following a documented knee injury was classified as a secondary problem. Additionally, little concern was given to the initial treatment and long-term management of the etiology, which would have slowed down the progression of the undesirable changes to the structural integrity. Typically, the athlete would remain active in sports, only expediting the "unavoidable" progression of the acute changes, resulting in a chronically painful and functionally deficient knee. Unfortunately, due to an avid desire to return an athlete to all activities rather than be realistic and make modifications in lifestyle that may prolong the life of the injured joint, too little progress has been made in the appropriate initial treatment and long-term management.

Two other factors came into play regarding OA in the late 1970s and early 1980s, the first being the sudden surge of adolescent and teenage girls into injury-producing sports. As the number of participants in sports dramatically increased, the number of significant acute injuries, not only to the knee but to other joints as well, resulted in a large increase of symptoms and findings compatible with OA in younger and middle-aged athletes. Additionally, it was noted that not only could the onset of OA [through findings noted on **arthroscopy, magnetic resonance imaging (MRI),** or symptoms compatible with OA] occur following an acute injury to a joint, but it could also occur following persistent microtrauma to the structural integrity of a joint, as seen in distance runners. In the early 2000s (approximately 20 to 25 years following the surge in female participation in sports), a dramatic increase in individuals with physical and radiographic findings compatible with significant osteoarthritic changes in the knees and hips began to appear. The following characteristics were common in this group:

- A female participating in sports that were only sparsely available to the female community prior to 1980, but sprang into popularity in the 1980s (e.g., basketball, volleyball, softball, soccer, and distance running)
- An individual incurring a knee/hip injury or simply having a history of following a compulsive daily running regimen
- An individual treated with one of the increasing number of surgical procedures designed to address these injuries, followed by aggressive rehabilitation programs

With emphasis placed on early surgical intervention and aggressive rehabilitation, the high rate of attrition from sports entirely due to injuries at an early age suddenly came more into focus. Experts had assumed that injured joints would naturally degenerate with time and that lifestyle modifications of young athletes would have little or no effect on the outcome of the process of degeneration.

It is slowly becoming understood that the progression of the initial changes to the structural integrity of a joint can be "slowed down" through alterations in the individual's daily lifestyle and through rehabilitation programs designed to regain and maintain normal strength and flexibility of the muscles surrounding the joint. These programs are designed to slow the progression of the degenerative changes already existing in the joint. Each exercise incorporated into a rehabilitation program for an individual with OA must be evaluated for the amount of force it places on the vulnerable joint, because, although the individual may be able to perform the exercise without any pain, this is no guarantee that the exercise is not doing more harm than good over an extended period of time.

Another factor in the increase in prevalence of OA was the changing of dietary and exercise habits. It soon became apparent that people were living longer and presenting with significant arthritic changes in the hips and/or knees, although they had never experienced acute trauma. This suggests that people are living longer with chronic conditions such as heart disease, diabetes, and obesity, allowing more time for non-traumatic osteoarthritis to develop. Although from this group it appeared that a primary form of OA was associated with normal aging, 52% of patients who required total knee **arthroplasty** and 36% of those who required total hip arthroplasty had overweight or obesity (Namba et al., 2005).

Although there are some individuals who will develop OA with no identifiable underlying causes, the vast majority of OA is secondary in nature—secondary to trauma and/or obesity. Therefore, exercise programs for individuals with OA must keep forces on the osteoarthritic joint to a minimum, as clients strive to retain the strength and flexibility necessary for a joint to function normally.

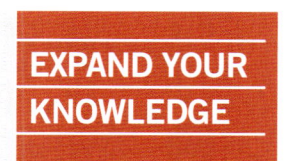

Rheumatoid Arthritis

About 1.5 million people (approximately 1% of the general population) in the U.S. have RA. It affects women two to three times as often as men, and mortality hazards are 60 to 70% higher for those with RA compared to the general population (Arthritis Foundation, 2019). Risk factors for RA include genetic susceptibly and being female. Lifestyle factors have also been associated with the development of RA. Smoking contributes up to 25% of the population burden of RA. Other less-definitive associations have also been found—prospective studies suggest that dietary **antioxidants** and breastfeeding may be protective and that high coffee consumption may increase RA risk. In addition, an increased risk with alcohol intake (especially in smokers), lower education/social class, and obesity has been noted (Lahiri et al., 2012).

EXPAND YOUR KNOWLEDGE

STAGES OF RHEUMATOID ARTHRITIS

RA is a chronic autoimmune disease that results in inflammation of the **synovium,** leading to long-term joint damage, chronic pain, and loss of function or disability (Arthritis Foundation, 2019). RA progresses in three stages, with the first being a swelling of the synovial lining, resulting in pain, warmth, stiffness, redness, and swelling of the joint. The second phase is a rapid division and growth of cells, which causes the synovium to thicken. In the third and final stage, the inflamed cells release **enzymes** that break down bone and cartilage, causing the affected joint to lose structure and alignment, leading to more pain and a further decrease in function. RA is a chronic disease that typically worsens with time, resulting in further physical limitations of the involved joints. In comparison to OA, RA—being an autoimmune disease and having a more systemic effect—may manifest itself in the development of heart and lung disease and diabetes. As with OA, the quality of life for individuals with RA can be improved with exercises that are designed to maintain muscle strength, joint ROM, and cardiovascular function. Certain modifications, such as the use of wrist straps or ankle or wrist weights and the performance of low-intensity and low-impact activities, may be needed to accommodate certain clients.

Juvenile Arthritis

JA is an umbrella term used to describe the many autoimmune and inflammatory conditions that can develop in youth. While arthritis typically affects joints, JA can involve the eyes, skin, and gastrointestinal tract as well (Arthritis Foundation, 2019). As prevalence rises, researchers are working to develop a more sophisticated understanding of the differences among the different forms. The most frequently diagnosed type of JA is juvenile idiopathic arthritis (JIA), which has an etiology of unknown origin with other known conditions excluded. To receive a diagnosis, a child must be younger than 16 and have initial swelling in one or more joints for at least six weeks. JIA is one of the more common chronic childhood diseases, with a prevalence of approximately one per 1,000. JIA often persists into adulthood and can result in significant long-term **morbidity,** including physical disability (Beukelman et al., 2011).

OVERVIEW

Arthritis is the leading cause of disability in the U.S., with more than 23 million people (i.e., approximately 44% of adults with arthritis) experiencing AAAL (CDC, 2019b). Accordingly, the economic, social, and psychological costs of arthritis-related conditions are significant.

Osteoarthritis

To understand the symptoms experienced with OA, the CMES must have knowledge of the anatomical structures of a joint. Furthermore, the CMES must understand the role each structure plays in normal joint functioning and the contributions each makes to the physical symptoms experienced and the physical findings noted on examination.

The role of a joint, or **articulation,** is to allow motion between bones at a specific site. Because of its high frequency of injury and because it is a common site of OA, the knee will be used in this discussion.

A **capsule** fully encloses each joint, so that fluid produced in the joint is retained in the joint. Lining the capsule is a **synovial membrane** that consists of **synovial cells.** There are two types of synovial cells, type A and type B. The lubrication system, which sounds very simplistic, is actually very sophisticated. The type A cells are secretory in that they produce the synovial fluid that acts as a lubricant for the joint. The natural viscosity of the synovial fluid minimizes the degenerative process normally seen between two healthy structures that repetitively articulate with each other. The type B cells are phagocytic, in that they are responsible for the debridement (removal) of the "worn out" synovial fluid and any excess fluid (synovial fluid and/or blood) that may have accumulated in the joint. The articular cartilage of the knee is entirely separate from the two **menisci,** which are made up of fibrocartilage and function to provide shock absorption and stability to the knee.

The articular cartilage is unquestionably a key anatomical structure. OA begins and ends with changes to the structural integrity of the articular cartilage. There are a few properties unique to articular cartilage:
- It has no blood supply and thus cannot heal if injured.
- Because it lacks a blood supply, the role of providing nourishment to the articular cartilage is carried out by the synovial fluid, which is able to enter and exit the articular cartilage at will through microscopic pores in the surface.
- The articular cartilage is void of pain receptors.

The contributions of the articular cartilage to a normal, healthy joint include the following:
- When the surface of the articular cartilage is pristine and covered with synovial fluid, the **coefficient of friction** between the two articulating surfaces is almost zero.
- Because it lacks pain receptors, the articular cartilage prevents the subchondral bone, which has an abundance of pain receptors, from experiencing pain related to the normal transmission of force across joints on a daily basis. Without articular cartilage, the joint would be basically bone on bone—which would be very painful.
- It has been determined clinically that healthy articular cartilage can tolerate approximately seven times the person's body weight before undesirable and often silent detrimental changes begin to compromise the structural integrity of the articular cartilage, which is why it is so important to avoid activities that place unnecessarily high forces on the joints (Repo & Finlay, 1977).

Initial changes to the articular cartilage involve the changing of the once pristine surface into an uneven, incongruous surface. These changes can occur quickly from acute trauma, such as a torn ACL, meniscal tear, or dislocated patella. Each of these injuries produces **shear forces** in the joint that damage the articular cartilage. The rating of the severity of damage is based on the amount of articular cartilage involved and the depth of the disruption, which ranges from grade 1 to grade 4. Grade 1 implies only superficial changes to the articular cartilage, while grade 4 implies damage to the point where subchondral bone is exposed. The loss of the pristine surfaces leads to an increase in the coefficient of friction, which hastens damage due to wear and tear on the remaining articular cartilage.

Along with the loss of the pristine surface, the once microscopic pores that allowed the synovial fluid to flow freely into the articular cartilage become enlarged, allowing the escape of chemicals from inside the articular cartilage into the joint. These chemicals are direct irritants to the synovial cells and cause them to become inflamed (chemical synovitis). Once inflamed, the cells produce soreness throughout the knee as well as an excessive amount of synovial fluid, which is experienced as tightness in the knee. The inflammation from the chemicals, with the resultant discomfort and excessive synovial fluid production, typically takes 10 to 14 hours. Thus, the individual can be physically active on the knee in the evening, but will note the diffuse discomfort and tightness the next day.

With the continuous wear-and-tear changes due to the increased coefficient of friction, the articular cartilage becomes thinner, allowing the subchondral bone to experience more of the forces transmitted across the joint. Forces experienced by the subchondral bone result in pain, the

amount and frequency of which is dependent on many factors:
- The location of the site of exposed subchondral bone (weight-bearing vs. non-weight-bearing areas)
- The amount of force placed on the site with physical activity (e.g., minimal with swimming and highest with weight-bearing activities)
- The weight of the individual, as higher body mass can increase joint **compressive forces** that are exacerbated by misalignment of the femoral-tibial joint (Felson et al., 2004)

The pain can start out as minimal following activity, but progresses in accordance with the amount and frequency of undesired forces placed on the site, typically to the point where the individual's lifestyle is greatly altered by the pain. Unfortunately, most individuals will not consider making changes in their level of physical activity until they are experihencing constant bone pain.

Normal Course of Symptoms in an Osteoarthritic Joint

In the earliest stages, there may be no symptoms or findings until continued forces are placed on the joint and the degenerative changes subsequently progress. Initial symptoms are next-day discomfort and/or stiffness of the joint from chemical synovitis.

As the changes to the structural integrity increase, the next-day discomfort and/or stiffness will increase in intensity and frequency. As the articular cartilage becomes thinner, forces are transmitted and experienced by the subchondral bone, resulting in bone pain during and after activity. Further progression leads to bone-on-bone contact and constant pain.

It is highly recommended that the CMES speak in detail with their client to get a full history before developing an exercise program. If the CMES or the client is unsure of the status or progression of OA, the client should be referred to a medical professional.

APPLY WHAT YOU KNOW

DETERMINING WHICH CLIENTS NEED EXERCISES FOR JOINT PROTECTION

The task for a CMES is to recommend specific exercises for clients with OA that will allow them to remain physically active without doing harm to their existing problem. The CMES must understand which individuals are at risk for OA and who will therefore need exercise programs designed to protect the joints.

- *Individuals who have had surgery on a joint involved in the exercise program:* The initial injury requiring surgical intervention in the vast majority of cases disrupts the structural integrity of the joint (i.e., the articular cartilage and subchondral bone). This situation must be recognized when developing their exercise program.
- *Individuals who state that they experience discomfort and/or tightness the day following physical activity:* Chemical synovitis is the number-one reason for these symptoms to occur and persist. Temporary relief can be achieved with over-the-counter anti-inflammatory medications, but the symptom and not the etiology itself is being treated. Also, the concern over the possible significant side effects of all anti-inflammatory medications often outweighs the palliative benefits. A safer route to control the discomfort may be the use of a glucosamine sulfate with a low-molecular chondroitin (only found in CosaminDS). A study by the National Institutes of Health (Clegg et al., 2006) reported better relief of pain and no known side effects with the use of the ingredients found only in CosaminDS when compared to Celebrex 200 mg a day or a placebo.
- *Individuals with overweight:* The excessive forces associated with overweight and obesity result in undesirable changes to the articular cartilage. The CMES must not do anything to hasten these changes. Reducing body weight with the assistance of other healthcare professionals should be considered, and resistance-training programs should be of a higher volume and lower intensity to reduce post-workout muscular and joint soreness (Strasser & Schobersberger, 2010).
- *Individuals who walk with an altered gait, especially following participation in a weight-bearing activity:* This can result in an asymmetrical loading of the joint, which increases the risk of joint degeneration (Buckwalter & Martin, 2006).
- *Individuals who feel the need to wear a brace with activity:* Bracing is often a result of a previous injury or current joint pain, which may have resulted in alterations of the articular structures and can increase the risk of the development of OA (Buckwalter & Martin, 2006).

Rheumatoid Arthritis

RA is a chronic inflammatory disease in which the body's immune system mistakenly attacks its own tissues. The abnormal immune response causes inflammation that can damage joints and organs, such as the heart. The severity of RA varies among individuals, and symptoms can change from one day to the next. Sudden increases in symptoms and illness are common and are called flares, which can last for days or months. Inflammatory periods are characterized by an unusual increase in synovial membrane cell size, a thickening of the synovial membrane, and subsequent further joint swelling. The progression of RA often results in degradation of the cartilage and bone of the affected joints, which in severe cases can lead to decreased joint spacing, a loss of cartilage, decreased joint mobility, increased pain, and irreversible deformity (Arthritis Foundation, 2019).

Key RA symptoms are pain, fatigue, and warm, swollen, reddish joints. Additionally, long periods of joint stiffness after waking are common. Inflammation in the small joints of the wrists, hands, feet, elbows, knees, and ankles is typical. Joints are typically affected bilaterally. That is, if a joint on one side of the body is affected, the same one on the other side is usually affected (Arthritis Foundation, 2019).

EXPAND YOUR KNOWLEDGE

RHEUMATOID ARTHRITIS AND CARDIOVASCULAR DISEASE

RA is associated with increased morbidity and reduced life expectancy, with standardized mortality rates ranging from 1.28 to 3.0. These increased morbidity and mortality rates in individuals with RA are notable, as **ischemic heart disease** and subsequent heart failure represent one of the most common causes of death in RA. In this regard, RA appears to be an independent risk factor for ischemic heart disease, similar to diabetes (Kaplan, 2010).

In a meta-analysis conducted by Avina-Zubieta and colleagues (2008), the risk of **cardiovascular disease (CVD)**–associated death was found to be as much as 50% higher among patients with RA compared to controls, with the risk of ischemic heart disease and cerebrovascular diseases being elevated to a similar degree. While the reasons for the dramatic rise in atherosclerotic disease in patients with RA are not completely understood, the disease is associated with chronic inflammation, which can promote endothelial cell activation and vascular dysfunction (Kaplan, 2010). These findings indicate that the CMES should take into account the potential presence of CVD in clients with RA and, as such, proceed with screening, referral, and exercise-testing strategies accordingly.

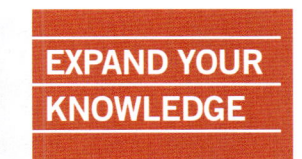

Juvenile Arthritis

JA consists of a heterogeneous group of arthritis-related conditions. The most frequently diagnosed is JIA, which has a large impact on patients, both physically and psychologically.

JIA typically affects joints—limiting or halting movement—but can involve the eyes, skin, and gastrointestinal tract as well. JIA can significantly affect quality of life, which includes disability, growth and development abnormalities, absence from school and extracurricular activities, identity and body image crises, and pain and loss of function (Cordingley et al., 2012). No known cause has been found for most forms of JA, nor is there evidence to suggest that substances—such as toxins or foods—or allergies cause children to develop the disease. Some research points toward a genetic predisposition when triggered by other factors (Arthritis Foundation, 2019).

DIAGNOSTIC CRITERIA

Arthritis can take many forms. This section covers diagnostic criteria for OA and RA, and concludes with a brief statement about JA, as the diagnosis for JA is less clearly defined.

Osteoarthritis

OA refers to a clinical syndrome of joint dysfunction accompanied by varying degrees of joint pain and reduced quality of life. It is defined by loss of articular cartilage, a variable subchondral bone reaction, and involvement of other associated joint structures (e.g., ligaments, meniscus, capsule, synovial membrane, and muscle). The knee, hip, spine, hands, and feet are the main joints affected by OA. The classic pathology is cartilage deterioration, with fibrillation, fissures, ulceration, and ultimate loss associated with hypertrophy of subchondral bone (Cooper et al., 2013).

Interestingly, more than 50% of people with diagnosed OA are younger than 65 and will live for many decades with arthritis, providing more time for disability to occur and sufficient progression to lead to knee replacement eligibility (Arthritis Foundation, 2019). Because of this variability, diagnosis is based on several different features, including laboratory and clinical tests, radiographic results, or purely clinical assessment. A conceptual model for the pathogenesis of OA is that systemic factors (e.g., age, gender, ethnicity, **metabolic syndrome,** and genetic factors) increase general susceptibility to OA, while local mechanical factors (e.g., obesity, joint injury or deformity, and muscle weakness) influence its site and severity (Cooper et al., 2013).

For the knee, diagnostic criteria used to identify individuals with OA are outlined by the Agency for Healthcare Research and Quality and consist of joint pain plus five of the following criteria (Samson et al., 2007):
- Client over 50 years of age
- More than 30 minutes of morning joint stiffness
- **Crepitus** (a crackling sound in the joints)
- Bony tenderness
- Bony enlargement
- Palpable warmth of synovium reflecting a long-held understanding of the potential relationship between joint temperature and clinical presence of arthritis (Horvath & Hollander, 1949)
- Erythrocyte sedimentation rate (ESR) >40 mm/hour, reflecting an increased level of inflammation
- Rheumatoid factor >1:40, indicating increased concentrations of antibodies that may contribute to the development of RA
- Non-inflammatory synovial fluid

The CMES should consult with medical professionals if they are interested in learning more about clinical criteria for the diagnosis of OA.

Rheumatoid Arthritis

RA is an autoimmune dysfunction characterized by the immune system attacking the joint capsule. The major symptoms are pain, swelling, stiffness, and reduced ROM. The classification of "definite rheumatoid arthritis" is based on the confirmed presence of synovitis in at least one joint, absence of an alternative diagnosis that better accounts for the synovitis, and a score of 6 or higher in four individual score domains (Table 16-1).

Juvenile Arthritis

JA is a chronic inflammatory condition of childhood. JIA is a category of JA, which represents an umbrella term summarizing the internationally recognized International League Against Rheumatism (ILAR) classification system for the various chronic pediatric arthritic conditions (Petty et al., 2004). The term "disease activity" refers to the overall burden of inflammatory disease at a particular point in time. However, the heterogeneous nature of JIA ensures that no single measure can reliably capture overall disease activity in all patients (McErlane et al., 2013). As such, the identification and classification of JIA remains unclear as researchers struggle to come to a consensus on mutually exclusive identifiers (Martini, 2012). A CMES who works with youth who suffer from JA should do so only after receiving medical clearance and physician's recommendations and guidelines for exercise.

Arthritis   CHAPTER 16

TABLE 16-1

THE 2010 AMERICAN COLLEGE OF RHEUMATOLOGY/EUROPEAN LEAGUE AGAINST RHEUMATISM CLASSIFICATION CRITERIA FOR RHEUMATOID ARTHRITIS (RA)

	Score
Target population (Who should be tested?): Patients who: 1. Have at least 1 joint with definite clinical synovitis (swelling)* 2. With the synovitis not better explained by another disease[†] Classification criteria for RA (score-based algorithm: add score of categories A–D; a score of ≥6/10 is needed for classification of a patient as having definite RA)[‡]	

A. Joint involvement**
   1 large joint[††]
   2–10 large joints
   1–3 small joints (with or without involvement of large joints)[‡‡]
   4–10 small joints (with or without involvement of large joints)
   >10 joints (at least 1 small joint)[a]
	0
	1
	2
	3
	5

B. Serology (at least 1 test result is needed for classification)[b]
   Negative RF and negative ACPA
   Low-positive RF or low-positive ACPA
   High-positive RF or high-positive ACPA
	0
	2
	3

C. Acute-phase reactants (at least 1 test result is needed for classification)[c]
   Normal CRP and normal ESR
   Abnormal CRP or abnormal ESR
	0
	1

D. Duration of symptoms[d] <6 weeks ≥6 weeks	0 1

* The criteria are aimed at classification of newly presenting patients. In addition, patients with erosive disease typical of RA with a history compatible with prior fulfillment of the 2010 criteria should be classified as having RA. Patients with longstanding disease, including those whose disease is inactive (with or without treatment) who, based on retrospectively available data, have previously fulfilled the 2010 criteria should be classified as having RA.

[†] Differential diagnoses vary among patients with different presentations, but may include conditions such as systemic lupus erythematosus, psoriatic arthritis, and gout. If it is unclear about the relevant differential diagnoses to consider, an expert rheumatologist should be consulted.

[‡] Although patients with a score of <6/10 are not classifiable as having RA, their status can be reassessed and the criteria might be fulfilled cumulatively over time.

** Joint involvement refers to any *swollen* or *tender* joints on examination, which may be confirmed by imaging evidence of synovitis. Distal interphalangeal joints, first carpometacarpal joints, and first metatarsophalangeal joints are *excluded from assessment*. Categories of joint distribution are classified according to the location and number of involved joints, with placement into the highest category possible based on the pattern of joint involvement.

[††] "Large joints" refers to shoulders, elbows, hips, knees, and ankles.

[‡‡] "Small joints" refers to the metacarpophalangeal joints, proximal interphalangeal joints, second through fifth metatarsophalangeal joints, thumb interphalangeal joints, and wrists.

[a] In this category, at least 1 of the involved joints must be a small joint; the other joints can include any combination of large and additional small joints, as well as other joints not specifically listed elsewhere (e.g., temporomandibular, acromioclavicular, and sternoclavicular).

[b] Negative refers to IU values that are less than or equal to the upper limit of normal (ULN) for the laboratory and assay; low-positive refers to IU values that are higher than the ULN but ≤3 times the ULN for the laboratory and assay; high-positive refers to IU values that are >3 times the ULN for the laboratory and assay. Where rheumatoid factor (RF) information is only available as positive or negative, a positive result should be scored as low-positive for RF. ACPA = Anti-citrullinated protein antibody.

[c] Normal/abnormal is determined by local laboratory standards. CRP = C-reactive protein; ESR = Erythrocyte sedimentation rate.

[d] Duration of symptoms refers to patient self-report of the duration of signs or symptoms of synovitis (e.g., pain, swelling, and tenderness) of joints that are clinically involved at the time of assessment, regardless of treatment status.

Reprinted with permission from Aletaha, D. et al. (2010). 2010 Rheumatoid arthritis classification criteria: An American College of Rheumatology/European League Against Rheumatism collaborative initiative. *Arthritis and Rheumatism, 62,* 9, 2569–2481. DOI: 10.1002/art.27584

TREATMENT OPTIONS

Non-pharmacological Treatment

Physical activity and weight management are important steps in dealing with the pain and stiffness from many forms of arthritis. Individuals with arthritis may suffer from deficits in strength, flexibility, and aerobic power, which make performing **activities of daily living** difficult. Unfortunately, because joints become stiff and painful from arthritis, this creates a challenge to performing physical activity, which is essential to manging arthritic conditions (ACSM, 2022). Ultimately, being inactive leads to even further reductions in overall function and joint ROM and fatigue, as well as weight gain, which places excess pressure on weight-bearing joints. Hence, the non-pharmacological treatments for individuals with arthritis include a focus on lifestyle factors such as increased physical activity, joint-protection strategies (e.g., teaching people how to move without pain and lift objects properly), and eating a healthy diet. Cognitive behavioral therapy has also been shown to benefit individuals with arthritis-related fatigue by enhancing self-management and reducing their sense of helplessness (Hewlett et al., 2011).

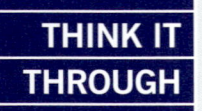

> **THINK IT THROUGH**
>
> Clients who suffer from arthritis have joints that become stiff and painful, which results in the tendency to decrease movement in hopes of not exacerbating the problem. Unfortunately, being inactive leads to even further reductions in overall function and joint ROM and fatigue, as well as weight gain, which places excess pressure on weight-bearing joints. How will you encourage your clients to remain active even though they might instinctively resist doing so? Think about exercise approaches and coaching strategies to help them overcome obstacles to being physically active due to arthritis pain.

Pharmacological Treatment

Acetaminophen and anti-inflammatory medications are popular forms of pharmacological treatment for OA. Specifically among OA patients, it is estimated that 70% take a prescription medication and 44 to 70% take an over-the-counter analgesic to control joint symptoms (Albert et al., 2008). The American College of Rheumatology recommends the use of acetaminophen for patients with OA to manage mild-to-moderate lower-limb pain. However, some data show that acetaminophen is not as efficacious as **nonsteroidal anti-inflammatory drugs (NSAIDs)** (e.g., aspirin, ibuprofen, and naproxen) for pain at rest and pain in motion (Hochberg & Dougados, 2001). Due to the risk of side effects (e.g., gastrointestinal bleeding, liver damage, and cardiovascular events), it has been suggested that individuals on these medications be continuously monitored by their physicians for signs of renal toxicity, **hypertension,** and limb edema (ACSM, 2014). A topical medication, capsaicin, is a preferred treatment for some arthritic patients because of its negligible side effects, although the pain relief it provides appears to be less effective than that seen with the oral analgesics (Fraenkel et al., 2004).

For treatment of RA, pharmacological therapies are the mainstay. These include NSAIDs, disease-modifying anti-rheumatic drugs (DMARDs), glucocorticoids (steroids), and biologic therapy (etanercept). The potential side effects of these drugs [NSAIDs (stomach bleeding and ulcers), DMARDs (liver and kidney damage), and glucocorticoids (increased risk of infection)] require that clients be carefully monitored by their physicians (ACSM, 2014). The CMES should communicate with their client's healthcare team to ensure appropriate exercise program design and implementation for anyone taking drugs to treat RA.

Surgical Treatment

Individuals with OA who fail to get relief from noninvasive treatments may consider surgery. Injections of hyaluronic acid have been shown to relieve pain in the knee (Zhang et al., 2010). Joint lavage (washing) and debridement (trimming and removing torn and damaged cartilage) are commonly performed surgical treatments for moderate-to-mild knee OA, with patients reporting pain relief about 50% of the time from either procedure (Moseley et al., 2002). In patients with severe knee OA, another surgical option is total knee replacement or arthroplasty. OA sufferers between 60 and 75 years of age are the most common candidates for total knee replacement, as those younger than age 55 experience more stress on the knee and have an increased likelihood for a second procedure (ACSM, 2014). Accordingly, younger patients typically undergo alternative surgical procedures such as a partial knee replacement.

For RA, orthopedic procedures such as synovectomy (removal of inflamed synovial tissue), tendon realignment, and arthroscopic debridement may be performed, but with less definitive outcomes. These approaches may prolong joint function and delay the need for joint-replacement procedures. After all other options have been exhausted, joint replacement may be considered (ACSM, 2014).

Exercise Treatment

Evidence suggests that both strengthening and aerobic exercise are associated with relief of pain in knee OA. Reduced pain in hip OA has been found with strength exercise, and water-based exercise has been associated with pain relief and improvement in function in both knee and hip OA (Zhang et al., 2010). By increasing muscular strength and endurance, enhancing the stability of the joints, improving ROM, and reducing passive tension of the soft tissue surrounding joints, a CMES can help their clients improve their quality of life, maintain normal function, and prevent deconditioning. One of the secondary outcomes of OA is a development of other diseases, such as **coronary artery disease,** diabetes, and hypertension, as physical activity becomes too painful to attempt, cardiovascular function declines, and the client becomes sedentary. For the high number of clients who have overweight or obesity as well as OA, a further reduction in physical activity can increase the risk for the development of comorbidities. By encouraging clients to maintain cardiovascular fitness by doing exercise that does not increase joint pain, combined with exercises and treatments to help reduce joint pain, a CMES can reduce the impact of OA on pain, day-to-day function, cardiovascular health, and quality of life.

EXPAND YOUR KNOWLEDGE

OSTEOARTHRITIS SYMPTOMS AND EXERCISE

Of the randomized, controlled trials exploring the effects of exercise on OA symptoms, some have used **hydrotherapy, tai chi,** or other low-impact exercises to reduce the stress on the joints (Lund et al., 2008; Fransen et al., 2007; Hinman, Haywood, & Day, 2007; Wang et al., 2007; Ettinger et al., 1997). This outcome is certainly recommended for individuals who experience pain throughout the day, but for those who are relatively pain-free, weight-bearing exercise and resistance training can be beneficial in not only reducing pain and disability, but also in maintaining normal everyday function. A study examining the effects of different exercise modes on pain, disability, and performance measures found that 60 minutes of light- to moderate-intensity walking three days per week [50 to 70% **heart-rate reserve (HRR)**], or light- to moderate-intensity resistance training three days per week (two sets of 12 repetitions of nine exercises) had significantly better results than those seen in the control group over an 18-month intervention (Ettinger et al., 1997). Similar results showed that individuals performing three days per week of light- to moderate-intensity resistance training (three sets of eight to 10 repetitions) had lower pain scores and higher functional abilities compared to those who performed only passive-ROM exercises (Mikesky et al., 2006). There was also a dose-response relationship between those who did more exercise (75 to 100% of programmed sessions) and those who did less activity (<40% of programmed sessions), with those in the former group experiencing lower pain and disability scores and having greater performance and fitness scores (Ettinger et al., 1997). However, as with all exercise programs for individuals with limitations, the CMES must always be cognizant of the client's needs. If the client is hurting, they will not do the exercise, so the CMES must base decisions on individual feedback, not general guidelines.

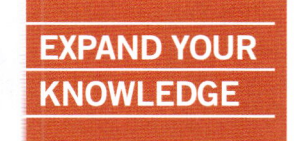

Unfortunately, exercise is not a cure for OA, but maintaining a regular exercise program of resistance and aerobic training can reduce the pain and rate of decline in functional capacity (Zhang et al., 2010; Mikesky et al., 2006). No evidence exists that properly programmed and managed exercise will increase the rate of joint degeneration, as measured by joint-space narrowing (Mikesky et al., 2006) or pain scores (van Baar et al., 1999; Ettinger et al., 1997). Exercise can help reduce some of the risk factors associated with the progression of OA, including weak quadriceps (Mikesky et al., 2006; Bennell & Hinman, 2005), **valgus** (knock-kneed) or **varus** (bow-legged) knee alignment, weak hip abductors, and obesity (Issa & Sharma, 2006). By selecting exercises or developing programs that address these conditions, a CMES can help reduce pain and functional limitations, as well as slow the progression of OA to keep clients active. Further reductions in quadriceps strength, as well as in the strength of the hip abductors and extensors, will accelerate the deterioration of the joint by reducing the ability of the individual to control anterior-posterior motion of the knee, while also exacerbating structural alignment problems that may lead to asymmetrical wear on the articular cartilage.

Like individuals with OA, those with RA also suffer from reduced muscle strength and joint function that reduces mobility and increases pain. Fortunately, regular exercise appears to minimize functional decline, reduce fall risk and joint stiffness, and attenuate pain (ACSM, 2022). Studies have shown that physically inactive patients with RA have a significantly worse CVD risk profile compared with physically active patients (Elkan et al., 2011; Metsios et al., 2010). Conversely, those with RA who perform high levels of physical activity have been shown to have a significantly better CVD risk profile than those with low levels of physical activity, even when adjusting for RA disease duration, activity and severity, and steroid use (Metsios et al., 2009). Aerobic training for those with stable RA has been shown to be safe (Baillet et al., 2010) and to improve aerobic power (Hurkmans et al., 2009). Furthermore, resistance training—both water-based and land-based—is recommended as routine practice for individuals with RA (Hurkmans et al., 2009).

Although OA and RA are different forms of arthritis, the FITT recommendations for both conditions are consistent with those established for apparently healthy adults. However, additional considerations should be given for functional limitations, pain, disease activity, joint integrity, and personal preferences while improving cardiorespiratory and muscular fitness with little or no joint pain or damage (ACSM, 2022).

NUTRITIONAL CONSIDERATIONS

The most effective nutrition therapy for both RA and OA serves to decrease inflammation and thus reduce overall disease morbidity. Additionally, any nutrition intervention that helps improve overall CVD risk profile (in particular for those with RA who tend to be at increased risk of heart disease due to their condition) and manage weight (especially for those with OA for which obesity is a major risk factor) is beneficial. While the scientific research aiming to understand the role of nutrition in arthritis continues to evolve, a recap of the current understanding on the role of nutrition in arthritis is described here.

A Key Role for Fatty Acids

The evidence is clear: consumption of **omega-3 fatty acids** reduces inflammation. This is especially beneficial for individuals with RA where inflammation is more pronounced and chronic. A literature review looking at the effects of omega-3 fatty acids on RA found that consumption may limit inflammatory responses and modulate disease activity on the number of tender and swollen joints (Kostoglou-Athanassiou, Athanassiou, & Athanassiou, 2020).

In contrast to omega-3 fatty acids, **omega-6 fatty acids** may worsen disease severity. These fatty acids are known for their proinflammatory effects, with the exception of γ-linolenic acid (GLA), which possesses anti-inflammatory properties. An optimal diet provides a 4:1 to 1:1 ratio of omega-6 fatty acids to omega-3 fatty acids. However, the typical American diet more closely resembles a 20:1 ratio, with overconsumption of omega-6 fatty acids and underconsumption of omega-3 fatty acids (Lopez, 2012a). Food sources of omega-3 fatty acids are shown in Table 16-2.

TABLE 16-2
SELECTED FOOD SOURCES OF ALA, DHA, AND EPA

FOOD	ALA	DHA	EPA
Flaxseed oil, 1 tbsp	7.26		
Chia seeds, 1 ounce	5.06		
English walnuts, 1 ounce	2.57		
Flaxseed, whole, 1 tbsp	2.35		
Salmon, Atlantic, farmed, cooked, 3 ounces		1.24	0.59
Salmon, Atlantic, wild, cooked, 3 ounces		1.22	0.35
Herring, Atlantic, cooked, 3 ounces*		0.94	0.77
Canola oil, 1 tbsp	1.28		
Sardines, canned in tomato sauce, drained, 3 ounces		0.74	0.45
Mackerel, Atlantic, cooked, 3 ounces*		0.59	0.43
Salmon, pink, canned, drained, 3 ounces	0.04	0.63	0.28
Soybean oil, 1 tbsp	0.92		
Trout, rainbow, wild, cooked, 3 ounces		0.44	0.40
Black walnuts, 1 ounce	0.76		
Mayonnaise, 1 tbsp	0.74		
Oysters, eastern, wild, cooked, 3 ounces	0.14	0.23	0.30
Sea bass, cooked, 3 ounces*		0.47	0.13
Edamame, frozen, prepared, ½ cup	0.28		
Shrimp, cooked, 3 ounces*		0.12	0.12
Refried beans, canned, vegetarian, ½ cup	0.21		
Lobster, cooked, 3 ounces*	0.04	0.07	0.10
Tuna, light, canned in water, drained, 3 ounces*		0.17	0.02
Tilapia, cooked, 3 ounces*	0.04	0.11	
Scallops, cooked, 3 ounces*		0.09	0.06
Cod, Pacific, cooked, 3 ounces*		0.10	0.04
Tuna, yellowfin, cooked, 3 ounces*		0.09	0.01
Kidney beans, canned, vegetarian, ½ cup	0.10		
Baked beans, canned, vegetarian, ½ cup	0.07		
Ground beef, 85% lean, cooked, 3 ounces**	0.04		
Bread, whole wheat, 1 slide	0.04		
Egg, cooked, 1 egg		0.03	
Chicken, breast, roasted, 3 ounces		0.02	0.01
Milk, low-fat (1%), 1 cup	0.01		

*Except as noted, the USDA database does not specify whether fish are farmed or wild caught.

**The USDA database does not specify whether beef is grass fed or grain fed.

Note: ALA = alpha-linolenic acid; DHA = docosahexaenoic acid; EPA = eicosapentaenoic acid

Reprinted from National Institutes of Health (2020). *Omega-3 Fatty Acids: Fact Sheet for Health Professionals.* https://ods.od.nih.gov/factsheets/Omega3FattyAcids-HealthProfessional/

Consumption of **monounsaturated fatty acids**—especially oleic acid (olive oil)—may help reduce pain and inflammation in individuals with RA, but the studies are inconclusive. It is uncertain whether the monounsaturated fat itself helps to reduce inflammation, or an increased consumption of monounsaturated fatty acids may replace omega-6 fatty acids in the diet, thus improving disease symptoms primarily by way of decreasing omega-6 intake (Rennie et al., 2003).

The Healthy Mediterranean-Style Dietary Pattern as Disease Modifier

Adoption of the **Healthy Mediterranean-Style Dietary Pattern** may provide multiple benefits for people with arthritis. Not only is this eating pattern associated with improved heart health (de Lorgeril, 2013) (those with RA are at particularly high risk of heart disease), improved weight management when combined with caloric restriction and physical activity (Esposito et al., 2011) (OA, old age, and obesity often go hand-in-hand), and improved cognitive function (Féart, Samieri, & Barberger-Gateau, 2010) (the elderly are disproportionately affected by arthritis), but controlled studies specifically looking at the Healthy Mediterranean-Style Dietary Pattern and disease outcomes with arthritis have shown promising results. For example, one study found that the adoption of a Mediterranean dietary pattern for 12 weeks was associated with improved function status and quality of life and decreased inflammation in individuals with RA (Sköldstam et al., 2005). A Mediterranean eating plan is high in vegetables, fruits, nuts, olive oils, whole grains, and fish; moderate in wine consumption (one to two glasses per day); and limited in full-fat milk products and meat (see Chapter 7 for more information on the Healthy Mediterranean-Style Dietary Pattern).

Nutrients in Question

Many nutrients have been suggested to play a role in arthritis, though in most cases the evidence is lacking. A summary of these nutrients is shown in Table 16-3.

Supplements Under Investigation

Many nutritional supplements are under investigation as possible disease modifiers. These supplements are highlighted in Table 16-4.

Elimination Diets: Help or Hype?

Many people with arthritis—in particular RA—feel that certain foods make their symptoms worse. The main culprits are purported to be red meat, dairy, gluten, and wheat. However, the blinded controlled studies that have been conducted to date have not found a consistent relationship between intake of these substances and symptoms or disease course (Rennie et al., 2003). Because many people with arthritis already have poor nutritional status, aiming to achieve dietary recommendations and follow a balanced meal pattern is more likely to ensure adequate nutritional status.

Ultimately, the most important nutritional plan for people with RA or OA is one that provides at least the recommended levels of the nutrients and micronutrients, with a particular emphasis on regular consumption of fatty fish or other omega-3-rich foods and vegetables and fruits. While many other nutrients and nutriceuticals are under investigation, in most cases the science to date is not conclusive. Those individuals interested in exploring nutritional supplementation or specific meal plans in an effort to modify their disease course should consult with their rheumatologist and a **registered dietitian** with knowledge of rheumatic diseases.

EXERCISE RECOMMENDATIONS

As noted earlier, the FITT guidelines for arthritis mirror those for all apparently healthy adults. Hence, the CMES should consider each client's unique situation and individual preferences when designing an exercise program to increase program adherence (ACSM, 2022). The following sections provide some important considerations for working with individuals who have OA and RA.

TABLE 16-3
NUTRIENTS SUGGESTED TO PLAY A ROLE IN ARTHRITIS

Nutrient	The Science	Recommendation
Antioxidants	The role of antioxidants, including vitamin C, E, and selenium, in RA has been studied with mixed results.	Avoiding deficiency may help improve arthritis symptoms, but consuming high doses is probably not efficacious. Aim to meet recommendations through consumption of fruits and vegetables, rather than supplements.
Folate (Vitamin B9)	For those with RA, a Cochrane Review concluded that taking methotrexate (MTX), supplementation with folic or folinic acid: • Probably improves some side effects of MTX such as nausea and abdominal pain • Probably reduces the chance of developing abnormal liver blood tests • Probably helps people continue on their MTX treatment • May improve some side effects of MTX such as mouth sores • May help prevent neutropenia (problems with producing white blood cells), but the research is inconclusive • Probably has no effect on how well MTX is able to treat RA	Individuals taking MTX should consult with their rheumatologist to discuss folic acid supplementation; this should occur prior to initiating supplementation, as overconsumption of folic acid may mask a vitamin B12 deficiency.
Zinc	While many people with RA have low serum zinc levels, studies have not supported a benefit from consuming zinc beyond the recommended amounts.	Aim to meet recommended amounts of zinc through dietary intake. There is no evidence that supplementation provides a benefit.
Iron	RA may increase the risk of iron-deficiency anemia due to any of a number of routes such as chronic inflammation, gastrointestinal blood loss from inflamed synovial tissue, or poor dietary intake.	Iron-deficiency anemia is relatively common in the general population, including among those with arthritis. Adequate dietary intake to meet recommended amounts should be encouraged, but there is no evidence of benefit for routine supplementation in those with arthritis.
Calcium and vitamin D	Steroids increase disease-associated bone loss and diminish intestinal calcium absorption. This may be moderated with adequate calcium and vitamin D intake. However, there is no evidence to support additional benefit from calcium and vitamin D supplementation.	Aim to meet calcium and vitamin D needs mostly through dietary intake. If this is not possible, consult with a rheumatologist to evaluate whether supplementation may provide benefit.

Note: RA = Rheumatoid arthritis

Sources: Shea, B. et al. (2013). Folic acid and folinic acid for reducing side effects in patients receiving methotrexate for rheumatoid arthritis. *Cochrane Musculoskeletal Group.* DOI: 10.1002/14651858.CD000951.pub2; Lopez, H.L. (2012a). Nutritional interventions to prevent and treat osteoarthritis. Part I: Focus on fatty acids and macronutrients. *PM&R,* 4, S145–S154; Rennie, K.L. et al. (2003). Nutritional management of rheumatoid arthritis: A review of the evidence. *Journal of Human Nutrition and Dietetics,* 16, 97–109.

TABLE 16-4
NUTRIENT SUPPLEMENTS THAT MAY MODERATE ARTHRITIS SEVERITY

Nutrient Supplement	Purported Mechanism of Action	Strength of Evidence	Recommendation
Fish oil	Reducing inflammation	Clear benefit	Fatty fish at least 2–3 times per week. Some may benefit from DHA and EPA (at least 2 grams and up to 4 grams) supplementation
Krill oil	A natural source of astaxanthin, a potent antioxidant that decreases inflammation, improves cardiac health, and may benefit athletic performance	Randomized double-blind controlled trial found significant decrease in CRP, pain, stiffness, and functional impairment (Deutsch, 2007)	300 mg of krill oil supplementation may be beneficial
γ-linolenic acid (GLA)	Upon metabolism, GLA preferentially generates PGE1, an eicosanoid with anti-inflammatory and immunoregulatory properties	Appears to suppress acute and chronic inflammation (Dawczynski et al., 2011)	Supplementation with 450–2,000 mg of GLA from borage seed or evening primrose oil may provide benefit to joint health
Glucosamine	As an important component of articular cartilage, believed to improve joint pain and function, reduce risk of total joint replacement, and encourage bone regeneration in OA	Limited scientific evidence to support beliefs, though beliefs continue to be widely held by clinicians	Discuss potential value of supplementation with rheumatologist
Chondroitin	As an important component of articular cartilage, thought to benefit joint health	Studies suggest it can slow progressive joint-space narrowing and inflammation associated with OA	Discuss potential value of supplementation with rheumatologist
Avocado-soybean unsaponifiable fractions	Shown to have anti-inflammatory properties on bone cells	Studies show supplementation helps to improve pain and decrease need for NSAIDs	300 mg daily supplementation could be beneficial. Discuss with doctor.
Methylsulfonylmethane (MSM)	Joints affected by OA tend to have lower sulfur content, which may be repleted with MSM supplementation	Associated with decreased pain and swelling and improved function in individuals with OA	May provide benefit. Discuss with doctor.
Hyaluronan	As an important component of articular cartilage, thought to play important role in improvement in pain and function	Shown to provide benefit when injected into knee joint for those with knee OA	Safety and efficacy yet to be firmly established

Arthritis CHAPTER 16

TABLE 16-4 (continued)

Nutrient Supplement	Purported Mechanism of Action	Strength of Evidence	Recommendation
S-adenosyl-methionine (SAMe)	Provides antioxidant protection in synovial cells	Benefits appear to be as strong as NSAIDs with fewer side effects in some studies	Typical doses of 800–1,600 mg per day have been used; should discuss with doctor before starting. Note that homocysteine is a by-product of metabolism of SAMe. May require vitamin B12, B6, and folate supplementation to handle possible elevation in homocysteine
Collagen preparations (undenatured type II collagen, hydrolyzed collagen products)	Help to improve immune response	May improve mobility, reduce pain, and improve functional status in both RA and OA	Discuss with doctor prior to supplementing
Phytoflavonoids and botanicals	Powerful antioxidants with free-radical scavenging properties	Studies suggest high potential for improvement of symptoms with low risk of toxicity	Supplementation up to 150–1,500 mg daily may improve symptoms; discuss with doctor
Proteolytic enzymes	May have anti-inflammatory, analgesic, antithrombotic, and antifibrinolytic properties	Studies are limited to preclinical and small pilot studies	Await further scientific evidence supporting high efficacy and low safety risk
Probiotics and prebiotics	May help to modulate immune response, especially in RA	Emerging evidence found addition to standard medication regimen decreased pain, CRP and improved function and walking capacity in OA (Mandel, Eichas, & Holmes, 2010)	Await further evidence
Cissus quadrangularis	A vine found in Asia and West Africa, it is thought to help heal bone fractures and joint pain	Some early data suggest bone-protecting properties	Await further evidence
Isothiocyanates	Found naturally in cruciferous vegetables like broccoli, kale, mustard greens, and Brussel sprouts, possess antioxidant and anti-inflammatory properties	A study of RA found improvement in biomarkers of joint disease	Await further evidence regarding value of supplementation. Encourage high intake of cruciferous vegetables to attain possible benefits of isothiocyanates as well as many other health-promoting effects

Note: RA = Rheumatoid arthritis; OA = Osteoarthritis; DHA = Docosahexanoic acid; EPA = Eicosapentaenoic acid; PGE1 = Prostaglandin E1; NSAID = Nonsteroidal anti-inflammatory drug; CRP = C-reactive protein

Unless otherwise specified, data from Lopez, H.L (2012a). Nutritional interventions to prevent and treat osteoarthritis. Part I: Focus on fatty acids and macronutrients. *PM&R*, 4, S145–S154; Lopez, H.L. (2012b). Nutrition interventions to prevent and treat osteoarthritis. Part II: Focus on micronutrients and supportive nutraceuticals. *PM&R*, 4, S155–S168.

Contraindications and Precautions

- Avoid vigorous exercise during acute flare-ups and periods of inflammation. However, gentle ROM exercises are appropriate during these conditions.
- Encourage clients to schedule workout sessions at a time of day when pain is the least and/or pain medications are at their peak effectiveness.
- Stop exercise if the client indicates joint pain that is too severe to continue.
- Explain to clients that a small amount of joint and/or muscle discomfort during exercise is normal, and that it does not necessarily mean that damage has occurred to the joints. However, reduce volume and intensity if pain is present at higher levels two hours after the exercise session than before the session.
- More frequent, lower-intensity exercise may be necessary, as long continuous bouts can be difficult for some individuals with arthritis.
- Perform an adequate warm-up (five to 10 minutes) to ensure joint lubrication and increased elasticity of tissues.
    - ✓ Start with light aerobic exercise to increase systemic blood flow and body temperature.
    - ✓ Perform activation exercises to target specific areas (e.g., knees and hips), such as unloaded knee **flexion** and **extension** focusing on full ROM.
    - ✓ Dynamic flexibility exercises should be performed to maintain elasticity and further increase lubrication (static stretching will cool the body down; the goal is to keep it warm and moving).
- Perform an adequate cool-down, gently taking the joints through their ROM.
- Water temperatures for aquatic exercise should be kept between 83 and 88° F (28 to 31° C) to help relax muscles and reduce pain.

Cardiorespiratory Endurance Exercise

- Three to five days per week of moderate- to vigorous-intensity training [40 to 59% $\dot{V}O_2$**reserve ($\dot{V}O_2R$)** or HRR] of activities with low joint stress (e.g., walking, swimming, and cycling) for at least 150 minutes per week
    - ✓ Multiple, shorter sessions per day may help reduce joint pain. Encourage clients to perform any amount of physical activity they are able to perform.
    - ✓ Aquatic exercise or swimming can reduce joint stress while maintaining cardiovascular function and muscular endurance.
    - ✓ Clients should gradually progress to longer sessions (increases of 5 to 10 minutes in duration) when able to comfortably exercise without any fatigue or increasing joint pain. High-impact activities may be used if well tolerated and can be introduced as cardiorespiratory fitness improves.
    - ✓ If exercising on consecutive days, clients should switch modes to avoid overuse and repetitive stress injuries.
    - ✓ The CMES should remind clients that proper footwear and softer terrain are important to reduce joint forces during weight-bearing exercise.

Resistance Exercise

- Two to three days per week
    - ✓ Perform one to three sets of eight to 12 repetitions at a lower intensity [e.g., 50 to 80% **one-repetition maximum (1-RM)**] for all the major muscle groups.
    - ✓ The program should include functional exercises to develop **synergists,** as well as overall coordination of the musculature to control and stabilize the joints.
    - ✓ Incorporate exercises to improve neuromuscular control, balance, and the ability to perform activities of daily living.
    - ✓ Exercising in the water allows for light resistances to help condition muscles through a full, pain-free ROM, while also reducing joint stresses.
    - ✓ Progress to light resistance (e.g., cuff weights, tubing/bands, and dumbbells) or bilateral exercises (e.g., body-weight squats).

Arthritis CHAPTER 16

✓ Work toward moderate-resistance exercises with as much ROM as can be tolerated, or to unilateral exercises (e.g., lunges and step-ups).

Flexibility Exercise

- ROM exercises daily to keep joints mobile and compliant
    ✓ Perform a combination of active, static, and **proprioceptive neuromuscular facilitation (PNF)** exercises for all the major joints, with an emphasis on affected joints and the muscles that cross them to increase ROM, keep joints lubricated, and decrease passive tension.
    ✓ Perform up to 10 repetitions for dynamic movements and hold static stretches for 10 to 30 seconds and repeat two to four times.

CONSIDERATIONS FOR CLIENTS WITH OA OF THE KNEE OR HIP

OA of the Knee

- Clients can begin with isometric exercises or light resistance (ankle weights) to strengthen the quadriceps, hamstrings, and gluteals without putting undue pressure on the joint. These exercises can be performed in a pool to further reduce joint pressures.
- Clients can move to body-weight bilateral exercises (e.g., squats) to develop overall muscular and joint control while encouraging full ROM.
    ✓ Clients can add external resistance to increase muscular strength and endurance if they are pain free
- Clients can progress to unilateral exercises (lunges, step-ups) to develop muscular control of the joint complex.
    ✓ They should focus on proper control and technique to make sure the patella and femur track correctly.

OA of the Hip

- Clients can begin with passive ROM exercises to increase circulation and synovial lubrication, which helps reduce joint compression. Also, aqua-therapy can be used to reduce pressure on the joint.
- Clients can perform exercises lying on the ground to avoid putting too much load on the hips. They should begin with limited-ROM lying hip abduction and extension exercises, plus ROM exercises to strengthen the hip and increase flexibility.
- Clients can progress to bilateral weight-bearing exercises with limited ROM (e.g., wall slides and body-weight squats) to develop the hip complex. They can perform ROM exercises at the end of the session to keep the joint flexible and reduce joint compression and passive tension.
- When the client is able to perform bilateral exercises with limited pain through a larger ROM, they can progress to unilateral exercises (e.g., single-leg squat) to further develop the gluteals and hamstrings.

APPLY WHAT YOU KNOW

SAMPLE EXERCISES

All programs should be tailored to meet the individual needs and experiences of each client, but free-weight or body-weight exercises are generally preferred for clients with OA, as they allow for the development of neuromuscular control and conditioning of **antagonists** and synergists to help control and stabilize the joint.

Note that this list of exercises is not meant to be a complete exercise program, but rather sample exercises that can be beneficial in reducing symptoms and ameliorating the progression of the disease.

It is important to identify any potential muscular dysfunctions that can contribute to the development of OA. By having the client perform calf raises to full **plantar flexion** (Figure 16-1), perform a standing single-leg balance (Figure 16-2), and walk on the heels and toes (Figure 16-3), a CMES can get a basic idea of any muscle-recruitment difficulties. If the client is unable to perform a full-ROM calf raise, they may have an underdeveloped gastrocnemius, which may limit the ability to control the knee joint during locomotion. Similarly, the performance of a standing single-leg balance exercise can identify any hip or pelvic stability problems, as there is increased demand on these muscles during unilateral support tasks. Often, weakness of the spine stabilizers will present itself as a leaning of the hips away from the stance leg, which results in the loss of balance. Weakness of the hip abductors will often result in a rotation of the hips. Any neurological troubles stemming from degeneration of the lumbar discs or nerve compression along the sciatic nerve can be identified if the client has difficulty walking on the heels and toes. Conditioning the rotator cuff muscles using the diagonal arm raise exercise (Figure 16-4), along with direct internal and external rotation of the humerus using exercise bands, can reduce the loss of shoulder function that may occur with later development of OA in the cervical spine.

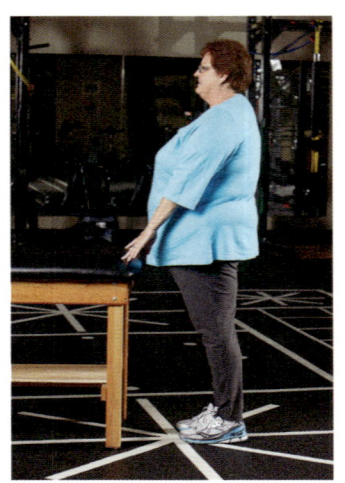

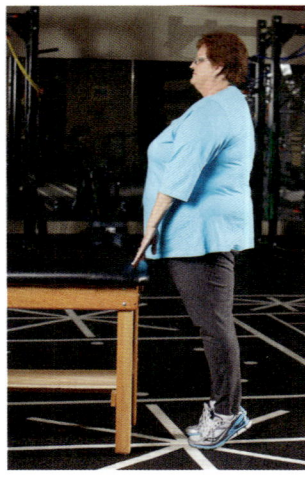

Figure 16-1
Calf raises. Using a chair or other stable object for support, the client rises onto the balls of the feet, coming to full plantar flexion and pausing to fully engage the gastrocnemius. Clients with stronger calves can perform this exercise on one leg at a time.

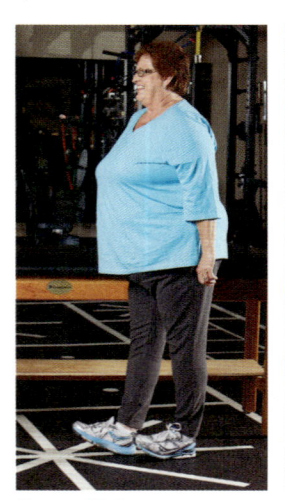

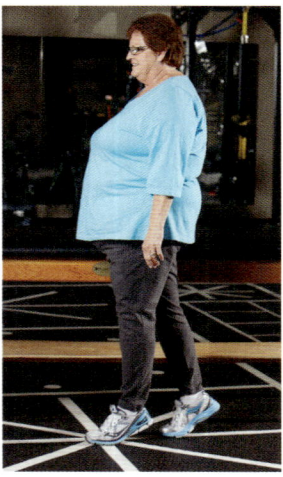

Figure 16-2
Standing single-leg balance. To test the ability of the client to engage the deep spinal stabilizers, obliques, and hip extensors and abductors, the CMES can have the client stand facing a table or other stable surface with the feet comfortably under the hips. The client lifts one leg at a time while trying to keep the pelvis level and then holds that position for as long as possible.

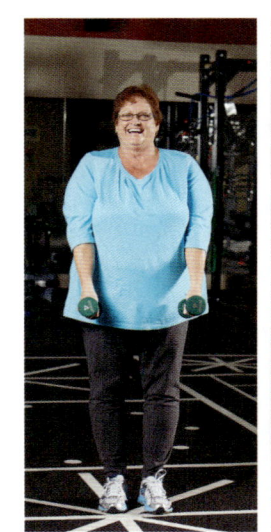

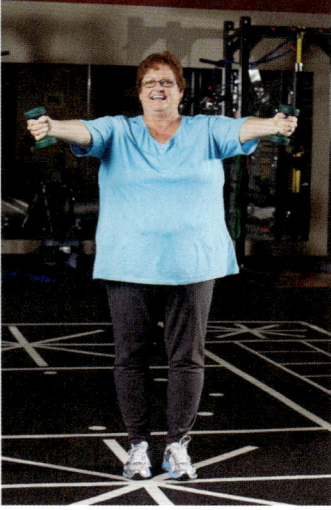

Figure 16-3
Heel and toe walking. To assess any potential neurological difficulties created by osteoarthritis of the spine or hip, the CMES can have the client walk on the heels and then on the toes. If the client is unable to walk in these positions, this may be evidence of muscle weakness that is caused by joint pain resulting in dysfunction. It may also be evidence of neurological disorders caused by degeneration of the intervertebral discs or the hip joint that leads to pressure on the nerve, resulting in muscular atrophy. These types of diagnoses should be made formally by a physician, but they can give a CMES an indication of whether there is some dysfunction.

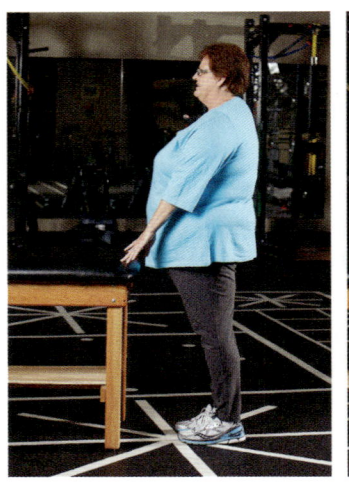

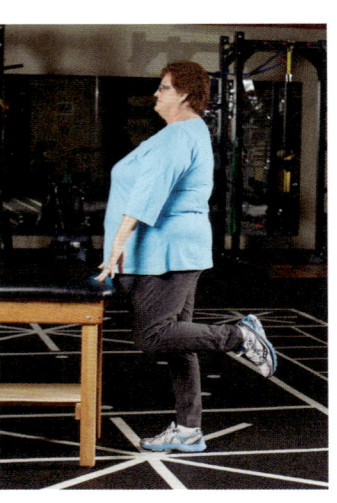

Figure 16-4
Diagonal arm raise. The client holds a dumbbell in each hand slightly below waist level. They then abduct and externally rotate the shoulder, with the arms at approximately 45 degrees in relationship to the torso until the arm reaches shoulder height. The client can then slowly return to the starting position.

Arthritis   CHAPTER 16

At the beginning stages of exercise, individuals need to increase quadriceps strength without increasing the risk of joint degeneration. The open-chain terminal 30-degrees knee extension exercise (Figure 16-5) is effective because it strengthens the knee extensors, and by performing only the final 30 degrees, the client avoids the high shearing forces of the full-ROM knee extension.

Once the client has progressed to where they can create adequate force and endurance to sustain the contraction shown in Figure 16-5 for 15 to 30 seconds, the client can progress to the closed-chain terminal knee extension (Figure 16-6). This exercise develops the quadriceps, but also develops the hip extensors and abductors in a stabilizing capacity.

As the client progresses, the addition of body-weight exercises to condition the lower body is recommended. The isometric or small-ROM wall slide or wall squat (Figure 16-7) is the first exercise that should be added to the program, as it develops the strength of the knee extensors, hip extensors, and abductors, and also helps the client develop the neuromuscular control to help move on to dynamic exercises.

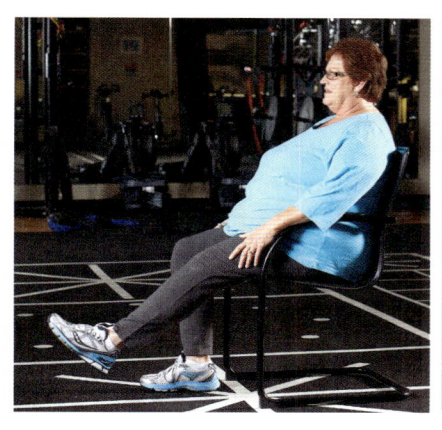

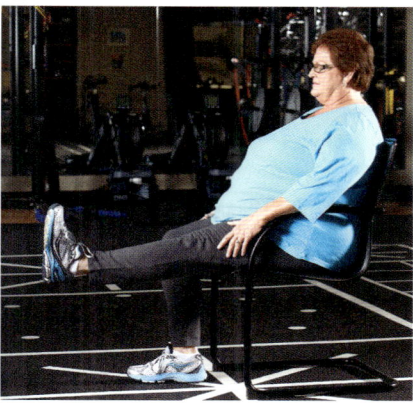

Figure 16-5
Terminal 30-degrees knee extension (open chain). Starting the knee at 30 degrees of flexion and moving to full extension reduces the shearing forces on the underside of the patella, minimizing wear and preventing further degeneration of the articular cartilage. This exercise can be performed with ankle weights or as an isometric hold at the terminal range of motion.

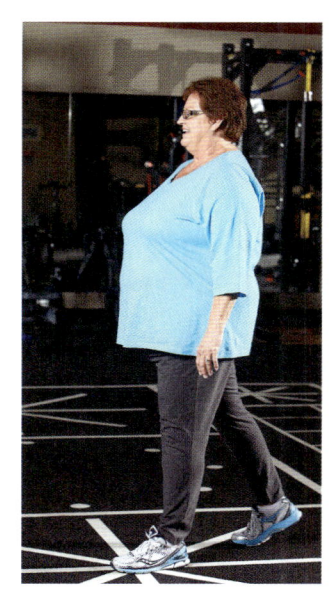

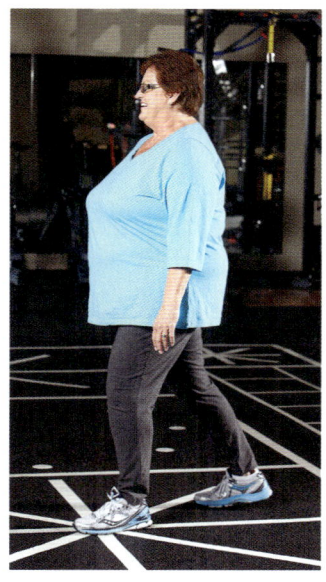

Figure 16-6
Terminal knee extensions (closed chain). The client starts by standing on one leg with the non-supporting leg resting toes-down for support. The client then moves the support leg into 30 degrees of flexion, keeping the shoulders and hips over the heel, and then presses the knee of the supporting leg backward, actively contracting the quadriceps to move into full extension. Resistance bands can be added to increase difficulty.

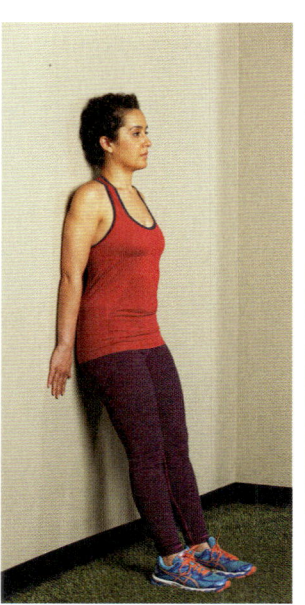

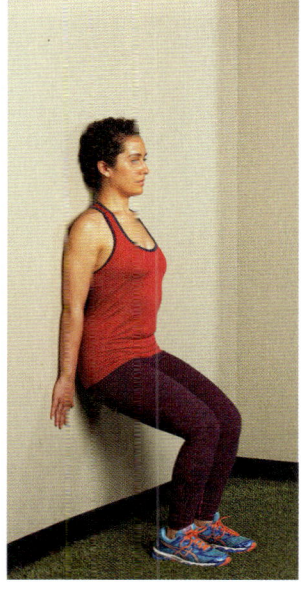

Figure 16-7
Wall slide/squat. The client begins with the feet comfortably under the hips and the back flat against the wall and slides down the wall until the knees are flexed (staying above 90 degrees or to tolerance) and holds for 2–30 seconds. The client presses through the heels and returns to the starting position.

After the client is able to perform the wall slide comfortably, they can progress to the body-weight squat to develop the musculature surrounding the hips and knees (Figure 16-8). The CMES must pay particular attention to the client's knees as they perform the exercise. Many clients will allow the knees to move medially (inward), which places strain on the joint and leads to uneven wear of the articular cartilage.

The next progression is the single-leg squat, which places greater demand on the client, especially on the quadriceps, to control the leg and the hip muscles to control and stabilize the pelvis and femur (Figure 16-9). Many people will have difficulty with this exercise, as they do not have the hip strength to maintain proper pelvic alignment or the strength and balance of the legs to maintain correct form. Two common errors are to allow the knees to move laterally (outward) during the eccentric phase of the exercise (descent) and medially (inward) during the concentric phase (ascent). *Note:* Individuals displaying medial motion of the knee often have poorly functioning external hip rotators and extensors (gluteal group) or tight adductors.

One factor that may contribute to both knee and hip pain is the inability to control the hips and pelvis, potentially leading to poor femur-tibia alignment, altered gait patterns, and weakness of the hip abductors. Therefore, development of the spinal, pelvic, and hip stabilizers is important. A simple exercise to accomplish this objective is the glute bridge (Figure 16-10). Particular emphasis should be placed on training the deep-spine stabilizers to provide adequate support of the spine and pelvis when engaging in single-leg balance or locomotion activities. Dysfunction in this region often prevents the appropriate recruitment of the prime movers, as the pelvis is unstable and does not provide a good foundation for movements.

Exercises such as the side bridge (Figure 16-11), prone plank (Figure 16-12), and prone hip extension (Figure 16-13) develop strength and endurance of these muscles. Stability, flexibility, and adequate ROM are important, as reducing passive tension along the kinetic chain can reduce tissue stress surrounding the joint, which may be contributing to uneven muscle-recruitment patterns. Using a foam roller or massage may be effective, but doing simple hip ROM exercises (Figure 16-14) can be beneficial as well.

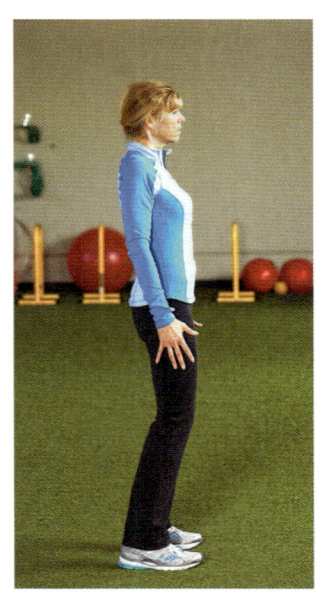

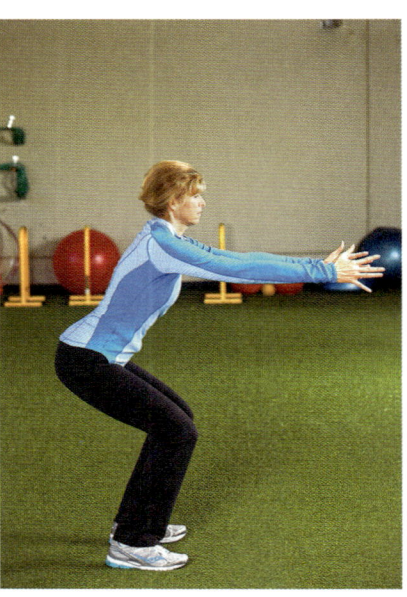

Figure 16-8
Body-weight squat. The client starts with the feet under the hips. The client begins the movement by contracting the glutes and hamstrings to pull the hips backward (i.e., hip hinge). The CMES should remind the client to allow the body to bend naturally at the hips and allow the knees to flex until comfortable. The client must keep the knees in line with the hips and ankles.

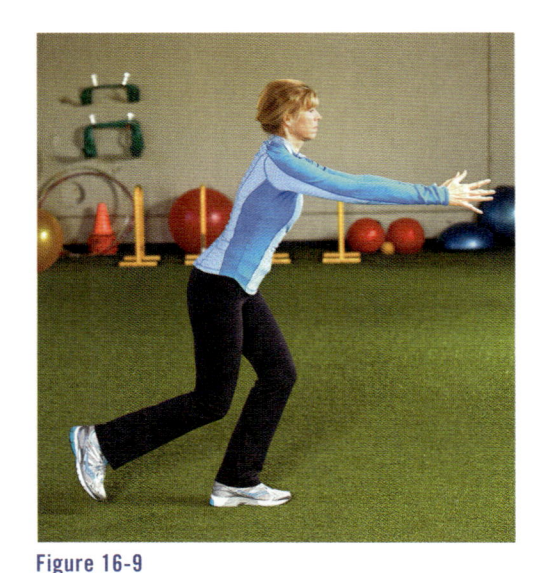

Figure 16-9
Single-leg squat. The client begins by balancing on one foot with the other leg flexed behind for counterbalance. The client initiates the movement by pulling the hips back (i.e., hip hinge), and then sinks the weight downward over the support-leg heel. It is essential that the patella tracks straight and the knee does not move medially or "cave in."

Arthritis   CHAPTER 16

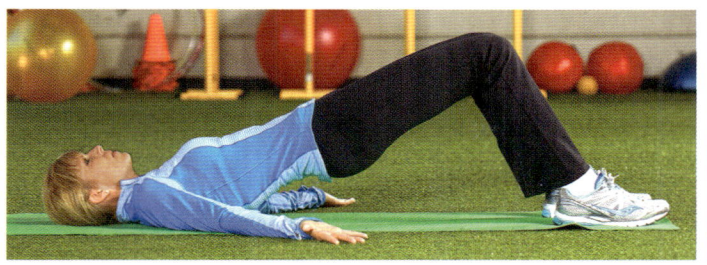

Figure 16-10
Glute bridge. The client lies supine with the feet about hip-width apart and the shoulders down with the arms out for support. The client presses through the heel and elevates the hips so that they are in a straight line with the knees and shoulders. The client engages the lower back, glutes, and hamstrings to help develop strength and endurance of the hip extensors.

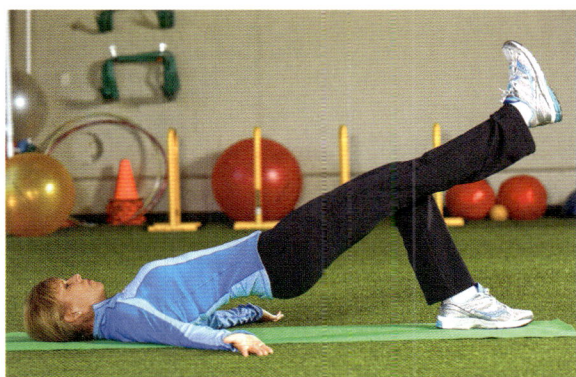

An advanced single-leg version of the glute bridge

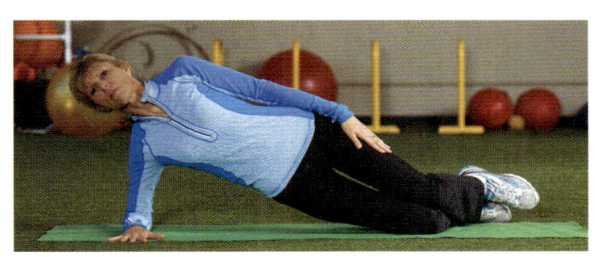

Figure 16-11
Side bridge. The client positions the elbow under the shoulder and the knees in line with the hips so that the body is straight, and then lifts the hips off the ground by engaging the deep muscles of the trunk. It is important the hips are straight and not "sagging" below the level of the shoulders.

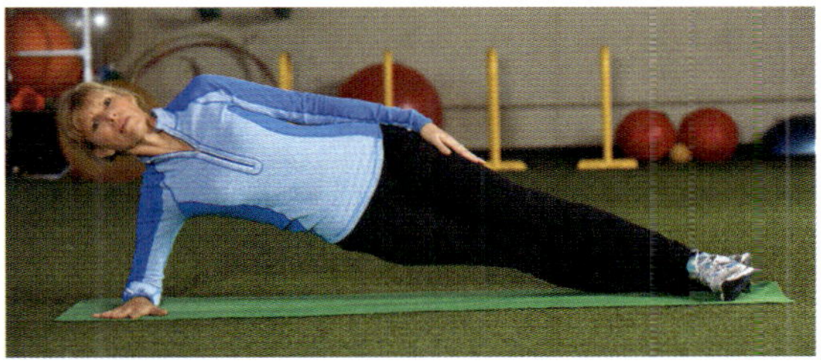

For a more advanced and challenging exercise, the client can support themself on the elbow and toes, again with the hips raised so that they are level with the line of the shoulders.

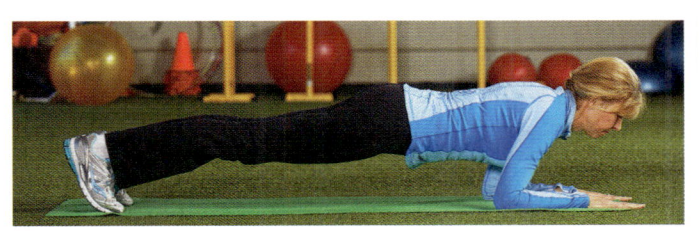

Figure 16-12
Prone plank. The client lies prone with the elbows on the floor and the feet flexed for support. They then lift the hips off the ground by engaging the abdominals, gluteals, hamstrings, and spinal extensor muscles so that the hips are level with the shoulders and knees.

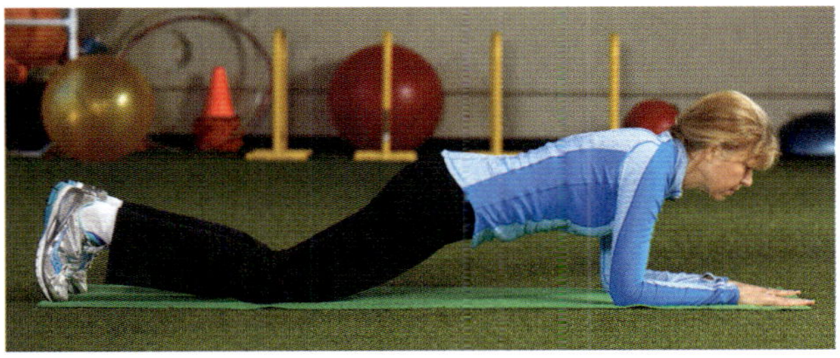

The CMES can modify this exercise by having the client put the knees down while keeping the hips level with the shoulders.

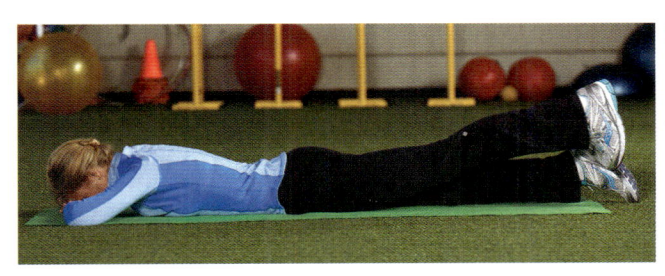

Figure 16-13
Prone hip extension. The client lies in a prone position with the hands under the forehead for support and then lifts the leg with the knee straight by engaging the gluteals and hamstrings. The CMES should watch for a "roll" of the torso away from the leg being lifted, as this is a sign of dysfunction of the hip extensors and of the pelvic/spine stabilizers.

Figure 16-14
Hip ROM complex
a. The client lies on their back and pulls the knee to the chest to feel the stretch in the gluteals, hamstrings, and opposite-side hip flexors.
b. The client pulls the knee to the same-side shoulder, stretching the hips and hamstrings while also targeting the adductors.
c. The foot is returned to the center and the knee is dropped to the outside to stretch the adductors. The CMES should ensure that the opposite hip is kept stable and does not roll toward the side being stretched.
d. The client pulls the leg across the body, stretching the lower back and hip abductors and extensors. Note that the shoulders are kept down and the arm is extended to the side for support.

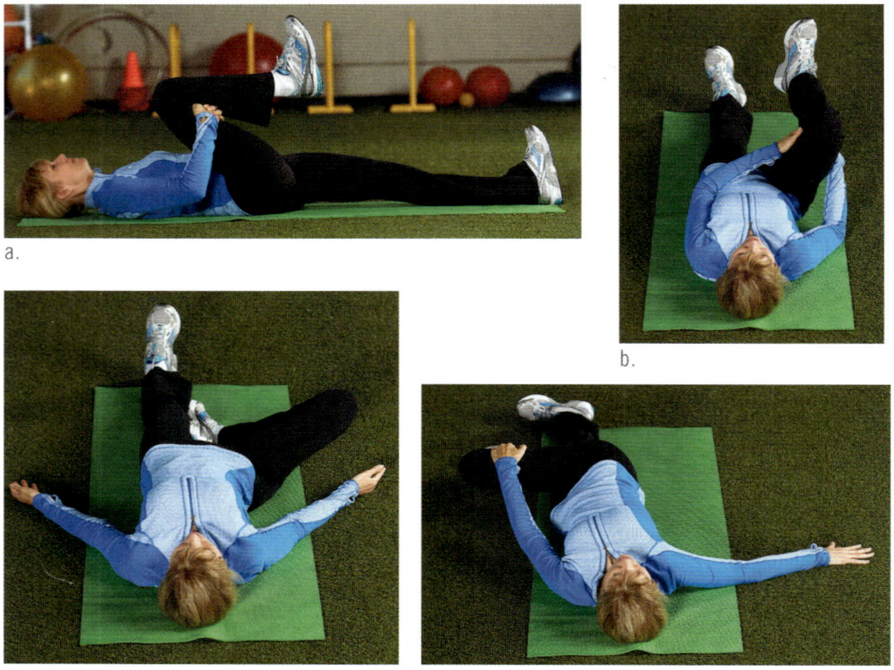

EXERCISE GUIDELINES SUMMARY FOR CLIENTS WITH ARTHRITIS

CARDIORESPIRATORY TRAINING	
Frequency	• 3–5 days per week
Intensity	• Below VT1 HR; can talk comfortably
	• Moderate (40–59% HRR or $\dot{V}O_2R$) to vigorous (≥60% HRR or $\dot{V}O_2R$) intensity*
	• Light intensity (e.g., 30–39% HRR or $\dot{V}O_2R$) may be necessary for deconditioned clients with arthritis.
Time	• Minutes per session will be dictated by the client's tolerance to exercise.
	• Accumulate 150 minutes per week of moderate intensity, 75 minutes of vigorous intensity, or a combination of the two in bouts of at least 10 minutes
Type	• A variety of rhythmic large-muscle-group exercises with low joint stress: ✓ Walking ✓ Cycling ✓ Swimming or aquatic exercise
	• High-impact activities such as running are not recommended for those with lower-extremity arthritis.
	• Balance training is recommended for individuals with lower-limb involvement to reduce the risk of falling.
Progression	• Progress following the ACE Integrated Fitness Training® Model based on client goals and availability.

MUSCULAR TRAINING	
Frequency	• 2–3 days per week
Intensity	• 50–80% 1-RM, with lower initial intensities
Time	• 1–3 sets of 8–12 repetitions
Type	• All major muscle groups
	• Include machines, free weights, resistance bands, tubing, and body weight
	• If an exercise is painful, select a new one targeting the same muscle groups and energy system.
Progression	• Progress following the ACE Integrated Fitness Training Model based on client goals and availability.

*Moderate intensity = Heart rates <VT1 where speech remains comfortable and is not affected by breathing; Vigorous intensity = Heart rates from ≥VT1 to <VT2 where clients feel unsure if speech is comfortable.
Note: HRR = Heart-rate reserve; $\dot{V}O_2R$ = Oxygen uptake reserve; 1-RM = One-repetition maximum; VT1 = First ventilatory threshold; VT2 = Second ventilatory threshold

Arthritis   CHAPTER 16

> **CMES FOCUS**
>
> The recommendations for exercise for healthy individuals generally apply to those with arthritis. However, a CMES who works with clients who have been diagnosed with arthritis must take into account individual factors, such as joint function and pain levels, and modify the exercise program accordingly. Low- to moderate-intensity aerobic exercise that does not place undue stress on the weight-bearing joints is appropriate for clients with arthritis. An adequate warm-up and cool-down and a focus on flexibility exercises are important for minimizing pain.
>
> Source: American College of Sports Medicine (2022). *ACSM's Guidelines for Exercise Testing and Prescription* (11th ed.). Philadelphia: Wolters Kluwer.

CASE STUDY

Client Information

A 46-year-old male Navy SEAL presents with a history of bilateral knee pain that has been increasing in intensity and frequency over the past four years. There is no history of a significant injury or surgery to either knee. At the time of initial evaluation, his daily activities of lifting weights and running in hard-soled boots on asphalt for 2 miles (3.2 km) [he was running 6 miles (9.7 km) a day but steadily decreased his distance over time due to increasing knee pain], were losing appeal to him due to the bilateral knee pain, with swimming being his only well-tolerated activity.

The client was well known among his fellow SEALs for more than 20 years for putting 40 pounds in a rucksack and running in the mountains, until bilateral knee pain forced him to stop. Although he attempted to keep running the mountains without the weighted rucksack, the pain was a persistent problem. The client had noted **atrophy** of his quadriceps for years and attempted to build them up with knee extension exercises, squats, and lunges, only to experience more knee pain and visible atrophy of his quadriceps. Finally, he sought medical attention. Examination revealed a disproportionate 6'3" 230-pound male (1.9 m; 103.5 kg) with an extremely well-developed upper body, while his lower extremities, most notably his quadriceps, showed significant atrophy. He has tight quadriceps, iliotibial band, adductors, hamstrings, and low-back muscles. The initial health-history interview revealed no history of injuries to his knees. The client revealed that he can walk short distances, but that he can no longer run due to knee pain. He admittedly avoids stairs and anything that requires him to squat. He is on permanent limited-duty status until his scheduled retirement date from the Navy due to chronic bilateral knee pain.

ACE IFT® MODEL AT A GLANCE

Cardiorespiratory Training

In this case study, the client's arthritis is the limiting factor for all movement. As a U.S. Navy SEAL, he would have achieved very high levels of cardiorespiratory fitness that would have allowed him to train in all phases of Cardiorespiratory Training, as his training cycles warranted programs at all intensity levels. Unfortunately, due to his arthritis and resultant knee issues, this client would be performing cardiorespiratory exercise at Base Training intensities and progressing to Fitness Training as tolerated based on pain levels during activity.

Muscular Training

The CMES developed a Functional Training program for this client, based almost entirely on rebuilding what had been lost due to pain, immobility, and atrophy associated with his arthritis. This program was put on hold when the client went for physical therapy sessions, and resumed six weeks later. As he regains muscular fitness, he can progress to Movement Training and eventually Load/Speed Training as his arthritis permits.

CMES Approach

In discussion with the client, he has no desire for total knee replacements except as a "last ditch measure." He has been on a plethora of anti-inflammatory drugs over the years with minimal relief from pain. His exercise program should factor in the many changes that have occurred to his daily lifestyle in accordance with recommendations from his physician, with the end goals of improving mobility as his pain decreases and regaining the size and the tone of his quadriceps via low-force, pain-free exercises, and enhancing the flexibility of the muscles of the lower extremities and lower back.

- In accordance with recommendations from his attending physician, he can manage the pain initially with Celebrex, 200 mg a day, along with CosaminDS, three tablets three times a day for the first two months. He and his physician have decided to discontinue the use of Celebrex after the initial two months over concerns of potential significant side effects, while continuing the CosaminDS at two tablets, three times a day.
- The client should eliminate boots whenever possible from his daily life and replace them with soft-soled shoes.
- The client should discontinue all running until he is 100% pain free, and then consider resuming a low-intensity, short-duration running program with input from his physician.
- He can use a bicycle with the seat in a high position for transportation around the base and for exercise.
- The client should avoid stairs and any activity that causes knee pain (such as full squats and lunges) due to the increased forces these movements place on the knee, especially during the descending, or eccentric, phase.
- The client should perform exercises with an emphasis on developing strength in the quadriceps and gluteal muscles. Terminal knee extension exercises are appropriate as long as the knee is kept within the final 30 degrees of extension. In this exercise, the client should hold the knee in full extension (while avoiding hyperextension) to see and feel the quadriceps and gluteal muscles contract for 10 seconds (see Figure 16-5). Squats should be performed within the 30-degree ROM with the back against the wall. The squats should be held for 10 seconds with an emphasis on an isometric quadriceps contraction. Exercising through a pain-free ROM on elliptical and step machines is acceptable, since both feet are on a surface (i.e., weight-bearing) at all times. He should not use a treadmill, as only one foot is on a surface at all times, thereby forcing one leg to accept the entire body weight with each step. The client should be encouraged to participate in **yoga** classes as frequently as possible, as long as they do not cause or increase knee pain.
- He should double the time spent in the pool, with a portion devoted to kicking on his back with fins, while not allowing the knees to break the surface of the water.
- The client should have a goal of weight reduction via a modification in dietary habits so that the weight will not simply be regained once his goal of 200 pounds (91 kg) is reached.
- The CMES should follow up in two weeks for reassessment specifically of the quadriceps and gluteal muscles.

The client was very cooperative due to frustration with prolonged and increasing pain, and his incredible focus and work ethic as a U.S. Navy SEAL. At the two-week follow-up, although his pain was significantly reduced, little gain had been made in the size and strength of his quadriceps and gluteal muscles, and thus the client was scheduled for physical therapy daily for 30 sessions of quadriceps electrical stimulation for 20 minutes per session.

After six weeks, the client comes back to the CMES to build on the work done during his physical therapy sessions. The CMES conducts new baseline assessments and notes that the client has much improved size and development of the quadriceps, and that he reports a decrease in pain and discomfort.

SUMMARY

Exercise is an essential tool for helping clients manage arthritis. When used in combination with medical interventions, exercise can help maintain function and reduce pain in an affected joint. Exercises that focus on developing the strength and endurance of muscles that surround the joint can reduce mechanical loading and lessen symptoms. Individual selection of progressive exercises that begin with unloaded **isometrics** and end with full weight-bearing exercises can be an effective method for maintaining joint ROM, strength, and endurance, and reducing joint pain. The CMES must take care to not introduce exercises or activities that have high loads or high strain rates, especially if the client has overweight.

REFERENCES

Albert, S.M. et al. (2008). Self-care and professionally guided care in osteoarthritis: Racial differences in a population-based sample. *Journal of Aging and Health,* 20, 198–216.

Aletaha, D. et al. (2010). 2010 Rheumatoid arthritis classification criteria: An American College of Rheumatology/European League Against Rheumatism collaborative initiative. *Arthritis and Rheumatism,* 62, 9, 2569–2481. DOI: 10.1002/art.27584

American College of Sports Medicine (2022). *ACSM's Guidelines for Exercise Testing and Prescription* (11th ed.) Philadelphia: Wolters Kluwer.

American College of Sports Medicine (2014). *ACSM's Resource Manual for Guidelines for Exercise Testing and Prescription* (6th ed.). Philadelphia: Wolters Kluwer/Lippincott Williams & Wilkins.

Arthritis Foundation (2019). *Arthritis by the Numbers: Book of Trusted Facts & Figures.* Atlanta, Ga.: Arthritis Foundation

Avina-Zubieta, J.A. et al. (2008). Risk of cardiovascular mortality in patients with rheumatoid arthritis: A meta-analysis of observational studies. *Arthritis and Rheumatism,* 59, 12, 1690–1697.

Baillet, A. et al. (2010). Efficacy of cardiorespiratory aerobic exercise in rheumatoid arthritis: Meta-analysis of randomized controlled trials. *Arthritis Care & Research (Hoboken),* 62, 984–992. DOI: 10.1002/acr.20146

Barbour, K.E. et al. (2017). Vital signs: Prevalence of doctor-diagnoses arthritis and arthritis-attributable activity limitation: United States, 2013–2015. *Morbidity and Mortality Weekly Report,* 66, 9, 246–253.

Bennell, K. & Hinman, R. (2005). Exercise as a treatment for osteoarthritis. *Current Opinion in Rheumatology,* 17, 5, 634–640.

Beukelman, T. et al. (2011). 2011 American College of Rheumatology recommendations for the treatment of juvenile idiopathic arthritis: Initiation and safety monitoring of therapeutic agents for the treatment of arthritis and systemic features. *Arthritis Care Research (Hoboken),* 63, 4, 465–482. DOI: 10.1002/acr.20460

Buckwalter, J.A. & Martin, J.A. (2006). Osteoarthritis. *Advanced Drug Delivery Reviews,* 58, 150–167.

Centers for Disease Control and Prevention (2020). *Osteoarthritis.* www.cdc.gov/arthritis/basics/osteoarthritis.htm#:~:text=OA%20affects%20over%2032.5%20million%20US%20adults

Centers for Disease Control and Prevention (2019a). *Arthritis: Comorbidities.* www.cdc.gov/arthritis/data_statistics/comorbidities.htm

Centers for Disease Control and Prevention (2019b). *Arthritis: Disabilities and Limitations.* www.cdc.gov/arthritis/data_statistics/disabilities-limitations.htm

Centers for Disease Control and Prevention (2018). *Arthritis: National Statistics.* www.cdc.gov/arthritis/data_statistics/national-statistics.html

Clegg, D.O. et al. (2006). Glucosamine, chondrointin sulfate, and the two in combination for painful knee osteoarthritis. *New England Journal of Medicine,* 35, 8, 795–808.

Cooper, C. et al. (2013). How to define responders in osteoarthritis. *Current Medical Research and Opinion,* 29, 6, 719–729. DOI: 10.1185/03007995.2013.792793

Cordingley, L. et al. (2012). Juvenile-onset inflammatory arthritis: A study of adolescents' beliefs about underlying cause. *Rheumatology* (Oxford), 51, 12, 2239–2245. DOI: 10.1093/rheumatology/kes216

Dawczynski, C. et al. (2011). Incorporation of n-3 PUFA and γ-linolenic acid in blood lipids and red blood cell lipics together with their influence on disease activity in patients with chronic inflammatory arthritis: A randomized controlled human intervention trial. *Lipids in Health and Disease,* 10, 130.

de Lorgeril, M. (2013). Mediterranean diet and cardiovascular disease: Historical perspective and latest evidence. *Current Atherosclerosis Reports,* 15, 12, 370.

Deutsch, L. (2007). Evaluation of the effect of Neptune Krill Oil on chronic inflammation and arthritic symptoms. *Journal of the American College of Nutrition,* 26, 39–48.

Elkan, A.C. et al. (2011). Low level of physical activity in women with rheumatoid arthritis is associated with cardiovascular risk factors but not with body fat mass: A cross sectional study. *BMC Musculoskeletal Disorders,* 12, 13. DOI: 10.1186/1471-2474-12-13

Esposito, K. et al. (2011). Mediterranean diet and weight loss: Meta-analysis of randomized controlled trials. *Metabolic Syndrome and Related Disorders,* 9, 1, 1–12.

Ettinger, W.H. et al. (1997). A randomized trial comparing aerobic exercise and resistance exercise with a health education program in older adults with knee osteoarthritis: The Fitness Arthritis and Seniors Trial (FAST). *Journal of the American*

Medical Association, 277, 1, 25–31.

Féart, C., Samieri, C., & Barberger-Gateau, P. (2010). Mediterranean diet and cognitive function in older adults. *Current Opinion in Clinical Nutrition and Metabolic Care,* 13, 1, 14–18.

Felson, D.T. et al. (2004). The effect of body weight on progression of knee osteoarthritis is dependent on alignment. *Arthritis and Rheumatism,* 50, 12, 3904–3909.

Fraenkel, L. et al. (2004). Treatment options in knee osteoarthritis: The patient's perspective. *Archives of Internal Medicine,* 164, 12, 1299–1304.

Fransen, M. et al. (2007). Physical activity for osteoarthritis management: A randomized controlled clinical trial evaluating hydrotherapy or Tai Chi classes. *Arthritis and Rheumatism,* 57, 3, 407–414.

Hewlett, S. et al. (2011). Self-management of fatigue in rheumatoid arthritis: A randomised controlled trial of group cognitive-behavioural therapy. *Annals of Rheumatic Disease,* 70, 6, 1060–1067.

Hinman, R.S., Haywood, S.E., & Day, A.R. (2007). Aquatic physical therapy for hip and knee osteoarthritis: Results of a single-blind randomized controlled trial. *Physical Therapy,* 87, 1, 32–43.

Hochberg, M.C. & Dougados, M. (2001). Pharmacological therapy of osteoarthritis. *Best Practice and Research Clinical Rheumatology,* 15, 4, 583–593.

Horvath, S.M., & Hollander, J.L. (1949). Intra-articular temperature as a measure of joint reaction. *Journal of Clinical Investigation,* 28, 3, 469.

Hurkmans, E. et al. (2009). Dynamic exercise programs (aerobic capacity and/or muscle strength training) in patients with rheumatoid arthritis. *Cochrane Database of Systematic Reviews,* Oct. 7, 4, CD006853. DOI: 1002/14651858.CD006853.pub2

Issa, S.N. & Sharma, L. (2006). Epidemiology of osteoarthritis: An update. *Current Rheumatology Reports,* 8, 1, 7–15.

Kaplan, M.J. (2010). Cardiovascular complications of rheumatoid arthritis: Assessment, prevention and treatment. *Rheumatic Disease Clinics of North America,* 36, 2, 405–426. DOI: 10.1016/j.rdc.2010.02.002

Kostoglou-Athanassiou, I., Athanassiou, L., & Athanassiou, P. (2020). The effects of omega-3 fatty acids on rheumatoid arthritis. *Mediterranean Journal of Rheumatology,* 31, 2, 190–194.

Lahiri, M. et al. (2012). Modifiable risk factors for RA: Prevention, better than cure? *Rheumatology (Oxford),* 51, 3, 499–512. DOI: 10.1093/rheumatology/ker299

Lopez, H.L (2012a). Nutritional interventions to prevent and treat osteoarthritis. Part I: Focus on fatty acids and macronutrients. *PM&R,* 4, S145–S154.

Lopez, H.L. (2012b). Nutrition interventions to prevent and treat osteoarthritis. Part II: Focus on micronutrients and supportive nutraceuticals. *PM&R,* 4, S155–S168.

Lund, H. et al. (2008). A randomized controlled trial of aquatic and land-based exercise in patients with knee osteoarthritis. *Journal of Rehabilitation Medicine,* 40, 2, 137–144.

Mandel, D.R., Eichas, K., & Holmes, J. (2010). Bacillus coagulans: A viable adjunct therapy for relieving symptoms of rheumatoid arthritis according to a randomized, controlled trial. *BMC Complementary and Alternative Medicine,* 10, 1.

Martini, A. (2012). Viewpoint: It is time to rethink juvenile idiopathic arthritis classification and nomenclature. *Annals of Rheumatic Disease.* DOI:10.1136/annrheumdis-2012-201388

McErlane F. et al. (2013). Validity of a three-variable Juvenile Arthritis Disease Activity Score in children with new-onset juvenile idiopathic arthritis. *Annals of Rheumatic Disease,* 72, 12, 1983–1988. DOI: 10.1136/annrheumdis-2012-202031

Metsios, G.S. et al. (2010). Vascular function and inflammation in rheumatoid arthritis: The role of physical activity. *The Open Cardiovascular Medicine Journal,* 4, 89–96.

Metsios, G.S. et al. (2009). Association of physical inactivity with increased cardiovascular risk in patients with rheumatoid arthritis. *European Journal of Cardiovascular Prevention and Rehabilitation,* 16, 188–194. DOI: 10.1097/HJR.0b013e3283271ceb

Mikesky, A.E. et al. (2006). Effects of strength training on the incidence and progression of knee osteoarthritis. *Arthritis and Rheumatism,* 55, 5, 690–699.

Moseley, J.B. et al. (2002). A controlled trial of arthroscopic surgery for osteoarthritis of the knee. *New England Journal of Medicine,* 347, 2, 81–88.

Namba, R.S. et al. (2005). Obesity and perioperative morbidity in total hip and total knee arthroplasty patients. *Journal of*

Arthroplasty, 20, 7, Suppl. 3, 46–50.

National Institutes of Health (2020). *Omega-3 Fatty Acids: Fact Sheet for Health Professionals.* https://ods.od.nih.gov/factsheets/Omega3FattyAcids-HealthProfessional/

Petty, R.E. et al. (2004). International League of Associations for Rheumatology classification of juvenile idiopathic arthritis: Second revision, Edmonton, 2001. *Journal of Rheumatology,* 31, 390–392.

Rennie, K.L. et al. (2003). Nutritional management of rheumatoid arthritis: A review of the evidence. *Journal of Human Nutrition and Dietetics,* 16, 97–109.

Repo, R.U. & Finlay, J.B. (1977). Survival of articular cartilage after controlled impact. *Journal of Bone & Joint Surgery,* 59, 3, 1068–1076.

Samson, D.J. et al. (2007). *Treatment of Primary and Secondary Osteoarthritis of the Knee.* Rockville, Md.: Agency for Healthcare Research and Quality, U.S. Department of Health and Human Services. Publication No. 07-E012.

Shea, B. et al. (2013). Folic acid and folinic acid for reducing side effects in patients receiving methotrexate for rheumatoid arthritis. *Cochrane Musculoskeletal Group.* DOI: 10.1002/14651858.CD000951.pub2

Sköldstam, L. et al. (2005). Weight reduction is not a major reason for improvement in rheumatoid arthritis from lacto-vegetarian, vegan or Mediterranean diets. *Nutrition Journal,* 4, 15–21.

Strasser, B., & Schobersberger, W. (2010). Evidence for resistance training as a treatment therapy in obesity. *Journal of Obesity,* Article ID 482564.

van Baar, M.E. et al. (1999). Effectiveness of exercise therapy in patients with osteoarthritis of the hip or knee: A systematic review of randomized clinical trials. *Arthritis and Rheumatism,* 42, 7, 1361–1369.

Wang, T.J. et al. (2007). Effects of aquatic exercise on flexibility, strength and aerobic fitness in adults with osteoarthritis of the hip or knee. *Journal of Advanced Nursing,* 57, 2, 141–152.

Zhang, W. et al. (2010). OARSI recommendations for the management of hip and knee osteoarthritis: Part III: Changes in evidence following systematic cumulative update of research published through January 2009. *Osteoarthritis and Cartilage,* 18, 4, 476–499. DOI: 10.1016/j.joca.2010.01.013

SUGGESTED READING

American College of Sports Medicine (2009). *ACSM's Exercise Management for Persons With Chronic Diseases and Disabilities* (3rd ed.). Champaign, Ill.: Human Kinetics.

Cooper, C. et al. (2013). How to define responders in osteoarthritis. *Current Medical Research and Opinion,* 29, 6, 719–729. DOI: 10.1185/03007995.2013.792793

Lahiri, M. et al. (2012). Modifiable risk factors for RA: Prevention, better than cure? *Rheumatology* (Oxford), 51, 3, 499–512. DOI: 10.1093/rheumatology/ker299

Zhang, W. et al. (2010). OARSI recommendations for the management of hip and knee osteoarthritis: Part III: Changes in evidence following systematic cumulative update of research published through January 2009. *Osteoarthritis and Cartilage,* 18, 4, 476–499. DOI: 10.1016/j.joca.2010.01.0139.

17 OSTEOPOROSIS AND OSTEOPENIA

IN THIS CHAPTER

EPIDEMIOLOGY

OVERVIEW OF OSTEOPOROSIS
FACTORS THAT AFFECT BONE

DIAGNOSTIC CRITERIA

TREATMENT OPTIONS FOR OSTEOPOROSIS AND OSTEOPENIA
NON-PHARMACOLOGICAL TREATMENT
PHARMACOLOGICAL TREATMENT
SURGICAL TREATMENT
EXERCISE TREATMENT

NUTRITIONAL CONSIDERATIONS FOR CLIENTS WITH OSTEOPOROSIS AND OSTEOPENIA

EXERCISE RECOMMENDATIONS FOR CLIENTS WITH OSTEOPOROSIS AND OSTEOPENIA
PHYSICAL ACTIVITY AND BONE RESPONSE IN CHILDREN AND ADOLESCENTS
PHYSICAL ACTIVITY AND BONE RESPONSE IN PREMENOPAUSAL WOMEN
PHYSICAL ACTIVITY AND BONE RESPONSE IN POSTMENOPAUSAL WOMEN
PHYSICAL ACTIVITY AND BONE RESPONSE IN MEN
PROGRAMMING AND PROGRESSION GUIDELINES

EXERCISE GUIDELINES SUMMARY FOR CLIENTS AT RISK FOR OSTEOPOROSIS

EXERCISE GUIDELINES SUMMARY FOR CLIENTS WITH OSTEOPOROSIS

CASE STUDIES

SUMMARY

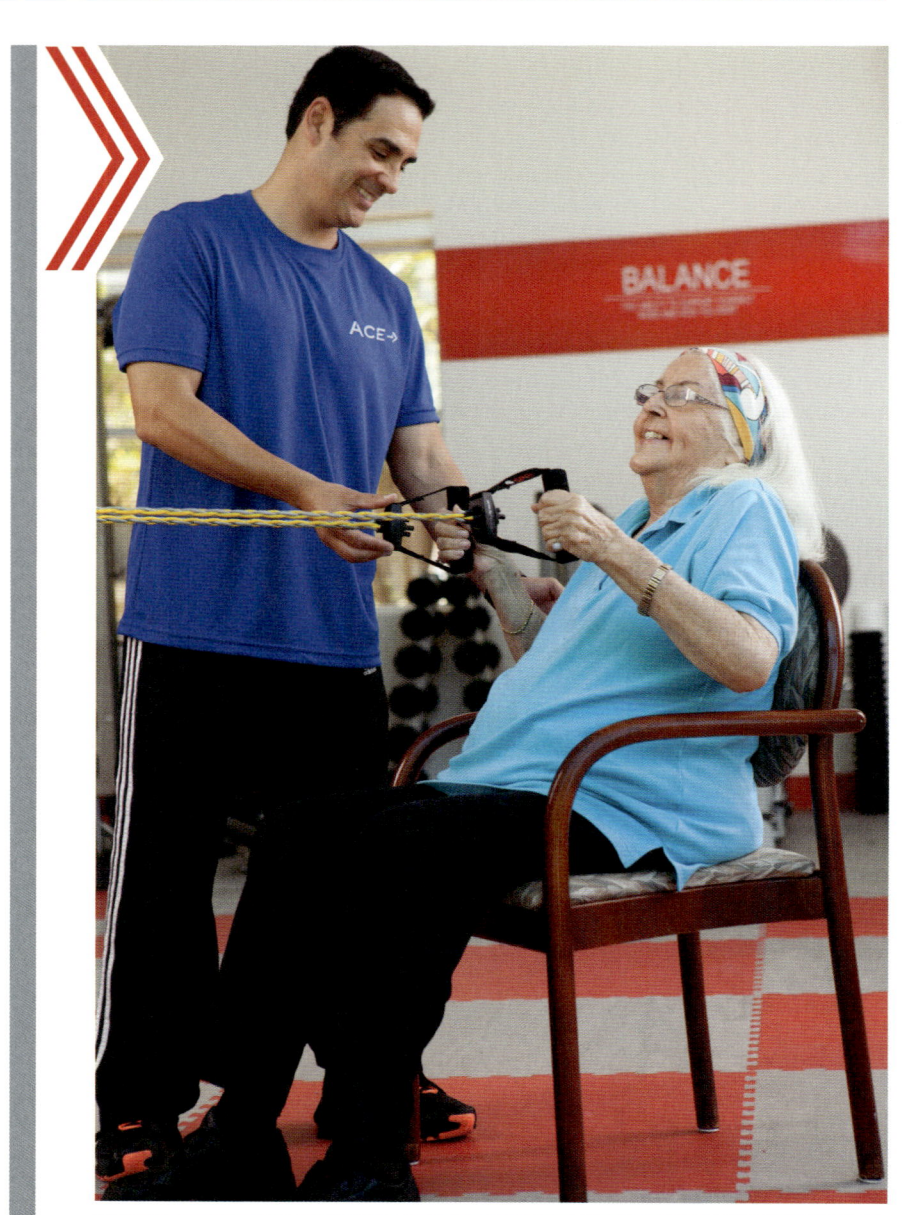

ABOUT THE AUTHOR

Kara A. Witzke, Ph.D., is program lead of the Kinesiology Department at Oregon State University-Cascades in Bend, Ore. She has worked in industry and various wellness venues around the country and has promoted wellness and lifestyle management to children and adults of all ages through education, research, and community involvement. Dr. Witzke serves as a subject matter expert for the ACE® certification and exam-development department and is an ACE media spokesperson. Her work focuses on the implementation of exercise for populations with chronic disease and the effects of exercise on bone health.

By Kara A. Witzke

OSTEOPOROSIS IS DEFINED CONCEPTUALLY AS a condition of generalized skeletal fragility (very low bone mass) that increases the risk of fracture with minimal trauma. **Osteopenia** refers to reduced skeletal mass (low bone mass) that, while not as severe as osteoporosis, may still warrant close monitoring to ensure that the condition does not worsen.

EPIDEMIOLOGY

Osteoporosis is the most prevalent disease affecting the skeleton. It is characterized by low bone mass and deterioration of the microarchitecture of the bone, resulting in structural weakness and an increased risk for fracture. It is one of the most important public health issues in America because of its prevalence. According to the National Osteoporosis Foundation (NOF), 10 million Americans aged 50 and older have osteoporosis, with the majority being women (77 to 80%), and in 2016 more than 1.6 million osteoporotic fractures occurred (Hansen et al., 2019). Interestingly, fracturing the hip increases the likelihood of later hospitalizations by 231% and increases the probability of death by 83% over the following eight years (Hansen et al., 2019).

Osteoporotic fractures are most common in the proximal femur (hip), vertebrae (spine), and **distal** forearm (wrist). However, osteoporosis is really a systemic disease, and individuals with low bone mass are at an increased risk of all types of fractures. Adults who fracture are 50 to 100% more likely to fracture again in a different location (Wu et al., 2002). Hip fractures are by far the most devastating type of fracture due to their strong association with low bone mass, the cost to repair, and the level of disability that often accompanies them even post-surgery. Hip fracture incidence rates increase exponentially with age in both men and women, due to both age-related declines in bone density (a surrogate measure for bone fragility) and an increase in falls, which are responsible for more than 90% of all hip fractures (Marks, 2010; Hayes et al., 1996).

An estimated 33.6 million Americans (80% of them women), have osteopenia, a condition of low, but not very low, bone mass. The usefulness of labeling such individuals, whose **bone mineral density (BMD)** may actually be within a "normal" range, has been questioned, but osteopenia can be viewed not unlike elevated blood pressure, impaired fasting **glucose,** and borderline high **cholesterol** in defining an intermediate-risk group with somewhat uncertain boundaries. Although fracture risk is still greater in individuals with osteoporosis rather than osteopenia, the much larger number of persons with osteopenia means that this group represents a substantial portion of the population at risk for fracture (Khosla & Melton, 2007).

Because women live longer and experience more age-related bone loss and falls than men, their incidence of hip fracture is also about two to three times that seen in men (Cummings & Melton, 2002). However, when men suffer a hip fracture due to osteoporosis, they do not fare as well as women afterward. Bass and colleagues (2007) found that in a large study of hip fractures in elderly individuals, 32% of men died within one year of the incident (compared to just 18% of women). Age-adjusted rates of hip fracture are highest in Scandinavian and North American populations, and seven times lower in southern European countries and in Asian or African populations (Melton & Cooper, 2001). It should be noted that although Asian populations are at an increased risk for osteoporosis, they suffer relatively few fractures, probably due to decreased rates of falling.

LEARNING OBJECTIVES:

» Describe the difference between osteoporosis and osteopenia.

» Explain the importance of proper nutrition and adequate physical activity throughout the lifespan and how these factors affect bone accumulation and/or loss.

» Describe how osteoporosis affects women versus men.

» Explain the basic diagnostic criteria and treatment options associated with osteoporosis and osteopenia.

» Design and implement safe and effective exercise programs for clients who are at risk for, and who have been diagnosed with, osteoporosis.

The epidemiology of vertebral fractures is different than that of hip fractures. While only about one-third of all vertebral fractures identified by x-ray come to a specialist's attention, less than 10% result in hospital admissions. These fractures can cause pain and disability. The occurrence of one vertebral fracture signifies a 20% risk for an additional vertebral fracture within one year and an increased risk for kyphosis of the thoracic spine (Bergstrom et al., 2011). Approximately 66% of patients who have vertebral compression fractures become asymptomatic after several months. However, these fractures heal in a malaligned position, so it is important for the patient to restore stability and anatomic alignment as soon as safely possible (Marcucci & Brandi, 2010). Most vertebral fractures do not result from falls, but rather from routine activities such as bending or lifting light objects (Cooper et al., 1992).

OVERVIEW OF OSTEOPOROSIS

Figure 17-1
Trabecular and cortical bone

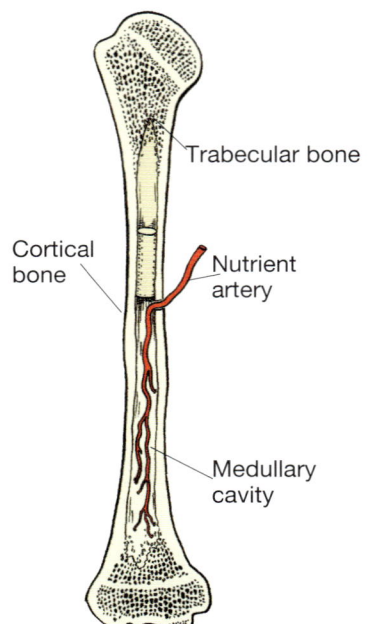

Bone is a unique tissue with enormous responsibilities. The simple task of supporting loads imposed on it requires that bone have incredible strength and resilience, while also being lightweight and adaptable so that locomotion is not a metabolic burden. Bone consists of an organic component (20 to 25% by weight), an inorganic component (70 to 75% by weight), and a water component (5% by weight). The organic component is primarily composed of type I collagen and some bone cells, while the inorganic component is almost all mineral (crystalline calcium hydroxyapatite).

The human skeleton is composed of two types of bone: cortical (compact) and trabecular (spongy). An important difference between **cortical bone** and **trabecular bone** is in the way the bone matrix and cellular components are arranged. Calcium comprises 80 to 90% of cortical bone volume, but only 15 to 25% of trabecular bone volume. Cortical bone forms a dense shell around all bones and constitutes the thick shafts of long bones, while trabecular bone is found in the vertebrae and in the ends of long bones (Figure 17-1). Trabecular bone forms a lattice-like network, which greatly increases its surface area for metabolic activity. As a result, trabecular bone undergoes far more remodeling cycles during an individual's lifetime than does cortical bone (Fonseca et al., 2014). A remodeling cycle consists of a bone **resorption** (removal) stage that is followed by a period of new bone formation. Through this coupled process, bone is constantly renewed.

During growth and young adulthood, the rate of bone formation is faster than the rate of bone resorption, leading to an overall gain in bone mineral. This is called **bone modeling.** Modeling improves bone strength not only by adding mass, but also by expanding the inner and outer diameters of bone. This allows bone to adapt its shape according to the loads imposed, which maximizes its strength and resistance to fracture. **Bone remodeling,** on the other hand, is a locally coordinated activity of **osteoclasts** (bone resorption cells) and **osteoblasts** (bone formation cells), whereby bone can both prevent and repair damage caused by everyday loading. A key feature of remodeling is that it replaces damaged tissue with an equal amount of new bone tissue.

Figure 17-2
Normal versus osteoporotic trabecular bone

© Fotosearch
www.fotosearch.com

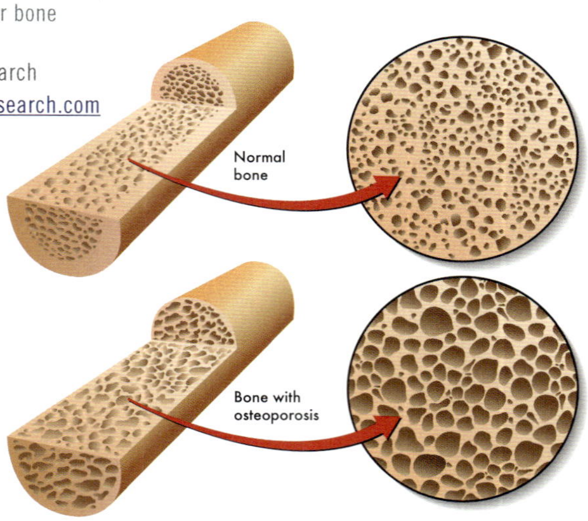

In the aging and osteoporotic skeleton, however, the balance between the amount of bone being resorbed and the amount being formed is unequal, favoring bone resorption. This causes a net loss of bone that eventually causes bone strength and integrity to be compromised (Figure 17-2).

Factors That Affect Bone

While the effects of physical activity on bone are undeniable, these positive effects account for only approximately 10% of bone mineral in the population as a whole. The remaining 90% of bone mineral is accounted for by a combination of other factors such as family history of fracture, gender, age, race, disorders associated with osteoporosis (e.g., **type 1 diabetes, hyperthyroidism,** and **rheumatoid arthritis**), hormones, lifestyle factors (e.g., smoking and alcohol), nutrition, medication, and soft-tissue composition (i.e., lean and fat mass). These factors interact with each other and their degree of influence varies based on the stage of life and the skeletal site.

Age, Sex, Genetics, and Race

Bone mineral is accrued at various rates throughout early childhood and adolescence, and then diminishes with aging. This normal, age-related process causes a net loss of approximately 5 to 10% of bone mineral per decade and begins some time after the cessation of longitudinal growth and the achievement of peak bone mass (in the third decade) (Snow-Harter & Marcus, 1991). Bone resorption in women is especially rapid during the first five years following menopause (if pharmacotherapy is not implemented), and may cause a loss of 3 to 5% of overall bone mass per year. These age-related bone mineral decrements are not as pronounced in men, primarily because men reach a higher peak BMD, have larger bones that afford a biomechanical resistance to fracture, and do not experience the same rapid postmenopausal bone loss as women. For individuals diagnosed with osteoporosis, it is often impossible to expect to build back significant amounts of bone mineral.

BMD appears to be controlled by a combination of several genes, which may also display important interactive effects with environmental factors (such as physical activity and calcium intake). Nevertheless, familial studies have shown that BMD is strongly influenced by parental bone mass (McKay et al., 1994; Tylavsky et al., 1989), and these assumptions are supported by research that shows very little variation between identical twins (Krall & Dawson-Hughes, 1993). Although various genes [such as those encoding the vitamin-D receptor, collagen Ia1, LDL receptor-related protein 5 (LRP5), and estrogen receptor] have some relation to BMD, attempts to relate them to fracture risk have generally been unsuccessful (Sambrook & Cooper, 2006).

Race implies similar genetic characteristics in a population, perhaps even among individuals in a similar environment, that interact with genes to cause the expression of a particular trait. Studies have confirmed that compared with whites, black adults have higher BMD at both the hip and spine and an increased cortical thickness. Lower fracture rates at both the hip and spine have also been reported in many studies (Aloia et al., 1996; Griffin et al., 1992). Although rates of bone loss appear similar for black and white individuals, it is estimated that African-American women have a 50% lower risk of fracture than Caucasian women (Eskridge et al., 2010). Similar lower fracture rates have also been shown for Hispanic and Asian populations (Maggi et al., 1991).

Hormones

The endocrine system is highly involved in the regulation of the biologic processes that control bone. The hormones involved in these processes belong to one of two classes, either "controlling" or "influencing" serum calcium levels and the levels of other agents related to bone. Controlling hormones include **parathyroid hormone (PTH),** vitamin D, and **calcitonin.** These hormones induce responses based on plasma concentrations of calcium. Influencing hormones, such as **estrogen, progesterone, testosterone, growth hormone, insulin-like growth factor I (IGF-I), corticosteroids,** and **thyroid hormone,** also modify calcium metabolism, but in response to other factors besides plasma calcium concentrations.

Estrogen has both direct and indirect effects on bone. Directly, estrogen decreases bone remodeling (turnover) through a complex interaction with the estrogen receptor on osteoblasts and by inhibiting other hormones that would normally stimulate osteoclast production. In this way, estrogen maintains bone mass by limiting resorption. Estrogen may also exhibit indirect effects on bone through the parathyroid gland, gut, and kidneys. Specifically, estrogen may lower the sensitivity of PTH to serum calcium levels that would promote mineralization by reducing bone turnover. It may also increase reabsorption of calcium via the kidneys by stimulating vitamin D and calcitonin production, which would also limit bone turnover.

Evidence has been presented about the influence of oral contraceptives on bone mass. In a systematic review of 86 studies published between 1966 and August 2005 that reported on fracture or BMD outcomes by use of combined hormonal contraceptives, researchers report that studies of adolescent and young adult women generally found lower BMD among users of combined oral contraceptives than among non-users. Evidence for premenopausal adult women suggested no differences in BMD between oral contraceptive users and non-users, and use in perimenopausal and postmenopausal women generally preserved bone mass, while non-users lost BMD (Martins, Curtis, & Glasier, 2006). Oral contraceptive pills are often prescribed to female athletes for treatment of menstrual irregularities, but it is still fairly unclear whether BMD improves in these women. It seems as though estrogen-containing pills are more beneficial (or less harmful) to bone in premenopausal women than progesterone-only derivations such as depot medroxyprogesterone acetate (Depo Provera) (Curtis & Martins, 2006).

During the third trimester of pregnancy, estrogen levels are high, but during lactation, mothers become hypoestrogenic as prolactin becomes a dominant hormone. A lactating mother secretes about 200 to 300 mg/day of calcium into her breast milk, which represents a considerable proportion of the calcium intake for many lactating women. Maternal bone lost as a result of breastfeeding seems to be recoverable upon weaning (Laskey et al., 2011).

Lifestyle Factors

Lifestyle factors such as smoking and alcohol consumption may adversely affect bone. Smoking seems to have a detrimental effect on both pre- and postmenopausal bone density via increased bone resorption and decreased calcium absorption (Tudor-Locke & McColl, 2000).

Excessive alcohol consumption also appears to exert a direct toxic effect on bone. While studies consistently show bone irregularities in alcoholics, moderate alcohol consumption may be associated with a slight increase in bone via increases in **estradiol** concentrations. It does not appear that moderate alcohol consumption (up to 1 drink per day for women and up to 2 drinks per day for men) is deleterious to bone density, but clients should be cautioned against the potential effects of an alcoholic lifestyle on bone (Tudor-Locke & McColl, 2000).

EXPAND YOUR KNOWLEDGE

WOMEN AND OSTEOPOROSIS

As noted earlier, osteoporosis disproportionately affects women [i.e., >50% of all women who live beyond 50 years of age will experience osteoporosis, compared to only 20% of men of the same age (NOF, 2014)]. Young athletic women and menopausal women have an elevated risk for developing osteoporosis due to hormonal and lifestyle factors.

The Female Athlete Triad

The term **female athlete triad** describes a condition consisting of a combination of energy deficiency, menstrual disturbances/**amenorrhea**, and decreased bone mass/osteoporosis in athletic women. This combination of factors may increase a woman's risk of a premature fracture. The pattern of the triad is more typical in athletes who believe that they will receive a performance advantage by having lower body weight (e.g., gymnasts, dancers, figure skaters, and long-distance runners). Dieting behavior usually becomes very restrictive and the pathogenic weight-control behaviors predispose a woman to menstrual dysfunction and eventually compromised bone mass. In this way, the triad disorders are interrelated and the existence of one component is linked, directly or indirectly, to the others (Beals & Meyer, 2007).

The mechanism of bone loss in athletic women with menstrual disturbances has been debated and the original position stand published in 1997 by the American College of Sports Medicine (ACSM) has been revised. ACSM's October 2007 position stand reflects newer evidence that estrogen deficiency is probably not the primary mechanism of bone loss in these athletes, but rather a combination of low estrogen and, more importantly, chronic undernutrition that reduces the rate of bone formation (Nattiv et al., 2007). A well-designed study by Zanker and Swaine (1998) evaluated biochemical markers of bone turnover in active women. Their work showed that women distance runners with long-term amenorrhea have reduced bone formation, compared to eumenorrheic runners and **sedentary** age-matched eumenorrheic women. Low BMD appears to be much less responsive to estrogen therapy in premenopausal amenorrheic women. This work helps explain why treatment with estrogen in amenorrheic women has not led to the same gains in bone mass as it has with postmenopausal women.

Screening for the triad requires an understanding of the relationships among the three components. Athletes who present with one of the components of the triad should always be evaluated for the others. If an ACE Certified Medical Exercise Specialist (CMES) suspects that a client may have an eating disorder (restrictive/purging behaviors) and/or menstrual dysfunction, the client should be referred to the appropriate healthcare provider for follow-up.

Menopause

Menopause marks a time of dramatic change in reproductive hormone secretion in women, characterized by estrogen and progesterone deficiency that causes menstrual cycles to cease. The average onset of natural menopause is about 45 to 50 years of age. Clinically, menopause is retrospectively diagnosed when a woman has not had a menstrual period for one year. Changes and symptoms, which usually start several years earlier, as marked by the "perimenopausal" period, include:

- A change in periods—shorter or longer, lighter or heavier, with more or less time in between
- Hot flashes and/or night sweats
- Trouble sleeping
- Vaginal dryness
- Mood swings
- Trouble focusing
- Less hair on the head and more on the face

The early phase of postmenopausal estrogen and progesterone withdrawal that occurs during the first three to five years after menopause is characterized by rapid bone loss (up to 3 to 5% of total bone mass per year), increased circulating plasma levels of calcium, and increased renal calcium excretion (Borer, 2005). Estrogen replacement therapy is most effective at reducing bone loss during this early menopausal period, while calcium supplementation is less effective. After the first five years following menopause, the rate of bone loss decreases back to premenopausal rates of loss (about 1% of total bone mass per year).

DIAGNOSTIC CRITERIA

The operational definitions of osteoporosis and osteopenia relate to BMD scores, which are usually measured by **dual-energy x-ray absorptiometry (DXA)**. In 1994, the WHO adopted the diagnostic criteria represented in Table 17-1. These criteria have been widely accepted as both diagnostic and intervention thresholds. However, because these criteria were developed primarily based on data from Caucasian postmenopausal women and took into consideration only bone

TABLE 17-1

DIAGNOSTIC CATEGORIES OF BONE MINERAL DENSITY

Diagnostic Category	Criterion
Normal	A value for BMD or BMC that is within 1.0 SD of the reference mean for young adults
Low bone mass (osteopenia)	A value for BMD or BMC that is more than 1.0 but less than 2.5 SD below the mean for young adults
Osteoporosis	A value for BMD or BMC that is 2.5 SD or more below the mean for young adults
Severe osteoporosis (established osteoporosis)	A value for BMD or BMC that is 2.5 SD or more below the mean for young adults in combination with one or more fragility (low-trauma) fractures

Note: The WHO BMD diagnostic classification should not be applied to premenopausal women, men <50 years old, or children. BMD = Bone mineral density; BMC = Bone mineral content; SD = Standard deviation

Source: World Health Organization (1994). *Assessment of Fracture Risk and Its Application to Screening for Postmenopausal Osteoporosis: Report of a WHO Study Group.* Geneva: WHO Technical Report Series, No. 843.

mineral density in the prediction of fracture risk, and the reality that DXA is not available to everyone, new criteria were developed by the WHO at a consensus meeting of experts in 2004. Published in 2007 (WHO, 2007), these proceedings introduced a new method of assessing fracture risk that includes BMD (when available) and other selected risk factors such as height, weight, fracture history, and behaviors known to affect bone. A tool called the Fracture Risk Assessment Tool, or FRAX (Figure 17-3), uses a regression model to assess one's risk for fracture. Soon after the release of the FRAX tool, the NOF developed a set of criteria for determining when U.S. Food & Drug Administration (FDA)–approved pharmaceutical treatment may be necessary. These criteria apply to postmenopausal women of any race or ethnicity and men over the age of 50 (NOF, 2010):

- History of fracture of the hip or spine
- BMD in the osteoporosis range: T-score less than –2.5
- BMD in the osteopenia range (T-score between –1.0 and –2.5) with a higher fracture risk determined by FRAX score for:
  ✓ Major osteoporotic fracture 10-year probability of 20% or higher OR
  ✓ Hip fracture 10-year probability of 3% or higher

The NOF (2014) guidelines indicate that BMD testing should be performed on:

- Women aged 65 and older
- Men aged 70 and older
- Anyone who breaks a bone after 50 years of age
- Younger postmenopausal women with risk factors
- Postmenopausal women under age 65 with risk factors
- Men aged 50 to 69 with risk factors

Note: Medicare covers BMD testing for the following individuals aged 65 and older and permits individuals to repeat BMD testing every two years:

- Estrogen-deficient women at clinical risk for osteoporosis
- Individuals with vertebral abnormalities
- Individuals receiving, or planning to receive, long-term glucocorticoid (steroid) therapy
- Individuals with primary hyperparathyroidism
- Individuals being monitored to assess the response or efficacy of an approved osteoporosis drug therapy

Scientists and researchers are interested in the measurement of bone's shape and size (anatomy), strength (biomechanics), and metabolic activity (biochemistry), and the development and adaptation capabilities of bone. Clinicians see bone a little differently, because they view bone as tissue that provides structure and permits the body to move. They generally are interested in preserving or reestablishing those functions and in predicting fracture risk. In this case, bone imaging *in vivo* provides the most important information about bone. The most commonly used methods for imaging bone for clinical purposes include DXA, **quantitative ultrasound (QUS),** and **quantitative computed tomography (QCT).**

DXA is probably the most widely used method of clinical evaluation of BMD and risk for fracture. DXA uses a low-dose x-ray that emits photons at two different energy levels. BMD is calculated based on the amount of photon energy attenuated (absorbed) by the different body tissues (bone, muscle, and fat). Bone attenuates the most energy, followed by muscle and then fat, based on their relative tissue densities. In this way, DXA can not only measure bone density, but also **body composition,** and is arguably the new "gold standard" against which other techniques are compared. Regional sites such as the lumbar spine, proximal femur (hip), and distal wrist are the most commonly measured sites for assessment of fracture risk. BMD is reported in units equal to bone mineral content divided by the area of the region of interest (g/cm^2). In this way, BMD is not a true "volumetric" density, but rather an "areal" density. The advantages of DXA, when compared to other methods, include its ease of measurement (five to 10 minutes), low radiation exposure (about equal to the amount received flying across the country), high accuracy and precision, and the ability to measure small changes in BMD over time. Disadvantages of DXA include the fact that it provides no measure of bone architecture, because it does not distinguish between trabecular and cortical bone. It is therefore difficult to determine material properties of bone, including bone strength, using DXA.

QUS is another popular method of determining bone status, especially as a "field test" due to its portability and the fact that no ionizing radiation is used. Two ultrasound transducers are positioned on each side of the tissue to be measured (commonly the heel). QUS does not measure bone density, but rather speed of sound (SOS) and broadband ultrasound attenuation (BUA). SOS is expressed as the quotient of the time taken to pass through the bone and the dimension that it passed through (expressed in m/s). Although the sensitivity of QUS is not enough for a clinical osteoporosis diagnosis, its advantages include low cost, no radiation, and the identification of comprehensive information on both bone mass and the microstructure of the bone. Hence, QUS has been recommended as an effective screening technique (Liu et al., 2012).

QCT provides two advantages over DXA in that it can provide a three-dimensional measure (true volumetric density; mg/cm^3) of trabecular and cortical bone. For this reason, it can also be used to study the trabecular structure, which makes it quite attractive for researchers in particular, though it is also useful for clinicians to monitor age-related bone loss and to follow patients with osteoporosis or other metabolic bone diseases. However, this technology has several disadvantages, including poor precision and accuracy, as well as radiation doses 125 times higher than a standard regional DXA scan. It is also limited to peripheral regions and the lumbar spine, so it not useful for determining qualities of bone at the hip. Newer peripheral quantitative computed tomography (pQCT) units that are typically used in research to measure bone in the tibia/fibula region have improved precision and accuracy, but still expose the patient to higher radiation doses than DXA and cannot be used at clinically relevant fracture sites such as the hip and spine.

EXPAND YOUR KNOWLEDGE

The World Health Organization has adopted a scientifically validated tool that predicts the 10-year probability of sustaining an osteoporosis-related fracture, called the WHO Fracture Risk Assessment Tool, or FRAX (www.shef.ac.uk/FRAX). This tool enhances patient assessment by integrating clinical risk factors alone or in combination with known BMD.

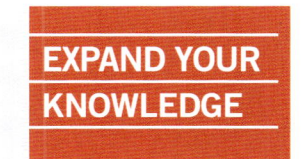

The FRAX models were developed after studying population-based cohorts from Europe, North America, Asia, and Australia. Figure 17-3 presents the calculation tool for the United States, which is presented on the website alongside country-specific notes and risk-factor information.

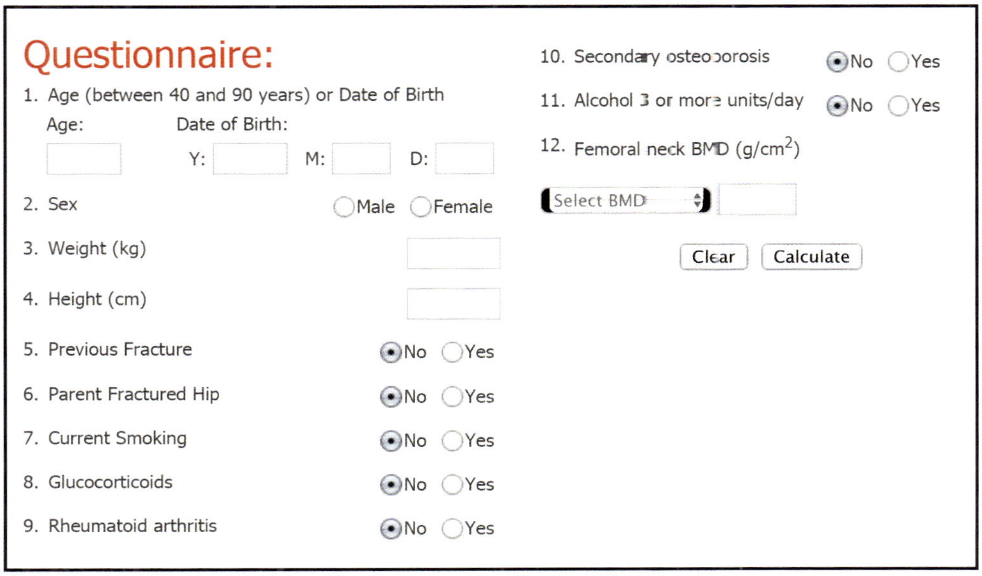

Figure 17-3
A screen shot of the FRAX tool. To assess your client's risk go to www.shef.ac.uk/FRAX/tool.aspx?country=9

Reprinted with permission from World Health Organization Collaborating Centre for Metabolic Bone Diseases, University of Sheffield, UK. www.shef.ac.uk/FRAX. FRAX® is a sophisticated risk-assessment instrument, developed by the University of Sheffield in association with the World Health Organization. It uses risk factors in addition to DXA measurements for improved fracture-risk estimation. It is a useful tool to aid clinical decision making about the use of pharmacologic therapies in patients with low bone mass. The International Osteoporosis Foundation (IOF) supports the maintenance and development of FRAX. Reprinted with permission from the IOF.

Questionnaire:
1. Age (between 40 and 90 years) or Date of Birth
   Age: Date of Birth: Y: M: D:
2. Sex   ○ Male ○ Female
3. Weight (kg)
4. Height (cm)
5. Previous Fracture   ● No ○ Yes
6. Parent Fractured Hip   ● No ○ Yes
7. Current Smoking   ● No ○ Yes
8. Glucocorticoids   ● No ○ Yes
9. Rheumatoid arthritis   ● No ○ Yes
10. Secondary osteoporosis ● No ○ Yes
11. Alcohol 3 or more units/day ● No ○ Yes
12. Femoral neck BMD (g/cm^2)
    [Select BMD ▼]

[Clear] [Calculate]

TREATMENT OPTIONS FOR OSTEOPOROSIS AND OSTEOPENIA

Since most fractures occur as a result of falls, a reduction in the risk for falls is an important goal of clinicians, as well as the CMES. Strategies to reduce fracture risk should emphasize lifestyle modifications such as optimal nutrition, smoking cessation, moderate alcohol and caffeine intake, and exercise that provides adequate bone loading. Emphasis should also be placed on reducing the risk of falls, including improving home safety by reducing tripping hazards; maintaining eyesight through regular vision check-ups and updates for prescription lenses; and improving muscle strength, power, and balance. Hip protector pads are sometimes used to help dissipate the forces sustained in a fall, although compliance in wearing the hip pads is an issue. On a mechanistic level, drugs can be used to help reduce bone resorption or increase bone formation, and, although they do nothing to mediate fall risk, they could help prevent a fracture in the case of a fall.

Non-pharmacological Treatment

Lifestyle modifications are central to decreasing the risk for osteoporosis and resultant fractures. An optimal diet to improve the prevention and management of osteoporosis includes adequate caloric intake (to avoid malnutrition), and adequate calcium and vitamin D intake (see Table 17-3, page 568). Regular exercise benefits bone health in children and adults as a result of increased bone density, volume, and strength and increased muscle strength. Exercise may also improve balance, which can help reduce osteoporotic fracture risk and falls (ACSM, 2022).

Pharmacological Treatment

Most of the drugs with current FDA approval for the management of postmenopausal osteoporosis are called "antiresorptives." These include estrogens, calcitonin, bisphosphonates, selective estrogen receptor modulators (SERMs), and receptor activator of nuclear factor kappa-beta ligand (RANKL) inhibitors (Table 17-2).

After the publication of the Women's Health Initiative study in 2002 (Rossouw et al., 2002), the role of long-term postmenopausal hormone therapy (both estrogen alone and estrogen and progesterone in combination) for the prevention and management of osteoporosis became controversial. The study population consisted of women 50 to 79 years old, many of whom had cardiovascular risk factors. Women were not specifically selected for low bone mass, as is the case in most osteoporosis trials. While both trials did find substantial reductions in subsequent osteoporotic fractures, controversy arose when the results showed an elevated risk for stroke and cardiovascular events with combined hormone therapy, especially if women over the age of 70 began treatment. Although the data suggest a different risk profile for combination therapy versus estrogen alone, the results support the recommendation that hormone therapy should be avoided in favor of alternative antiresorptive agents, and that hormone therapy should remain an option only for short-term early use around menopause in symptomatic women at risk for fracture (Sambrook & Cooper, 2006).

Calcitonin is a hormone that inhibits osteoclastic activity, thus reducing bone resorption. Calcitonin derived from human, pig, salmon, and eel have all been used in studies of osteoporosis and have shown effectiveness in both increasing low bone mass and decreasing fracture risk in postmenopausal women (Iwamoto et al., 2002). Side effects may include headaches and flushing. Calcitonin is commonly administered via nasal spray in 200 IU dosages.

Bisphosphonates, another class of antiresorptives, arguably represent one of the most significant advances in the treatment of osteoporosis since the mid-1990s. Oral bisphosphonates are generally well tolerated, although they may cause gastrointestinal intolerance in some individuals. It is very important that clients remain upright for at least 30 minutes following oral dosing to avoid esophageal discomfort. This class of drugs has been shown to reduce the risk of vertebral fractures

TABLE 17-2
MEDICAL THERAPIES AVAILABLE FOR THE TREATMENT OR PREVENTION OF OSTEOPOROSIS

Class	Generic Name	Brand Name
Estrogens	Conjugated estrogens	Premarin
	Estradiol transdermal	Estraderm
	Estropipate	Ogen, Ortho-Est
	Esterified estrogens	Estratab
	Conjugated estrogens, medroxyprogesterone	Premphase, Prempro
	Estradiol, norethindrone	Activella
Bisphosphonates	Alendronate	Fosamax
	Risedronate	Actonel
	Etidronate	Didronel
	Ibandronate	Boniva
	Zoledronic acid	Reclast
	Pamidronate	Aredia
	Tiludronate	Skelid
RANKL inhibitor	Denusomab	Prolia, Xgeva
Anabolic agent	Teriparatide	Forteo
Antiresorptive and anabolic	Strontium	Protelos, Prolos
SERMs	Raloxifene	Evista
	Tamoxifen	Nolvadex
Others		
Calcitonin	Calcitonin-salmon	Miacalcin
	Calcitriol or other vitamin D metabolites	
	Sodium fluoride	

Note: RANKL = Receptor activator of nuclear factor kappa-B ligand; SERM = Selective estrogen receptor modulator
Source: American College of Sports Medicine (2014). *ACSM's Resource Manual for Guidelines for Exercise Testing and Prescription* (7th ed.). Philadelphia: Wolters Kluwer/Lippincott Williams & Wilkins.

by 40 to 50% and non-vertebral fractures (including hip fractures) by 20 to 40% (Guyatt et al., 2002). They function by inhibiting the action of osteoclasts (formation remains the same), thereby slowing bone resorption. Despite their impressive potential to reduce fractures, long-term use of bisphosphonates is controversial (ACSM, 2014). These drugs remain in the skeleton for decades, and bone turnover can be affected for up to five years after the drugs are discontinued. Since the natural purpose of bone remodeling is to repair microdamage sustained as a result of everyday wear and tear, it is suspected that bone not permitted to resorb and renew may become brittle. While the fracture data is positive, studies have followed patients only three to five years into treatment and the optimal duration of therapy remains unclear (Keen, 2007). Furthermore, there have been reports of the rare but serious disorder of **osteonecrosis** (the death of bone tissue) of the jaw associated with bisphosphonate use, mainly in patients receiving high doses in combination with cancer treatment, as well as atypical fractures of the femur. This area needs more investigation to understand the mechanism of this disease.

SERMs represent a class of agents that, while similar in structure to estrogen, exert their effects only on target tissues. The most studied is raloxifene (Evista) and its effects on markers of bone turnover have been more modest than with bisphosphonates, and its effect on non-vertebral fractures such as the hip has not been marked. For this reason, it is recommended for use in women with milder osteoporosis or in those with osteoporosis primarily in the spine. Side effects include hot flashes and an increased risk of venous thrombosis similar to that associated with hormone therapy.

Strontium ranelate is an antiosteoporotic agent that increases bone formation while also reducing bone resorption and has been recommended for use in postmenopausal women with osteoporosis (Roux, 2008). Vertebral fracture rates are reduced by about 50% and non-vertebral rates by about 16%, with even higher rates of fracture reduction seen in individuals with the weakest bones (Reginster et al., 2005).

PTH is an **anabolic** hormone that acts mainly to stimulate bone formation. PTH works by helping to regulate blood calcium levels through: (1) stimulating bone resorption in the presence of adequate vitamin D, (2) increasing intestinal calcium absorption, and (3) enhancing reabsorption of calcium in the kidneys (ACSM, 2014). Although clinical trials showed a 65% risk reduction for new vertebral fractures and a 53% reduction for non-vertebral fractures, benefits to BMD receded after discontinuation. Therefore, this drug is recommended for short durations of less than two years (Sambrook & Cooper, 2006).

Surgical Treatment

While surgical procedures to treat osteoporosis are not available, once a fracture has occurred, surgery is often needed to repair damage to the bones. Despite advances in orthopedic surgery, anesthesia, and perioperative care, hip fracture surgery is still associated with complications in up to one-third of patients. The risk of nonunion (failure of the fracture to heal) and osteonecrosis are of particular concern. Data from well-designed outcome studies indicate that the most predictable, durable, and cost-effective procedure for an active older patient with a femoral neck fracture is total joint **arthroplasty.** However, not all patients are candidates for this procedure. In addition, the potential complications of such an invasive surgery, including increased mortality, may be more difficult to manage and more severe than those associated with less radical procedures (Schmidt et al., 2005).

A newer treatment option for vertebral fractures involves the injection of a special bone cement into the compressed body of the vertebrae. Studies have shown increased bone strength (Steens et al., 2007) and pain relief (Afzal et al., 2007; Steens et al., 2007) in patients treated with this technique. A treatment called balloon kyphoplasty has also shown positive results. This process involves the insertion of an inflatable balloon into the vertebral body, which creates a cavity to elevate the vertebral end plates. Bone cement is then inserted in this cavity. The balloon used in this procedure may allow for improved height restoration, cavity creation, and decreased cement leakage rates (Marcucci & Brandi, 2010).

Exercise Treatment

Weight-bearing exercise provides one of the most viable, potent tools for both prevention and management of osteopenia and/or osteoporosis. Of all of the lifestyle behaviors used to prevent and treat osteoporosis, exercise is the only one that can simultaneously improve low BMD, increase muscular strength, and augment balance—all of which are independent risk factors for fracture (ACSM, 2022). In addition, properly planned weight-bearing exercises also provide a direct stimulus to bone that improves its strength and structure. Clearly, a well-planned exercise program should provide the foundation from which the disease can be effectively addressed.

NUTRITIONAL CONSIDERATIONS FOR CLIENTS WITH OSTEOPOROSIS AND OSTEOPENIA

Nutrition plays an important role both in the prevention and treatment of osteoporosis. The most critical nutrients in helping to optimize and maintain bone health are calcium and vitamin D. Calcium comprises about half of bone mass (and 99% of the body's calcium is stored in bone) and adequate calcium intake is important to help keep bones strong [Institute of Medicine (IOM), 2011]. Inadequate calcium intake triggers a rise in the release of PTH, which causes calcium to be removed from bone to maintain normal blood levels of calcium. This weakens bones and increases risk of bone disease like osteopenia and eventually osteoporosis. Vitamin D is critical due largely to its important role in facilitating calcium absorption. Even with the highest intakes of calcium, if vitamin D levels are low, the body will not be able to most effectively use the calcium. Vitamin D is also important for maintaining muscle strength and may play other roles that are not yet well defined (Avenell et al., 2009).

The nutrients that have been implicated in helping to maintain bone health in addition to calcium and vitamin D are described here, though it is important to note that this is an area of ongoing research and investigation. It may turn out that other nutrients not listed here are important for bone health, or that some of the nutrients described here promote health for other reasons but may not play a key role in bone health.

- *Vitamin K* may help decrease fracture risk by activating important bone proteins (Cockayne et al., 2006). Both the Nurses' Health Study (Feskanich et al,. 1999) and the Framingham Heart Study (Booth et al., 2000) found that low vitamin K intakes were associated with increased risk of hip fracture in women.
- *Protein* is important for building bone mass during childhood and adolescence and for preserving bone mass with aging. While a high-protein diet can increase urinary calcium losses, a moderate protein diet (1 to 1.5 g/day for each kg of body weight) does not appear to contribute to weakened bones as long as sufficient calcium is consumed in the diet (Heaney & Layman, 2008).
- *Magnesium and potassium* may protect bone by buffering bone-harming acidic metabolic by-products to create a more alkaline environment. Magnesium also helps to build bone strength while potassium can help to decrease calcium excretion, particularly in postmenopausal women with high-sodium diets (IOM, 2011).
- *Vitamin C* is necessary for synthesis of collagen, the main protein in bone.
- *Omega-3 fatty acids* may help improve bone strength by tempering inflammatory mediators during bone remodeling (Mangano et al., 2013). This is an ongoing area of investigation.
- *Fruits and vegetables* contain a variety of nutrients and phytochemicals, which help to maintain strong bones. Studies support that a diet high in fruits and vegetables is associated with increased bone density in older adults and adolescent boys and girls (Prynne et al, 2006).

The following nutrients may harm bone health:

- *Sodium* consumed in excess causes the body to excrete calcium (rather than use it to help maintain bone strength).
- *Phosphorus* competes with calcium, and too much phosphorus and not enough calcium causes bone weakening. Phosphorus is present in moderate amounts in sodas and soft drinks, raising concern that if people consume too many soft drinks, bone health may be compromised (Tucker et al., 2006). However, this could be because people who drink large amounts of soft drinks are unlikely to consume calcium-containing drinks like milk (IOM, 2011).
- *Caffeine* has been implicated in disrupting bone health due to it causing a modest increase in urinary excretion of calcium and a modest decrease in calcium absorption. However, it is unlikely to have a negative effect in those who consume at least 800 mg of

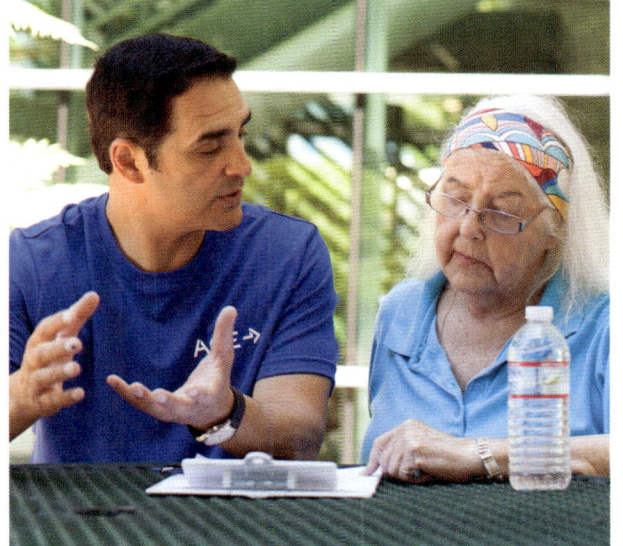

calcium per day, equivalent to about 2.5 cups of milk, 4 ounces of cheese, or just under 2 cups of yogurt (IOM, 2011).
- *Alcohol* may reduce calcium absorption, although the amount at which this occurs and whether alcohol may also have beneficial effects on bone are unknown (IOM, 2011).
- *Vitamin A* in excessive amounts (typically from vitamin A supplementation or fortification of foods) may contribute to bone loss and increase the risk of fracture (Feskanich et al., 2002).
- *Oxalates* and *phytates* can interfere with calcium absorption. Oxalates are found in spinach, rhubarb, beet greens, and some beans. Phytates are found mostly in beans and wheat bran. For beans, the phytate level can be decreased by soaking the beans for several hours and then cooking in fresh water. Note that the phytates in 100% whole grain will decrease calcium absorption from calcium-containing foods consumed at the same time (such as milk with 100% whole-grain cereal).

Table 17-3 presents the recommended intakes of bone-protecting nutrients, as well as excellent food sources for each nutrient.

TABLE 17-3
NUTRIENTS IMPORTANT FOR BONE HEALTH

	Recommended Amount	Sources
Calcium	Males >50 years: 1,000 mg/day Females >50 years: 1,200 mg/day Adults <50 years: 1,000 mg/day	Dairy products (milk, yogurt, cheese) Canned sardines, canned salmon Calcium-fortified foods (e.g. orange juice, ready-to-eat cereals, soy milk) Certain green leafy vegetables such as kale, collard greens, mustard greens, and broccoli Dietary supplements (calcium carbonate and calcium citrate)
Vitamin D	Adults <50 years: 600 IU Adults >50 years: 600 IU	Sunshine Fortified dairy products, juices, and cereals Fatty fish including salmon, mackerel, tuna, and sardines
Vitamin K	Adult males: 120 µg/d Adult females: 90 µg/d	Dark green, leafy vegetables including spinach, kale, and brussel sprouts
Vitamin C	Adult males: 90 mg/d Adult females: 75 mg/d	Citrus fruits (including oranges, grapefruits, and lemons), as well as strawberries, papaya, and pineapple Vegetables including red, yellow, and green peppers, broccoli, and brussel sprouts
Potassium	All adults: 4.7 g/day	Vegetables and fruits, especially bananas, tomatoes, spinach, sweet potatoes, and oranges Dairy products Meat Nuts
Magnesium	Adult males: 400–420 mg/d Adult females: 310–320 mg/d	Vegetables and fruits, especially spinach, artichokes, tomatoes, sweet potatoes, and raisins Nuts including almonds, cashews, and peanuts Fortified cereals
Omega-3 Fatty Acids	Adult males: 1.6 g/d Adult females: 1.1 g/day	Fatty fish such as salmon, tuna, and mackerel Nuts and seeds Vegetable oils such as soybean, canola, and flax seed

Source: Institute of Medicine's Dietary Reference Intakes. Available at www.nap.edu

EXERCISE RECOMMENDATIONS FOR CLIENTS WITH OSTEOPOROSIS AND OSTEOPENIA

In general, physically active individuals of all ages enjoy better skeletal mass than their inactive peers. The magnitude of this difference depends on the mode and intensity of the activity, when the activity was initiated during the lifetime, and for how many years it is performed. The data clearly show that loading exercises performed prior to puberty have the greatest influence on bone. Likewise, increases in bone mass of pre- and postmenopausal women have usually been modest, and the best adaptations occur in those with the lowest starting bone-mass values.

Physical Activity and Bone Response in Children and Adolescents

Childhood (prior to puberty) appears to be the time when the skeleton is most responsive to bone-loading activities. Thus, optimizing bone mineral accumulation during the growing years is crucial for the prevention of osteoporosis later in life. It is reported that as much bone mineral is laid down during the adolescent years as an adult will lose from ages 50 to 80 years (ACSM, 2014).

Sports that require participants to begin physical training at an early age provide useful information about the role of physical activity in bone growth and mineral accretion. The volume and intensity of training performed by highly motivated young athletes often exceeds five to 24 hours per week. Studies on young gymnasts, whose bodies regularly experience **ground reaction forces** of 15 times their body weight, confirm that these types of forces can induce a change in BMD that is between 30 and 85% higher than that seen in controls for the whole body, spine, and legs (Bass et al., 1998). Randomized controlled trials in prepubescent children have similarly shown that jumping exercises performed for as little as seven months can confer large differences in bone mineral content of 3 to 4% at the spine and hip between exercise and control groups (Fuchs, Bauer, & Snow, 2001). Furthermore, there is evidence that impact exercise performed during the years before puberty may produce changes in bone that are sustained into adulthood (Fuchs & Snow, 2002). Even weightlifting activities that produce high skeletal loads via muscular pull in the absence of impact have the potential to positively influence bone. In a cross-sectional study of 15- to 20-year-old Olympic weightlifters, forearm bone mineral content was 40 to 50% higher in these athletes versus levels seen in controls (Virvidakis et al., 1990).

Longitudinal studies also support the observation that children who are generally more physically active than their sedentary counterparts, even in the absence of targeted bone-loading exercise, display higher BMD. A six-year study following the bone mineral accrual in children passing from childhood into adulthood found a 9% and 17% greater total body bone mineral content for active boys and girls, respectively, over their inactive peers (Bailey et al., 1999).

Physical Activity and Bone Response in Premenopausal Women

Not unlike active children, active adults tend to have higher BMD than sedentary adults. These differences have been observed for all regions of the skeleton, regardless of the measurement device used. Some activities may not incorporate loads that apply a sufficient stimulus to bone to produce an adaptive response. Those who participate in activities with high force and load magnitudes, such as gymnastics, jumping, and power lifting, display higher BMD than those who participate in low-intensity or non-weight-bearing activities like swimming and cycling. Even though swimming provides muscular pull on bones, it does not appear that this level of loading is adequate to offset the many hours of skeletal *unloading* individuals experience while buoyant in the water (Bellew & Gehrig, 2006).

The most successful exercise interventions in this age group have incorporated jumping exercises that create ground reaction forces of up to six times body weight. These data also suggest that exercises must be performed for a minimum of six months to elicit a significant bone response, but it may take up to nine months or longer (Khan et al., 2001). Another important feature of bone-loading exercises done during the adult years is that unlike results observed in children, these activities must be continued if the individual is to maintain the increases in bone mass. The principle of **reversibility** definitely applies to adult bone mass. There are no studies in premenopausal women that have demonstrated permanent bone gain as a result of short-term training.

Physical Activity and Bone Response in Postmenopausal Women

Bone mineral density of the hip predicts an individual's risk for fracture, and most intervention studies in postmenopausal women have found small, positive effects on hip BMD. Many of the "benefits" to bone described in these studies are due to an observed maintenance of bone in the exercise group with a concomitant decrease in bone in the control group. In this age group, however, even maintenance of bone is a very positive thing, as it may translate into a reduced fracture risk. Intervention studies using only strength training in postmenopausal women have shown mixed results. Nelson and colleagues (1994) had 50- to 70-year-old, previously untrained, estrogen-depleted women train at 80% of **one-repetition maximum (1-RM)** for one year. They showed a 0.9% and 1% gain in BMD in the strength-training group for the hip and spine, respectively, compared to changes of –2.5% and –1.8% in BMD controls. Furthermore, they showed that indices of falling, such as muscle mass, muscle strength, and dynamic balance, also improved, which may have implications for fracture risk as well, especially if the exercises are maintained. These results have since been replicated by others and suggest that exercise intervention in this age group can maintain BMD, but rarely serves to add substantial amounts of bone. Similar results have been found for hip BMD using high-impact exercises. Kohrt, Ehsani, and Birge (1997) conducted a study comparing the effects of strength training versus high-impact training on bone. They found that while both programs improved lumbar spine BMD, only the impact group augmented hip BMD. They concluded that it may be better to recommend exercises that generate impact forces on bone over those that generate muscle forces. However, because strength training reduces risk factors for falling, both types of activities should be considered when designing programs for individuals at risk for fracture.

During the late postmenopausal years, when the rate of bone loss has slowed compared to early postmenopause (if estrogen is not replaced), calcium supplementation becomes more important as a way to compensate for reduced estrogenic actions on intestinal calcium absorption and renal calcium excretion (Borer, 2005). There is also evidence that exercise has a synergistic effect on calcium retention in the skeleton and may help to ameliorate bone loss (Specker, 1996). Clients over the age of 50 years should be encouraged to obtain at least 1,200 mg of calcium per day, through either dietary or supplement sources.

Physical Activity and Bone Response in Men

Men have larger bones compared with women, resulting in greater bone strength. A main difference between male and female osteoporosis concerns bone microarchitecture. The patterns of bone loss in men seem to be different from those in women such that earlier trabecular loss is observed in men, with cortical loss starting after the age of 50 years, possibly linked to gonadal steroid decline. Men have a higher trabecular bone volume/tissue volume, which declines at a similar rate to that seen in women, with men showing a relative preservation of trabecular number, but more trabecular thinning (Kaufman et al., 2013).

There is a surprising lack of intervention studies on the effects of exercise on bone in men. This is unfortunate, since the number of men with osteoporosis and related fractures is increasing. The few intervention studies that do exist indicate that the response of the male skeleton to exercise is similar to that of women, but is not complicated by the abrupt withdrawal of reproductive hormones in late adulthood. Similar to the results of studies in women, more rigorous training conveys more benefit to the skeleton, while low-intensity exercises, such as walking and moderate-intensity running, afford little benefit (Fonseca et al., 2014; Beck & Snow, 2003).

EXPAND YOUR KNOWLEDGE

SUMMARY OF BONE'S RESPONSE TO LOADING, HORMONAL INTERVENTION, AND DIETARY INTERVENTION

The literature in this area supports eight basic principles related to how bone responds to exercise loading, hormonal intervention, and dietary intervention, which are summarized as follows (Borer, 2005):

- The best time to load bone is prior to puberty. Improvements in bone mass during this time are more dramatic and evidence suggests that they may cause an increase in peak bone mass that persists into adulthood.
- Bone requires dynamic, rather than static, loads to improve its size, shape, and/or density.
- Bone requires loads over and above normal daily loading to improve its size, shape, and/ or density. Bone must sense an overload stimulus if it is to adapt. Higher stresses produce higher bone strains, and these can be accomplished by higher force magnitudes and/or faster application of force. This may partially explain the ineffectiveness of walking programs and low-to-moderate intensity weight-training programs in producing positive gains in bone mass.
- Bone's response is proportional to strain frequency. Bone is maintained both with less frequent mechanical loads of higher intensity and with higher frequency loads at lower intensity.
- Bone's response is improved with brief, intermittent exercise, and may require six to eight hours of recovery between intense loading sessions. The number of loads need not be high (anywhere from five to 50 impacts can be beneficial) to produce the desired response.
- Bone requires an unusual loading pattern to improve. Exercise that loads the skeleton in unusual, uncustomary ways, produces more dramatic responses than those using normal loading patterns. In other words, performing the same activity exclusively (e.g., running) will have less impact on improving bone than will performing various types of training simultaneously (e.g., running, martial arts, and aerobic dancing).
- Bone requires abundant available nutrient energy if it is to respond. Caloric restriction negatively impacts bone via suppression of key anabolic hormones.
- Bone requires abundant calcium and vitamin D availability. This is more important before puberty and after menopause, when the antiresorptive effects of estrogen are suppressed and vitamin D intake may be inadequate. Evidence also suggests synergistic effects of exercise and calcium and vitamin D on bone during these times.

Programming and Progression Guidelines

Recommendations for Children and Young Adults

- Choose weight-bearing activities such as basketball, soccer, volleyball, and gymnastics over non-weight-bearing activities such as swimming and cycling. Although these weight-bearing activities specifically target bone, it should be understood that a well-rounded program should also contain activities to promote cardiovascular health.
- Emphasize activities and movements that develop muscular strength and power, such as running, hopping, skipping, and jumping. These activities are easily incorporated into games and regular physical-activity classes and should maximize movement and minimize inactive time.
- Remember the principles of **specificity** and **overload.** The skeletal response to exercise is greatest at the site of maximal stress, and the training load must be greater than that encountered on an everyday basis.
- Adequate energy intake is essential for proper growth and bone development. Girls especially should be educated about the importance of a healthy diet and the dangers of menstrual dysfunction.
- Youth should avoid substituting soft drinks for milk. Calcium intake during growth is essential for healthy bones.

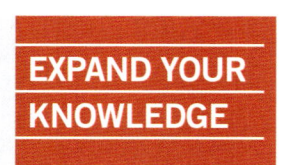

Recommendations for Premenopausal Women and Middle-aged Adult Men

- Choose weight-bearing activities such as running, group fitness classes (including aerobic and/or muscle-conditioning classes), basketball, soccer, volleyball, and martial arts over non-weight-bearing activities such as swimming, cycling, and rowing. Although these weight-bearing activities specifically target bone, it should be understood that a well-rounded program also includes activities to promote cardiovascular health.
- Emphasize activities and movements that develop muscular strength and power, such as running, hopping, skipping, and jumping. These are easily incorporated into games and regular physical-activity classes and should maximize movement and minimize inactive time.
- Remember the principles of specificity and overload. The skeletal response to exercise is greatest at the site of maximal stress, and the training load must be greater than that encountered on an everyday basis.
- Simple jumping seems to provide an adequate stimulus for bone, and is a safe and appropriate loading modality for younger women and older nonosteoporotic women (Heikkinen et al., 2007; Winters & Snow, 2000; Bassey et al., 1998; Bassey & Ramsdale, 1994). Studies in premenopausal women using 50 daily jumps (two-footed, using arms for propulsion, bare/stocking feet, bent-knee landing) have shown positive gains in bone mass at the hip. This is a very simple, yet effective method for incorporating high-impact activity into an existing exercise program (Bassey & Ramsdale, 1994).
- High-intensity strength-training exercises (5- to 6-RM) should also be included in a well-rounded exercise program, as they have been shown to benefit bone and multiple indices of falling and fracture risk.

These clients should perform strength-training exercises in a standing (weight-bearing) position, using free weights and/or a weighted vest when possible. Doing so will challenge the **vestibular system,** involve stabilizing muscles, and translate to **activities of daily living (ADL)** much more effectively than seated activities. Weighted vest loads of 7 to 15% of the client's body weight are an effective means of loading the skeleton during exercises performed while standing (e.g., lunges, squats, stair steps, and calf raises).

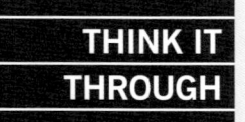

> **THINK IT THROUGH**
>
> Premenopausal women are prime candidates for high-intensity resistance training to improve bone health. However, this population can be resistant to engage in lifting heavy loads due to lack of experience or cultural views. What would you say to a female client who could benefit from starting a resistance-training program to enhance bone, but who expresses the opinion that "weight training is not for me"?

Recommendations for Non-osteoporotic Postmenopausal Women and Older Men

Based on the available research, it is not only advisable to recommend exercises that will directly benefit bone, but also those that will reduce the risk for falling. Because falls cause more than 90% of hip and 50% of spine fractures, fall prevention should be central to an exercise program for older adults in general. Muscle weakness, postural instability, and poor functional mobility are important risk factors for falls.

- Any program should be individualized based on the physician's recommendations and the client's current health/fitness status, joint concerns, medication use, and ability level. Having the results from a bone density test is valuable to help determine risk for osteoporosis and fracture.
- Low-intensity activities, such as walking, impart very low bone loads and are not recommended as an effective strategy for the prevention of osteoporosis in postmenopausal women. If walking is performed as a primary exercise modality, it should definitely be accompanied by high-intensity strength training (using 8-RM as a guide).
- Older adults can perform high-intensity strength-training exercises (8-RM), as they have been shown to benefit bone and multiple indices of fracture risk.

Osteoporosis and Osteopenia   CHAPTER 17

- These clients can perform strength-training exercises in a standing (weight-bearing) position, using free weights and/or a weighted vest when appropriate and possible. Doing so will challenge the vestibular system, involve stabilizing muscles, and translate to improvements in ADL much better than seated activities. Heavy loads (>10% of body weight) in a weighted vest should be avoided if spine BMD status is unknown.
- Clients should focus on lower-body muscle groups, but must not neglect the upper body, as these muscles are important for daily living and maintaining independence.
- High-impact jumping (>2.5 times body weight) and other plyometric exercises should probably be avoided in these individuals, especially if bone status is unknown.

PLYOMETRICS

Plyometric exercises provide a means for incorporating a variety of different movements, including medial/lateral movements that overload the skeleton. **Plyometrics** are specialized jumping exercises associated with high-impact loads and forceful muscular takeoffs, and include various exercises specifically designed to increase muscular strength and power. They are based on the premise that increasing eccentric preload on a muscle will induce the **myotatic stretch reflex,** thereby causing a more forceful concentric contraction. Plyometrics range in difficulty and intensity level from simple stationary jumping to traveling drills, such as hopping and bounding, to high-intensity box jumps (Chu, 2011; Radcliffe & Farentinos, 1999). An inherent benefit of utilizing these types of activities is that they require little equipment, small blocks of time, and are generally safe for adolescents and healthy adults to perform. Care should be taken to make sure clients have adequate leg strength to land properly before incorporating these types of high-intensity plyometric activities.

A proper progression of plyometric exercises is important to ensure adequate muscular strength to maintain proper body mechanics during execution and landing. A plyometric program should begin with one to two sets of 10 repetitions of five to seven different exercises and progress slowly to the more strenuous activities, adding sets and repetitions as tolerated. All exercises should be performed on a medium-hard surface such as grass (preferred), a group fitness room floor, or carpet.

It is important to note that plyometrics should not be performed by osteoporotic individuals or by older adults with joint concerns. Clients can perform the sample exercises presented in Figures 17-4 through 17-10 in succession, minimizing time spent on the floor. This method maximizes muscle preload and ensures optimal gains in power.

There are also several more advanced plyometric exercises that can be used with more fit clientele. When performing alternating leg bounds, the knee on the lead leg drives up and forward, lands, and then the opposite knee drives up and forward. The client should emphasize maximal height and distance, and move the bent arms in a backward circular motion for added propulsion. This exercise also can be performed as a same-leg bound, where the lead leg cycles around and is the only leg to touch the ground.

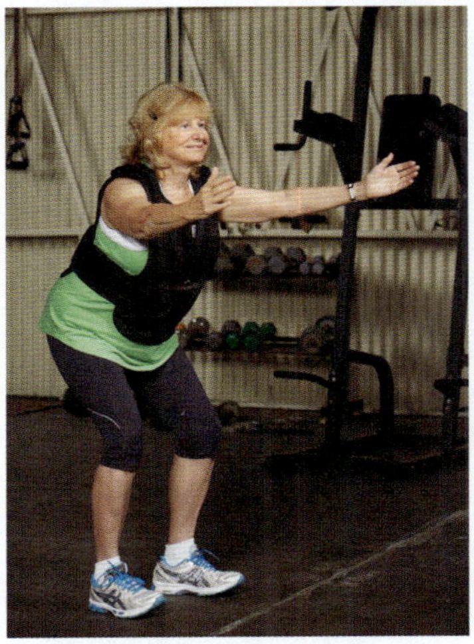

APPLY WHAT YOU KNOW

Figure 17-4
Squat with weighted vest

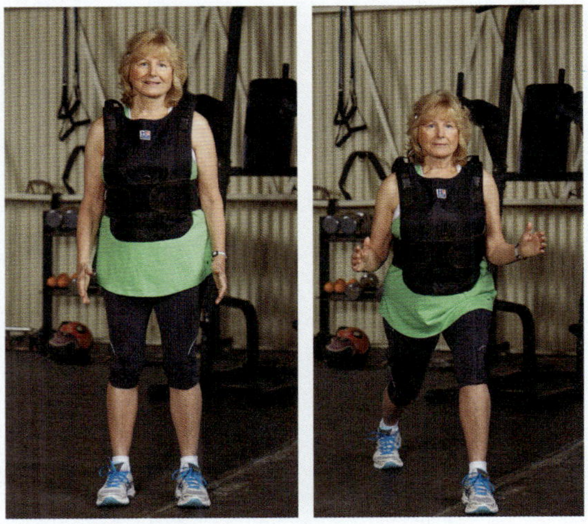

Figure 17-5
Backward lunge with weighted vest

A variety of advanced plyometric exercises can be performed on a flight of stairs, ranging from standard running and "bounding" (skipping several stairs at a time) to using a sideways approach to ascend the stairs. To perform a sideways stair exercise, the client stands sideways on two successive steps, with the trailing leg straight, and pushes the lead leg up to the next step. They then move the trailing leg up to the next step, push off, and so on. This exercise represents a sort of "seesaw" motion and strengthens the hip abductors and adductors.

Figure 17-6
Sideways lunge with weighted vest

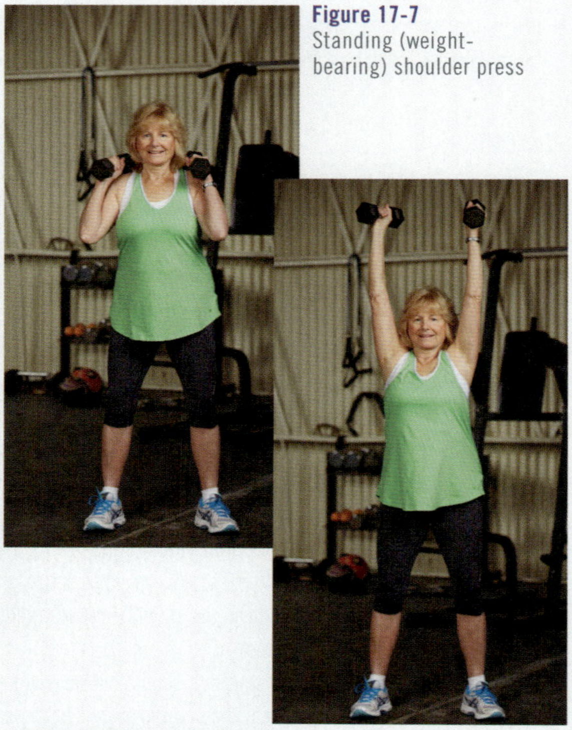

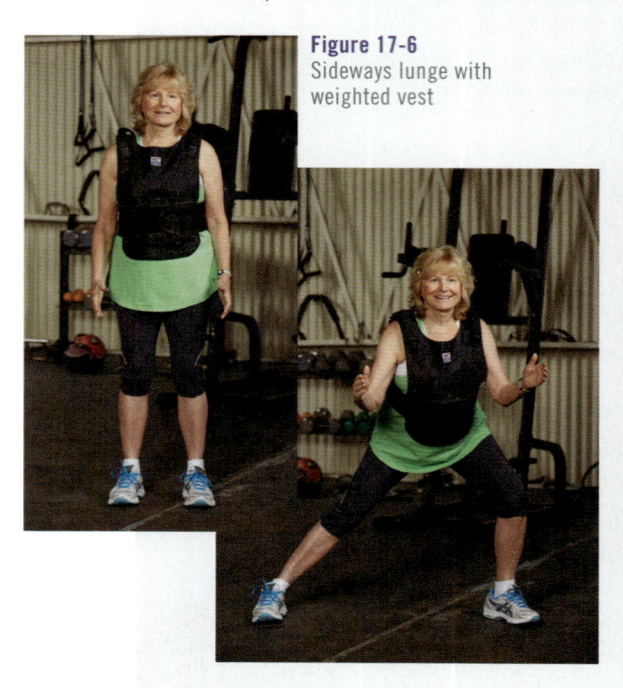

Figure 17-7
Standing (weight-bearing) shoulder press

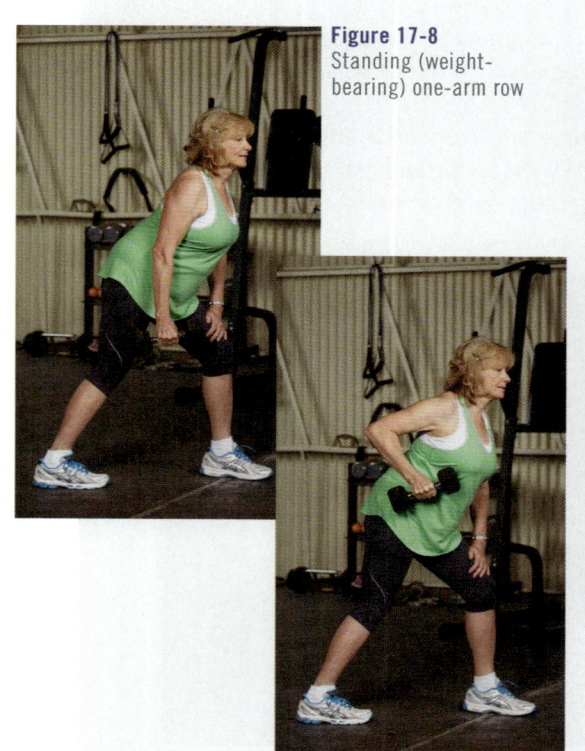

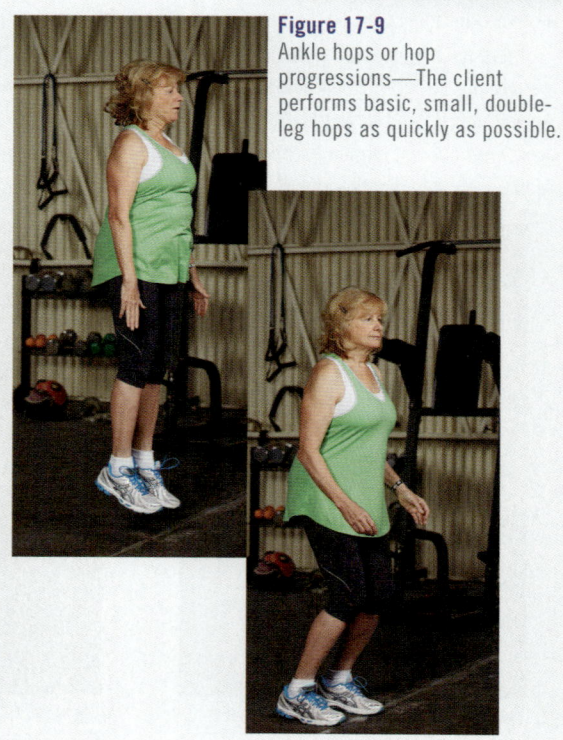

Figure 17-8
Standing (weight-bearing) one-arm row

Figure 17-9
Ankle hops or hop progressions—The client performs basic, small, double-leg hops as quickly as possible.

Osteoporosis and Osteopenia

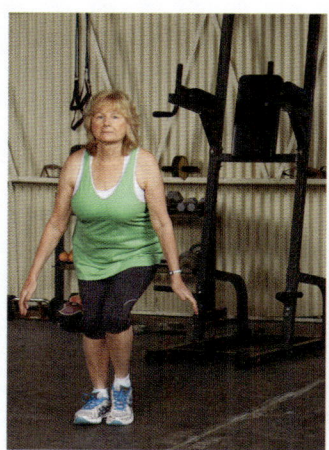

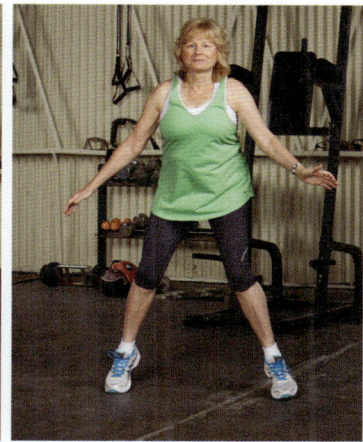

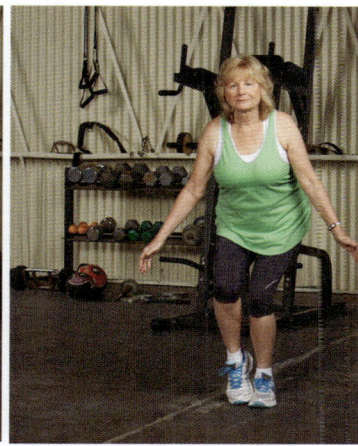

CHAPTER 17

Figure 17-10
Side leap

Recommendations for the Osteoporotic Client

Currently, there are no established guidelines for specific contraindications to exercise for individuals with osteoporosis. The general recommendation is for individuals with, or at risk for, osteoporosis to engage in weight-bearing aerobic exercise in combination with some form of higher-velocity, higher-intensity, and higher-impact muscular training (ACSM, 2022). To date, there have been very few intervention studies in people with osteopenia or osteoporosis, so specific recommendations are difficult for this group. Clients diagnosed with osteoporosis, with or without a history of vertebral fractures, should not engage in jumping activities or deep forward trunk flexion exercises such as rowing, toe touches, and full sit-ups (ACSM, 2014). In this group of individuals, a regular walking program that may include hills to increase intensity, combined with resistance training that targets balance and upper- and lower-body muscle strength, may help to improve muscle strength and coordination, thereby reducing fall risk. Specialized balance-training programs to prevent falls are also recommended for this population and can be found at many local recreational and gym facilities, senior centers, and university extension programs.

The body-weight resistance exercises shown in Figures 17-11 through 17-20 may be useful for osteoporotic clients. The exercise session should begin with an eight- to 15-minute warm-up of gentle dynamic stretching and range-of-motion exercises, followed by five to 10 minutes of aerobic activity at 60 to 75% of maximum predicted heart rate.

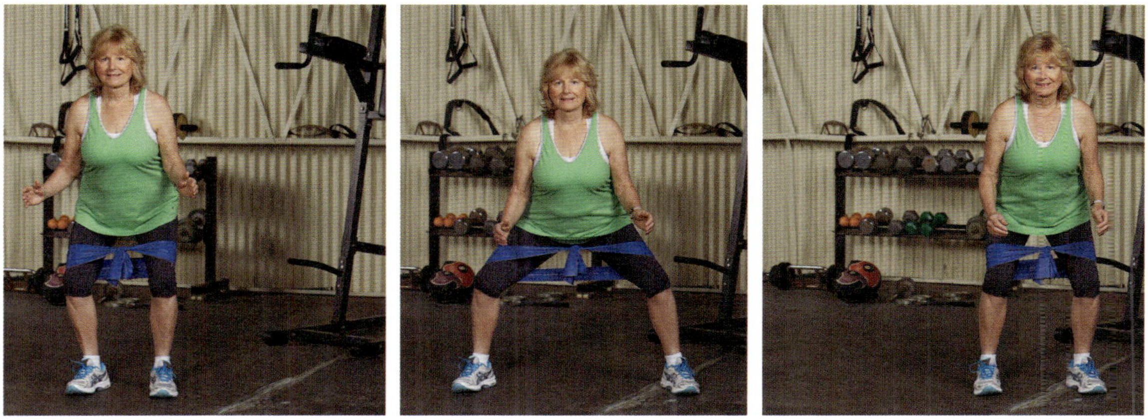

Figure 17-11
Thoracic mobility

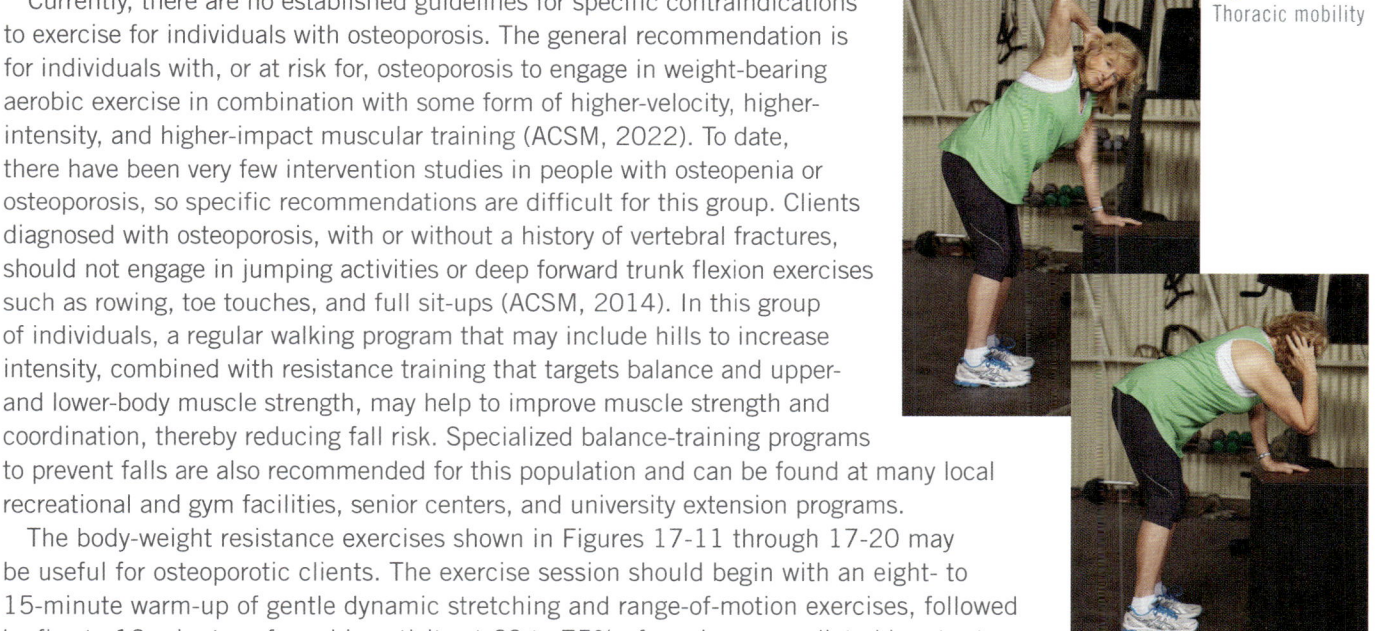

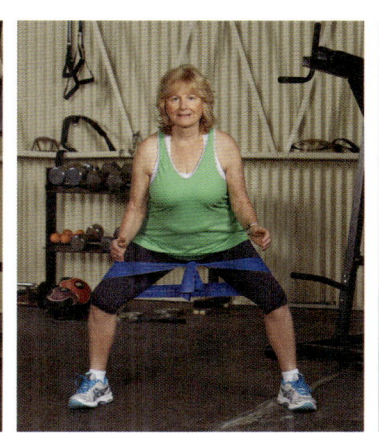

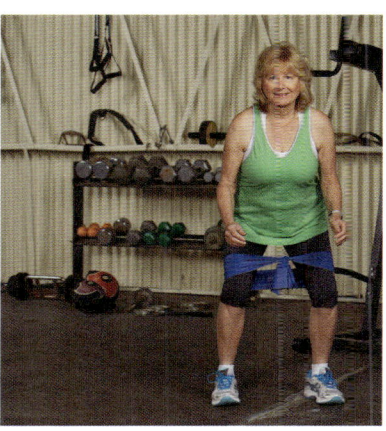

Figure 17-12
Banded lateral step

If osteoporotic clients are limited by severe pain, exercise options may be limited. It may be advantageous to begin exercise with a warm pool-based program, which, while non-weight-bearing, can improve flexibility and muscle strength in deconditioned clients. These clients may also want to discuss with their physicians the use of calcitonin (a hormone beneficial to bone, administered via nasal spray, that has been shown to help reduce pain).

Figure 17-13
Banded monster walk

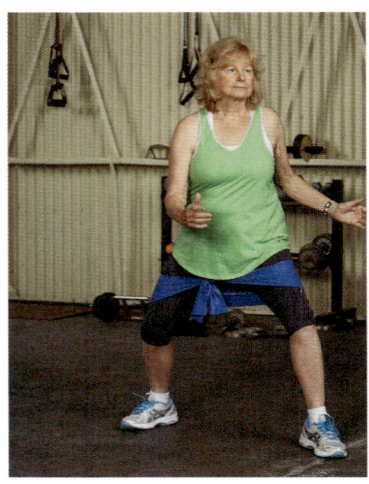

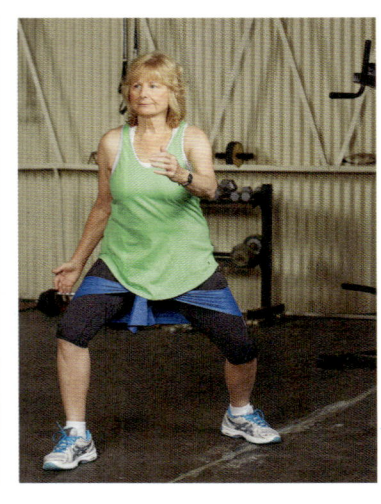

Figure 17-14
Hover squat

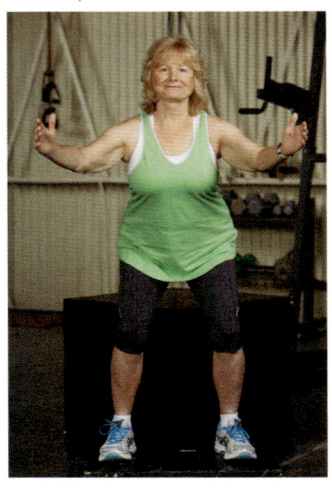

Figure 17-15
Seated posture correction

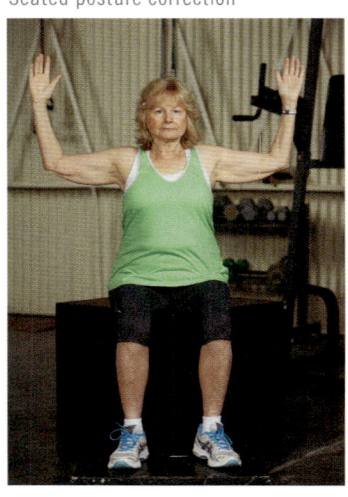

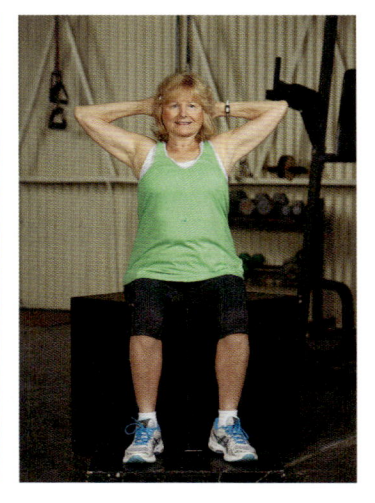

Figure 17-16
Prone trunk lift

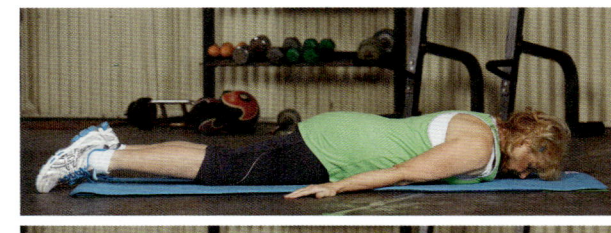

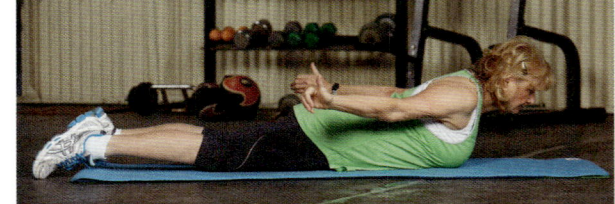

Figure 17-17
Chest press

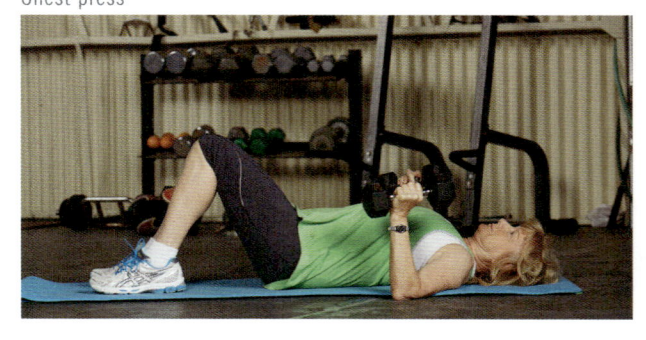

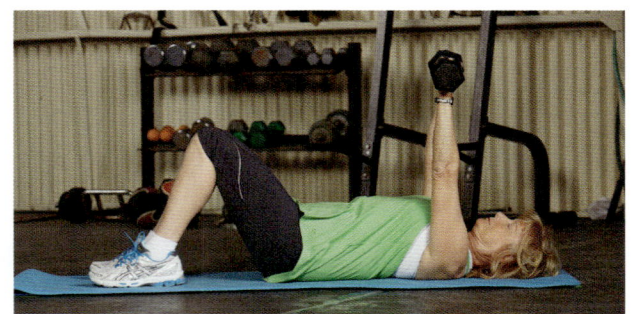

Osteoporosis and Osteopenia

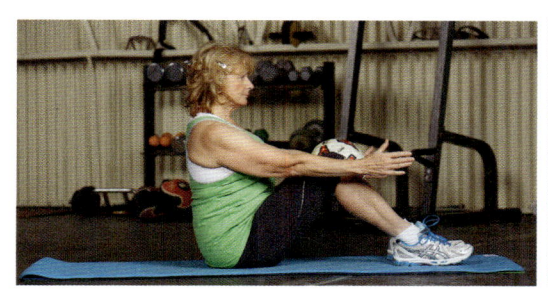

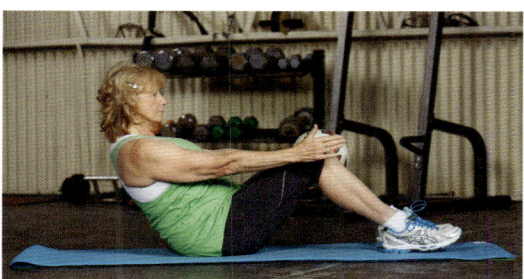

CHAPTER 17

Figure 17-18
Half roll back

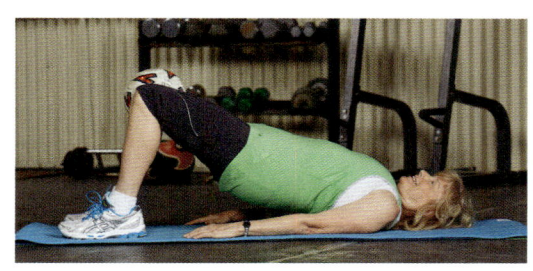

Figure 17-19
Glute bridge

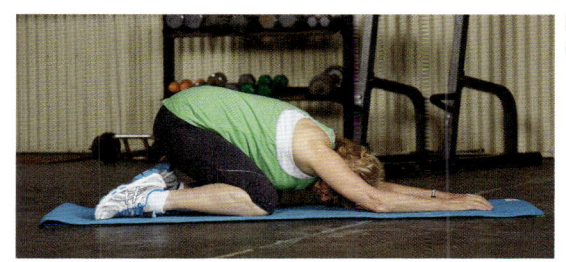

Figure 17-20
Child's pose

EXERCISE GUIDELINES SUMMARY FOR CLIENTS AT RISK FOR OSTEOPOROSIS

	CARDIORESPIRATORY EXERCISE
Frequency	• At least 3 days per week
Intensity	• Moderate (40 to 59% HRR or $\dot{V}O_2R$) or vigorous (60–89% HRR or $\dot{V}O_2R$) intensity
Time	• Accumulate 30–60 minutes per day of a combination of weight-bearing aerobic and resistance activities
Type	• Emphasis should be placed on weight-bearing, large-muscle-group activities, such as: ✓ Walking with intermittent jogging ✓ Tennis ✓ Stair climbing/descending ✓ Jumping
Progression	• Progression should be individualized depending on tolerance and following the ACE Integrated Fitness Training® Model.
	RESISTANCE EXERCISE
Frequency	• 2–3 days per week
Intensity	• Moderate (60–80% 1-RM, 8–12 repetitions) to vigorous (80–90% 1-RM, 5–6 repetitions) intensity
Time	• 30–60 minutes per day of a combination of weight-bearing and resistance activities
Type	• Exercises involving each major muscle group with an emphasis on bone-loading forces • Exercises while standing that emphasize functional movements
Progression	• Progression should be individualized depending on tolerance and following the ACE Integrated Fitness Training Model.

Note: HRR = Heart-rate reserve; $\dot{V}O_2R$ = Oxygen uptake reserve; 1-RM = One-repetition maximum

EXERCISE GUIDELINES SUMMARY FOR CLIENTS WITH OSTEOPOROSIS

CARDIORESPIRATORY TRAINING	
Frequency	• 4–5 days per week
Intensity	• Moderate (40–59% HRR or $\dot{V}O_2R$) intensity,* although some clients may be able to tolerate more intense exercise • Below VT1 HR; can talk comfortably
Time	• Begin with 20 minutes and gradually progress to a minimum of 30 minutes and a maximum of 45–60 minutes

Type	• Emphasize weight-bearing, large-muscle-group activities, such as:
	  ✓ Walking
	  ✓ Stair climbing/descending
	• Impact loading exercises such as bench stepping and jumping can be used with individuals with moderate or low fracture risk.

Progression	• Progress following the ACE Integrated Fitness Training® Model based on client goals and availability.

MUSCULAR TRAINING	
Frequency	• Start with 1–2 nonconsecutive days and possibly progress to 2–3 days per week
Intensity	• Adjust resistance so that the last 2 repetitions are challenging to perform. • High-intensity, high-velocity training is beneficial for those who can tolerate it.
Time	• Begin with 1 set of 8–12 repetitions and increase to 2 sets after approximately 2 weeks; no more than 8–10 exercises per session
Type	• Exercises involving each major muscle group with an emphasis on bone-loading forces • Exercises while standing that emphasize balance, gait, and functional movements • Compound exercises are best.
Progression	• Progress following the ACE Integrated Fitness Training Model based on client goals and availability.

*Moderate intensity = Heart rates <VT1 where speech remains comfortable and is not affected by breathing; Vigorous intensity = Heart rates from ≥VT1 to <VT2 where clients feel unsure if speech is comfortable.

Note: HRR = Heart-rate reserve; $\dot{V}O_2R$ = Oxygen uptake reserve; VT1 = First ventilatory threshold; VT2 = Second ventilatory threshold

CMES FOCUS

Weight-bearing aerobic and resistance exercise are crucial for individuals at risk for and with osteoporosis. To preserve musculoskeletal integrity and prevent bone loss, even the frailest of elderly individuals should remain as physically active as their health permits. Exercise programming for clients at risk for developing osteoporosis should focus on preserving bone health, whereas programming for clients with osteoporosis should focus on preventing disease progression.

Source: American College of Sports Medicine (2022). *ACSM's Guidelines for Exercise Testing and Prescription* (11th ed.). Philadelphia: Wolters Kluwer.

CASE STUDIES

Case Study 1

Client Information

Rhonda is a thin, fair-skinned, 35-year-old marathon runner who has come to a CMES for a strength-training program after finding out that her 60-year-old mother has osteoporosis. She currently runs about 50 to 70 miles per week (80 to 113 km/week), and would like to add a weightlifting regimen if it will help reduce her risk for osteoporosis. In the pre-screening assessment, the CMES asks Rhonda to utilize the FRAX tool (see Figure 17-3), which shows that she is at high risk for sustaining a fracture in the next 10 years. The CMES also discovers that Rhonda has not had a menstrual period for two years (since she increased her training volume to compete in marathons) and only had a period every other month for three years

Osteoporosis and Osteopenia
CHAPTER 17

prior to that. She has had two stress fractures in the past 12 months, but managed to continue her physical activity with non-weight-bearing exercise while they healed. She is very concerned about her dietary fat intake, and claims that she consumes about 1,200 calories per day. She is very eager to begin her strength-training program.

CMES Approach

Rhonda is displaying characteristics of the female athlete triad. The CMES should immediately be concerned that she has not menstruated in two years, and had irregular periods for some time before that. Her high training volume and low caloric intake probably have contributed to her amenorrhea due to low energy availability. A visit to her physician is definitely in order before the CMES can begin working with her. The CMES should talk to Rhonda about concern over her training volume and associated stress fractures, and discuss amenorrhea, but must not diagnose the problem. The CMES should also educate Rhonda on the usefulness of a bone-density assessment so that she may talk with her physician about getting one. The CMES should also ask Rhonda about her dietary intake and recommend that she consult with a qualified nutritionist.

Once Rhonda returns with her medical clearance and the results from her bone-density assessment, the CMES is ready to design a training program for Rhonda. Initial assessments should be performed to identify any inadequacies with stability, mobility, balance, or movement patterns. Once any deficiencies have been addressed, external loads can be added to increase the positive stress on the musculoskeletal system.

If her bone mass is below normal (osteopenic), the CMES should implement a conservative program that begins with strength training and then adds stationary jumping once she has shown adequate strength, range of motion, and ability to land properly during jumping. Additional plyometric exercises should not be added for at least three months to ensure that Rhonda tolerates the jumping without injury. She can begin with upper- and lower-body resistance exercises for all major movements and muscle groups using a weighted vest or dumbbells for resistance. Since she is in good physical condition, she can begin with two sets of 10 repetitions, using 8% of her body weight in the vest, or 75% of her 1-RM. Every two to three weeks, Rhonda can gradually increase her resistance. The CMES should recommend that Rhonda weight train two days per week, substituting one or two of her running days for weight-training days.

ACE IFT® MODEL AT A GLANCE

Cardiorespiratory Training

Given Rhonda's training volume and performance goals, she should be following a well-developed Performance Training program. This case study specifically calls for the CMES to review her current running program to make any modifications necessary to optimize training and recovery, while limiting additional fatigue and overuse injuries. Taking this step will provide Rhonda with a solid training program based on her current health, fitness, and performance goals.

Muscular Training

After addressing any issues with postural stability, kinetic-chain mobility, and balance (Functional Training), or Movement Training, the CMES will develop a Load/Speed Training program to help Rhonda to create a positive stress on the musculoskeletal system that promotes strength and stimulates bone tissue. This program will gradually introduce plyometric exercises to support the client's bone health and performance goals.

Case Study 2

Client Information

Fiona is a 70-year-old, postmenopausal woman with a small build who does not exercise regularly and has just been told by her physician that she has osteoporosis. She has lost 1.5 inches (3.8 cm) in height and has upper-back pain, but has been cleared by her physician to begin an exercise program. She performed some upper-body rubber tubing exercises with a physical therapist, but is more concerned about a hip fracture. She is otherwise sedentary and has chosen not to use estrogen replacement therapy, although she has heard positive things about "these new bone drugs" from her friends. She wants the CMES to tell her which bone drug she should begin taking, and to start her on a strength-training program to help slow her bone loss. She is on an antidepressant drug that sometimes makes her dizzy, especially when she forgets to wear her

ACE IFT® MODEL AT A GLANCE

Cardiorespiratory Training

Fiona's cardiorespiratory training will be focused initially on moving more consistently and establishing basic cardiorespiratory endurance (Base Training) for improved cardiorespiratory health, fitness, and function, to support her Muscular Training program. Once she can perform 20 minutes or more of continuous cardiorespiratory exercise on three to five days each week, she can be progressed to Fitness Training.

Muscular Training

After addressing any issues with postural stability, kinetic-chain mobility, and balance (Functional Training), or postural control during movement patterns (Movement Training), the CMES will develop a Load/Speed Training program to help Rhonda to create a positive stress on the musculoskeletal system that promotes strength and stimulates bone tissue. This program may be progressed to high-intensity, high-impact, high-velocity exercises at an appropriate rate of progression based on the client's ability levels and comfort.

glasses. She took a bad fall in her home last month when she tripped over her small dog, and is concerned that she is having trouble climbing the stairs in her home.

CMES Approach

Since Fiona has a physician's release to begin working with the CMES, she is ready for screening and program development. Although the CMES can educate Fiona about the new anti-resorptive drugs, all questions about whether or not they are right for her should be directed to Fiona's physician. The regimen her physical therapist prescribed for her to help maintain upper-back flexibility should be the starting point for her upper-body muscular-training program, with appropriate modifications introduced by the CMES based on Fiona's challenges and successes. Since she has a recent history of falling and experiences episodes of dizziness, the CMES should assess her functional mobility using an older adult fitness battery (Rikli & Jones, 2013). The CMES also should help Fiona assess safety in her home and suggest that she wear stable shoes and her glasses while inside to prevent another tripping incident. A bell on her dog might also be a good idea. She also should secure all area rugs in her house and might consider installing handrails in the bathroom. Fiona definitely needs lower-body strength training, especially if she is to continue to climb the stairs in her home. The CMES should implement the exercises presented in this chapter for osteoporotic adults, but should not include any jumping activities, since Fiona's osteoporosis is already established. The CMES should also introduce weight-bearing cardiorespiratory exercise performed at a moderate intensity following the guildelines in this chapter with a focus on balance, movement, and increasing duration to improve fitness, function, and endurance. It is important to make sure that Fiona has her eyeglasses on while training to maximize her safety and minimize her fear and risk of falling.

SUMMARY

Bone is a dynamic, metabolically active tissue that responds to both use and disuse by adapting the amount of mineral to accommodate daily loading patterns. Of the two types of bone in the human body, trabecular bone is more susceptible to the deleterious effects of osteoporosis. Because of its high trabecular content, the neck of the femur is a common osteoporotic fracture site; hip fractures often cause a loss of independence and death in many cases. Osteoporosis prevention and treatment strategies include estrogen replacement therapy or other pharmacological agents, increased calcium and vitamin D intake, and exercise.

Bone is most responsive to mechanical loading during growth, and is progressively less responsive as an individual ages. Bone-loading exercises are beneficial to the skeleton at all stages of life and should be incorporated into a well-rounded program for all clients, especially those at risk for osteoporosis. The types of exercise that are most beneficial to bone are those that sufficiently overload bone using high-force magnitude rather than a high number of low-force repetitions. High-force magnitude can be produced through direct impact loading of the bone, as with jumping, or through strong muscular contractions that bend bone, as with strength training. Non-weight-bearing, non-impact exercises such as swimming and rowing do not sufficiently overload bone to increase bone formation or slow bone loss. Similarly, weight-bearing exercises that are not significantly different from daily loading patterns (in normally ambulating individuals), such as walking, also do not provide a stimulus for new formation.

Osteoporosis and Osteopenia CHAPTER 17

The frequency and intensity of the exercises should take into account the client's bone status (preferably from a bone-density scan), physical and functional status, medication use, and hormonal status, as well as the overall goals for the program. If the client is at risk for osteopenia or osteoporosis, it is wise for the CMES to obtain a medical clearance for strength-training exercises and/or any type of impact exercise prior to beginning a program.

REFERENCES

Afzal, S. et al. (2007). Percutaneous vertebroplasty for osteoporotic fractures. *Pain Physician,* 10, 4, 559–563.

Aloia, J.F. et al. (1996). Risk for osteoporosis in black women. *Calcified Tissue International,* 59, 6, 415–423.

American College of Sports Medicine (2022). *ACSM's Guidelines for Exercise Testing and Prescription* (11th ed.). Philadelphia: Wolters Kluwer.

American College of Sports Medicine (2014). *ACSM's Resource Manual for Guidelines for Exercise Testing and Prescription* (7th ed.). Philadelphia: Wolters Kluwer/Lippincott Williams & Wilkins.

Avenell, A. et al. (2009). Vitamin D and vitamin D analogues for preventing fractures associated with involutional and postmenopausal osteoporosis. *Cochrane Database of Systematic Reviews,* CD000227

Bailey, D.A. et al. (1999). A six-year longitudinal study of the relationship of physical activity to bone mineral accrual in growing children: The University of Saskatchewan bone mineral accrual study. *Journal of Bone Mineral Research,* 14, 10, 1672–1679.

Bass, E. et al. (2007). Risk-adjusted mortality rates of elderly veterans with hip fractures. *Annals of Epidemiology,* 17, 7, 514–519.

Bass, S. et al. (1998). Exercise before puberty may confer residual benefits in bone density in adulthood: Studies in active prepubertal and retired female gymnasts. *Journal of Bone Mineral Research,* 13, 3, 500–507.

Bassey, E.J. & Ramsdale, S.J. (1994). Increase in femoral bone density in young women following high-impact exercise. *Osteoporos International,* 4, 2, 72–75.

Bassey, E.J. et al. (1998). Pre- and postmenopausal women have different bone mineral density responses to the same high-impact exercise. *Journal of Bone Mineral Research,* 13, 12, 1805–1813.

Beals, K.A. & Meyer, N.L. (2007). Female athlete triad update. *Clinical Sports Medicine,* 26, 1, 69–89.

Beck, B.R. & Snow, C.M. (2003). Bone health across the lifespan: Exercising our options. *Exercise and Sport Science Review,* 31, 3, 117–122.

Bellew, J.W. & Gehrig, L. (2006). A comparison of bone mineral density in adolescent female swimmers, soccer players, and weight lifters. *Pediatric Physical Therapy,* 18, 1, 19–22.

Bergstrom, I. et al. (2011). Back extensor training increases muscle strength in postmenopausal women with osteoporosis, kyphosis and vertebral fractures. *Advances in Physiotherapy,* 13, 3, 110–117.

Booth, S.L. et al. (2000). Dietary vitamin K intakes are associated with hip fracture but now with bone mineral density in elderly men and women. *American Journal of Clinical Nutrition,* 71, 1201–1208.

Borer, K.T. (2005). Physical activity in the prevention and amelioration of osteoporosis in women: Interaction of mechanical, hormonal and dietary factors. *Sports Medicine,* 35, 9, 779–830.

Chu, D.A. (2011). *Jumping into Plyometrics* (2nd ed.). Champaign, Ill.: Human Kinetics.

Cockayne, S. et al. (2006). Vitamin K and the prevention of fractures: Systematic review and meta-analysis of randomized controlled trials. *Archives of Internal Medicine,* 166, 12, 1256–1261.

Cooper, C. et al. (1992). Incidence of clinically diagnosed vertebral fractures: A population-based study in Rochester, Minnesota, 1985–1989. *Journal of Bone Mineral Research,* 7, 2, 221–227.

Cummings, S.R. & Melton, L.J. (2002). Epidemiology and outcomes of osteoporotic fractures. *Lancet,* 359, 9319, 1761–1767.

Curtis, K.M. & Martins, S.L. (2006). Progesterone-only contraception and bone mineral density: A systematic review. *Contraception,* 73, 5, 470–487.

Eskridge, S.L. et al. (2010). Estrogen therapy and bone mineral density in African-American and Caucasian women. *American Journal of Epidemiology,* 171, 7, 808–816. DOI: 10.1093/aje/kwp460

Feskanich, D. et al. (2002). Vitamin A intake and hip fractures among postmenopausal women. *Journal of the American Medical Association,* 287, 1, 47–54.

Feskanich, D. et al. (1999). Vitamin K intake and hip fractures in women: A prospective study. *American Journal of Clinical Nutrition,* 69, 74–79.

Fonseca, H. et al. (2014). Bone quality: The determinants of bone strength and fragility. *Sports Medicine,* 44, 1, 37–53.

Fuchs, R.K., Bauer, J.J., & Snow, C.M. (2001). Jumping improves hip and lumbar spine bone mass in prepubescent children: A randomized controlled trial. *Journal of Bone Mineral Research,* 16, 1, 148–156.

Fuchs, R.K. & Snow, C.M. (2002). Gains in hip bone mass from high-impact training are maintained: A randomized controlled trial in children. *Journal of Pediatrics,* 141, 3, 357–362.

Griffin, M.R. et al. (1992). Black-white differences in fracture rates. *American Journal of Epidemiology,* 136, 11, 1378–1385.

Guyatt, G.H. et al. (2002). Summary of meta-analyses of therapies for postmenopausal osteoporosis and the relationship between bone density and fractures. *Endocrinology Metabolism Clinics of North America,* 31, 3, 659–679, xii.

Hansen, D. et al. (2019). *Medicare Cost of Osteoporotic Fractures.* https://static1.squarespace.com/static/5c0860aff793924efe2230f3/t/5d76b949deb7e9086ee3d7dd/1568061771769/Medicare+Cost+of+Osteoporotic+Fractures+20190827.pdf

Hayes, W.C. et al. (1996). Etiology and prevention of age-related hip fractures. *Bone,* 18, 77S–86S.

Heaney, R.P. & Layman, D.K. (2008). Amount and type of protein influences bone health. *American Journal of Clinical Nutrition,* 87, 5, 1567S–1570S.

Heikkinen, R. et al. (2007). Acceleration slope of exercise-induced impacts is a determinant of changes in bone density. *Journal of Biomechanics,* 40, 13, 2967–2974.

Institute of Medicine (2011). *Dietary Reference Intakes for Vitamin D and Calcium.* Washington, D.C.: National Academies Press.

Iwamoto, J. et al. (2002). Effects of five-year treatment with elcatonin and alfacalcidol on lumbar bone mineral density and the incidence of vertebral fractures in postmenopausal women with osteoporosis: A retrospective study. *Journal of Orthopedic Science,* 7, 6, 637–643.

Kaufman, J.-M. et al. (2013). Treatment of osteoporosis in men. *Bone,* 53, 1, 134–144. DOI: 10.1016/j.bone.2012.11.018

Keen, R. (2007). Osteoporosis: Strategies for prevention and management. *Best Practice & Research Clinical Rheumatology,* 21, 1, 109–122.

Khan, K. et al. (2001). *Physical Activity and Bone Health.* Champaign, Ill.: Human Kinetics.

Khosla, S. & Melton III, L.J. (2007). Clinical practice: Osteopenia. *New England Journal of Medicine,* 356, 22, 2293–2300.

Kohrt, W.M., Ehsani, A.A., & Birge, Jr., S.J. (1997). Effects of exercise involving predominantly either joint-reaction or ground-reaction forces on bone mineral density in older women. *Journal of Bone Mineral Research,* 12, 8, 1253–1261.

Krall, E.A. & Dawson-Hughes, B. (1993). Heritable and life-style determinants of bone mineral density. *Journal of Bone Mineral Research,* 8, 1, 1–9.

Laskey, M.A. et al. (2011). Proximal femur structural geometry changes during and following lactation. *Bone,* 48, 4, 755–759. DOI: 10.1016/j.bone.2010.11.016

Liu, C-R. et al. (2012). The effect of physical loading on calcaneus quantitative ultrasound measurement: A cross-section study. *BMC Musculoskeletal Disorders,* 13, 70. DOI: 10.1186/1471-2474-13-70

Maggi, S. et al. (1991). Incidence of hip fractures in the elderly: A cross-national analysis. *Osteoporosis International,* 1, 4, 232–241.

Mangano, K.M. et al. (2013). Polyunsaturated fatty acids and their relation with bone and muscle health in adults. *Current Osteoporosis Reports,* 11, 3. DOI: 10.1007/s11914-013-0149-0

Marcucci, G. & Brandi, M.L. (2010). Kyphoplasty and vertebroplasty in the management of osteoporosis with subsecuent vertebral compression fractures. *Clinical Cases in Mineral and Bone Metabolism,* 7, 1, 51–60.

Marks, R. (2010). Hip fracture epidemiological trends, outcomes, and risk factors, 1970–2009. *International Journal of General Medicine,* 3, 1–17.

Martins, S.L., Curtis, K.M., & Glasier, A.F. (2006). Combined hormonal contraception and bone health: A systematic review. *Contraception,* 73, 5, 445–469.

McKay, H.A. et al. (1994). Familial comparison of bone mineral density at the proximal femur and lumbar spine. *Bone and Mineral,* 24, 2, 95–107.

Melton, L.J. & Cooper C. (2001). Magnitude and impact of osteoporosis and fractures. In: Marcus, R., Feldman, D., & Kelsey, J. (Eds.) *Osteoporosis.* San Diego, Calif.: Academic Press.

National Osteoporosis Foundation (2014). *Bone Health Basics: Get the Facts.* www.nof.org/learn/basics

National Osteoporosis Foundation (2010). *Clinician's Guide to Prevention and Treatment of Osteoporosis.* Washington, D.C.: National Osteoporosis Foundation.

Nattiv, A. et al. (2007). American College of Sports Medicine position stand: The female athlete triad. *Medicine & Science in Sports & Exercise,* 39, 10, 1867–1882.

Nelson, M.E. et al. (1994). Effects of high-intensity strength training on multiple risk factors for osteoporotic fractures: A randomized controlled trial. *Journal of the American Medical Association,* 272, 24, 1909–1914.

Prynne, C.J. et al. (2006). Fruit and vegetable intakes and bone mineral status: A cross-sectional study in 5 age and sex cohorts. *American Journal of Clinical Nutrition,* 83, 6, 1420–1428.

Radcliffe, J.C. & Farentinos, R.C. (1999). *High-powered Plyometrics.* Champaign, Ill.: Human Kinetics.

Reginster, J.Y. et al. (2005). Strontium ranelate reduces the risk of nonvertebral fractures in postmenopausal women with osteoporosis: Treatment of Peripheral Osteoporosis (TROPOS) study. *Journal of Clinical Endocrinology Metabolism,* 90, 5, 2816–2822.

Rikli, R.E. & Jones, J.C. (2013). *Senior Fitness Test Manual* (2nd ed.). Champaign, Ill.: Human Kinetics.

Rossouw, J.E. et al. (2002). Risks and benefits of estrogen plus progestin in healthy postmenopausal women: Principal results From the Women's Health Initiative randomized controlled trial. *Journal of the American Medical Association,* 17, 3 321–333.

Roux, C. (2008). Strontium ranelate: Short- and long-term benefits for post-menopausal women with osteoporosis. *Rheumatology (Oxford),* 47, Suppl. 4, iv20–iv22. DOI: 10.1093/rheumatology/ken166

Sambrook, P. & Cooper, C. (2006). Osteoporosis. *Lancet,* 367, 9527, 2010–2018.

Schmidt, A.H. et al. (2005). Femoral neck fractures. *Instructional Course Lectures,* 54, 417–445.

Snow-Harter, C. & Marcus, R. (1991). Exercise, bone mineral density, and osteoporosis. *Exercise and Sport Science Review,* 19, 351–388.

Specker, B.L. (1996). Evidence for an interaction between calcium intake and physical activity on changes in bone mineral density. *Journal of Bone Mineral Research,* 11, 10, 1539–1544.

Steens, J. et al. (2007). The influence of endplate-to-endplate cement augmentation on vertebral strength and stiffness in vertebroplasty. *Spine,* 32, 15, E419–E422.

Tucker, K.L. et al. (2006). Colas, but not other carbonated beverages, are associated with low bone mineral density in older women: The Framingham Osteoporosis Study. *American Journal of Clinical Nutrition,* 84, 936–942.

Tudor-Locke, C. & McColl, R.S. (2000). Factors related to variation in premenopausal bone mineral status: A health promotion approach. *Osteoporosis International,* 11, 1, 1–24.

Tylavsky, F.A. et al. (1989). Familial resemblance of radial bone mass between premenopausal mothers and their college-age daughters. *Calcified Tissue International,* 45, 5, 265–272.

Virvidakis, K. et al. (1990). Bone mineral content of junior competitive weightlifters. *International Journal of Sports Medicine,* 11, 3, 244–246.

Winters, K.M. & Snow, C.M. (2000). Body composition predicts bone mineral density and balance in premenopausal women. *Journal of Women's Health and Gender-Based Medicine,* 9, 8, 865–872.

World Health Organization (2007). *WHO Scientific Group on the Assessment of Osteoporosis at the Primary Health Care Level: Summary Meeting Report.* Brussels, Belgium (May 5–7, 2004).

World Health Organization (1994). *Assessment of Fracture Risk and Its Application to Screening for Postmenopausal Osteoporosis: Report of a WHO Study Group.* Geneva: WHO Technical Report Series, No. 843.

Wu, F. et al. (2002). Fractures between the ages of 20 and 50 years increase women's risk of subsequent fractures. *Archives of Internal Medicine,* 162, 1, 33–36.

Zanker, C.L. & Swaine, I.L. (1998). Relation between bone turnover, oestradiol, and energy balance in women distance runners. *British Journal of Sports Medicine,* 32, 2, 167–171.

SUGGESTED READING

Fonseca, H. et al. (2014). Bone quality: The determinants of bone strength and fragility. *Sports Medicine,* 44, 1, 37–53.

Institute of Medicine (2011). *Dietary Reference Intakes for Vitamin D and Calcium.* Washington, D.C.: National Academies Press.

Nattiv, A. et al. (2007). American College of Sports Medicine position stand: The female athlete triad. *Medicine & Science in Sports & Exercise,* 39, 10, 1867–1882.

United States Public Health Service, Office of the Surgeon General. (2004). *Bone Health and Osteoporosis: A Report of the Surgeon General.* Rockville, Md., U.S. Department of Health and Human Services, Public Health Service, Office of the Surgeon General.

18 MUSCULOSKELETAL INJURIES OF THE LOWER EXTREMITY

IN THIS CHAPTER

PRINCIPLES OF RESTORATIVE EXERCISE
FUNCTIONAL TRAINING
MOVEMENT TRAINING

HIP PATHOLOGIES
TROCHANTERIC BURSITIS
ILIOTIBIAL BAND FRICTION SYNDROME
HIP OSTEOARTHRITIS
TOTAL HIP REPLACEMENT

KNEE PATHOLOGIES
PATELLOFEMORAL PAIN SYNDROME
MENISCAL INJURIES
ANTERIOR CRUCIATE LIGAMENT INJURIES
TOTAL KNEE REPLACEMENT

LOWER LEG, ANKLE, AND FOOT PATHOLOGIES
SHIN SPLINTS
ANKLE SPRAINS
ACHILLES TENDINOPATHY
PLANTAR FASCIITIS

CASE STUDIES

SUMMARY

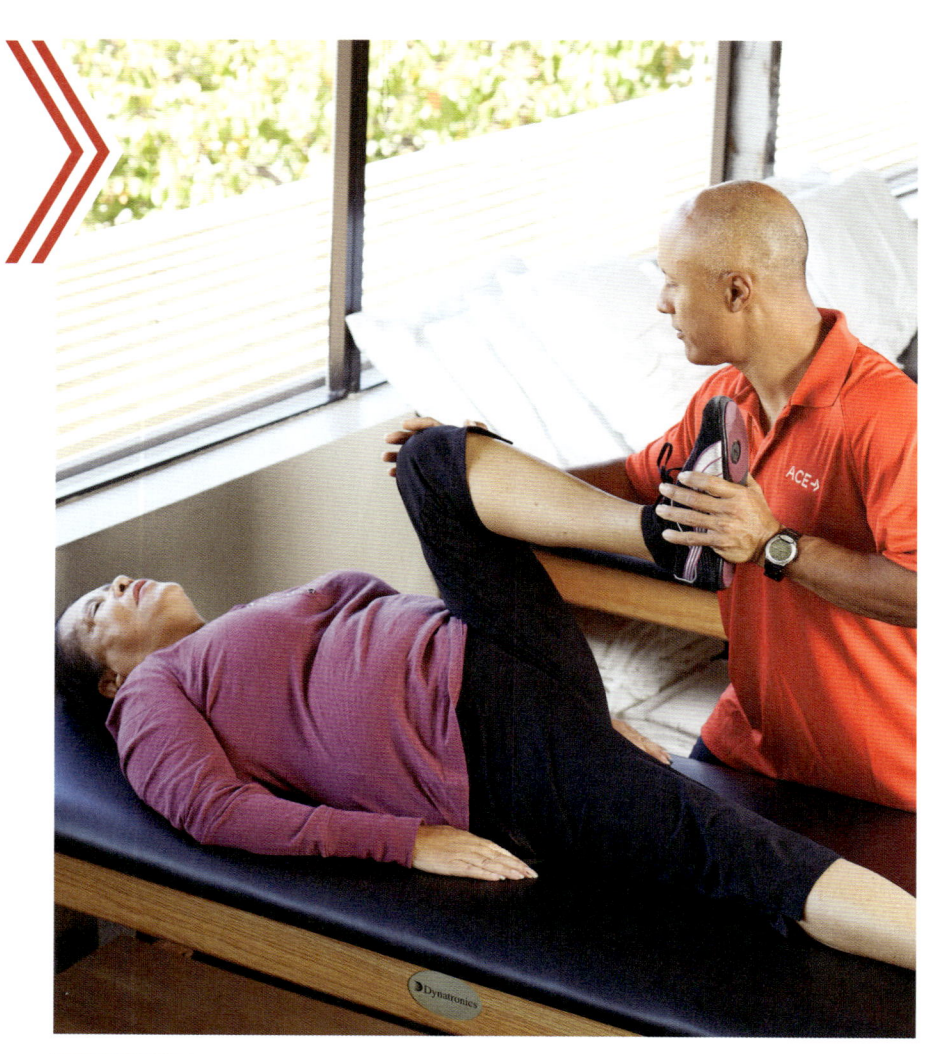

ABOUT THE AUTHOR
Scott Cheatham, Ph.D.(C), PT, DPT, OCS, ATC, CSCS, is an assistant professor in the Division of Kinesiology at California State University Dominguez Hills. He is also owner of the National Institute of Restorative Exercise, where he provides continuing education to medical and exercise professionals. Dr. Cheatham received his Doctor of Physical Therapy from Chapman University and is currently a Ph.D. candidate in Physical Therapy at Nova Southeastern University. Dr. Cheatham is a Certified Athletic Trainer (ATC) and a board-certified specialist in orthopedics (OCS). He also holds several fitness certifications and is a certified ergonomic specialist. He is a national presenter for various organizations and has authored more than 40 peer-reviewed publications, textbook chapters, and home study courses on the topics of orthopedics, health and fitness, and sports medicine. Dr. Cheatham's professional responsibilities include being an associate editor for the *International Journal of Athletic Therapy and Training* and a reviewer for the *Journal of Athletic Training, NSCA Strength & Conditioning Journal,* and *NSCA's Personal Training Quarterly.*

By Scott Cheatham

> **THE FITNESS INDUSTRY HAS EVOLVED** tremendously in recent years due to changes in America's healthcare system. Patients are being discharged from rehabilitation early and are being referred to exercise professionals for further guidance.

The current demands require the ACE® Certified Medical Exercise Specialist (CMES) to have a broad base of knowledge about common medical and post-operative conditions to create safe and effective programs.

This chapter focuses on common musculoskeletal injuries of the lower extremity. Particular attention is placed on recognition, management, and restorative exercise guidelines for the selected topics. A thorough understanding of common non-operative and post-operative musculoskeletal conditions is necessary to make accurate assessments and to know when to refer to other healthcare professionals.

LEARNING OBJECTIVES:

» Describe the principles of restorative exercise, including flexibility, strengthening, and functional integration.

» Explain the three main phases of tissue healing.

» Differentiate between various pathologies of the hip, knee, lower leg, ankle, and foot.

» Describe basic signs, symptoms, and treatment options associated with different pathologies of the lower extremity.

» Design and implement safe and effective exercise programs for clients who have various musculoskeletal injuries of the lower extremity while staying within the ACE Certified Medical Exercise Specialist's scope of practice.

SCREENING THE CLIENT

In addition to the general health information obtained from questionnaires such as the Physical Activity Readiness Questionnaire for Everyone (PAR-Q+) (see Figure 3-1, pages 74 to 77), more specific screening questions are needed to obtain a complete history from the client. It is important to understand what interventions have been done and at what stage in the healing process the client is currently. The following screening questions are recommended prior to designing a restorative program:

- How did the injury happen (i.e., the mechanism of injury)?
- Did the client see their physician? If yes, what treatment has been done (e.g., surgery, physical therapy, oral medications, or cortisone injection)?
- Did the physician issue any exercise precautions or contraindications (e.g., limit walking to 15 minutes)?
- What type of symptoms is the client feeling (e.g., "sharp" pain when walking on the treadmill)?
- Does the client have any functional limitations (e.g., unable to lift objects overhead)?
- What is the client's tolerance to activity (e.g., "feeling fatigued" after 10 minutes of treadmill walking)?

APPLY WHAT YOU KNOW

These questions will help guide the CMES in answering the single most important question: Is exercise appropriate for this client at this time?

PRINCIPLES OF RESTORATIVE EXERCISE

The design of a restorative exercise program needs to be specific to the client's goals and functional abilities. Typically, when a client is recovering from an injury or is post-surgery, restorative exercise programs can help them regain flexibility, strength, **proprioception,** and endurance, and provide positive progress toward more functional or sport-specific activities. There are many different approaches to designing a restorative exercise program. The most effective programs take into account the individual's functional abilities, recovery status (e.g., stage of healing) (Table 18-1), prior activity level, comorbidities (e.g., diabetes), and goals (Houglum, 2010). If a post-injury or post-surgery client undergoes rehabilitation, the physical therapist usually addresses these principles. Typically, the role of the CMES is to progress what has been done in rehabilitation and help the client transition back to full function. The timelines given for returning to fitness activities are general recommendations and may be different among individuals due to the doctor's guidelines. In fact, the CMES may see these clients earlier in the timeline based on their unique situation. For each topic discussed in this chapter, exercise recommendations are categorized into flexibility, strengthening, and functional integration. These categories are given for organization and ease of reference.

TABLE 18-1
PHASES OF TISSUE HEALING

Phase	Description	Objective	Duration
Inflammation	Immediately post-injury, the area shows signs of warmth, redness, swelling, and pain	Care for injury and control inflammation	1 day–1 week
Proliferation	Development of scar tissue that lays down with random orientation; increased girth due to edema	Clear necrotic tissue; begin tissue and cell regeneration to improve circulation	1–4 weeks
Remodeling	Scar tissue edema decreases, but density increases; signs and symptoms reduce; tissue fully fuses	Reestablish function of tissue, skeletal muscle, and joint in the area	1–12 months

Source: Denegar, C.R., Saliba, E., & Saliba, S. (2009). *Therapeutic Modalities for Musculoskeletal Injuries* (3rd ed.). Champaign, Ill.: Human Kinetics.

> The phases of training discussed in association with each of the injuries covered in this chapter refer to the ACE Integrated Fitness Training® (ACE IFT®) Model (see Chapter 2). While the ACE IFT Model provides guidelines for proper progression in a training program, the CMES should always be sure to adhere to the instructions of the client's physician or other healthcare provider.

Functional Training

The program focus during Functional Training is to establish postural stability and kinetic-chain mobility using exercises to improve joint and core function, flexibility, muscular endurance, and balance. This phase of training helps the post-rehabilitation client safely progress to Movement Training and then eventually to more demanding modes of physical activity during Load/Speed Training.

Flexibility is defined as the **range of motion (ROM)** of a joint, which can be limited by joint structure, neuromuscular coordination, muscle strength of opposing groups, and the mobility of the soft tissues (e.g., muscles, ligaments, and connective tissue) associated with the joint. Most flexibility programs utilize various forms of stretching and **myofascial release** to achieve the desired level of flexibility. Common techniques include static stretching, **proprioceptive neuromuscular facilitation (PNF),** and myofascial release using a foam roller.

Strengthening of the post-injury or post-surgery client is very important to the success of the program. When an individual is recovering, there may be a decline in neuromuscular control, muscular strength, and local muscular endurance. When appropriate, the introduction of **progressive resistive exercises** will ensure adequate progression of muscular fitness. This technique uses the **overload** principle to challenge the client as they get stronger. Increasing the weight by 5% with each set is an example. The goal is to safely overload the tissue in a progressive fashion.

Strengthening exercises can be classified into two main categories: open-kinetic-chain (OKC) and closed-kinetic-chain (CKC). OKC exercises for the lower extremities are non-weight-bearing, with the **distal** end (e.g., the foot) free, and involve isolating a specific muscle group. The leg extension machine and side-lying hip abduction are examples of OKC activities. CKC exercises have the distal end fixed and are typically more functional. Examples include squats and lunges. CKC exercises are often thought to be superior due to joint compression, muscle co-contraction, and increased functionality (Begalle et al., 2012).

Movement Training

During Movement Training, the program shifts focus to helping clients develop good movement patterns while maintaining postural and joint stability. Exercises included at this time feature the five primary movement patterns and emphasize the proper sequencing of movements and controlling the body's **center of gravity (COG)** throughout the normal range of motion.

It is important to focus on the maintenance and improvement of postural stability and kinetic-chain mobility throughout Movement Training to restore proper strength, flexibility, and proprioception. Proprioception can be defined as a person's awareness of their body in space. This awareness is part of the sensory system that detects joint movement (**kinesthesia**) and joint position (proprioception). Balance is dependent on sensory receptors, which are located in muscles, skin, tendons, ligaments, joints, and inner ear. The **central nervous system (CNS)** receives input from these receptors along with visual and vestibular input, which are used to control body position and balance. When injury occurs, these pathways can be diminished due to trauma or disuse, which leads to poor balance and increased risk for injury. Retraining these pathways is necessary to maintain adequate neuromuscular control during functional and athletic activities. Proprioceptive exercises must be specific to the activity and should follow a graduated progression that includes the following principles: slow to fast, low force to high force, and controlled to uncontrolled movement.

Therefore, functional integration represents exercises that are specific to the activity or sport and reflect the client's physical abilities and performance goals. Specific functional-integration strategies are discussed along with cardiovascular recommendations for the various topics covered in this chapter.

STRAINS

The term "strain" is one of the most frequently used words to describe exercise-related muscle injury, but it is used with high variability. For the purposes of this chapter, strains are injuries in which a muscle works beyond its capacity, resulting in a tear of the muscle fibers or associated tendons, leading to loss of continuity and contractile properties (Mueller-Wohlfahrt et al., 2013). In mild strains, the client may report tightness or tension (Anderson & Parr, 2013). In more severe cases, the client may report feeling a sudden "tear" or "pop" that leads to immediate pain and weakness in the muscle. Swelling, discoloration (**ecchymosis**), and loss of function often occur after the injury (Houglum, 2010). Strains of the lower extremity primarily occur in the hamstrings, groin muscles, and calves.

Strains of the hamstring group are often caused by a severe stretch to the muscle or a rapid, forceful **eccentric** contraction (e.g., during sprinting). The hamstrings have the highest frequency of strains in the body; hamstring strains are common in running and jumping sports (Houglum, 2010). The client will often report a "sharp" **posterior** thigh pain that occurs after insult. Pain may also be felt with contraction or stretching of the muscle. Risk factors include poor flexibility; poor posture; muscle imbalance among the gluteals, quadriceps, and hamstrings; improper warm-up; errors in training; and prior injury (Anderson & Parr, 2013).

Groin or adductor strains are common in sports such as ice hockey and figure skating that require explosive acceleration, deceleration, and change of direction. With injury, the client may report an initial "pull" of the groin muscles, followed by intense pain and loss of function. Pain may be felt with contraction of the muscles with the hip in adduction, passive stretching with the hip in abduction, or when crossing the leg over the midline of the body. In more severe cases, increased pain and weakness occurs, which may limit specific motions. Jogging straight may be tolerable, but any side-to-side motion tends to elicit pain. Muscle imbalance between the adductors and abductors is the most prevalent risk factor for this type of injury (Cheatham et al., 2014).

Calf strains are common in most running and jumping sports. With injury, the client will often report a sudden and painful "tearing" sensation in the medial muscle belly or at the junction between the muscle belly and the Achilles tendon. Pain, swelling, ecchymosis, and loss of function often occur after the injury. Risk factors include muscle weakness and advanced age (McHugh, 2004).

Management

If a muscle strain does occur, all aggravating activity should be stopped and the RICE principle (i.e., rest or restricted activity, ice, compression, and elevation) can be applied immediately (see page 617). The CMES should administer basic first-aid procedures and then refer the client to the appropriate healthcare professional. It is beyond the **scope of practice** for the CMES to attempt to diagnose a client's problem and to make decisions regarding their care.

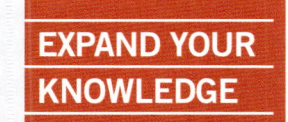

EXPAND YOUR KNOWLEDGE

> **THINK IT THROUGH**
>
> When working with a client who has recently recovered from a musculoskeletal injury, a CMES must be careful to program exercises that do not provoke pain. As such, the CMES must rely on the client to communicate how an exercise feels. Spend some time thinking about how you will explain the importance of pain avoidance during exercise activities and how you and your client will communicate about pain.

HIP PATHOLOGIES

The hip is unique from other joints in its structure and function. It is secured by a deep bony socket and is supported by strong muscles. Hence, the hip is more likely to experience repetitive, microtraumatic injuries rather than acute, major traumas. Further, the hip is a common site of pain referral from other conditions such as lumbar disc disruption, organ disease, sacroiliac dysfunction, and knee injury (Houglum, 2010). Thus, clients presenting with hip pain should be evaluated by their healthcare providers to rule out other conditions and to be cleared for physical activity.

The iliotibial band (ITB) complex is a band of fibrous connective tissue (**fascia**) on the outside of the femur that goes from the hip to the knee. Proximally, the gluteals and tensor fasciae latae (TFL) both blend into the upper fibers of the ITB (Figure 18-1). This is the region where **trochanteric bursitis** occurs. The lower fibers of the ITB attach distally to the proximal anterolateral tibia (Gerdy's tubercle) and also attach to the patella and biceps femoris via fascial connections (Fairclough et al., 2006). This is also the region where **iliotibial band friction syndrome (ITBFS)** occurs. The function of the ITB complex is to serve as a shock absorber and lateral stabilizer. Problems in this complex are common among both active and **sedentary** individuals. Acute or repetitive overuse can tighten the ITB complex, resulting in microtears of the fascia that can lead to scar tissue and functional shortening of the ITB over time (Houglum, 2010; Foye & Stitik, 2006).

Figure 18-1
Posterior musculature of the hip and knee, prime movers for hip extension (gluteus maximus and hamstrings) and knee flexion (hamstrings and gastrocnemius)

Labels: Iliac crest; Gluteus medius; Gluteus maximus; Gracilis; Iliotibial band; Long head / Short head — Biceps femoris; Lateral head (gastrocnemius); Semitendinosus; Semimembranosus; Popliteal space; Medial head (gastrocnemius)

Trochanteric Bursitis

Trochanteric bursitis is characterized by painful inflammation of the trochanteric bursa between the greater trochanter of the femur and the gluteus medius/iliotibial complex. Inflammation of the bursa may be due to an acute incident or repetitive (cumulative) trauma. Acute incidents may include trauma from falls, contact sports (e.g., football), and other sources of impact. Repetitive trauma may be due to excessive friction by the ITB. Factors such as prolonged running, an increase or change in activity, leg-length discrepancy, and lateral hip surgery have been described as causes of repetitive trauma (Foye & Stitik, 2006). Research shows a higher prevalence rate of trochanteric bursitis with low-back pain and **osteoarthritis (OA)** of the hip (Lievense, Bierma-Zeinstra, & Schouten, 2005; Foye & Stitik, 2006). Tears in the gluteus medius, also referred to as the "rotator cuff tears of the hip," are found in up to 22% of elderly patients and may also be an underlying cause of lateral hip pain in this population. Although the incidence of trochanteric bursitis is highest in middle-aged to elderly adults, the **etiology** is multifactorial and it can affect patients of all ages (Lustenberger et al., 2011).

Iliotibial Band Friction Syndrome

When the concept of ITBFS was first developed, the presumed model was that with activities involving repetitive knee **flexion** (such as running), the iliotibial band repetitively shifted forward and backward over the lateral femoral condyle, causing friction and thus inflammation of the ITB. However, Fairclough and colleagues suggested that the ITB is not a distinct anatomical structure but merely a thickened zone within the lateral fascia. Based on these anatomical considerations they believe that anterior–posterior glide of the ITB is impossible, and instead proposed that an illusion of anterior–posterior movement of the ITB results from repetitive cycles of tightening within which the lateral fascia exerts a repetitive compression effect on connective tissues lying deep to the ITB (Fairclough et al., 2007). The actual etiology of the ITBFS remains controversial (Lavine, 2010).

Regardless of the cause, it is generally accepted that ITBFS is the most common running injury of the lateral knee (with an incidence between 1.6 and 12% in runners) and also commonly diagnosed in cyclists (with a reported incidence of 15% of all overuse injuries of the knee region in cyclists) (Lavine, 2010). Biomechanical factors that have been linked with ITBFS include increased landing forces, increased knee internal rotation, low hamstring strength as compared to the quadriceps strength on the same side, and genu recurvatum (i.e., a deformity of the knee, such that the knee bends backward or hyperextends) (Lavine, 2010). Signs and symptoms, precautions, and restorative exercise strategies for both pathologies are discussed in the following sections.

Signs and Symptoms of Trochanteric Bursitis and ITBFS

Trochanteric bursitis pain and/or **paresthesias** (i.e., tingling, prickling, and numbness) often radiate from the greater trochanter to the posterior lateral hip, down the iliotibial tract, to the lateral knee. Symptoms are most often related to an increase in activity or repetitive overuse. Aggravating activities may include lying on the affected side, prolonged walking/running, and certain hip movements (internal and external rotation) (Houglum, 2010). Deficits in hip strength, ROM, and gait may be present secondary to the pain. The client may walk with a limp (i.e., **Trendelenburg gait**) due to pain or weakness. They may develop a compensation pattern through the painful limb that directly affects the lower kinetic chain. This may result in decreased muscle length (e.g., in the quadriceps and hamstrings) and myofascial tightness (Rothschild, 2013).

Clients with ITBFS often report a gradual onset of tightness, burning, or pain at the lateral aspect of the knee during activity. The pain may be localized, but generally radiates to the outside of the knee and/or up the outside of the thigh. Snapping, popping, or pain may be felt at the lateral knee when it is flexed and extended. Aggravating factors may include any repetitive activity such as running (especially downhill) or cycling. During downhill running, more time is spent in knee flexion, increasing ITB stress (Houglum, 2010). Symptoms often resolve with rest but can increase in intensity and frequency if not properly treated. The client may present with weakness in the hip abductors, ITB shortening, and tenderness throughout the ITB complex (Martinez & Honsik, 2006).

Precautions

There are no direct precautions for either trochanteric bursitis or ITBFS. Clients are advised to avoid any aggravating activities and return to activity in a slow, systematic manner. When a client is ready to return to fitness activities, a written clearance from their physician may be necessary. More specifically, clarification from the physician or physical therapist regarding what the client can and cannot do would help guide the CMES when designing the restorative exercise program.

Early Intervention

Conservative treatment of trochanteric bursitis and ITBFS often includes avoiding aggravating activities, physical therapy, modalities (e.g., ice and heat), assistive devices (e.g., a cane), oral anti-inflammatory medication, cortisone injections, or surgery (Houglum, 2010). Once the client is cleared for more advanced activity, the restorative exercise program should progress from what has already been done in treatment and rehabilitation.

Restorative Exercise Program for Trochanteric Bursitis and ITBFS

When designing the program, the CMES should include client education. Important components include proper training techniques, appropriate footwear, and early injury recognition. The client should be pain-free with activity and should be reminded to use ice after the workouts to prevent any latent discomfort or inflammation. The following restorative exercise principles are recommended.

Functional Training

For trochanteric bursitis and ITBFS, muscle tightness and myofascial restrictions should be addressed to restore proper length and symmetry to the hip and thigh region. Particular emphasis should be placed on the ITB complex and the surrounding muscles. Due to their fascial connections, tightness or decreased length in the biceps femoris, vastus lateralis, and gluteus medius can directly impair mobility. Tightness often leads to friction over the proximal greater trochanteric bursa or the lateral femoral epicondyle. These muscle and fascial connections are often called the mechanical interface to the ITB complex. Stretching should target these areas and may include static stretching, assisted PNF stretching, and myofascial release of the ITB complex using a foam roller (Figure 18-2).

Figure 18-2
Self–myofascial release of the iliotibial band (ITB) complex with a foam roller

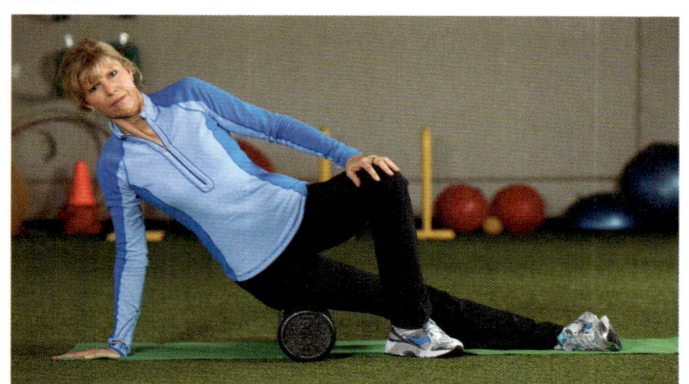

For both conditions, the focus of strengthening should be to restore proper neuromuscular control throughout the hip region and abdominal core. The gluteals, hip abductors, adductors, and external rotators should be the focus of strengthening. At this point, isolated OKC strengthening may still be necessary due to local weakness, endurance deficits, and poor muscle recruitment. Examples of isolated hip exercises include abduction and adduction (Figures 18-3 and 18-4), and "clams" lying on a stability ball (Figure 18-5).

Figure 18-3
Standing abduction

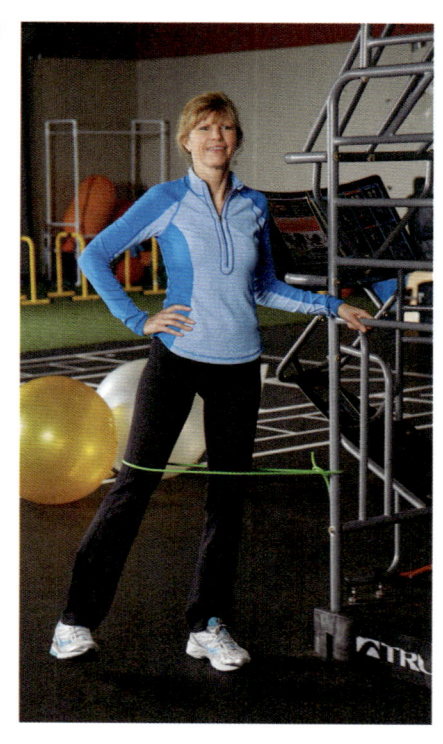

Figure 18-4
Standing adduction

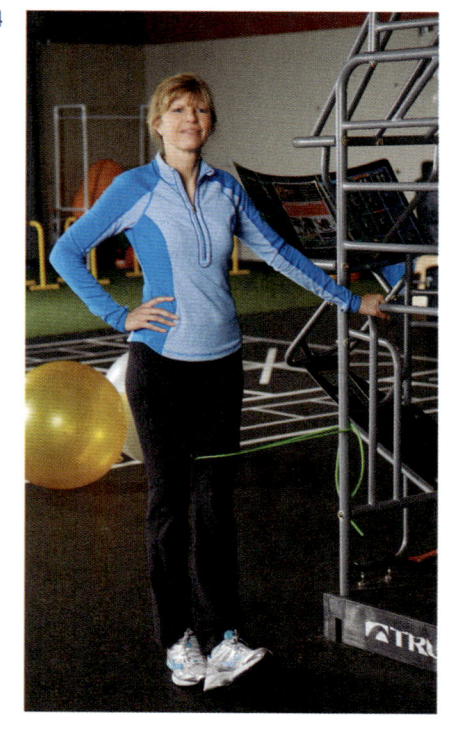

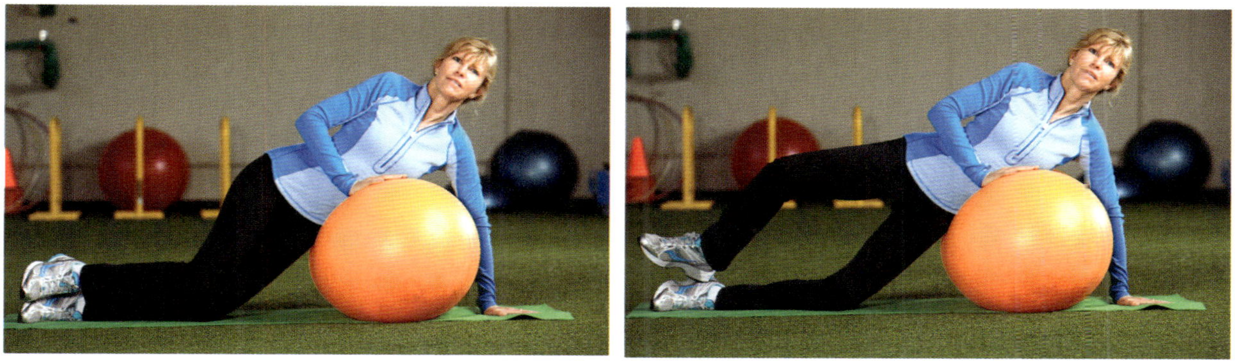

Figure 18-5
Side-lying "clams" for hip external rotator muscles

Movement Training

For both pathologies, the functional program should focus on challenging the core and hip complex. CKC exercise can be introduced to integrate more functional activity, which can be progressed in all planes of motion (Table 18-2). Challenging the client through specific Functional and Movement Training exercises will help to prepare them for more advanced activity or sport-specific training.

Deficits in general balance may be evident due to disuse of the kinetic chain. Basic progression of balance activities can be combined with CKC activities to challenge the client. For example, a single-leg squat on an air-filled disc combines CKC and proprioceptive exercise. Simply combining an unstable surface with different modes of exercise can be an efficient way to challenge a client (Table 18-3).

Cardiovascular conditioning is essential for recovery and overall health. The client should return to cardiovascular activity in a slow, progressive manner. Running, prolonged walking, and cycling have been associated with both trochanteric bursitis and ITBFS. Cardiovascular activities such as riding a stationary bike or using an elliptical trainer can be alternatives until the client is cleared to continue with higher-loading activities.

TABLE 18-2
SUGGESTED CLOSED KINETIC CHAIN PROGRESSION FOR THE LOWER EXTREMITY

Plane of Motion	Exercise Progression (Easy → Hard)
Sagittal plane	Leg press machine → wall squats with ball → forward lunges → stair stepping → bilateral squats on a foam pad → bilateral squats on air-filled discs or a BOSU → single-leg squats on the ground → single-leg squats on a foam pad → single-leg squats on an air-filled disc or BOSU
Frontal plane	Side stepping on a level surface → side stepping up onto a step → side stepping with bands → side stepping (fast) with ball passing → slide board
Combined planes	Multidirectional lunges → single-leg balance with multidirectional toe touch → single-leg reach → multidirectional hops (bilateral) → multidirectional hops (single-leg)

TABLE 18-3
SUGGESTED BALANCE PROGRESSIONS

Difficulty Level	Exercise Progression (Easy → Hard)
Level I (bilateral balance)	Ground → mini-trampoline → foam pad → air-filled discs → BOSU → wobble board
Level II (single limb—basic)	Ground → mini-trampoline → foam pad → air-filled discs → BOSU → wobble board
Level III (single limb—advanced)	Level II progression with ball tossing → head turning (up/down or side/side) → head diagonals → eyes closed Manipulate time and speed of movement

Hip Osteoarthritis

Osteoarthritis Facts

OA, or **degenerative joint disease,** is the most common form of arthritis (see Chapter 16). OA is most common among individuals with other chronic conditions, such as obesity, diabetes, and heart disease, and affects one in seven U.S. adults, or 32.5 million people, with over half of all diagnosed adults being of working age (18 to 64 years of age) [Osteoarthritis Action Alliance (OAAA), 2020]. This estimate matches future total arthritis projected prevalence estimates of 78 million by the year 2040. Further, 23.7 million (42.5% of adults with arthritis) have activity limitations because of their arthritis [Centers for Disease Control and Prevention (CDC), 2019].

OA develops from the degeneration of joint cartilage and supporting structures, and changes in the underlying bone structure. These changes often develop slowly, and progressively get worse over time, leading to stiffness, pain, mobility problems, and limited physical activity (OAAA, 2020). This degeneration is caused by a physiologic imbalance between the stress applied to the joint and the ability of the joint to endure the stress. Simply put, OA develops when breakdown (i.e., **catabolism**) exceeds regrowth (i.e., cartilage synthesis).

OA commonly affects joints of the hand, knee, hip, foot, and spine. The true cause of OA is unknown. A conceptual model for the pathogenesis of OA is that systemic factors (e.g., age, gender, ethnicity, **metabolic syndrome,** and genetic factors) increase general susceptibility to the disease, while local mechanical factors (e.g., obesity, joint injury or deformity, and muscle weakness) influence its site and severity (Cooper et al., 2013).

Signs and Symptoms of Hip Arthritis

A client with hip arthritis may complain of a "deep aching" pain in the anterior hip with weight-bearing activity and "stiffness" after inactivity (less than 30 minutes). The client may have activity limitations due to restricted, painful motion, or a feeling of instability (Zhang & Jordan, 2010).

Precautions

These clients must limit prolonged weight-bearing activities, shock loading (e.g., running), and repetitive squatting. Specific activities to avoid include deep squats or lunges, knee extensions, and plyometric activity. Light-to-moderate activity is recommended due to the diminished shock-absorbing capacity of the joint.

Early Intervention

Early intervention includes patient education, physical therapy (e.g., ROM exercises and strengthening), weight loss, supportive devices (e.g., cane or bracing), oral anti-inflammatory medication, cortisone injections, and modalities (e.g., heat and ice) (Houglum, 2010).

Restorative Exercise Program

Management of hip OA includes progressing what was done in the early intervention. The focus of the program should be on light- to moderate-loading exercises that are specific to the client's needs.

Functional Training

Due to the stiffness of the hip joint and surrounding tissues, clients may have global restrictions, as opposed to restrictions related to one specific movement such as hip internal or external rotation. Flexibility exercises should be done at a level that does not elicit pain and within a comfortable ROM. Stretching should focus on the surrounding hip muscles, including the gluteals, hamstrings, hip adductors, hip abductors, and hip external rotators.

The focus of strengthening should be to restore proper strength throughout the hip region and core. Specific OKC exercises, such as abduction (see Figure 18-3), adduction (see Figure 18-4), clams (see Figure 18-5), prone hip extension (Figure 18-6), and seated internal or external rotation with a band, can help to isolate the muscles that control the hip (Figures 18-7 and 18-8). CKC exercises should be progressed with caution. As mentioned earlier, light- to moderate-loading exercises are best for these clients. Exercises such as deep squatting or lunging can excessively load the joint and elicit pain. Midrange activity such as partial squats or lunges may be tolerable and can be progressed to single-leg movements.

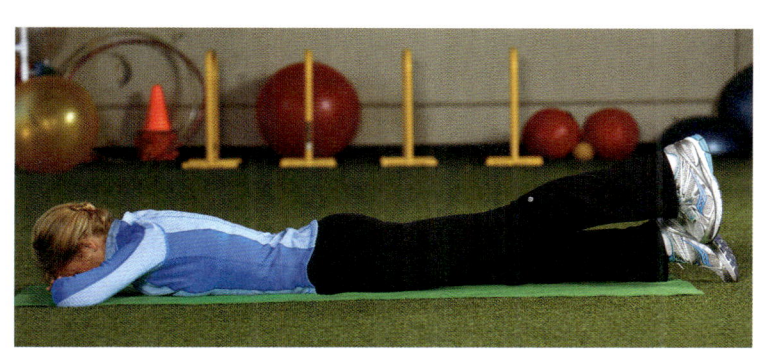

Musculoskeletal Injuries of the Lower Extremity — CHAPTER 18

Figure 18-6
Prone hip extension

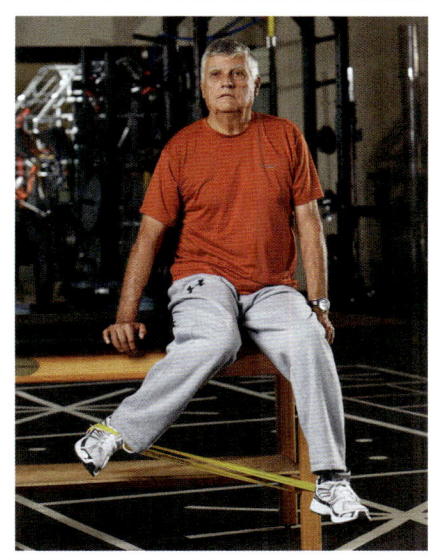

Figure 18-7
Seated hip internal rotation

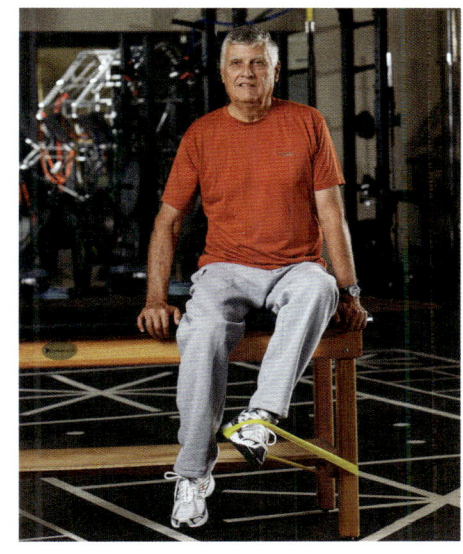

Figure 18-8
Seated hip external rotation

Movement Training

The combination of adequate flexibility, strength, and aerobic conditioning is vital for the success of the program. Functional and Movement Training should integrate all of these principles, but needs to follow the precautions mentioned earlier. Aquatic exercise is a great way to integrate basic functional activity while de-weighting the joint. The warmth and buoyancy of the water creates a great medium for exercise for these clients. A greater understanding of the science behind aquatic exercise is essential for the CMES when working with individuals who have arthritis (visit www.aeawave.com to learn more).

Deficits in general balance may be evident due to disuse of the kinetic chain. Basic progression of balance activities would be appropriate if no pain is elicited. Table 18-3 highlights a progressive program for balance.

Cardiovascular activity should be included to build cardiovascular and local muscular endurance. The bike or elliptical trainer is preferred over treadmill walking due to their mild-to-moderate joint loading. Other low-loading activities include swimming and water walking.

Total Hip Replacement

Total hip replacement or total hip arthroplasty is a surgical procedure where the head of the femur and the surface of the acetabulum are replaced with a prosthetic "ball and socket." The "ball" replaces the head of the femur and the "socket" is the cup-shaped form of the acetabulum. Total hip replacement is one of the most common surgical procedures performed in the United States. More than 1 million hip arthroplasties are done every year worldwide, a number that is expected to double within the next two decades. Symptomatic OA is the primary indication for surgery in more than 90% of patients, and its incidence is increasing because of an aging population and the obesity epidemic (Pivec et al., 2012).

This procedure is done to correct intractable damage from OA, **rheumatoid arthritis,** hip fractures, **avascular necrosis,** and **cerebral palsy** (Maxey & Magnusson, 2013). Contraindications, or factors that would prevent the surgical procedure, may include **osteoporosis,** ligament **laxity,** infection, medical risk factors (e.g., diabetes), and poor patient motivation (Maxey & Magnusson, 2013). It is important for the CMES to understand that a total hip replacement is an end-stage procedure for the client. Total hip replacement is indicated for patients who failed to respond to non-surgical management options such as pharmaceutical treatments (e.g., analgesics, anti-inflammatory agents, steroid injections, and topical treatments), self-management, patient education, acupuncture, exercise, physical therapy, or manual therapy (Tsertsvadze et al., 2014). When these conservative approaches have failed, replacing the joint is often the best option. The primary goals of the procedure are to replace the diseased joint and to decrease or eliminate pain.

There are three commonly used procedures conducted by surgeons. First, primary total hip replacement is when the whole joint is replaced with three components: a synthetic cup that replaces the acetabulum (plastic, ceramic, or metal); a ball that replaces the femoral head (highly polished metal or ceramic material); and a metal stem that is secured in the medullary canal of the proximal femur (Maxey & Magnusson, 2013). Second, a **hemiarthroplasty,** or partial hip replacement, involves only half of the joint and includes replacing the ball portion of the joint, but not the socket portion. This procedure is commonly used to treat hip fractures or avascular necrosis of the hip (Maxey & Magnusson, 2013). Third, for younger active individuals (less than 55 years of age), hip resurfacing can be done. This procedure includes resurfacing and reshaping only the femoral head with a shell or cap. Hip resurfacing is a common alternative to primary total hip replacement because it leaves more of the bone in place and does not remove the femoral neck shaft. Therefore, the procedure may give the patient more time before having to replace the whole joint (Cioppa-Mosca et al., 2006).

Primary total hip replacement is the most common among the three procedures. The success of the surgery depends on factors such as surgical technique, patient selection, type of implant, and method of fixation (Cioppa-Mosca et al., 2006). There are three main surgical procedures for primary total hip replacement currently used by surgeons. It is important for the CMES to have a working knowledge of these procedures.

Posterior Lateral Approach

This technique includes cutting the hip external rotators (i.e., piriformis, gemelli, obturators, quadratus femoris, and gluteus maximus) and posterior hip capsule with an incision between the gluteus maximus and medius (Figure 18-9; see Figure 18-1) (Maxey & Magnusson, 2013). This technique spares the hip abductors but makes the hip susceptible to posterior dislocation, because the posterior supporting structures are cut to perform the surgery. Due to this trauma, surgeons require individuals to follow specific movement precautions. In general, the individual should avoid the following (Maxey & Magnusson, 2013):

- Hip flexion greater than 90 degrees
- Hip adduction past the midline of the body
- Hip internal rotation past neutral

Typically, these precautions are followed for the first eight weeks, but can last up to one year depending on the individual and the surgeon's preference (Cioppa-Mosca et al., 2006). The reported benefits of this approach include preservation of the hip abductors and surgeon familiarity. The primary risk of this procedure is posterior dislocation (Maxey & Magnusson, 2013).

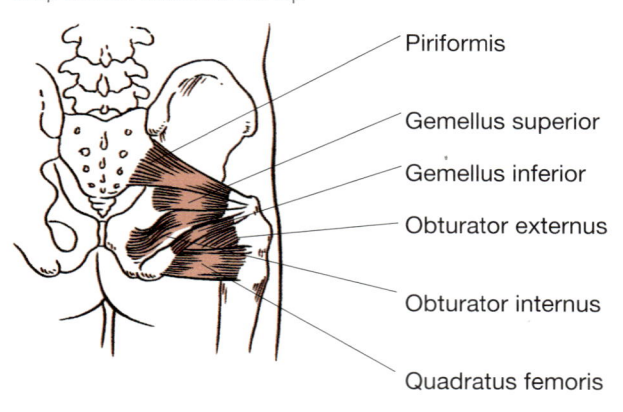

Anterior Lateral Approach

This surgical procedure utilizes a lateral curved incision that cuts through the gluteus minimus, gluteus maximus, tensor fasciae latae, vastus lateralis, and anterior capsule.

Figure 18-9
Deep external rotators of the hip

- Piriformis
- Gemellus superior
- Gemellus inferior
- Obturator externus
- Obturator internus
- Quadratus femoris

The technique spares the posterior elements of the hip (i.e., hip external rotators and posterior capsule), but does violate the hip abductors (Maxey & Magnusson, 2013). Movement restrictions also apply with this procedure. In general, the patient should avoid the following (Maxey & Magnusson, 2013):
- Combined hip external rotation and flexion
- Hip adduction past the midline of the body
- Hip internal rotation beyond neutral

As with the posterior lateral approach, these restrictions are followed for the first eight weeks, but can last up to one year depending on the individual and the surgeon's preference (Maxey & Magnusson, 2013). The reported benefits of this procedure are preservation of the posterior elements and a decreased dislocation rate (Maxey & Magnusson, 2013). However, the risks include the onset of a post-operative limp due to disruption of the abductor tendon or injury to the superior gluteal nerve (Maxey & Magnusson, 2013).

Anterior Approach

This surgical procedure is more current and has fewer post-operative restrictions. The procedure utilizes an anterior incision between the tensor fasciae latae and sartorius, which affects only the anterior capsule (Matta, Shahrdar, & Ferguson, 2005; Kennon et al., 2004). The anterior incision does not violate the contractile (e.g., hip external rotators and abductors) and connective tissues (e.g., hip capsule) around the hip, except for the surgical site. The procedure is done on a special table that positions the patient **supine,** allowing clear access to the hip joint. This procedure has two general movement precautions. The patient should avoid the following (Matta, Shahrdar, & Ferguson, 2005; Kennon et al., 2004):
- Hyperextension of the hip
- Extreme hip external rotation

These precautions may only be relative, depending on the surgeon. In fact, some surgeons have given no post-operative precautions with this procedure. The reported benefits include preservation of the hip muscles, decreased dislocation rate, normal hip mechanics, and true pelvic and leg alignment. Negligible post-operative complications have been reported with this procedure (Matta, Shahrdar, & Ferguson, 2005; Kennon et al., 2004).

Precautions

High-impact activities such as running, football, basketball, soccer, karate, waterskiing, and racquetball should be avoided following total hip replacement (Maxey & Magnusson, 2013). These activities may cause abnormal stress to the prosthetic joint. As mentioned earlier, there may be certain movement restrictions, depending on the procedure.

Early Intervention

Typically, the client has been discharged from the hospital and is transitioning from home therapy to outpatient rehabilitation. Outpatient physical therapy will help the client move back to more functional activities. It is not uncommon for clients to be severely deconditioned and have post-operative pain during this phase. The focus is on improving basic strength, functional ability, ROM, and endurance within the precautions prescribed by the physician. Management of the scar and soft-tissue restrictions will often be addressed through massage, stretching, and myofascial release.

Restorative Exercise Program

A restorative program needs to progress systematically to avoid unnecessary pain or possible re-injury. When the client is still under movement restrictions, it is important to program exercises that do not violate the prescribed hip precautions (Table 18-4). If precautions are lifted, the client may be progressed as tolerated. The client should be monitored for surgical-site pain during and after training sessions. This pain is often described as "sharp or stabbing" rather than the typical low-grade "muscle ache" [i.e., **delayed-onset muscle soreness (DOMS)**] that is often felt following a vigorous workout session.

TABLE 18-4
MOVEMENT RESTRICTIONS FOLLOWING TOTAL HIP REPLACEMENT

Hip Precautions	Posterior Lateral Approach	Anterior Lateral Approach	Anterior Approach
Flexion >90 degrees	Deep squats, lunges, yoga poses	Deep squats, lunges, yoga poses	—
Adduction (past midline)	Side-lying adduction, stretching the leg across midline	Side-lying adduction, stretching the leg across midline	—
Internal rotation	Yoga poses	Yoga poses	—
External rotation	—	Yoga poses, seated groin stretch, sitting with legs crossed	Yoga poses, seated groin stretch, sitting with legs crossed
Hyperextension	—	—	Lunges, prone hip extension

APPLY WHAT YOU KNOW

QUESTIONS FOR PHYSICIANS OF CLIENTS WITH JOINT REPLACEMENT

The CMES may begin to see the client between six and 12 weeks after surgery. Typically, the client may do a combination of physical therapy and fitness activities. Prior to working with clients who have had joint-replacement surgery, it is important for the CMES to talk with the physician and/or physical therapist to find out the client's status. Specific questions to ask include the following:

- Does the client have any movement restrictions or medical precautions?
- Did the client attend physical therapy? If yes, what types of exercises were performed for aerobic and anaerobic activity?
- Does the client have any functional limitations?

The CMES must remember that factors such as age, pre-existing medical conditions, nutritional status, prior fitness level, and client motivation will influence the client's program. There are many published post-operative protocols for primary total hip replacement. However, most surgeons have developed their own protocols based on the type of surgery, their own preferences, and available research. Reviewing specific protocols is beyond the scope of this text. The specific recommendations presented here for each category are based on the idea that the client has no motion restrictions and is cleared for fitness activities.

Functional Training

General stretching should be included to address any muscle tightness or myofascial restrictions. Static stretching, assisted PNF stretching, and self–myofascial release may be done at a mild-to-moderate level that does not stress the surgical site or hip prosthesis. A good rule is for the client to stretch into "slight or mild discomfort" but not into "pain." Particular emphasis should be placed on the gluteals, ITB complex, hamstrings, and quadriceps. Self–myofascial release should not cause "pain" that is more intense than the typical "discomfort" that is felt with this technique. Muscle groups that should be targeted include the gluteals/external rotators (Figure 18-10), ITB complex (see Figure 18-2), hamstrings (Figure 18-11), and quadriceps (Figure 18-12).

These clients are generally deconditioned and may need an initial program that focuses on building local strength and endurance throughout the hip region and abdominal core. Early fitness activity may include isolated hip OKC strengthening using lighter resistance with higher repetitions to improve local strength, endurance, and muscle recruitment. The goal should be to restore proper strength and neuromuscular control prior to advancing to functional activity.

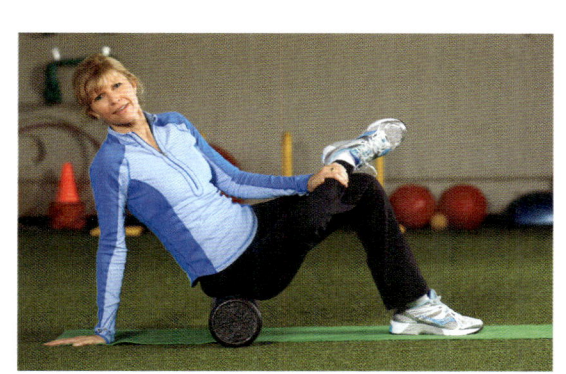

Musculoskeletal Injuries of the Lower Extremity   CHAPTER 18

Figure 18-10
Myofascial release for gluteals/external rotators

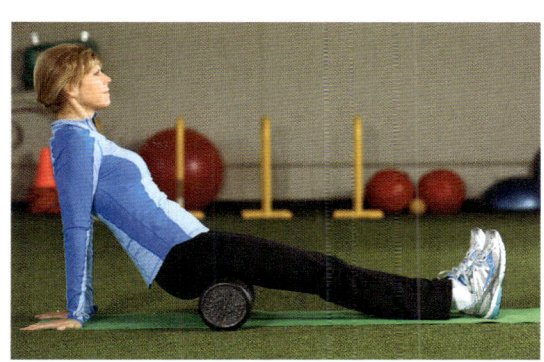

Figure 18-11
Myofascial release for the hamstrings

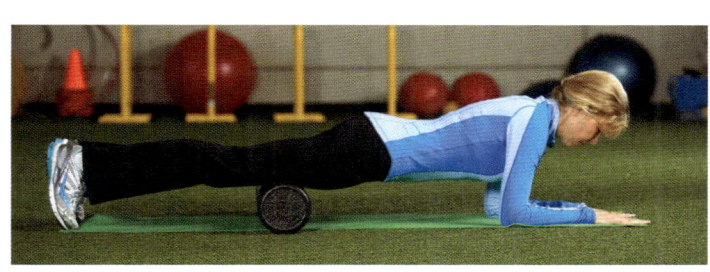

Figure 18-12
Myofascial release for the quadriceps

Movement Training

The Movement Training program should challenge the abdominal core and lumbo-pelvic-hip complex in all planes of motion, but must be progressed from basic Functional Training activities. The post-operative client may be at a lower functional level than a relatively healthy client. Basic functional tasks such as sit-to-stand, rolling in bed, stair climbing, and picking up objects may still be difficult. The client may need to master these basic skills prior to progressing with the CKC exercises.

Deficits in general balance may be evident due to disuse of the kinetic chain. Remember, basic functional ability should be obtained prior to implementing balance activity. Early balance activity can be combined with basic functional tasks. For example, the client can do the sit-to-stand exercise with a foam pad under their feet or pick up objects while standing on two air-filled discs. When appropriate, the client can be progressed with balance activity.

Cardiovascular conditioning is essential for recovery in the post-operative client. Cardiovascular activity should be within physician guidelines and general precautions. Low-loading activities such as water aerobics, stationary cycling, and elliptical training are all good alternatives to higher-loading activities such as running.

EXPAND YOUR KNOWLEDGE

THE MINIMALLY INVASIVE APPROACH TO TOTAL HIP REPLACEMENT

Total hip arthroplasty is considered one of the most successful operations in orthopedic surgery due to its positive clinical outcomes. Over the past decade, considerable interest has been devoted to the development of minimally invasive surgical techniques. Minimally invasive total hip arthroplasty, defined as the use of a 4-inch (10-cm) or even smaller incision [as opposed to the 8- to 10-inch (20- to 25-cm) incision typically used in the standard method], has become a popular approach (Yang et al., 2012).

The advantages of minimally invasive surgeries include less soft-tissue trauma (e.g., smaller skin incision and less muscle damage), reduced blood loss, and fewer blood transfusion requirements. Postoperative benefits include less pain, shorter hospital stay, quicker return to function, and a better cosmetic appearance.

It remains controversial whether minimally invasive techniques benefit patients in total hip arthroplasty. Proponents of minimally invasive total hip arthroplasty claim that it leads to a faster functional recovery, quicker hospital discharge, and increased patient satisfaction. Opponents believe that compared with traditional methods, minimally invasive total hip arthroplasty leads to increased risk of nerve injury, prosthesis malposition, and revision rate, because of the limited field of vision during the surgery (Yang et al., 2012).

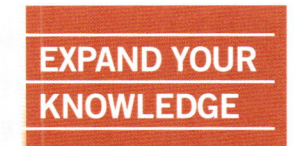

> To date, there are very few well-designed trials available based on high-level evidence regarding whether the minimally invasive approach is superior to the standard approach for total hip arthroplasty. Two meta-analyses revealed that the posterior approach in minimally invasive total hip arthroplasty is a safe surgical procedure, without increased operative complication rates and component malposition rates. These findings showed a significant decrease in surgical duration, blood loss, and hospital stay (Xu et al., 2013; Yang et al. 2012).
>
> Although more clinical evidence must be gathered to make any definitive conclusions regarding the use of minimally invasive total hip arthroplasty, the CMES will likely work with clients who have had this newer procedure. Accordingly, these clients' healing rates and return to function may be sooner than for those who receive the standard method of total hip replacement. Regardless of the procedure performed, the CMES must communicate with the client's healthcare providers and follow the specific recommendations and guidelines for returning to physical activity given by the client's medical professionals.

KNEE PATHOLOGIES

The knee is one of the most frequently injured weight-bearing joints, as it sits between the two long levers made up of the lower leg and thigh. It consists of two distinct articulations, the tibiofemoral and the patellofemoral joints. The tibiofemoral joint is one of the most complex articulations of the body—its main structures are the femur, tibia, fibula, articular cartilages, menisci, and ligaments. The tibiofemoral joint enables the relative motion of the femur and tibia, which is facilitated through contacts between the cartilages and menisci. The patellofemoral joint consists of the patella as it sits in the femoral groove surrounded by the quadriceps tendon. The tendon attachment from the patella to the tibial tubercle is sometimes called the patellar ligament because it travels from bone to bone. This structure is also known as the patellar tendon. The patellofemoral joint adds to the stability of the knee and protects the knee from anterior blows.

Patellofemoral Pain Syndrome

Patellofemoral pain syndrome (PFPS) is often called "anterior knee pain" or "runner's knee." This syndrome has been found to be the most common knee diagnosis in the outpatient setting and to have the highest prevalence among runners. In fact, PFPS makes up 16 to 25% of all running injuries (Dixit et al., 2007). Prevalence is estimated to be between 8 and 40%, with a higher incidence in females (Roush & Curtis Bay, 2012; Boling et al., 2010). Sufferers generally present with patellar pain aggravated by activities stressing the patellofemoral joint, such as squatting, prolonged sitting, stair climbing, and running (Crossley et al., 2012). The exact etiology of PFPS remains unknown, but is linked with three primary categories: overuse, biomechanics, and muscle dysfunction.

Mechanism of Injury

Overuse

PFPS is often classified as an overuse syndrome when repetitive loading activities (e.g., climbing and/or descending stairs or hills) or sports (e.g., running) are the cause of symptoms. These repetitive activities cause abnormal stress to the knee joint, which leads to pain and dysfunction. The excessive loading exceeds the body's physiological balance, which leads to tissue trauma, injury, and pain (Dixit et al., 2007). Recent increase in intensity, frequency, or duration or a change in the training environment (e.g., surface) may contribute to this condition.

Biomechanical Abnormalities

Biomechanical abnormalities can alter tracking of the patella and/or increase patellofemoral joint stress. **Pes planus,** or flat foot, has been associated with PFPS because it alters the alignment of the knee. Loss of the medial arch flattens the foot, causing a compensatory internal rotation of the tibia or femur that alters the dynamics of the patellofemoral joint (Dixit et al., 2007). Conversely, **pes cavus,** or high arches, causes less cushioning compared to a normal foot. This leads to excessive stress to the patellofemoral joint, particularly with loading activities such as running (Dixit et al., 2007). Another popular belief regarding PFPS etiology is that an increased **Q-angle** causes the quadriceps to exert a greater lateral force and predispose the patella to excessive lateral tracking. The Q-angle is the angle formed by lines drawn from the anterior superior iliac spine (ASIS) to the central patella and from the central patella to the tibial tubercle (Figure 18-13). The Q-angle is an estimate of the effective angle at which the quadriceps group pulls on the patella. A normal Q-angle is considered to be below 12 degrees, and angles greater than 15 degrees are considered pathological (Houglum, 2010; Dixit et al., 2007). On average, the Q-angle is several degrees greater in women than in men. Although it is believed that this increased Q-angle places more stress on the knee joint and leads to increased foot pronation in women (Naslund et al., 2006), this theory is not supported by the research findings, and many studies have found no relationship between an increased Q-angle and PFPS (Bolgla & Boling, 2011). It could be that the static nature of the Q-angle measurement does not accurately relate to movement at the knee, as many of PFPS patients exhibit faulty lower-extremity **kinematics** during dynamic activities like running, jumping, or single-leg landing.

Figure 18-13
Q-angle

Muscle Dysfunction

Muscle tightness and length deficits have been associated with PFPS. Tightness in the ITB complex (e.g., gluteals) causes an excessive lateral force to the patella via its fascial connection. Limited quadriceps and gastrocnemius flexibility and knee extension weakness may predict PFPS development. A knee **valgus** moment at initial contact during landing from a jump may also be a predictor of PFPS, especially in female athletes (Pappas & Wong-Tom, 2012). Tightness in the hamstrings and gastrocnemius can cause a posterior force on the knee, leading to increased contact between the patella and femur. Also, tightness in the gastrocnemius/soleus complex can lead to compensatory pronation and excessive posterior force that result in increased patellofemoral contact pressure (Houglum, 2010).

Muscle weakness in the quadriceps and hip external rotators has been associated with PFPS. In particular, quadriceps weakness has been associated with patellofemoral maltracking. For years, weakness of the vastus medialis oblique (VMO) muscle has been thought to cause patellar maltracking and increased patellofemoral contact pressure. This theory of VMO weakness has been questioned based on more recent evidence. The current thought points to training the quadriceps as a group, versus isolated training of the VMO, and is considered the "gold standard" treatment (Bolgla & Boling, 2011). Also, weakness of the hip external rotators can cause femoral internal rotation, abnormal knee valgus, and compensatory foot pronation (Robinson & Nee, 2007). Weakness in the external rotators and all of the resultant malalignments can affect patellofemoral tracking, which may lead to pain and dysfunction. Accordingly, evidence supports strengthening exercises of the hip to benefit individuals with PFPS. The use of hip abductor and external rotator strengthening, which may be further enhanced with the inclusion of exercises targeting hip flexion and hip extension, has been shown to improve hip function and reduce symptoms in individuals with this condition (Bolgla & Boling, 2011).

Signs/Symptoms

Commonly reported symptoms include pain with running, stair climbing, squatting, or prolonged sitting. The client will typically describe a gradual "achy" pain that occurs behind or underneath the knee cap and may be immediate if trauma has occurred. Clients may also report knee stiffness, giving way, clicking, or a popping sensation during movement (Houglum, 2010).

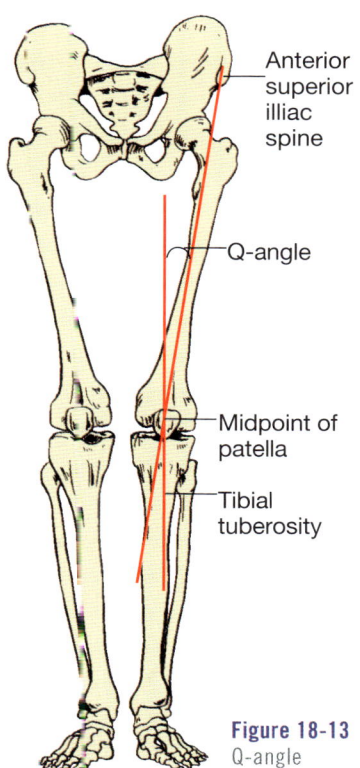

Precautions

The client is encouraged to avoid high-stress activities such as running, repetitive squatting, prolonged sitting, and stair climbing. Also, certain OKC exercises (e.g., leg extensions) have been known to cause abnormal stress on the patellofemoral joint.

Early Intervention

Evidence is inconclusive as to which particular regimen seems to demonstrate significantly better results than the others. Reports of early intervention strategies for PFPS have included the following (Al-Hakim et al., 2012; Dixit et al., 2007):
- Avoiding aggravating activities (e.g., prolonged sitting, deep squats, and running)
- Modifying training techniques (e.g., decreasing frequency and intensity)
- Proper footwear
- Physical therapy
- Patellar taping
- Knee bracing
- Arch supports
- Foot orthotics
- Patient education
- Oral anti-inflammatory medication
- Modalities (e.g., ice and heat)

If non-surgical intervention fails, surgery to correct patellar alignment would be the next option but is often considered the last resort, as the surgical outcome often fares no better than exercise treatment (Houglum, 2010).

Restorative Exercise Program

With regard to the knee, the choice between CKC and OKC activity has been debated for years. The primary concern is the stresses that are imposed on the knee joint and patella during exercise. With CKC exercises, the patellofemoral contact pressure increases as the knee bends closer to 90 degrees of flexion. In fact, the joint force begins to rise between 30 and 60 degrees and peaks at 90 degrees of flexion (Manske, 2006). These findings support the current standard of avoiding exercises that force the knee to bend beyond 90 degrees of flexion (e.g., squats). Extreme ranges of knee flexion can put the client at risk for injury due to the increased joint stress. Thus, CKC exercises between 0 and 45 degrees have been suggested as a safe range for clients with knee pathology (Kisner & Colby, 2012).

Consequently, when the foot is not fixed (as in OKC activity) the opposite occurs—the lowest force across the patella is at 90 degrees of flexion. As the knee moves toward extension, the joint forces increase and the patellar contact area decreases, producing a large increase in joint stress. The joint stress peaks between 25 and 0 degrees (Manske, 2006). These findings also support the standard that OKC exercises, such as the leg extension, need to be done with caution for certain knee pathologies [e.g., PFPS, post-operative anterior cruciate ligament (ACL) injury]. Some experts have suggested that an exercise range between 90 and 60 degrees may be safe due to low joint stress (Manske, 2006). OKC exercises that are done with the knee straight are the best option. Examples include the straight-leg raise (Figure 18-14) and prone hip extension (see Figure 18-6). These exercises isolate the muscle groups that cross the knee but do not impose any abnormal stress.

There has been some debate in the literature regarding the application of OKC and CKC exercises. A study by Cohen et al. (2001) measured the knee joint forces in subjects while they were doing OKC exercises (i.e., knee extension 90 to 0 degrees) and CKC exercises (partial squat 20 to 60 degrees). The authors found that during OKC exercises, joint stresses were not significantly higher than with CKC exercises. Another study series by Witvrouw et al. (2000) looked at subjects with patellofemoral pain after a five-week intervention program, and again at a five-year follow-up. The goal was to assess the efficacy of OKC versus CKC exercises. At five weeks, both groups showed improved function and decreased pain. At the five-year follow-up, both groups still reported functional improvements and

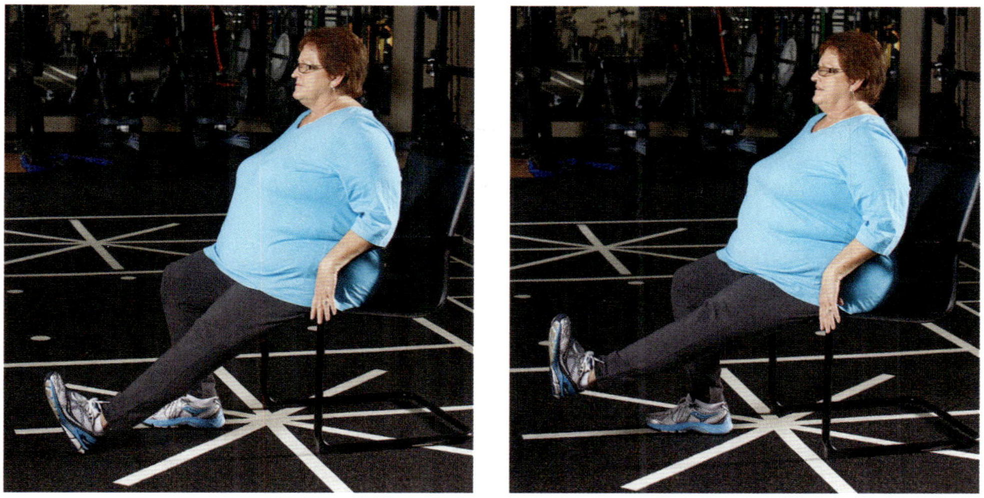

Figure 18-14
Straight-leg raise

decreased pain. The authors concluded that both OKC and CKC exercises have long-term benefits in individuals with patellofemoral pain. These studies lack clear-cut evidence regarding which type of exercise is better. The choice to use CKC or OKC exercises should be based on a thorough assessment, the client's physical abilities, exercise tolerance, and physician clearance. Further studies are needed to confirm which exercises are safer and more effective for specific populations.

The focus of the restorative program is to progress what was done in the early stages and avoid activities that aggravate the patellofemoral joint. The CMES must remember that restoring proper strength and flexibility is the key with PFPS.

Functional Training

Deficits in muscle length and myofascial mobility have been associated with PFPS. More specifically, addressing tightness in the ITB complex through stretching and myofascial release (e.g., on a foam roller) can have a major impact on the dynamics of the patellofemoral joint. Stretching of the hamstrings and calves will also help to restore muscle-length balance across the knee joint. Clients with PFPS may have tightness in these muscle groups from compensatory patterns that developed in response to pain. For example, the client may limp or avoid certain movements due to pain. This results in a tight, shortened muscle group that is unable to contract or relax through a full range of joint motion.

The focus should be to restore proper strength and neuromuscular control throughout the hip, knee, and ankle. Strengthening the quadriceps group should be the priority. The CMES should use a combination of OKC and CKC exercises to train the quadriceps group. OKC exercises can be used to isolate the quadriceps muscle group and are often utilized in the early stages. Examples of OKC exercises include straight-leg raises and leg extensions from 90 to 60 degrees. Once local strength is obtained, CKC exercises can be introduced to progress toward more functional movements. Examples of CKC exercises include bilateral quarter squats, single-leg squats, step-ups, and side-stepping. The CMES is again reminded to have the client do these exercises in a pain-free ROM to avoid re-injury.

Exercises for the hip and ankle complex should be included due to their effects on the knee joint. A systematic review by Peters and Tyson (2013) found that exercise interventions that focused on regaining function in the hip resulted in clinical improvements in pain and function in patients with PFPS. Presumably, these exercises improve proximal and distal alignment and reduce load on the patellofemoral joint, which may be especially important for individuals wherein increasing the load on the patellofemoral joint (e.g., exercises that focus specifically on flexion and extension of the knee) initially could increase symptoms such as pain and swelling. The muscles that control the ankle complex may need to be strengthened if they are to have distal control. See "Lower Leg, Foot, and Ankle Pathologies" on page 614 for further discussion.

Movement Training

For a client with PFPS, the return to function should be a systematic process that follows the precautions mentioned earlier in this chapter and the phases of the ACE IFT Model. The client should have adequate flexibility, strength, and neuromuscular control prior to progressing toward more advanced Movement Training. Slowly returning to full activity while monitoring for changes in symptoms (e.g., pain) is recommended. Refer to Table 18-2 for further examples of functional CKC exercises.

Deficits in general balance may be evident due to disuse of the kinetic chain. Basic progression of balance activities would be appropriate if no pain is elicited. Table 18-3 highlights a progressive program for balance. Low-loading cardiovascular activity such as water aerobics, riding a stationary bike, and using an elliptical trainer is preferred over higher-loading activities such as running or treadmill walking.

Meniscal Injuries

Meniscal tears are one of the most commonly reported knee injuries. Meniscal tears can be either acute or degenerative. Studies have reported that the mean annual incidence of acute meniscal tears is about 60 to 70 per 100,000, with a male to female ratio ranging from 2.5:1 to 4:1 (Maffulli et al., 2010). In individuals older than 65 years, the prevalence of degenerative meniscal tears is 60%. The primary age range for meniscal tears for males is 31 to 40 years and for females is 11 to 20 years (Baker & Lubowitz, 2006; Bhagia et al., 2006). Meniscal pathology in younger patients is likely due to an acute traumatic event, while degenerative changes are more frequent at an older age.

The menisci have an important role within the knee through their multiple functions (Figure 18-15). First, both the medial and lateral menisci act as shock absorbers and assist with load bearing of the joint. Second, the menisci work together to assist with joint congruency of the femur and tibia during motion. Third, they act as secondary restraints to give the joint more stability. Fourth, the menisci assist with joint lubrication by helping to maintain a synovial layer inside the joint. Fifth, nerve endings within the menisci are thought to give proprioceptive feedback during motion and compression (Baker & Lubowitz, 2006; Bhagia et al., 2006; Manske, 2006). It is important to note that the menisci receive blood only in 10 to 25% of the outer periphery, which is called the vascular zone. Due to its blood supply, this region may heal better than the non-vascular inner region of the meniscus (Bhagia et al., 2006; Manske, 2006). This can be a factor in determining when surgery is necessary.

Mechanism of Injury

Meniscal injuries often occur from trauma or degeneration. Traumatic injuries can occur from a combination of loading and twisting of the joint. For example, a tear can occur when an individual suddenly decelerates and twists on a flexed knee during running. The combination of axial loading with pivoting of the femur on the tibia causes a **shear force** across the meniscus that exceeds the strength of the tissue, resulting in injury (Manske, 2006). Older individuals with degenerative menisci are more predisposed to meniscal tears, and degenerative types of meniscal tears are commonly seen in men aged between 40 and 60 years (Maffulli et al., 2010). Meniscal tears can also occur with other traumatic injuries such as acute ACL tears (e.g., lateral meniscus) or medial collateral ligament injury (e.g., medial meniscus) (Manske, 2006).

Signs and Symptoms

When a client has a meniscal tear, they may complain of symptoms during activity. Commonly reported symptoms include stiffness, clicking or popping with joint loading, giving way, catching,

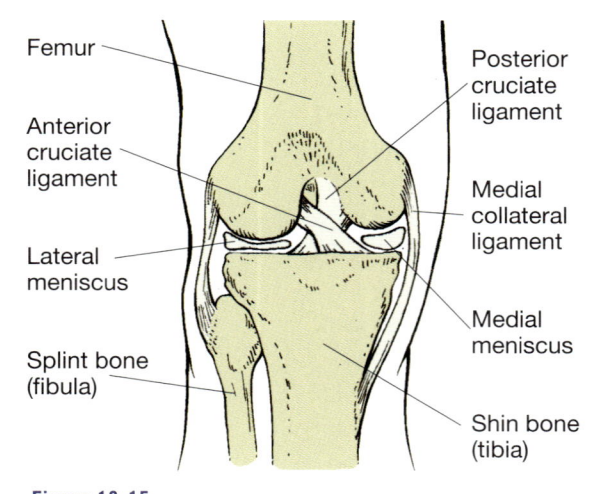

Figure 18-15
Knee joint anatomy depicting the anterior cruciate ligament (ACL), the medial collateral ligament (MCL), the posterior cruciate ligament (PCL), and the medial and lateral menisci

and locking (in more severe tears). Other signs include joint pain, swelling, and muscle weakness (e.g., quadriceps) (Baker & Lubowitz, 2006; Manske, 2006).

Precautions

Frequently with non-operative management, clients will be cleared to resume activity once symptoms have diminished, but they are encouraged to avoid deep squats, cutting, pivoting or twisting for as long as symptoms are present (Manske, 2006).

Non-operative Management

Indications for non-operative management include absent or diminished symptoms, and small or degenerative tears (Manske, 2006). Typically, the client will be sent to physical therapy to improve strength and ROM. Modalities (e.g., ice and heat), compression, bracing, and oral anti-inflammatory medication often accompany physical therapy. If conservative management fails, surgical intervention may be the next step. For degenerative tears, current evidence suggests that although non-operative management can be beneficial initially, around a third of patients will go on to have a **meniscectomy** to achieve satisfactory pain relief and improved function (Mordecai et al., 2014).

Surgical Considerations

In the past, total meniscectomy (removal of the greater part of the meniscus) was commonly done to relieve symptoms. Over time, this procedure has become less popular due to the progressive joint degeneration that it causes. Arthroscopic (e.g., with a camera) partial meniscectomy and meniscal repairs are now the two most common procedures. When choosing which procedure is appropriate, the surgeon must consider several factors, including age, location, severity, associated ligament injury, and type of tear (Houglum, 2010).

With a partial meniscectomy, the surgeon removes only the unstable, torn fragments and leaves the viable, healthy tissue intact—especially in the peripheral rim, which is mostly responsible for the biomechanical function of the knee (Jeong, Lee, & Ko, 2012). This is typically done when there is a large tear that enters the avascular inner zone (Maxey & Magnusson, 2013). The goal is to preserve as much of the meniscus as possible and allow the remaining meniscus to still serve its function without causing early degeneration. Short-term results following partial meniscectomy are positive, with studies reporting around 90% satisfactory clinical results. With regard to arthritic changes in the knee, several long-term studies show that partial meniscectomy may delay degeneration but not prevent it (Mordecai et al., 2014).

A meniscal repair involves suturing the torn fragment back in place. The ideal location for repair is a tear that occurs in the outer vascular zone. This procedure preserves the meniscal tissue, but requires a slower rehabilitation due to healing of the repair versus extracting the torn tissue. For the patient and clinician, the potential benefits of meniscal repair must be weighed against significant differences in post-operative rehabilitation. Patients having a simple meniscectomy can usually return to full work after a couple of weeks. However, following meniscal repair, patients are required to wear a brace for up to six weeks and will have precautions related to weight-bearing movements and ROM, followed by extensive physiotherapy (Mordecai et al., 2014). Common candidates include active individuals under the age of 50 who have a small tear in the outer vascular zone (Baker & Lubowitz, 2006).

Early Intervention

Early intervention after partial meniscectomy or meniscal repair may involve specific precautions for the first two to eight weeks, depending on the surgeon's preference. With partial meniscectomy, there is no anatomical structure that needs to be protected, so rehabilitation can be progressed more aggressively with immediate partial or full weight-bearing. The client may still have to use crutches and a brace. The meniscal repair often involves a slower progression with partial or non-weight-bearing activities with crutches and a brace. The client may also have ROM restrictions for knee flexion (e.g., OKC knee flexion to 90 degrees,

OKC knee extension to 30 degrees, and leg press to 10 degrees of extension) for the first four to six weeks to protect the healing tissue (Houglum, 2010).

For both procedures, the patient is typically sent to outpatient physical therapy for six to 12 weeks, depending on the physician's plan of care and the patient's insurance constraints. During this time, the goal is to increase ROM, improve lower-extremity strength, control pain and swelling, and progress to more functional activity.

> **EXPAND YOUR KNOWLEDGE**
>
> **PROTOCOL FOR REHABILITATION AFTER AN ARTHROSCOPIC PARTIAL MENISCECTOMY**
>
> This feature provides a sample of how the important phases of healing are considered and integrated into the clinical practice of rehabilitation. Note that the CMES will likely see the client only in the last phase (Phase III), and as such, this information is intended only to give the reader a glimpse into the practice of early clinical intervention with a specific musculoskeletal pathology.
>
> *Overview*
>
> Typically, damage to the meniscus results in a tear. As the torn piece begins to move in an abnormal fashion inside the joint, it can cause a great deal of pain and limitation in the knee, thereby limiting activity tolerance. Depending on the type and size of the tear, arthroscopic surgery may be recommended. The options are to perform a repair of the meniscus or a meniscectomy, where the damaged meniscus is removed to prevent further irritation. Since the meniscus has such a poor blood supply, a meniscectomy is often performed. Generally, following knee arthroscopy, a fairly aggressive approach can be taken and ROM and strength are progressed as tolerated.
>
> *Phase I (Weeks 1–4)*
>
> The emphasis is on regaining full knee extension so the patient can ambulate with a normal gait pattern. This requires facilitating neuromuscular control of the quadriceps, controlling swelling, emphasizing normal gait pattern, and achieving knee ROM of 0 to 90 degrees.
>
> *Strengthening:* Quad sets (**isometric** quadriceps contractions); straight-leg raise (SLR) in all planes of motion; standing heel raises on a step; stretching (pain-free range) of the hamstrings, gastrocnemius, ITB, and piriformis
>
> *ROM:* Manual patellar mobilizations; heel slides using a towel or wall if needed; prone hangs as needed to gain full extension
>
> *Balance:* Weight shifting; single-limb stance
>
> *Gait:* Move to single crutch when the patient is able and then discontinue the use of crutches when the patient is able to ambulate with a normal gait pattern
>
> *Modalities:* **Electrical muscle stimulation (EMS)** may be needed to facilitate the quadriceps if voluntary muscle contraction is difficult. Ice should be used following exercise and initially every hour for 20 minutes. A clinically directed home exercise program should be performed three times a day.
>
> *Phase II (Weeks 5–11)*
>
> The criteria to progress to this phase are minimal pain and swelling to allow sufficient healing, full weight-bearing with normalized gait mechanics, and good control of lower-extremity musculature. By the end of this phase, the patient should independently ambulate with a normal gait, have good quadriceps control and controlled swelling, and be able to ascend and descend stairs.
>
> *Strengthening:* Quad sets should be continued until swelling is gone and quadriceps tone is restored. SLR in all planes should be continued with progression to ankle weights when ready. Leg presses, both bilateral and unilateral, should be performed with the body weight on the heels to avoid too much load on the patellar tendon. Step-ups, step-overs, wall slides, mini squats, calf raises, and hamstring curls are also appropriate strengthening exercise choices.
>
> *ROM:* Biking should not be performed until 110 degrees of knee flexion is achieved. Patients must not use the bike to gain ROM. Biking should be performed daily with a focus on increasing resistance as the patient is able to work the quadriceps.

Stretching: Continue with hamstring, calf, ITB, and piriformis stretching. The goal for ROM is 0 to 125 degrees. Additionally, aggressive scar massage at incision sites, prone hangs, and seated or supine heel slides are appropriate for stretching enhancement.

Balance: Single-leg stance on even and uneven surfaces focusing on knee flexion; medicine ball toss; lateral cone walking with single-leg balance between each cone; foam roller or biomechanical ankle platform system (BAPS) board balance work

Gait: Cone walking forward and lateral; discontinue the use of crutches when normal gait pattern is achieved

Modalities: Continue to use ice after exercise

Phase III (Weeks 12–18)

The criteria to progress to this phase includes a good tolerance for the previous phase, full ROM, normal muscle strength, good closed-chain control in linear and multidirectional activities, and **isokinetic** strength of 70% of the uninvolved extremity. Goals for this phase are full quadriceps control and good quadriceps tone, ability to perform **activities of daily living (ADL)** without difficulty, a return to pre-injury sport and recreational activities, and the establishment of an ongoing training program. *Note:* Exercises will be progressed based on the patient's quadriceps tone. A client who continues to have poor quadriceps tone must not be advanced to activities that require high quadriceps strength, such as squats and lunges.

Strengthening: Continue with the previous exercises, increasing the intensity as much as the client can tolerate. Appropriate exercises during this phase include slow and controlled forward and lateral step-ups using dumbbells as needed to increase intensity; free squats or squats using the Smith machine; forward and reverse lunges using dumbbells as needed to increase intensity; hip flexion with elastic resistance; single-leg squats and single-leg wall squats; and Russian deadlifts (unilateral and bilateral).

Restorative Exercise Program

The CMES may begin to see the client for fitness activities as soon as four weeks after a meniscectomy and eight to 12 weeks after a meniscal repair (Houglum, 2010). The client may do a combination of physical therapy and fitness activities. As noted earlier, it is important to consult with the doctor or physical therapist regarding exercise precautions or contraindications. The strategies presented in the following sections take into account clearance by the physician and the client's ability to load the knee with no symptoms.

Functional Training

At this point, the client will have done stretching for a period of time. However, fitness activities can be more demanding than general rehabilitation on a weakened lower extremity. With both the partial meniscectomy and meniscal repair, progressive stretching of the muscle groups that cross the knee should be done. Specifically, stretching of the quadriceps and hamstrings should be emphasized to help maintain adequate flexibility.

When recommending exercises after both the meniscectomy and meniscal repair, exercises that require deep squatting, cutting, or pivoting should be avoided until cleared by the client's physician. Examples of exercises to avoid include bar squats, leg presses or lunges with greater than 90 degrees of flexion, full ROM on the leg-extension machine, and plyometric or agility drills that include cutting or pivoting. These exercises may impart high shear forces to the healing tissues, which can result in re-injury. In fact, deep squatting and hyperflexion of the knee are discouraged for the first six months following a meniscal repair (Manske, 2006).

Movement Training

Most exercises are safe if progressed appropriately by the CMES. After a client demonstrates movement efficiency in all three planes, CKC activities such as squats, leg presses, and lunges can be performed initially from 0 to 45 degrees and progressed to 90 degrees once the client is cleared by their physician. OKC activities such as the straight-leg raise (see Figure 18-14), abduction (see Figure 18-3), and adduction (see Figure 18-4) are encouraged to isolate the hip musculature.

Initially, knee extensions are advised from 90 to 60 degrees and progressed once cleared. More advanced, double- and single-leg multiplanar activity should be safe once adequate healing has taken place and proper clearance is obtained.

Functional integration back into athletic activity should be relatively easy for these clients. In general, a client with a partial meniscectomy can return to basic activity after two to four weeks and return to athletic and sports activity between six and 12 weeks after surgery. For a client with a meniscal repair, running may begin at three to four months after surgery, and full return to athletic and sports activity may begin five to six months after surgery (Manske, 2006).

Deficits in general balance may be evident due to disuse of the kinetic chain. Basic progression of balance activities would be appropriate at this stage (see Table 18-3).

Anterior Cruciate Ligament Injuries

ACL injuries are among the most common and devastating sports-related injuries of the knee. ACL injury frequently affects young, active individuals, with females having a reported two- to tenfold greater risk than males playing the same sport. High risk of injury, along with a high rate of sports participation among girls and young women over the last 30 years, has led to a rapid rise in ACL injuries in females (Hewett, Di Stasi, & Myer, 2014). Seventy to 80% of ACL injuries are non-contact and occur as a result of improper landing from a jump or lateral cutting maneuvers that are common in different athletic activities such as basketball, volleyball, and soccer (Levine et al., 2013).

Because the bony relationship between the tibia and femur offers little bony stability, the ACL is of primary importance as a stabilizer of the knee, with its main role of preventing anterior translation of the tibia on the femur (see Figure 18-15). The ACL and posterior cruciate ligament (PCL) work together to control excessive rotary motion. An intact ACL handles around 454 Newtons (N) of force in daily activities, and can tolerate forces up to 1,730 N prior to rupturing (Houglum, 2010). Typical running and cutting maneuvers create approximately 1,700 N of force (Brotzman & Manske, 2011; Manske, 2006). However, injury will occur if the forces imposed on the knee exceed its strength.

Mechanism of Injury

A lack of neuromuscular control during dynamic movements has been hypothesized to be the primary cause for ACL injury risk and re-injury following ACL reconstruction. This deficit in dynamic control is thought to result in excessive joint loads that lead to detrimental ACL stress/strains and ultimate failure (Figure 18-16). The mechanism of injury often involves a maneuver of deceleration combined with twisting, pivoting, or side-stepping. The combined multiplanar movements cause a traumatic shearing force that exceeds the tensile strength of the ACL, resulting in injury (Hewett, Di Stasi, & Myer, 2013).

Signs/Symptoms

An ACL injury is often traumatic. The client will often report hearing a "pop" during the activity, followed by immediate swelling, instability, decreased ROM, and pain. This typically requires immediate medical care to immobilize and protect the joint, followed by a visit to the orthopedic doctor for further diagnosis and intervention (e.g., non-operative versus operative approaches) (Houglum, 2010).

Non-operative Management

Non-operative treatment may be beneficial for older, sedentary individuals, but it may be problematic for younger, active individuals. The ACL-deficient knee may still cause instability with activity and may lead to further injury to knee structures such as the menisci or articular cartilage (Houglum, 2010). The focus of treatment is to maintain adequate ROM, gait, proprioception, and strength of the muscles around the knee. Modalities including ice and compression wrapping may be used to control swelling.

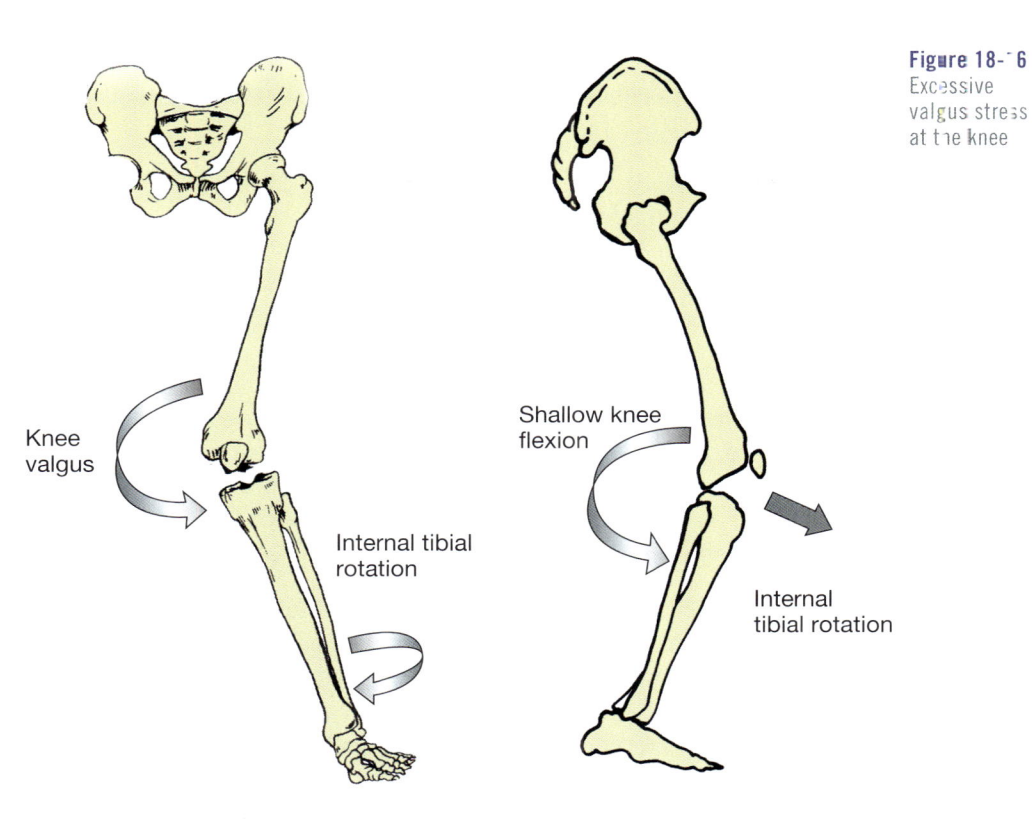

Musculoskeletal Injuries of the Lower Extremity CHAPTER 18

Figure 18-16
Excessive valgus stress at the knee

Knee valgus
Internal tibial rotation
Shallow knee flexion
Internal tibial rotation

Non-operative Precautions

With non-operative management, the client may be cleared to slowly resume activity once symptoms have diminished, but may be restricted from performing jumping, cutting, pivoting, or twisting motions. Wearing a protective knee brace is recommended to protect the deficient knee during activity. After rehabilitation, some individuals attempt to return to their activity or sport despite the presence of instability. If this proves unsuccessful, surgery may be the next option. Prior to surgery, the physician may prescribe pre-operative rehabilitation to restore ROM, muscle strength, and proper gait.

Surgical Considerations

There are several procedures currently used by surgeons to repair the ACL. Surgery to reconstruct the ACL involving the medial third of the patellar tendon and the medial hamstring (i.e., semitendinosus) are the two most common procedures. There are good data to support all the different types of grafts used in current practice for the reconstruction of a ruptured ACL. There is no clear "best" graft to use, and the surgeon's decision to choose one approach over another is multifactorial, with an emphasis on each patient's unique situation (Shaerf et al., 2014). Although ACL reconstruction has become the current gold standard for restoring the stability of a symptomatic ACL-deficient knee, researchers report that conventional ACL reconstruction fails to restore the normal joint kinematics and **kinetics** (Hoshino et al., 2013; Hall, Stevermer, & Gillette, 2012). Remarkably, patients remain at high risk (i.e., between 66 and 100%) for development of early onset OA even after surgical reconstruction (Kiapour & Murray, 2014). These findings should alert the CMES to the importance of an effective post-operative restorative exercise program to help mitigate the effects of potential OA.

The Patellar Tendon Graft

This procedure involves taking the middle third of the patellar tendon (autograft) to replace the damaged ACL. The procedure is recommended for athletes in high-demand sports and individuals with occupations that do not require large amounts of kneeling or squatting. This procedure may not be indicated for people with a history of patellofemoral pain, arthritis, or patellar tendinitis, or for smaller individuals with a narrow patellar tendon (Allen, 2007). Reported problems with the procedure include post-operative pain behind the kneecap, pain with squatting, and a low risk of patellar fractures (Houglum, 2010).

The Hamstring Tendon Graft

With this procedure, the surgeon typically harvests strands of tendons from the medial semitendinosus to reconstruct the ACL. Surgeons also use additional tendons from the gracilis muscle, which creates a combined four-strand tendon graft (Houglum, 2010). This procedure may be especially beneficial for younger patients who still have open growth plates. With the hamstring tendon graft, there are no graft bone ends that could violate the growth plate and stimulate early closure, as may occur with a patellar graft (Brown, 2007). This procedure has fewer problems with pain behind the knee cap, better **cosmesis** (no anterior incision), decreased post-operative stiffness, and faster recovery (Manske, 2006). Reported problems with the procedure include increased laxity of the new ligament due to graft elongation (stretching), slower healing of the tendon graft, and loosening of the graft at the anchoring site in the bone (Manske, 2006).

The Allograft

Surgeons also use cadaveric or **allograft** grafts from the Achilles tendon, tibialis anterior, and patellar tendon to replace the torn ACL. The allograft procedure may be beneficial for patients who have failed prior ACL reconstruction or who have multiple ligaments that need repair. Advantages include decreased morbidity at the donor site, decreased surgical time, and less post-operative pain. Problems with the allograft procedure include risk of infection and graft elongation (Houglum, 2010). *Note:* The client's physician is always in the best position to make the most appropriate recommendation regarding the choice of a given surgical technique.

Post-operative Precautions

It is common for clients who return to higher-level activity to develop anterior knee pain. The prevalence ranges from 15 to 25%, with reported incidences as high as 55% (Manske, 2006). The healing patellar graft has been linked to anterior knee pain. The knee should be gradually introduced to activity to allow adaptation and adequate healing. To protect the graft, the physician may have the client wear a protective brace for the first year after surgery or permanently during activity. Activity should be stopped if any of the following occurs: increased pain at the surgical site, increased swelling, loss of ROM, or increased exercise pain.

Early Intervention

Typically, the client will be in physical therapy for the first three to four months, depending on the physician's preferences and the client's insurance constraints. The client is generally able to perform full weight-bearing with crutches and a brace for the first two to six weeks. The client may also get a custom brace later on to wear during workouts and athletic activity.

During the first six to 12 weeks after surgery, the fixation of the graft into the bone is the weakest point. Exercise programming during this time must take this weakness into account. Also, the graft goes through a sequence of avascular necrosis (i.e., breakdown), revascularization, and remodeling. This sequential process helps to change the properties, or "ligamentize," the graft so that it will eventually resemble the original ACL that was replaced. The implanted graft begins to resemble the original ACL after around six months to one year. Full maturation has been reported to occur after one year (Houglum, 2010).

There are a vast amount of published protocols on ACL rehabilitation. Early protocols developed in the 1970s and 1980s stressed more protection of the knee, limited weight-bearing, and immobilization with a cast or brace for the first six to 12 weeks. The client was then slowly progressed with strength and ROM, and then began running between nine and 12 months post-surgery. As researchers began to understand more about the ACL, the protocols began to mature between the late 1980s and the 1990s with the development of the "accelerated protocol" in which early mobility is stressed while still protecting the graft through bracing. Researchers found that early, safe activities that loaded the graft site helped to stimulate healing (Kruse, Gray, & Wright, 2012). Most current protocols are based on milestones that the individual must meet before continuing to the next phase. For example, the individual needs to have adequate quadriceps strength, proprioception, and ROM before being able to unlock the brace and walk without crutches. Common among protocols is a return to functional activity between 12 and 16 weeks after surgery and a return to sporting activities around six months (Houglum, 2010). Most orthopedic surgeons have developed their own protocols based on the type of surgery, personal preferences and experience, and available research. Reviewing specific protocols is beyond the scope of this text, though the following sections cover specific recommendations within each category that are based on the idea that the client is cleared to do fitness activities.

Restorative Exercise Program

The CMES may begin to see the client as soon as 12 to 16 weeks after surgery. The client may do a combination of physical therapy and fitness activities. It is important for the CMES to consult the physician or physical therapist regarding what procedure was done and the post-operative protocol, as well as to obtain clearance for fitness activities.

Functional Training

Stretching the muscles around the knee is a priority for the client. One important principle is that weak muscles can become tight and tight muscles can become weak. Weakened muscles may not be able to generate adequate force due to poor strength and endurance. This may create tightness due to the inability to generate the needed force for movement. A tight muscle has a poor length-tension relationship and cannot generate adequate force for movement. Specifically, the quadriceps, hamstrings, and calves should be targeted to maintain adequate flexibility around the knee.

The choice between CKC and OKC activity is of utmost importance for the client who is post-surgery. The goal is to progressively strengthen the leg without risking injury to the graft site. CKC exercises have been used preferentially because they tend to be safer for the patellofemoral joint, replicate functional tasks, and do not contribute to increased risk of anterior tibial displacement. CKC exercises are mainly used to train the quadriceps to improve muscle strength, coordination, and proprioception, while putting the least amount of tensile strain on the ACL (Glass, Waddell, & Hoogenboom, 2010). In their systematic review, Glass, Waddell, and Hoogenboom found that CKC and OKC exercises seem to have similar outcomes on knee laxity, pain, and function, and therefore can both be used during the rehabilitation of a patient with ACL deficiency or post–ACL reconstruction. The authors concluded that the conservative approach would be to use CKC exercises primarily, at least at the start of rehabilitation (for the first six weeks), and then incorporate OKC exercises as an additional method.

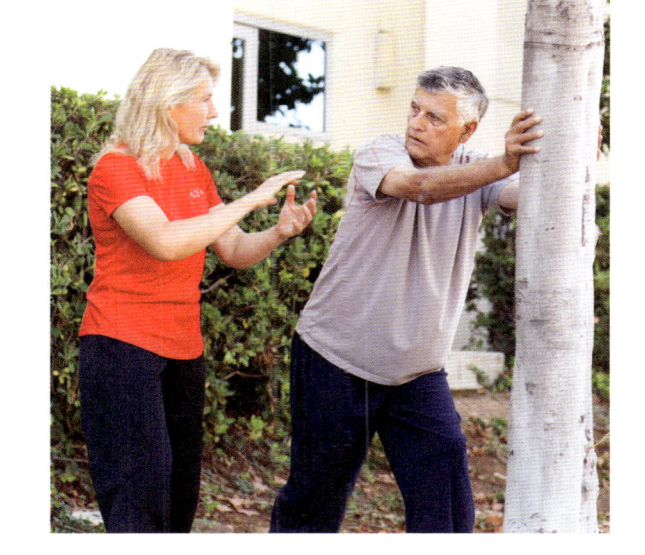

Immediate postoperative weight-bearing, range of knee motion from 0 to 90 degrees of flexion, and strengthening with CKC exercises appear to be safe (Kruse, Gray, & Wright, 2012). It is important to understand that limiting the ROM helps protect the healing graft by preventing excessive force to the joint. OKC exercises with the knee straight and CKC exercises within the appropriate ranges are recommended to protect the surgical site. The ROM precautions can be lifted once adequate healing has taken place.

Strengthening of the quadriceps, hamstrings, and hip musculature is important. Both the hamstrings and quadriceps play a key role in prevention of further injury. Hip strengthening should be implemented due to its effect on the knee joint during CKC exercises.

Movement Training

Integration of neuromotor, flexibility, and muscular conditioning exercises may begin with basic activity as early as 12 weeks post-surgery and can be progressed toward athletic activity between four and six months. The goal during this time (i.e., 12 weeks to six months) is to safely load the knee in all planes of motion without compromising the graft site. Refer to Table 18-2 for a description of CKC progression.

Clients who have undergone ACL reconstruction will have deficits in balance. Balance activity should have been implemented in the early stages of rehabilitation. At the time of fitness activity, the client should have good balance with basic single-leg activities. Progressively challenging the knee in multiple planes will help prepare the joint for higher-level activity (see Table 18-3).

Low-loading cardiovascular activity, such as water aerobics, stationary cycling, and elliptical training, is preferred over higher-loading activity until the client is cleared by their physician.

Total Knee Replacement

Total knee replacements (TKR), or total knee arthroplasty, were first performed in 1968. Since then, improvements in surgical materials and procedures have greatly increased its success. TKR is currently the international standard of care for treating degenerative and rheumatologic knee joint disease, as well as certain knee joint fractures. In the U.S., the use of this procedure has increased substantially in the past decade and this growth is expected to continue (Kurtz et al., 2011). TKR is indicated when conservative treatment fails to restore mobility or reduce arthritic pain, chronic knee inflammation, or swelling. Similar to a client coping with an arthritic hip, the TKR client has suffered with a painful joint for some time and may have tried conservative treatment such as oral medication, injections, and physical therapy. When these conservative approaches have failed, replacing the joint is often the best option. With joint replacement, the primary goals are to replace the diseased joint and eliminate knee pain (Zanasi, 2011). Contraindication to the procedure may include osteoporosis, ligament laxity, infection, medical risk factors, extreme or severe obesity, and poor patient compliance (Maxey & Magnusson, 2013; Kerkhoffs et al., 2012). There are two common procedures conducted for total knee replacement: primary TKR and partial knee replacement.

Primary Total Knee Replacement

Primary TKR commonly consists of three components: the femoral component (e.g., highly polished metal), the tibial component (e.g., durable plastic often held in a metal tray), and the patellar component (e.g., durable plastic). The aggregate of these components make up the prosthetic knee joint. Primary TKR is recommended for candidates who have arthritis throughout the knee joint, as well as for young people. TKR success is dependent mainly upon the implant alignment and post-operative activity level of the recipient, so is often used in elderly patients with limited activities or in younger, low-demand patients who have limited function because of systemic disease in multiple joints (Zanasi, 2011). It is the treatment of choice in patients over age 55 with progressive and painful OA in whom nonsurgical and less-invasive treatments have failed (Rosneck et al., 2007).

Partial Knee Replacement

Another alternative to primary TKR is the partial, or unicompartmental, knee replacement. The knee joint consists of three compartments: the medial compartment, the lateral compartment, and the patellofemoral compartment. This procedure is used for a knee joint that is relatively healthy with only one damaged (e.g., arthritic) compartment. If two or more compartments are damaged, partial knee replacement is not recommended [American Academy of Orthopedic Surgeons (AAOS), 2007]. Although generally considered a more difficult procedure than TKR, partial knee replacement is thought to allow preservation of the uninvolved soft tissue and bone, reduced operating time, better post-operative ROM, less pain, better stair-climbing ability, improved gait due to proprioception maintenance, and increased patient satisfaction compared to TKR (Dalury et al., 2009). This technique is used to replace the medial or lateral compartment, but not the patellar component.

This procedure is generally not recommended for younger, active individuals because the partal components tend to have less durability than the primary components and can break down faster. Candidates tend to be older individuals with a fairly sedentary lifestyles. Only six to eight out of 100 patients with arthritic knees are appropriate candidates for this procedure (AAOS, 2007).

Precautions

There are no specific movement precautions for these procedures. The client is encouraged to avoid high-stress activities such as jogging, skiing, tennis, racquetball, jumping, repetitive squatting, and contact sports (e.g., football and basketball). Until cleared, lifting is typically limited to no more than 40 pounds (18 kg) and heavy weightlifting is discouraged (Maxey & Magnusson, 2013; AAOS, 2007).

Early Intervention

Patients who receive TKR experience a loss of approximately 80% of their knee-extension strength over the two to three days of their hospitalization (Holm et al., 2010), which is caused by failure of the CNS to activate the quadriceps muscle (Rice & McNair, 2010). The mechanisms underlying post-operative quadriceps muscle inhibition appear to be altered afferent signaling from the affected knee due to swelling, inflammation, and damage to joint afferents. Hence, rehabilitation modalities that are known to increase CNS activation of the quadriceps muscle are indicated after TKR (Bandholm et al., 2014). The client is typically sent to outpatient physical therapy for six to 12 weeks, depending on the physician's plan of care and the client's insurance constraints. During this time, the goal is to increase ROM, improve lower-extremity strength, enhance balance, control pain and swelling, and progress to more functional activity (Maxey & Magnusson, 2013; AAOS, 2007). It is not uncommon for these clients to still have post-surgical knee pain and be deconditioned. The recommendations in the following sections are based on the idea that the client has been cleared for fitness activities.

Restorative Exercise Program

The client may be cleared to return to progressive fitness activities as soon as six to eight weeks after surgery. The client may still be attending physical therapy during this time. It is important to consult the physician or physical therapist regarding any post-operative guidelines and obtain clearance for exercise.

Functional Training

Post-operative muscle tightness is common with patients who underwent TKR. Stretching the muscles around the knee will be important to restore adequate flexibility. In particular, the quadriceps group can become tight at the incision site and throughout the muscle group. General stretching and myofascial release of the hip muscles, hamstrings, and calves may also help to maintain flexibility throughout the kinetic chain (Bedekar et al., 2012). Flexibility exercises should be done at a level that does not elicit pain and is within a comfortable ROM.

Most exercises are safe, if they are gradually progressed. OKC exercises can still be implemented for isolated strengthening. Particular attention should be placed on the quadriceps and hamstrings to regain knee stability. Basic guidelines for OKC exercises can be applied. The CMES must remember that even though the client has a prosthetic knee, they still have a patella. Therefore, OKC exercises with the knee straight or from 90 to 60 degrees will prevent excessive loading of the patella. CKC exercises (see Table 18-2) can be progressed appropriately within the acceptable range of 0 to 45 degrees with a progression to 90 degrees. General conditioning of the hip and ankle muscles should be included to address any deficits.

Movement Training

The client should have adequate strength, ROM, and basic proprioception before progressing to Movement Training. Functional Training should progress what has been done in rehabilitation and must follow any precautions. The client should master basic functional skills before progressing to Movement Training and higher-level activity. For these clients, aquatic exercise is a great way to progress functional activity while de-weighting the joint. Aquatic exercise often is used to transition clients to higher-intensity land-based activity. The buoyancy of the water unloads the joint, allowing for more activity with lower amounts of pain.

Deficits in general balance may be evident due to disuse of the kinetic chain. Basic progression of balance activities would be appropriate if no pain is elicited (see Table 18-3). Low-level cardiovascular activity is indicated for these clients. Exercising on a bike or elliptical trainer is preferred over jogging or walking long distances.

LOWER LEG, ANKLE, AND FOOT PATHOLOGIES

There are 26 bones and 33 joints in the lower leg, ankle, and foot, along with numerous intrinsic and extrinsic muscles. As such, injuries to this area of the body are often complex and have the potential to affect mechanics of joints further up the kinetic chain. The lower leg is comprised of the tibia and fibula, which are held together by strong ligamentous attachments. The ankle joint complex is defined as the talocrural and subtalar joints, along with their numerous associated ligaments. With a loss of ankle function, hip flexors and extensors are more heavily utilized during gait, increasing the energy required for locomotion. Further, those with better ankle function have higher mobility and functional status relative to those with poor ankle function (Rao, Riskowski, & Hannan, 2012). The foot is formed by numerous bones and joints that are fastened together by the three layers of ligaments, which are arranged to form three strong arches. From the biomechanical viewpoint, the foot is typically considered a "functional unit" with two important aims: to support the body weight and to serve as a lever to propel the body forward in walking and running (Wright, Ivanenko, & Gurfinkel, 2012).

Shin Splints

"Shin splints" is a general term used to describe exercise-related leg pain. Shin splints are typically classified as two specific conditions: **medial tibial stress syndrome (MTSS)** and **anterior shin splints** (Figure 18-17).

Figure 18-17
Site of pain for anterior and posterior shin splints

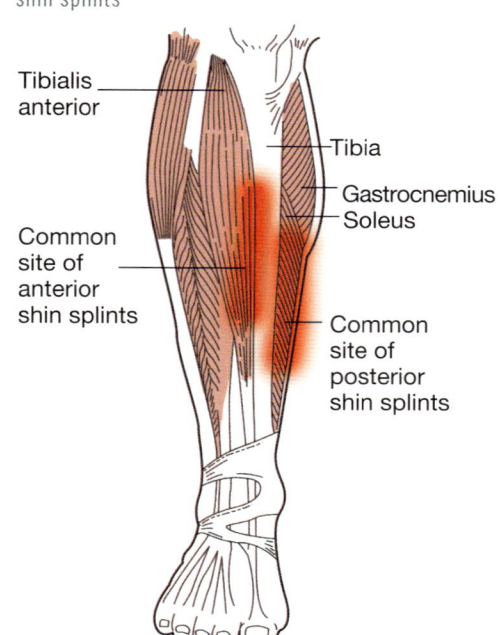

MTSS, also called posterior shin splints, is an overuse injury that occurs in the active population, and is an exercise-induced condition that is often triggered by a sudden change in activity. MTSS is actually **periostitis,** or inflammation of the periosteum (connective tissue covering) of the bone. It is the most frequently diagnosed injury in runners and is associated with training errors, improper shoes, and a tight Achilles tendon. It has a higher prevalence in female runners than male runners (Newman et al., 2013).

Anterior shin splints are also common in the active population and pain often occurs in the anterior compartment. The anterior compartment muscles (i.e., tibialis anterior, extensor digitorum longus, and extensor hallucis longus), fascia, and periosteal attachments are most commonly affected. Anterior shin splints are also common in runners and among military personnel (Brotzman & Manske, 2011).

Mechanism of Injury

MTSS has been most frequently associated with pes planus, or flat foot. Excessive overpronation of the foot during activity produces an eccentric stress to the muscles that results in a painful periostitis. The etiology of anterior shin splints is not completely known, but the condition is often associated with exertional activity (Houglum, 2010). Both MTSS and anterior shin splints have been associated with overtraining, poor footwear, changes in running surface, muscle weakness, and poor flexibility (Anderson & Parr, 2013).

Signs and Symptoms

Clients commonly complain of a "dull ache" along the distal two-thirds of the posterior medial tibia for MTSS and the distal anterior shin for anterior shin splints. The pain is elicited by initial activity, but diminishes as activity continues. The pain typically returns hours after activity. If the condition progresses, the pain becomes constant and tends to restrict performance (Anderson & Parr, 2013).

Precautions

Clients are encouraged to stop all aggravating activity and to rest. Repetitive loading activities such as running and jumping are discouraged until symptoms have resolved. The client should be referred to their physician if this condition has not resolved within one or two months after initiation of modified activity and proper intervention. It is important for the CMES to monitor symptoms during activity and refer the client to the doctor if there is no improvement, as a stress fracture must be ruled out. Stress fractures of the tibia can have similar signs and symptoms as shin splints (e.g., pain along the posterior medial tibia) (Metzl, 2005).

Early Intervention

Management of both conditions includes modifying training with lower-impact conditioning and **cross-training** (e.g., aquatic exercise). However, the best intervention may just be to rest. Five to seven days of rest have been suggested to help relieve acute symptoms (Anderson & Parr, 2013). Modalities (e.g., ice and ultrasound), stretching of tight muscles and structures (e.g., Achilles tendon and soleus) throughout the day, performing exercises for weak muscle groups (e.g., muscles of the hips and core), soft-tissue massage, and the use of foot orthotics may also be beneficial to relieve symptoms (Houglum, 2010). The client may need to be referred to physical therapy to address these issues.

Restorative Exercise Program

The client may be restricted with activity or may be limited due to pain. The role of the CMES should be to slowly progress the client back to full unrestricted activity without exacerbating the symptoms. Cross-training to maintain adequate levels of fitness is indicated in the early stages. Consulting the client's physician and physical therapist can give key information about how the client is responding to treatment and what they are currently doing for exercise. The following sections summarize strategies for management of this condition.

Functional Training

Pain-free stretching of the calf muscles, especially the soleus, has been shown to be effective in relieving symptoms related to MTSS (Figure 18-18). Stretching the anterior compartment may also help to relieve the symptoms of anterior shin splints (Figures 18-19 and 18-20). The goal of

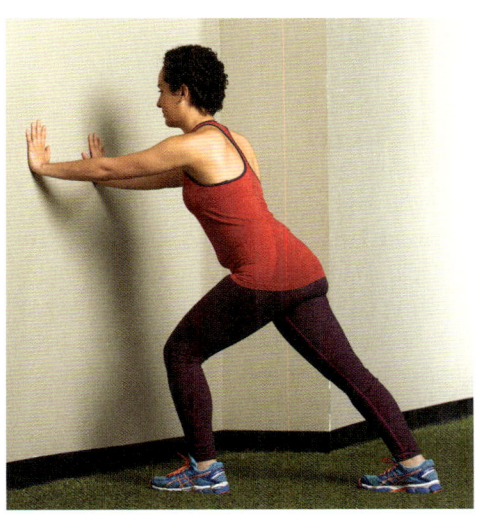

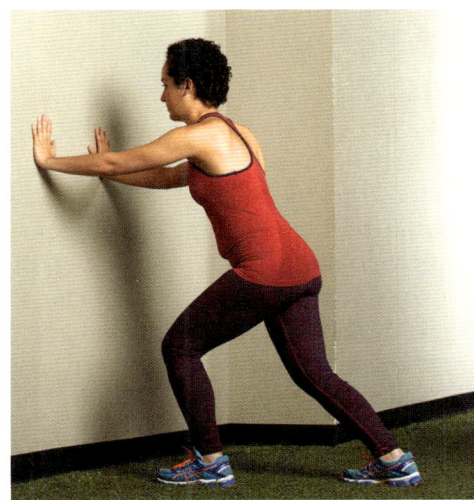

Figure 18-18
Calf wall stretch
a. Gastrocnemius/soleus stretch
b. Soleus stretch

a.

b.

Figure 18-19
Sitting stretch for the anterior compartment

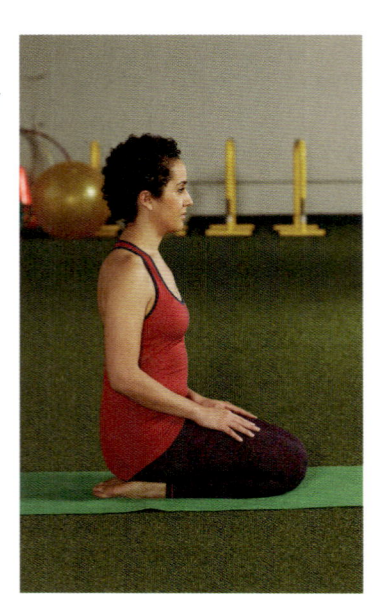

Figure 18-20
Standing "toe drag" stretch for the anterior compartment

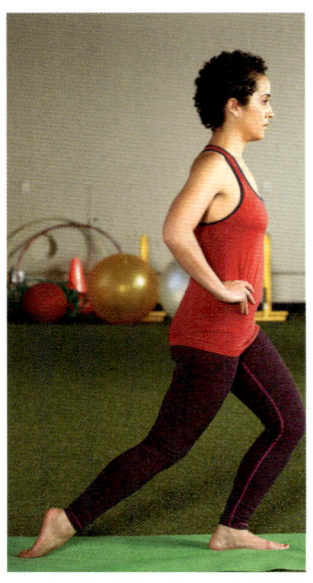

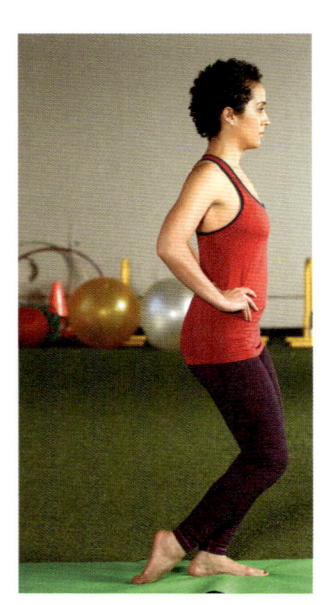

stretching should be to restore proper length and elasticity to the muscle and reduce strain in the muscle-tendon unit. A general lower-body stretching program should accompany more specific stretching to address any secondary muscle-length deficits that may affect the foot and ankle.

Rest and modified activity are the primary interventions for symptom relief. However, there may be some residual strength deficits in the muscles that control the ankle. Targeting the muscles that control the ankle is the goal, especially the calf and anterior tibialis muscles. Exercises for the hip and knee should be added as needed.

Movement Training

A gradual return to athletic and sports activity is best for these clients. Strengthening exercises should be related to the client's functional goals, correct training errors, and be low-impact to avoid any excessive stress. Both OKC and CKC exercises can be integrated throughout the program as tolerated by the client. Movement Training should begin with developing good movement patterns and progress to low-loading activities and then to higher-loading activities such as jumping or running, as long as the client is pain-free. Balance exercises can also be integrated into the program as needed.

Cross-training can be utilized throughout the program to maintain adequate cardiovascular fitness. Examples of low-impact activities include water jogging, stationary biking, and elliptical training. Clients should avoid running, jumping, and shock-loading activities that stress the affected region.

Ankle Sprains

Ankle sprains are one of the most common musculoskeletal injuries. Ankle sprains are common injuries that affect people of all ages and in all sporting activities. An estimated 28,000 ankle injuries occur in the United States each day (Adams et al., 2008). In sport, ankle injuries are the most common injury, with some estimates attributing upward of 45% of all athletic injuries to ankle sprains (Ferran & Maffulli, 2006). Ankle sprains are most common in sports such as basketball, volleyball, soccer, and ice skating (Kaminski et al., 2013). There is little data regarding risk factors for ankle sprains, though a history of ankle sprains has been found to be a risk factor. Foot type, general laxity, and gender have also been linked to the incidence of ankle sprains (Ivins, 2006).

Mechanism of Injury

Lateral, or **inversion,** ankle sprains are the most common type of ankle sprain. The mechanism is typically inversion with a plantar flexed foot. Landing from jumps, landing or stepping on another athlete's foot, trauma at heel strike during running, and stressing the foot while in a fixed position are common causes of ankle sprains (Ferran & Maffulli, 2006). The lateral ankle ligaments are the most common structures involved, including the anterior talofibular ligament (ATFL), calcaneofibular ligament (CFL), and posterior talofibular ligament (Petersen et al., 2013).

Medial, or **eversion**, ankle sprains account for approximately 10 to 15% of all ankle injuries and result from forced dorsiflexion and eversion of the ankle. The medial deltoid ligament is the most common structure involved and injury often requires further examination to rule out a fracture (Anderson & Parr, 2013).

Signs/Symptoms

With lateral ankle sprains, the individual can often recall the mechanism and hearing a "pop" or "tearing" sound. Specific signs and symptoms for lateral ankle sprains are described in the next section. Medial ankle sprains rarely happen in isolation. The individual is often unable to recall the specific mechanism, but can reproduce discomfort by dorsiflexing and everting the ankle. There may be medial swelling with tenderness over the deltoid ligament (Anderson, Hall, & Parr, 2008).

Classification

Lateral ankle sprains are often described using a specific grading system (Table 18-5). A grade I ankle sprain involves the ATFL ligament, with pain and mild swelling over the lateral aspect of the ankle. Typically, weight-bearing is tolerable after injury. A grade II ankle sprain involves both the ATFL and CFL ligaments, with more severe pain and swelling over the lateral ankle. Weight-bearing may be limited due to pain. A grade III ankle sprain is considered a complete tear of one or more of the lateral ligaments. Rapid, severe pain, swelling, and discoloration occur and individuals are unable to bear weight (Anderson & Parr, 2013).

Medial ankle sprains are often associated with fibular fractures, severe lateral ankle sprains, and fractures to the medial malleolus. To date, there is no specific grading system for medial ankle sprains (Anderson & Parr, 2013).

TABLE 18-5
GRADING SYSTEM FOR LATERAL ANKLE SPRAINS

	Grade I	Grade II	Grade III
Ligament involved	ATFL	ATFL and CFL	One or more
Stretched or ruptured	Stretched	Stretched	Ruptured
Pain/swelling	Mild	Moderate	Severe
Weight-bearing	Full	Partial	Unable

Note: ATFL = Anterior talofibular ligament; CFL = Calcaneofibular ligament

Precautions

The client may be cleared to slowly resume activity once symptoms have diminished. They are encouraged to wear the appropriate ankle bracing and to avoid lateral and multiplanar movements until cleared by a physician. These movements may put the client at risk for further injury and should be introduced when appropriate (Petersen et al., 2013).

Early Intervention

Early intervention often includes medical management. The acronym RICE—rest or restricted activity, ice, compression, and elevation—describes a common early-intervention strategy for an acute ankle sprain. This method is almost universally accepted as best practice by athletic trainers and other healthcare professionals immediately after acute ankle sprains, with the goals of protecting the injured ankle from further injury, controlling pain, limiting swelling, and reducing the secondary hypoxic injury that results from the acute inflammatory reaction. However, limited evidence from high-quality randomized clinical trials actually supports the use of these interventions. Typically, components of RICE are applied simultaneously in both clinical practice and research studies, making it impossible to determine which components are truly effective or potentially deleterious (Kaminski et al., 2013). Nonetheless, the following list describes the practical application for RICE for an acute ankle sprain:

- Restricted activity includes limiting weight-bearing activity and ROM until the client is cleared by the physician.
- Ice should be applied every two hours for 10 to 15 minutes.

- Compression can be done by applying an elastic wrap to the area. This helps to minimize local swelling.
- Elevating the ankle 6 to 10 inches (15 to 25 cm) above the level of the heart will also help control swelling. This is done to reduce hemorrhage, inflammation, swelling, and pain.

Most often, individuals with lateral and medial ankle sprains are referred to a medical doctor for further diagnosis and treatment. The standard of care for grade I and II lateral ankle sprains is functional rehabilitation, which consists of ankle stabilization (via elastic bandage, bracing, taping, or external support or a combination of these) with progressive weight-bearing and exercise. As with grade I and II sprains, grade III sprains are often managed by functional rehabilitation, but the optimal management of grade III ankle sprains is less clear (Kaminski et al., 2013).

Early intervention can begin one to three weeks after injury, unless a severe ankle sprain has occurred that may require further immobilization (Houglum, 2010). The client may be sent to physical therapy to improve strength, flexibility, proprioception, and endurance, as well as to control swelling.

Restorative Exercise Program

The CMES may begin to see the client for fitness training as soon as one to two weeks post-injury for grade I ankle sprains, two to three weeks post-injury for grade II ankle sprains, and three to six weeks for grade III ankle sprains (Houglum, 2010). During this time, the client may still be in physical therapy and be ready to transition to fitness activities. The client should be progressed according to their tolerance to exercise. In other words, pain should be the guide. It is common for the injured ankle to have mild to moderate discomfort and swelling after increased activity.

Functional Training

After a sprain, dorsiflexion ROM may be impaired, which can lead to functional limitations in gait and contribute to re-injury or a compensation-related injury to the unaffected leg. Historically, clinicians have employed ROM exercises for the ankle and foot (i.e., dorsiflexion, **plantar flexion,** inversion, and eversion) during the acute and subacute phases of injury, but no evidence exists to suggest that one type of exercise is superior or even efficacious for improving patient outcomes (Kaminski et al., 2013). For the CMES, ROM exercises should be limited to only those that do not provoke pain. Stretching of the gastrocnemius and soleus may be beneficial if the client has tightness and decreased length after immobilization. Stretching the ankle in motions that stress the injured ligaments is not recommended. For example, stretching the ankle into inversion or eversion can stretch the healing ligaments, resulting in local pain and irritation. General stretches for the lower extremity should be included to maintain adequate flexibility throughout the whole kinetic chain.

Evidence supports the need to strengthen all muscles around the ankle after injury, as **concentric** and eccentric strength deficits for the ankle evertors, invertors, and plantar flexors have been reported. Muscle inhibition may also occur from joint and ligamentous trauma and effusion after a lateral ankle sprain (Kaminski et al., 2013). Strengthening the muscles of the kinetic chain will also be beneficial, with particular emphasis on the muscles that control the foot and ankle (Figures 18-21 and 18-22). OKC exercises using resistive bands are a good way to isolate the muscles that control the ankle (Figures 18-23 through 18-26). Finally, towel crunches with the toes effectively target the foot intrinsic muscle group (Figure 18-27).

Targeting the peroneal group for inversion ankle sprains is essential for prevention. The peroneal reflex with muscle contraction has been considered the first mechanism for dynamic joint stability. Therefore, with sudden inversion ankle movements, the peroneals will be the first muscles to contract and attempt to stabilize the ankle. Delayed action of this mechanism has been associated with inversion ankle sprains. Experts recommend training these muscle groups eccentrically to improve the stabilizing effect. Eccentric loading creates higher tension levels versus isometric or concentric activities at specific joint ranges. Strength gains have been reported as soon as six weeks after initiation of a program of progressive resistive exercise (Kaminski et al., 2013).

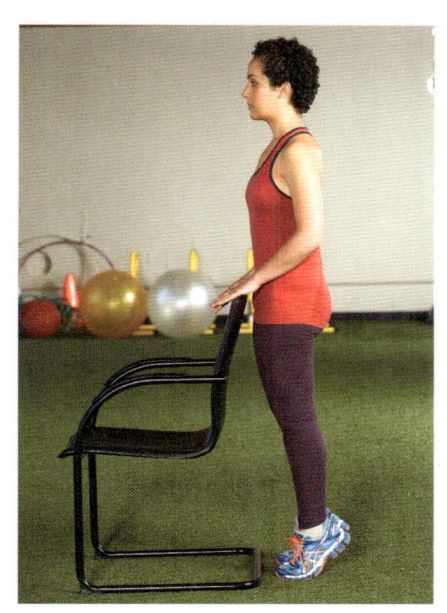

Musculoskeletal Injuries of the Lower Extremity   CHAPTER 18   619

Figure 18-21
Calf raise with knee straight

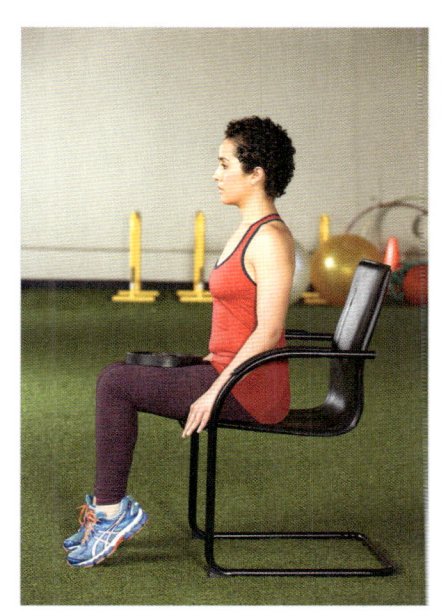

Figure 18-22
Calf raise with knee bent for added intensity add weight to lap

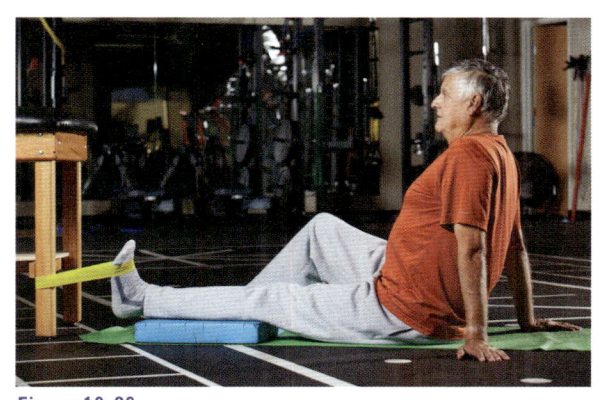

Figure 18-23
Resistive ankle dorsiflexion

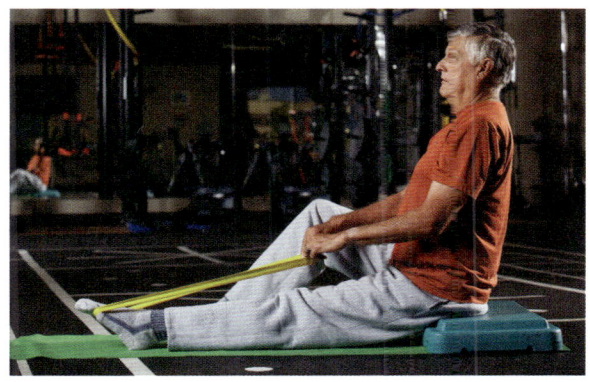

Figure 18-24
Resistive ankle plantar flexion

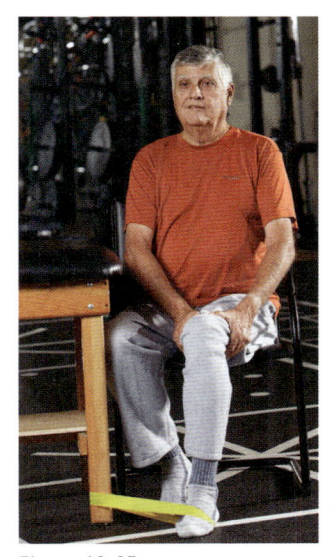

Figure 18-25
Resistive ankle eversion

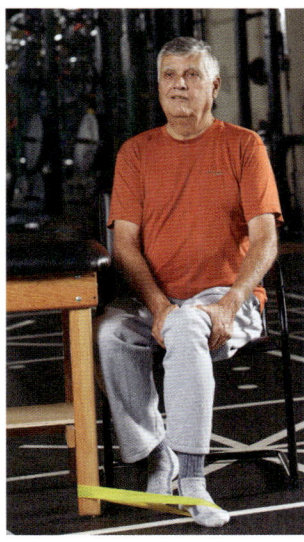

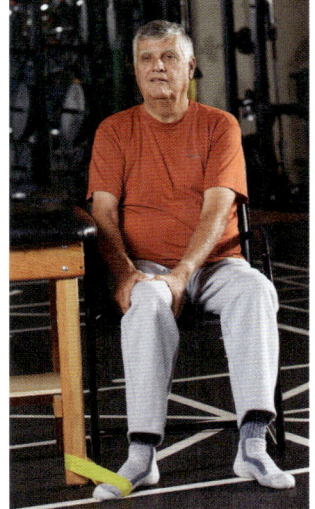

Figure 18-26
Resistive ankle inversion

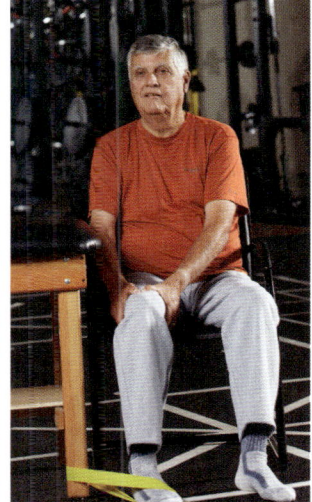

ACE MEDICAL EXERCISE SPECIALIST MANUAL   AMERICAN COUNCIL ON EXERCISE

Figure 18-27
Towel crunches

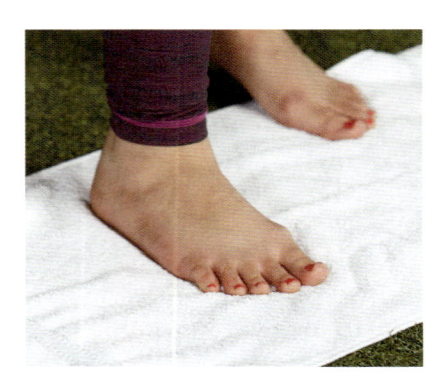

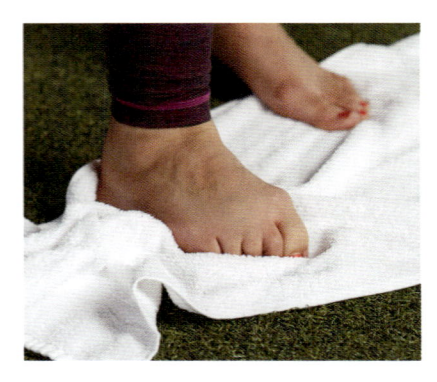

Clients with eversion ankle sprains may have more global deficits due to the fact that eversion ankle sprains are rarely seen in isolation; often they follow other trauma such as a fracture. CKC exercise progression should emphasize dynamic single-leg strengthening activities that challenge the lower kinetic chain. Strengthening programs for these injuries are often individualized and are determined by the injury. As mentioned in previous sections, exercises for the hip and knee should be included to address any strength deficits and to help maintain control of the kinetic chain during activity.

Movement Training

Movement Training can begin once the client has adequate strength, ROM, joint function, and most importantly, proprioception. Clients who have suffered ankle sprains may have deficits in balance. The ligaments are a major source of proprioceptive feedback for balance and joint position sense throughout the kinetic chain. If ligament trauma occurs, the feedback can be lost, which results in a higher risk of re-injury (Petersen et al., 2013). In fact, chronic lateral ankle sprains have been associated with muscle weakness (e.g., in the hip abductors and peroneal group), delayed activation patterns in the hip and knee, and diminished postural control (Van Deun et al., 2007; Friel et al., 2006; Evans, Hertel, & Sebastianelli, 2004). Based on this evidence, one can appreciate the interaction between the muscular and proprioceptive systems. If injury occurs in the lower extremity, the information to the CNS from the lower-extremity changes, which results in delayed muscle activation patterns, weakness, and overall compensation.

Movement Training progression for these clients should include a combination of CKC and balance activities to achieve the optimal benefits. The client should be safely progressed through the program while wearing their protective bracing. OKC exercises can still be used to isolate specific muscle groups as needed. CKC exercises that integrate balance are a key element in challenging the kinetic chain and reestablishing the reactive feedback loop that is required for multiplanar activity (see Tables 18-2 and 18-3). A commonly used progression is challenging the kinetic chain with double- or single-leg activity in the **sagittal plane** first, the **frontal plane** second, and combined planes last (Figure 18-28). The frontal and combined plane activities may need to be slowly introduced to prevent re-injury.

Cardiovascular activity such as biking and elliptical training can be added to the program to build or maintain basic cardiovascular fitness. Higher-level activity such as running, sprints, or agility drills should follow the progression just described.

Achilles Tendinopathy

Injury to the Achilles tendon is common in athletes and the active population. The prevalence of the condition is highest among runners, gymnasts, and dancers. Other sports where this injury is common include track and field, volleyball, basketball, and soccer. Typically, older athletes are more affected by the condition than teens or children (Mazzone, 2002). This condition can eventually lead to rupture if not addressed appropriately. Achilles ruptures primarily occur in males 30 to 50 years of age. The prevalence rate has increased in recent years due to the fact that more people are exercising (Mazzone, 2002).

Musculoskeletal Injuries of the Lower Extremity   CHAPTER 18

The classification of Achilles injuries has been quite confusing due to the many names given to the condition. Terms commonly used in the past, including Achilles tendinitis, tenosynovitis, and tendonosis, have become questionable due to subsequent findings. Histology studies indicate that the pathology is predominantly of tendon degeneration (tendinosis), as opposed to the historically hypothesized inflammation (tendinitis) and can develop long before the onset of symptoms (Sussmilch-Leitch et al., 2012). This confusion has led to the term **Achilles tendinopathy.** Maffulli, Khan, and Puddu (1998) suggested this term to describe the combination of pain, swelling, and poor function that accompanies this condition. Thus, Achilles tendinopathy may include both an inflammatory and degenerative process of the tendon.

Mechanism of Injury

Various intrinsic and extrinsic factors are associated with this condition. Intrinsic factors include age, body weight, pes cavus, pes planus, leg-length discrepancies, and lateral ankle instability. Extrinsic factors include poor foot mechanics. increased frequency of training sessions, improper footwear, improper training surfaces, and a lack of flexibility and strength (Houglum, 2010). The extrinsic factors are typically responsible for acute tendon trauma. Overuse and chronic injuries are often multifactorial and include a combination of intrinsic and extrinsic factors.

Signs and Symptoms

Individuals often complain of pain that is 0.75 to 2.25 inches (2 to 6 cm) above the tendon insertion into the calcaneus. The typical pattern is initial morning pain that is "sharp" or "burning," as well as pain with more vigorous activity. Rest will often alleviate the pain, but as the condition becomes worse the pain becomes more constant and begins to interfere with ADL (Houglum, 2010).

Precautions

Clients with this condition are encouraged to stop all aggravating activity and seek proper treatment for the condition. High-loading activities such as jumping, running, and stair climbing should be avoided until the condition has improved.

Early Intervention

Early intervention includes controlling pain and inflammation by using modalities (e.g., ice and ultrasound), rest, and oral anti-inflammatory medication (Houglum, 2010). Management of the condition may include modified rest and the addressing of specific risk factors. Modified rest allows the injured body part to rest while the client is exercising the uninjured parts of the body (e.g., using an upper-body ergometer). Proper training techniques, losing weight, proper footwear, orthotics, strengthening, and stretching can help alleviate pain and prevent progression of the condition. Also, the client may be sent to physical therapy to address the factors mentioned earlier.

Restorative Exercise Program

The client may be cleared to exercise immediately to tolerance, or they may have some activity restrictions. The role of the CMES is to design a program that helps to meet the client's overall goals but does not exacerbate the condition. Consulting the medical doctor and physical therapist can give key information about how the client is responding to treatment and what they are currently doing for exercise. The following sections summarize strategies for management of this condition.

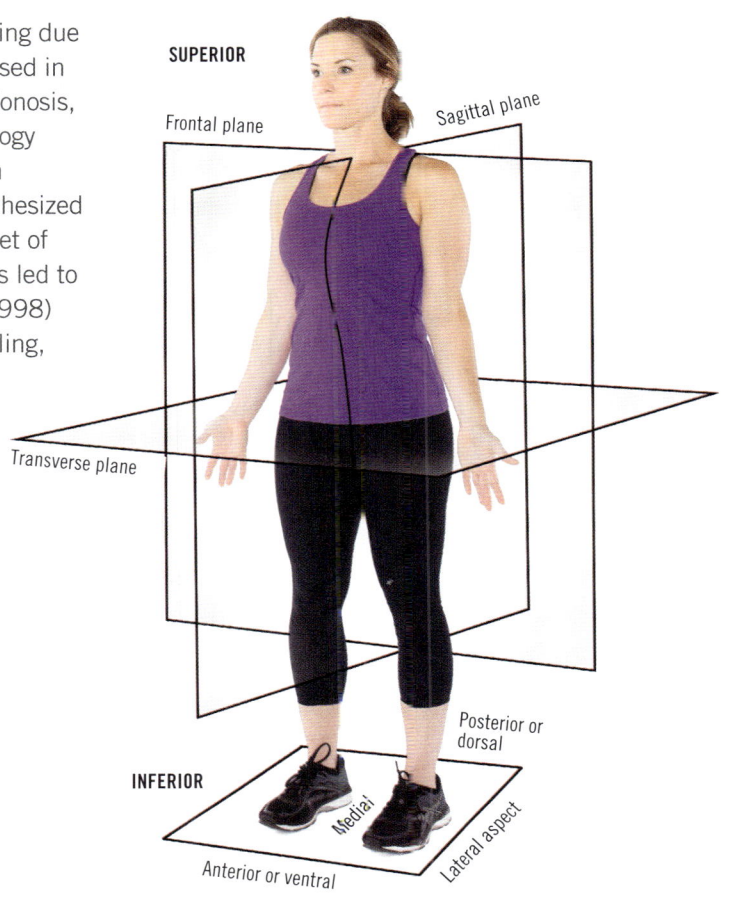

Figure 18-28
Anatomical position and planes of motion

Functional Training

Functional Training should begin with flexibility exercises for the restricted area to improve joint function (Houglum, 2010). The goal of stretching should be to restore general lower-body flexibility, with an emphasis on calf mobility. The client should be cautioned to stretch to tolerance and avoid overexertion. Overstretching of the Achilles tendon can cause irritation to the muscle-tendon unit and should be avoided.

Eccentric strengthening of the calf complex has been shown to be beneficial for relieving symptoms. In fact, Wasielewski and Kotsko (2007) conducted a systematic review of research from 1980 to 2006 on eccentric strengthening of the calf muscles. Their analysis revealed that eccentric exercise may reduce pain and improve strength in Achilles tendinopathy. However, eccentric training has not been shown to be superior over other forms of therapeutic interventions for this condition (Wasielewski & Kotsko, 2007). Therefore, progressively loading the Achilles tendon with eccentric activity can benefit the client, but may be even more beneficial when combined with other interventions. Examples of eccentric activity include slowly lowering the calf while standing on a step or performing a single-leg squat with an emphasis on slowly lowering the leg.

Movement Training

Returning to normal and sports activities may be challenging for these clients. The nature of the condition can bring changes in symptoms with activity. A gradual, pain-free return to activity is indicated for this condition. Modifications in training techniques and the training environment should be addressed, with an emphasis on client education. CKC exercise combined with eccentric loading can progressively challenge the Achilles tendon, but should not create pain. Any deficits in balance should be addressed as needed. Simply adding an unstable surface such as a foam pad to CKC exercises can challenge the client's balance (see Tables 18-2 and 18-3). Cardiovascular activity should be progressed with caution. Low-loading activity should precede higher-loading activity to avoid pain or re-injury.

Plantar Fasciitis

Plantar fasciitis is a painful condition of the plantar aponeurosis, or fascia, of the foot. The plantar fascia is a broad, flat, fibrous, tendon-like structure, which consists of noncontractile irregularly ordered collagen fibers with minimal elastic properties. Plantar fasciitis is commonly described as an inflammatory condition, but there is controversy in this respect, as some researchers have questioned the presence of inflammation in this condition. Current literature suggests that plantar fasciitis is more correctly termed "fasciosis" because of the chronicity of the disease and the evidence of degeneration rather than inflammation (Schwartz & Su, 2014). Plantar fasciitis is reported to commonly occur in runners and those who have overweight. The condition affects both athletic and sedentary people, and does not seem to be influenced by gender. Research indicates that 10% of the general population will experience this pathology at least once in their lifetime (Uden, Boesch, & Kumar, 2011). The prevalence is highest among individuals 40 to 60 years old. Up to one-third of injured individuals have pain in both feet (Cole, Seto, & Gazewood, 2005; Buchbinder, 2004).

Mechanism of Injury

There have been several intrinsic and extrinsic risk factors associated with this condition. Intrinsic factors include pes planus (excessive pronation or low arch height), pes cavus (high arch height), and decreased strength and poor flexibility of the calf muscles. Extrinsic factors include overtraining, improper footwear, obesity, and unforgiving and hard surfaces (Cutts et al., 2012). Any of these factors can cause excessive loading of the plantar fascia, leading to pain and dysfunction.

Signs and Symptoms

Typically, individuals report pain on the plantar, medial heel at its calcaneal attachment that worsens after rest, but improves after 10 to 15 minutes of activity. In particular, clients will commonly report excessive pain during the first few steps in the morning. During sleep, the foot usually falls into a plantar flexed position, and when the individual rises from bed in the morning, the foot moves into dorsiflexion during walking. The plantar fascia slightly contracts in bed and the initial stretching associated with early morning waking is probably responsible for initiation of pain (Cutts et al., 2012). Clients may also have stiffness and muscle spasms in the lower leg with tightness in the Achilles tendon (Buchbinder, 2004).

Precautions

Individuals with plantar fasciitis may be limited in their activity due to pain. Activities that excessively load the fascia, such as running or jumping, should be avoided due to exacerbation of the condition. The condition can be challenging due to the pain relief that occurs with basic activity and the recurrence of symptoms after rest. The CMES needs to monitor changes in symptoms and refer the client to the appropriate medical professional, if necessary.

Early Intervention

Management of this condition may include modalities (e.g., ice), oral anti-inflammatory medication, heel pad or plantar arch, stretching, and strengthening exercises. The medical doctor may prescribe physical therapy, a night splint, or orthotics, or inject the area with cortisone (Cutts et al., 2012). Conservative treatment of this condition has shown good long-term outcomes. A study by Wolgin and colleagues (2004) found that 80% of patients treated with conservative therapies had complete resolution of symptoms after a four-year follow-up. Some individuals may require surgery f conservative treatment fails after six to 12 months of intervention (Houglum, 2010).

Restorative Exercise Program

The client may be cleared to exercise immediately to tolerance or they may have some restrictions. The role of the CMES is to design a program that helps to meet the client's overall goals but does not excessively load the foot. Integrating specific foot exercises into the general fitness program often provides the best results, as this allows the client to work toward their fitness goals, as well as address the foot problems.

Functional Training

Stretching of the gastrocnemius, soleus, and plantar fascia is beneficial and has been shown to help relieve symptoms (Houglum, 2010). In fact, a study by DiGiovanni et al. (2006) found that specific plantar fascia stretching (Figure 18-29) had excellent results (94% satisfaction) in a group of 66 subjects after an eight-week program and at a two-year follow-up. Proper stretching of the calf complex will restore adequate muscle length and prevent compensatory pronation at the ankle. During gait, tight calf muscles prevent the tibia from gliding forward on the ankle, forcing the foot to excessively pronate to achieve the needed ROM for movement. Self–myofascial release techniques, including rolling the foot over a baseball, golf ball, or dumbbell, may help to break up myofascial adhesions in the plantar fascia.

Strengthening the intrinsic foot muscles may help to improve arch stability of the feet and help to unload the stresses imposed across the plantar fascia. Some examples of effective exercises include towel crunches (see Figure 18-27) and marble pick-up (Figure 18-30). Strengthening of the gastrocnemius, soleus, peroneals, tibialis anterior, and tibialis posterior may be needed to help improve strength at the ankle. The client may have done similar exercises in physical therapy and may need to be progressed accordingly. Exercises for the hip and knee should be included as needed.

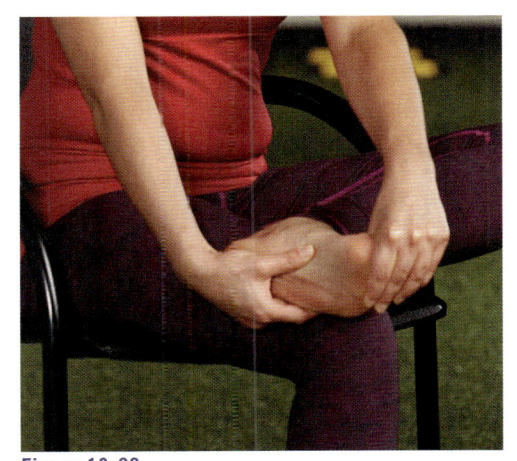

Figure 18-29
Plantar fascia stretching

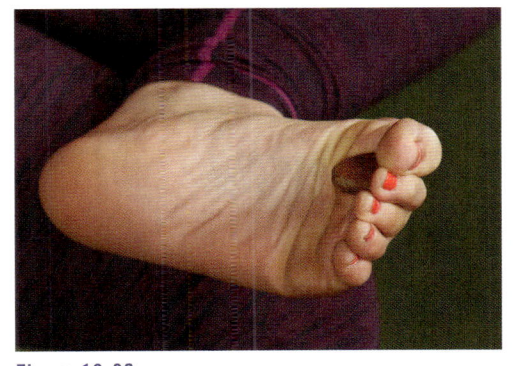

Figure 18-30
Marble pick-up for intrinsic foot muscles

Movement Training

Returning to normal physical activity may be a challenge for these clients. The nature of the condition can bring false hope due to the changes in symptoms with activity. A slow, pain-free return to activity is indicated. As mentioned earlier, high-loading activities should be limited to avoid further exacerbation of the injury. With these clients, balance may be an issue and should be addressed, if needed. Low-loading cardiovascular activities such as biking, elliptical training, or water aerobics are preferred over higher-loading activities such as running.

EXPAND YOUR KNOWLEDGE

STRUCTURAL ABNORMALITIES

Certain structural changes in the lower-extremity kinetic chain have been associated with various musculoskeletal conditions. First, pes planus, or overpronation, is considered to be a flat mobile foot, which offers little structural support. It has been associated with plantar fasciitis, Achilles tendinopathy, posterior tibial tendinitis, shin splints, ITBFS, and patellofemoral pain. Second, pes cavus, or high arches, is considered to be a rigid foot that offers little shock absorption. It has been associated with ITBFS, plantar fasciitis, stress fractures of the tarsal and metatarsal bones of the foot, and peroneal tendinitis. Third, leg-length discrepancies have been associated with hip problems such as trochanteric bursitis and ITB syndrome (Anderson & Parr, 2013; Manske, 2006).

It is important for the CMES to note any structural deviations, as they may be contributing factors to the pathologies discussed in this chapter. Attempting to correct these biomechanical deviations is beyond the scope of the CMES. If a CMES suspects that a deviation may be contributing to an undiagnosed problem, then referral to the appropriate medical professional is indicated.

CASE STUDIES

Case Study 1

Client Information

A CMES was referred a 32-year-old male recreational soccer player who had a right knee ACL repair 12 weeks ago with a patellar tendon graft. The mechanism of injury was a planting and twisting maneuver. The client has been in physical therapy for the past 12 weeks and treatment has included a combination of strengthening, cardiovascular, and balance exercises. The physical therapist has also been doing massage, stretching, and myofascial release. The physical therapist reports that the client has responded well to physical therapy and is highly motivated. He is on schedule with the physician's protocol, but because of insurance constraints has been transitioned to fitness activity. Review of medications reveals the following: Vicodin (pain) and Advil as needed.

Upon meeting with the client for initial assessment, the CMES notices that he is highly motivated and immediately talks about returning to soccer. The client does have written clearance by the medical doctor, with the precautions of wearing a brace during activity and no running until 16 weeks. His health history reveals no major medical problems or comorbidities. The client does have a history of recurrent right ankle sprains and occasional low-back pain. The client is an engineer and works at a desk most of the day. His fitness goals are to return to soccer, running, and weightlifting.

When asked about his knee, the client reveals that he has been getting anterior knee pain with increased swelling for the past two weeks while working out at the gym. The client is doing 45 minutes of cardiovascular exercise several days per week on the elliptical trainer and general upper-body strengthening. Further questioning reveals that he has been doing lunges, leg presses, and leg extensions three to five times per week, including during his physical-therapy program.

At the time of the fitness assessment, the client demonstrated problems with basic movements. In particular, the client demonstrated immediate pain with getting out of the chair and walking down stairs. At this time, the session was stopped and no further action was taken.

Musculoskeletal Injuries of the Lower Extremity   CHAPTER 18

CMES Approach

Observation of the knee revealed it to be swollen and painful to bend. The client was immediately referred back to the medical doctor for further evaluation. The CMES recommended that the client use the RICE principle until he sees the doctor and receives proper clearance to resume activity. The goal was to make sure the client did not re-injure the ACL or damage any other structures. Upon hearing back from his patient, the doctor diagnosed him as having patellar tendinitis and general joint irritation. The client is restricted from fitness activity for two weeks. Upon clearance to resume activity, the following actions should be taken with this client:

- Client education: CKC vs. OKC exercises, overtraining, and injury recognition
- Training modification: Reestablish program goals and training schedule, incorporating and building on the exercises performed in physical therapy
- Fitness assessments: Baseline data for flexibility, muscular strength and endurance, and body composition
- Exercise program: Slow progression of sets, repetitions, and time
- Flexibility: Focus on stretching and self–myofascial release for the ITB complex, quadriceps, hamstrings, and calves
- Strengthening: Focus on strengthening the quadriceps and hamstrings, and agonists for primary hip movements
- Balance: Progress to multiplanar activity with a knee brace
- Functional: Focus on CKC exercises within pain-free limits with a progression toward sport-specific movements. After 16 weeks, begin basic agility and sport-specific movements as tolerated.
- Incorporate a focus on safety into all exercises and all exercise sessions.
- The client should wear his knee brace during all workouts, with the CMES and on his own.
- Recommend icing after workouts.
- Monitor for increased symptoms: redness, pain, and swelling.
- Monitor for signs and symptoms of overtraining.

ACE IFT® MODEL AT A GLANCE

Cardiorespiratory Training

Prior to his setback, this client was performing cardiorespiratory exercise for 45 minutes several days per week. Even if the CMES reduces training volume to 20 to 30 minutes per session following the two weeks with restricted physical activity, this client will still be exercising in the Fitness Training phase. He can progress his Fitness Training program for quite some time, and will only move to Performance Training when his knee, fitness, and goals meet the requirements for this transition.

Muscular Training

The initial focus of this client's training program is on Functional Training to establish adequate knee stability, while increasing hip and ankle range of motion and strengthening the muscles that create and control these movements. Once the lower kinetic-chain stability and mobility is reestablished, the CMES can progress the primary focus of this client's program to be on movement pattern before adding heavier resistance in Load/Speed Training. Upper-body movement should be assessed to determine if Functional or Movement Training is needed to address any inequities in the upper body before moving on to Load/Speed Training.

Case Study 2

Client Information

A CMES is working with a 72-year-old female who is three months post-operative after a left total hip replacement via the posterior lateral approach. The woman has a history of hip arthritis and finally elected to have the procedure. She has been attending physical therapy for strengthening, endurance, and balance activities. The physical therapist reports that the client is doing well with ROM but still has hip weakness that makes functional and balance activities difficult. Due to insurance constraints, the client has been transitioned to fitness activity.

The client provides written clearance from the medical doctor with precautions noted to avoid high-impact activity such as running. Her health history reveals **hypertension,** osteoporosis, and OA. The client did have a left TKR three years ago with no reported problems. Review of medications is as follows: diuretic (hypertension), Fosamax (osteoporosis), and Celebrex (OA). The client is retired but volunteers at the local school, where she is on her feet most of the day. Her fitness goals are to return to walking and swimming.

When asked about her left hip, the client reveals having mild to moderate pain after physical therapy that goes away after icing. The client reports being cleared by the medical doctor to resume full ROM of the hip with no restrictions. Further questioning reveals that she is still having trouble with certain movement patterns, such as sit-to-stand actions and picking up objects.

At this time, the fitness assessment was limited due to the global hip weakness that the client was having. The following information was obtained from the modified assessment:

- Movement screens: Not performed due to weakness and fall risk
- Flexibility: Tightness in the ITB complex, hamstrings, and calves
- Functional testing: Weakness noted in the hip with sit-to-stand, side-stepping, quarter lunges, and partial-ROM step-ups
- Cardiorespiratory fitness: Unable to do submaximal testing on the bike or step due to weakness and deconditioning
- Muscular strength: Able to establish baseline weights on exercise machines and resistive bands

CMES Approach

Due to the client's low functional level, a modified restorative program should be created that focuses on hip and abdominal core strengthening, balance, and cardiorespiratory endurance. The following actions should be taken with this client.

- Client education: Basic training principles, CKC vs. OKC exercises, and injury recognition
- Precautions and program modifications for osteoporosis and hypertension
- Training modification: Establish program goals and training schedule
- Exercise program: Slow progression of sets, repetitions, and time
- Flexibility: Focus on stretching and self–myofascial release for the hip muscles, ITB complex, quadriceps, hamstrings, and calves
- Strengthening: Focus on the gluteals, hip external rotators, quadriceps, and hamstrings
- Balance: Slowly progress multiplanar activity under close supervision
- Functional: Focus on CKC exercises within pain-free limits with a progression toward multiplanar functional activities
- Basic movements: Focus on improving the sit-to-stand movement
- Gait: Walking over even and uneven terrain (e.g., cement vs. grass)
- Incorporate a focus on safety into all exercises and all exercise sessions.
- Always account for and follow precautions for osteoporosis and hypertension.
- Recommend icing after workouts and monitor for change in symptoms.

ACE IFT® MODEL AT A GLANCE

Cardiorespiratory Training

This client wants to return to walking and swimming for regular exercise. However, she was unable to perform basic cardiorespiratory fitness assessments due to deconditioning. The CMES should design a Functional Training program to help this client build basic cardiorespiratory endurance for improved health, function, and fitness. Once established, the CMES and client can assess the situation and determine the appropriate time to transition her to Fitness Training.

Muscular Training

The initial focus of this client's training program is on Functional Training to establish adequate postural stability and mobility of the kinetic chain, and then Movement Training to improve her performance of primary movement patterns (e.g., sit-to-stand). Additional emphasis is placed on improving balance and function for activities of daily living. Light loads are applied to movement patterns as Movement Training is progressed. Future progressions would move this client into Load/Speed Training when appropriate.

SUMMARY

Due to the changes in the healthcare system, the role of exercise professionals has expanded. The CMES is required to have a deeper knowledge about non-operative and post-operative musculoskeletal conditions. This chapter has focused on the recognition, management, and restorative exercise guidelines for common musculoskeletal injuries and post-operative conditions of the lower extremity. The reader is encouraged to continue the study of these conditions to effectively design safe restorative programs for different conditions and populations.

REFERENCES

Adams, J. et al. (2008). *Emergency Medicine*. Philadelphia: Saunders.

Allen, C. (2007). *ACL Injury: Does It Require Surgery?* American Academy of Orthopedic Surgeons. www.orthoinfo.aaos.org

Al-Hakim, W. et al. (2012). The non-operative treatment of anterior knee pain. *Open Orthopaedics Journal*, 6, 320–326. DOI: 10.2174/1874325001206010320

American Academy of Orthopedic Surgeons (2007). *Your Orthopedic Connection: Total Knee Replacement*. www.orthoinfo.aaos.org

Anderson, M.K. & Parr, G.P. (2013). *Foundations of Athletic Training: Prevention, Assessment, and Management* (5th ed.). Philadelphia: Lippincott Williams & Wilkins.

Baker, B. & Lubowitz, J. (2006). Meniscal injuries. *E-Medicine Online Journal* (Web MD), 1–14. www.emedicine.com

Bandholm, T. et al. (2014). Knee pain during strength training shortly following fast-track total knee arthroplasty: A cross-sectional study. *PLoS One*, 9, 3, e91107. DOI: 10.1371/journal.pone.0091107

Bedekar, N. et al. (2012). Comparative study of conventional therapy and additional yogasanas for knee rehabilitation after total knee arthroplasty. *International Journal of Yoga*, 5, 2, 118–122. DOI: 10.4103/0973-6131.98226

Begalle, R.L. et al. (2012). Quadriceps and hamstrings coactivation during common therapeutic exercises. *Journal of Athletic Training*, 47, 4, 395–405.

Bhagia, S.M. et al. (2006). Meniscal tears. *E-Medicine Online Journal* (Web MD), 1–14. www.emedicine.com

Bolgla, L.A. & Boling, M.C. (2011). An update for the conservative management of patellofemoral pain syndrome: A systematic review of the literature from 2000 to 2010. *International Journal of Sports and Physical Therapy*, 6, 2, 112–125.

Boling, M. et al. (2010). Gender differences in the incidence and prevalence of patellofemoral pain syndrome. *Scandinavian Journal of Medicine & Science in Sports*, 20, 5, 725–730.

Brotzman, B. & Manske, R.C. (2011). *Clinical Orthopedic Rehabilitation* (3rd ed.). St. Louis, Mo.: Mosby.

Brown, D.W. (2007). *Anterior Cruciate Ligament Reconstruction Techniques*. Orthopedic Associates. www.orthoassociates.com

Buchbinder, R. (2004). Plantar fasciitis. *New England Journal of Medicine*, 350, 21, 2159–2167.

Centers for Disease Control and Prevention (2019). *Arthritis: Disabilities and Limitations*. www.cdc.gov/arthritis/data statistics/disabilities-limitations.htm

Cheatham, S.W. et al. (2104). Adductor related groin pain in the athlete: A review of the literature. *Physical Therapy Reviews*, 19, 5, 328–337.

Cioppa-Mosca, J.M. et al. (2006). *Postsurgical Rehabilitation Guidelines for the Orthopedic Clinician*. St. Louis, Mo.: Mosby

Cohen, Z. et al. (2001). Patellofemoral stresses during open and closed kinetic chain exercises: An analysis using computer simulation. *American Journal of Sports Medicine*, 29, 480–487.

Cole, C., Seto, C., & Gazewood, J. (2005). Plantar fasciitis: Evidence-based review of diagnosis and therapy. *American Family Physician*, 72, 11, 2237–2243.

Cooper, C. et al. (2013). How to define responders in osteoarthritis. *Current Medical Research and Opinion*, 29, 6, 719–729. DOI: 10.1185/03007995.2013.792793

Crossley, K. et al. (2012). Anterior knee pain. In: Brukner, P. & Khan, K. (Eds.) *Brukner & Khan's Clinical Sports Medicine* (4th ed.). North Ryde, N.S.W.: McGraw-Hill Australia, pp. 684–714.

Cutts, S. et al. (2012). Plantar fasciitis. *Annals of the Royal College of Surgeons of England*, 94, 8, 539–542. DOI: 10.1308/003588412X13171221592456

Dalury, D.F. et al. (2009). Unicompartmental knee arthroplasty compares favorably to total knee arthroplasty in the same patient. *Orthopedics*, www.orthoassociates.com

Denegar, C.R., Saliba, E., & Saliba, S. (2009). *Therapeutic Modalities for Musculoskeletal Injuries* (3rd ed.). Champaign, Ill.: Human Kinetics.

DiGiovanni, B.F. et al. (2006). Chronic plantar fasciitis: A prospective clinical trial with two-year follow-up. *Journal of Bone & Joint Surgery,* 88-A, 8, 1–15.

Dixit, S. et al. (2007). Management of patellofemoral pain syndrome. *American Family Physician,* 75, 194–204.

Evans, T., Hertel, J., & Sebastianelli, W. (2004). Bilateral deficits in postural control following lateral ankle sprain. *Foot & Ankle International,* 25, 11, 833–839.

Fairclough, J. et al. (2006). The functional anatomy of the iliotibial band during flexion and extension of the knee: Implications for understanding iliotibial band syndrome. *Journal of Anatomy,* 208, 3, 309–316. DOI: 10.1111/j.1469-7580.2006.00531.x

Ferran, N.A. & Maffulli, N. (2006). Epidemiology of sprains of the lateral ankle ligament complex. *Foot and Ankle Clinics,* 11, 3, 659–662.

Foye, P.M. & Stitik, T.P. (2006). Trochantaric bursitis. *E-Medicine Online Journal* (Web MD), Dec. 21, 1–14. www.emedicine.com

Friel, K. et al. (2006). Ipsilateral hip abductor weakness after inversion ankle sprain. *Journal of Athletic Training,* 41, 1, 74–78.

Glass, R., Waddell, J., & Hoogenboom, B. (2010). The effects of open versus closed kinetic chain exercises on patients with ACL deficient or reconstructed knees: A systematic review. *North American Journal of Physical Therapy,* 5, 2, 74–84.

Hall, M., Stevermer, C.A., & Gillette, J.C. (2012). Gait analysis post anterior cruciate ligament reconstruction: Knee osteoarthritis perspective. *Gait and Posture,* 36, 56–60.

Hewett, T.E., Di Stasi, S.L., & Myer, G.D. (2013). Current concepts for injury prevention in athletes after anterior cruciate ligament reconstruction. *American Journal of Sports Medicine,* 41, 216–224.

Holm, B. et al. (2010). Loss of knee-extension strength is related to knee swelling after total knee arthroplasty. *Archives of Physical Medicine and Rehabilitation,* 91, 1770–1776. DOI: 10.1016/j.apmr.2010.07.229

Hoshino, Y. et al. (2013). Can joint contact dynamics be restored by anterior cruciate ligament reconstruction? *Clinical Orthopaedics and Related Research,* 471, 2924–2931.

Houglum, P.A. (2010). *Therapeutic Exercise for Musculoskeletal Injuries* (3rd ed.). Champaign, Ill.: Human Kinetics.

Ivins, D. (2006). Acute ankle sprains: An update. *American Family Physician,* 74, 1714–1720.

Jeong, H.J., Lee, S.H., & Ko, C.S. (2012). Meniscectomy. *Knee Surgery and Related Research,* 24, 129–136.

Kaminski, T.W. et al. (2013). National Athletic Trainers' Association position statement: Conservative management and prevention of ankle sprains in athletes. *Journal of Athletic Training,* 48, 4, 528–545. DOI: 10.4085/1062-6050-48.4.02

Kennon, R. et al. (2004). Anterior approach for total hip arthroplasty: Beyond the minimally invasive technique. *Journal of Bone and Joint Surgery,* 86, 91–97.

Kerkhoffs, G.M. et al. (2012). The influence of obesity on the complication rate and outcome of total knee arthroplasty: A meta-analysis and systematic literature review. *Journal of Bone and Joint Surgery,* 94, 20, 1839–1844. DOI: 10.2106/JBJS.K.00820

Kiapour, A.M. & Murray, M.M. (2014). Basic science of anterior cruciate ligament injury and repair. *Bone and Joint Research,* 3, 2, 20–31. DOI: 10.1302/2046-3758.32.2000241

Kisner, C. & Colby, L. (2012). *Therapeutic Exercise: Foundations and Techniques* (6th ed.). Philadelphia: F.A. Davis Company.

Kruse, L.M., Gray, B., & Wright, R.W. (2012). Rehabilitation after anterior cruciate ligament reconstruction: A systematic review. *Journal of Bone and Joint Surgery,* 94, 19, 1737–1748. DOI: 10.2106/JBJS.K.01246

Kurtz, S.M. et al. (2011). International survey of primary and revision total knee replacement. *International Orthopaedics,* 35, 12, 1783–1789. DOI: 10.1007/s00264-011-1235-5

Lavine, R. (2010). Iliotibial band friction syndrome. *Current Reviews in Musculoskeletal Medicine,* 3, 1–4, 18–22. DOI: 10.1007/s12178-010-9061-8

Levine, J.W. et al. (2013). Clinically relevant injury patterns after an anterior cruciate ligament injury provide insight into injury mechanisms. *American Journal of Sports Medicine,* 41, 385–395.

Lievense, A., Bierma-Zeinstra, S., & Schouten, B. (2005). Prognosis of trochantaric pain in primary care. *British Journal of General Practice,* 55, 512, 199–204.

Lustenberger, D.P. et al. (2011). Efficacy of treatment of trochanteric bursitis: A systematic review. *Clinical Journal of Sports Medicine,* 21, 5, 447–453. DOI: 10.1097/JSM.0b013e318221299c

Maffulli, N., Khan, K.M., & Puddu, G. (1998). Overuse tendon conditions: Time to change a confusing terminology. *Arthroscopy,* 14, 840–843.

Maffulli, N. et al. (2010). Meniscal tears. *Open Access Journal of Sports Medicine,* 1, 45–54.

Manske, R.C. (2006). *Postsurgical Orthopedic Sports Rehabilitation: Knee and Shoulder.* St. Louis, Mo.: Mosby.

Martinez, J.M. & Honsik, K. (2006). Iliotibial band syndrome. *E-Medicine Online Journal* (Web MD), Dec. 6, 1–14. www.emedicine.com

Matta, J.M., Shahrdar, C., & Ferguson, T. (2005). Single-incision anterior approach for total hip arthroplasty on an orthopedic table. *Clinical Orthopedics and Related Research,* 441,115–124.

Maxey, L. & Magnusson, J. (2013). *Rehabilitation for the Postsurgical Orthopedic Patient* (3rd ed.). St. Louis, Mo.: Mosby.

Mazzone, M. (2002). Common conditions of the achilles tendon. *American Family Physician,* 65, 1805–1810.

McHugh, M.P. (2004). The prevention of muscle strains in sport: Effective pre-season interventions? *International Sports Medicine Journal,* 5, 3, 177.

Metzl, J. (2005). A case-based look at shin splints. *Patient Care,* Nov, 39–46.

Mordecai, S.C. et al. (2014). Treatment of meniscal tears: An evidence based approach. *World Journal of Orthopedics,* 5, 3, 233–241. DOI: 10.5312/wjo.v5.i3.233

Mueller-Wohlfahrt, H-W et al. (2013). Terminology and classification of muscle injuries in sport: The Munich consensus statement. *British Journal of Sports Medicine,* 47, 6, 342–350. DOI: 10.1136/bjsports-2012-091448

Naslund, J. et al. (2006). Comparison of symptoms and clinical findings in subgroups of individuals with patellofemoral pain. *Physiotherapy Theory & Practice,* 22, 5, 105–118.

Newman, P. et al. (2013). Risk factors associated with medial tibial stress syndrome in runners: A systematic review and meta-analysis. *Open Access Journal of Sports Medicine,* 4, 229–241. DOI: 10.2147/OAJSM.S39331

Osteoarthritis Action Alliance (2020). *A National Public Health Agenda for Osteoarthritis: 2020 Update.* https://oaaction.unc.edu/wp-content/uploads/sites/623/2020/05/OA-Agenda-Final_04302020.pdf

Pappas, E. & Wong-Tom, W.M. (2012). Prospective predictors of patellofemoral pain syndrome: A systematic review with meta-analysis. *Sports Health,* 4, 2, 115–120.

Peters, J.S. & Tyson, N.L. (2013). Proximal exercises are effective in treating patellofemoral pain syndrome: A systematic review. *International Journal of Sports and Physical Therapy,* 8, 5, 689–700.

Petersen, W. et al. (2013). Treatment of acute ankle ligament injuries: A systematic review. *Archives of Orthopaedic and Trauma Surgery,* 133, 8, 1129–1141. DOI: 10.1007/s00402-013-1742-5

Pivec, R. et al. (2012). Hip arthroplasty. *The Lancet,* 380, 1768–1777.

Rao, S., Riskowski, J., & Hannan, M.T. (2013). Musculoskeletal conditions of the foot and ankle: Assessments and treatment options. *Best Practice and Research Clinical Rheumatology,* 26, 3, 345–368. DOI: 10.1016/j.berh.2012.05.009

Rice, D.A. & McNair, P.J. (2010). Quadriceps arthrogenic muscle inhibition: Neural mechanisms and treatment perspectives. *Seminars in Arthritis and Rheumatism,* 40, 250–266. DOI: 10.1016/j.semarthrit.2009.10.001

Robinson, R.L. & Nee, R.J. (2007). Analysis of hip strength in females seeking physical therapy treatment for unilateral patellofemoral pain syndrome. *Journal of Orthopedic and Sports Physical Therapy,* 37, 5, 232–238.

Rosneck J. et al. (2007). Managing knee osteoarthritis before and after arthroplasty. *Cleveland Clinic Journal of Medicine,* 74, 663–671.

Rothschild, B. (2013). Trochanteric area pain, the result of a quartet of bursal inflammation. *World Journal of Orthopedics,* 4, 3, 100–102. DOI: 10.5312/wjo.v4.i3.100

Roush, J.R. & Curtis Bay, R. (2012). Prevalence of anterior knee pain in 18–35 year-old females. *International Journal of Sports and Physical Therapy,* 7, 4, 396–401.

Schwartz, E.N. & Su, J. (2014). Plantar fasciitis: A concise review. *The Permanente Journal,* 18, 1, e105–e107. DOI: 10.7812/TPP/13-113

Shaerf, D.A. et al. (2014). Anterior cruciate ligament reconstruction best practice: A review of graft choice. *World Journal of Orthopedics,* 5, 1, 23–29. DOI: 10.5312/wjo.v5.i1.23

Sussmilch-Leitch, S.P. et al. (2012). Physical therapies for Achilles tendinopathy: Systematic review and meta-analysis. *Journal of Foot and Ankle Research,* 5, 1, 15. DOI: 10.1186/1757-1146-5-15

Tsertsvadze, A. et al. (2014). Total hip replacement for the treatment of end stage arthritis of the hip: A systematic review and meta-analysis. *PLoS One,* 9, 7, e99804. DOI: 10.1371/journal.pone.0099804

Uden, H., Boesch, E., & Kumar, S. (2011). Plantar fasciitis - to jab or to support? A systematic review of the current best evidence. *Journal of Multidisciplinary Healthcare,* 4, 155–164. DOI: 10.2147/JMDH.S20053

Van Deun, S. et al. (2007). Relationship of chronic ankle instability to muscle activation patterns during the transition from double-leg to single-leg stance. *American Journal of Sports Medicine,* 35, 274–281.

Wasielewski, N.J. & Kotsko, K.M. (2007). Does eccentric exercise reduce pain and improve strength in physically active adults with symptomatic lower extremity tendinosis? A systematic review. *Journal of Athletic Training,* 42, 3, 409–422.

Witvrouw, E. et al. (2000). Open versus closed kinetic chain exercises for patellofemoral pain: A prospective, randomized study. *The American Journal of Sports Medicine,* 28, 687–694.

Wolgin, M. et al. (2004). Conservative treatment of plantar heel pain: Long-term follow-up. *Foot & Ankle International,* 5, 97–102.

Wright, W.G., Ivanenko, Y.P., & Gurfinkel, V.S. (2012). Foot anatomy specialization for postural sensation and control. *Journal of Neurophysiology,* 107, 5, 1513–1521. DOI: 10.1152/jn.00256.2011

Xu, C.P. et al. (2013). Mini-incision versus standard incision total hip arthroplasty regarding surgical outcomes: A systematic review and meta-analysis of randomized controlled trials. *PLoS One,* 8, 11, e80021. DOI: 10.1371/journal.pone.0080021

Yang, B. et al. (2012). Minimally invasive surgical approaches and traditional total hip arthroplasty: A meta-analysis of radiological and complications outcomes. *PLoS One,* 7, 5, e37947. DOI: 10.1371/journal.pone.0037947

Zanasi, S. (2011). Innovations in total knee replacement: New trends in operative treatment and changes in peri-operative management. *European Orthopaedics and Traumatology,* 2, 1–2, 21–31. DOI: 10.1007/s12570-011-0066-6

Zhang, Y. & Jordan, J.M. (2010). Epidemiology of osteoarthritis. *Clinical Geriatric Medicine,* 26, 3, 355–369. DOI: 10.1016/j.cger.2010.03.001

SUGGESTED READING

Cheatham, S.W. (2013). Do patient factors and prehabilitation improve outcomes after total knee arthoplasty? *Topics in Geriatric Rehabilitation,* 29, 1, 17–24. DOI: 10.1097/TGR.0b013e318275c288

Cheatham, S.W. (2013). Hip resurfacing: Current concepts and clinical considerations. *Topics in Geriatric Rehabilitation,* 29, 4, 246–252.

Cheatham, S. & Kreiswirth, E. (2014). The regional interdependence model: A clinical examination concept. *International Journal of Athletic Therapy & Training,* 19, 3, 8–14.

Cheatham, S.W. et al. (2014). Adductor-related groin pain in the athlete. *Physical Therapy Reviews,* 19, 5, 328–337.

Kaminski, T.W. et al. (2013). National Athletic Trainers' Association position statement: Conservative management and prevention of ankle sprains in athletes. *Journal of Athletic Training,* 48, 4, 528–545. DOI: 10.4085/1062-6050-48.4.02

Kiapour, A.M. & Murray, M.M. (2014). Basic science of anterior cruciate ligament injury and repair. *Bone and Joint Research,* 3, 2, 20–31. DOI: 10.1302/2046-3758.32.2000241

Levine, J.W. et al. (2013). Clinically relevant injury patterns after an anterior cruciate ligament injury provide insight into injury mechanisms. *American Journal of Sports Medicine,* 41, 385–395.

Mueller-Wohlfahrt, H-W et al. (2013). Terminology and classification of muscle injuries in sport: The Munich consensus statement. *British Journal of Sports Medicine,* 47, 6, 342–350. DOI: 10.1136/bjsports-2012-091448

Rao, S., Riskowski, J., & Hannan, M.T. (2013). Musculoskeletal conditions of the foot and ankle: Assessments and treatment options. *Best Practice and Research Clinical Rheumatology,* 26, 3, 345–368. DOI: 10.1016/j.berh.2012.05.009

19 MUSCULOSKELETAL INJURIES OF THE UPPER EXTREMITY

IN THIS CHAPTER

ACROMIOCLAVICULAR JOINT PATHOLOGY
ACROMIOCLAVICULAR JOINT SPRAIN

SHOULDER PATHOLOGIES
ANTERIOR SHOULDER INSTABILITY
POSTERIOR SHOULDER INSTABILITY
SHOULDER IMPINGEMENT SYNDROME

ELBOW PATHOLOGIES
LATERAL EPICONDYLITIS
MEDIAL EPICONDYLITIS

WRIST AND HAND PATHOLOGIES
CARPAL TUNNEL SYNDROME
DE QUERVAIN'S TENOSYNOVITIS

CASE STUDIES

SUMMARY

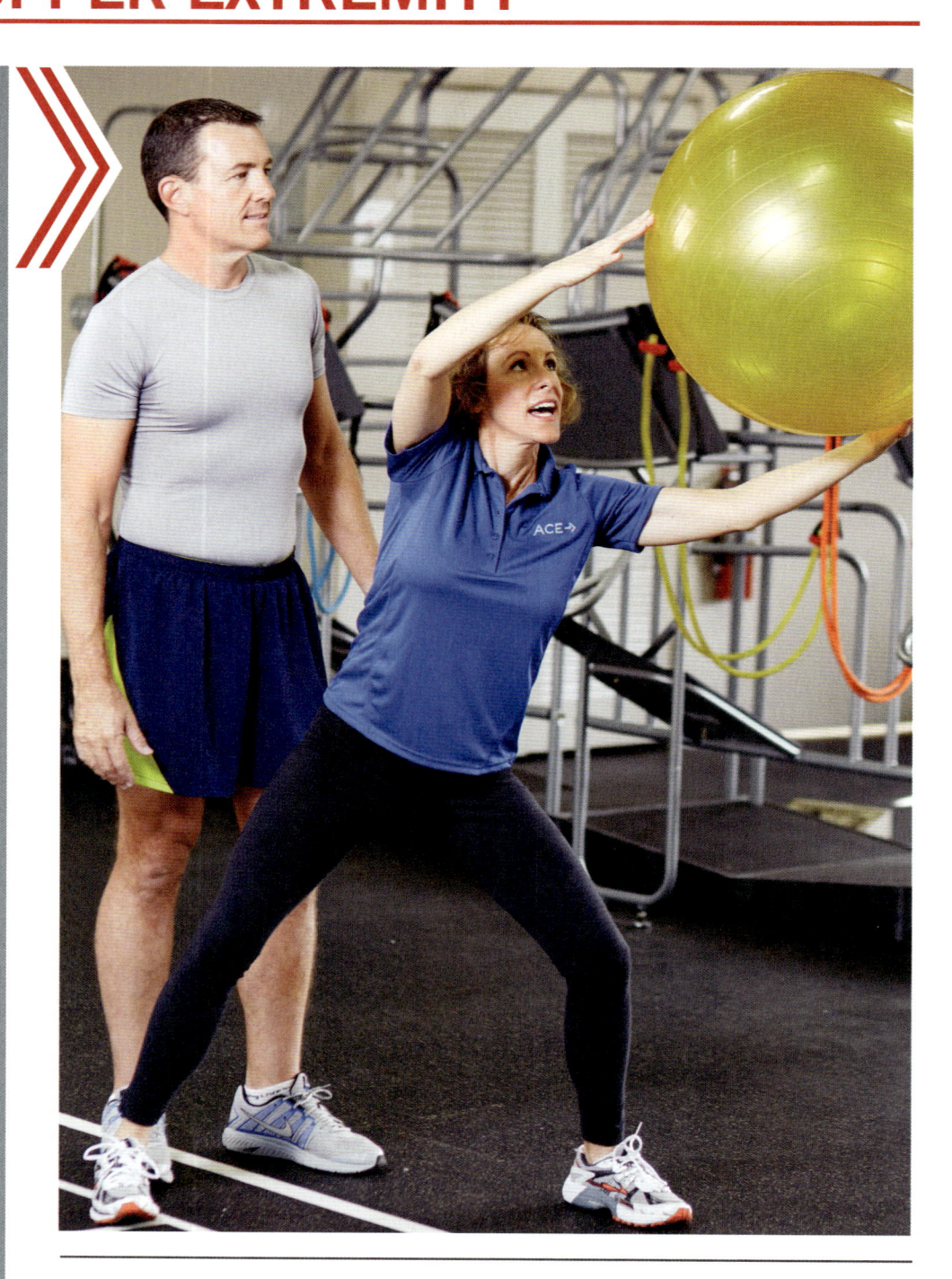

ABOUT THE AUTHOR
Michael Levinson, P.T., CSCS, has been at the Hospital for Special Surgery since 1984, where he is a clinical supervisor of the Rehabilitation Department. Levinson is also a physical therapist for the New York Mets Baseball Club. He is certified by the National Strength and Conditioning Association as a Strength and Conditioning Specialist.

By Michael Levinson

WHEN TRAINING AN INDIVIDUAL FOLLOWING AN upper-extremity musculoskeletal injury, it is important that the ACE® Certified Medical Exercise Specialist (CMES) is aware of several factors, including the mechanism of injury, the structures involved, the healing constraints of the structures involved (see Table 18-1, page 588), exacerbating activities, and **range of motion (ROM)** issues. Pain is the most important guideline when designing a training program. Communication with the client's physical therapist and physician can be extremely valuable in preventing re-injury. Symptoms such as recurrent pain, instability, or loss of ROM should be communicated.

ACROMIOCLAVICULAR JOINT PATHOLOGY

The acromioclavicular joint consists of the **articulation** of the **distal** end of the clavicle and the acromion, which is a portion of the scapula (Figure 19-1). The joint is covered with cartilage and is stabilized by the coracoclavicular and acromioclavicular ligaments. The clavicle rotates upward 40 to 50 degrees as the arm is fully elevated. Without **rotation** of the clavicle, the arm can be elevated to only approximately 110 degrees. Injuries to the acromioclavicular joint can present as either traumatic or chronic.

Acromioclavicular Joint Sprain

Acromioclavicular joint sprains are common and can occur across different age groups. Although a typical athletic injury, acromioclavicular joint separation is often diagnosed after road traffic accidents and a fall on the side of the body. Traditionally, the condition was seen as a shoulder issue, as noted by Hippocrates (460–377 BC) in 400 BC, and acromioclavicular separation often was misdiagnosed as a glenohumeral injury (Babhulkar & Pawaskar, 2014).

Mechanism of Injury

The most common mechanism of injury is a direct force on the point of the shoulder or a fall on an outstretched arm. If the clavicle does not fracture, the acromion is driven inferiorly and medially in relation to the clavicle. The ligaments are then stretched or torn, depending on the severity of the injury. This injury is often referred to as a "separated shoulder." The sports with the highest incidence of acromioclavicular joint dislocation are bicycling (29%) and skiing/snowboarding (10%), which are associated with falls onto the shoulder (Tischer et al., 2009). The injury is classified by six different degrees of severity. A type I sprain indicates a mild stretching of the ligaments. In type II and III sprains, the acromioclavicular ligament is torn and some deformity can be seen. In types IV, V, and VI, ligaments are torn and significant damage to the structures around the joint occurs (Figure 19-2) (Rockwood & Matsen, 2009).

Signs and Symptoms of Acromioclavicular Joint Sprain

Patients with acromioclavicular joint pathology often present with pain during passive horizontal **adduction** or have pain during an O'Brien active compression test, which consists of resistance of the shoulder in **flexion**, internal rotation, and horizontal adduction (O'Brien et al., 1998) (Figure 19-3). More severe cases will present with a "step" deformity where the separation of the clavicle and the acromion can be seen.

LEARNING OBJECTIVES:

» Identify important anatomical features of and movement-related dysfunctions that commonly occur in the joints of the upper extremity.

» Differentiate between various pathologies of the acromioclavicular joint, shoulder, elbow, hand, and wrist.

» Describe basic signs, symptoms, and treatment options associated with different pathologies of the upper extremity.

» Design and implement safe and effective exercise programs for clients who have various musculoskeletal injuries of the upper extremity while staying within the ACE Certified Medical Exercise Specialist's scope of practice.

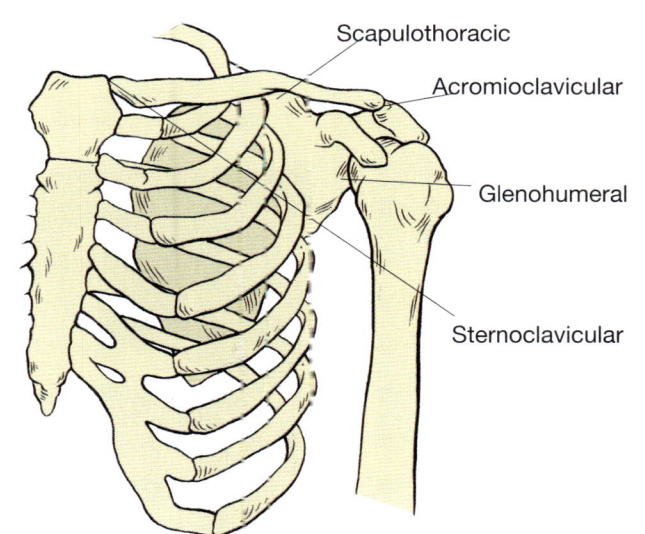

Figure 19-1
The four articulations of the shoulder joint complex

CHAPTER 19 — Musculoskeletal Injuries of the Upper Extremity

Figure 19-2
Classification of acromioclavicular joint injuries

Reprinted with permission from Beim, G. (2000). Acromioclavicular joint injuries. *Journal of Athletic Training*, 35, 3, 261–267.

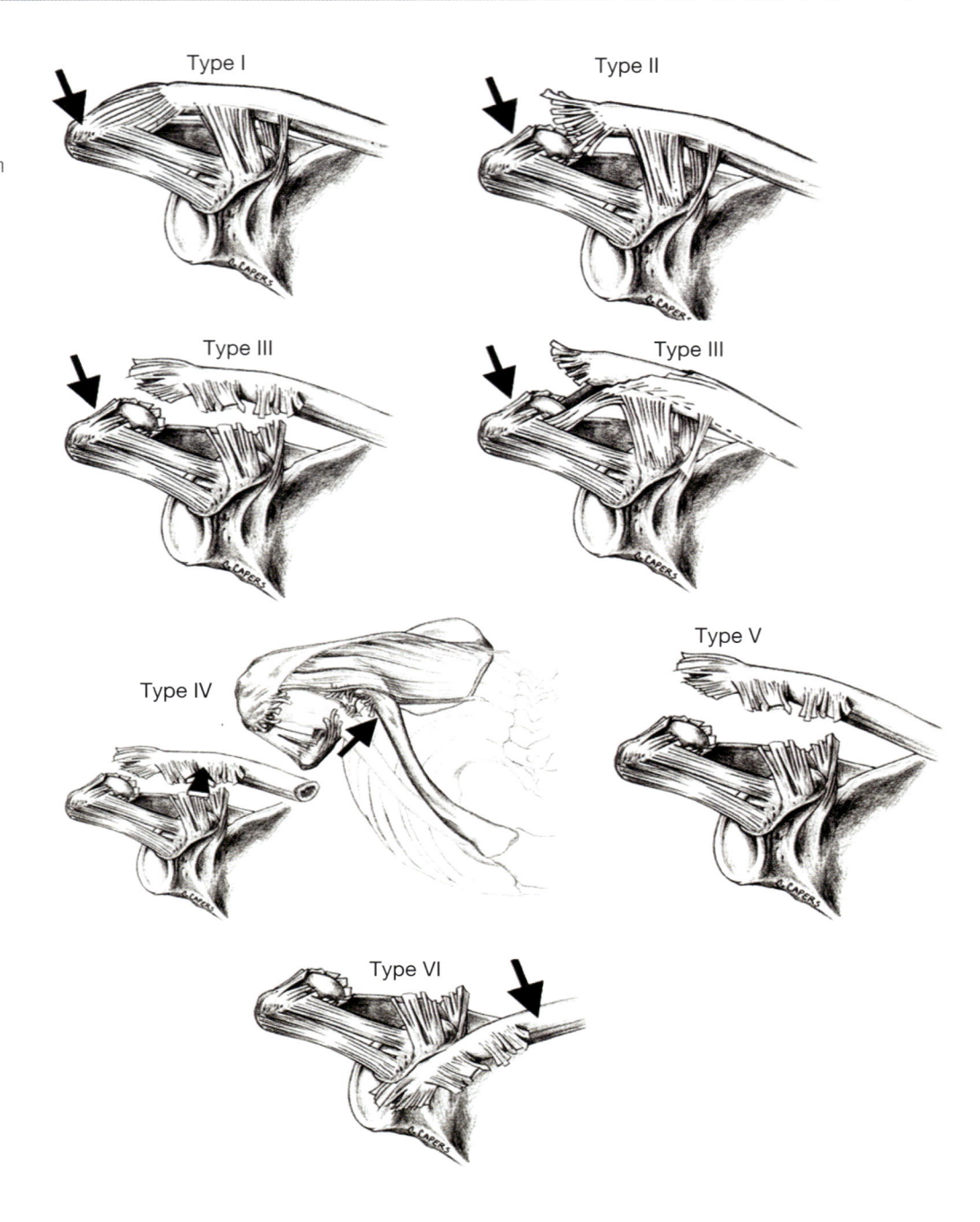

Figure 19-3
O'Brien active compression test

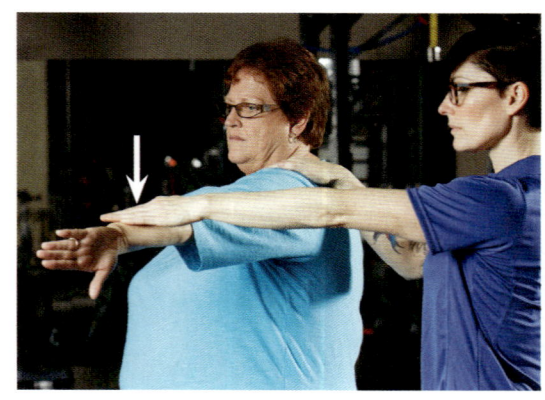

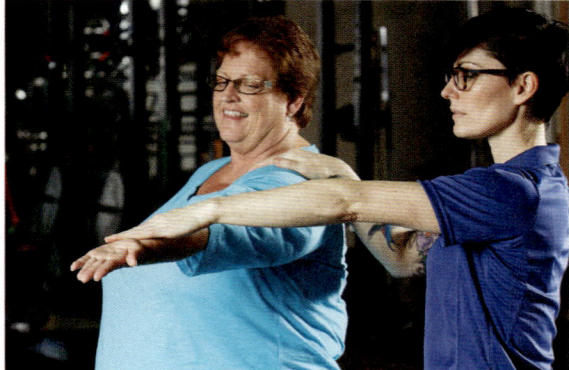

Precautions

Strengthening can be initiated with submaximal **isometrics** for **abduction,** flexion, **extension,** internal rotation, and external rotation. When progressing a strengthening program, several precautions should be followed:

- **Traction** through the shoulder joint should be avoided or minimized. For example, when a client is performing shrugs or curls, the CMES should provide a weight that can be controlled. Also, weights should not be carried around the gym. Beginning exercise with elastic resistance or tubing is often the safest choice.
- Resistive exercises in horizontal abduction or adduction should be avoided or minimized secondary to stress on the joint.
- When performing scapular muscle strengthening exercises, extremes of scapular **retraction** and **protraction** should be avoided.
- Internal and external rotation exercises for the rotator cuff are tolerated best with the arm in adduction.
- Overhead resistive activity, such as the military press and incline bench press, should be minimized or avoided. These activities should be initiated only when the client is asymptomatic and has a good proximal strength base.

PATHOMECHANICS OF THE ACROMIOCLAVICULAR JOINT AFTER SHOULDER INJURY

Injury to the acromioclavicular joint can lead to chronic degenerative changes at the joint. Abnormal mechanics or instability at the joint can result in a wearing away of the cartilage and **arthrosis.** In addition, people with poor mechanics who have done a great deal of bench pressing or push-ups can cause degenerative changes at the joint.

Pathomechanics following injury to this joint vary. First, there may be a loss of clavicle rotation, which can result in a loss of shoulder **elevation.** Secondly, the structural suspension of the entire shoulder girdle may be compromised. Most critical are the pathomechanics of the scapula. The scapula provides a stable platform for shoulder motion and any deviation may result in other shoulder problems. Inferior and medial rotation of the scapula is often a consequence of this injury. Hence, working to restore normal ROM and function in the scapulothoracic joint is a primary focus of exercise treatment.

APPLY WHAT YOU KNOW

Early Intervention

Treatment varies greatly and is partially dependent on the severity of the injury. The current trend is toward conservative treatment without surgery (Smith et al., 2011). However, in certain severe cases, a surgical procedure is the treatment of choice. Surgical procedures vary greatly and are utilized for individuals who present with persistent pain, joint instability, or an undesirable and visible deformity at the joint sight. Especially among the female population, **cosmesis,** or a concern for appearance, is often a rationale for surgery. In addition, athletes who perform overhead movements and individuals who perform a great deal of highly physical work may find conservative treatment unsatisfactory. There are numerous surgical techniques available. However, there is no true "gold standard." Surgical treatment includes resection of the distal clavicle, ligament transfer, ligament reconstruction, and internal fixation. Patients undergoing clavicle resection often must modify certain activities such as push-ups and the bench press. Reconstructions that are successful can theoretically return the individual to a normal exercise level.

Conservative treatment of this injury varies, but the trend is moving away from extended periods of immobilization. Initially, an immobilizer may be utilized for pain control, reduction of muscle spasm, and reduction of soft-tissue damage for a few days for type I sprains and the first one to three weeks for types II and III. Reduction of the injury with strict immobilization for extended periods has not been demonstrated to be an effective treatment plan. Patient compliance has often been a limiting factor. **Cryotherapy** for reduction of pain, swelling, and spasm is a key component of the early stages of recovery.

The goal of the initial stages of recovery is to restore pain-free ROM. Manske (2006) advises avoiding active-ROM and passive-ROM exercises in the supine position. The rationale is that the client's body weight prevents scapular ROM and thus results in greater clavicle rotation, which may result in exacerbation of the injury. Seated or standing is the preferred position.

Restorative Exercise Program for Acromioclavicular Joint Sprain

When designing the program, the CMES should include client education. Important components include proper training techniques, awareness of precautions, and early injury recognition. The client should be pain-free with activity and should be reminded to use ice after the workouts to prevent any latent discomfort or inflammation.

Functional Training

The focus of the initial training sessions should be to restore proper neuromuscular control throughout the scapulothoracic and shoulder regions and abdominal core. The rotator cuff, deltoids, pectorals, trapezius, rhomboids, and latissimus dorsi should be the focus of strengthening. At this point, isolated open-kinetic-chain (OKC) strengthening may still be necessary due to local weakness, endurance deficits, and poor muscle recruitment. Shoulder exercises can include flexion, extension, internal and external rotation, and abduction (below 90 degrees) with a light weight or elastic resistance.

Movement Training

The Movement Training program should focus on maintaining and improving neuromuscular control and kinetic-chain mobility while challenging the abdominal core and shoulder complex. This could include a variety of planks and light medicine-ball tosses. Again, the focus should be on proper stabilization and movement in the scapulothoracic and shoulder joints.

SHOULDER PATHOLOGIES

The glenohumeral joint consists of the head of the humerus and the glenoid fossa, which is a portion of the scapula (see Figure 19-1). Together, they form a "ball and socket." Unlike the true ball-and-socket joint of the hip formed primarily by bony structures, the motion at the glenohumeral joint is controlled by the capsule and ligaments that surround the joint and the four rotator cuff muscles. In fact, less than one-third of the humeral head actually articulates with the glenoid fossa, allowing a great deal of ROM to perform many athletic activities. For this reason, the glenohumeral joint is an inherently unstable joint, and is the most commonly dislocated joint in the body (Farrar et al., 2013).

Anterior Shoulder Instability

Shoulder instability is a symptomatic abnormal motion of the glenohumeral joint, which presents as a spectrum of symptoms from chronic pain to a sense of, or actual, displacement (**subluxation/dislocation**). Shoulder instability has been associated with athletic injuries, the majority of which are traumatic in nature (Jaggi et al., 2012).

Mechanism of Injury

Shoulder instability can be a result of an acute, traumatic event such as a dislocation. It can also be a chronic condition that results from overuse activities, especially overhead activities such as when throwing or playing tennis or volleyball, where the shoulder experiences various forces related to acceleration and deceleration. These powerful repetitive activities can cause excessive **laxity** in the capsule and ligaments that surround the shoulder joint. In addition, certain individuals are born with congenital joint laxity, which may predispose them to shoulder instability.

When the head of the humerus actually comes out of the socket, it is considered a dislocation. At times, it will go back in by itself. However, it often has to be **reduced** by a physician in the emergency room or on the field. Resultant trauma can cause soft-tissue damage and muscle spasm. The shoulder capsule and a structure called the **labrum** are often injured. The labrum is fibrocartilage that helps to increase the stability of the shoulder joint. Bony damage or loss can also result from recurrent instability. In addition, with instability, the humerus may **translate** excessively, but not completely come out of the socket. This is referred to as a subluxation, which is often a chronic condition. The most common instability is **anterior.** It usually occurs during some combination of shoulder external rotation, abduction, and extension. Common mechanisms of injury are falling on an outstretched arm, planting a ski pole and falling forward, or trying to arm-tackle someone. In each case, the humeral head is levered out the front of the shoulder. The recurrence rate for shoulder dislocations is extremely high, especially in younger people (Farrar et al., 2013).

Signs and Symptoms of Anterior Shoulder Instability

Clients may complain of point tenderness at the anterior and posterior glenohumeral joint, acromioclavicular joint, and sternoclavicular joint (Dumont, Russell, & Robertson, 2011). Further, clients with anterior shoulder instability may present with a positive apprehensive sign. That is, the client may become apprehensive about, or not allow the joint to be brought into, abduction and external rotation (Figure 19-4). When performing this test, the CMES must be cautious to avoid dislocating the joint.

Precautions

When initiating a strengthening program, submaximal, pain-free isometrics are performed for the rotator cuff and the deltoid to help reestablish stability of the shoulder joint. Precautions should be taken for the rotator cuff when performing internal and external rotation (IR/ER) exercises. The rotator cuff is often inflamed with a shoulder dislocation or instability. Isolated IR/ER exercises can increase the inflammation and thus reflexively inhibit the rotator cuff. As external-rotation ROM improves and inflammation is reduced, **isotonic** IR/ER exercises may be incorporated using elastic resistance.

Early Intervention

Following an initial dislocation, there is a period of immobilization in a sling. This allows for soft-tissue healing and reduction of pain and spasm. The trend is moving toward shorter periods of immobilization to prevent loss of ROM and excessive muscle **atrophy.**

During the initial phase of recovery, the goals are to decrease pain, inflammation, and spasm and gradually restore shoulder ROM in a safe manner. Positions of abduction, external rotation, and extension are avoided. Elevation of the arm is initiated in the plane of the scapula, which is 30 to 45 degrees anterior to the **frontal plane** (Figure 19-5). This plane provides the greatest amount of joint congruity and the least amount of stress to the shoulder capsule (Saha, 1983).

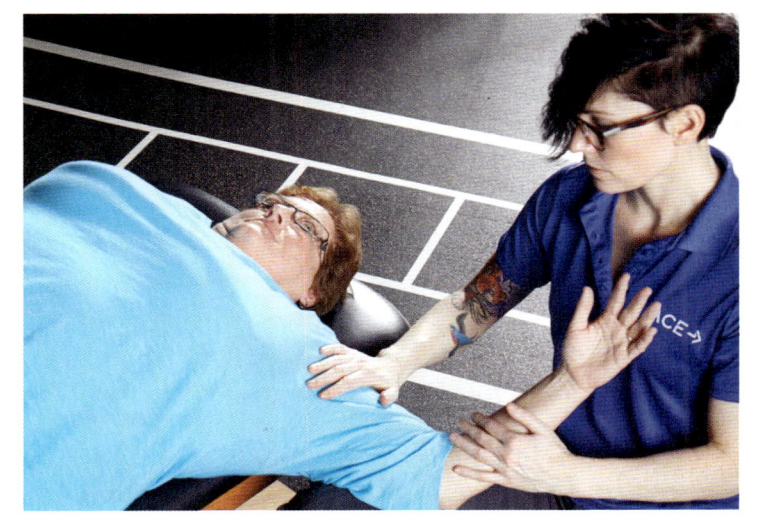

Figure 19-4
Anterior apprehension test

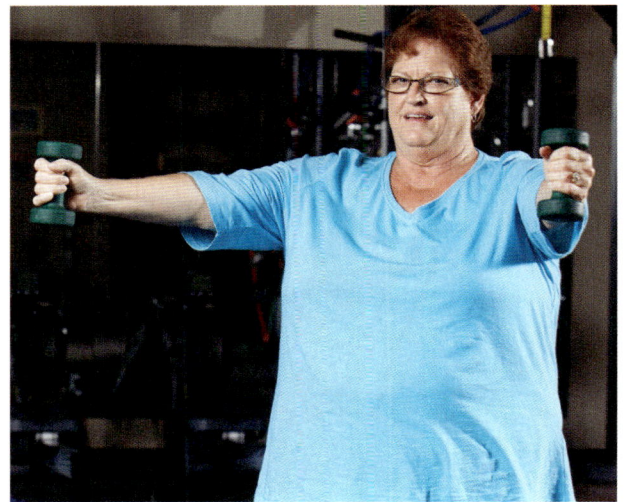

Figure 19-5
Diagonal arm raise in the plane of the scapula

Restorative Exercise Program for Anterior Shoulder Instability

A key component of restoring shoulder stability is to restore the strength of the muscles associated with the scapula. A stable scapula provides a stable base for shoulder rotation and maintains the proper length-tension relationship of the rotator cuff and deltoid muscles. The main stabilizers are the serratus anterior, rhomboid major and minor, levator scapulae, and trapezii (Figures 19-6 and 19-7). The glenohumeral stabilizers include the muscles of the rotator cuff: the supraspinatus, infraspinatus, teres minor, and subscapularis (Figure 19-8). These muscle groups function through synergistic co-contraction to anchor the scapula and guide movement (Paine & Voight, 2013).

Figure 19-6
Superficial and deep muscles that act at the scapulothoracic articulation

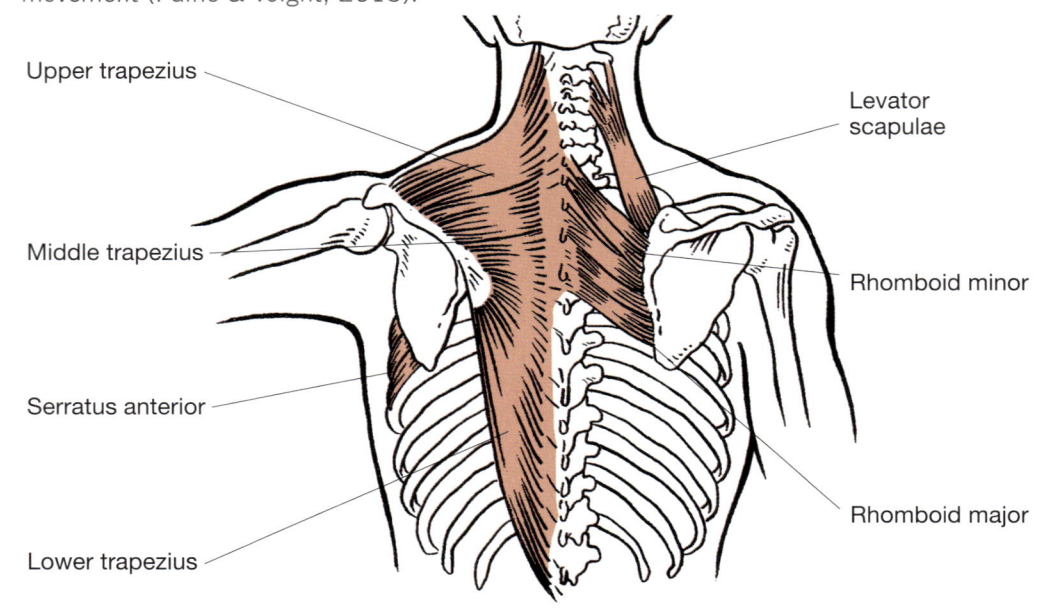

Figure 19-7
Anterior shoulder-girdle muscles

Figure 19-8
Rotator cuff muscles

Functional Training

When initiating scapula musculature strengthening, the CMES should continue to protect the shoulder capsule and labrum. External rotation and extension should be limited to neutral. For individuals with anterior instability, closed-kinetic-chain (CKC) exercises are often utilized. These exercises are performed with the distal end of the limb fixed and provide a compressive load to the shoulder joint and promote stability. Examples include ball stabilization, wall push-ups, quadruped stabilization, and dips or seated press-ups (Figures 19-9 through 19-12).

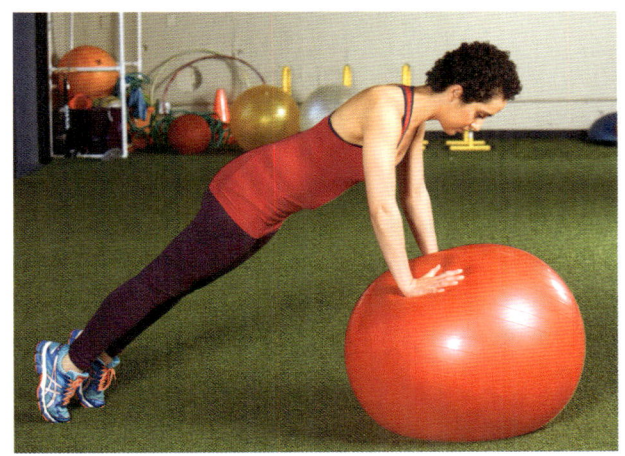

Figure 19-9
Shoulder stablization on stability ball

Figure 19-10
Wall push-ups

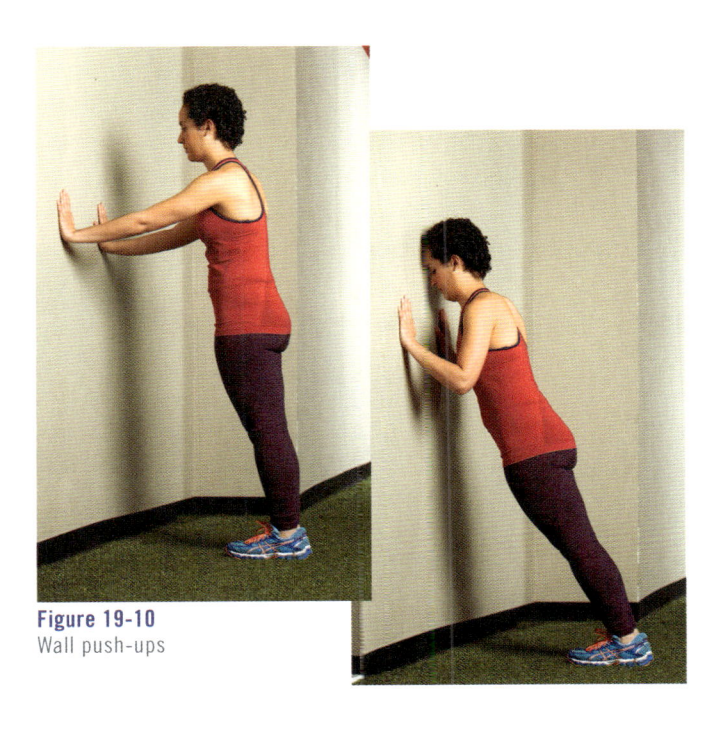

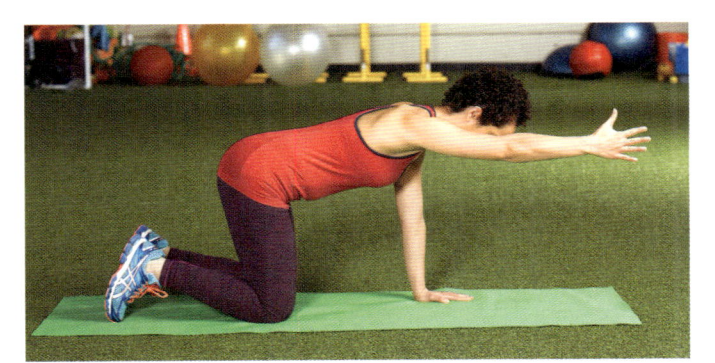

Figure 19-11
Quadruped shoulder stablization

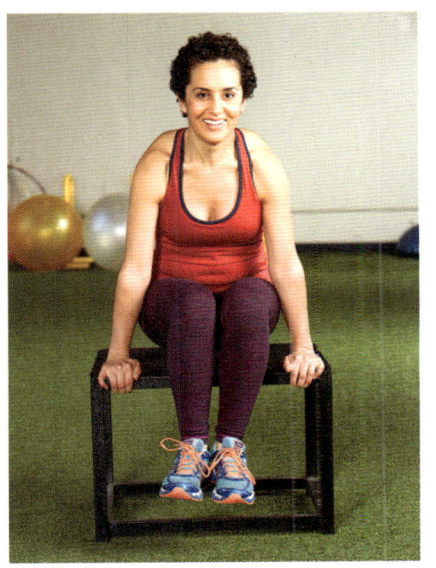

Figure 19-12
Seated press-ups

Movement Training

As the client improves postural stability and kinetic-chain mobility, OKC exercises are incorporated for scapula musculature strengthening. These exercises are performed with the distal end of the limb free and can be considered more functional, as most **activities of daily living (ADL)** take place in this mode. Scapula-muscle exercises may include rowing (retraction), shrugs (elevation), and serratus punches (protraction) (Figures 19-13 through 19-15). In addition, these exercises have been shown to indirectly strengthen the rotator cuff. The scapula initially sets during the first 60 degrees of elevation of the arm. Following this phase, there should be a 2:1 ratio of glenohumeral motion to scapulothoracic motion. Any deviation from this ratio may manifest itself as shoulder pathology.

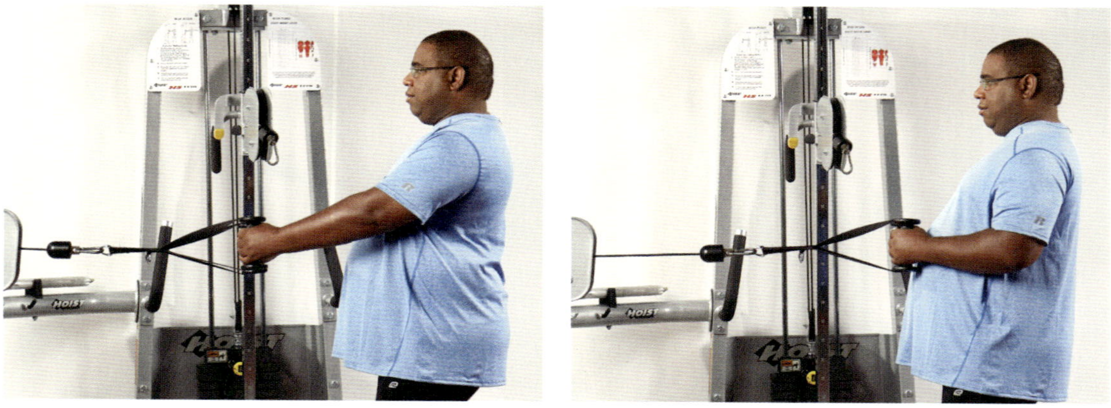

Figure 19-13
Standing rows

Figure 19-14
Shoulder shrugs

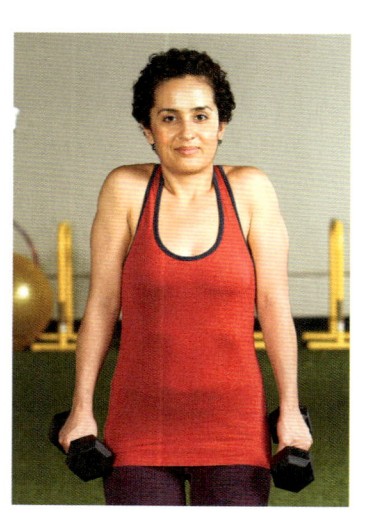

Figure 19-15
Serratus punches

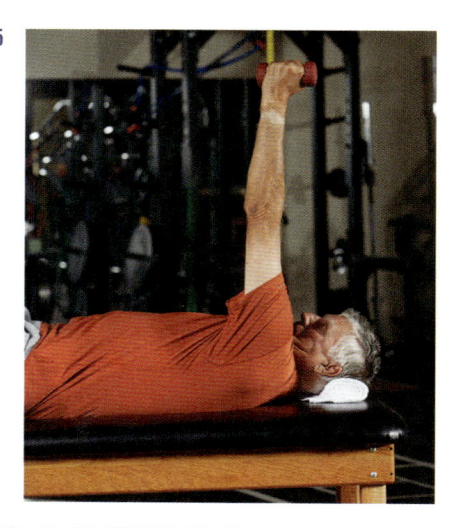

APPLY WHAT YOU KNOW

CONCERNS WITH COMMON WEIGHT-LIFTING EXERCISES FOR CLIENTS WITH SHOULDER INSTABILITY

The latissimus dorsi also contributes to the stability of the shoulder by providing a compressive force to the glenohumeral joint. When initiating strengthening, the CMES should limit the ROM from below 90 degrees of forward flexion to neutral extension. This may be accomplished with elastic resistance or a cable column (Figure 19-16). When progressing, the latissimus pull-down in the behind-the-neck position should be avoided (Reinold & Curtis, 2013). This position places the shoulder in abduction and external rotation, thus increasing the stress on the shoulder capsule and ligaments by producing a more anteriorly directed joint-reaction force that could result in anterior **translation** (Jaggi et al., 2012). The pull-down should be performed in front and in a reclined position with the trunk in slight extension (Figure 19-17). The bar is pulled down to the chest. Aside from reducing the chance of injury, this position provides a greater mechanical advantage for the latissimus dorsi and the scapular retractors.

Musculoskeletal Injuries of the Upper Extremity   CHAPTER 19

Figure 19-16
Shoulder extension

Figure 19-17
Lat pull-down

A client with shoulder instability may return to performing biceps curls, a very popular exercise in most health clubs and gyms. However, the CMES must be aware that the long head of the biceps has an attachment at the labrum. One particular labral tear is referred to as a SLAP lesion (superior labrum from anterior to posterior) (Houglum, 2010). This injury occurs in the region where the biceps originate. If there has been any damage to the labrum, excessive biceps activity may cause traction and exacerbate the injury. In addition, the CMES should monitor the client for any increased anterior/superior shoulder pain. Pain in this region with resistive forearm **supination** or resistive shoulder forward flexion with the forearm in supination may be an indication of **bicipital tendinitis** (Figure 19-18). In this case, the activity should be stopped and the physician or physical therapist should be informed. Biceps curls performed in a seated, supported position may reduce the chances of exacerbation. Avoiding end ranges of elbow extension may reduce the traction on the labrum. In addition, performing curls with a neutral forearm position will reduce the load on the biceps.

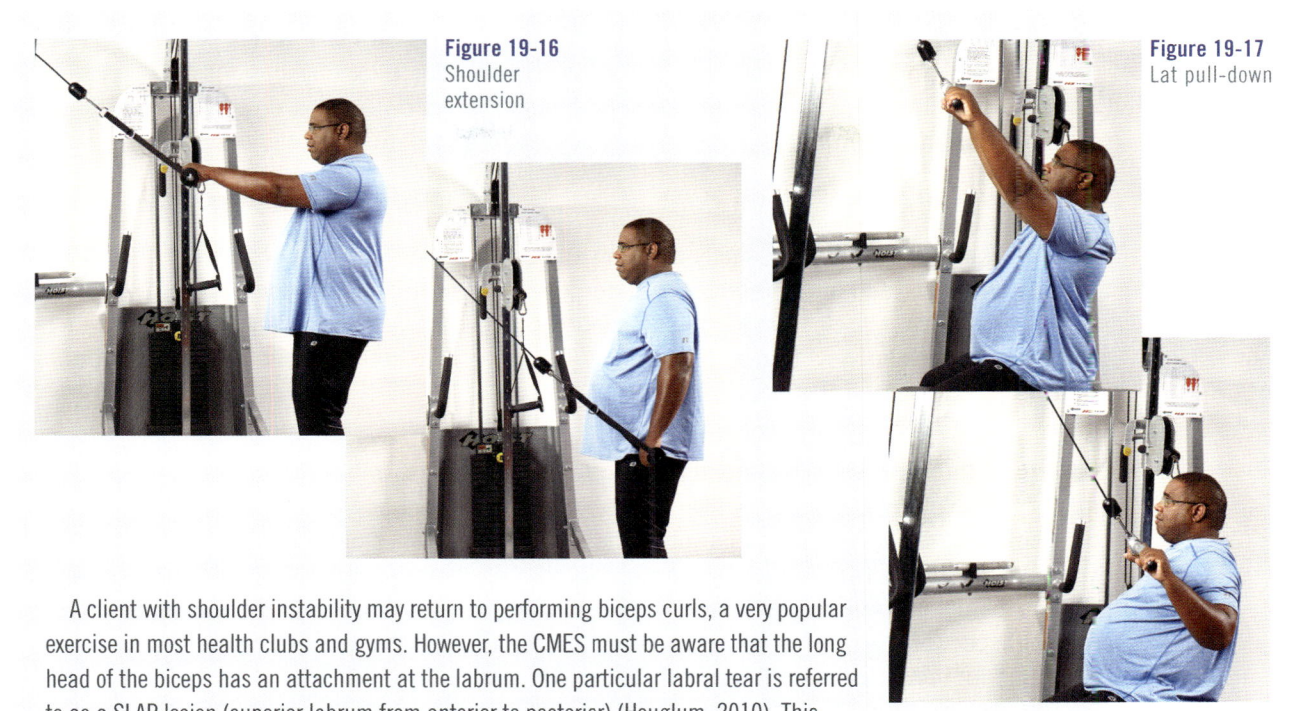

Modifications should be made for a client who wants to return to the bench press, as an overactive pectoralis major has been associated with an anterior translation of the glenohumeral joint, which could result in a destabilizing effect (Jaggi et al., 2012). First, there should be a mandatory "handoff" and spot. Second, shoulder position should be limited to below 90 degrees of forward flexion, 45 degrees of abduction, and neutral external rotation (Fees et al., 1998). These restrictions eliminate performance of the incline bench press, which would increase the stress on the capsule and ligaments. Repetitions should also be limited to avoid excessive fatigue, which can result in a loss of dynamic shoulder stability. Finally, weight machines such as a chest press, in which ROM can be controlled, may be a safer option.

The shoulder press or military press is another popular exercise. It is best to discourage clients with shoulder instability from performing this exercise.

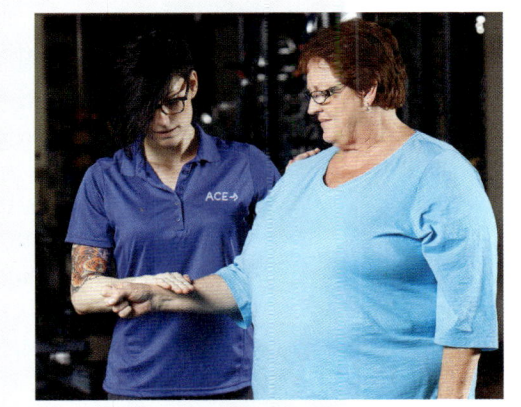

Figure 19-18
Resistive forearm supination

An effective initial strategy for the CMES is to advise the client to substitute other exercises in its place. Those who want to continue the shoulder press should avoid the behind-the-neck position (Reinold & Curtis, 2013). This position places significant stress on the shoulder capsule and ligaments and places the shoulder in a tenuous position for instability. Bringing the shoulder into a more anterior position or closer to the scapular plane significantly reduces the stress to the shoulder capsule and ligaments and provides better joint conformity between the humeral head and the glenoid fossa. Again, weight machines may provide a safer alternative to free weights.

Posterior Shoulder Instability

Posterior instability is less common, but it does occur. Posterior dislocations are rare. Competitive athletes are among the most common sufferers owing to overuse or a single traumatic episode resulting in posterior subluxation or dislocation (Tannenbaum & Sekiya, 2011).

Mechanism of Injury

The mechanism of injury is usually a fall on an outstretched hand in a position of shoulder flexion, adduction, and internal rotation. Other mechanisms include seizures, car accidents, and electric shock. More common are subluxations, or excessive translation, often related to overhead activities such as throwing or tennis. Also, repetitive activities such as bench pressing or push-ups can stretch the posterior shoulder capsule.

Signs and Symptoms of Posterior Shoulder Instability

Overhead throwers; volleyball, football, and tennis players; swimmers; and weight lifters are among the athletes at highest risk for developing posterior shoulder instability. Athletes commonly report shoulder pain that intensifies in the later stages of their sporting events when dynamic stability decreases because of muscle fatigue. Clients with posterior shoulder instability primarily complain of aching pain and weakness along the posterior shoulder, biceps tendon, or superior aspect of the rotator cuff. Symptoms intensify with the arm in 90 degrees of forward flexion, adduction, and internal rotation (Tannenbaum & Sekiya, 2011).

Precautions

Contrary to anterior instability, CKC or weight-bearing activities must be minimized or modified to avoid excessive stretch to the posterior capsule. Activities such as push-ups, which drive the humeral head posteriorly, are often contraindicated. Any exercises that may force the humeral head posteriorly should be performed with posterior support or in the plane of the scapula to avoid excessive stretching of the capsule (Figure 19-19).

Figure 19-19
Supine serratus punch or chest press with a towel roll under the shoulder to avoid excessive posterior translation

Bench pressing is often contraindicated. However, clients who want to continue performing this exercise should use a wider grip and avoid full elbow extension. This will limit the amount of horizontal adduction and decrease stress on the posterior capsule.

Early Intervention

During the early stages of rehabilitation, the goals and treatment are similar to those used when working with a client with anterior instability. Again, the rotator cuff may be inflamed and care should be taken in restoring IR/ER strength. Conversely, positions of shoulder flexion, internal rotation, and horizontal adduction must be avoided or minimized. Typically, at least six months of therapy is common before consideration for surgical repair. In postoperative rehabilitation, for the first month, the shoulder is kept in relative external or neutral rotation to relax the posterior capsule. Between the first and second months post-surgery, the clinician can employ passive and active assisted ROM in a protected fashion while still limiting end ROMs.

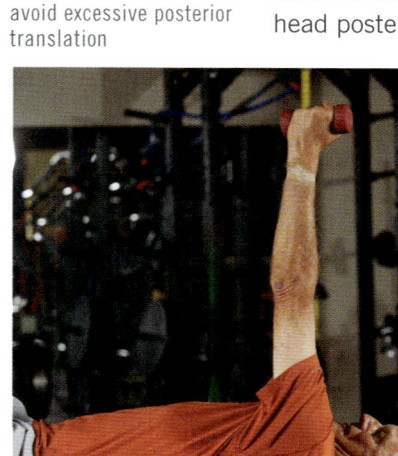

Restorative Exercise Program for Posterior Shoulder Instability

Restorative exercise for posterior shoulder instability aims to improve rotator cuff and scapular strength, endurance, and neuromuscular control. By increasing cuff and scapular strength, there is a return of important force couples that allow for dynamic stabilization of the shoulder. Because the rotator cuff muscles blend into the glenohumeral ligaments and joint capsule, increasing dynamic ligament tension during cuff activity through exercise training is beneficial to those with shoulder instability (Manske, Grant-Nierman, & Lucas, 2013).

Functional Training

For the CMES, the exercise protocol focuses on strengthening the rotator cuff and the scapular stabilizers through resisted external-rotation exercises. It is important to balance the strengthening program with internal-rotation exercises to reestablish synchronous scapulohumeral rhythm. Further, clients should modify their activity levels to avoid pain and prevent further injury.

Movement Training

When restoring efficient movement patterns and strength, the program is often biased to the posterior musculature to provide secondary restraints to the posterior stabilizers of the shoulder. Rowing with scapular retraction, external rotation, shoulder extension, and horizontal abduction are important exercises with posterior instability.

Shoulder Impingement Syndrome

The rotator cuff is a group of four muscles that surround the glenohumeral joint. The muscles function to rotate the shoulder and contribute to stability by forming a dynamic "sling" for the joint. They consist of the subscapularis (anteriorly), the supraspinatus (superiorly), and the infraspinatus and teres minor (posteriorly) (see Figure 19-8). Injuries of the rotator cuff are common and may be chronic conditions or the result of trauma.

Mechanism of Injury

Traumatic injuries are more common in the older population and are often related to a fall with an indirect force on an abducted arm. **Tendinitis** of the rotator cuff is very common and can be a result of repetitive overhead activities or incorrect body mechanics during weight training. Activities such as tennis, swimming, and throwing can eccentrically overload the rotator cuff and cause tendinitis. Carrying and lifting heavy bags in daily life is another common mechanism of injury. In addition, excessive shoulder laxity or instability can predispose a person to this pathology by making the rotator cuff work much harder.

A common diagnosis of the rotator cuff is referred to as **impingement syndrome.** This refers to the impingement of the soft tissues between the humeral head and the archway that is formed by the acromion and the coracoacromial ligament (Figure 19-20). Conditions that narrow this archway, such as soft-tissue swelling, bone spurs, or arthritic changes, can predispose an individual to impingement. For some individuals, the acromion is congenitally hooked or curved in shape—as opposed to flat—which may predispose the client to an impingement syndrome as the acromion rubs on the rotator cuff.

The most common structures affected are the supraspinatus, the infraspinatus, the long head of the biceps (and their associated tendons), and the subacromial **bursa.** A bursa is a sac of fluid that is present in areas of the body that are potential sites of friction. With overuse, a bursa can become swollen and inflamed, resulting in **bursitis.** As the tendons become inflamed, they may rub on the bone and become frayed and eventually lead to chronic rotator cuff tears, which can vary greatly in terms of size, thickness, and location. These tears may continue to get larger until surgical intervention is required. Surgical intervention is determined by several factors such as pain, loss of function, activity level, and the amount of repairable tissue available.

Figure 19-20
Anatomical structures associated with shoulder impingement syndrome
© Fotosearch
www.fotosearch.com

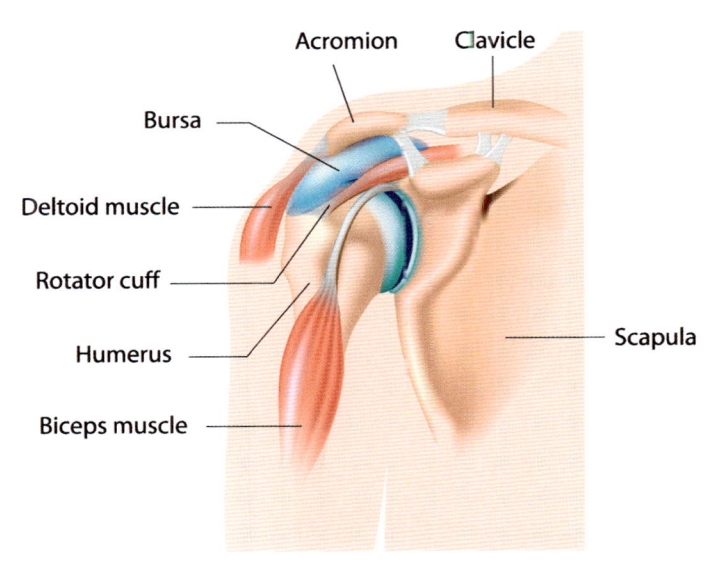

Signs and Symptoms of Shoulder Impingement Syndrome

The presentation of clients with shoulder impingement will vary greatly depending on the location and severity of the injury. The duration of the injury is also often a factor. A person with a torn or inflamed rotator cuff may present with pain or weakness with resistive external rotation. Supraspinatus pathology is often consistent with pain and/or weakness in resistive flexion with internal rotation in the plane of the scapula (i.e., the "empty can" position; see page 645) (Jobe & Jobe, 1983). In addition, passive full-forward flexion (Neer test) and passive forward flexion and internal rotation (Hawkins-Kennedy test) may elicit pain (Hawkins & Kennedy, 1980). Weakness is sometimes a function of the severity of the injury, but there is a great deal of variability. Individuals with massive tears of the rotator cuff may have difficulty initiating elevation of the arm or maintaining it in an abducted position, but this is not always the case. These clients may not be appropriate for training and need to be referred back to their therapist or physician. Finally, individuals with rotator cuff pathology may describe a "painful arc" of ROM. As they approach 90 degrees of elevation of the shoulder, they reach the impingement zone and complain of pain that then resolves as they move beyond that zone.

Precautions

Common causes of injury are overhead sports, military press, incline bench press, and lateral raises in the frontal plane. As always, the CMES should have the client avoid ranges that are painful.

Early Intervention

The primary emphasis of the treatment program is to reduce the mechanical irritation to the rotator cuff and promote a restoration in tendon vascularity that can result from muscle guarding, mechanical compression, and abnormal shoulder mechanics.

Restorative Exercise Program for Shoulder Impingement Syndrome

The initial stages of training individuals with rotator cuff injuries focus on reducing inflammation and promoting healing. This is a stage of "active rest" in which the exacerbating activities are eliminated or modified. Restoring flexibility is also an important goal of this phase (Escamilla, Hooks, & Wilk, 2014). Individuals with rotator cuff pathology often lose flexibility of the posterior structures of the shoulder. Loss of horizontal adduction is often an indication of a contracture of the posterior capsule, while loss of internal rotation is often an indication of a contracture of the posterior rotator cuff. Both of these situations can contribute to an increased chance of rotator cuff impingement. Flexibility exercises are initiated to restore ROM (Figures 19-21 and 19-22).

Figure 19-21 Posterior capsule stretch

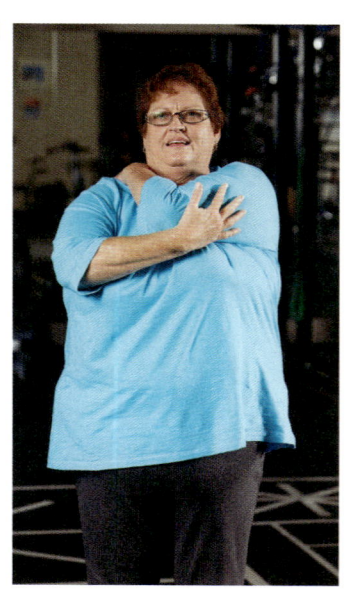

Figure 19-22 Medial rotation stretch using a towel or strap

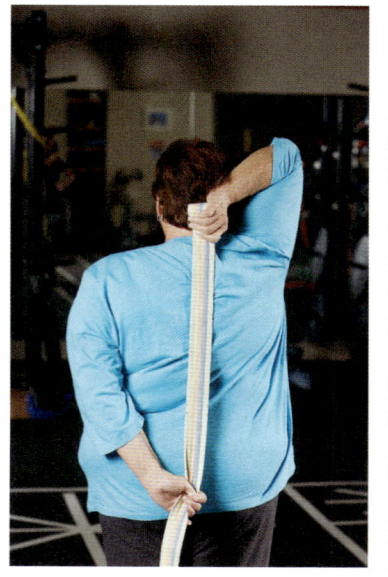

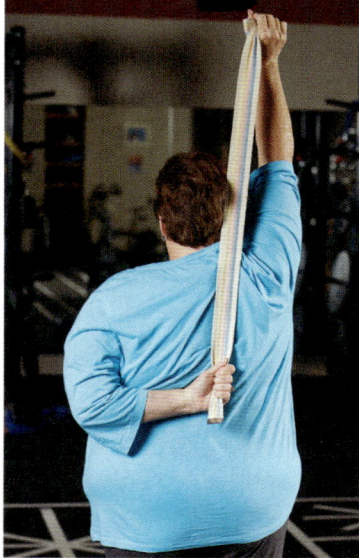

Musculoskeletal Injuries of the Upper Extremity CHAPTER 19

Functional Training

As in the case of shoulder instability, strengthening should be initiated with the scapula, especially in the case of a significantly inflamed rotator cuff. Any deviation in scapular function can have a negative effect on the shoulder. For example, if the scapula is elevated too high, the mechanical advantage of the rotator cuff is altered. By restoring normal scapular function, the proper length-tension relationship of the rotator cuff is restored. In addition, many of the scapular muscle-strengthening exercises [(e.g., rowing, shrugs, serratus punches, and push-ups with a plus (i.e., push-ups with exaggerated scapular protraction performed at the top position)] indirectly strengthen the rotator cuff. Hence, the scapular retractors, protractors, and depressors are commonly emphasized with isolation strengthening exercises because of weakness associated with these muscle groups commonly noted in patients with shoulder impingement syndrome (Escamilla, Hooks, & Wilk, 2014). In addition, stabilization and strengthening exercises for the abdomen and lower-back region can be initiated. Athletes can be encouraged to perform lower-extremity strengthening and conditioning activities specific for their sport.

As inflammation decreases, IR/ER exercises may be cautiously introduced. As mentioned previously, the CMES should carefully monitor symptoms to avoid an inhibition of the rotator cuff. It should be noted that not everyone can tolerate these exercises. Strengthening can be introduced as submaximal isometrics. Clients can then progress to using elastic resistance. When performing external rotation exercises, the client can position a towel roll at their side, which places the shoulder in a slightly abducted position (Figure 19-23). This will improve the blood supply to the shoulder and enhance the mechanical advantage of the external rotators.

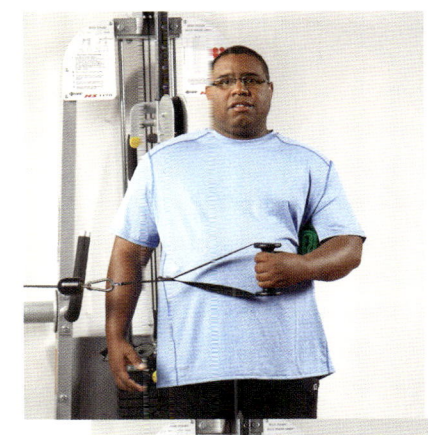

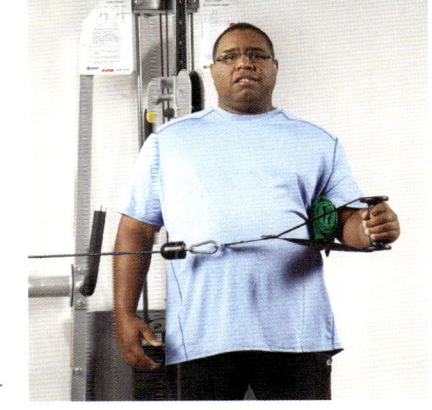

Figure 19-23
External rotation

Movement Training

During Movement Training, the focus shifts to performing the five primary movement patterns more efficiently in all three planes of motion. For those who want to continue deltoid strengthening, shoulder flexion in the scapular plane is preferred to performing lateral raises in the frontal plane (Figure 19-24). The exercise in the scapular plane affords the least amount of stress on the shoulder. It is also a more functional plane in which to work. Finally, this exercise also recruits much of the scapula musculature, and to some extent the supraspinatus (Moseley, Jobe, & Pink, 1994). The "empty can" position described by Jobe and Jobe (1983) for strengthening the supraspinatus is not advised, as the internally rotated position significantly increases the chance of shoulder impingement and is a common source of shoulder pain (Figure 19-25) (Escamilla, Hooks, & Wilk, 2014).

When designing a strength-training program, the CMES should consider that many athletic or functional demands require a significant amount of **eccentric** muscle activity. Therefore, the eccentric

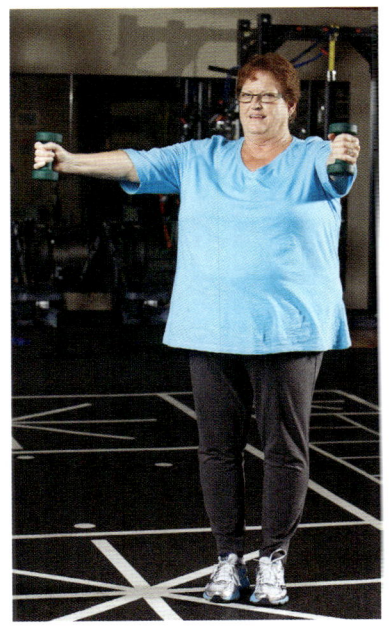

Figure 19-24
Shoulder flexion in the scapular plane

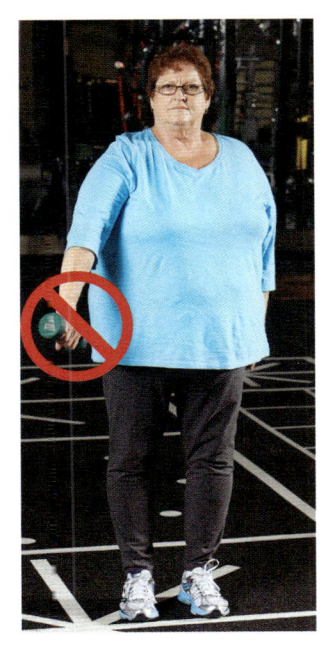

Figure 19-25
The "empty can" position increases the chance of shoulder impingement and is a common source of shoulder pain

Figure 19-26
D2 flexion pattern

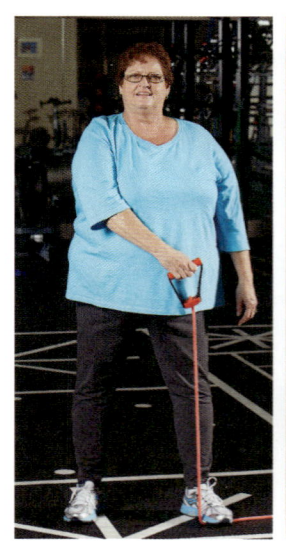

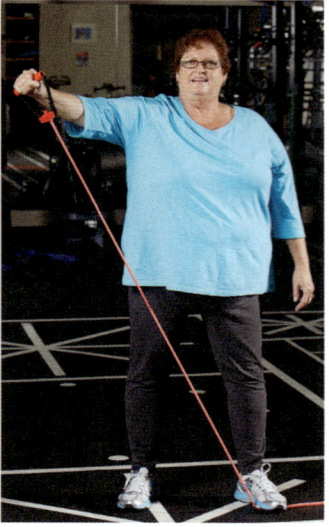

or negative phase of each exercise should also be emphasized. However, the CMES should closely monitor these exercises, as they are often a cause of **delayed-onset muscle soreness (DOMS).** Many clients with rotator cuff injuries will want to return to overhead activities such as tennis, swimming, or throwing. In such cases, multijoint activities such as **proprioceptive neuromuscular facilitation (PNF)** patterns are useful to reproduce these demands. In particular, the D2 flexion pattern, which consists of shoulder flexion, abduction, and external rotation, reproduces the neuromuscular demands of many overhead activities (Figure 19-26).

When a client is returning to performing a bench press, a narrower hand spacing should be utilized to minimize the peak shoulder torque in the pressing motion and reduce the rotator cuff and biceps tendon requirements to stabilize the humeral head (Fees et al., 1998).

ELBOW PATHOLOGIES

The activities required during overhead sports produce large forces at the elbow joint. Injuries to the elbow joint frequently occur in the overhead athlete because of the large amount of forces observed during the act of throwing, playing tennis, or playing golf. In nonathletic populations, elbow pathologies are common among working-aged adults who are exposed to repetitive bending/straightening of the elbow for more than one hour per day, such as construction workers and auto-assembly workers (Walker-Bone et al., 2012). Injuries may result because of repetitive overuse, leading to tissue failure. The elbow is a hinge joint allowing flexion and extension. The proximal radioulnar joint permits rotation, which involves both **pronation** and supination. The elbow also allows frontal plane motion when valgus and varus stresses are applied to it, such as those experienced in throwing and racquet sports.

Lateral Epicondylitis

Lateral epicondylitis is often referred to as "tennis elbow." It results from the repetitive tension overloading of the wrist and finger extensors that originate at the lateral epicondyle. Although originally described as an inflammatory process, the current consensus is that lateral epicondylitis is initiated as a microscopic tear of the extensor carpi radialis brevis tendon (Figure 19-27) (Inagaki, 2013).

Figure 19-27
Lateral epicondylitis, or "tennis elbow"

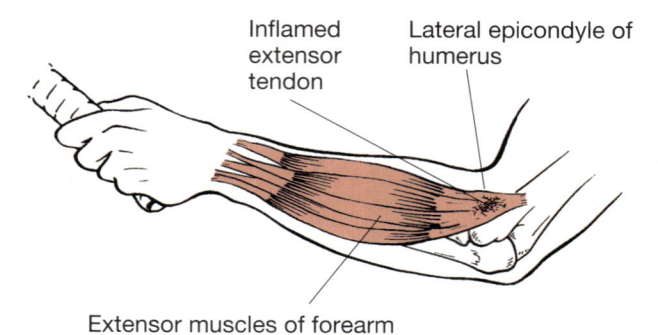

Mechanism of Injury

Traditionally, the mechanism of injury takes place during the backhand of a novice tennis player who has poor mechanics. For example, not getting the racquet back fast enough and hitting the ball in front of the body or having a poor weight shift can result in greater stresses on the lateral aspect of the elbow. A change in the frequency of activity or a poorly fitted racquet can also contribute to injury. Tennis players who have a deficit in their proximal strength, such as in the scapula muscles or the rotator cuff, may be more susceptible to developing lateral epicondylitis. A lack of proximal stability may manifest itself further down the chain at the elbow. In addition, poor mechanics reduces the use of the lower body and core in the tennis stroke. This can result in increased stress on the elbow.

"Tennis elbow" is often a misnomer, as this injury it is not always a result of tennis. Carrying heavy bags or performing manual labor, especially with the elbow in extension, can result in lateral epicondylitis. In addition, excessive computer work can lead to increased stress to the extensor tendons. Ergonomic adjustments are often a key aspect of treatment.

Signs and Symptoms of Lateral Epicondylitis

Regardless of the mechanism of injury, the overload can result in inflammation and pain at the lateral epicondyle. In later stages, a mass may form in the tendon and even result in a tear. This injury is often very resistant to treatment, as it is not often detected until latter stages of the pathology. At those stages, clients will complain about activities such as shaking hands, holding a coffee cup, or carrying something with the elbow in extension. Pain is elicited with resistive wrist extension and forearm supination, especially with the elbow in extension and passive wrist flexion (Figure 19-28).

Figure 19-28
Resistive wrist extension

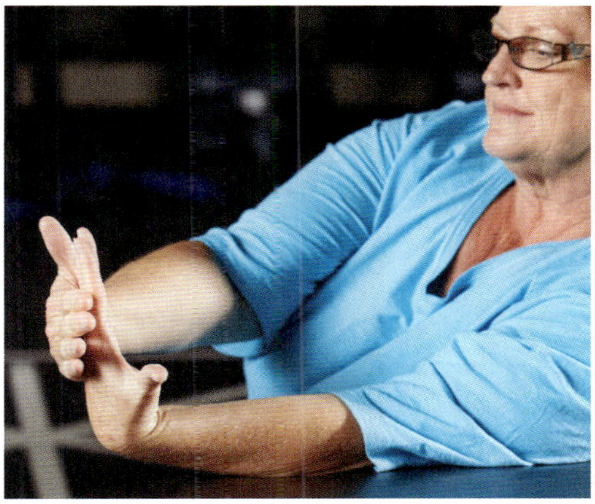

Precautions

Any causative activity that provokes pain or the injury mechanism must be eliminated or modified. For example, a client may be encouraged to avoid tennis or make ergonomic adjustments. In the gym, lifting weights is avoided or modified, depending on the severity of symptoms. Lifting weights with the elbow extended is certainly to be avoided. A wrist splint may be used to rest the extensor mechanism. In addition, a counterforce brace may be used around the elbow to dissipate forces away from the injured site and reduce pain.

Early Intervention

The goals of the initial stage of treatment are to reduce the symptoms and promote healing. Various modalities are utilized to reduce symptoms and a period of active rest is encouraged.

Restorative Exercise Program for Lateral Epicondylitis

As symptoms begin to subside, the client can work toward restoring normal flexibility. Loss of passive wrist flexion is a common finding, and can be restored with passive wrist flexion with the elbow in extension (Figure 19-29). As always, stretching should be performed slowly and gradually, and be maintained in a pain-free range. Slow, progressive stretching allows the muscle to relax instead of reflexively guarding the area. These types of stretches have a longer-lasting effect.

Figure 19-29
Passive wrist flexion

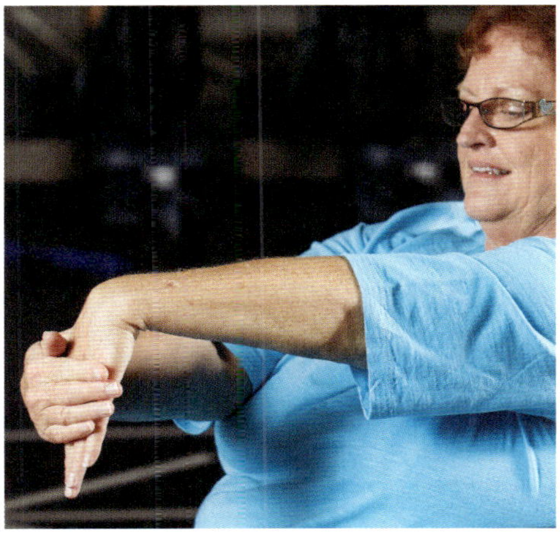

Functional Training

When initiating a training program, the CMES should assess the shoulder and scapula for any underlying functional deficits. With tennis elbow, proximal strength deficits, especially in the shoulder rotators, are often found. Figure 19-30 illustrates proximal exercise options for clients who have elbow pathologies, for whom distal isolation exercises might prove painful. A low-resistance, high-repetition exercise format (e.g., three sets of 15 to 20 repetitions) can be followed to improve strength and local muscular endurance. Consider using cuff weights above the elbow to allow rotator cuff and scapular exercises to be performed while minimizing overload at the elbow and forearm (Ellenbecker, Nirschl, & Renstrom, 2013). Initially, attempting to isolate the wrist extensors can exacerbate the symptoms. The client should be relatively asymptomatic in normal ADL prior to performing wrist-extension exercises. Tolerance to a firm handshake has been described as a prerequisite to these exercises. When initiating wrist-extension strengthening, the elbow should be supported and be in flexion to reduce the stress (Figure 19-31).

Figure 19-30
Proximal exercises used to strengthen periscapular muscles in elbow tendon injury

a. Side-lying external rotation

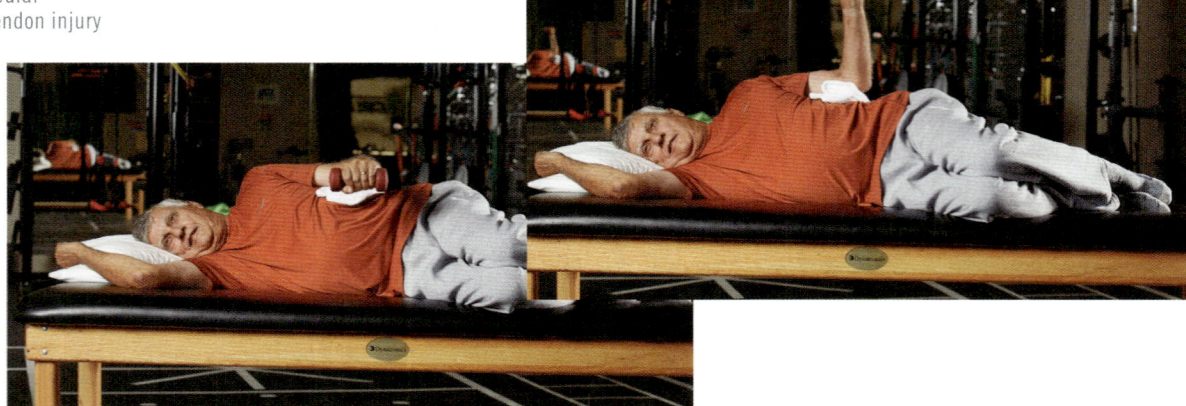

b. Prone extension with external humeral rotation (thumb-out position)

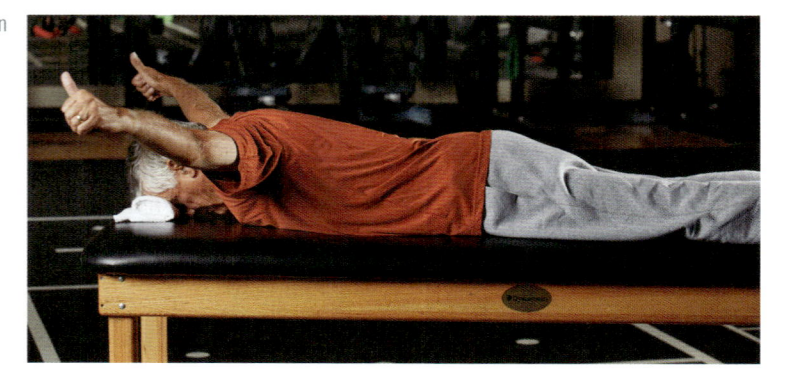

c. Prone horizontal abduction with external humeral rotation (thumb-out position)

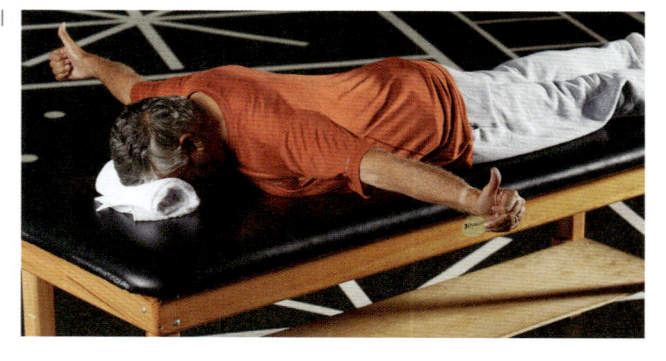

d. Prone external rotation with scapular retraction

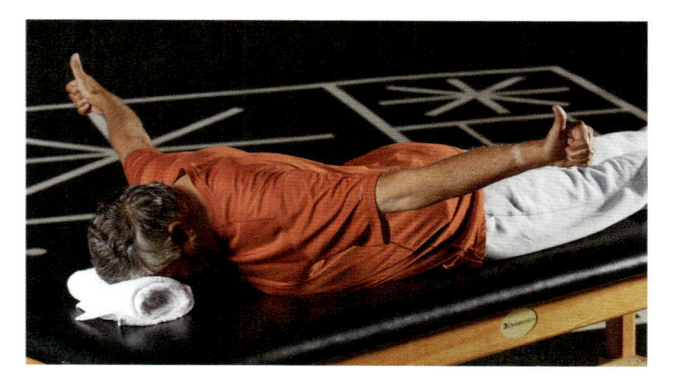

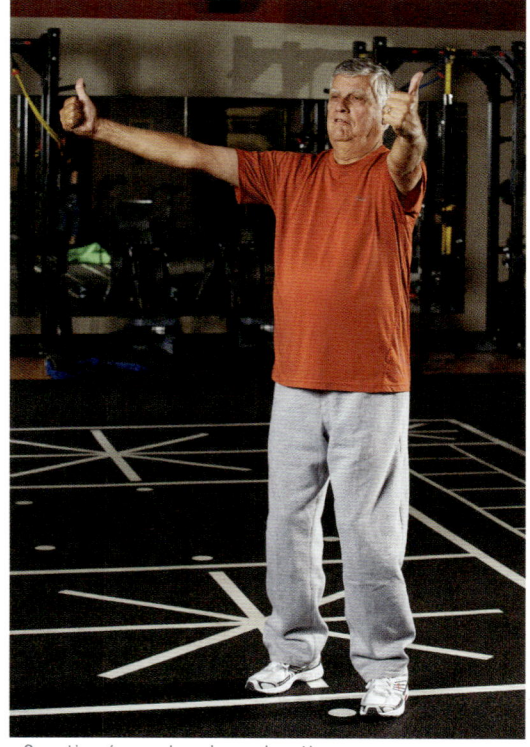

e. Scaption (scapular plane elevation with thumb-up position)

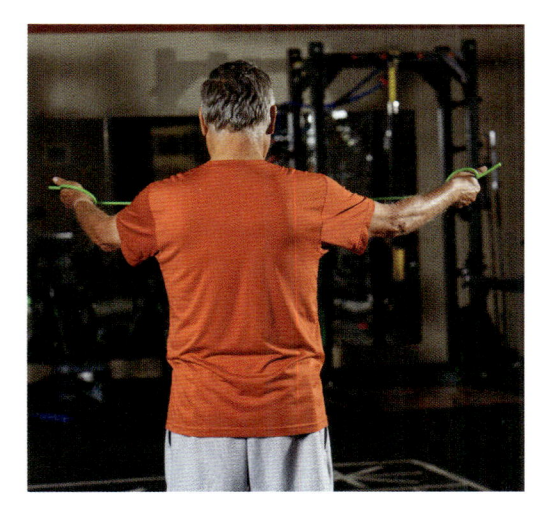

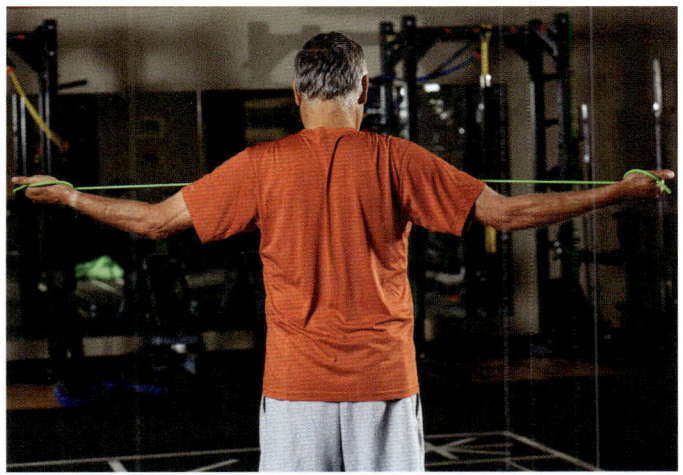

Musculoskeletal Injuries of the Upper Extremity

CHAPTER 19

f. External rotation with scapular retraction (standing with elastic resistance)

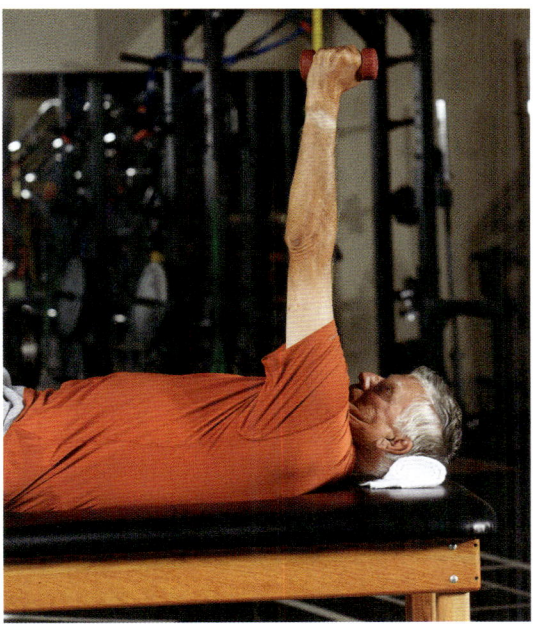

g. Supine serratus punch

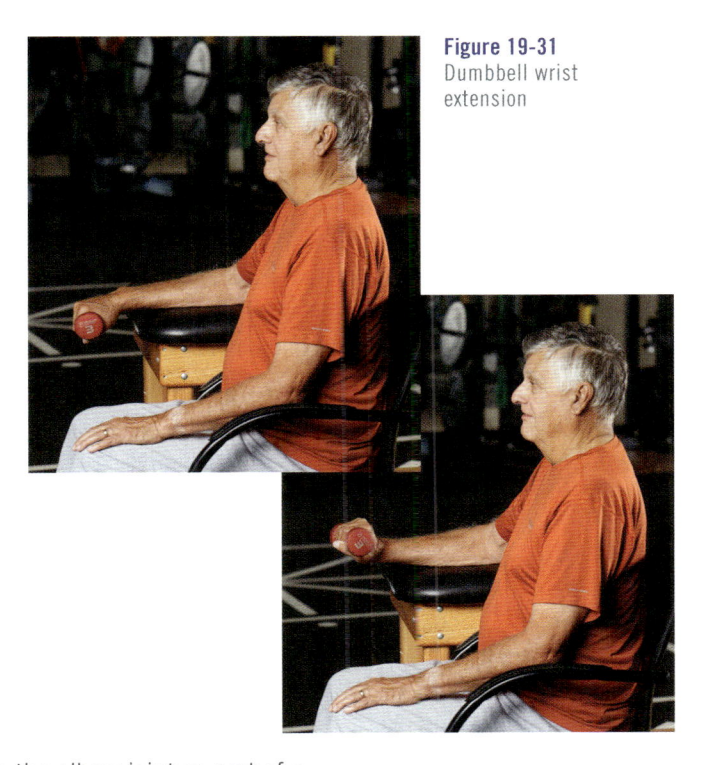

Figure 19-31
Dumbbell wrist extension

Movement Training

One approach to strengthening the musculature that supports the elbow joint as part of a Movement Training program is to use multijoint exercises such as rowing, shrugs, latissimus pulldowns, and PNF patterns. These exercises allow some strengthening of the wrist and forearm without trying to isolate them. They also provide a more global approach to strengthening the entire upper extremity and establishing proximal strength. These exercises should be performed while avoiding the end-ranges of elbow extension. When a client is performing any activity, increasing the grip size of resistive equipment or a tennis racquet can reduce the amount of wrist-extensor activity and the amount of stress on the lateral epicondyle.

As symptoms subside, the wrist extensors and forearm supinators can gradually be exercised in greater degrees of elbow extension. Movement patterns such as a tennis stroke or a golf swing can be reproduced using elastic resistance. Novice tennis players are encouraged to take lessons to improve mechanics. As weight training is progressed, the CMES should continue to closely monitor the client for any recurrence of lateral elbow pain. Finally, when performing cardiovascular activities, the client should avoid gripping the apparatus too tightly with the affected hand.

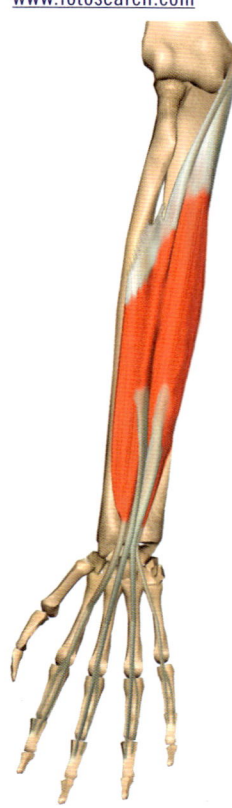

Figure 19-32
Flexor digitorum superficialis

www.fotosearch.com

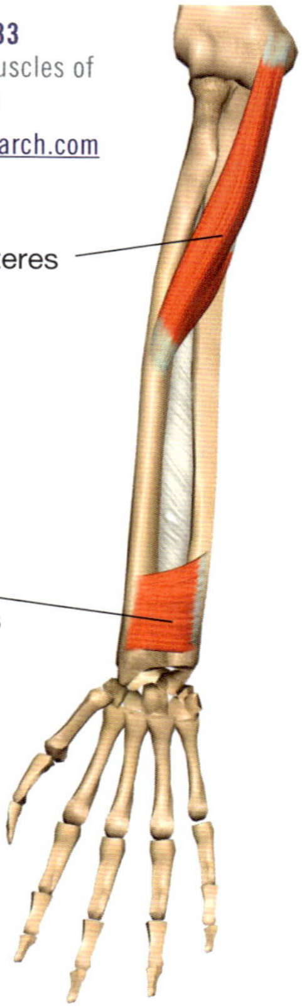

Figure 19-33
Pronator muscles of the forearm

www.fotosearch.com

Pronator teres

Pronator quadratus

Medial Epicondylitis

Medial epicondylitis is a disorder similar to lateral epicondylitis affecting the medial elbow in the region of the flexor digitorum superficialis (Figure 19-32). The injury is a result of tendinous microtearing owing to muscle-tendon overload. Following the overload, tendon degeneration occurs instead of repair (Rineer & Ruch, 2009). Medial epicondylitis presents as pain at the medial epicondyle, aggravated by activities that resist the flexor muscles of the wrist. Medial epicondylitis can cause pain and weakness throughout the upper extremity and can result in impairment or disability.

Mechanism of Injury

Medial epicondylitis occurs due to an overload of the wrist flexors and forearm pronators. Golf, throwing, and swimming are common mechanisms of injury. Overuse or poor mechanics may lead to tendinitis or small tears of these muscles near the origin at the medial epicondyle. "Golfer's elbow" refers to an injury to the medial side of the right elbow (for a right-handed golfer). Novice golfers who fail to use their larger body parts and do not weight shift correctly are more susceptible. Beginners tend to throw the club down at the ball or hit too far behind the ball and put greater stress on the medial aspect of the elbow. Participating in throwing sports also tends to place a great deal of stress on the medial aspect of the elbow. In throwing, the medial aspect of the elbow undergoes tremendous tension (distraction) forces, while the lateral aspect is forcefully compressed. Further, the posterior compartment is subject to tensile, compressive, and torsional forces during both the acceleration and deceleration phases of throwing, which may result in valgus extension overload within the posterior compartment. These forces may cause a variety of specific elbow injuries in this athletic population (Wilk et al., 2012). The CMES must be aware that injuries to the ulnar nerve are often associated with this area. Any numbness or tingling along the ulnar aspect of the forearm or the fourth and fifth fingers should alert the CMES to this possibility.

Signs and Symptoms of Medial Epicondylitis

Clients will present with tenderness over the medial epicondyle or the proximal wrist flexors and pronator teres (Figure 19-33). Resistive wrist flexion or forearm pronation may elicit symptoms. In addition, performing high-load biceps curls often exacerbates symptoms.

Precautions

Exercises such as biceps curls may be better tolerated in a neutral forearm position than in a supinated position. Full elbow extension should be avoided when performing resistive exercises. Note that repetitive activity at the computer can result in medial epicondylitis. The **etiology** of this injury is rapid, repetitive finger flexion with a fixed wrist as the individual clicks and drags the mouse. Hence, educating clients on the importance of frequent breaks from computer use and maintaining proper shoulder and wrist alignment while at work can be helpful.

Early Intervention

Treatment of medial epicondylitis includes anti-inflammatory drugs, massages, elbow braces, steroid injections, and in severe cases, surgery (Lee & Lee-Robinson, 2010). The goals of the early stages of rehabilitation are to reduce symptoms and promote healing. This includes reestablishing nonpainful ROM, decreasing pain and inflammation, and retarding muscular atrophy (Wilk et al., 2012). During these stages, causative activities are modified or eliminated, golfers are encouraged to take lessons, throwing mechanics are reviewed, and swimming strokes are assessed. Proximal shoulder and scapular strength are assessed for any underlying deficits.

Restorative Exercise Program for Medial Epicondylitis

The restorative exercise program should focus on progressively restoring strength and neuromuscular control while gradually incorporating client-specific activities to successfully return them to the previous level of function as safely as possible. For athletes, the program focus should include the entire kinetic chain (i.e., scapula, shoulder, hand, core/hips, and legs) to ensure the athlete's return to high-level sports participation (Wilk et al., 2012).

Functional Training

Initially, the focus is on the rotator-cuff and scapular musculature (see Figure 19-8). A low-resistance, high-repetition exercise format (e.g., three sets of 15 to 20 repetitions) can be used. Again, using cuff weights above the elbow minimizes overload at the elbow and forearm (Ellenbecker, Nirschl, & Renstrom, 2013). Gradual introduction of elbow flexion and extension, wrist flexion and extension, and forearm pronation and supination can be added as long as the ROM is pain-free.

Flexibility can be initiated by stretching into wrist extension and forearm supination (Figure 19-34). Once again, the range should be basically pain-free. When initiating these exercises, they should be done with the elbow supported and in flexion. The CMES should proceed cautiously with isolated pronation exercises, as they can often be a source of pain or injury, in addition to an overall program to improve flexibility, muscular conditioning, and movement efficiency.

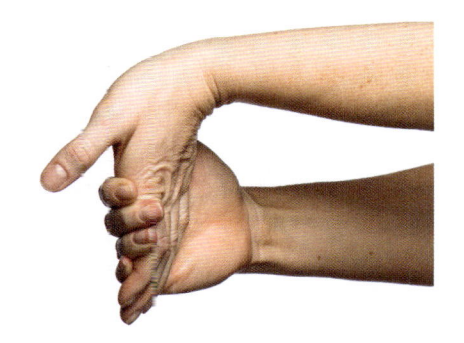

Figure 19-34
Passive wrist extension

Movement Training

Strengthening can be continued with multijoint, functional exercises, as opposed to isolating the wrist flexors and forearm pronators (see Figures 19-9 through 19-12). Prior to a return to activity, functional exercises such as PNF patterns may be helpful.

> **THINK IT THROUGH**
>
> Elbow injuries are often associated with abnormal mechanics of the scapulothoracic and glenohumeral joints. Thus, restorative exercise often focuses on these more proximal joints when addressing elbow pathologies. Think about how you would explain the relationship between scapula and shoulder movement and elbow function to a client who is learning these concepts for the first time.

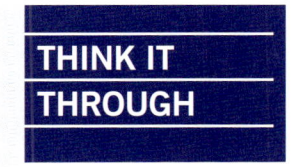

WRIST AND HAND PATHOLOGIES

There are numerous types of pathologies of the wrist and hand. Two of the most common injuries are **carpal tunnel syndrome (CTS)** and **de Quervain's tenosynovitis.** These conditions are overuse pathologies, as trauma accumulates over a period of time and produces stress at a greater rate than the soft tissues can accommodate.

Carpal Tunnel Syndrome

CTS is the most common form of work-related peripheral neuropathy among workers who perform hand-intensive tasks. In addition to grip force and hand repetition, sustained or repeated extension or flexion may lead to an increased risk of CTS among workers (You, Smith, & Rempel, 2014). This disorder impacts the quality of workers' lives and may lead to job change. In addition, CTS is associated with certain systemic conditions, such as rheumatoid arthritis, hypothyroidism, diabetes mellitus, gout, and pregnancy.

Mechanism of Injury

The carpal tunnel is formed by ligaments and bones at the base of the hand. CTS occurs when the median nerve, which extends from the forearm into the hand, becomes compressed at the wrist. Thickened tendons or other swelling can cause the nerve to become impinged or compressed (Figure 19-35). Forceful, hand-intensive work can lead to elevated pressures within the carpal tunnel and persistent tissue edema and painful nerve compression. Some people are congenitally predisposed to this condition. However, common causes are wrist trauma, arthritis, work stress, and fluid retention.

Figure 19-35

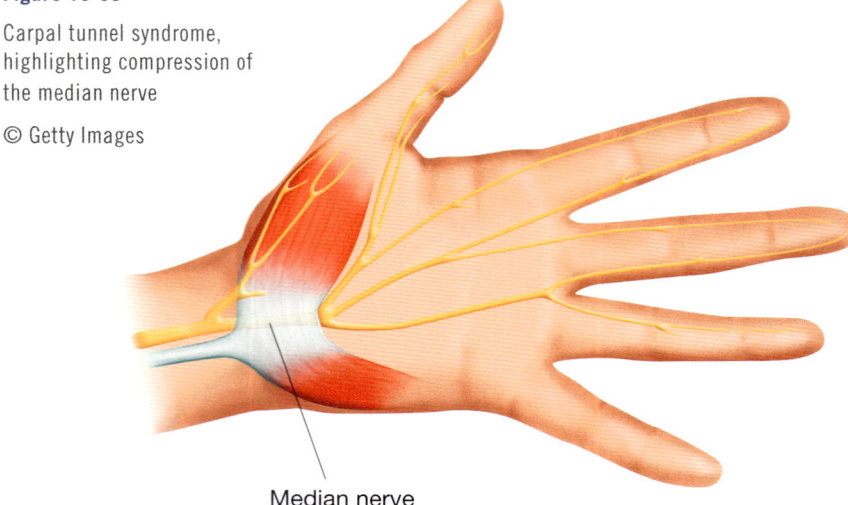

Carpal tunnel syndrome, highlighting compression of the median nerve

© Getty Images

Median nerve

Signs and Symptoms of Carpal Tunnel Syndrome

Classic symptoms include numbness, tingling, burning, or pain in at least two of the three digits supplied by the median nerve (i.e., the thumb and the index and middle fingers). Provocative factors include sustained arm or hand positions and repetitive actions of the hand or wrist. Relieving factors include changes in hand posture and shaking the hand (Ashworth, 2010). As the condition worsens, grip strength may be affected. When a client presents with any of these symptoms, the CMES should refer them to a hand specialist.

Precautions

Some general precautions and adjustments for the injured hand and wrist are as follows:
- Any point tenderness at one of the small bones of the wrist or hand may indicate a fracture. If these symptoms persist, a referral to a hand specialist is advised.
- A change in positioning is often helpful for individuals with hand or wrist pain. When exercising, the wrist is often most comfortable in a neutral position. A good guideline is to avoid wrist flexion and extension greater than 30 degrees. In addition, avoid radial or ulnar deviation. Pain on the ulnar side of the wrist is often exacerbated by forearm pronation or supination.
- The grip size of exercise equipment can be adjusted. The CMES may add padding to a piece of exercise equipment to create a larger grip. Often, a larger grip will reduce stress on the wrist, hand, or fingers.

Early Intervention

Both conservative and surgical treatments are used to manage CTS. The non-surgical treatment options include splinting, steroids, activity modification, **nonsteroidal anti-inflammatory drugs (NSAIDs), diuretics,** vitamin B-6, and others. However, of the conservative approaches, only splinting and steroids are supported by high-quality evidence (Shi & MacDermid, 2011). If conservative treatment does not resolve the problem, surgical intervention that releases the transverse carpal ligament may be necessary (Houglum, 2010).

Restorative Exercise Program for Carpal Tunnel Syndrome

Restoring ROM and avoidance of aggravating activities are the primary foci of a restorative exercise program for CTS. Some clinical practitioners employ nerve and tendon gliding exercises in their rehabilitation treatment. However, these assisted stretches typically involve some degree of stretching of the median nerve, which could exacerbate symptoms of CTS (Ashworth, 2010). Thus, it is always prudent to follow the guidelines and limitations provided by the client's healthcare provider before working with a client who is recovering from CTS and not to attempt therapy-based practices unless otherwise specifically credentialed to do so.

Functional Training

Initial resistive exercises for all wrist, finger, and thumb movements (i.e., starting with isometrics, and advancing to isotonics, eccentric exercises, and then **concentric** exercises) are appropriate only after inflammation is under control (Houglum, 2010). Figure 19-36 demonstrates exercises that can be used for these purposes.

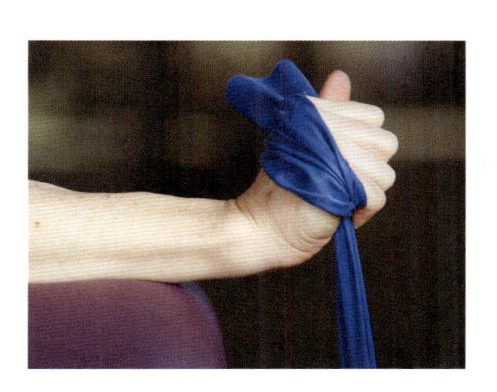

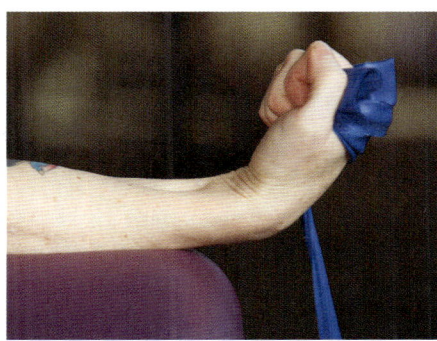

Musculoskeletal Injuries of the Upper Extremity CHAPTER 19

Figure 19-36
a. Wrist extension/flexion

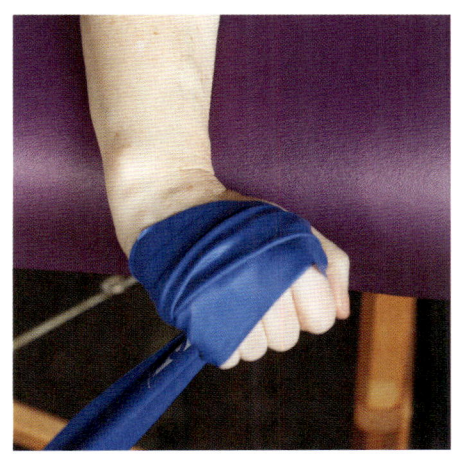

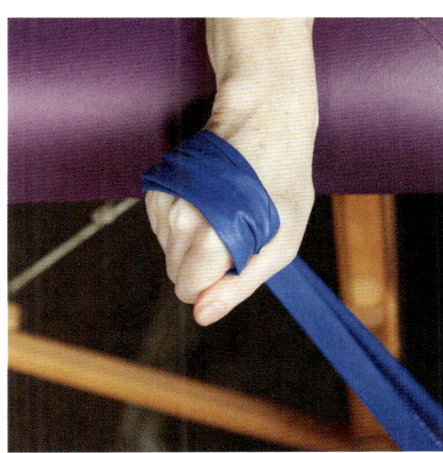

b. Radial/ulnar deviation

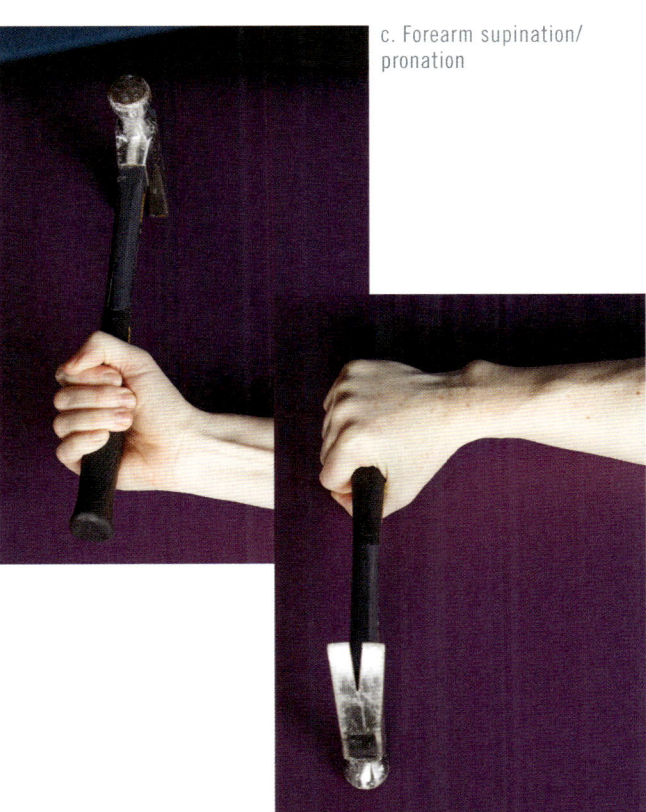

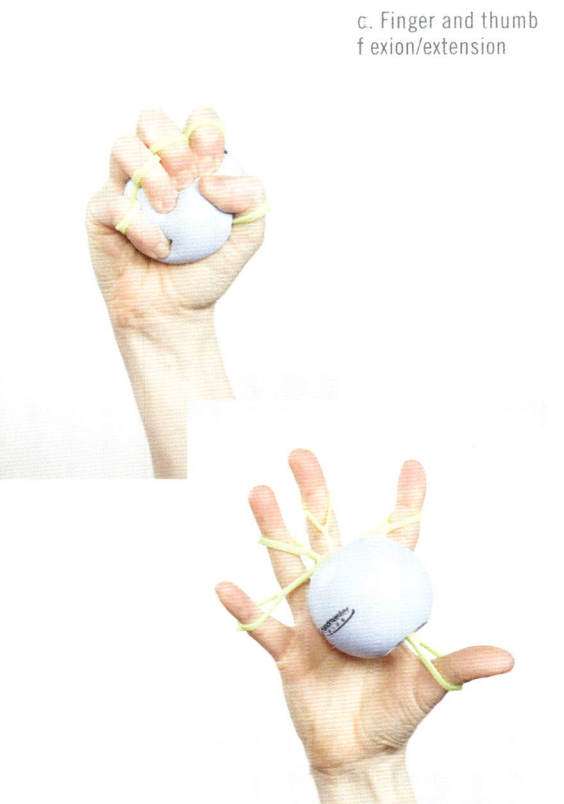

c. Forearm supination/pronation

c. Finger and thumb flexion/extension

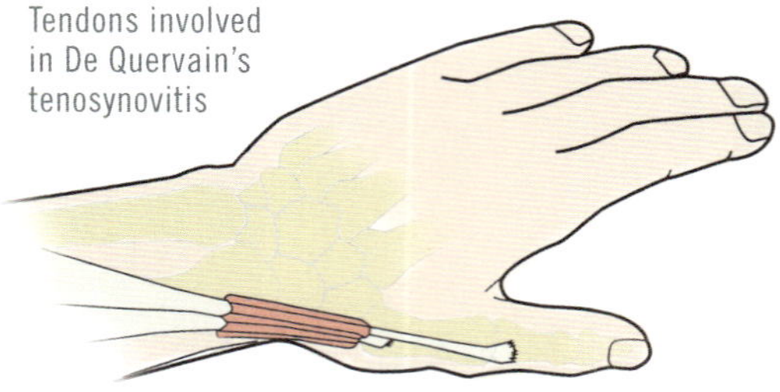

Figure 19-37
Tendons involved in De Quervain's tenosynovitis

Figure 19-38
Dorsal view of the wrist and hand

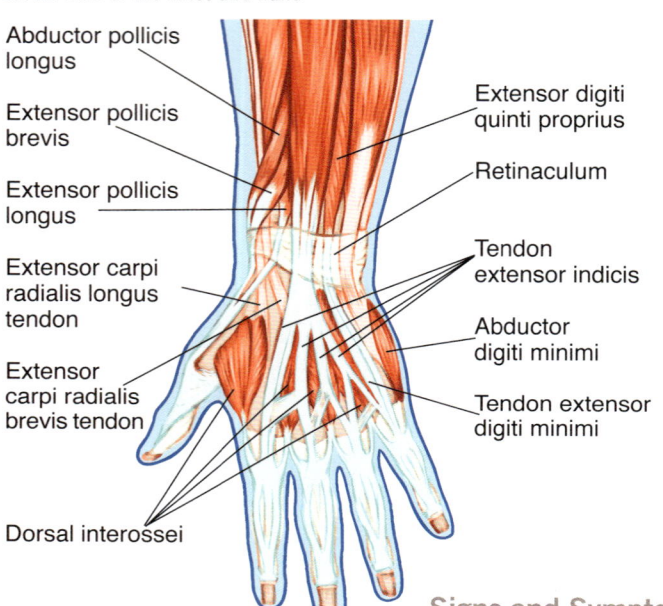

- Abductor pollicis longus
- Extensor pollicis brevis
- Extensor pollicis longus
- Extensor carpi radialis longus tendon
- Extensor carpi radialis brevis tendon
- Dorsal interossei
- Extensor digiti quinti proprius
- Retinaculum
- Tendon extensor indicis
- Abductor digiti minimi
- Tendon extensor digiti minimi

Figure 19-39
Finkelstein's test

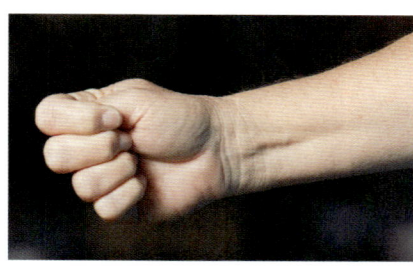

Movement Training

Once initial stability and mobility are restored, pain-free functional exercises using the hands for gripping objects can be introduced. These exercises could include anything from traditional resistance training to daily or occupational activities required by the client.

De Quervain's Tenosynovitis

De Quervain's tenosynovitis is a common pathological condition that affects the two tendons that move the thumb away from the hand (Figure 19-37). In the literature, this condition has various synonyms, including first dorsal compartment tenosynovitis, texting tenosynovitis, Blackberry Thumb, and Washer Woman's Sprain (Ali et al., 2014). More commonly found in perimenopausal and pregnant women, de Quervain's tenosynovitis has been linked to overuse, although no clear evidence has supported this notion (Patel, Tadisina, & Gonzalez, 2013). It is a mechanical disorder related to **hypertrophy** of the retinaculum that covers the first dorsal compartment of the wrist.

Mechanism of Injury

De Quervain's tenosynovitis is thought to be caused by overuse or an increase in repetitive activity, resulting in shear microtrauma from repetitive gliding of the first dorsal compartment tendons (abductor pollicis longus and extensor pollicis brevis) beneath the sheath of the first compartment over the styloid of the radius (Figure 19-38). This eventually leads to thickening of the extensor retinaculum of the wrist (and not related to inflammation, as was once thought) (Howell, 2012).

Predisposing movements include forceful grasping with ulnar deviation or repetitive use of the thumb, which includes many athletic pursuits, such as golf, fly-fishing, and racquet sports. De Quervain's tenosynovitis has also been shown to typically present in the fifth and sixth decades of life, as well as being more common in pregnant and lactating women (Howell, 2012).

Signs and Symptoms of De Quervain's Tenosynovitis

Symptoms may include pain and/or swelling over the thumb side of the wrist. Gripping may also become difficult. When testing for this syndrome, the thumb is tightened as in a closed fist and the hand is tilted toward the ulna side (Finkelstein's test) (Figure 19-39). If the condition is present, this position will produce pain at the wrist below the thumb. Any of these symptoms that last for one to two weeks should be addressed by the client's healthcare provider.

Precautions

See general precautions for the wrist and hand on page 652.

Early Intervention

Conservative treatment for De Quervain's tenosynovitis includes corticosteroids, NSAIDs, and splinting. There is limited evidence showing any benefits to NSAIDs or splinting except in those patients with only minimal symptoms (Ilyas, 2009). Surgical decompression is reserved for patients who have failed conservative treatment.

Restorative Exercise Program for De Quervain's Tenosynovitis

Similar to CTS, restoring ROM and avoidance of aggravating activities are the primary foci of a restorative exercise program for de Quervain's tenosynovitis.

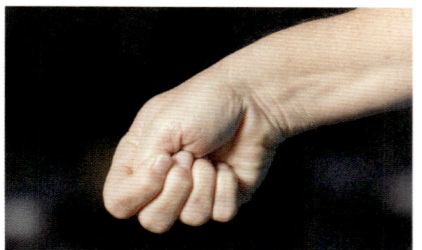

Functional Training

After inflammation is controlled, the same initial resistive exercises for all wrist, finger, and thumb movements are appropriate for de Quervain's tenosynovitis as for CTS (see Figure 19-36) (Papa, 2012).

Movement Training

Once initial stability and mobility are restored, pain-free functional exercises using the hands for gripping objects can be introduced. These exercises could include anything from traditional resistance training to daily or occupational activities required by the client.

CASE STUDIES

Case Study 1

Client Information

John is a 49-year-old recreational tennis player who has been unable to play for approximately six months after developing lateral elbow pain. Upon seeing an orthopedist, he was diagnosed with lateral epicondylitis. He was treated with NSAIDs and physical-therapy sessions for three months. Since his release from physical therapy, he has been following a home-based exercise program given to him by his physical therapist. He has consistently performed these exercises and is relatively asymptomatic. His occupation requires him to perform a great deal of computer work and travel often. He comes to work with a CMES to get himself back into "tennis shape," as this is his preferred exercise activity.

CMES Approach

The CMES should contact John's physical therapist to discuss his home-exercise program and any ergonomic precautions he was given. The CMES should incorporate the exercises into a comprehensive general program that addresses the entire kinetic chain. Shoulder and scapular strength and flexibility should be emphasized, using functional, multijoint exercises. John's lateral elbow symptoms should be monitored regularly to identify any exacerbating exercises. This is especially important if John is performing wrist-extension exercises. When designing John's exercise program, the CMES should avoid resistance training in the end ranges of elbow extension. John should also avoid carrying weights around the gym whenever possible. When performing conditioning exercises such as cycling or treadmill walking, John should avoid excessive gripping on the handles or handrails.

Prior to returning to tennis, John should be encouraged to begin hitting with a tennis professional or taking some lessons. This will reinforce the need for him to use his entire body when hitting and develop a good weight shift to reduce the forces at the elbow. He should also be advised to have his tennis pro check his racquet for the proper tension and grip size to help limit any chances of exacerbating the injury. In addition, John should be advised to use roller bags and avoid carrying heavy bags when traveling.

ACE IFT® MODEL AT A GLANCE

Cardiorespiratory Training

This case study does not provide a specific cardiorespiratory program for the client, as it is focused on helping him to build on the work done during physical therapy with a goal of playing recreational tennis again. As a recreational tennis player, it is likely that he would be able to perform 20 or more minutes of moderate-intensity cardiorespiratory exercise. This would allow the CMES to start John either directly in a Fitness Training program, or to start him in Base Training and then progress him once it is determined that an adequate training volume can be achieved.

Muscular Training

The initial movement-based workout that the CMES designs for John builds off the work that he completed in his physical-therapy sessions and the home-based program he has performed since his release from physical therapy. The primary aims of the initial program are on developing strength and flexibility in the shoulder and scapula, making his first program based on Functional Training. As he progresses, John will begin training movement patterns across the whole kinetic chain, and then will work with a coach to improve his sport-specific movements. This progression to Movement Training and eventually Load/Speed Training is based on sport-specific goals.

ACE IFT® MODEL AT A GLANCE

Cardiorespiratory Training

This case study does not provide a specific cardiorespiratory program for the client, as it is focused on helping him to transition from physical therapy to a medical exercise program. As a recreational skier, Steve would benefit from having good cardiorespiratory fitness that would allow him to ski repeated runs with limited fatigue. This could be developed through a program focused on enhancing aerobic efficiency through Fitness Training. Whether Steve could start in Fitness Training or would have to start in Base Training and progress accordingly, would need to be evaluated through appropriate client interview questions.

Muscular Training

Steve's initial program is focused on Functional Training to build on the work he has performed in physical therapy to further develop stability of the AC and scapulothoracic joints, while maintaining and possibly improving ROM. Progression to Movement training occurs as scapular and AC joint stability improve without exacerbating the injury, with early resistance introduced only in the middle of the ROM to help prevent exacerbation of the injury.

Case Study 2

Client Information

Steve is a 32-year-old recreational skier who suffered a grade II separation of his acromioclavicular joint while skiing six weeks ago. He was immobilized for two weeks and then underwent a four-week course of physical therapy that restored his shoulder ROM. He presents with mild, intermittent acromioclavicular joint discomfort and a slight palpable defect at the joint. Prior to the injury, Steve lifted weights three times a week and is eager to resume his exercise program. He comes to the CMES to begin a safe exercise program and avoid exacerbation of the injury.

CMES Approach

The CMES should contact Steve's physical therapist to discuss the exercises performed in physical therapy, progress to date, and any contraindications or safety precautions. When initiating a strength-training program, the CMES should carefully monitor Steve's symptoms at his acromioclavicular joint. Steve should be encouraged to ice after his workout, even if he is asymptomatic at the time. This may help to prevent any residual symptoms. When using free weights, Steve should be encouraged to begin with weights that he can control well to avoid any traction at the acromioclavicular joint. He should also be advised to not carry the weights around the gym. Strengthening exercises for the scapular muscles should be performed in the middle of the ROM to avoid excessive retraction and protraction. This will prevent excessive stress to the acromioclavicular joint. Steve should be extremely cautious with exercises that create a great deal of stress at the acromioclavicular joint, such as bench pressing or push-ups. He should never perform any bench presses without a spotter.

SUMMARY

The key to working with the post-injury client is to understand the pathology and structures involved, as well as the underlying mechanism of injury. In addition, the CMES should understand the positions and activities that may exacerbate the condition. Listening to the subjective complaints and symptoms and being proactive in communicating with the client's clinician are critical to preventing re-injury.

REFERENCES

Ali, M. et al. (2014). Frequency of De Quervain's tenosynovitis and its association with SMS texting. *Muscles, Ligaments and Tendons Journal,* 4, 1, 74–78.

Ashworth, N.L. (2010). Carpal tunnel syndrome. *Clinical Evidence (Online),* March 23.

Babhulkar, A. & Pawaskar, A. (2014). Acromioclavicular joint dislocations. *Current Reviews in Musculoskeletal Medicine,* 7, 1, 33–39. DOI: 10.1007/s12178-013-9199-2

Beim, G. (2000). Acromioclavicular joint injuries. *Journal of Athletic Training,* 35, 3, 261–267.

Dumont, G.D., Russell, R.D., & Robertson, W.J. (2011). Anterior shoulder instability: A review of pathoanatomy, diagnosis and treatment. *Current Reviews in Musculoskeletal Medicine,* 4, 4, 200–207. DOI: 10.1007/s12178-011-9092-9

Ellenbecker, T.S., Nirschl, R., & Renstrom, P. (2013). Current concepts in examination and treatment of elbow tendon injury. *Sports Health,* 5, 2, 186–194.

Escamilla, R.F., Hooks, T.R., & Wilk, K.E. (2014). Optimal management of shoulder impingement syndrome. *Open Access Journal of Sports Medicine,* 5, 13–24. DOI: 10.2147/OAJSM.S36646

Farrar, N.G. et al. (2013). An overview of shoulder instability and its management. *The Open Orthopedics Journal,* 7, 338–346. DOI: 10.2174/1874325001307010338

Fees, M. et al. (1998). Upper extremity weight-training modifications for the injured athlete. *American Journal of Sports Medicine,* 26, 5, 732–742.

Hawkins, R.J. & Kennedy, J.C. (1980). Impingement syndrome in athletes. *American Journal of Sports Medicine,* 8, 151–158.

Houglum, P.A. (2010). *Therapeutic Exercise for Musculoskeletal Injuries* (3rd ed.). Champaign, Ill.: Human Kinetics.

Howell, E.R. (2012). Conservative care of De Quervain's tenosynovitis/tendinopathy in a warehouse worker and recreational cyclist: A case report. *Journal of the Canadian Chiropractic Association,* 56, 2, 121–127.

Ilyas, A.M. (2009). Nonsurgical treatment for de Quervain's tenosynovitis. *Journal of Hand Surgery,* 34, 5, 928–929.

Inagaki, K. (2013). Current concepts of elbow-joint disorders and their treatment. *Journal of Orthopedic Science,* 18, 1, 1–7. DOI: 10.1007/s00776-012-0333-6

Jaggi, A. et al. (2012). Muscle activation patterns in patients with recurrent shoulder instability. *International Journal of Shoulder Surgery,* 6, 4, 101–107. DOI: 10.4103/0973-6042.106221

Jobe, F.W. & Jobe, C.M. (1983). Painful athletic injuries of the shoulder. *Clinical Orthopedics,* 173, 117–125.

Lee, A.T. & Lee-Robinson, A.L. (2010). The prevalence of medial epicondylitis among patients with C6 and C7 radiculopathy. *Sports Health,* 2, 4, 334–336. DOI: 10.1177/1941738109357304

Manske, R.C. (2006). *Postsurgical Orthopedic Sports Rehabilitation: Knee and Shoulder.* St. Louis, Mo.: Mosby Elsevier.

Manske, R.C., Grant-Nierman, M., & Lucas, B. (2013). Shoulder posterior internal impingement in the overhead athlete. *International Journal of Sports and Physical Therapy,* 8, 2, 194–204.

Moseley, J.B., Jobe, F.W., & Pink, M. (1994). EMG analysis of scapular muscles during a shoulder rehabilitation program. *American Journal of Sports Medicine,* 20, 128–134.

O'Brien, S.J. et al. (1998). The active compression test: A new and effective test for diagnosing labral tears and acromioclavicular joint abnormality. *American Journal of Sports Medicine,* 26, 610–613.

Paine, R. & Voight, M.L. (2013). The role of the scapula. *International Journal of Sports and Physical Therapy,* 8, 5, 617–629.

Papa, J.A. (2012). Conservative management of De Quervain's stenosing tenosynovitis: A case report. *Journal of the Canadian Chiropractic Association,* 56, 2, 112–120.

Patel, K.R., Tadisina, K.K., & Gonzalez, M.H. (2013). De Quervain's disease. *Eplasty,* 13, ic52.

Reinold, M.M. & Curtis, A.S. (2013). Microinstability of the shoulder in the overhead athlete. *International Journal of Sports and Physical Therapy,* 8, 5, 601–616.

Rineer, C.A. & Ruch, D.S. (2009). Elbow tendinopathy and tendon ruptures: Epicondylitis, bicep, and triceps ruptures. *Journal of Hand Surgery,* 34, 3, 566–576.

Rockwood, C.A. & Matsen, F.A., III. (Eds.) (2009). *The Shoulder* (4th ed.). Philadelphia: Saunders.

Saha, K. (1983). Mechanism of shoulder movements and plea for recognition of the zero position of the glenohumeral joint. *Clinical Orthopedics,* 173, 3–10.

Shi, Q. & MacDermid, J.C. (2011). Is surgical intervention more effective than non-surgical treatment for carpal tunnel syndrome? A systematic review. *Journal of Orthopedic Surgery Research,* 6, 17. DOI: 10.1186/1749-799X-6-17

Smith, T.O. et al. (2011). Operative versus non-operative management following Rockwood grade III acromioclavicular separation: A meta-analysis of the current evidence base. *Journal of Orthopedics and Traumatology,* 12, 1, 19–27. DOI: 10.1007/s10195-011-0127-1

Tannenbaum E. & Sekiya, J.K. (2011). Evaluation and management of posterior shoulder instability. *Sports Health,* 3, 3, 253–263. DOI: 10.1177/1941738111400562

Tischer, T. et al. (2009). Incidence of associated injuries with acute acromioclavicular joint dislocations types III through V. *American Journal of Sports Medicine,* 37, 136–141.

Walker-Bone, K. et al. (2012). Occupation and epicondylitis: A population-based study. *Rheumatology (Oxford)*, 5, 2, 305–310. DOI: 10.1093/rheumatology/ker228

Wilk, K.E. et al. (2012). Rehabilitation of the overhead athlete's elbow. *Sports Health*, 4, 5, 404–414. DOI: 10.1177/1941738112455006

You, D., Smith, A.H., & Rempel, D. (2014). Meta-analysis: Association between wrist posture and carpal tunnel syndrome among workers. *Safety and Health at Work*, 5, 1, 27–31. DOI: 10.1016/j.shaw.2014.01.003

SUGGESTED READING

Escamilla, R.F., Hooks, T.R., & Wilk, K.E. (2014). Optimal management of shoulder impingement syndrome. *Open Access Journal of Sports Medicine*, 5, 13–24. DOI: 10.2147/OAJSM.S36646

Farrar, N.G. et al. (2013). An overview of shoulder instability and its management. *The Open Orthopedics Journal*, 7, 338–346. DOI: 10.2174/1874325001307010338

Inagaki, K. (2013). Current concepts of elbow-joint disorders and their treatment. *Journal of Orthopedic Science*, 18, 1, 1–7. DOI: 10.1007/s00776-012-0333-6

Paine, R. & Voight, M.L. (2013). The role of the scapula. *International Journal of Sports and Physical Therapy*, 8, 5, 617–629.

Walker-Bone, K. et al. (2012). Occupation and epicondylitis: A population-based study. *Rheumatology* (Oxford), 5, 2, 305–310. DOI: 10.1093/rheumatology/ker228

20 LOW-BACK PAIN

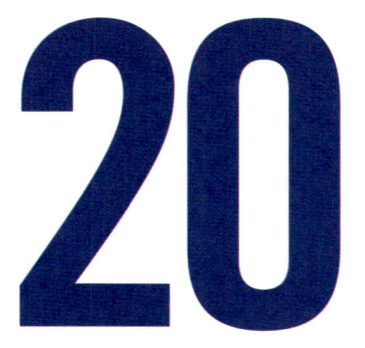

IN THIS CHAPTER

EPIDEMIOLOGY

OVERVIEW
INDIVIDUAL FACTORS
ACTIVITY-RELATED FACTORS
PSYCHOLOGICAL FACTORS

OVERVIEW OF CONDITIONS

DIAGNOSTIC CRITERIA

TREATMENT OPTIONS
NON-PHARMACOLOGICAL TREATMENT
PHARMACOLOGICAL TREATMENT
SURGICAL TREATMENT
EXERCISE TREATMENT

EXERCISE RECOMMENDATIONS FOR CLIENTS WITH A HISTORY OF LOW-BACK PAIN
EXERCISE PROGRAM PROGRESSIONS

CASE STUDY

SUMMARY

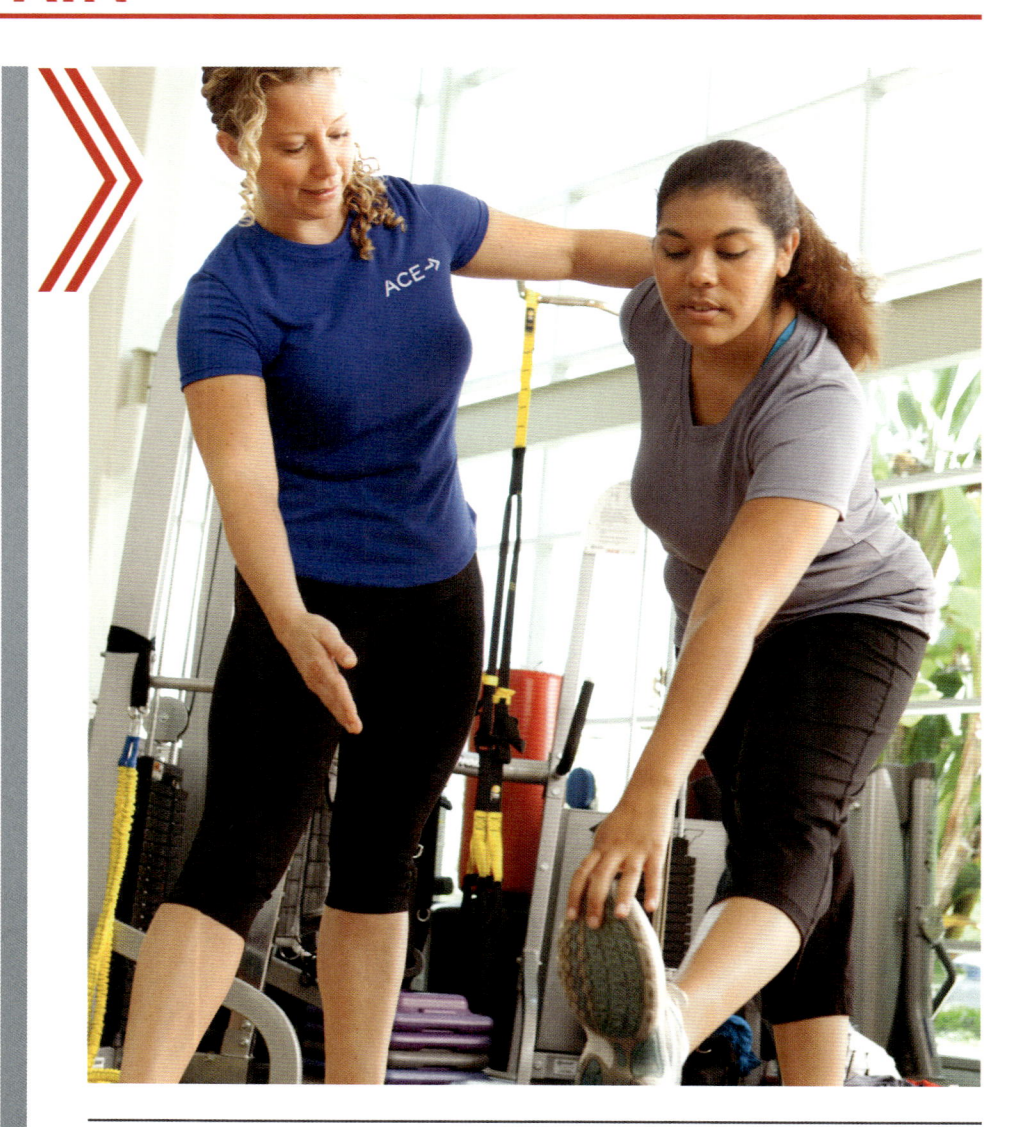

ABOUT THE AUTHOR

Jennifer Solomon, M.D., is board certified in Physical Medicine and Rehabilitation and fellowship-trained in Spine and Sports Medicine. She specializes in non-operative treatments for sports and spine injuries, including electrodiagnostics. Dr. Solomon is assistant attending physiatrist at the Hospital for Special Surgery's Women's Sports Medicine Center and clinical instructor at the Weill Medical College of Cornell University. She serves as team physician for St. Peter's College and has covered several sporting events, including the NYC Marathon, tennis tournaments, and various races. Dr. Solomon is also a team physician for the United States Federation Cup Tennis Team and a medical consultant for La Palestra Center for Preventative Medicine. Dr. Solomon is a member of the American Academy of Physical Medicine and Rehabilitation, the North American Spine Society, and the American Association of Electrodiagnostic Medicine. She has published more than 15 articles and chapters on a variety of spine and sports medicine topics.

By Jennifer Solomon

LOW-BACK PAIN (LBP) IS A COMMON CONDITION, which until recently has been depicted as self-resolving and transient. Traditionally, it has been assumed that spontaneous recovery occurs in the majority of cases. However, emerging evidence contradicts this notion, with back pain being neither insignificant nor self-limiting (Amorin-Woods et al., 2014).

EPIDEMIOLOGY

LBP plagues modern society and is a significant source of cost and disability. Clinically, **chronic** LBP has been defined as pain lasting for more than three months in the area below the inferior border of the twelfth rib and above the gluteal folds (Sloan et al., 2008). Estimates from the CDC reveal that about 25% of adults in the U.S. experience LBP [Centers for Disease Control and Prevention (CDC), 2020a]. Estimates for the lifetime prevalence range from 11 to 84%, while those for one-year prevalence range from 22 to 65% (Walker, 2000). While these episodes vary in length and intensity, historical records estimate that at any one time there are 1.2 million adults disabled as a result of their LBP (Wong & Transfeltd, 2007). A significant proportion of these individuals seek assistance from a healthcare professional. In fact, back pain is the second most common complaint heard in doctors' offices.

Until recently, it was common to classify LBP according to the duration of the pain (i.e. **acute, subacute,** or chronic) with chronicity being considered relatively uncommon. Currently, LBP is considered to be a recurring or persistent condition with a fluctuating course over time (Lemeunier, Leboeuf-Yde, & Gagey, 2012). LBP is reported to run a recurrent course in the majority of patients, which means that following an episode of LBP, it is likely that a patient will have future episodes of pain, causing suffering for the patient and time loss from work (Stanton et al., 2010). Individuals with LBP not only have individual physiologic mechanisms, but there may also be varying psychological, societal, and economic implications. People with LBP report symptoms of **depression, anxiety,** and insomnia more frequently than those without it (Morris, 2006). LBP is the second leading cause of work absenteeism, following upper-respiratory infections (Wong & Transfeltd, 2007), and the estimates of the direct cost burden in the United States show $86 billion in incremental healthcare costs (Ivanova et al., 2011; Dagenais, Caro, & Haldeman, 2008).

BIOPSYCHOSOCIAL MODEL APPLIED TO LOW-BACK PAIN

Pain is a multidimensional experience influenced by many environmental and personal factors. Over the past several decades, researchers investigating LBP have applied the biopsychosocial model, which states that biological, psychological, and social factors all play a significant role in the context of disease or illness (Valencia, Robinson, & George, 2011).

Biological factors are discovered through a clinical analysis of the patient's physical condition, which could uncover patho-anatomical or biomechanical concerns directly influencing injury and pain in the lumbar area. Low-back **sprains, strains, compression fractures,** or disc problems could be diagnosed upon a clinical examination, for example.

LEARNING OBJECTIVES:

» Identify important individual, activity-related, and psychological factors related to low-back pain.

» Differentiate between various pathologies that may contribute to the occurrence of low-back pain.

» Describe basic signs, symptoms, and treatment options associated with low-back pain.

» Design and implement safe and effective exercise programs for clients who have a history of low-back pain.

EXPAND YOUR KNOWLEDGE

Related to psychology, the development of chronic LBP has been associated with a fear-avoidance model (FAM) of musculoskeletal pain. The FAM refers to fear due to catastrophic thoughts followed by the avoidance of movement due to the fear of pain and re-injury. The FAM has highlighted the importance of pain catastrophizing and pain-related fear in the development of chronic LBP from an acute episode (Leeuw et al., 2007). A psychological factor that appears particularly influential is work-related fear-avoidance, whereby an individual exhibits pain-related fear specific to occupational activities, which accentuates anxiety and the long-term negative functional impact. Specifically, work-related fear-avoidance beliefs have been found to be predictive of disability, reduced work-related physical capacity, and a longer period before returning to work for patients with LBP (Dupeyron et al., 2011).

The social aspect takes into account the social pressures and constraints on an individual's ability to function. The prevalence of chronic pain has been reported to vary with socioeconomic levels, such that low socioeconomic status is related to an adverse health outcome. Theoretically, individuals are exposed to more demands as socioeconomic status decreases, and psychosocial responses to such stress may be harmful to health over time as it exhausts an individual's reserve capacity to respond to the challenges of the environment, making them more vulnerable to different diseases and chronic conditions (Valencia, Robinson, & George, 2011).

The biopsychosocial model emphasizes the value of an integrated approach to clinical, psychological, and social factors, and highlights the importance of multidisciplinary strategies for dealing with LBP. As such, the ACE® Certified Medical Exercise Specialist (CMES) should also consider these factors when working with clients who have suffered from LBP. Understanding that physical activity is only one part of the multidisciplinary approach for helping individuals overcome their troubles with pain will help the CMES recognize the potential for appropriate referral to other healthcare specialists that may be necessary to benefit their clients.

OVERVIEW

Specific causes of LBP are difficult to discern, accounting for less than 15% of all back pain, whereas approximately 85% of patients with isolated LBP cannot be given a precise patho-anatomical diagnosis and are considered to have back pain from a nonspecific origin (Franke, Franke, & Fryer, 2014). Nonspecific LBP has been defined as tension, soreness, and/or stiffness in the lower-back region for which it is not possible to identify a specific cause of the pain. Moreover, this definition conveys the limitations of the medical community's knowledge of the pathological source of most people's LBP (Hancock et al., 2011). Nonetheless, researchers have attempted to organize risk factors for LBP into individual, activity, and psychological categories.

Individual Factors

Age

Aging affects the spine. In fact, degenerative changes of the lumbar spine that are visible by **magnetic resonance imaging (MRI)** become more common with age and are present in nearly 100% of persons over age 60 (Cheung et al., 2009). Clinical evidence suggests that the incidence of LBP is highest in the third decade, and overall prevalence increases with age until the early 60s, at which point it gradually declines (Hoy et al., 2010). Interestingly, self-reported back pain in the general population does not get worse with old age. In fact, in their review of the literature, Fejer and Leboeuf-Yde (2012) found that the prevalence of LBP appears to decline with age. The researchers reported that back pain is no more common in the elderly population (>60 years) when compared to the middle-age population. They concluded that back pain does not increase with increasing age, but seems to decline in the oldest people. A likely explanation for this trend could be a decreased need to be physically active in old age, thus reducing pain-provoking circumstances.

Smoking

Tobacco smoking remains the leading preventable cause of morbidity and mortality in the United States, accounting for approximately 480,000 deaths each year (CDC, 2020b). Despite known health consequences, an estimated 34.2 million people in the United States smoke cigarettes. According to the CDC (2020b), 13.7% of U.S. adults were classified as current cigarette smokers in 2018. Researchers have examined associations between smoking status (i.e., never, former, or current) and chronic LBP, and concluded that smoking should be considered a risk factor for the incidence and prevalence of LBP (Ditre et al., 2011). Further, a seminal meta-analysis on this topic revealed that both current and former smokers have a higher prevalence and incidence of LBP than those who were never smokers (Shiri et al., 2010).

It is thought that smoking may decrease blood flow to the intervertebral discs, leading to a deficit of nutrients and/or a lack of sufficient oxygen, which may lead to accelerated cell death. Other effects of smoking may include an increase in the rate of development of **osteoporosis,** fractures, and degenerative changes in the spine. There is, however, reason to believe that smoking-induced intervertebral disc degeneration may be repaired by cessation of smoking (Ditre et al., 2011).

Activity-related Factors

Occupation

Certain types of occupational activities appear to predispose individuals to LBP, including heavy lifting, exposure to awkward positions (e.g., bending and twisting), carrying, pulling, pushing, prolonged walking or standing, and driving (Heneweer et al., 2011). High exposure to whole-body vibration is also a risk factor for back pain (Griffith et al., 2012). Specific professions that are at higher risk include sales, clerical work, repair service, transportation, and healthcare (e.g., emergency medical technician and nurse) (Bahr et al., 2004; Heneweer et al., 2011).

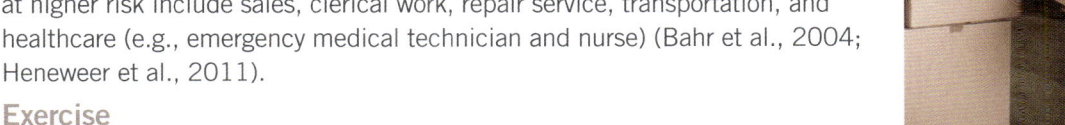

Exercise

Inconsistent findings have been found for leisure-time physical activities, sports, and exercise related to LBP (Heneweer et al., 2011). Studies that surveyed athletes to determine which sports have higher rates of back pain have yielded conflicting results. However, athletes involved in certain activities, such as gymnastics, diving, American football, weight lifting, wrestling, ice hockey, cross-country skiing, rowing, and rotation-related sports (e.g., tennis, racquet ball, and golf) may have higher rates of LBP than non-athletes (Chimenti, Scholtes, & Van Dillen, 2013; Petering & Webb, 2011; Baranto et al., 2009; Borenstein, Wiesel, & Boeden, 2004).

The protective role of specific exercise regimens in preventing LBP is less clear, as are associations with **overweight** and **obesity.** In general, those who engage in regular recreational physical activity appear to be less likely to have back pain at any given time and are less likely to develop future pain (Rubin, 2007). While physical fitness does not completely prevent LBP, it may improve functional outcomes by decreasing recovery time. Unfortunately, many people with LBP choose not to exercise and actually believe that doing so would be detrimental to their condition.

Psychological Factors

In general, depression, anxiety, and insomnia are strongly correlated with back pain. They can be both predisposing (e.g., psychogenic muscle tension and work distress) and resulting factors of existing back pain. Depression may affect an individual's ability to cope with pain. The inability to determine an exact cause of pain or to effectively relieve symptoms may result in further depression. It has been reported that between 26 and 46% of patients with LBP in physical-therapy settings exhibit depressive signs or symptoms (George et al., 2011). Studies have also demonstrated that patients with chronic LBP accompanied by depressive symptoms show significantly higher subjective pain compared to LBP patients without depression (Ha et al., 2011).

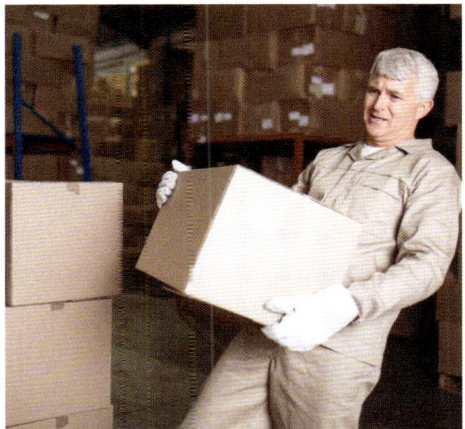

Fear-avoidance personality variables (exaggerated pain or fear that activity will cause permanent damage) and passive coping techniques (e.g., avoidance, withdrawal, and wishful thinking) are positive predictors of chronic back-pain symptoms (Darlow et al., 2013). Further, evidence suggests that patients' beliefs about LBP are associated with their clinicians' beliefs, and moderate evidence suggests that patient and clinician fear-avoidance beliefs are also associated (Darlow et al., 2012).

APPLY WHAT YOU KNOW

TALKING TO CLIENTS ABOUT LOW-BACK PAIN CAN HAVE FAR-REACHING EFFECTS

Research on patients' beliefs about LBP has revealed that recovery expectations can be heavily influenced by statements from treating clinicians. This finding is important given that low recovery expectations are a strong predictor of poor outcome (Iles et al., 2009). For example, study participants who reported being advised to adopt certain postures and strengthen specific muscles to manage their LBP claimed that this approach reinforced their belief that their spine was vulnerable. They saw muscles as being important to limit movement, reduce spinal load, maintain structural alignment, and prevent injury. Ultimately, these participants focused on their backs and maintained constant vigilance because of the perceived benefits of pain relief or a feeling of control. Interestingly, Darlow and colleagues (2013) found that these protection strategies resulted in increased vigilance, worry, frustration, and guilt for patients with LBP.

Another example of practitioner influence is related to prognosis expectations. Participants who believed that their problem would fully resolve perceived new episodes of LBP as being unrelated problems that would also resolve. In contrast, those who had received negative expectations saw new episodes as recurrences of the previous problem. For example, one participant was told, "Unfortunately, because you've done this, you have a very high chance of doing it again" (Darlow et al., 2013).

In clinical settings, physicians and other healthcare providers are advised to reassure patients that recovery is to be expected, and to manage fear-avoidance and psychosomatic issues by letting them know that hurt does not equal harm (Amorin-Woods et al., 2014). Darlow and colleagues (2013) found that giving unambiguous activity advice can be very empowering, and that appropriate reassurance and positive prognostic expectations can have a very beneficial effect, as these approaches positively influence participants' beliefs about their current and subsequent episodes of LBP. To avoid unwittingly creating fear-avoidance behaviors in the management of LBP, the CMES should consider educating clients on the positive aspects of movement to empower them in their efforts to remain active. For example, encouraging clients to keep active in their daily activities and to engage in daily walking could influence their views about the importance of movement and activity and provide reassurance about being physically active, even with LBP.

THINK IT THROUGH

It is important for the CMES who works with clients with LBP to use appropriate language when discussing restorative exercise principles. Comments about limiting movement can cause fear-avoidance behaviors in clients who are concerned about further injuring their backs through exercise or daily activities. Think about what kind of language you will use to support and encourage clients with LBP in their efforts to restore back health and resume or maintain physical activity.

OVERVIEW OF CONDITIONS

Back pain is a symptom and the possible etiologies are numerous. Muscle strains, ligament sprains, and soft-tissue contusions account for as much as 97% of back pain in the general adult population. In adolescents, the clinical spectrum of **spondylolysis, spondylolisthesis,** and **pars interarticularis** stress fractures may be the most common cause of LBP (Petering & Webb, 2011). Two percent of cases are "visceral disease," or disease of the internal organs and structures, such as **pancreatitis, prostatitis,** and **aortic aneurysm.** The remaining 1% of back pain results from non-mechanical spinal conditions such as tumors, infections, and rheumatologic disorders (Deyo & Weinstein, 2001). This section describes some of the most common mechanical back pain diagnoses, along with their causes and typical symptoms.

Lumbar strain or sprain is a non-specific term often used to describe mechanical LBP. Typically, a strain refers to a muscle injury in which the fibers are abnormally stretched, while a sprain refers to a torn ligament. A more descriptive and accurate term for most of these cases is **discogenic back pain**, which refers to dysfunction or degeneration of lumbar intervertebral discs. This phenomenon is a universal process of aging that leads to chemical and physical changes in the disc. Discs are comprised of an outer ring, the **annulus fibrosus,** and an inner gel, the **nucleus pulposus** (Figure 20-1). Over time, discs lose their water content and acquire gradual fibrotic changes that limit mobility.

While these changes occur in everyone, the presence of symptomatic back pain is multifactorial. Microtrauma may lead to small tears or cracks in the annulus and result in inflammation and pain around annular nerves. Also, gradual narrowing of the disc height may cause an unstable surface where the facet joints articulate, leading to an overloading of those structures and, ultimately, pain. Generally, discogenic pain is caused by activities that increase pressure within the disc, such as coughing, sneezing, sitting, and bending forward. Discogenic pain can be acute or chronic.

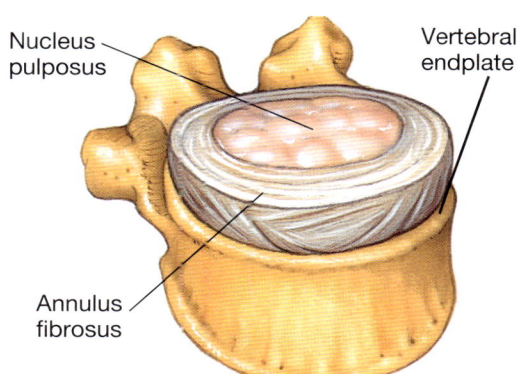

Figure 20-1
Anatomy of a vertebral disc
© Fotosearch
www.fotosearch.com

Herniated discs account for approximately 4% of all mechanical LBP (Deyo & Weinstein, 2001) and occur when there is a displacement of disc material (nucleus pulposus or annulus fibrosis) beyond the intervertebral disc space. The highest prevalence is among people aged 30 to 50 years, with a male to female ratio of 2:1. In people aged 25 to 55 years, about 95% of herniated discs occur at the lower lumbar spine (L4/5 and L5/S1 level), whereas disc herniation above this spinal level is more common in people aged over 55 years (Jordan, Konstantinou, & O'Dowd, 2011). As previously noted, aging affects discs by decreasing the nearly 80% water content of the nucleus and making the annulus more prone to tears. Individuals with herniated discs may complain of sharp or throbbing LBP, which is worse with movement but improved with lying down. Herniated material may extend out far enough to compress the nerve roots that exit the spinal cord at that level, causing pain, numbness, tingling, or weakness. These are signs and symptoms of lumbar **radiculopathy,** or nerve root impairment. Disc herniation diagnosis can be confirmed by radiological examination. However, it is interesting to note that MRI findings of herniated disc are not always accompanied by clinical symptoms (Jordan, Konstantinou, & O'Dowd, 2011).

Sciatica refers to radicular symptoms that follow the path of the sciatic nerve, down the posterior aspect of the thigh, lower leg, and foot. In approximately 90% of the cases, sciatica is caused by a herniated disc involving nerve root compression. However, lumbar canal **stenosis** or foraminal stenosis and (less often) tumours or cysts are other possible causes (Valat et al., 2010). Generally, there is no acute event associated with the onset of sciatica, which may be exacerbated by standing, sitting, sneezing, heavy lifting, or having a bowel movement. In some cases, the sciatic symptoms may be equivalent to, or worse than, the LBP itself. The symptoms of sciatica resolve spontaneously in more than 50% of patients during the first month. Consequently, guidelines generally recommend conservative treatment initially because more intensive therapy could hinder rehabilitation and prolong disability (Scott, Moga, & Harstall, 2010).

Another form of mechanical pain is secondary to spinal stenosis, which results from narrowing of the central spinal canal, either by bone or soft tissue. Although the prevalence of lumbar spinal stenosis is unknown, there has been a steady, dramatic rise in spine surgery rates over recent decades, with spinal stenosis being the most common diagnosis associated with spinal surgery in adults over 60 years of age (Macedo et al., 2013). Degenerative changes of the facet joints and intervertebral discs are largely responsible for this process. Thus, spinal stenosis typically arises in persons over age 50. Symptoms arise when the narrowing causes compression of the spinal cord or spinal nerves. Most commonly, spinal stenosis sufferers complain of cramping, pain, numbness or weakness in their back or legs. However, some will report leg pain only. The typical pattern is termed **pseudoclaudication,** which refers to pain in the buttock, thigh, or leg that occurs with standing or walking and is relieved by rest in a lying or sitting position, or by flexing forward at the waist.

Approximately 4% of mechanical LBP occurs from osteoporotic compression fractures (Deyo & Weinstein, 2001). Spinal fractures generally result from major trauma, such as a fall from a great height or a motor vehicle accident. However, individuals with **osteopenia** or osteoporosis, in which bone density is reduced, can acquire compression fractures from less significant trauma, even from something as simple as a sneeze or cough. It is estimated that 750,000 new vertebral fractures occur in the United States each year. Although only about one-third of these fractures become symptomatic, they can result in height loss, spinal deformity, acute and chronic pain, restriction of thoracic and abdominal contents, impaired mobility, and disability (Han et al., 2011).

Spondylolysis is a bony defect, possibly a stress fracture, of one or both pars interarticularis and most commonly occurs in the lower lumbar spine. Prevalence of spondylolysis is estimated to range from approximately 6 to 11.5% in the general population and approximately 7 to 8% in elite athletes, but is thought to be grossly underreported (Garet et al., 2013). Repetitive microtrauma from lumbar hyperextension combined with rotation and loading has been associated with spondylolysis. These injuries have been observed in dancers, gymnasts, figure skaters, weight lifters, and football players. Symptoms can be unilateral or bilateral, acute or chronic, and range in severity from mild to immobilizing.

Spondylolysis can lead to spondylolisthesis, which is an anterior displacement of a vertebra relative to the one below it. The most common symptom is LBP, which may or may not be associated with an acute injury and is worse with **flexion** but relieved by **extension.** Leg pain can also occur with spondylolisthesis if spinal nerve roots are irritated as they leave the canal.

DIAGNOSTIC CRITERIA

Generally, all clients with back pain should receive a thorough physical exam from a physician. The exclusion of specific pathologies is step one of the clinical assessment. Approximately 10% of all malignancies have symptomatic spine involvement as the initial manifestation of the disease, including multiple myeloma, non-Hodgkin's lymphoma, and carcinoma of the lung, breast, and prostate. Early detection and treatment of spinal malignancies are important to prevent further spread of metastatic disease and the development of complications such as vertebral fracture and spinal cord compression (Amorin-Woods et al., 2014). In all of the previously described conditions, there are common warning signs that necessitate immediate attention, including fever, loss of bowel or bladder control, unexplained weight loss, history of cancer or recent infection, and intravenous drug use.

After careful evaluation, the physician may choose to pursue further evaluation with an imaging study. Plain radiographs or x-rays are often used as an initial test, as they are the best option for evaluating bony changes such as fracture, tumor, spondylolisthesis, and disc-space narrowing. **Computed tomography (CT)** and MRI are used to visualize spinal stenosis and herniated discs and may be used to rule out conditions such as infection or cancer. However, CT and MRI may also detect asymptomatic abnormalities. Therefore, careful correlation with the individual's subjective history and physical exam is essential when using any imaging technique.

TREATMENT OPTIONS

Because the natural history of LBP is variable, treatment goals depend on the specific condition. While the majority of people with an episode of acute LBP improve enough to return to work within the first two weeks, the probability of recurrence within the first year ranges from 30 to 60%. In as many as one-third of people, the initial episode of LBP persists for a year (Amorin-Woods et al., 2014). Thus, a significant proportion of back-pain patients experience a relapsing and remitting course of pathology. Still others may develop a chronic disabling or persistent condition. Multiple factors may determine the overall prognosis, but each diagnosis also inherently includes general expectations for the extent and timing of recovery.

Treatment options for patients with LBP have evolved and, in some cases, become a source of much debate. Because of the ubiquitous nature of LBP in modern society, many patients approach their diagnosis with several preconceived ideas about treatment, formed from a combination of lay-press articles and recounted experiences from friends and relatives. However, for almost all conditions, current thinking among health professionals is one of active recovery. Most clinical LBP guidelines emphasize the importance of considering psychosocial risk factors for developing chronic pain, reassuring patients that their condition is not serious, and encouraging them to remain active within the limits of their pain (Scott, Moga, & Harstall, 2010). Bed rest is contraindicated, as it has been shown to not only delay recovery, but also worsen symptoms. Understanding a client's condition is essential for them to actively participate in improving current symptoms and preventing future recurrences.

Non-pharmacological Treatment

In the acute setting, clients often fear that the pain they feel with activity is a sign of further injury, or even permanent disability. However, clients can be reassured that returning to daily activities has actually been shown to be an integral part of treatment and recovery. Basic recommendations include avoiding specific movements or activities that provoke pain and limiting bed rest to times of severe pain only. Because there is little evidence that specific back exercises are useful in the acute setting (Petering & Webb, 2011), clients are generally encouraged to engage in low-stress aerobic activities such as walking. Heavy lifting and prolonged sitting and standing should be avoided. In cases of subacute (duration of greater than six weeks after injury but no longer than 12 weeks after onset of symptoms) and chronic LBP, a physical therapist can design specific exercises that focus on conditioning the core musculature in an attempt to improve current symptoms and avoid future recurrences. Physical therapy serves to reeducate patients on proper posture and alignment, as well as correct current muscle imbalances. Using popular exercise modalities, such as **yoga** and **Pilates,** as maintenance therapy may be appropriate for certain individuals. Exercise is covered in more depth later in the chapter.

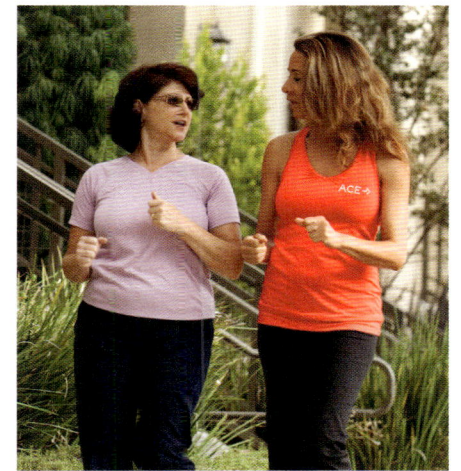

Passive interventions such as electrotherapies are often used in the clinical treatment of LBP, even though the evidence for use of such approaches is lacking. According to Seco, Kovacs, and Urrutia (2011), the available evidence does not support the effectiveness of ultrasound or **transcutaneous electrical nerve stimulation (TENS)** for treating LBP. In the absence of such evidence, the researchers concluded that clinical use of these forms of treatment is not justified and should be discouraged. The evidence for the use of specific back exercise therapy, back education, joint mobilization (with therapeutic intent), massage (with therapeutic intent), physical agents (heat and cold), and traction/lumbar supports is either insufficient, equivocal, or negative (Amorin-Woods et al., 2014).

Spinal manipulation refers to adjustment of the spine using twisting, pushing, or pulling movements and is performed predominantly by chiropractors. Individuals interested in chiropractic services should have a thorough evaluation of their symptoms by their primary care physician and have an understanding of their diagnosis before choosing to try this modality.

Pharmacological Treatment

Pain relievers such as acetaminophen (Tylenol) and **nonsteroidal anti-inflammatory drugs (NSAIDs)** are often used in the short-term for acute cases of LBP. Narcotics and muscle relaxants are also options for pain, especially night-time symptoms, but their side effects and dependence profiles make them more appropriate for cases of severe pain. Given the pathway to misuse and abuse and the known illicit market for these drugs, this is of significant concern and has become a major issue for health care (Mafi et al., 2013).

Neuropathy or neuropathic pain, which clients may experience as burning, "pins and needles," or "electric shock" sensations, can be treated with two newer drugs, gabapentin (Neurontin) and pregabalin (Lyrica). These medications work directly on the **central nervous system** and serve as nerve stabilizers. The mechanisms of action of gabapentin and pregabalin are unknown, but it is believed that they involve binding to voltage-dependent calcium-ion channels.

Spinal injections, another option for chronic pain relief, can also be used as a diagnostic tool to localize symptoms. If the patient responds to the steroid injection, it may allow them to advance in a non-surgical treatment program and avoid surgery (Goertz et al., 2012). Typically, local anesthetics and/or **corticosteroids** are used to relieve pain and decrease inflammation. Injections can target several different structures:

- Trigger-point injections target areas of muscle that are painful and fail to relax.
- Facet injections target facet joints on the posterior aspect of the spine that form where one vertebra overlaps another. Pain from facet joints can cause localized spinal pain or refer pain to adjacent structures.
- Epidural injections target the epidural space inside the spinal canal that contains, among other structures, spinal nerve roots.

These injections are thought to be particularly helpful for patients with radicular signs and symptoms such as sciatica. Sacroiliac joints are also occasionally injected in patients with accompanying buttock and thigh pain or sacroiliac dysfunction. Both facet and epidural injections can be done under **fluoroscopy,** or x-ray guidance, to ensure that the medications reach the correct location.

Surgical Treatment

Rarely, if conservative treatments have failed or patients develop progressive and limiting neurologic symptoms, spinal surgery is considered. The two most common types of lumbar surgery are decompression and spinal fusion. Decompression surgery, either a **laminectomy** or a **microdiscectomy,** aims to relieve impingement of the nerve root by removing a small piece of bone and/or disc material. These procedures, which are most commonly used for spinal stenosis or herniated discs, create a wider spinal canal and, therefore, more space for the spinal nerves. Spinal fusion surgery uses a bone graft to fuse two vertebral segments together. This, in turn, stops abnormal or excessive motion at the joint that is thought to be generating pain. Fusion is most often used for degenerative disc disease, spondylolysis, and spondylolisthesis.

Exercise Treatment

For most individuals with LBP, exercise will be the cornerstone of their treatment program. However, clients with LBP, especially chronic sufferers, may have developed fear-avoidance behaviors and negative beliefs about their abilities to exercise or perform certain activities. Therefore, clear communication between the CMES and the client is essential for facilitating a positive outcome from the exercise program. The overall goals of symptom relief and return to function must be discussed, and expectations must be set prior to beginning exercise. In some cases, complete resolution of all symptoms is not a realistic goal. In such cases, clients must view exercise as a way of overcoming their LBP rather than eradicating it. Discussing specific physical-activity objectives [e.g., work duties, **activities of daily living (ADL),** and sport skills] allows the client and CMES to create long-term goals.

Exercise is recommended to reduce the recurrence of pain. However, no specific exercise is preferred for acute LBP (Goertz et al., 2012). Instead, the exercise program for those with acute pain focuses on walking and resuming normal daily activities as soon as possible. While modifications to avoid strenuous activities such as running and heavy-lifting are reasonable, periods of immobility, including bed rest and prolonged sitting or standing, are not recommended.

Creating an individualized exercise program for a person with a history of LBP requires consideration of their specific clinical diagnosis. Initially, an assessment of the client's overall

Low-back Pain — CHAPTER 20

fitness level is also important, as an athlete will have a different starting point than a **sedentary** person. Additionally, understanding the duration and severity of symptoms, as well as any activity limitations, will allow the CMES to establish a baseline from which to observe progress.

The following are contraindications and modifications to consider when designing an exercise program for clients with a history of LBP:

- Clients should be encouraged to obtain clearance from their physicians before beginning a program, as exercise may not be appropriate for certain individuals with serious conditions such as tumor, fracture, or progressive neurologic deficits.
- Although walking is generally a good choice for aerobic fitness in clients with LBP because it places low compressive loads on the lumbar structures, it may not be suitable for all clients. Because walking places the lumbar spine in a more extended position, clients with spinal stenosis who have symptoms while walking that are relieved with rest, should avoid prolonged walking.
- As previously described, the progression of exercises can be as important as the exercises themselves. In general, the CMES should consider working on the muscles that stabilize the spine prior to the muscles that move the spine, to decrease the likelihood that unsupported exercises will cause damage to ligaments.
- Keep in mind that clients in beginning stages may not need additional weight added to exercises. Initially, the weight of their limbs may provide enough of a challenge.
- Know each client's limitations as set forth by their physician or physical therapist prior to designing the exercise program. Avoid extreme postures or actions that take the individual beyond their normal **range of motion (ROM).** Although creativity is an important motivational factor when designing a program, performing exercises outside of normal body mechanics is not useful and may be detrimental.
- Respect the client's normal spinal curvature when performing trunk exercises. Avoid hyperextension of the spine, which would cause clients to exceed their normal lordosis.
- Many of the exercises used in LBP rehabilitation require only subtle movements, such as abdominal hollowing. Using extreme movements or momentum is usually unwarranted for individuals with a history of LBP.
- Although a hands-on approach can be beneficial to provide adjustments and guidance, the CMES must never physically force a client into a position. Providing extra force to bring a client "deeper" into a stretch can cause serious injury.

EXERCISE RECOMMENDATIONS FOR CLIENTS WITH A HISTORY OF LOW-BACK PAIN

The balance of this chapter is based on the work of Stuart M. McGill, Ph.D., a renowned expert in spine biomechanics and kinesiology whose books *Low Back Disorders,* 3rd Edition (2016), and *Ultimate Back Fitness and Performance,* 6th Edition (2017), can be purchased through his website: www.backfitpro.com.

Clients with a history of back troubles may desire pain relief and spinal stability (a health objective), while others may seek a performance objective (which may be counterproductive to optimal back health). Some clients may need more stability, while others may need more mobility. Certain exercises will exacerbate the back troubles of some people but may help others. Because each individual has different needs, proficient exercise professionals will need an understanding of the issues, and of the myths and realities pertaining to each issue, to form a foundation for the decision-making process.

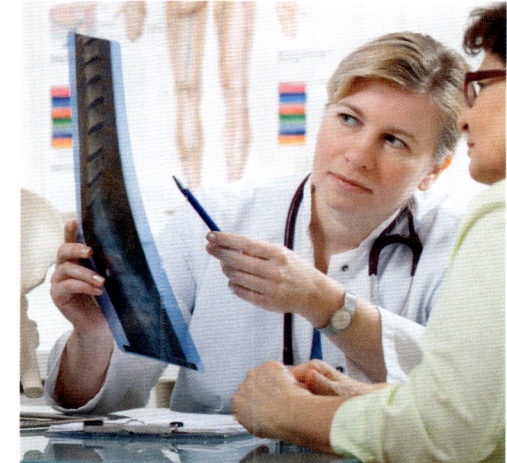

The scientific foundation for many "common sense" recommendations offered for back health yield no, or very thin, evidence. For example, it is widely believed that stretching the back and increasing the ROM is beneficial and reduces back problems—however, the scientific evidence shows that, on average, those who have more ROM in their backs have a greater risk of future troubles (Biering-Sorensen, 1984). Clearly, there is a tradeoff between mobility and stability; the optimal balance is a very personal and individual variable. Indeed, the "stability/mobility balance" may shift during a progressive exercise program as symptoms resolve, with advancing age, or as rehabilitation or training objectives change.

Another generally perceived goal of training the back is to increase strength. Strength has little association with low-back health (Biering-Sorensen, 1984). In fact, many people hurt their backs in an attempt to increase strength. It could be argued that this is an artifact, in that some exercise programs intended to enhance strength contained poorly chosen exercises such as sit-ups. Performing sit-ups both replicates a potent injury mechanism (i.e., posterior disc herniation) and results in high loads on the spine. On the other hand, muscle endurance, as opposed to strength, has been shown to be protective against future back troubles (Luoto et al., 1995). Further, for many people, it is better to train for stability rather than stretching to increase ROM (Saal & Saal, 1989). Investigations into injury mechanisms have revealed that many back-training practices actually replicate the loads and motions that cause parts of the low back to become injured (Axler & McGill, 1997). For example, disc herniations need not have excessive loading on the back to occur; rather, repeated forward flexion motion of the spine is a more potent mechanism. Thus, if full flexion or deviation is avoided in the spine, the risk of herniation is remote.

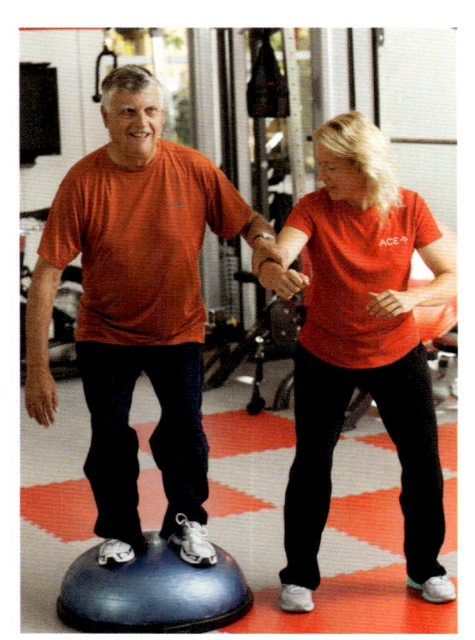

Injury is caused by damage to supporting tissues. This damage reduces the normal stiffness in the spine, resulting in unstable joints. Thus, while injury results in joint instability, an event characterized by improper muscle activation can cause the spine to "buckle" or become unstable. There is no question that excessive loading can lead to back injury, but instability at low loads is also possible and problematic. For example, it is possible to damage the passive tissues of the back while bending down and picking up a pencil, if sufficient stability is not maintained. Some people recommend that when training, the client should exhale upon exertion. In terms of reinforcing stabilizing motor patterns for all tasks, this is a mistake. Breathing in and out should occur continuously, and not be trained to a specific exertion effort. This continuous breathing helps the client maintain constant abdominal muscle activation and ensure spine stability during all possible situations.

Further, specific muscle-activation patterns are essential to avoid injury, but have also been documented to become perturbed following injury (Hodges & Richardson, 1996). Pain is a powerful instigator in the deprogramming of normal/healthy motor patterns and the creating of perturbed patterns. The exercises and programs described in this section are based on the latest scientific knowledge of how the spine works and how it becomes injured. In addition, they have been quantified for spine load, resultant spine stability, and muscle oxygenation. These are only a few examples to begin a program. The goals are to enhance spine stability by grooving motion and muscle-activation patterns to prepare for all types of challenges. Of course, other exercises may be required subsequently to enhance daily functioning, but once again, these will depend upon the characteristics and objectives of the individual.

Two other concepts must be emphasized. First, training approaches intended to enhance athletic performance are often counterproductive to the approaches used when training for health. Too many patients are rehabilitated using athletic philosophies or, worse yet, "bodybuilding" approaches designed primarily to isolate and **hypertrophy** specific muscles, and progress is thwarted. Many bad backs are created due to inappropriate performance philosophies. Identifying the training objectives is paramount.

The emphasis should be on enhancing spine health; training for performance is another topic. Second, many of the training approaches that are used at joints such as the knee, hip, or shoulder are mistakenly applied to the back. The back is a very different and complex structure, involving a flexible column with complex muscle and ligamentous support. The spine contains the spinal cord and lateral nerve roots, and musculature intimately involved in several other functions, including breathing mechanics, to give just one example. Many of the traditional approaches for training other joints in the body are not appropriate for the back—either they do not produce the desired result or they create new LBP patients.

EXPAND YOUR KNOWLEDGE

CAVEATS FOR DESIGNING EXERCISE PROGRAMS FOR BACK HEALTH
- While there is a common belief that exercise sessions should be performed at least three times per week, it appears low-back exercises have the most beneficial effect when performed daily.
- The "no pain, no gain" axiom does not apply when exercising the low back in pained individuals, particularly when applied to weight training.
- General exercise programs that combine cardiovascular components (like walking) with specific low-back exercises have been shown to be more effective in both rehabilitation and injury prevention. The exercises shown in this chapter comprise only a component of the total program.
- Diurnal variation in the fluid level of the intervertebral discs (i.e., discs are more hydrated early in the morning after rising from bed) changes the stresses on the discs throughout the day. Specifically, they are highest following bed rest and diminish over the subsequent few hours. It would be very unwise to perform full-range spine motion while under load shortly after rising from bed.
- Low-back exercises performed for maintenance of health need not emphasize strength; rather, more repetitions of less-demanding exercises will assist in the enhancement of endurance and strength. There is no doubt that back injury can occur during seemingly low-level demands (such as picking up a pencil) and that motor-control error can increase the risk of injury. While it appears that the chance of motor-control errors, which can result in inappropriate muscle forces, increases with fatigue, there is also evidence documenting the changes in passive tissue loading with fatiguing lifting. Given that endurance has more protective value than strength, strength gains should not be overemphasized at the expense of endurance.
- There is no such thing as an ideal set of exercises for all individuals. An individual's training objectives must be identified (be they rehabilitation specifically to reduce the risk of injury, optimize general health and fitness, or maximize athletic performance), and the most appropriate exercises chosen. While science cannot evaluate the optimal exercises for each situation, the combination of science and clinical experiential "wisdom" must be utilized to enhance low-back health.
- Clients should be encouraged to be patient and stick with the program. Increased function and pain reduction may not occur for three or more months.

Exercise Program Progressions

In Dr. McGill's *Ultimate Back Fitness and Performance*, 6th Edition, a variety of LBP-prevention solutions and training progressions are presented. This evidence-based approach for enhancing back health involves five distinct stages, beginning with corrective exercise and building a foundation and ultimately progressing to high-performance training. According to McGill, the training process that ensures a foundation for eventual strength, speed, and power for building the ultimate back is as follows:
- Ingrain motion/motor patterns, and corrective exercise
- Build whole-body and joint stability
- Increase muscle endurance
- Build muscle strength
- Develop speed, power, and agility

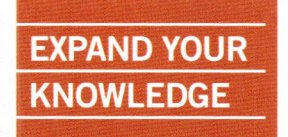

Stage 1: Ingrain Motion/Motor Patterns and Corrective Exercise

The first stage involves identifying disrupted motion patterns and developing appropriate corrective exercises. Determining where to begin the process of finding the most appropriate and suitable exercises for a client with a history of LBP starts with an assessment of the client's current fitness status and an evaluation of which, if any, movements produce pain.

A natural consideration when selecting appropriate exercises is to determine a course of action if an exercise or movement produces pain. Any exercise that causes pain is inhibiting and detracts from proper exercise technique or form. Attempting to "work through the pain" with the back is almost never beneficial. If an individual has pain, they are probably doing the exercise incorrectly, or more likely, doing the wrong exercise. The CMES should prompt clients to describe tasks, postures, and movements that exacerbate their LBP. After determining which movements are problematic for a client, the CMES should develop an exercise program to minimize the exacerbating movements.

Proper motor patterns of the muscles that support the spine enhance the back's ability to withstand the various loads and directional forces that it encounters during daily activities and physical exertion. A client's awareness of their lumbar spine, **abdominal bracing,** and gluteal complex activation are all elements in improving motor patterns for appropriate spine function.

An awareness of proper spine position allows a client to adopt a neutral spine wherein the tissues supporting the vertebrae have minimal elastic stress. Teaching clients how to adopt and maintain a neutral spine is one of the first important lessons for those with LBP. Neutral spine may be modified by clients who find relief with slightly more lumbar flexion or extension. This modified position becomes their neutral spine.

Abdominal bracing, or maintaining a mild contraction of the abdominal wall, can help ensure sufficient spine stability. Many exercise professionals mistakenly believe that activating the transverse abdominis and intentionally sucking in the abdominal wall toward the spine (a technique known as hollowing) increases spinal stability and is therefore helpful for back-pain sufferers. However, training the transverse abdominis in this manner actually compromises stability and creates spine dysfunction.

It is not uncommon for individuals to possess sufficient levels of torso flexion and extension strength, but fail tests indicative of torsional, or rotational, control. A simple, low-level test for torsional control starts in a modified push-up position with the hips above the shoulders (Figure 20-2a). One hand is then placed directly over the other hand (Figure 20-2b). The client's pelvis and rib cage should remain locked throughout the movement. An elevated pelvis, as illustrated in Figure 20-2c, is indicative of poor lumbar torsional control. It would be contraindicated to recommend a rotational cable-pulling exercise, such as the high-to-low cable chop exercise, to a client with poor torsional control because of the high level of twisting torque it produces.

For many individuals, learning to "lock" the rib cage on the pelvis is essential for enhancing torsional control (i.e., the ability to limit rotation), resulting in a reduced potential for injury and optimal functional performance during rotational or twisting movements. Locking the rib cage on the pelvis involves abdominal bracing—or the co-contraction of the abdominal wall muscles without pulling in the navel.

To enhance lumbar torsional control, Dr. McGill developed and used an exercise progression that begins with the wall-roll exercise to improve an individual's level of torsional control. The wall roll begins with the client in the plank position with both elbows planted on the wall (Figure 20-3a). The abdominals are braced and the rib cage is locked on the pelvis. The client pivots on the balls of their feet while pulling one elbow off the wall (Figure 20-3b). No spine motion should occur throughout the movement.

The torsional-control exercise progression continues with the floor roll and scramble-up exercise. This exercise begins with the client in contact with the floor with both hands and feet (Figure 20-4a). The rib cage is locked to the pelvis with an abdominal brace. The client pivots, rolls completely (360 degrees), and eventually moves into a sprinting or bounding

Low-back Pain   CHAPTER 20

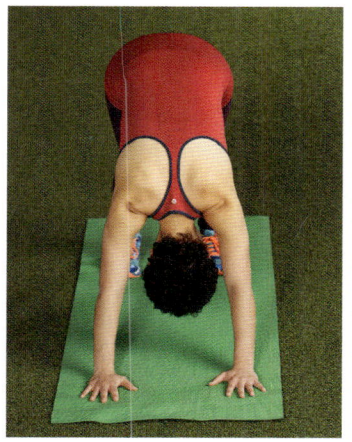

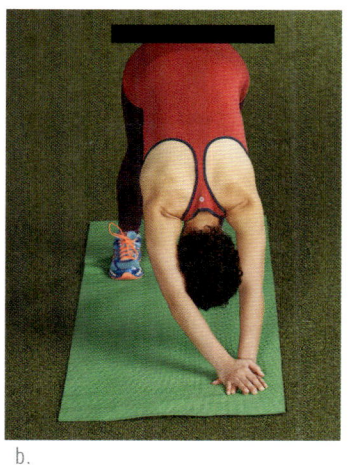

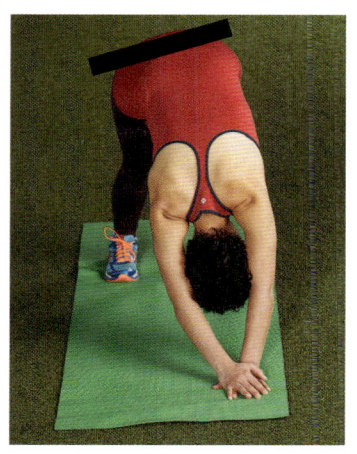

Figure 20-2
Test for lumbar torsional control

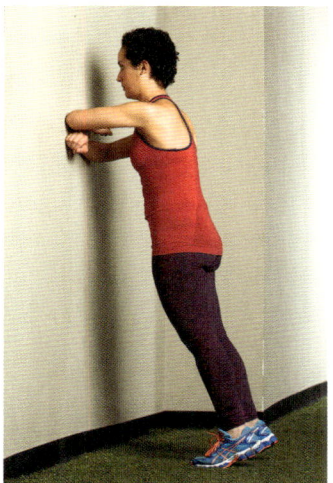

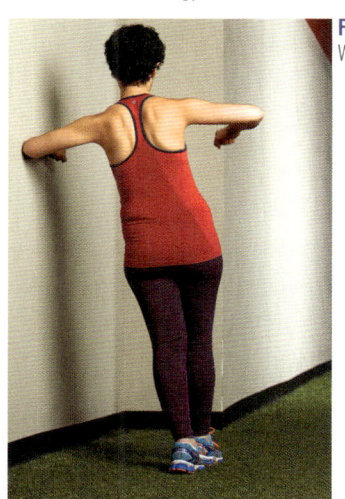

a.   b.   c.

Figure 20-3
Wall roll

a. Starting position   b. Ending position

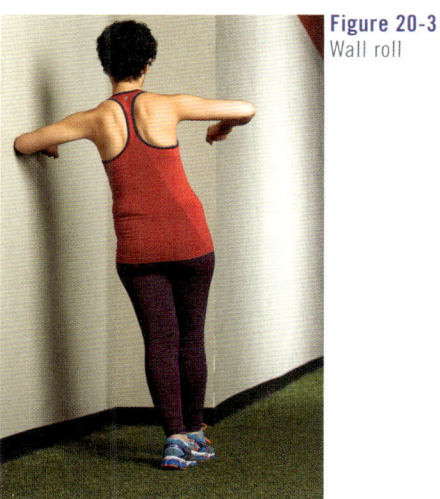

Figure 20-4
Floor-roll and scramble-up exercise

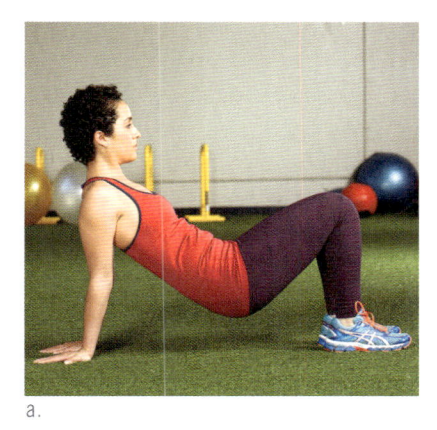

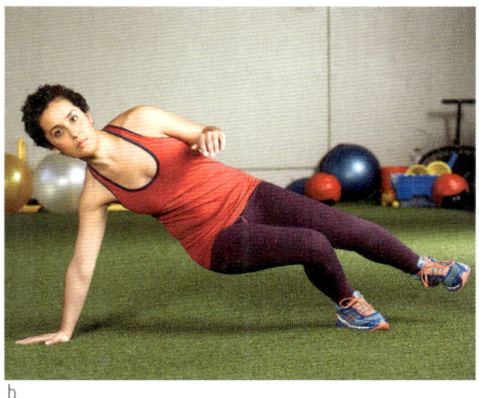

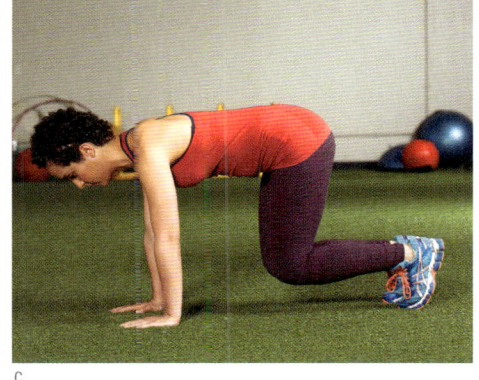

a.   b.   c.

motion (Figures 20-4b & c). A neutral spine should be maintained throughout the floor-roll and scramble-up movements—no spine motion should occur.

A healthy back also requires healthy gluteal muscle function, since the performance and safety of many movements are dependent on balanced hip-power production. The "crossed-pelvis syncrome" is a phenomenon that occurs when the gluteal complex is inhibited during squatting patterns. It is very common in individuals with a history of back problems. Interestingly, it is not known if the crossed-pelvis syndrome exists prior to back problems or is a consequence of having back problems. Regardless of whether the syndrome is a cause or an outcome, individuals with impaired gluteal motor patterns are unable to spare their backs during squatting patterns since they rely on their hamstrings and erector spinae to drive the extension motion. In turn, the erector spinae forces create loads that compress the lumbar spine. It is impossible to achieve optimal squat performance without well-integrated hip-extensor or gluteal patterns. One of the more common reasons individuals fail to properly rehabilitate their backs is due to an emphasis on strength development without first effectively addressing the impaired gluteal patterns.

Retraining of the gluteals cannot be achieved with conventional barbell squat exercises. Performing a conventional squat requires relatively little hip abduction. As a result, gluteus medius activation is minimized and activation of the gluteus maximus is delayed during the traditional barbell squat until lower squat angles are reached. McGill argues, as many other experts do, that the barbell squat is primarily a quadriceps exercise and not a gluteal exercise in the truest sense. Unlike the conventional barbell squat, the single-leg squat elicits almost immediate activation of the gluteus medius and more rapid integration of the gluteus maximus during the squat descent to assist in the **frontal plane** hip drive needed for common activities such as running and jumping.

The CMES should begin by instructing unfit clients to learn how to activate the gluteus medius by performing the clamshell exercise. During the clamshell exercise, the client lies on their side while anchoring the thumb on the anterior superior iliac spine and reaching around with the fingertips, positioning them to land on the gluteus medius. Opening the knees like a clamshell will allow the individual to feel the gluteus medius activation (Figure 20-5).

The single-leg squat matrix is an example of a more advanced corrective exercise for retraining the gluteals. During the single-leg squat matrix progressions with the leg to the front (Figure 20-6a), side (Figure 20-6b), and rear (Figure 20-6c), the abdominals are braced, the lumbar spine is neutral, and the mental focus of the individual should be on the development of hip torque.

Stage 2: Build Whole-body and Joint Stability—The "Big Three"

McGill recommends that after individuals successfully ingrain motion and motor patterns, they should begin focusing on developing whole-body and joint stability. An exercise program consisting of the "big three" (modified curl-ups, side bridge, and bird dog) is an excellent choice for spine stabilization during the early stages of training or rehabilitation and for simply enhancing low-back health.

The modified curl-up is an exercise for the rectus abdominis. In a supine position, the client places the hands or a rolled towel under the lumbar spine and flexes one knee. They then raise the head and shoulders off the floor while maintaining a neutral spine, pause, and then return to the starting position (Figure 20-7). Clients should not flatten the back to the floor, as flattening the back flexes the lumbar spine, eliminates the neutral spine, and increases the loads on the discs and ligaments. By flexing one knee and keeping the other one straight, a neutral lumbar spine is maintained throughout the exercise movement. The bent leg should be alternated midway through each set of repetitions.

The lateral muscles of the torso (quadratus lumborum and abdominal obliques) are important for optimal spinal stability, and are targeted with the side-bridge exercise. The beginner level of this exercise involves bridging the torso between the elbow and the knees (Figure 20-8a). Once this is mastered and well tolerated, the challenge can be increased by bridging between the elbow and the feet (Figure 20-8b). An even more advanced variation involves placing the upper leg and foot in front of the lower leg and foot to facilitate longitudinal "rolling" of the torso (Figures 20-9). This variation is far superior to exercises such as performing a sit-up with a twist because it produces greater levels of muscle activation with lower tissue loads.

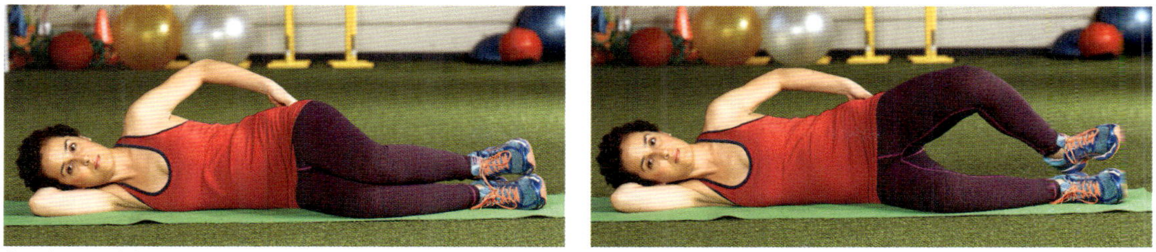

Low-back Pain

CHAPTER 20

Figure 20-5
Clamshell exercise—Beginner-level corrective exercise for retraining the gluteals

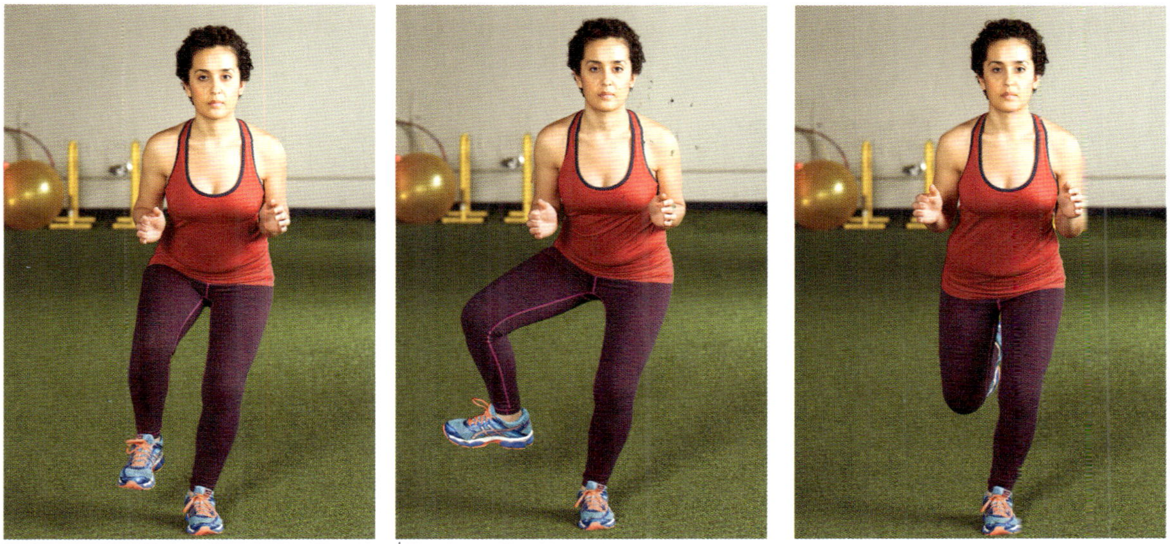

Starting position

Ending position

Figure 20-6
Single-leg squat matrix—Advanced-level corrective exercise for retraining the gluteals

a.

b.

c.

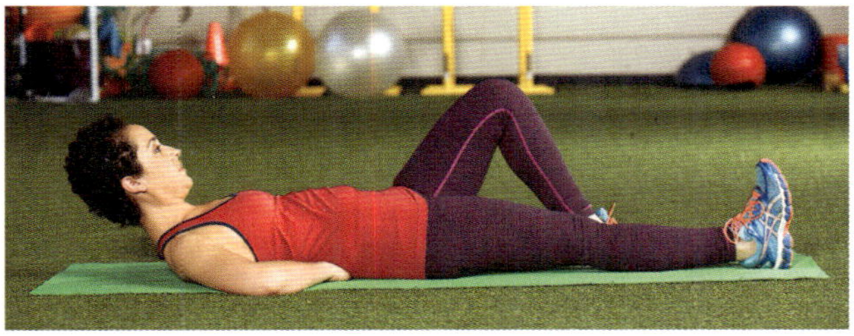

Figure 20-7
Modified curl-up

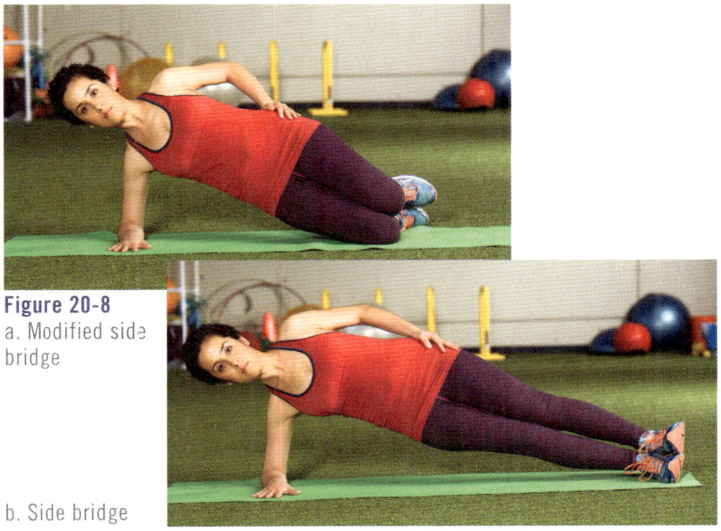

Figure 20-8
a. Modified side bridge

b. Side bridge

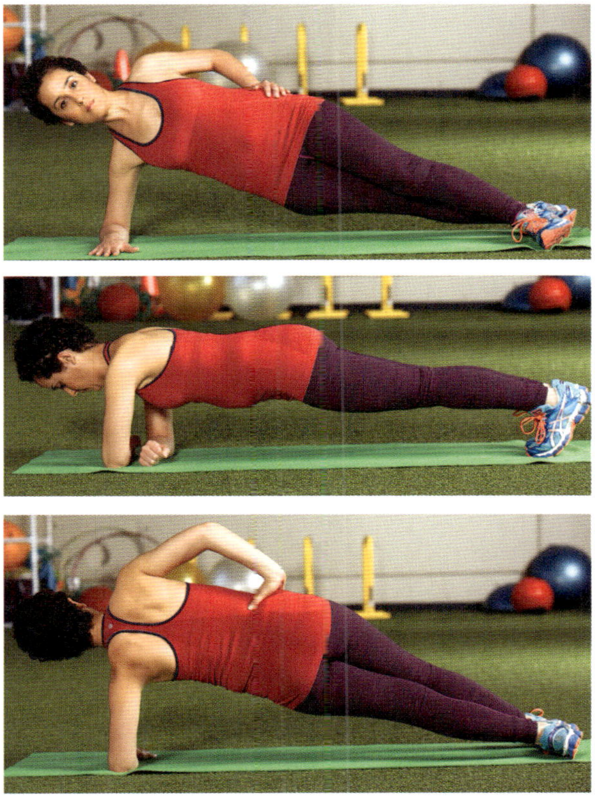

Figure 20-9
Rolling bridge

The bird dog is a safe and effective exercise for developing the spinal extensors. It is performed by extending one leg and the opposite arm, from an all-fours position, so that they are parallel to the floor (Figure 20-10). The extended position should be held for seven to eight seconds, and then repeated with the opposite arm and leg.

More challenging exercise progressions for developing whole-body and joint stability include performing the conventional push-up with a staggered hand placement or with labile surfaces under the hands (Figures 20-11 and 20-12). These advanced exercises facilitate torso stabilization. As with any exercise, abdominal bracing and good torsional control should be maintained throughout the activity.

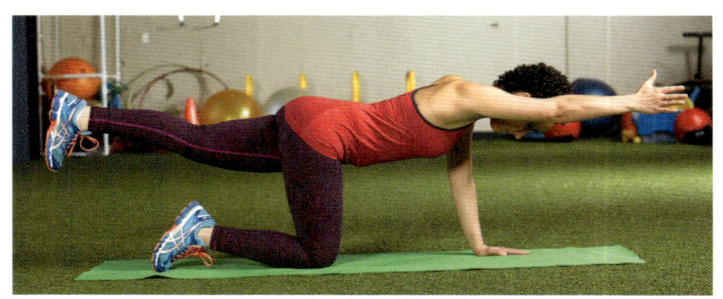

Figure 20-10
Bird dog

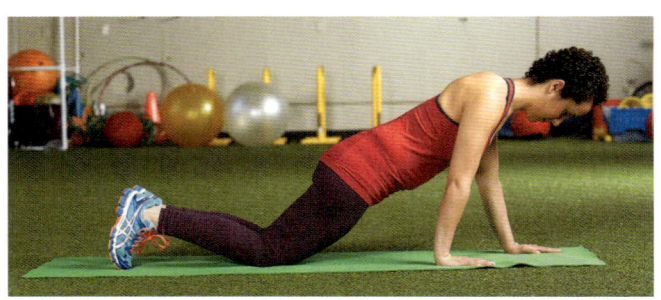

Figure 20-11
Performing the push-up with staggered hand placement (one hand forward of the shoulder and one hand beside the lower ribs) enhances shoulder and abdominal muscle activation, thereby promoting the stabilizing functions of these muscles.

Figure 20-12
Placing both hands on a single BOSU or each hand on a BOSU while performing a push-up significantly enhances the rectus abdominis and internal and external obliques activation on both sides of the torso.

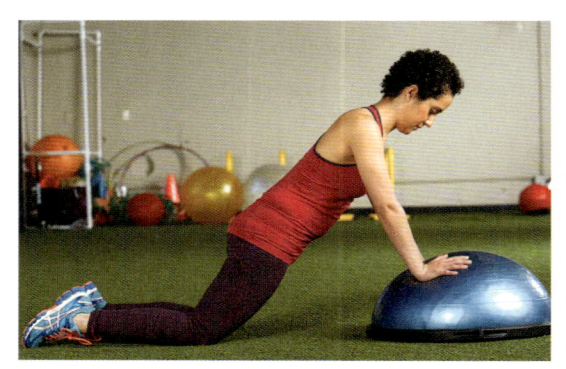

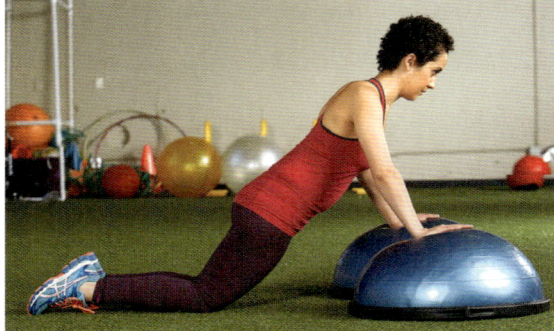

Stage 3: Increase Muscle Endurance

During stage 3, the focus is on improving muscle endurance. Endurance is typically developed first with repeated sets or repetitions of exercises. The client then progresses to longer-duration workouts for an overall increase in total work volume. Endurance progression should generally begin with isometric holds, such as curl-ups, side bridges, and birddog exercises. It is recommended that individuals continue to progress by increasing the number of repetitions completed rather than extending the "hold time."

The "reverse pyramid for endurance training" is an approach to designing endurance sets based on the Russian tradition of maintaining excellent exercise technique and form. For example, an endurance workout involving the side bridge exercise might consist of:
- Five repetitions on the right side followed by five on the left
- Rest
- Four repetitions on the right side followed by four on the left
- Rest
- Three repetitions on the right side followed by three on the left

The basic rationale behind this approach is that the exerciser does as much as possible while they are least fatigued. That is, it is easier to maintain proper exercise technique as the repetitions are reduced with each fatiguing set.

Low-back Pain
CHAPTER 20

Stage 4: Build Strength

The fourth stage in the progression to building the ultimate back emphasizes strength development. Training for maximal back strength without injury is a difficult challenge that requires a delicate balance. A one-size-fits-all recipe for back-strength development does not exist. However, several basic considerations exist for strengthening the back:

- Develop general fitness and balancing ability to train safely and effectively
- Consider the matching of a client's fitness level and motor abilities to the skill demands of the planned training program
- Develop the foundation of proper motor and motion patterns to protect any potential weak links
- Consider the balance of strength around a joint and between adjacent joints, as well as the balance of strength to endurance
- Consider the ROM required by the task and whether the client's motion capability is appropriately matched

Stage 5: Speed, Power, and Agility

Power development represents the fifth and final stage in Dr. McGill's recommended progression to building the ultimate back. Developing spine power can potentially compromise both safety and performance. Power can be defined as both the velocity of force production and the rate of performing work:

POWER EQUATIONS
Power = Force x Velocity
or
Power = Work/Time
Where:
Force = Mass x Acceleration
Velocity = Distance/Time
Work = Force x Distance

Therefore, if either force or velocity is high, then the other should generally be kept low. Power is developed in the extremities and transferred through the torso. Efficient and effective power transfer through the torso requires spine posture control, spine stiffness and stability, and strength.

For clients who have successfully progressed through the first four stages, abdominal plyometric exercises can be incorporated into the training programs to enhance their abilities to effectively and efficiently transfer power through their torsos. The medicine ball toss, performed either while standing or while supine on the floor or a stability ball, is an example of an effective abdominal plyometric exercise that provides excellent progression to power (Figure 20-13).

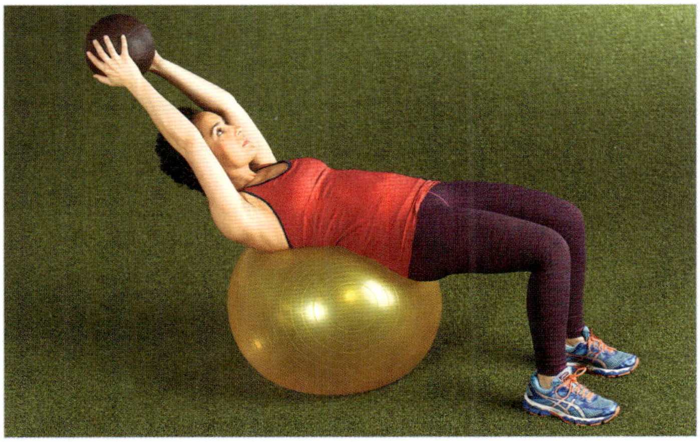

Figure 20-13
Medicine ball toss. The client and CMES softly toss the ball back and forth.

CASE STUDY

Client Information

Amy is a 37-year-old woman with overweight and has chronic low-back pain. She has decided to begin an exercise program to improve her overall fitness and lose weight on the advice of her physician and physical therapist. She has limited experience with exercise programs and has become increasingly inactive due to her low-back pain. Physical therapy reduced her symptoms to localized discomfort and she is afraid of making her back worse again by doing the wrong things at the gym. Amy was released from therapy with a home exercise program that includes supine pelvic tilts, modified curl-ups, several dynamic stabilization exercises (e.g., modified side bridge and modified bird dog), wall squats, hamstring and piriformis stretches, and 10 minutes of cycling. She has hired a CMES to help her achieve her weight-loss goal without exacerbating her low-back pain.

CMES Approach

All the exercises on Amy's home-exercise program are clearly described with illustrations, verbal cues, and intensity and frequency guidelines. Additional programming is developed by the CMES to address Amy's conditioning and weight-loss goals. Amy initially tries cardiorespiratory exercise on a recumbent cycle; however, she reports some increased pain with prolonged sitting. Several other modes of activity are then tested, including stair climbers and elliptical trainers. Treadmill walking on a cushioned deck provides the most comfortable cardiorespiratory exercise for Amy and is chosen as the primary modality. The speed is kept below Amy's stride maximum to ensure that she can maintain postural alignment throughout her workout. Incline is introduced as tolerated by her conditioning as well as her low back.

Amy's home-based exercise program is progressed with the introduction of resistance-training exercises for all major movements. The focus of her resistance training is on improved postural stability, increased muscular fitness, and enhanced caloric expenditure to promote progress toward her weight-loss goal. Initially, resistance is kept low and repetitions are moderate to high due to Amy's deconditioned state and to promote her learning of exercise technique. Supine or standing exercises replace seated exercises whenever possible. In the event that a seated exercise is used, posture is closely monitored. Strengthening of the core muscles is emphasized, along with stability of the lower back. Any complaints of pain, weakness, radicular symptoms, or increased low-back discomfort indicate that a given exercise should be discontinued.

Stretching concentrates on the iliopsoas, hamstrings, piriformis, gluteal complex, quadriceps, and quadratus lumborum.

As Amy progresses, the frequency, intensity, and duration will increase as tolerated. Her low-back comfort is continuously monitored. More functional exercises can be introduced as her fitness improves. Proper exercise technique and postural maintenance are always a critical concern during Amy's workouts.

ACE IFT® MODEL AT A GLANCE

Cardiorespiratory Training

Amy has very little experience with regular exercise and has become increasingly inactive due to her low-back issues. The CMES starts her with a Base Training program focused on moderate-intensity exercise, as tolerated, on a variety of modalities to find the best options for successful exercise and low-back health. While there is no progression to Fitness Training in this case study, that would be the normal progression for Amy as fitness improves and her low-back stability and health improve.

Muscular Training

The CMES implements a post-rehabilitative exercise program that builds directly on the work that Amy did with her physical therapist. The program is focused primarily on Functional Training exercises, with additional exercises focused on proper movement patterns (Movement Training) introduced as she progresses. The seated-to-standing progression allows Amy to safely progress from segmental to full-kinetic-chain exercises. Whether Amy progresses to Load/Speed Training will depend on her success with the program and the response of her lower back.

SUMMARY

LBP is a significant source of cost and disability, as more than 80% of Americans suffer from at least one episode of back pain during their lifetimes. A significant proportion of these individuals seek assistance from a healthcare professional. While the majority of acute back pain improves over time, some people develop recurrences, and still others experience continuous pain. The onset and persistence of LBP is related to individual, activity, and psychological factors.

Mechanical causes account for the majority of LBP cases. Discogenic pain can be attributed to conditions such as a herniated disc, sciatica, spinal stenosis, spondylolysis, and spondylolisthesis. Treatment options for individuals with LBP have evolved and, in some cases, become a source of much debate. However, for almost all conditions, current thinking among health professionals is one of active recovery. Remaining physically active is a central focus in the treatment of LBP.

The back is a very unique and complex structure involving a flexible column with complex muscle and ligamentous support. The spine contains the spinal cord and lateral nerve roots, and musculature intimately involved in several other functions (e.g., breathing mechanics). Many of the traditional approaches used to train other joints in the body are not appropriate for the back—either they fail to produce positive results or they result in injury. The CMES can play a vital role in the prevention of LBP and maintenance of back health through designing evidence-based exercise programs that address the important structures and functions of the spine.

REFERENCES

Amorin-Woods, L.G. et al. (2014). Adherence to clinical practice guidelines among three primary contact professions: A best evidence synthesis of the literature for the management of acute and subacute low back pain. *Journal of the Canadian Chiropractic Association,* 58, 3, 220–237.

Axler, C. & McGill, S.M. (1997). Low back loads over a variety of abdominal exercises: Searching for the safest abdominal challenge. *Medicine & Science in Sports & Exercise,* 29, 6, 804–811.

Bahr, R. et al. (2004). Low back pain among endurance athletes with and without specific back loading: A cross-sectional survey of cross country skiers, rowers, orienteers, and nonathletic controls. *Spine,* 29, 449–454.

Baranto, A. et al. (2009). Back pain and MRI changes in the thoraco-lumbar spine of top athletes in four different sports: A 15-year follow-up study. *Knee Surgery, Sports Traumatology, Arthroscopy,* 17, 9, 1125–1134. DOI: 10.1007/s00167-009-0767-3

Biering-Sorensen, F. (1984). Physical measurements as risk indicators for low-back trouble over a one-year period. *Spine,* 9, 106–119.

Borenstein, D., Wiesel, S., & Boeden, S. (2004). *Low Back and Neck Pain: Comprehensive Diagnosis and Management* (3rd Ed.). Philadelphia: Elsevier.

Centers for Disease Control and Prevention (2020a). *Acute Low Back Pain.* www.cdc.gov/acute-pain/low-back-pain/index.html#:~:text=25%25%20of%20U.S.%20adults%20report,back%20pain%2C%20were%20prescribed%20opioids

Centers for Disease Control and Prevention (2020b). *Smoking and Tobacco Use: Fast Facts.* www.cdc.gov/tobacco/data_statistics/fact_sheets/fast_facts/index.htm

Cheung, K.M. et al. (2009). Prevalence and pattern of lumbar magnetic resonance imaging changes in a population study of one thousand forty-three individuals. *Spine,* 34, 934–940.

Chimenti, R.L. Scholtes, S.A., & Van Dillen, L.R. (2013). Activity characteristics and movement patterns in people with and people without low back pain who participate in rotation-related sports. *Journal of Sport Rehabilitation,* 22, 3, 161–169.

Dagenais, S., Caro, J., & Haldeman, S. (2008). A systematic review of low back pain cost of illness studies in the United States and internationally. *The Spine Journal,* 8, 1, 8–20.

Darlow, B. et al. (2013). The enduring impact of what clinicians say to people with low back pain. *Annals of Family Medicine,* 11, 6, 527–534. DOI: 10.1370/afm.1518

Darlow, B. et al. (2012). The association between health care professional attitudes and beliefs and the attitudes and beliefs, clinical management, and outcomes of patients with low back pain: A systematic review. *European Journal of Pain,* 16, 1, 3–17.

Deyo, R.A. & Weinstein, J.N. (2001). Primary care: Low back pain. *New England Journal of Medicine,* 344, 363–370.

Ditre, J.W. et al. (2011). Pain, nicotine, and smoking: Research findings and mechanistic considerations. *Psychological Bulletin,* 137, 6, 1065–1093. DOI: 10.1037/a0025544

Dupeyron, A. et al. (2011). Education in the management of low back pain: Literature review and recall of key recommendations for practice. *Annals of Physical and Rehabilitative Medicine,* 54, 5, 319–335. DOI: 10.1016/j.rehab.2011.06.001

Fejer, R. & Leboeuf-Yde, C. (2012). Does back and neck pain become more common as you get older? A systematic literature review. *Chiropractic and Manual Therapy,* 20, 1, 24. DOI: 10.1186/2045-709X-20-24

Franke, H., Franke, J.D., & Fryer, G. (2014). Osteopathic manipulative treatment for nonspecific low back pain: A systematic review and meta-analysis. *BMC Musculoskeletal Disorders,* 30, 15, 286. DOI: 10.1186/1471-2474-15-286

Garet, M. et al. (2013). Nonoperative treatment in lumbar spondylolysis and spondylolisthesis: A systematic review. *Sports Health,* 5, 3, 225–232. DOI: 10.1177/1941738113480936

George, S.Z. et al. (2011). Depressive symptoms, anatomical region, and clinical outcomes for patients seeking outpatient physical therapy for musculoskeletal pain. *Physical Therapy,* 91, 3, 358–372. DOI: 10.2522/ptj.20100192

Goertz, M. et al. (2012). *Adult Acute and Subacute Low Back Pain. Institute for Clinical Systems Improvement.* www.icsi.org/_asset/bjvqrj/LBP.pdf

Griffith, L.E. et al. (2012). Individual participant data meta-analysis of mechanical workplace risk factors and low back pain. *American Journal of Public Health,* 102, 2, 309–318. DOI: 10.2105/AJPH.2011.300343

Ha, J.Y. et al. (2011). Factors associated with depressive symptoms in patients with chronic low back pain. *Annals of Rehabilitative Medicine,* 35, 5, 710–718. DOI: 10.5535/arm.2011.35.5.710

Han, S. et al. (2011). Percutaneous vertebroplasty versus balloon kyphoplasty for treatment of osteoporotic vertebral compression fracture: A meta-analysis of randomised and non-randomised controlled trials. *International Orthopaedics,* 35, 9, 1349–1358. DOI: 10.1007/s00264-011-1283-x

Hancock, M.J. et al. (2011). Discussion paper: What happened to the 'bio' in the bio-psycho-social model of low back pain? *European Spine Journal,* 20, 12, 2105–2110. DOI: 10.1007/s00586-011-1886-3

Heneweer, H. et al. (2011). Physical activity and low back pain: A systematic review of recent literature. *European Spine Journal,* 20, 6, 826–845. DOI: 10.1007/s00586-010-1680-7

Hodges, P.W. & Richardson, C.A. (1996). Inefficient muscular stabilization of the lumbar spine associated with low back pain. *Spine,* 21, 2640–2650.

Hoy, D. et al. (2010). The epidemiology of low back pain. *Best Practice and Research: Clinical Rheumatology,* 24, 6, 769–781. DOI: 10.1016/j.berh.2010.10.002

Iles, R.A. et al. (2009). Systematic review of the ability of recovery expectations to predict outcomes in non-chronic non-specific low back pain. *Journal of Occupational Rehabilitation,* 19, 1, 25–40.

Ivanova, J.I. et al. (2011). Real-world practice patterns, health-care utilization, and costs in patients with low back pain: The long road to guideline-concordant care. *The Spine Journal,* 11, 7, 622–632.

Jordan, J., Konstantinou, K., & O'Dowd, J. (2011). Herniated lumbar disc. *Clinical Evidence (Online),* June 28.

Leeuw, M. et al. (2007). The fear-avoidance model of musculoskeletal pain: Current state of scientific evidence. *Journal of Behavioral Medicine,* 30, 77–94.

Lemeunier, N., Leboeuf-Yde, C., & Gagey, O. (2012). The natural course of low back pain: A systematic critical literature review. *Chiropractic and Manual Therapies,* 20, 1, 33. DOI: 10.1186/2045-709X-20-33

Luoto, S. et al. (1995). Static back endurance and the risk of low back pain. *Clinical Biomechanics,* 10, 323–324.

Macedo, L.G. et al. (2013). Physical therapy interventions for degenerative lumbar spinal stenosis: A systematic review. *Physical Therapy,* 93, 12, 1646–1660. DOI: 10.2522/ptj.20120379

Mafi, J.N. et al. (2013). Worsening trends in the management and treatment of back treatment trends. *JAMA Internal Medicine,* 173, 17, 1573–1581.

McGill, S. (2017). *Ultimate Back Fitness and Performance* (6th ed.). Gravenhurst, Ont.: Backfitpro Inc.

McGill, S. (2016). *Low Back Disorders* (3rd ed.). Champaign, Ill.: Human Kinetics.

Morris, C. (2006). *Low Back Syndromes.* New York: McGraw-Hill.

Petering, R.C. & Webb, C. (2011). Treatment options for low back pain in athletes. *Sports Health,* 3, 6, 550–555. DOI: 10.1177/1941738111416446

Rubin, D. (2007). Epidemiology and risk factors for spine pain. *Neurologic Clinics,* 25, 353–371.

Saal, J.A. & Saal, J.S. (1989). Nonoperative treatment of herniated lumbar intervertebral disc with radiculopathy: An outcome study. *Journal of Biomechanics,* 14, 431–437.

Scott, N., Moga, C., & Harstall, C. (2010). Managing low back pain in the primary care setting: The know-do gap. *Pain Research & Management,* 15, 6, 392.

Seco, J., Kovacs, F.M., & Urrutia, G. (2011). The efficacy, safety, effectiveness, and cost-effectiveness of ultrasound and shock wave therapies for low back pain: A systematic review. *The Spine Journal,* 11, 10, 966–977.

Shiri, R. et al. (2010). The association between smoking and low back pain: A meta-analysis. *American Journal of Medicine,* 123, 1, 87.e7–87.e35.

Sloan, T.J. et al. (2008). Beliefs about the causes and consequences of pain in patients with chronic inflammatory or noninflammatory low back pain and in pain-free individuals. *Spine,* 33, 9, 966–972.

Stanton, T.R. et al. (2010). How do we define the condition 'recurrent low back pain'? A systematic review. *European Spine Journal,* 20, 533–539. DOI: 10.1007/s00586-009-1214-3

Valat, J.P. et al. (2010). Sciatica. *Best Practice and Research: Clinical Rheumatology,* 4, 241–252. DOI: 10.1016/j.berh.2009.11.005

Valencia, C., Robinson, M.E., & George, S.Z. (2011). Socioeconomic status influences the relationship between fear-avoidance beliefs work and disability. *Pain Medicine,* 12, 2, 328–336. DOI: 10.1111/j.1526-4637.2010.01024.x

Walker, B.F. (2000). The prevalence of low back pain: A systematic review of the literature from 1966 to 1998. *Journal of Spinal Disorders,* 13, 205–217. DOI: 10.1097/00002517-200006000-00003

Wong, D. & Transfeltd, E. (2007). *Macnab's Backache* (4th ed.). Philadelphia: Lippincott Williams & Wilkins.

SUGGESTED READING

Amorin-Woods, L.G. et al. (2014). Adherence to clinical practice guidelines among three primary contact professions: A best evidence synthesis of the literature for the management of acute and subacute low back pain. *Journal of the Canadian Chiropractic Association,* 58, 3, 220–237.

Darlow, B. et al. (2013). The enduring impact of what clinicians say to people with low back pain. *Annals of Family Medicine,* 11, 6, 527–534. DOI: 10.1370/afm.1518

Lemeunier, N., Leboeuf-Yde, C., & Gagey, O. (2012). The natural course of low back pain: A systematic critical literature review. *Chiropractic and Manual Therapies,* 20, 1, 33. DOI: 10.1186/2045-709X-20-33

Petering, R.C. & Webb, C. (2011). Treatment options for low back pain in athletes. *Sports Health,* 3, 6, 550–555. DOI: 10.1177/1941738111416446

PART VI
PERINATAL CONSIDERATIONS

CHAPTER 21
PRENATAL AND POSTPARTUM EXERCISE

21 PRENATAL AND POSTPARTUM EXERCISE

IN THIS CHAPTER

EXERCISE DURING PREGNANCY
PHYSICAL-ACTIVITY PARTICIPATION RATES
MATERNAL FITNESS

SPECIAL CONSIDERATIONS
GESTATIONAL DIABETES MELLITUS
PREECLAMPSIA
MATERNAL OBESITY

MATERNAL EXERCISE AND THE FETAL RESPONSE
CONTRAINDICATIONS AND RISK FACTORS

PHYSIOLOGICAL CHANGES DURING PREGNANCY
MUSCULOSKELETAL SYSTEM
CARDIOVASCULAR SYSTEM
RESPIRATORY SYSTEM
THERMOREGULATORY SYSTEM

PROGRAMMING GUIDELINES AND CONSIDERATIONS FOR PRENATAL EXERCISE

BIOMECHANICAL CONSIDERATIONS DURING PREGNANCY
LOW-BACK AND POSTERIOR PELVIC GIRDLE PAIN
PUBIC PAIN
CARPAL TUNNEL SYNDROME
DIASTASIS RECTI
STRESS URINARY INCONTINENCE

EXERCISE TECHNIQUES FOR PREGNANT WOMEN
LOWER-EXTREMITY EXERCISES
UPPER-EXTREMITY EXERCISES
CORE EXERCISES
STRETCHES

NUTRITIONAL CONSIDERATIONS
NUTRITION FOR LACTATION

PSYCHOLOGICAL CONSIDERATIONS

POSTPARTUM EXERCISE

PHYSIOLOGICAL CHANGES FOLLOWING PREGNANCY

PROGRAMMING GUIDELINES AND CONSIDERATIONS FOR POSTPARTUM EXERCISE
EXERCISE CONSIDERATIONS FOR THE LACTATING MOTHER

EXERCISE GUIDELINES SUMMARY FOR PRENATAL CLIENTS

CASE STUDY

SUMMARY

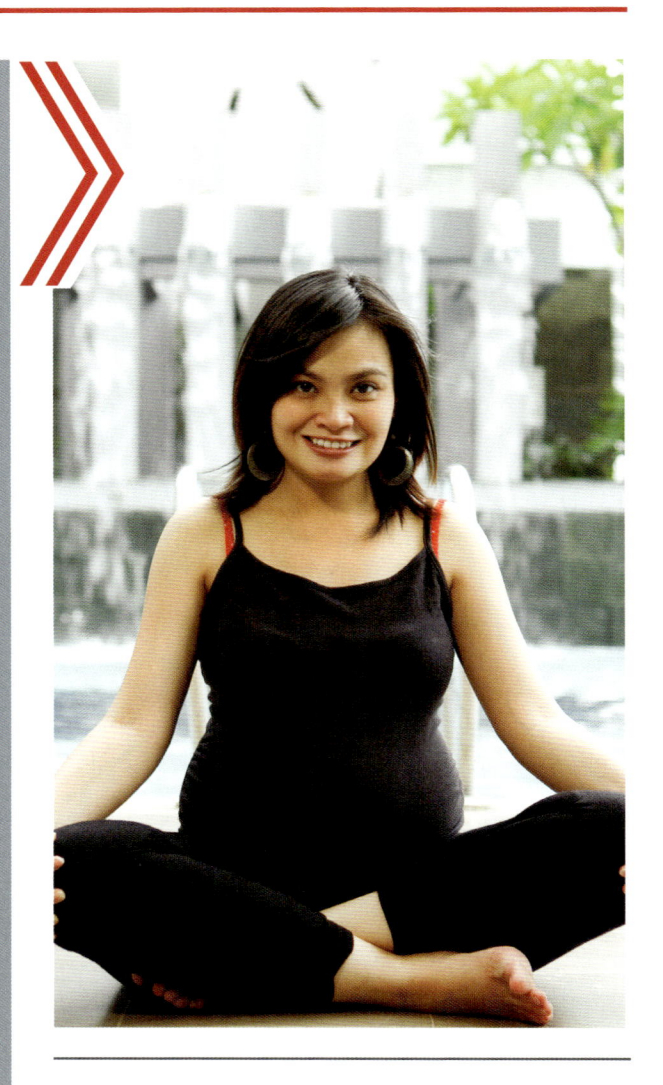

ABOUT THE AUTHOR
Sabrena Jo, MS, is the Director of Science and Research for the American Council on Exercise and ACE Liaison to the Scientific Advisory Panel. Jo has been actively involved in the fitness industry since 1987. As an ACE Certified Group Fitness Instructor, Personal Trainer, and Health Coach, she has taught group exercise and owned her own personal-training and health-coaching businesses and is a relentless pursuer of finding ways to help people start and stick with physical activity. Jo is a former full-time faculty member in the Kinesiology and Physical Education Department at California State University, Long Beach. She has a bachelor's degree in exercise science, a master's degree in physical education/biomechanics, and is pursuing a PhD in exercise psychology from the University of Kansas.

By Sabrena Jo

RESEARCH ESTABLISHING THE HEALTH BENEFITS of regular exercise has prompted healthcare professionals to broadly recommend physical activity as a component of a healthy lifestyle across the lifespan.

Although exercise during pregnancy was once discouraged by the medical community, it is now recommended as an important part of a healthy pregnancy and postpartum period. In fact, the U.S. Department of Health & Human Services (2018) recommends that during pregnancy and the postpartum period healthy women with uncomplicated pregnancies should engage in 150 minutes of moderate-intensity aerobic activity spread throughout the week. In addition, the American College of Obstetricians and Gynecologist (ACOG, 2020) recommends 30 to 60 minutes of moderate-intensity exercise on at least three to four days per week and up to daily. Interestingly, physical inactivity during pregnancy has now been shown to be an independent risk factor for maternal **obesity, gestational diabetes mellitus (GDM),** and pregnancy-related complications (ACOG, 2020). Similarly, the Society of Obstetricians and Gynecologists of Canada (SOGC), the Canadian Society for Exercise Physiology (CSEP), and the UK Chief Medical Officers currently recommend regular exercise for pregnant women based on maximal heart rate target zones and the talk test (SOCG/CSEP, 2018; UK Chief Medical Officers, 2019). As research in obstetrics has evolved, an historical perceived increased risk of preterm delivery and fetal growth impediment associated with women who exercise during pregnancy (Clapp & Capeless, 1990; Launer et al., 1990) has given way to physicians recommending regular physical activity to all healthy women during pregnancy, even to those who, at time of conception, were **sedentary.**

This chapter presents the current knowledge on exercise training during pregnancy, including the risks and benefits of regular physical activity, nutritional and psychological considerations, and exercise programming guidelines. Postpartum fitness concerns are also covered.

EXERCISE DURING PREGNANCY

For healthy pregnant women, physical activity is a safe and effective way of reducing adverse health risks. Expectant mothers can maintain or even improve cardiovascular and muscular fitness. Additionally, regular exercise is associated with reduced rates of **preeclampsia**, length of labor and postpartum recovery, gestational hypertension, postpartum depression, GDM, **Cesarean birth,** excessive gestational weight gain, and other pregnancy-related complications (ACOG, 2020; U.S. Department of Health & Human Services, 2018).

Physical-activity Participation Rates

With increased attention given to the health benefits of exercise in the past two decades, along with recommendations by physicians for all adults to engage in regular physical activity, the number of active pregnant women is on the rise. Although estimates show that between 42% and 66% of pregnant women engage in some form of regular leisure-time physical activity, less than 20% adhere to a physician-recommended level of exercise (Shivakumar et al., 2011; Evenson, Savitz, & Huston, 2004) and physical-activity participation is often lower in pregnant women than in the general population. Cross-sectional population studies using self-report measures of physical activity across the United Kingdom and United States estimate that only 3 to 15% of pregnant women were meeting current guidelines, compared with 24 to 26% of non-pregnant women (Currie et

LEARNING OBJECTIVES:

» Describe the research pertaining to both the mother and fetus relating to exercise during pregnancy and the postpartum period.

» List the benefits and potential risks for exercise during pregnancy for both the mother and unborn baby.

» Explain the important physiological and biomechanical changes that occur in the course of a woman's pregnancy and how those changes affect the performance of exercise.

» Describe basic nutritional requirements for pregnancy and the postpartum period.

» Give basic information on the psychological changes that may occur during pregnancy and the postpartum period and how exercise might play a role in relieving psychological symptoms.

» Explain the important physiological and biomechanical changes that occur during the postpartum period and how those changes affect the performance of exercise.

» Design and implement a safe and effective prenatal and postpartum exercise program.

al., 2013). Given the current epidemic of obesity and its associated comorbidities, as well as the apparent health risks of not exercising, exercise professionals who are competent to work with this population can provide safe and effective exercise programming to promote a healthy pregnancy, as well as healthy prenatal and postpartum lifestyles.

Maternal Fitness

Healthy women who consistently exercise throughout their non-complicated pregnancies can maintain or improve overall fitness and cardiovascular function and promote muscular endurance and strength (Sui & Dodd, 2013; Kawabata et al., 2012). Over time, they also gain less weight [7.5 vs 21.8 lb (3.4 vs. 9.9 kg)], deposit less fat [4.8 vs. 14.7 lb (2.2 vs. 6.7 kg)], have increased fitness, and have a lower cardiovascular risk profile than those who discontinue exercise (Clapp, 2008). Further, women who continue weight-bearing exercise (e.g., running and dance aerobics) during pregnancy tend to maintain their long-term fitness and have a low cardiovascular risk profile in the **perimenopausal** period (Clapp, 2008).

SPECIAL CONSIDERATIONS

Although exercise during pregnancy and the postpartum period can be an effective health-promoting activity, there are certain conditions to consider that may pose additional stress on the pregnant mother. Gestational diabetes, preeclampsia, and maternal obesity are potential complicating factors that could influence the course of a prenatal exercise program.

Gestational Diabetes Mellitus

Glucose intolerance that is first recognized or diagnosed during pregnancy and usually resolves not long after delivery is called GDM. Maternal muscular **insulin resistance** is a normal response to hormonal adaptations that occur to ensure adequate glucose regulation for fetal growth and development. In women with GDM, this **insulin** increase is exacerbated, resulting in maternal **hyperglycemia.** In the third trimester, a healthy pregnant woman has to increase her insulin secretion by two to four times to maintain glucose levels within normal limits. Pregnant women who develop GDM are unable to enhance insulin production to compensate for their increased resistance to insulin (Golbidi & Laher, 2013).

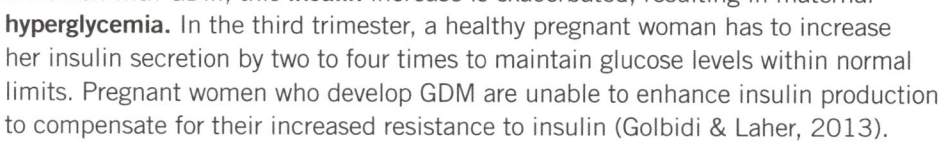

Of the nearly 4 million women who give birth each year in the United States, approximately 6 to 9% develop GDM [Centers for Disease Control and Prevention (CDC), 2018]. The condition is increasing as obesity and older age at pregnancy become more common. Other risk factors include having a family history of **type 2 diabetes** or belonging to an ethnic group at increased risk for the condition (such as African American, Hispanic/Latino American, American Indian, Alaska Native, Native Hawaiian, or Pacific Islander). Women with GDM are at higher risk for gestational **hypertension,** preeclampsia, and Cesarean birth, and have a 50% increased risk of developing type 2 diabetes later in life (CDC, 2019; ACOG, 2020).

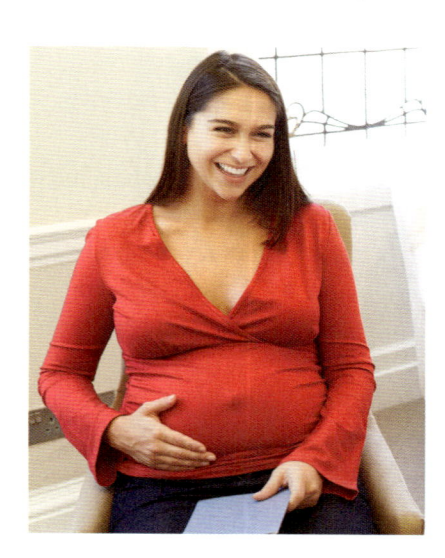

Once diagnosed, women with GDM are primarily treated through nutritional management by a **registered dietitian,** along with moderate-intensity exercise as an adjunct therapy (CDC, 2019). The American Diabetes Association suggests that women diagnosed with GDM should perform either aerobic or resistance exercise to improve insulin action and glycemic control. In addition, it is also recommended that women with overweight or obesity may benefit from vigorous-intensity exercise during pregnancy to reduce the risk of excess gestational weight gain (Colberg et al., 2016). Participation in regular physical activity also appears to have a protective effect against the development of GDM, as the available evidence suggests that women who exercise have a considerably lower chance of developing it (Golbidi & Laher, 2013). Preliminary studies have found that women who participated in any type of recreational activity within the first 20 weeks of gestation decreased their risk of GDM by almost half (Golbidi & Laher, 2013; Dempsey et al., 2004). Other data suggests that women who engage in intense physical activity before pregnancy have a 44% and 24% risk reduction for GDM and abnormal glucose tolerance, respectively (Oken et al., 2006). GDM itself is not considered a contraindication for exercise during pregnancy, and all women without contraindications are encouraged to be physically active throughout pregnancy in consultation with their healthcare provider [American College of Sports Medicine (ACSM), 2022].

Preeclampsia

Affecting 3 to 4% of all pregnancies worldwide, preeclampsia is a serious maternal-fetal syndrome that is usually diagnosed after 20 weeks of gestation and characterized by persistent hypertension (>140/90 mmHg) and **proteinuria** (24-hour urinary protein level ≥300 mg). Risk factors include primiparity (first pregnancy), previous preeclampsia, increased maternal **body mass index (BMI)** before pregnancy, ethnicity (black women are more at risk), multiple gestations, and underlying medical conditions such as renal disease and diabetes (Trogstad, Magnus, & Stoltenberg, 2011). Complications associated with preeclampsia include premature delivery and fetal growth retardation and death. Treatment of severe hypertension is necessary to prevent cerebrovascular, cardiac, and renal complications in the mother. Currently, the only definitive treatment of preeclampsia is delivery (Brown & Garovic, 2011).

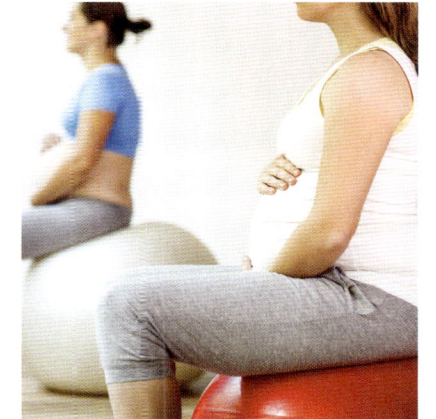

A review of the literature examining physical activity and preeclampsia risk reveals several epidemiological studies indicating that regular leisure-time physical activity in early pregnancy is associated with a reduced incidence of preeclampsia (Weissgerber et al., 2004). Several protective mechanisms associated with exercise are thought to play a role in preeclampsia prevention, including enhanced placental growth and vascularity, enhanced antioxidant defense systems, reduction of the systemic inflammatory response, and improved endothelial function (Weissgerber et al., 2006). However, at present there is insufficient evidence from randomized trials evaluating aerobic exercise in healthy pregnant women and in women at increased risk of preeclampsia (Moura et al., 2012).

Early-onset preeclampsia (less than 34 weeks) requires careful administration of antihypertensive medications, bed rest, and in-hospital monitoring of both the mother and fetus (Mustafa et al., 2012; Turner, 2010). Exercise in women with high-risk pregnancy conditions, such as preeclampsia, should be closely monitored and supervised by their physicians in a clinical setting, as these situations are outside the **scope of practice** for an ACE Certified Medical Exercise Specialist (CMES).

Maternal Obesity

With the World Health Organization (WHO) estimating that 1.4 billion adults have overweight and 500,000 have obesity, maternal obesity—both prior to conception and throughout pregnancy—is an increasing public health concern (WHO, 2013). Some estimates have shown that 20% of Americans have obesity at the start of pregnancy, representing a 70% increase over the course of a decade (Nelson, Matthews, & Poston, 2010). Estimates suggest the prevalence of obesity in pregnancy in the UK is at least 20%, with 5% having severe or extreme obesity (Oteng-Ntim et al., 2012). Maternal **overweight** and obesity is associated with numerous adverse maternal and neonatal outcomes, including GDM, hypertensive disease (including preeclampsia), **thromboembolism,** infection, C-section, congenital fetal anomalies, **macrosomia** (excessive birth weight), induction, stillbirth, shoulder dystocia (delivery in which the fetal anterior shoulder gets caught in the birth canal), and preterm delivery (Oteng-Ntim et al., 2012).

The extent to which being physically active during pregnancy affects maternal body weight in women who have obesity remains unclear. Physical activity, along with healthy lifestyle modification, during pregnancy is encouraged for women with overweight and obesity. Women with obesity during pregnancy are encouraged to start low and slow when it comes to exercise intensity and to gradually increase duration and intensity when able to do so. Research suggests that there are no adverse outcomes for exercise during pregnancy in women with obesity (ACOG, 2020). Women who are pregnant and have extreme or severe obesity should consult their physicians before beginning an exercise program (ACSM, 2022). The CMES should follow the client's physician recommendations for physical activity when developing exercise programs for pregnant women who have obesity to ensure that the exercise takes into account any comorbidities, symptoms, and physical-fitness level.

EXPAND YOUR KNOWLEDGE

GESTATIONAL WEIGHT GAIN PREDICTS LONG-TERM OBESITY

Maternal obesity prior to becoming pregnant is a public health concern. In addition, the impact of excessive weight gain during pregnancy has significant health consequences. In their 2009 report on revised guidelines for weight gain during pregnancy, the Institute of Medicine (IOM) stated, "Women today are heavier; a greater percentage of them are entering pregnancy with overweight or obesity, and many are gaining too much weight during pregnancy." Importantly, excessive weight gain in pregnancy is a predictor of long-term obesity that has far-reaching effects for mothers and their children.

A certain amount of weight gain during pregnancy is normal and required to promote fetal growth. In general, healthy gestational weight gain can be broken down as follows: approximately 27% resides in the fetus; 20% includes the placenta, amniotic fluid, and uterus; 3% comprises breast weight; 23% is related to blood volume and extravascular fluid; and the remaining 27% consists of maternal fat stores (IOM, 2009). The IOM recommends that normal-weight women should gain between 25 and 35 lb (11.4 and 15.9 kg) during pregnancy, while pregnant women who have overweight should gain between 15 and 25 lb (6.8 and 11.4 kg) (Table 21-1) (IOM, 2009). Weight gains within these guidelines are associated with healthy fetal and maternal outcomes, such that weight gains below these goals are associated with low infant birth-weight, and higher gains are associated with fetal macrosomia, which is associated with increased risks of C-section, trauma to the birth canal and the fetus, and risk of other pregnancy complications (IOM, 2009).

TABLE 21-1
INSTITUTE OF MEDICINE'S RECOMMENDATIONS FOR WEIGHT GAIN DURING PREGNANCY

Pre-pregnancy Weight	BMI (kg/m^2)	Total Weight Gain Range
Underweight	<18.5	28–40 lb (13–18 kg)
Normal weight	18.5–24.9	25–35 lb (11–16 kg)
Overweight	25.0–29.9	15–25 lb (7–11 kg)
Obese	≥30.0	11–20 lb (5–9 kg)

Data from: Institute of Medicine (2009). *Weight Gain During Pregnancy: Reexamining the Guidelines* Washington, D.C.: National Academies Press.

When it comes to gestational weight gain, excessive gain is more common than inadequate gain (Olson, 2008). Women who gain more than the recommended gestational increase are at risk for retaining more weight after pregnancy than women who gain within the recommendations. Further compounding this problem is evidence demonstrating that women who have overweight or obesity are nearly two times more likely to exceed IOM recommended gains compared to normal-weight women (Herring, Rose, & Oken, 2012). Obesity aside, even normal-weight women who gain excessive gestational weight tend to retain extra pounds. Nelson, Matthews, and Poston (2010) have reported that mothers with large gestational weight gains experience increased postpartum weight retention, which is maintained up to three years after pregnancy, independent of pre-pregnancy BMI. In one observational study, Fraser et al. (2011) reported women with average gains of 38.9 lb vs. 28.8 lb (17.7 kg vs. 13.1 kg) had higher BMI and more central adiposity that persisted 16 years after the referenced pregnancy, even after adjusting for parity, total caloric intake, physical activity, smoking, breastfeeding, and pre-pregnancy BMI. Further, mothers who gain excess weight during pregnancy have been found to have children at higher risk for having overweight in early childhood, during adolescence, and as adults (Herring, Rose, & Oken, 2012).

A CMES can be a valuable resource for pregnant women who are seeking safe and effective exercise programs to perform during the prenatal period. Although definitive research on the effects of physical activity in limiting excess gestational weight gain is lacking, the numerous benefits of exercise during pregnancy as described in this chapter can contribute to improved health of the mother and the fetus. In their extensive literature review on aerobic training during pregnancy, which included 1,177 subjects from 11 studies, Lamina and Agbanusi concluded that the regular practice of aerobic exercise by active, low-risk, and previously sedentary expectant mothers has a beneficial effect on maternal weight gain in pregnancy (Lamina & Agbanusi, 2013). Currently, however, meta-analyses of randomized trials indicate that while prenatal exercise interventions do not appear to be associated with harm, they have only a moderate effect on limiting gestational weight gain (Sui & Dodd, 2013). More investigation into the precise exercise programming guidelines for healthy weight gain during pregnancy needs to be conducted.

Obesity among pregnant women is highly prevalent and is associated with a markedly increased risk of adverse outcomes for both mother and infant. Although excessive gestational weight gain is associated with long-term obesity, the CMES should keep in mind that pregnancy is not a time for weight loss, as a certain amount of weight gain is necessary for the health of the fetus.

MATERNAL EXERCISE AND THE FETAL RESPONSE

In uncomplicated pregnancies, fetal injuries are highly unlikely, as most of the potential fetal risks are hypothetical. However, there are several areas of theoretical concern surrounding maternal exercise and its effects on the fetus. First, the selective redistribution of blood flow away from the fetus during regular or prolonged exercise in pregnancy may interfere with the transplacental transport of oxygen, carbon dioxide, and nutrients. To address this concern, experts have recommended aquatic exercise as a favorable mode of aerobic training during pregnancy. The hydrostatic pressure due to immersion in water can potentially decrease maternal edema and blood pressure, while maintaining uterine and placental blood flow (da Silva et al., 2013).

A second concern is that during exercise, transient **hypoxia** could result in fetal **tachycardia** and an increase in fetal blood pressure. These responses are protective mechanisms that occur during obstetric events and allow the fetus to facilitate the transfer of oxygen and decrease the carbon dioxide tension across the placenta. However, there are no reports to link such adverse events with maternal exercise. A review of a majority of studies examining fetal responses to exercise indicates that exercise during pregnancy causes "no harm" to several pregnancy outcomes, including rate of preterm delivery, birth weight, or early pregnancy loss (U.S. Department of Health & Human Services, 2018). Subsequent data has shown that both moderate- and vigorous-intensity exercise [i.e., 40 to 59% of **heart-rate reserve (HRR)** and 60 to 89% HRR, respectively] is well tolerated by both the mother and the fetus, as indicated by a variety of commonly used tests of fetal well-being (e.g., umbilical artery Doppler indices, fetal heart tracing, and fetal **heart rate**) (Szymanski & Satin, 2012).

A third concern is intrauterine growth restriction due to strenuous physical activity. Studies on the effect of exercise during pregnancy and resultant birth weights are inconclusive. It has been reported that pregnant women who participated in moderate-to-high intensity occupational physical activities had a higher risk of intrauterine growth restriction than women who participated in low-intensity activities (Spinillo et al., 1996). However, subsequent data has *not* indicated an increased risk related to low- and moderate-intensity physical activity. Tomić and colleagues (2013) have reported that participation in moderate-intensity aerobic exercise did not show any increased risk of intrauterine growth restriction. The researchers noted that they did not investigate participation in high-intensity physical activities (Tomić et al., 2013). More investigation is warranted in this area.

Contraindications and Risk Factors

Research from the past several decades has produced valid and reliable evidence that supports participation in a regular exercise program during pregnancy because of the important maternal-fetal benefits it provides, which outweigh any risks. National groups such as ACOG, ACSM, the Canadian Society for Exercise Physiology (CSEP), SOGC, and the UK Chief Medical Officers have provided guidelines and recommendations for exercise during pregnancy and the postpartum period indicating that, in uncomplicated pregnancies, women with or without a previously sedentary lifestyle should be encouraged to participate in aerobic and strength-conditioning exercises as part of a healthy lifestyle (ACSM, 2022; ACOG, 2020; UK Chief Medical Officers, 2019; Davies et al., 2003). However, it is recommended that women with complicated pregnancies be discouraged from participating in exercise activities for fear of impacting the underlying disorder or maternal or fetal outcomes.

It is imperative that a CMES performs routine health screenings prior to initiating an exercise program during pregnancy or the postpartum period (Figure 21-1). Healthy women without contraindications can begin an exercise program without the need for medical clearance but should be under the care of a obstetrician-gynecologist or other obstetric care provider. For women with medical complications (e.g., severe obesity, gestational diabetes, or hypertension) or contraindications for exercise, medical clearance is recommended before beginning or continuing physical activity (Figure 21-2).

Visit csep.ca/Getactivequestionnaire-pregnancy to download free PDFs of this questionnaire and consultation form.

In general, participation in a wide range of recreational activities appears safe during and after pregnancy. Overly vigorous activity in the third trimester, activities that have a high potential for contact, and activities with a high risk of falling should be avoided (Table 21-2). Additionally, women should refrain from activities with a risk of abdominal trauma, activities that may cause a loss of balance, and scuba diving (ACSM, 2022; ACOG, 2020).

Absolute Contraindications

ACOG (2020) has established that there are some women for whom exercise during pregnancy is absolutely contraindicated, while those with medical comorbidities should follow a personalized exercise program. For example, hemodynamically significant heart disease and restrictive lung disease are absolute contraindications. In addition, the following pregnancy-related conditions would prevent women from exercising: incompetent cervix/cerclage, multiple gestation at risk for premature labor, premature labor during the current pregnancy, ruptured membranes, or preeclampsia/pregnancy-induced hypertension. Finally, women with persistent second-or third-trimester bleeding or placenta previa after 26 weeks of gestation should avoid exercise as well.

Relative Contraindications

There are also certain women with comorbidities for whom the potential benefits of exercising may outweigh the risks (ACSM, 2022). For example, extreme obesity, or a BMI of ≥ 40 kg/m^2, is considered a relative contraindication to exercise during pregnancy. In addition, the CMES should be cautious when working with pregnant women with anemia, unevaluated maternal cardiac arrhythmia, chronic bronchitis, orthopedic limitations, a history of an extremely sedentary lifestyle, intrauterine growth restriction in the current pregnancy, or a heavy smoking habit. Poorly controlled hypertension, poorly controlled seizure disorder, eating disorder, malnutrition or extreme underweight, recurrent pregnancy loss, cardiovascular disease, history of spontaneous preterm birth, premature labor, miscarriage, and hyperthyroidism are also considered relative contraindications to exercise during pregnancy.

Signs to Terminate Exercise

The CMES and any pregnant clients should also familiarize themselves with specific signs and symptoms that indicate a reason to terminate exercise and immediately follow up with a medical professional, including vaginal bleeding, dyspnea prior to exertion, dizziness, headache, chest pain, and muscle weakness. Additional reasons to terminate exercise include calf pain or swelling (in which case, it is important to rule out thrombophlebitis), preterm labor, decreased fetal movement, and amniotic fluid leakage (ACOG, 2020).

GET ACTIVE QUESTIONNAIRE FOR PREGNANCY

CSEP | SCPE

Figure 21-1
Get Active Questionnaire for Pregnancy

Reprinted with permission from Canadian Society for Exercise Physiology, 2021. All rights reserved.

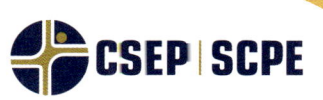

NAME (+ NAME OF PARENT/GUARDIAN IF APPLICABLE) [PLEASE PRINT]:

TODAY'S DATE (DD/MM/YYYY):   YOUR DUE DATE (DD/MM/YYYY):   NO. OF WEEKS PREGNANT: AGE:

Physical activity during pregnancy has many health benefits and is generally not risky for you and your baby. But for some conditions, physical activity is not recommended. This questionnaire is to help decide whether you should speak to your Obstetric Health Care Provider (e.g., your physician or midwife) before you begin or continue to be physically active.

Please answer YES or NO to each question to the best of your ability. **If your health changes as your pregnancy progresses you should fill in this questionnaire again.**

1.	In this pregnancy, do you have:		
	a. Mild, moderate or severe respiratory or cardiovascular diseases (e.g., chronic bronchitis)?	Y	N
	b. Epilepsy that is not stable?	Y	N
	c. Type 1 diabetes that is not stable or your blood sugar is outside of target ranges?	Y	N
	d. Thyroid disease that is not stable or your thyroid function is outside of target ranges?	Y	N
	e. An eating disorder(s) or malnutrition?	Y	N
	f. Twins (28 weeks pregnant or later)? Or are you expecting triplets or higher multiple births?	Y	N
	g. Low red blood cell number (anemia) with high levels of fatigue and/or light-headedness?	Y	N
	h. High blood pressure (preeclampsia, gestational hypertension, or chronic hypertension that is not stable)?	Y	N
	i. A baby that is growing slowly (intrauterine growth restriction)?	Y	N
	j. Unexplained bleeding, ruptured membranes or labour before 37 weeks?	Y	N
	k. A placenta that is partially or completely covering the cervix (placenta previa)?	Y	N
	l. Weak cervical tissue (incompetent cervix)?	Y	N
	m. A stitch or tape to reinforce your cervix (cerclage)?	Y	N
2.	In previous pregnancies, have you had:		
	a. Recurrent miscarriages (loss of your baby before 20 weeks gestation two or more times)?	Y	N
	b. Early delivery (before 37 weeks gestation)?	Y	N
3.	Do you have any other medical condition that may affect your ability to be physically active during pregnancy? What is the condition? Specify:	Y	N
4.	Is there any other reason you are concerned about physical activity during pregnancy?		

Go to Page 2 *Describe Your Physical Activity Level*

Continued on next page

Figure 21-1
Get Active Questionnaire for Pregnancy *(continued)*

Describe Your Physical Activity Level

CSEP | SCPE

During a typical week, what types of physical activities do you take part in (e.g., swimming, walking, resistance training, yoga)?

_____

_____

During the same week, please describe ON AVERAGE how often and for how long you engage in physical activity of a light, moderate or vigorous intensity. See definitions for intensity below the box.

ON AVERAGE	FREQUENCY (times per week)	INTENSITY (see below for definitions)	DURATION (minutes per session)
How physically active were you in the **six months before pregnancy**?	☐ 0 ☐ 3-4 ☐ 1-2 ☐ 5-7	☐ light ☐ moderate ☐ vigorous	☐ <20 ☐ 31-60 ☐ 20-30 ☐ >60
How physically active have you been **during this pregnancy**?	☐ 0 ☐ 3-4 ☐ 1-2 ☐ 5-7	☐ light ☐ moderate ☐ vigorous	☐ <20 ☐ 31-60 ☐ 20-30 ☐ >60
What are your physical activity goals for the **rest of your pregnancy**?	☐ 0 ☐ 3-4 ☐ 1-2 ☐ 5-7	☐ light ☐ moderate ☐ vigorous	☐ <20 ☐ 31-60 ☐ 20-30 ☐ >60

Light intensity physical activity: You are moving, but you do not sweat or breathe hard, such as walking to get the mail or light gardening.

Moderate intensity physical activity: Your heart rate goes up and you may sweat or breathe hard. You can talk, but could not sing. Examples include brisk walking.

Vigorous intensity physical activity: Your heart rate goes up substantially, you feel hot and sweaty, and you cannot say more than a few words without pausing to breathe. Examples include fast stationary cycling and running.

General Advice for Being Physically Active During Pregnancy

Follow the advice in the 2019 Canadian Guidelines for Physical Activity throughout Pregnancy: **csepguidelines.ca/pregnancy**

It recommends that pregnant women get at least 150 minutes of moderate-intensity physical activity (resistance training, brisk walking, swimming, gardening), spread over three or more days of the week. **If you are planning to take part in vigorous-intensity physical activity, or be physically active at elevations above 2500 m (8200 feet), then consult with your health care provider.** If you have any questions about physical activity during pregnancy, consult a Qualified Exercise Professional or your health care provider beforehand. This can help ensure that your physical activity is safe and suitable for you.

Declaration

To the best of my knowledge, all of the information I have supplied on this questionnaire is correct. **If my health changes, I will complete this questionnaire again.**

☐ **I answered NO to all questions on Page 1.**
  Sign and date the declaration below.
  Physical activity is recommended.

I answered YES to one or more questions on Page 1 and I will speak with my health care provider before beginning or continuing physical activity. *The Health Care Provider Consultation Form for Prenatal Physical Activity can be used to start the conversation (**www.csep.ca/getactivequestionnaire-pregnancy**).*

☐ **I have spoken with my health care provider who has recommended that I take part in physical activity during my pregnancy.**
  Sign and date the declaration below.

NAME (+ NAME OF PARENT/GUARDIAN IF APPLICABLE) [PLEASE PRINT]:	SIGNATURE (OR SIGNATURE OF PARENT/GUARDIAN IF APPLICABLE):
TODAY'S DATE (DD/MM/YYYY): TELEPHONE (OPTIONAL):	EMAIL (OPTIONAL):

Prenatal and Postpartum Exercise — CHAPTER 21

Figure 21-2
Health Care Provider Consultation Form for Prenatal Physical Activity

Reprinted with permission from Canadian Society for Exercise Physiology, 2021. All rights reserved.

HEALTH CARE PROVIDER CONSULTATION FORM FOR PRENATAL PHYSICAL ACTIVITY

CSEP | SCPE

PATIENT NAME: DUE DATE (DD/MM/YYYY):   TODAY'S DATE (DD/MM/YYYY):

Your patient wishes to begin or continue to be physically active during pregnancy. Your patient answered "Yes" to one or more questions on the Get Active Questionnaire for Pregnancy and has been asked to seek your advice (**www.csep.ca/getactivequestionnaire-pregnancy**).

Physical activity is safe for **most** pregnant individuals and has many health benefits. However, a **small number of patients** may need a thorough evaluation before taking part in physical activity during pregnancy.

The Society of Obstetricians and Gynaecologists of Canada/Canadian Society for Exercise Physiology *2019 Canadian Guideline for Physical Activity throughout Pregnancy* recommends that pregnant women get at least 150 minutes of moderate intensity physical activity each week (see next page or **csepguidelines.ca/pregnancy**). But there are contraindications to this goal for some conditions (see right).

Specific concern from your patient and/or from a Qualified Exercise Professional:

To ensure that your patient proceeds in the safest way possible, they were advised to consult with you about becoming or continuing to be physically active during pregnancy. Please discuss potential concerns you may have about physical activity with your patient and indicate in the box below any modifications you might recommend:

☐ Unrestricted physical activity based on the *SOGC/CSEP 2019 Canadian Guidelines for Physical Activity throughout Pregnancy*.
☐ Progressive physical activity
  ☐ Recommend avoiding:
  ☐ Recommend including:
☐ Recommend supervision by a Qualified Exercise Professional, if possible.
☐ Refer to a physiotherapist for pain, impairment and/or a pelvic floor assessment.
☐ Other comments:

Absolute contraindications

Pregnant women with these conditions should continue activities of daily living, but not take part in moderate or vigorous physical activity:

☐ ruptured membranes,
☐ premature labour,
☐ unexplained persistent vaginal bleeding,
☐ placenta previa after 28 weeks gestation,
☐ preeclampsia,
☐ incompetent cervix,
☐ intrauterine growth restriction,
☐ high-order multiple pregnancy (e.g. triplets),
☐ uncontrolled Type I diabetes,
☐ uncontrolled hypertension,
☐ uncontrolled thyroid disease,
☐ other serious cardiovascular, respiratory or systemic disorder.

Relative contraindications

Pregnant women with these conditions should discuss advantages and disadvantages of physical activity with you. They should continue physical activity, but modify exercises to reduce intensity and/or duration.

☐ recurrent pregnancy loss,
☐ gestational hypertension,
☐ a history of spontaneous preterm birth,
☐ mild/moderate cardiovascular or respiratory disease,
☐ symptomatic anemia,
☐ malnutrition,
☐ eating disorder,
☐ twin pregnancy after the 28th week,
☐ other significant medical conditions.

Continued on next page

Figure 21-2
Health Care Provider Consultation Form for Prenatal Physical Activity *(continued)*

SOGC/CSEP 2019 CANADIAN GUIDELINE FOR PHYSICAL ACTIVITY THROUGHOUT PREGNANCY

The evidence-based guideline outlines the right amount of physical activity women should get throughout pregnancy to promote maternal, fetal, and neonatal health.

Research shows the health benefits and safety of being active throughout pregnancy for both mother and baby. Physical activity is now seen as a critical part of a healthy pregnancy. Following the guideline can reduce the risk of pregnancy-related illnesses such as depression, by at least 25%, and of developing gestational diabetes, high blood pressure and preeclampsia by 40%.

Pregnant women should get at least 150 minutes of moderate-intensity physical activity each week over at least three days per week. But even if they do not meet that goal, they are encouraged to be active in a variety of ways every day. Please visit **csepguidelines.ca/pregnancy** for more information. The guideline makes six recommendations:

1 All women without contraindication should be physically active throughout pregnancy. Specific subgroups were examined:
- Women who were previously inactive.
- Women diagnosed with gestational diabetes mellitus.
- Women categorized as overweight or obese (pre-pregnancy body mass index ≥25kg/m^2).

2 Pregnant women should accumulate at least 150 minutes of moderate-intensity physical activity each week to achieve clinically meaningful health benefits and reductions in pregnancy complications.

3 Physical activity should be accumulated over a minimum of three days per week; however, being active every day is encouraged.

4 Pregnant women should incorporate a variety of aerobic and resistance training activities to achieve greater benefits. Adding yoga and/or gentle stretching may also be beneficial.

5 Pelvic floor muscle training (e.g., Kegel exercises) may be performed on a daily basis to reduce the risk of urinary incontinence. Instruction in proper technique is recommended to obtain optimal benefits.

6 Pregnant women who experience light-headedness, nausea or feel unwell when they exercise flat on their back should modify their exercise position to avoid the supine position.

No. 367-2019 Canadian Guideline for Physical Activity throughout Pregnancy
JOINT SOGC/CSEP CLINICAL PRACTICE GUIDELINE | Volume 40, ISSUE 11, P1528-1537, November 01, 2018

TABLE 21-2
HIGH-RISK EXERCISES

• Snow- and waterskiing • Rock climbing • Snowboarding • Diving • Scuba diving • Bungee jumping	• Horseback riding • Ice skating/hockey • Road or mountain cycling • Vigorous exercise at altitude (non-acclimated women)	• Soccer • Basketball • Rollerblading, • Vigorous-intensity racquet sports

Note: Risk of activities requiring balance is relative to maternal weight gain and morphologic changes; some activities may be acceptable early in pregnancy but risky later on.

PHYSIOLOGICAL CHANGES DURING PREGNANCY

During pregnancy, a woman's endocrine system signals changes in virtually every part of her body to prepare her and the fetus for gestation, delivery, and lactation. This section covers the adaptations related to exercise performance. Understanding these factors and how they impact a woman's ability to engage in prenatal physical activity is essential for safe and effective exercise programming.

Musculoskeletal System

With the average weight gain during pregnancy in the range of 25 to 40 pounds (11 to 18 kg) (15 to 25% of pre-pregnancy weight), forces across joints are significantly increased. Such large forces may cause discomfort to normal joints and increase damage to arthritic or previously unstable joints. A woman's enlarging abdomen increases the mechanical stress on the joints of the back, pelvis, hips, and legs as her **center of gravity** moves upward and out. A condition called pregnancy-related pelvic girdle pain has been associated with pain (stabbing, dull, shooting, and/or burning) near the sacroiliac joints and extending to the gluteal area or anteriorly to the vicinity of the symphysis pubis. It may radiate to the groin, perineum, or posterior thigh and may also change during the course of the pregnancy. Incidence of back pain (i.e., combined pelvic girdle pain and lumbar pain) during pregnancy has been reported to be as high as 76% (Kanakaris, Roberts, & Giannoudis, 2011).

During the first trimester, increased amounts of the hormones **relaxin** and **progesterone** are released to expand the uterine cavity. These **hormones** allow expansion by softening the ligaments surrounding the joints of the pelvis (hips and lumbosacral spine), thereby increasing mobility and joint laxity. Whether or not joint laxity occurs in other joints, such as the neck, shoulder, or periphery, is unclear. Theoretically, increased mechanical stress combined with joint laxity would predispose pregnant women to an increased incidence of strains and sprains. However, with the exception of low-back pain, data on the effects of the increased weight of pregnancy on joint injury and pathology are lacking. While an increased incidence of falling during pregnancy has not been reported, a woman's balance may be affected by changes in posture, predisposing her to loss of balance and increased risk of falling. Despite a lack of clear evidence that musculoskeletal injuries are increased during pregnancy, these possibilities should be considered when designing prenatal exercise programs.

Cardiovascular System

During pregnancy, the entire cardiovascular system experiences dramatic changes as hormonal signals initiate relaxation and reduced responsiveness in most, if not all, of the smooth muscle cells in a woman's blood vessels. In addition to causing many of the unpleasant early symptoms of pregnancy (e.g., lightheadedness, nausea, fatigue, cravings, constipation, bloating, and frequent urination), these hormonal changes result in an increase in the elasticity and volume of the entire circulatory system (i.e., a decrease in systemic vascular resistance). Initially, this creates a vascular "underfill" problem where the amount of blood returning to the heart decreases. To correct the underfill, the body triggers the release of several hormones, which cause a decrease in the excretion of salt and water by the kidneys. Ultimately, the retained extra salt and water expand plasma volume, allowing more venous return to the heart, thereby increasing **cardiac output** and improving arterial pressure and blood flow to the organs. Eventually, hormonal signals cause increases in heart volumes (chamber volume and **stroke volume**), blood volume, heart rate, and cardiac output.

By mid-pregnancy, cardiac outputs are 30 to 50% greater than before pregnancy due to an increase in both stroke volume and heart rate (Rossi et al., 2011). Maternal resting heart rate can be up to 15 beats per minute (bpm) higher than pre-pregnancy rates near the third trimester. Mean arterial pressure decreases 5 to 10 mmHg by the middle of the second trimester before gradually increasing back to pre-pregnancy levels. These hemodynamic changes appear to establish a circulatory reserve necessary to provide nutrients and oxygen to both mother and fetus at rest and during moderate exercise. Since heart-rate response among pregnant exercisers is variable, **rating of perceived exertion (RPE)** should be used to assess intensity instead of traditional heart rate–based methods.

As pregnancy progresses, a woman's body position can affect her cardiovascular system both at rest and during exercise. After the first trimester, the **supine** position results in relative obstruction of venous return (as a result of the fetus pressing on the veins), which leads to decreased cardiac output. For this reason, supine positions should be avoided as much as possible during rest and exercise. In addition, motionless standing is associated with a significant decrease in cardiac output and should be avoided.

Respiratory System

The delivery of oxygen to the mother and fetus is enhanced through improvements in lung function during pregnancy. At rest, an increase in the depth of each breath increases the amount of air inhaled by up to 50% (ACOG, 2020). This increase is the result of elevated levels of progesterone, which stimulates "overbreathing" by increasing the brain's sensitivity to carbon dioxide. As a result, oxygen tension is increased and carbon dioxide tension is decreased in the alveoli. Ultimately, these directional changes in breathing gases widen the pressure gradients, which improve the efficiency of oxygen uptake from the lungs and the elimination of carbon dioxide from maternal and fetal blood and tissues. The CMES should take into account that some estimates report perceived respiratory discomfort (breathlessness)

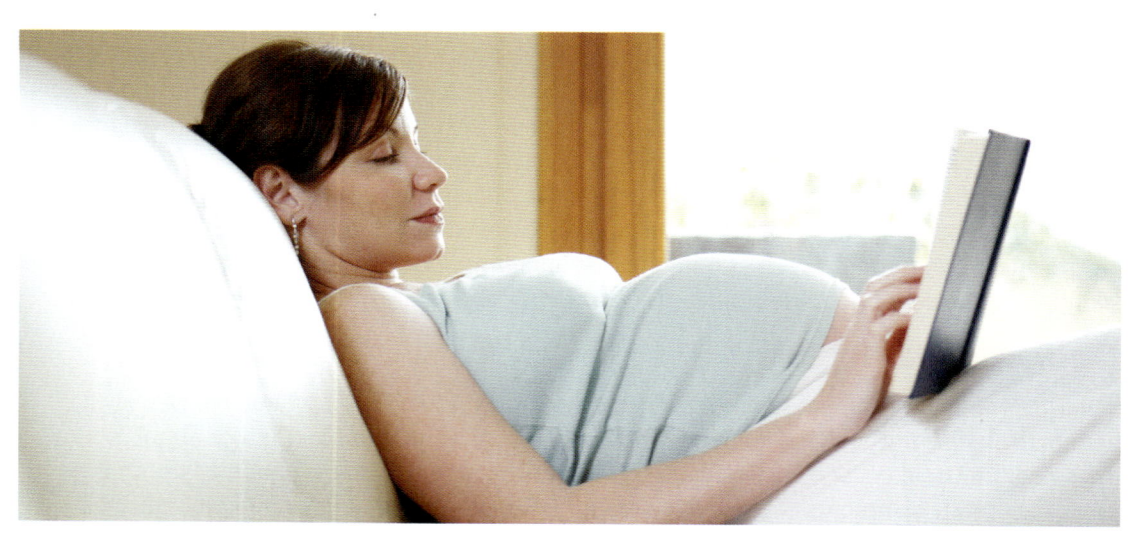

during **activities of daily living** in up to 75% of healthy pregnant women (Jensen et al. 2008). Physical activity during perceived respiratory discomfort may have to be reduced to match a pregnant client's tolerance.

Prenatal adaptations (including extra weight and possibly inefficient movements during the latter stages) of the respiratory system cause women to experience an associated increase in oxygen uptake during weight-bearing exercise (ACSM, 2022). Peak ventilation and maximal aerobic power are maintained during pregnancy. As a result of this maintained function and the pregnancy-induced increase in alveolar ventilation, gas transfer at the tissue level may improve. This causes a "training effect" of pregnancy in women who maintain moderate-to-intense exercise programs throughout gestation, and may explain anecdotal reports of women who experience an improvement in competitive endurance performance after giving birth.

Thermoregulatory System

A woman's ability to dissipate heat improves during pregnancy. The improved ability to eliminate body heat is most likely due to a decrease of the body's set point for normal temperature in early pregnancy and a significant increase in blood flow to the skin, which increases the rate of heat loss directly into the air. Additionally, an increase in tidal volume as described above, allows a pregnant woman to increase heat loss through exhalation.

During moderate-intensity aerobic exercise in thermoneutral conditions, the core temperature of non-pregnant women rises an average of 1.5° C during the first 30 minutes of exercise, and then reaches a plateau if exercise is continued for an additional 30 minutes (Soultanakis, Artal, & Wiswell, 1996). If heat production exceeds heat-dissipation capacity, as is commonly the case during exercise in hot, humid conditions or during very high-intensity exercise, a woman's core temperature will continue to rise. During prolonged exercise, loss of fluid as sweat may compromise heat dissipation. Given that fetal body core temperatures are naturally about 1° C higher than maternal temperatures, maintenance of proper hydration, and therefore blood volume, is critical to heat balance.

Research examining the effects of exercise on core temperature during pregnancy is limited. The results of some human studies suggest that **hyperthermia** in excess of 100° F (39° C) during the first 45 to 60 days of gestation may be **teratogenic** (disruptive to the growth and development of an embryo or fetus) in humans. Existing data support a possible association of neural-tube defects with hot tub and sauna use during early pregnancy, but not with hot environments (Van Zutphen et al., 2012). There have been no reports that hyperthermia associated with exercise causes malformations of the embryo or fetus in humans.

PROGRAMMING GUIDELINES AND CONSIDERATIONS FOR PRENATAL EXERCISE

Exercise programming guidelines for prenatal activity include the same elements as guidelines for non-pregnant women. The *Physical Activity Guidelines for Americans* (U.S. Department of Health & Human Services, 2018) recommend that pregnant women who are not already highly active get at least 150 minutes of moderate-intensity aerobic activity per week during pregnancy. Participating in vigorous-intensity exercise is not recommended for previously inactive women or women who engage in only moderate-intensity exercise. Women who are currently vigorously active may continue this level of activity during pregnancy according to the guidelines.

Aerobic exercise consisting of any activity that uses large muscle groups in a continuous rhythmic manner (e.g., walking, hiking, jogging/running, aerobic dance, swimming, cycling, rowing, dancing, and rope skipping) may be appropriate. Some activities, such as scuba diving and prolonged exertion in the supine position after 20 weeks of gestation, should be avoided due to the potential for decreased venous return as a result of aortocaval compression from the gravid uterus. Activities that increase the risk of falls, such as downhill snow skiing, or those that may result in excessive joint stress or musculoskeletal injury as a result of quick changes in direction or jumping should also be avoided (ACSM, 2022).

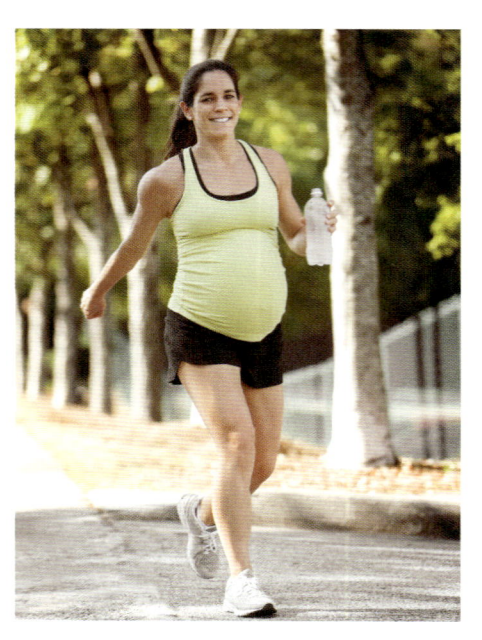

Musculoskeletal conditioning appears to be safe and effective during pregnancy when low weights and multiple repetitions (i.e., 12 to 15 repetitions) through a dynamic, controlled **range of motion** are performed. While research is lacking, it would be prudent to limit repetitive **isometric** or heavy-resistance weightlifting, as well as any exercises that result in a large **pressor response** (i.e., a disproportionate rise in blood pressure during resistance training resulting from **autonomic nervous system** reflex activity). Additionally, maintenance of normal joint range of motion through individualized stretching exercises is acceptable. However, pregnant exercisers should be aware of increased ligamentous laxity and strive to limit excessive stretching or ballistic stretching movements during pregnancy.

Several national health and medical organizations have published recommendations and guidelines on exercise and pregnancy. Not surprisingly, the content in the guidelines from the different organizations is similar. Specifically, the ACOG Committee Opinion on physical activity and exercise during pregnancy and the postpartum period recommends that women with uncomplicated pregnancies engage in 20 to 60 minutes of moderate-intensity exercise at least three days per week (ACOG, 2020). Guidelines from the United States and Canada jointly support recommendations stating that the mode, frequency, duration, and overload principles for cardiorespiratory, resistance, and flexibility exercise are the same for pregnant women as for non-pregnant women (ACSM, 2022; ACOG, 2020; Mottola et al., 2018). Pregnancy-specific issues to consider when designing prenatal exercise programs focus on attaining additional calories to maintain **homeostasis,** avoiding motionless standing, preventing maternal hyperthermia and **hypoglycemia,** and avoiding high-risk exercises (Table 21-3).

TABLE 21-3

SPECIAL CONSIDERATIONS FOR PRENATAL EXERCISE PROGRAMMING

- Drink water before, during, and after exercise following guidelines for fluid replacement.
- Women who are pregnant should avoid exercising in a hot and humid environment, be well hydrated at all times, and dress appropriately to avoid heat stress.
- Women experiencing low-back pain may consider water-based exercise.
- Women may need to modestly increase caloric intake to meet the increased caloric demands of pregnancy and exercise. To avoid excessive weight gain, women should discuss appropriate levels with their healthcare provider.
- Lowlanders should avoid exercising at elevations above 6,000 ft (~1,829 m) and consult with a knowledgeable obstetrician before exercising at high elevations.

Source: American College of Sports Medicine (2022). *ACSM's Guidelines for Exercise Testing and Prescription* (11th ed.). Philadelphia: Wolters Kluwer.

The sole use of heart-rate monitoring to assess exercise intensity is not recommended for pregnant exercisers due to the natural physiological influences of the cardiovascular system during pregnancy and the fact that maximal exercise testing is rarely performed with pregnant women. The "category" RPE scale (6–20) or the "category-ratio" Borg scale (0–10) may be used in conjunction with heart-rate measures. Ratings of "fairly light" to "very hard" are the recommended intensity ranges for prenatal exercise.

ACSM (2022) and ACOG (2020) offer specific guidelines when it comes to exercise during pregnancy and the postpartum period. Additionally, the *Physical Activity Guidelines for Americans* offer three guidelines to help women to begin being, or continue to be, physically active (Table 21-4). These guidelines suggest using an RPE of 5 to 6 on the 0 to 10 scale or the talk test (can carry on a conversation but not sing) to monitor intensity. The various recommendations from leading organizations offer a great deal of consistency and alignment, and it is helpful to think about how the CMES might communicate this information to clients in an easy-to-understand format, upon request, as part of a healthy lifestyle in conjunction with an individualized exercise plan.

TABLE 21-4
KEY GUIDELINES FOR WOMEN DURING PREGNANCY AND THE POSTPARTUM PERIOD

- Women should do at least 150 minutes (2 hours and 30 minutes) of moderate-intensity aerobic activity a week during pregnancy and the postpartum period. Preferably, aerobic activity should be spread throughout the week.
- Women who habitually engaged in vigorous-intensity aerobic activity or who were physically active before pregnancy can continue these activities during pregnancy and the postpartum period.
- Women who are pregnant should be under the care of a healthcare provider who can monitor the progress of the pregnancy. Women who are pregnant can consult their healthcare provider about whether or how to adjust their physical activity during pregnancy and after the baby is born.
- Women without medical reasons to avoid physical activity during pregnancy and postpartum period can begin or continue with light-to-moderate intensity muscle-strengthening physical activity.

Source: U.S. Department of Health & Human Services (2018). *Physical Activity Guidelines for Americans* (2nd ed.). www.health.gov/paguidelines

BIOMECHANICAL CONSIDERATIONS DURING PREGNANCY

Due to the wide range of postural and physiological adaptations that occur during pregnancy, the CMES must be proficient at designing exercise programs geared toward making physical activity more comfortable for this population. Physiological adaptations include a profound increase in body mass, retention of fluid, and laxity in supporting structures. Postural adaptations correspond with these physiological changes and usually entail an alteration in the loading and alignment of, and muscle forces along, the spine and weight-bearing joints. During the tenth to twelfth week of pregnancy, production of the hormone relaxin significantly increases (Aldabe et al., 2012). Relaxin creates joint laxity, which not only allows the pelvis to accommodate the enlarging uterus, but also is believed to weaken the ability of static supports in the lumbar spine to withstand shearing forces. In the pelvis, joint laxity is most prominent in the symphysis pubis and the sacroiliac joints. Interestingly, experimental studies have not shown a direct relationship between high levels of relaxin and increased pelvic mobility or peripheral joint mobility in pregnant women (Aldabe et al., 2012).

Typically, advancing pregnancy produces a forward shift in the center of gravity followed by an anterior pelvic tilt and subsequent increase in lumbar **lordosis** and thoracic **kyphosis**.

As pregnancy progresses, the biomechanical alterations of increased abdominal girth and weakened abdominal muscles may increase lumbar lordosis. It has been suggested that lordosis in the lower-back region might minimize the external moment of the center of mass of the upper body, while retaining a stable hip joint position (Wagner et al., 2012).

As noted previously, a large majority of women complain of low-back pain during pregnancy (Kanakaris, Roberts, & Giannoudis, 2011). Prenatal low-back and pelvic pain appear to be more related to pre-pregnancy postural habits that are exaggerated during gestation than to postural adaptations to pregnancy. Laxity in the supporting tissues, either pre-existing or enhanced by the hormone relaxin, becomes greater in the direction of habitual posture (Dumas et al., 1995). In other words, pronated feet may become flatter, hyperextended knees may become more pronounced, and spinal curves may soften. During the term of their pregnancies, most women adapt to these postural and physiological changes and, following the baby's delivery, return to their pre-pregnant states.

To alleviate the postural discomforts of exercise, many pregnant women choose to work out in the water. Evidence suggests that therapeutic aquatic exercise is potentially beneficial to women suffering from pregnancy-related low-back pain (Waller, Lambeck, & Daly, 2009). Warm-water exercise, usually termed hydrotherapy or aquatic therapy, is a popular treatment with a pain-relief effect for many individuals suffering from painful neurologic or musculoskeletal conditions. The warmth and buoyancy of water may block nociception (perception of pain) and facilitate muscle relaxation. The hydrostatic effect may also relieve pain by reducing peripheral edema and by dampening sympathetic nervous system activity (Kamioka et al., 2011). Thus, water exercise is a valuable option for women to consider, especially as advancing pregnancy makes other forms of physical activity uncomfortable or stressful on the joints.

In addition to low-back pain, common musculoskeletal complaints that arise during pregnancy include sacroiliac (SI) joint dysfunction, pubic pain, nerve compression syndromes, **diastasis recti,** and **stress urinary incontinence (SUI).** The remainder of this section covers each of these conditions in more detail.

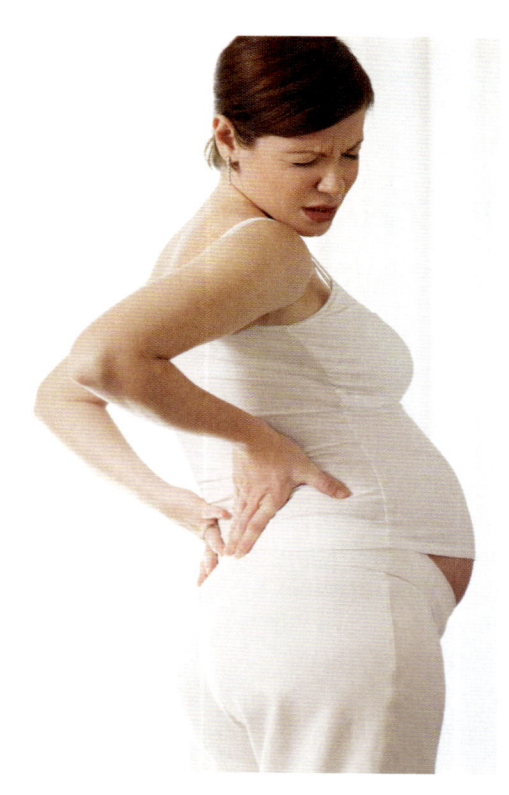

Low-back and Posterior Pelvic Girdle Pain

The two most common sites of back pain in pregnancy are the lumbar and posterior pelvic areas. Back pain occurs most commonly after the sixth month and can last until the sixth month postpartum. After 12 weeks of pregnancy, the uterus can no longer be contained within the pelvis and the mass moves superiorly and anteriorly. As the abdominal muscles are stretched and tone is diminished, they lose their ability to contribute effectively to the maintenance of neutral posture. In the lumbar spine, joint laxity is most notable in the anterior and posterior longitudinal ligaments. This weakens the ability of static supports in the lumbar spine to withstand the shearing forces. As a result, there may be an increase in discogenic symptoms and/or pain coming from the facet joints.

Lumbar pain during pregnancy is defined as back pain from the lumbar area only, with or without radiation to the legs (**sciatica**). In their review of the literature, Al-Khodairy, Bovay, and Gobelet (2007) reported that the lumbosacral trunk is vulnerable to pressure from any abdominal mass originating from the uterus and the ovaries. In pregnant women, direct pressure on nerve roots and ischemia of neural elements due to uterine pressure on the aorta and vena cava when lying on the back may result in back pain with radiation to the legs (Al-Khodairy, Bovay, & Gobelet, 2007).

Prenatal and Postpartum Exercise

CHAPTER 21

Exercises appropriate for pregnant women with lumbar pain include mobility and stretching movements that emphasize relaxing and lengthening the back extensors, hip flexors, scapular protractors, shoulder internal rotators, and neck flexors. Strengthening exercises should focus on the abdominals, gluteals, and scapular retractors to reinforce their ability to support proper alignment.

Posterior pelvic girdle pain is defined as pain experienced between the posterior iliac crest and the gluteal fold, particularly in the vicinity of the sacroiliac joint. The pain may radiate in the posterior thigh and can also occur in conjunction with, or separately, in the pubic symphysis. The prevalence of women suffering from posterior pelvic girdle pain during pregnancy is approximately 20% (Vleeming et al., 2008). Women with sacroiliac pain as their primary complaint tend to have low-back pain for a longer duration than those who simply have lumbar pain and it tends to persist postpartum (Aldabe, Milosavljevic, & Bussey, 2012). Further, women with pregnancy-related posterior pelvic girdle pain are three times more likely to have postpartum depressive symptoms (Aldabe et al., 2012). Unlike other forms of low-back pain during pregnancy, a previous high level of fitness does not necessarily prevent this problem, as risk factors for developing posterior pelvic girdle pain during pregnancy appear to be a history of previous low-back pain and previous trauma to the pelvis (Vleeming et al., 2008).

The hypothetical origins of SI joint dysfunction during pregnancy focus on decreased stability of the pelvic girdle. It is assumed that the stability of the pelvic girdle is provided, in part, by the coarse texture of the SI cartilage surfaces, the undulated shape of the joint, and the compressive forces of the muscles, ligaments, and thoracolumbar fascia. Muscles that generate a force perpendicular to the SI joints or increase tension on the sacroiliac ligaments or thoracolumbar **fascia** generate forces that may act to stabilize the SI joint. These include the internal and external abdominal obliques, the latissimus dorsi, the transversospinal parts of the erector spinae muscle (especially the multifidus), and the gluteus maximus. Therefore, functional exercise programs that target this musculature may benefit women with prenatal pelvic pain, partly by increasing muscle force and endurance (Aldabe et al., 2012).

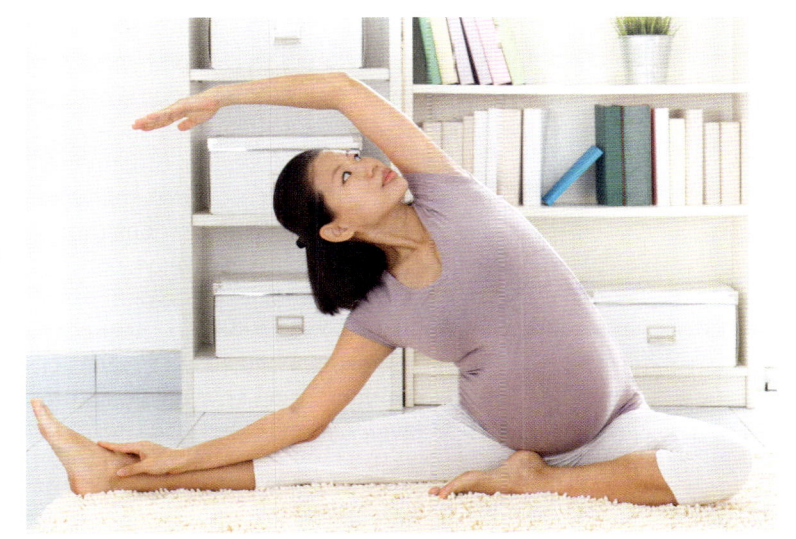

Pubic Pain

The irritation of the pubic symphysis caused by increased motion at the joint is called **symphysitis.** Symptoms include mild to severe pain in the pubic region, groin, and medial aspect of the thigh (unilateral or bilateral), frequently accompanied by sacroiliac, low-back, and suprapubic pain. Weight-bearing activities, particularly those that involve lifting one leg, intensify the pain. Women also may hear or feel a clicking or grinding sensation in the joint, and there is often difficulty walking, so that a "waddling" gait is adopted.

As noted previously, it has been suggested that pelvic instability is the primary cause of pelvic (sacroiliac and symphysis pubis) joint pain during pregnancy (Aldabe, Milosavljevic, & Bussey, 2012). Pregnancy-related connective tissue changes and the change in the center of gravity result in lengthening, and thus weakening, of the ligaments of the pelvic joints, the thoracolumbar fascia, and the surrounding muscles, all of which provide stability to the pelvic ring. Normally, the pre-pregnancy width of the pubic symphysis is 0.5 mm. As pregnancy progresses, the symphysis pubis continues to widen to a maximum of approximately 12 mm.

With this widening, there is the risk of vertical displacement of the pubis, and the possibility of rotatory stress on the sacroiliac joints. During delivery, partial symphyseal separations and complete dislocations are possible, resulting in a greater concern for postpartum exercisers.

Treatment of pubic symphysis dysfunction includes avoidance of weight-bearing activities that intensify pain, a physician evaluation, and physical therapy. Pelvic belts, which compress the pelvis and minimize motion in the symphysis pubis and SI joint, may be prescribed.

Carpal Tunnel Syndrome

The most common neurological disorder during pregnancy is **carpal tunnel syndrome,** with some estimates reporting an incidence of up to 70% in pregnant women (Padua et al., 2010). Symptoms include pain and **paresthesias** in the median nerve distribution (thumb, index, and middle fingers), as the nerve becomes depressed as it passes through the carpal tunnel in the wrist (see page 651). Emergence or worsening of carpal tunnel syndrome may occur during pregnancy, with some reports indicating that symptoms persisted in more than 50% of the subjects after 1 year and in about 30% after 3 years (Padua et al., 2010). The presumed mechanism is pressure on the median nerve within the carpal compartment at the wrist as a result of tissue swelling, secondary to the fluid retention that occurs during pregnancy.

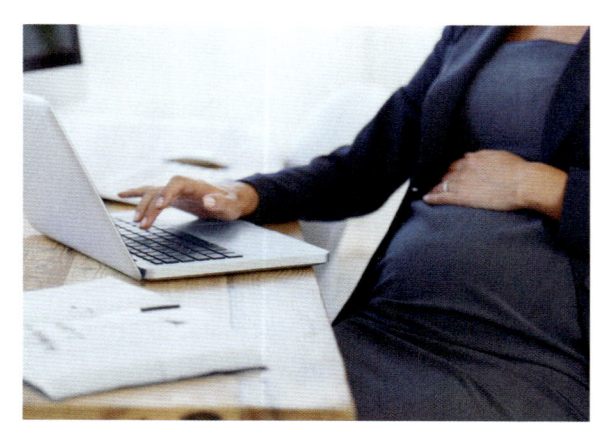

Treatments include ergonomic improvements, analgesia, splinting, and sometimes corticosteroid injection or surgery. Since activities or jobs that require repetitive **flexion** and **extension** of the wrist may contribute to carpal tunnel syndrome, these activities should be minimized. Care should be taken to avoid loading the wrist in hyperextension, grasping objects tightly, and repetitive flexion and extension of the wrist during exercise. Keeping the wrist in its neutral position during physical activities such as weightlifting should provide a comfortable, non-aggravating option.

Diastasis Recti

Diastasis recti is a partial or complete separation between the left and right sides of the rectus abdominis muscle. During pregnancy, the maternal inferior thoracic diameter is increased, thus altering the spatial relationship between the superior and inferior abdominal muscle attachments. In addition, anterior and lateral dimensions of the abdomen during pregnancy increase the distance between muscle attachments, producing increases in muscle length. In some women, the rectus abdominis muscles move laterally and may remain separated in the immediate post-delivery period.

Diastasis recti is commonly seen in women who have multiple pregnancies, because the muscles have been stretched many times. Extra skin and soft tissue in the front of the abdominal wall may be the only signs of this condition in early pregnancy. In late pregnancy, the top of the pregnant uterus is often seen bulging out of the abdominal wall. Three main factors contribute to the incidence and severity of diastasis recti during pregnancy: maternal hormones (relaxin, estrogen, and progesterone), mechanical stress within the abdominal cavity due to increasing girth, and weak abdominal muscles (strong abdominal muscles are more likely to resist this condition).

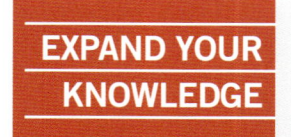

EXPAND YOUR KNOWLEDGE

FINGER-WIDTH TEST FOR DIASTASIS RECTI

While some rectus abdominis separation (Figure 21-3) is a normal part of every pregnancy, too much separation may lead to diminished muscular force production and even more separation during physical exertion. The most common test for diastasis recti is performed by placing two fingers horizontally on the suspected location while the client lies supine with the knees bent and performs a curl-up. If the fingers can penetrate at the location, there is probably a split. The degree of separation is measured according to the number of finger-widths of the split. One to two finger-widths is considered normal, whereas greater than three finger-widths is excessive and care should be taken to avoid placing a direct line of stress on the area.

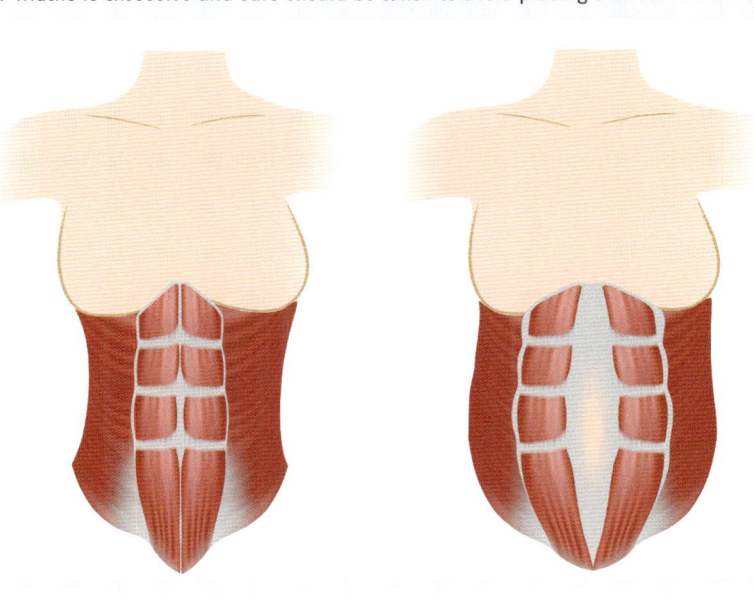

Figure 21-3
Diastasis recti
©Alila Medical Media

Abdominal-compression exercises and curl-ups in a semirecumbent position may be helpful for strengthening the rectus abdominis in this situation. A literature review revealed that exercise during the prenatal period reduced the presence of diastasis recti by 35%, and suggested that diastasis recti width may be reduced by exercising during the prenatal and postpartum periods. The interventions reviewed included some form of targeted abdominal/core strengthening. However, the authors stated that the overall quality of the available research studies was poor, indicating the need for more research (Benjamin, van de Water, & Peiris, 2013).

Stress Urinary Incontinence

SUI is the involuntary loss of urine that occurs with physical exertion and a rise in abdominal pressure. Coughing, sneezing, straining, laughing, and impact activities such as jumping and running are events commonly associated with SUI. The pelvic-floor muscles are considered important in maintaining pelvic organ support and bowel and bladder continence. Several studies have shown that women with urinary incontinence have decreased pelvic floor muscle thickness and electromyographic activity, and less muscle strength compared with control subjects without urinary incontinence (Hoyte et al., 2004; Morkved, Schei, & Salvesen, 2003; Morin et al., 2004). Further, pregnancy may be associated with reduced pelvic floor muscle strength (Sangsawang & Sangsawang, 2013).

During pregnancy and delivery, the prolonged stretching and trauma sustained by the pelvic floor musculature and the concomitant neural damage thought to accompany this stretching can reduce the strength of the pelvic floor. These changes can interfere with the normal transmission of information regarding changes in abdominal pressure to the proximal urethra, thereby predisposing the woman to SUI. Although the exact cause of pregnancy-related SUI is unknown, six risk factors predispose a woman to postpartum SUI: multiple pregnancies, vaginal delivery, high infant birth weight (>8.1 lb; 3.7 kg), large infant cranial circumference (>13.8 inches; 35.1 cm), high maternal weight gain during pregnancy (>28.6 lb; 13.0 kg), and tearing of the perineum during delivery (Sangsawang & Sangsawang, 2013). Women experiencing SUI during pregnancy and/or childbirth are generally thought to have a greater risk of developing the condition later in life.

Treatment of SUI during and after pregnancy includes the performance of **Kegel exercises** to strengthen the pelvic-floor muscles. Since the introduction of Kegel exercises in 1948, the efficacy of pelvic-floor muscle strengthening in the treatment of SUI has been supported by the findings of several randomized controlled studies and systematic reviews (Park et al., 2013; Sangsawang & Sangsawang, 2013). The benefits of an effective Kegel exercise regimen include providing support for the pelvic organs; preventing prolapse (falling) of the bladder, uterus, and rectum; supporting proper pelvic alignment; reinforcing sphincter control; enhancing circulation to the pelvic floor muscles; and providing a healthy environment for the healing process after labor and delivery. Women who exercise during pregnancy and resume it early in the postpartum period have a shorter duration of SUI than those who do not (Morkved & Bo, 2000) and there is some evidence that for prenatal and postpartum women, Kegel exercise can prevent SUI (Park et al., 2013; Sangsawang & Sangsawang, 2013).

EXERCISE TECHNIQUES FOR PREGNANT WOMEN

Although by no means comprehensive, the following exercises may be good options for pregnant clients because they take into account the physiological and biomechanical changes that occur as pregnancy progresses. That is, these exercises focus on important postural muscles (e.g., thighs, hips, trunk, and shoulders) and avoid the supine position. Further, clients should be encouraged to breathe deeply and to avoid the **Valsalva maneuver.**

Lower-extremity Exercises

Perform 12 to 15 repetitions of each of the following exercises (Figures 21-4 through 21-8). Progress the intensity only after the first movement is mastered.

Figure 21-4
Sit-to-stand squat

- Stand over the corner of a bench or box with the feet shoulder-width apart.
- Keeping the spine neutral, lower the hips down to the box to sit.
- Pushing through the heels, and keeping the spine neutral, return to stand.

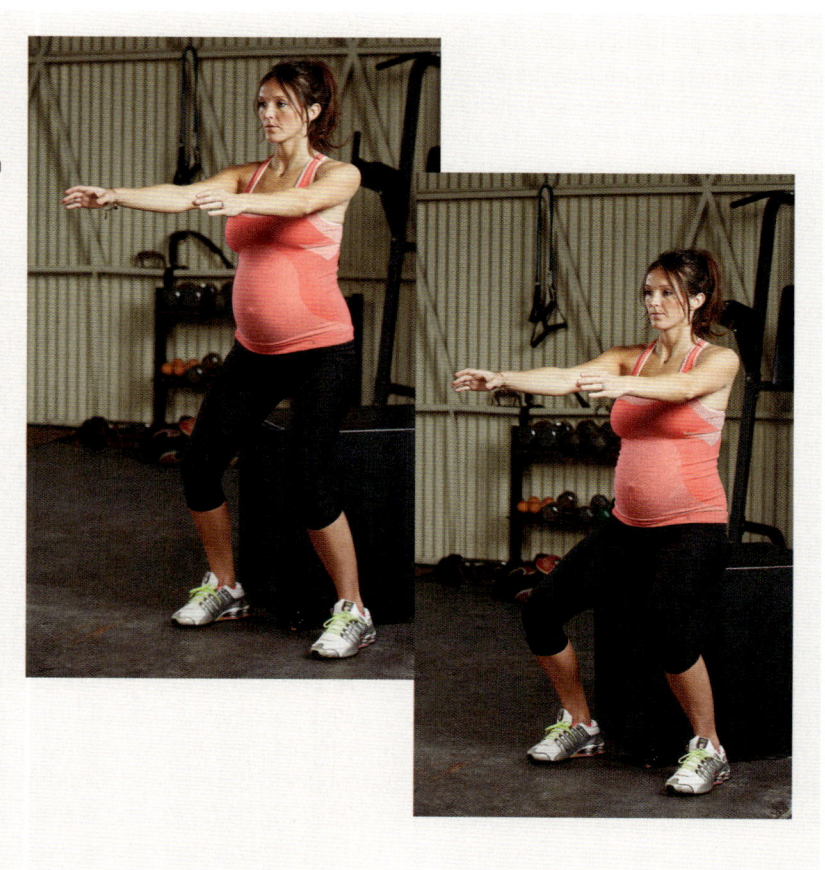

Prenatal and Postpartum Exercise CHAPTER 21 705

Figure 21-5
Single-leg squat

- Stand on one leg, lightly grasping onto something for support.
- Concentrating on the gluteal and thigh muscles, lower the hips downward into a squat position as far as is comfortable/tolerable for the supporting knee.
- Stand up, fully straightening the supporting knee and hip, and return to the starting position.

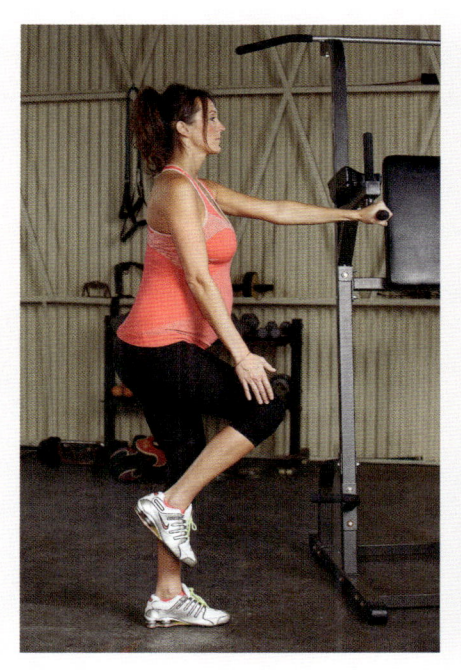

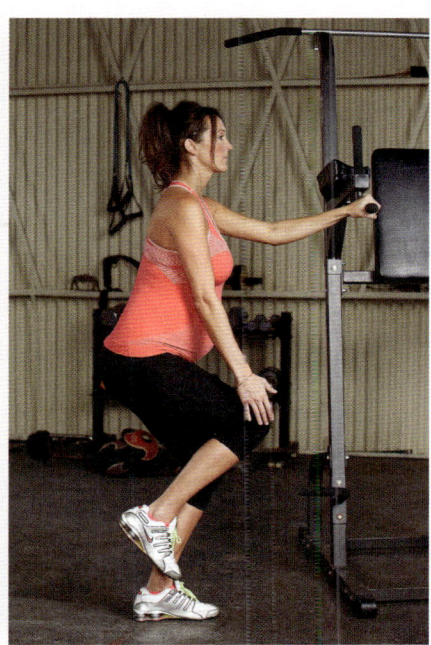

Figure 21-6
Lateral lunge

- Stand with the feet hip-width apart.
- Step out to the side, hinging at the hips and keeping the planted leg straight.
- Return to the starting position.
- Alternate legs.

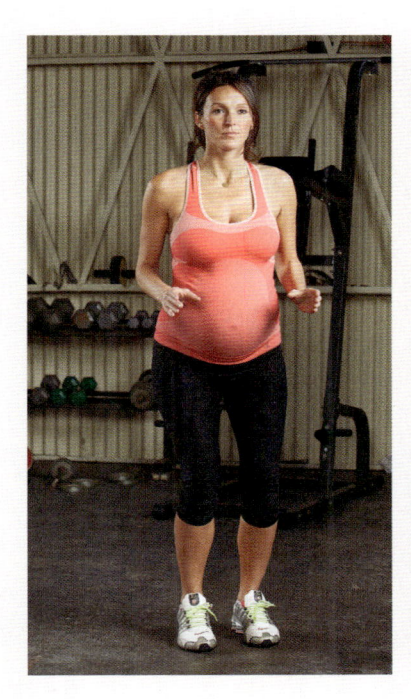

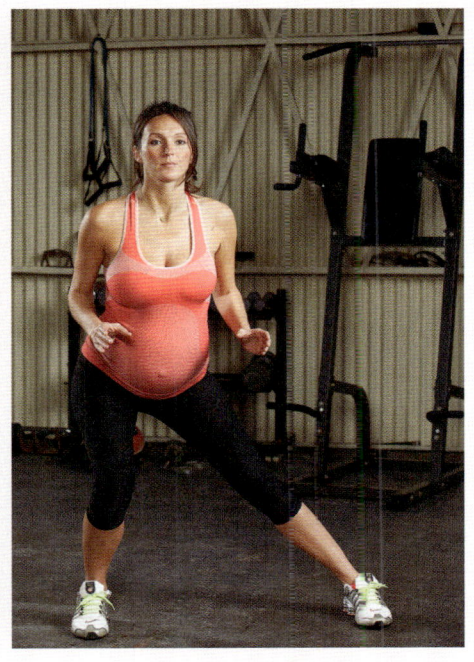

Figure 21-7
Single-leg hip abduction with band

- Place a resistance band above the ankles and stand alongside something to lightly grasp onto for support.
- Keep the spine in good alignment and maintain a slight bend in the knee of the supporting leg.
- Abduct one leg (however, avoid lifting the leg so high that the pelvis/hips start to shift).
- Return the leg to the starting position.

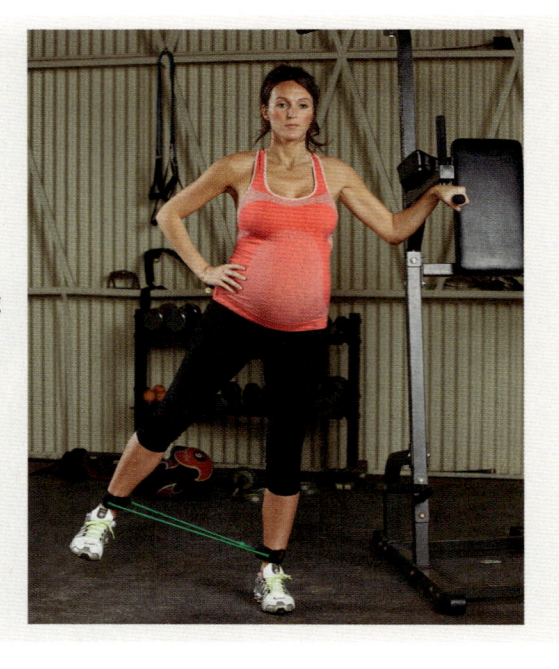

Figure 21-8
Single-leg lateral hip rotation with band

- Place a resistance band above the knees and stand alongside something to lightly grasp onto for support.
- Keep the spine in good alignment and maintain a slight bend in the knee of the supporting leg.
- Position one foot so that only the tip of the shoe is in contact with the floor.
- Contract the lateral rotators of the hip to externally rotate the thigh outward.
- Return the leg to the starting position.

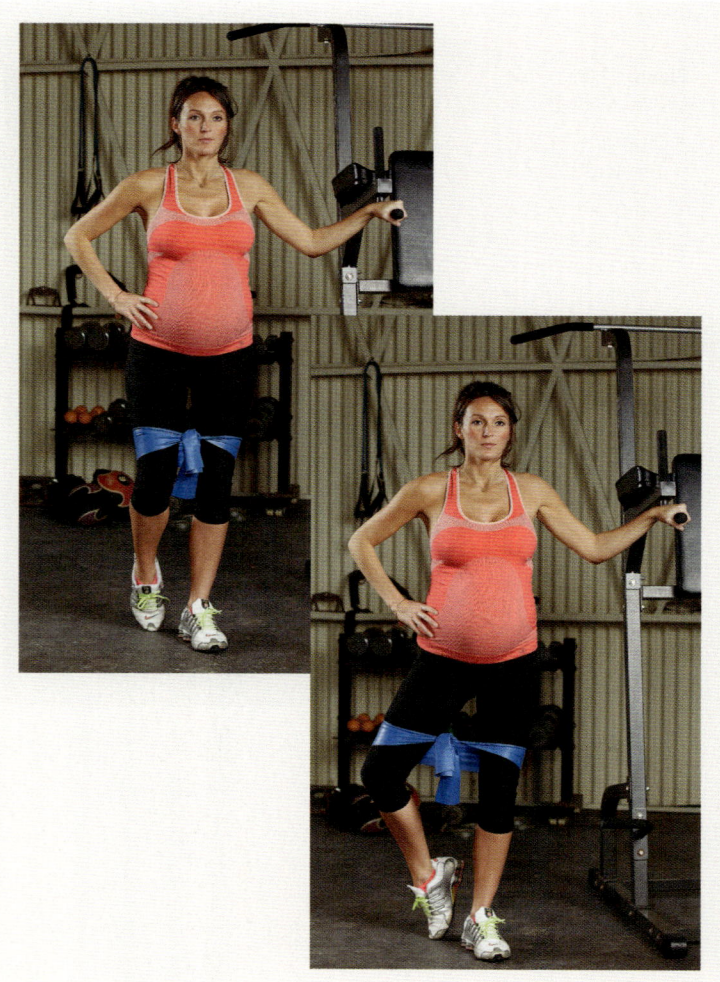

Prenatal and Postpartum Exercise — CHAPTER 21

Upper-extremity Exercises

Perform 12 to 15 repetitions of each of the following exercises (Figures 21-9 through 21-12). Progress the intensity only after the first movement is mastered. All of the dumbbell exercises can be performed with one arm at a time or with both arms simultaneously. It is typically more challenging to use both extremities at the same time versus one at a time. All of the dumbbell exercises can be progressed by adding small increments of weight (e.g., 2½ to 5 lb; 1 to 2 kg) when original weight becomes easy on the fifteenth repetition.

Figure 21-9
Standing chest press

- Stand with the back toward the anchor point of the resistance tube in a split-stance position (one foot in front of the other).
- Grasp the handles so that the tube rests underneath the arms.
- Push the handles forward until the elbows are extended.
- Return to the starting position.

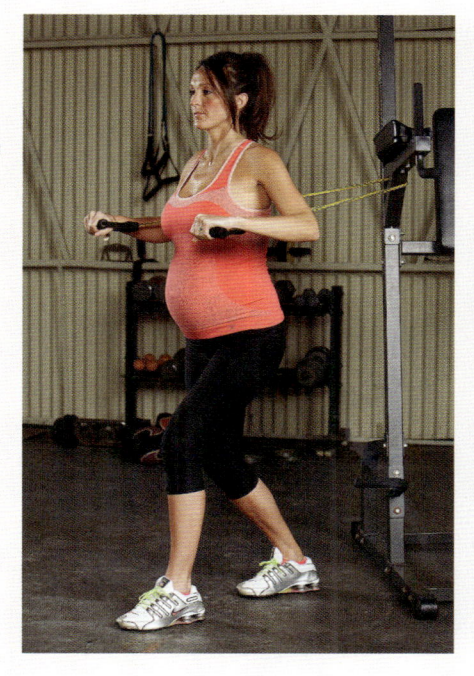

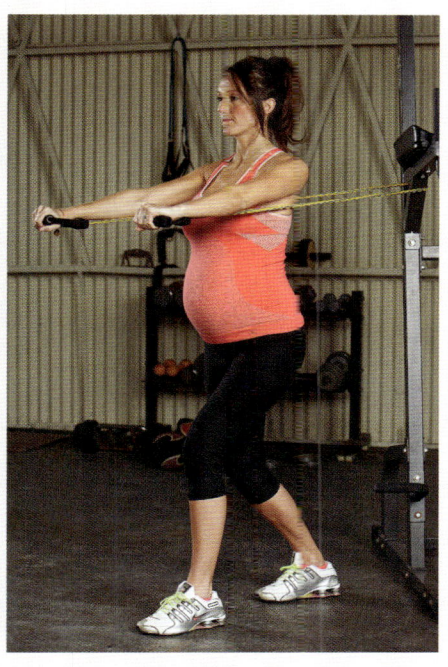

Figure 21-10
Biceps curl

- Stand with the feet shoulder-width apart, holding the dumbbells with the palms facing forward.
- Lift the weights toward the shoulders and then lower them to the starting position, moving only at the elbows (i.e., keep the shoulders still during the movement).

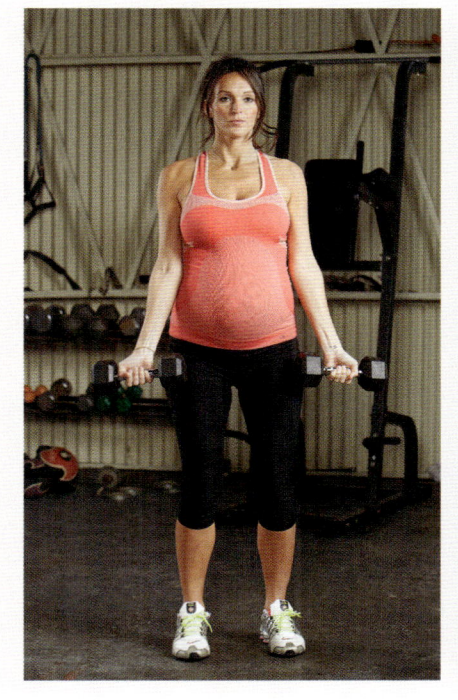

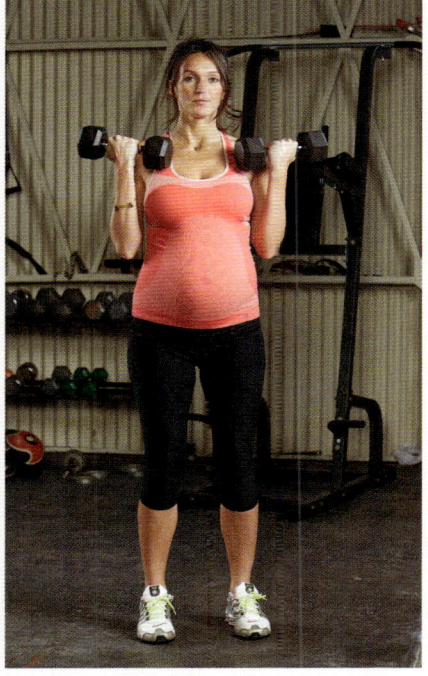

Figure 21-11
Overhead press

- Holding dumbbells, keep the elbows bent and close to the body, and position the hands in front of shoulders with the palms facing each other.
- Lift the arms overhead, trying to achieve full elbow extension at the top of the movement.
- Lower the weights, returning the arms to the starting position.

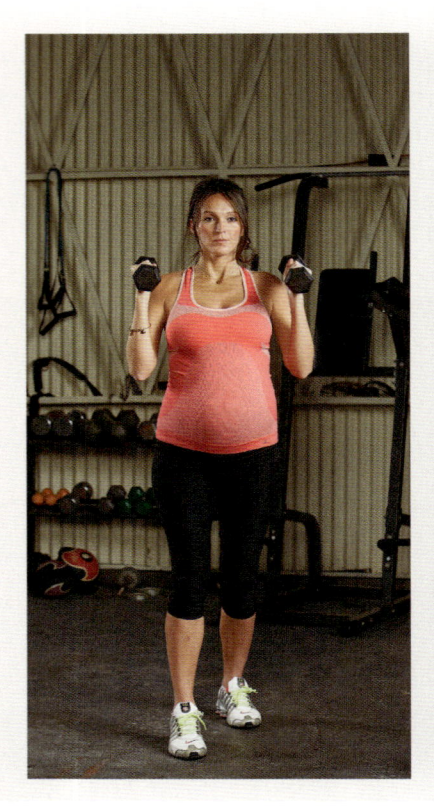

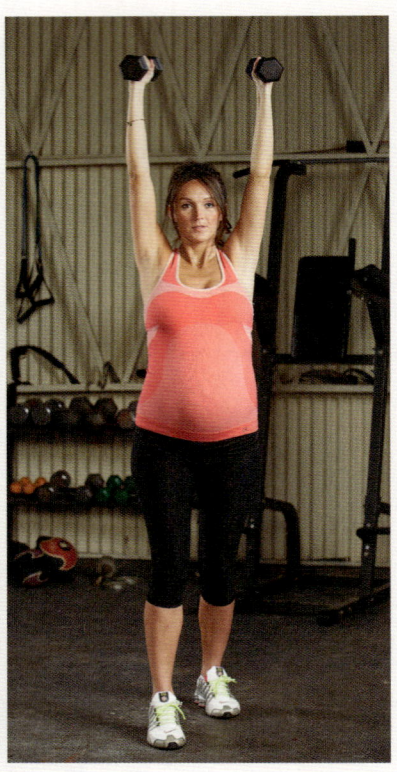

Figure 21-12
Standing bilateral row

- Stand facing the resistance tube with the feet in a split-stance position, keeping a slight bend in the knees.
- Keeping the spine in good alignment, maintain a slight bend in the knees.
- Pull the handles toward the ribs by flexing the elbows while squeezing the muscles of the upper/mid back, being sure that the elbows move behind the body in the end position.
- Return the arms to the starting position.

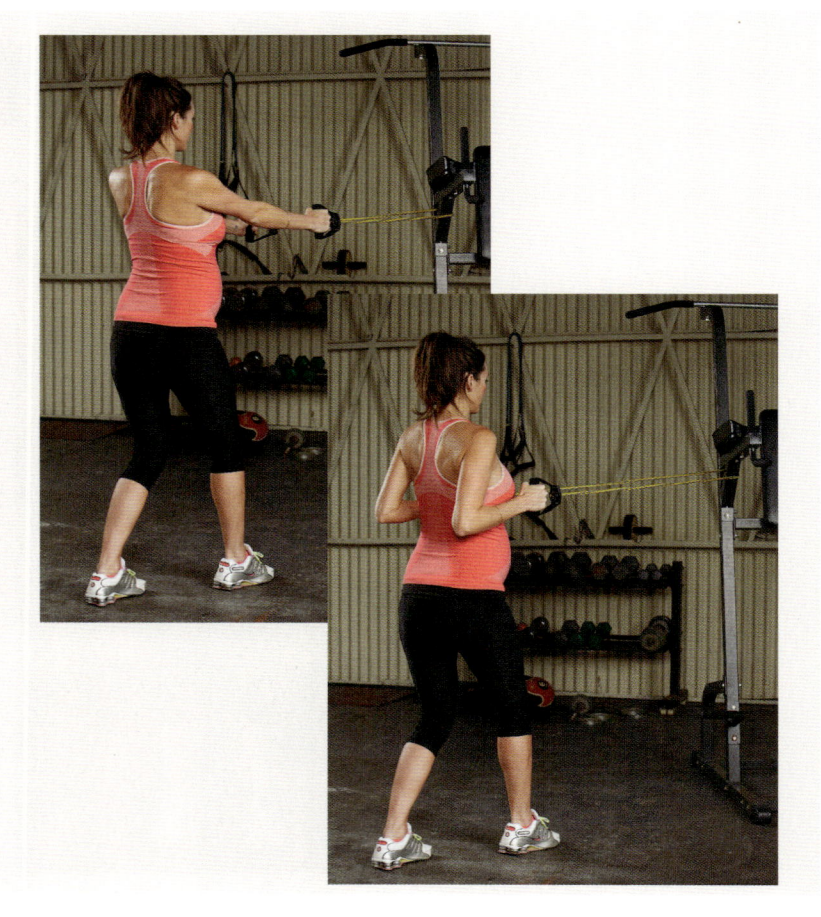

Prenatal and Postpartum Exercise   CHAPTER 21

Core Exercises

Perform 12 to 15 repetitions of each of the following exercises (Figures 21-13 through 21-16). Progress the intensity only after the first movement is mastered.

Figure 21-13
Crossover crunch

- Sit on a chair or bench, leaning back slightly with one arm on the seat for support.
- Raise the opposite arm to place the hand behind the head with the elbow pointing out to the side.
- Lightly contract the abdominals and move the opposite knee and elbow toward each other.
- Return to the starting position.

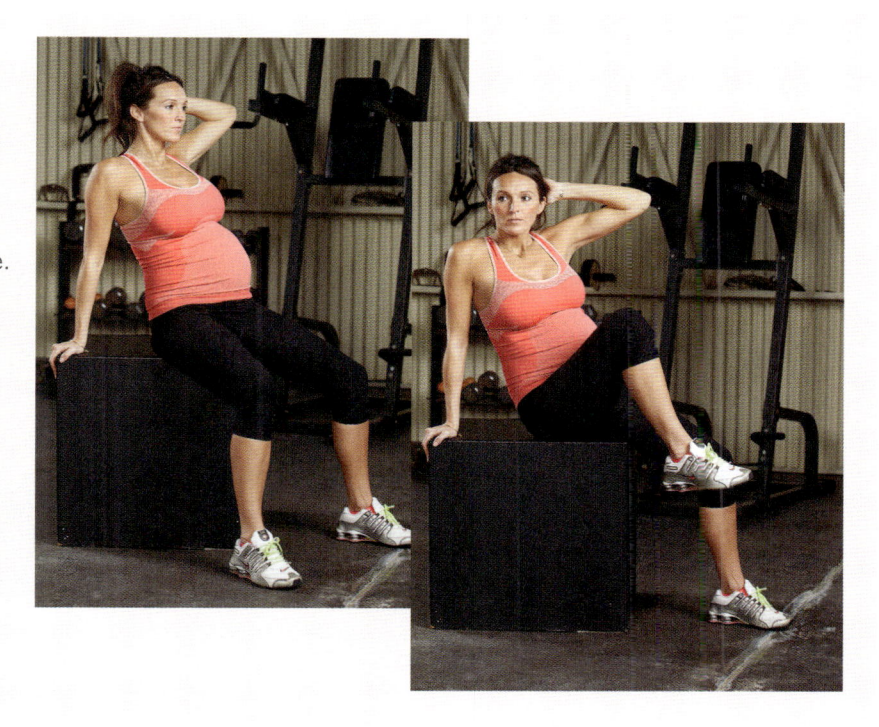

Figure 21-14
Diagonal hay baler

- Stand with the feet slightly wider than shoulder-width apart with the left foot on top of a resistance tube.
- Grasp the nylon portion of one of the tube handles (underneath the actual handle) with both hands and place the hands in front of the left hip.
- Press the arms upward across the body in a diagonal motion until both elbows reach full extension at the top of the movement while simultaneously shifting the body weight to the right foot.
- Return to the starting position.

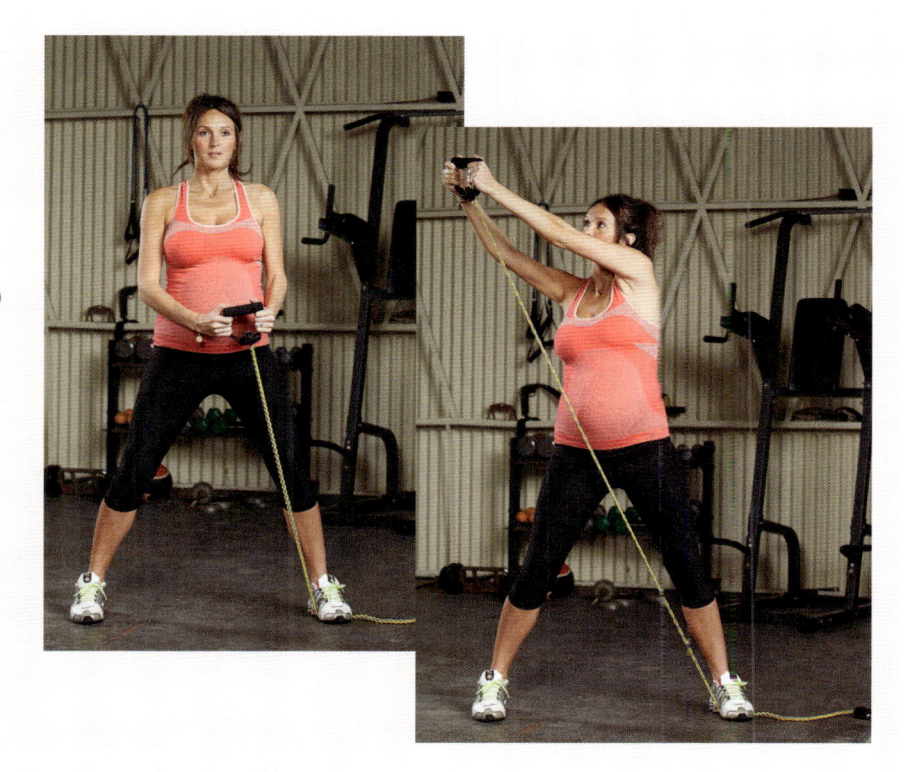

Figure 21-15
Bird dog

- Adopt a hands-and-knees position with the hands directly under the shoulders and the knees underneath the hips. For clients with painful wrists, a fist position may be used or the hands may be placed over dumbbells to keep the wrists in neutral rather than in weight-bearing extension.
- Slightly contract the abdominals and extend one leg at a time. Next, slightly contract the abdominals and extend one arm at a time.
- Slightly contract the abdominals and simultaneously flex the right shoulder and extend the left hip, while keeping the spine in good alignment.
- Hold for 5 seconds and return to the starting position, being sure to avoid the Valsalva maneuver by breathing deeply.
- Progression: Remove the 5-second hold and add arm and leg abduction and adduction to each shoulder flexion and hip extension before returning to the starting position. This requires stabilizing against an even more dynamic periphery.

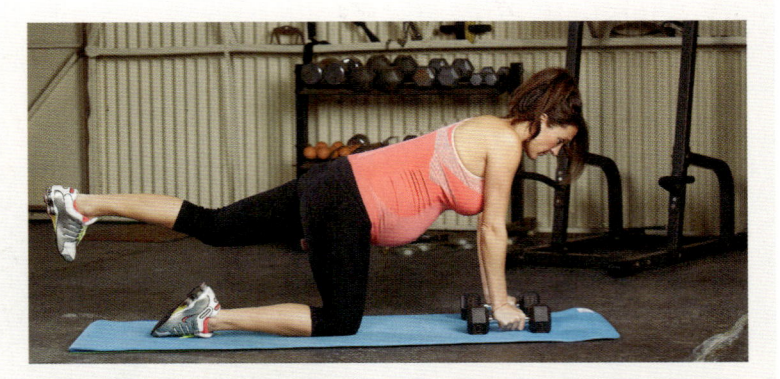

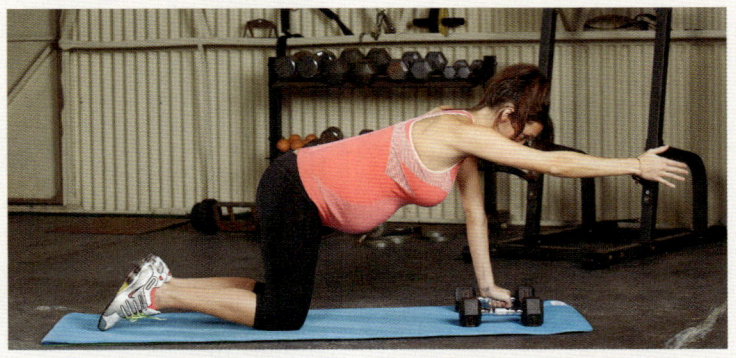

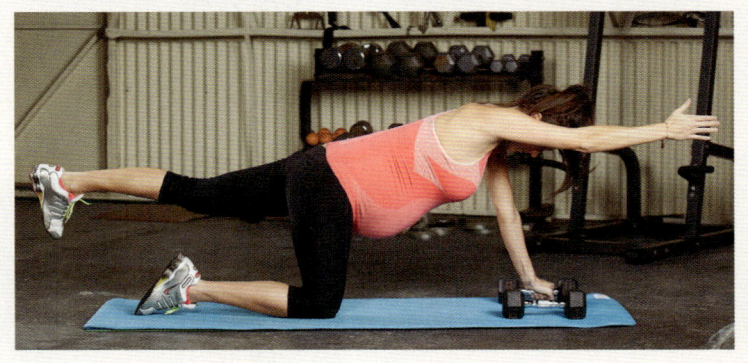

Figure 21-16
Side bridge

- Adopt a three-point side-plank position with the elbow, knee, and edge of the foot on the floor.
- Reach the hand upward with full elbow extension.
- Hold for up to 30 seconds and return to the starting position, being sure to avoid the Valsalva maneuver by breathing deeply.
- Progression: Add slight torso rotation by reaching the top arm under the rib cage and then returning to the starting position. This requires stabilizing against a dynamic periphery.

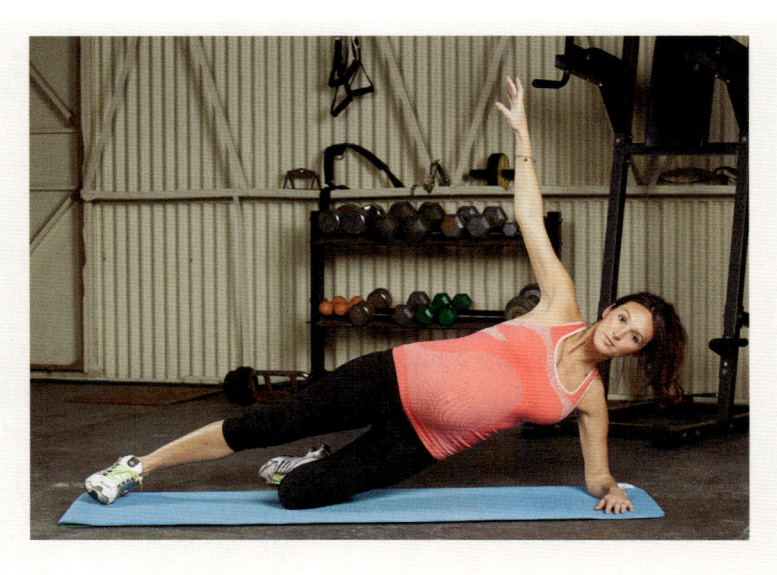

Prenatal and Postpartum Exercise   CHAPTER 21

Stretches

Each of the following stretches should be held in position for 15 to 60 seconds, with a focus on deep breathing to avoid the Valsalva maneuver (Figures 21-17 through 21-20). Further, although there is no evidence to support an increased risk of stretching injury due to increased circulating relaxin levels, pregnant women should be mindful of enhanced laxity in the joints and avoid extreme ranges of motion during flexibility exercises.

Figure 21-17
Modified downward-facing dog

- Place the arms on a chair or countertop with the thumbs turned up.
- Lower the chest toward the floor and bring the head between the arms.
- The stretch should be felt in the shoulders, back, and hamstrings.

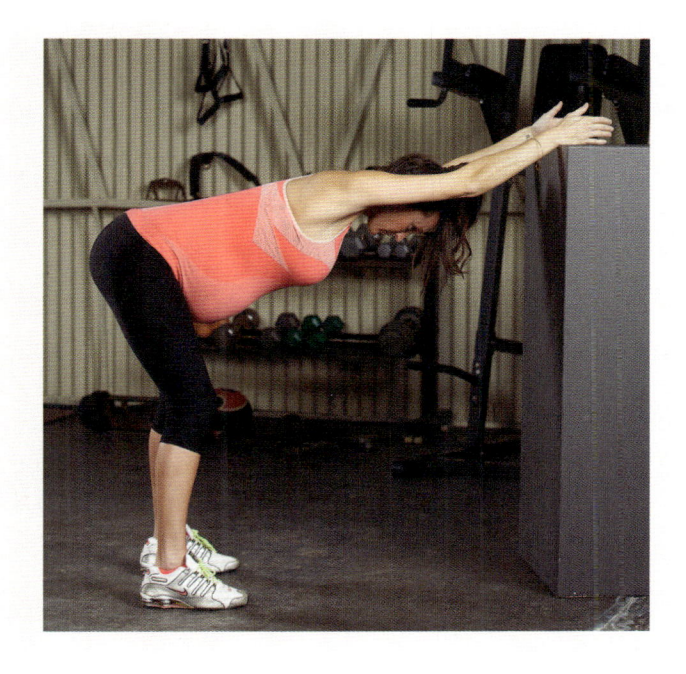

Figure 21-18
Calf stretch

- Stand on a step with the hands lightly touching a wall or chair for support.
- Drop one heel off the back of the step, keeping the knee straight and stretching the calf.

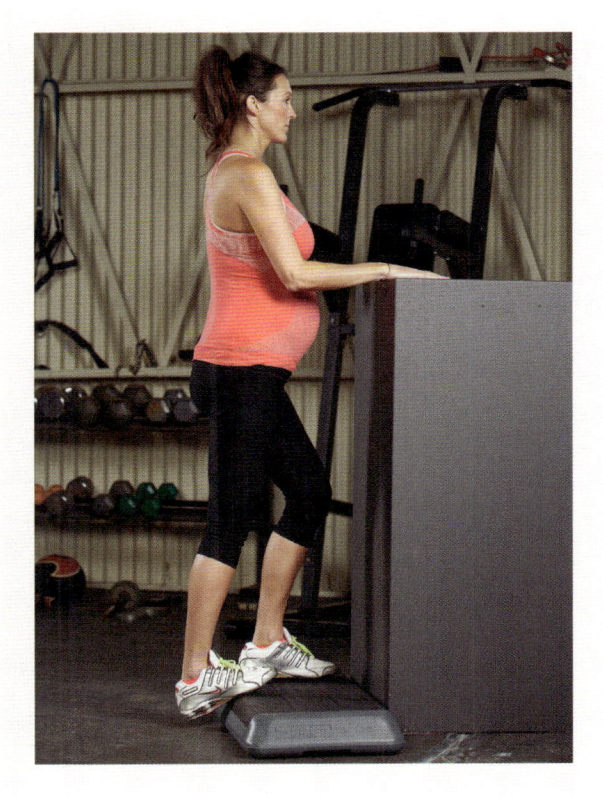

Figure 21-19
Leaning side-bend

- Stand with the left side of the body alongside the back of the chair or a countertop with the feet together. Cross the left foot behind the right foot.
- Lightly grasp onto the top of the chair or countertop with the left hand.
- Reach the right arm up overhead and bend the torso to the left side, leaning toward the countertop or chair.
- The stretch should be felt in the right side of the body.
- Repeat on the opposite side.

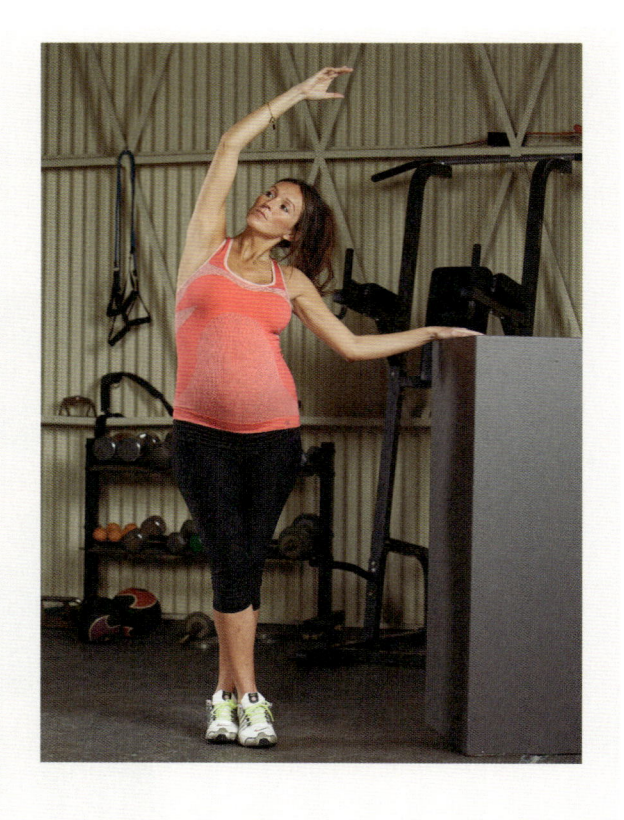

Figure 21-20
Chest/shoulder stretch

- Stand with the left side of the body alongside a wall with the feet hip-width apart.
- Lightly touch the wall with the left hand and take a step or two to the side away from the wall so that the left arm is bent 90 degrees.
- Gently rotate the torso away from the left arm.
- The stretch should be felt in the chest, shoulder, and upper arm of the left side.
- Repeat on the opposite side.

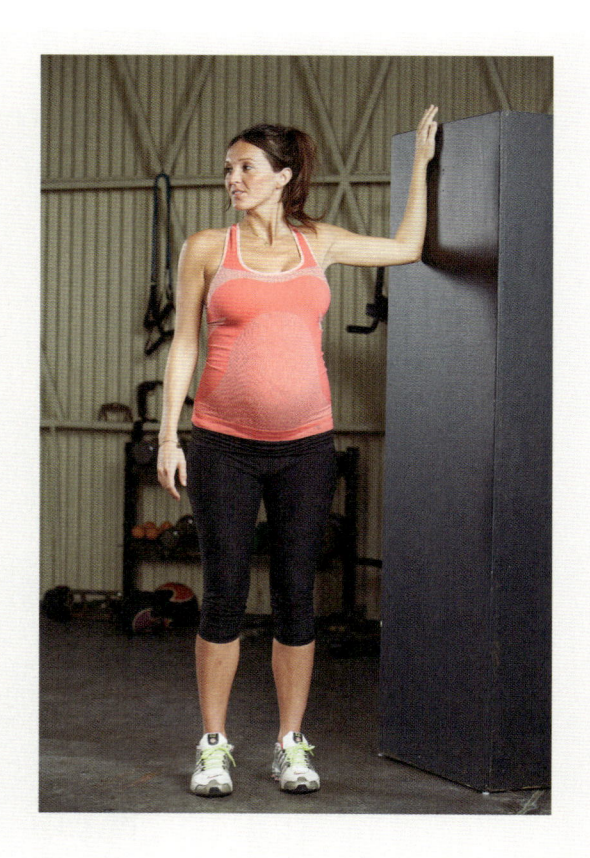

NUTRITIONAL CONSIDERATIONS

Good nutrition habits during pregnancy optimize maternal health and reduce the risk for some birth defects, suboptimal fetal growth and development, and chronic health problems in the developing child (Kaiser, 2014).

The key recommendations for nutrition during pregnancy include:

- *Consumption of a variety of foods and appropriate calories in accordance with the* Dietary Guidelines for Americans: The USDA's MyPlate offers specialized guidance for optimal nutrition for pregnant and breastfeeding women (www.myplate.gov). A healthy nutrition plan in pregnancy begins with eating small, frequent meals. Three meals are best replaced by five small meals per day, including breakfast, lunch, an afternoon snack, dinner, and a bedtime snack. Pregnant women should avoid fasting (longer than 13 hours) and should never skip breakfast due to a risk of **ketosis,** an increased acidity of the blood due to incomplete oxidation of fats, that can lead to a heightened increased risk of preterm delivery. Importantly, dieting is never healthy during pregnancy. An abundance of fruits, vegetables, whole grains, and high-calcium foods are recommended throughout pregnancy.

- *A moderate increase in calories:* In general, women do not have increased caloric needs until the second trimester, at which time needs increase by about 300 calories per day. The typical woman needs an additional 450 calories above baseline in the third trimester (Kaiser, 2014). Notably, caloric needs vary considerably among women, with one study finding a range of 25 calories to 800 calories more than pre-pregnancy (Pitkin, 1999). Women should be cautious not to gain excessive weight during pregnancy, as risks to mother and infant increase substantially (Kaiser, 2014).

- *Appropriate and timely vitamin and mineral intake or supplementation:* Pregnant women need 600 μg of **folic acid** daily from fortified foods or supplements in addition to food forms of folate from a varied diet (Kaiser, 2014). Folic acid reduces the risk of neural tube defects if taken prior to conception through the sixth week of pregnancy and may reduce birth defects if taken later in pregnancy. Because many pregnant women suffer from iron-deficiency anemia, most are advised to begin supplementation of 30 mg/day iron starting early in pregnancy. Vitamins and minerals that are needed in larger quantities during pregnancy and lactation are highlighted in Table 21-5. A woman considering pregnancy should consult with her primary care physician prior to becoming pregnant to discuss vitamin and mineral supplement needs. If this is not possible, a visit as soon as pregnancy is suspected or confirmed is advisable.

- *Avoidance of alcohol, tobacco, and energy drinks:* The CDC urges pregnant women not to drink alcohol any time during pregnancy. Alcohol passes readily through the placenta and can cause a variety of problems with an exposed fetus, including learning disabilities; low intelligence quotient (IQ); poor judgment; problems with the heart, kidney, or bones; and many others. Risks of smoking during pregnancy include preterm birth, stillbirth, and birth defects (such as some heart defects and cleft lip/palate), and sudden infant death syndrome (CDC, 2020). Energy drinks contain many ingredients that have not been well studied during pregnancy and may pose health risk to mother and fetus (Procter et al., 2014).

The Nutritional Considerations section is adapted from Muth, N.D. (2014). *Sports Nutrition for Health Professionals.* Philadelphia: F.A. Davis.

TABLE 21-5

NUTRIENT NEEDS THAT INCREASE DURING PREGNANCY AND LACTATION, FEMALES 19–50 YEARS

Nutrient	Non-pregnant	Pregnancy	Lactation
Carbohydrate (g/d)	130	175	210
Fiber (g/d)	25	28	29
Linoleic acid (g/d)	12	13	13
Linolenic acid (g/d)	1.1	1.4	1.3
Protein (g/d)	46	71*	71
Vitamin A (ug/d)	700	770	1,300
Vitamin E (mg/d)	15	15	19
Thiamin (mg/dl)	1.1	1.4	1.4
Riboflavin (mg/d)	1.1	1.4	1.6
Niacin (mg/d)	14	18	17
Pantothenic acid (mg/d)	5	6	7

*Increased protein needs during pregnancy are only for the second half of pregnancy. Needs are the same as non-pregnant women during the first half.

- *Caffeine in moderation:* Pregnant women are advised to consume no more than 200 mg of caffeine per day (equivalent to about a 12-oz cup of coffee). However, higher amounts do not appear to increase risk of poor fetal outcomes such as birth defects, miscarriage, preterm birth, or growth restriction (Procter et al., 2014).
- *Fluid intake to meet hydration and water needs:* Women are advised to consume 2.3 liters (about 10 cups) of beverages per day (Procter, et al., 2014).
- *Fish and seafood intake to boost fetal health:* Consumption of at least 8 oz of seafood per week may improve infant visual and cognitive development. This benefit generally outweighs the risk of mercury intake. However, fish should come from low mercury sources (Procter et al., 2014).
- *Safe food handling:* Pregnant women and their fetuses are at higher risk of developing foodborne illness and should take extra precautions to prevent consumption of contaminated foods by avoiding:
  - Soft cheeses not made with pasteurized milk
  - Deli meats, unless they have been reheated to steaming hot
  - Raw or unpasteurized milk or milk products, raw eggs, raw or undercooked meat, unpasteurized juice, raw sprouts, and raw or undercooked fish
  - Cat litter boxes
  - Handling pets when preparing foods
  - Shark, swordfish, king mackerel, or tilefish. Pregnant women can safely consume 12 ounces or less of fish or shellfish per week, provided that it is low in mercury, such as shrimp, canned light tuna, salmon, pollock, and catfish. Consumption of albacore tuna should be limited to 6 ounces or less per week.

Nutrition for Lactation

Prior to a child's birth, most women will decide whether they plan to breastfeed. Exclusive breastfeeding provides optimal nutrition and health protection for the first six months of life. From six to 12 months, breastfeeding combined with the gradual introduction of solid foods is optimal. Breastfeeding is nature's perfect source of nutrition for a newborn, providing the ideal nutrient mix, increased protection against a variety of infections, increased bonding, higher IQ, stronger bones, and many other benefits [American Academy of Pediatrics (AAP), 2012]. All mothers who are motivated and capable to breastfeed are highly encouraged to do so, not only for the significant benefits to the child, but also for maternal benefits, which include accelerated postpartum weight loss, decreased risk of breast and ovarian cancer, increased bonding, and decreased cost.

Women who breastfeed require approximately 500 additional calories per day for weight maintenance (AAP, 2012). Health professionals can help women return to pre-pregnancy weight by reinforcing the positive nutrition changes made during pregnancy, such as increased fruit, vegetable, and whole-grain consumption. Referral to a registered dietitian may be warranted if the woman requests or requires more extensive nutritional intervention such as meal planning.

PSYCHOLOGICAL CONSIDERATIONS

Pregnancy is associated with increased psychological distress for some women, which may include anxiety and **depression**. The onset of depression during pregnancy, also known as antenatal depression, has an estimated prevalence rate of 10 to 13% (Gavin et al., 2005). Antenatal depression has been associated with a number of adverse outcomes for both mothers and infants, including poor self-care, premature labor, low birth weight, longer hospital stays, and compromised mother-child bonding. Further, depression during pregnancy is one of the strongest predictors of postpartum depression (Shivakumar et al., 2011).

EXPAND YOUR KNOWLEDGE

PSYCHOLOGICAL STRESS DURING PREGNANCY MAY AFFECT THE CHILD

In their review on the impact of maternal stress, depression, and anxiety on fetal neurobehavioral development, Kinsella and Monk (2009) reported that women's antenatal psychological distress affects fetal behavior and child development. Exposure to a range of traumatic, as well as chronic and common, life stressors (e.g., bereavement and daily hassles), has been linked to significant alterations in children's neurodevelopment, such as increased risk for autism, affective disorders, and reduced cognitive ability. Maternal antenatal anxiety and/or depression have been associated with an increased risk for neurodevelopmental disorders in children and risk for future mental illness. Also, elevated levels of antenatal depression and anxiety are associated with poor emotional adjustment in young children (Kinsella & Monk, 2009).

Since physically active pregnant women tend to experience less insomnia, stress, anxiety and depression (Shivakumar et al., 2011; Daley et al., 2008), the CMES can play an important role in promoting health and psychological well-being in their pregnant clients.

After giving birth, a psychological disorder called postpartum depression is a risk for some women. Postpartum depression is estimated to affect 10 to 15% of women and is characterized by sadness, fatigue, irritability, and disinterest in life events (Fitelson et al. 2011; Yonkers, Vigod, & Ross, 2011). Women with postpartum depression often experience feelings of guilt, worthlessness and anxiety related to birth and parenting, and may also think of suicide or harm toward the baby. Postpartum depression is a serious mood disorder comparable with major depressive disorder that can develop as an extension of postpartum blues (i.e., a less severe form of depression characterized by tearfulness, irritability, **hypochondriasis,** sleeplessness, impairment of concentration, and headache that occurs in the 10 days or so postpartum) or arise independently in a mother whose mood has been stable until that point. Risk factors for postpartum depression include previous mental illness, recent psychological stress, inadequate social or economic support, and a difficult birth experience (Ellsworth-Bowers & Corwin, 2012).

Depression in the postpartum period has significant negative effects on a mother's ability to interact appropriately with her child. For example, depressed women have been found to have poorer responsiveness to infant cues and more negative, hostile, or disengaged parenting behaviors (Fitelson et al., 2011). Further, maternal depression increases the risk for negative infant feeding outcomes, including lower rates of initiating or maintaining breastfeeding, lower levels of breastfeeding self-efficacy, and more difficulties while breastfeeding (Dennis & McQueen, 2009).

Given the known links between physical inactivity and reduced mental health, it is plausible that a relationship exists between pregnancy-related reductions in physical activity and psychological distress. Evidence suggests a positive relationship between regular physical activity and mood during pregnancy such that pregnant women who maintained an active lifestyle experienced relatively lesser severity of mood states such as fatigue, depression, and tension (Shivakumar et al., 2011). In a study that measured physical activity and mood during pregnancy, it was shown that healthy women who maintain an above-average level of physical activity during the second and third trimesters enjoy more mood stability (Poudevigne & O'Connor, 2005). In women experiencing mild-to-moderate postpartum depression, exercise may be considered as a management strategy. In concordance with the established general recommendations for exercise for all adults, a review of the effects of exercise on postpartum depression defined moderate-intensity activities for at least 30 minutes per day, five days per week, including walking in the form of stroller pushing, as "feasible and effective" (Daley et al., 2008). These findings support the theory that regular endurance exercise throughout pregnancy not only improves maternal and fetal physical health, but may enhance psychological health as well.

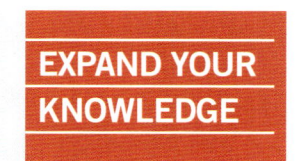

POSTPARTUM EXERCISE

Regular exercise is as beneficial in the postpartum period as it is at other times in a woman's life. The health benefits include improved cardiovascular health, support of healthy weight, increased fitness, and improved mental health (UK Chief Medical Officers, 2019; Davies et al., 2003; ACOG, 2020). Furthermore, a mother's participation in regular exercise after childbirth may encourage regular physical activity in her children.

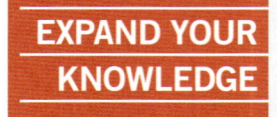

EXPAND YOUR KNOWLEDGE

POSTPARTUM WEIGHT LOSS

Pregnancy-related weight retention is a known contributor to overweight and obesity among women (Durham et al., 2011). For many women, returning to prepregnancy weight is a challenge. Approximately 14 to 25% of women are at least 11 lb (5 kg) heavier one year after delivery, placing them at increased risk for obesity and its comorbidities. Identified risk factors for retaining at least 11 lb (5 kg) at one year postpartum include higher pre-pregnancy weight and gestational weight gain, and behaviors including inadequate sleep, low physical activity, high **trans fat** intake, and frequent television viewing (Herring et al., 2008). During the postpartum period, women often reduce physical activity because of physiological, behavioral, and psychosocial changes. Factors such as limited childcare, more children in the home, and working full-time significantly contribute to inactivity during the postpartum period (Durham et al., 2011).

Similar to non-pregnant adults, overall lifestyle interventions focused on weight loss, including exercise plus intensive diet, are the most effective intervention strategies for postpartum women (Nascimento et al., 2013). With less than 20 to 30% of pregnant and postpartum women adhering to a physician-recommended level of exercise (Durham et al., 2011; Shivakumar et al., 2011), special emphasis should be placed on reducing sedentary time and on increasing moderate-intensity physical activity. The *Physical Activity Guidelines for Americans* recommend specifically that pregnant and postpartum women attain at least 150 minutes of moderate-intensity aerobic activity spread over a week if not already highly active or doing vigorous-intensity activity (U.S. Department of Health & Human Services, 2018). These recommendations should be encouraged to further health and weight loss in postpartum clients.

Research is lacking on maternal aerobic fitness and strength during the postpartum period. However, two randomized controlled trials have found a significant increase in aerobic power resulting from an endurance-exercise intervention during the first 10 to 12 weeks postpartum (Lovelady et al., 2000; Dewey et al., 1994). To date, studies have not assessed the effect of strength training (with or without aerobic exercise) during the postpartum period on muscle strength and endurance or the preservation of lean body mass. It seems reasonable to state, however, that the possible benefit of maternal fitness on the daily physical activities of mothering, including lifting, carrying, or running after a child, is worth the effort of beginning or maintaining regular exercise during the postpartum period.

With regard to exercising after childbirth, a major consideration is the method of delivery. Women who have undergone C-section deliveries have had major abdominal surgery that results in pain and tenderness in the abdomen, as well as considerable fatigue. Rehabilitation after C-section includes walking as soon as possible after the surgery to help minimize muscle wasting, increase circulation, and speed the healing process. Additionally, deep breathing, abdominal compression exercises, and Kegels can be resumed early in the recovery process. Vigorous exercise is contraindicated after a C-section until the recovery and rehabilitation process is complete.

Since deconditioning typically occurs during the early postpartum period, women should be encouraged to gradually increase physical-activity levels until pre-pregnancy fitness levels are achieved. Gradual exercise in the postpartum period may begin approximately four to six weeks after delivery for a normal vaginal birth or about eight to 10 weeks (with medical clearance) after a Cesarean birth. Women should not be concerned with physical activity interfering with breastfeeding, as light-to-moderate intensity exercise does not pose a problem with lactation, as long as an adequate food and fluid intake are maintained (ACSM, 2022).

PHYSIOLOGICAL CHANGES FOLLOWING PREGNANCY

As in pregnancy, the physiological changes following pregnancy are primarily determined by the endocrine system, with many of the pregnancy adaptations persisting into the postpartum period. The hormones that dominate during pregnancy gradually return to pre-pregnancy levels after childbirth, which results in concomitant changes in the musculoskeletal, cardiovascular, and respiratory systems.

Levels of the hormone relaxin, responsible for producing laxity in the collagenous structures of the pelvis and other areas in preparation for childbirth, rise dramatically during pregnancy. While the research is not clear on how long it takes for relaxin's effects to subside, it is undetectable in the serum within the first few days after delivery (Aldabe et al., 2012). Since ligamentous overstretching can remain in a new mother for up to eight months postpartum, she should learn how to correctly lift and carry her baby, put the baby in the crib, and take the baby out of the crib to reduce the potential risk of back pain due to the relaxed soft-tissue structures supporting the joints.

During pregnancy, the cardiovascular system adapts by increasing blood volume, heart rate, and cardiac output. Plasma volume increases by as much as 30 to 50% (West et al., 2010) to maintain the increased circulatory need of the enlarging uterus and fetoplacental unit, fill the ever-increasing venous reservoir, and protect the mother from the blood loss at the time of delivery. It takes about eight weeks after delivery for the blood volume to return to pre-pregnancy levels. Cardiac output increases by 30 to 50% during pregnancy (Rossi et al., 2011). The increase in heart rate lags behind the increase in cardiac output initially, and then ultimately increases by 10 to 15 bpm by 28 to 32 weeks of gestation. Cardiac output, heart rate, and stroke volume decrease to pre-labor values 24 to 72 hours after birth and return to non-pregnant levels within six to eight weeks after delivery.

The respiratory system exhibits adaptations to pregnancy starting as early as the fourth week of gestation. A woman can expect **minute ventilation** to increase by about 50% above nonpregnant values and tidal volume and respiratory rate to also increase during pregnancy. Within six to 12 weeks postpartum, all respiratory parameters return to non-pregnant values.

Because of the gradual return to pre-pregnancy musculoskeletal, cardiovascular, and respiratory parameters, and the detraining effect that occurs for most women during pregnancy, postpartum exercise programs should be individualized and resumed gradually. Furthermore, moderate weight reduction while nursing is considered safe and does not compromise neonatal weight gain (ACOG, 2020; McCrory et al., 1999).

PROGRAMMING GUIDELINES AND CONSIDERATIONS FOR POSTPARTUM EXERCISE

Exercise guidelines during pregnancy and the postpartum period are similar among many organizations, including ACSM, ACOG, and the UK Chief Medical Officers. A more detailed set of guidelines for postpartum exercise has been developed by Clapp and Cram (2012), who suggest that the initial goal of exercise (within the first six weeks) is to obtain personal time and redevelop a sense of control. This can be accomplished by doing the following:
- Beginning slowly and increasing gradually
- Avoiding excessive fatigue and dehydration
- Supporting and compressing the abdomen and breasts
- Stopping to evaluate if it hurts
- Stopping exercise and seeking medical evaluation if the postpartum client is experiencing bright red vaginal bleeding that is heavier than a menstrual period

Clapp and Cram (2012) go on to suggest that after six weeks postpartum, the goal of the exercise regimen in the remainder of the first year following birth is to improve physical fitness. Other reports suggest that exercise levels often diminish after childbirth, frequently leading to overweight and obesity, making the postpartum period an opportune time for the CMES and obstetric care providers to reinforce the importance of resuming exercise routines to support lifelong healthy habits (ACOG, 2020).

One area of concern for many women after childbirth is strengthening the pelvic floor. The pelvic-floor muscles form the pelvic basin and help maintain continence by actively supporting the pelvic organs and closing the pelvic openings when contracting. The pelvic-floor muscles are composed of the pelvic diaphragm muscles (together known as the levator ani), which can be referred to as the deep layer; the urogenital diaphragm muscles (together known as the perineal muscles), which can be referred to as the superficial layer; and the urethral and anal sphincter muscles (Figure 21-21). The pelvic-floor muscles are encased in fascia, which is connected to the endopelvic (parietal) fascia surrounding the pelvic organs and assists in pelvic organ support.

Figure 21-21
Pelvic floor muscles (inferior view)

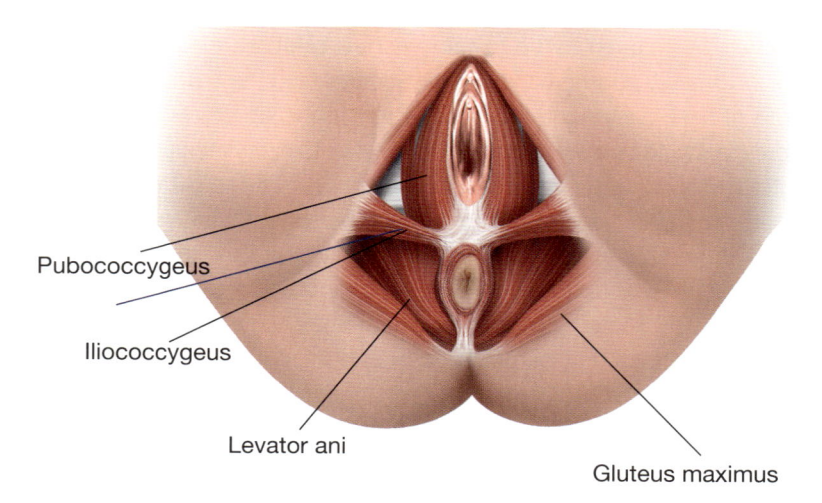

APPLY WHAT YOU KNOW

PRENATAL AND POSTPARTUM KEGEL EXERCISES

Correct action of the pelvic-floor muscles has been described as a squeeze around the pelvic openings and an inward lift (such as the action performed during a Kegel exercise). Pelvic-floor muscle training can increase the strength of the pelvic-floor muscles, thereby enhancing the structural support, timing, and strength of automatic contraction and resulting in the reduction or elimination of leakage. Initially, Kegel exercises can be performed utilizing the following three steps:

- Tightening the pelvic floor muscles and holding a static contraction for a count of 10
- Relaxing the muscles completely for a count of 10
- Performing 10 Kegel exercise sets, three times per day

Another option is to perform the Kegel exercises quickly (tighten, lift up, and let go) to work the muscles in a way that mimics shutting off the flow of urine to help prevent accidents. Many women prefer to do these exercises while lying down or sitting in a chair, but they can be performed anywhere. After four to six weeks, there is usually some improvement, but it may take up to three months to see a significant change.

Training the pelvic-floor musculature goes hand-in-hand with performing exercises to strengthen the core. Research findings have shown that maximal pelvic-floor muscle contractions are not possible without a co-contraction of the abdominal muscles, specifically the transversus abdominis and internal oblique muscles (Bordoni & Zanier, 2103). This abdominal contraction can be observed as a small inward movement of the lower abdomen. Prior to any strenuous abdominal exercise, postnatal clients should perform transversus abdominis work (i.e., a drawing-in maneuver), pelvic tilts, and spinal stabilization exercises. Since traditional abdominal crunches compress the abdominal space and increase pressure on the pelvic floor, they should be reserved for exercise regimens after the postpartum client has had time to re-educate the pelvic floor muscles through Kegel training and core stabilization work.

Prenatal and Postpartum Exercise

Exercise Considerations for the Lactating Mother

Increased weight in the breasts from lactation, coupled with the forward-rounded postures associated with holding, feeding, and cuddling the baby, may lead to upper-back pain in a new mother. Additionally, lifting car seats and pushing strollers with handles that are set too low can contribute to the back pain often reported after childbirth. Stretches for the anterior shoulder girdle, followed by scapular retraction and external shoulder rotation exercises, are appropriate for new mothers looking to improve posture post-delivery and ease the pain associated with these biomechanical concerns.

Good breast support is important for comfort during postpartum exercise. It is recommended that postnatal exercisers wear a very supportive exercise bra, or two bras together if necessary. Furthermore, breastfeeding women are advised to avoid exercise with a breast abscess or with painful, engorged breasts. Nursing or expressing milk before exercise has also been suggested to increase comfort during exercise.

THINK IT THROUGH

As described in this chapter, pregnancy is a time of significant anatomic and physiologic change for the expectant mother. Pregnant clients will undoubtedly have many questions for the CMES regarding sound practices for exercise during pregnancy. In addition to their obstetrician, the CMES will likely be an important resource for fitness-related topics throughout pregnancy. To better prepare for training prenatal and postpartum clients, come up with evidence-based answers to the following questions:

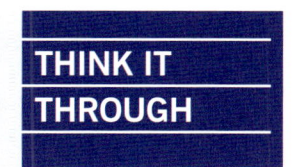

- How does exercise benefit the expecting mother?
- How does exercise affect the developing fetus?
- Does exercise affect weight gain during pregnancy?
- How much exercise is recommended?
- Which exercises or activities should be avoided?
- How late into pregnancy can an expecting mother exercise?
- Does postpartum exercise affect milk production?
- How soon after giving birth can a new mother begin to exercise?

While this list may seem extensive, the answers to these questions are important concepts for guiding prenatal and postpartum clients through safe and effective exercise programs.

FITT RECOMMENDATIONS FOR WOMEN WHO ARE PREGNANT

	Society of Obstetricians and Gynaecologists of Canada and Canadian Society for Exercise Physiology*	American College of Obstetricians and Gynecologists†	U.S. Department of Health & Human Services‡ and World Health Organization**
Frequency	• At least 3 days per week • Being active every day is encouraged	• At least 3–4 days per week	• Spread throughout the week
Intensity	• Moderate intensity ✓ Below VT1 ✓ Can carry on a conversation but not sing ✓ RPE 12–13 (6–20 scale) ✓ RPE 3–4 (6–10 scale) ✓ 3–5.9 METs	• Moderate intensity ✓ Less than 60–80% of age-predicted maximal maternal heart rate ✓ RPE 13–14 (6–20 scale) ✓ Can carry on a conversation while exercising (below VT1)	• Moderate intensity ✓ Below VT1 ✓ Can carry on a conversation but not sing ✓ RPE 12–13 (6–20 scale) ✓ RPE 5–6 (6–10 scale) ✓ 3–5.9 METs ✓ Women who habitually engaged in vigorous-intensity aerobic activity before pregnancy can continue these activities during pregnancy and the postpartum period, with uncomplicated pregnancies.

FITT RECOMMENDATIONS FOR WOMEN WHO ARE PREGNANT

(continued)

	Society of Obstetricians and Gynaecologists of Canada and Canadian Society for Exercise Physiology*	American College of Obstetricians and Gynecologists[†]	U.S. Department of Health & Human Services[‡] and World Health Organization**
Time	• Accumulate at least 150 minutes per week	• 30–60 minutes per day	• At least 150 minutes per week • Doing some physical activity is better than none • Limit the amount of time being sedentary and replace with physical activity of any intensity

Type	• Cardiorespiratory training
	• Muscular training
	• Yoga and gentle stretching
	• Daily Kegel exercise
		• Cardiorespiratory training
		  ✓ Walking
		  ✓ Stationary cycling
		  ✓ Dancing
		  ✓ Aquatic exercise
		• Muscular training
		  ✓ Resistance machines, free weights, and elastic bands
		  ✓ Pelvic floor exercises initiated in the immediate postpartum period
			• Cardiorespiratory training
			• Muscular training
			  ✓ Daily pelvic floor muscle training
			• Gentle stretching
			• Avoid contact and collision sports and activities with a high risk of falling or abdominal trauma

Progression	• Previously inactive women should begin gradually at a lower intensity and increase duration and intensity as pregnancy progresses • Progress based on medical recommendations, client goals, and the ACE Integrated Fitness Training® Model	• Progress based on medical recommendations, client goals, and the ACE Integrated Fitness Training Model • If sedentary before pregnancy, follow a more gradual progression	• Progress based on medical recommendations, client goals, and the ACE Integrated Fitness Training Model • Previously inactive women should start with small amounts of physical activity and gradually increase frequency, intensity, and duration over time

Note: VT1 = First ventilatory threshold; RPE = Rating of perceived exertion; METs = Metabolic equivalents

*Mottola, M.F. et al. (2018). 2019 Canadian guideline for physical activity throughout pregnancy. *British Journal of Sports Medicine*, 52, 1339–1346.

[†]American College of Obstetricians and Gynecologists (2020). Physical activity and exercise during pregnancy and the postpartum period, ACOG Committee Opinion No. 804. *Obstetrics & Gynecology,* 135, 4, e178–e188.73.

[‡]U.S. Department of Health & Human Services (2018). *Physical Activity Guidelines for Americans* (2nd ed.). www.health.gov/paguidelines/

**World Health Organization (2020). *WHO Guidelines on Physical Activity and Sedentary Behavior.* https://www.who.int/publications/i/item/9789240015128

CMES FOCUS

For healthy, pregnant women, exercise is encouraged throughout pregnancy with modifications to frequency, intensity, and duration applied as needed according to symptoms, discomforts, and abilities. Exercise recommendations for women who have overweight or obesity pre-pregnancy are modified slightly compared to women with a BMI <25 kg/m² prior to conception. Women who are pregnant and sedentary or pregnant with a medical condition (e.g., severe obesity, gestational diabetes, and hypertension) should receive a physician's clearance before beginning a new exercise program.

CASE STUDY

Client Information

Jacki is 37 years old and recently discovered she is pregnant. She is in her first trimester and would like to continue her exercise program. Currently, Jacki runs 3 to 4 miles (5 to 6 km) per workout for a total of about 12 to 15 miles (19 to 24 km) per week, and lifts weights two days a week. She has been cleared by her physician to continue her current routine as long as she reduces her exercise as overall discomfort dictates as her pregnancy progresses. Jacki has two children already, and during both pregnancies suffered from mild diastasis recti and low-back pain.

CMES Approach

Frequency: Jacki may continue to exercise at least three times per week following her typical exercise routine.

Intensity: Jacki should use RPE to monitor the intensity of her workout and aim for a rating of "fairly light" to "very hard" (3 to 6 on the 0 to 10 scale, or 12 to 17 on the 6 to 20 scale). She should also be instructed to avoid hot and humid conditions and remain properly hydrated.

Time: Jacki should be encouraged to exercise in accordance with her regular exercise program. However, she should be instructed not to continue an exercise session to the point of fatigue or exhaustion.

Type: Jacki may continue to perform weight-bearing exercise, including running, as long as she is comfortable. As her pregnancy progresses, she may want to perform non-weight-bearing exercise such as cycling or water aerobics, especially if she notices a recurrence of the low-back pain she experienced in her first two pregnancies. Jacki may continue her resistance-training program, but may find lighter resistance and higher repetitions more comfortable than a higher-intensity program. She should be instructed to avoid prolonged exercise in the supine position after the first trimester.

Exercises appropriate for Jacki that will help her avoid low-back pain include mobility and stretching movements that emphasize relaxing and lengthening the back extensors, hip flexors, scapular protractors, shoulder internal rotators, and neck flexors. Strengthening exercises should focus on the abdominals, gluteals, and scapular retractors to reinforce their ability to support proper alignment. Specifically, abdominal-compression exercises and curl-ups in a semirecumbent position may be helpful for strengthening the rectus abdominis without exacerbating her diastasis recti.

ACE IFT® MODEL AT A GLANCE

Cardiorespiratory Training

Jacki is a regular exerciser. Her pre-pregnancy running program would be categorized as a Fitness Training program, as she is training regularly at moderate and vigorous intensities, but she is not following a periodized program designed for peak performance that would be seen in Performance Training. As her pregnancy progresses, she will actually reduce her exercise intensity to primarily low-to-moderate. Following delivery, she may need to resume cardiorespiratory exercise in Base Training and then progress back to Fitness Training.

Muscular Training

Jacki is performing Load/Speed Training two days per week when she discovers that she is pregnant. She is cleared by her physician to continue training at this level initially, with regression as her pregnancy progresses. The CMES introduces a combination of Functional and Movement Training exercises to help Jacki maintain good mobility and movement patterns, while enhancing postural stability and kinetic-chain mobility as her pregnancy advances. Her postpartum program would start with Functional Training to address any stability and mobility issues before progressing to Load/Speed Training.

SUMMARY

An increasing amount of research on exercise in pregnancy has led to less debate regarding the maternal and fetal risks of regular physical activity during pregnancy. Women entering pregnancy with regular aerobic and strength-conditioning activities as a part of their daily routines is a growing trend, and many women who are not physically active view pregnancy as a time to modify their lifestyles to include more health-conscious activities.

Evidence that regular prenatal exercise is an important component of a healthy pregnancy is increasing. The positive effects of exercise during pregnancy on the musculoskeletal, cardiovascular, respiratory, and thermoregulatory systems have been reported. Several national health and medical organizations have published recommendations and guidelines on exercise and pregnancy (ACOG, 2020; ACSM, 2022; Mottola et al., 2018; ROCG, 2017). According to ACSM (2022), there are some women for whom exercise during pregnancy is absolutely contraindicated, and others for whom the potential benefits associated with exercise may outweigh the risks.

Due to the wide range of postural and physiological adaptations that occur during and after pregnancy, the CMES must be proficient at designing exercise programs geared toward making physical activity more comfortable for this population. Physiological adaptations include a profound increase in body mass, retention of fluid, and laxity in supporting structures. Postural adaptations correspond with these physiological changes and usually entail an alteration in the loading and alignment of, and muscle forces along, the spine and weight-bearing joints.

REFERENCES

Aldabe, D., Milosavljevic, S., & Bussey, M.D. (2012). Is pregnancy related pelvic girdle pain associated with altered kinematic, kinetic and motor control of the pelvis? A systematic review. *European Spine Journal*, 21, 9, 1777–1787.

Aldabe, D. et al. (2012). Pregnancy-related pelvic girdle pain and its relationship with relaxin levels during pregnancy: A systematic review. *European Spine Journal*, 21, 9, 1769–1776.

Al-Khodairy, A.T., Bovay, P., & Gobelet, C. (2007). Sciatica in the female patient: Anatomical considerations, aetiology and review of the literature. *European Spine Journal*, 16, 6, 721–731.

American Academy of Pediatrics, Section on Breastfeeding (2012). Breastfeeding and the use of human milk. *Pediatrics*, 129, 3, e827–e841.

American College of Obstetricians and Gynecologists (2020). Physical activity and exercise during pregnancy and the postpartum period, ACOG Committee Opinion No. 804. *Obstetrics & Gynecology*, 135, 4, e178–e188.73.

American College of Sports Medicine (2022). *ACSM's Guidelines for Exercise Testing and Prescription* (11th ed.). Philadelphia: Wolters Kluwer.

Benjamin, D.R., van de Water, A.T., & Peiris, C.L. (2013). Effects of exercise on diastasis of the rectus abdominis muscle in the antenatal and postnatal periods: A systematic review. *Physiotherapy*, S0031-9406(13)00083-7.

Bordoni, B. & Zanier, E. (2013). Anatomic connections of the diaphragm: Influence of respiration on the body system. *Journal of Multidisciplinary Healthcare*, 6, 281–291.

Brown, C.M. & Garovic, V.D. (2011). Mechanisms and management of hypertension in pregnant women. *Current Hypertension Reports*, 13, 5, 338–346.

Centers for Disease Control and Prevention (2020). *Pregnant? Don't Smoke!* www.cdc.gov/pregnancy/features/pregnantdontsmoke.html#:~:text=Smoking%20during%20pregnancy%20can%20cause,herself%20and%20her%20developing%20baby.

Centers for Disease Control and Prevention (2019). *Gestational Diabetes.* www.cdc.gov/diabetes/basics/gestational.html#:~:text=However%2C%20about%2050%25%20of%20women,your%20levels%20are%20on%20target.

Centers for Disease Control and Prevention (2018). *Diabetes During Pregnancy.* www.cdc.gov/reproductivehealth/maternalinfanthealth/diabetes-during-pregnancy.htm#:~:text=develops%20during%20pregnancy.-,How%20Common%20Is%20Diabetes%20During%20Pregnancy%3F,pregnant%20women%20develop%20gestational%20diabetes.

Clapp, J.F. (2008). Long-term outcome after exercising throughout pregnancy: Fitness and cardiovascular risk. *American Journal of Obstetrics & Gynecology*, 199, 5, 489.e1–489.e6.

Clapp, J.F., & Capeless, E.L. (1990). Neonatal morphometrics after endurance exercise during pregnancy. *American Journal of Obstetrics & Gynecology*, 163, 1805–1811.

Clapp, J.F. & Cram, C. (2012). *Exercising Through Your Pregnancy* (2nd ed.). Omaha, Nebr.: Addicus Books.

Colberg, S.R. et al. (2016). Physical activity/exercise and diabetes: A position statement of the American Diabetes Association. *Diabetes Care*, 39, 11, 2065–2079.

Currie, S. et al. (2013). Reducing the decline in physical activity during pregnancy: A systematic review of behavior-change interventions. *PLoS One*, 8, 6, e66385.

Daley, A. et al. (2008). Feasibility of an exercise intervention for women with postnatal depression: A pilot randomised controlled trial. *British Journal of General Practice*, 58, 178–183.

da Silva, J.R. et al. (2013). Effects of an aquatic physical exercise program on glycemic control and perinatal outcomes of gestational diabetes: Study protocol for a randomized controlled trial. *Trials*, 14, 390.

Davies, G.A. et al. (2003). Joint SOGC/CSEP clinical practice guideline: Exercise in pregnancy and the postpartum period. *Canadian Journal of Applied Physiology*, 28, 329–341.

Dempsey, J.C. et al. (2004). A case-control study of maternal recreational physical activity and risk of gestational diabetes mellitus. *Diabetes Research and Clinical Practice*, 66, 203–215.

Dennis, C.L. & McQueen, K. (2009). The relationship between infant-feeding outcomes and postpartum depression: A qualitative systematic review. *Pediatrics*, 123, 736–751.

Dewey, K.G. et al. (1994). A randomized study of the effects of aerobic exercise by lactating women on breast-milk volume and composition. *New England Journal of Medicine*, 330, 449–453.

Dumas, G.A. et al. (1995). Exercise, posture, and back pain during pregnancy—part 1: Exercise and posture. *Clinical Biomechanics*, 10, 2, 98–103.

Durham, H.A. et al. (2011). Postpartum physical activity in overweight and obese women. *Journal of Physical Activity & Health*, 8, 7, 988–993.

Ellsworth-Bowers, E.R. & Corwin, E.J. (2012). Nutrition and the psychoneuroimmunology of postpartum depression. *Nutrition Research Review*, 25, 1, 180–192.

Evenson, K., Savitz, D., & Huston, S. (2004). Leisure-time physical activity among pregnant women in the US. *Paediatric and Perinatal Epidemiology*, 18, 6, 400–7.

Fitelson, E. et al. (2011). Treatment of postpartum depression: Clinical, psychological and pharmacological options. *International Journal of Women's Health*, 3, 1–14.

Fraser, A. et al. (2011). Associations of gestational weight gain with maternal body mass index, waist circumference, and blood pressure measured 16 years after pregnancy: The Avon Longitudinal Study of Parents and Children (ALSPAC). *American Journal of Clinical Nutrition*, 93, 1285–1292.

Gavin, N.I. et al. (2005). Perinatal depression: A systematic review of prevalence and incidence. *Obstetrics & Gynecology*, 106, 1071–1083.

Golbidi, S. & Laher, I. (2013). Potential mechanisms of exercise in gestational diabetes. *Journal of Nutrition & Metabolism*, 2013, Article ID: 285948.

Herring, S.J., Rose, M.Z., & Oken, E. (2012). Optimizing weight gain in pregnancy to prevent obesity in women and children. *Diabetes & Obesity Metabolism*, 14, 3, 195–203.

Herring, S.J., et al. (2008). Association of postpartum depression with weight retention 1 year after childbirth. *Obesity*, 16, 6, 1296–1301.

Hoyte, L. et al. (2004). Levator ani thickness variations in symptomatic and asymptomatic women using magnetic resonance-based 3-dimensional color mapping. *American Journal of Obstetrics and Gynecology*, 191, 856–861.

Institute of Medicine (2009). *Weight Gain During Pregnancy: Reexamining the Guidelines*. Washington, D.C.: National Academies Press.

Jensen, D. et al. (2008). Mechanical ventilatory constraints during incremental cycle exercise in human pregnancy: Implications for respiratory sensation. *Journal of Physiology*, 586 (Pt 19), 4735–4750.

Kaiser, L.L. et al. (2014). Practice paper of the Academy of Nutrition and Dietetics: Nutrition and lifestyle for a healthy pregnancy outcome. *Journal of the Academy of Nutrition and Dietetics*. www.eatright.org

Kamioka, H. et al. (2011). A systematic review of nonrandomized controlled trials on the curative effects of aquatic exercise. *International Journal of General Medicine*, 4, 239–260.

Kanakaris, N.K., Roberts, C.S., & Giannoudis, P.V. (2011). Pregnancy-related pelvic girdle pain: An update. *BioMed Central Medicine*, 9, 15.

Kawabata, I. et al. (2012). The effect of regular exercise training during pregnancy on postpartum brachial-ankle pulse wave velocity, a measure of arterial stiffness. *Journal of Sports Science Medicine*, 11, 3, 489–494.

Kinsella, M.T. & Monk, C. (2009). Impact of maternal stress, depression, and anxiety on fetal neurobehavioral development. *Clinical Obstetrics & Gynecology*, 52, 3, 425–440.

Lamina, S. & Agbanusi, E.C. (2013). Effect of aerobic exercise training on maternal weight gain in pregnancy: A meta-analysis of randomized controlled trials. *Ethiopian Journal of Health Sciences*, 23, 1, 59–64.

Launer, L.H. et al. (1990). The effect of maternal work on fetal growth and duration of pregnancy: A prospective study. *British Journal of Obstetrics and Gynaecology*, 97, 62–70.

Lovelady et al. (2000). The effect of weight loss in overweight, lactating women on the growth of their infants. *New England Journal of Medicine*, 342, 449–453.

McCrory, M.A. et al. (1999). Randomized trial of short-term effects of dieting compared with dieting plus aerobic exercise on lactation performance. *American Journal of Clinical Nutrition*, 69, 959–967.

Morin, M. et al. (2004). Pelvic floor muscle function in continent and stress urinary incontinent women using dynamometric measurements. *Neurourology and Urodynamics*, 23, 668–674.

Morkved, S. & Bo, K. (2000). Effect of postpartum pelvic floor muscle training in prevention of urinary incontinence: A one-year follow up. *British Journal of Obstetrics and Gynaecology*, 107, 8, 1022–1028.

Morkved, S., Schei, B., & Salvesen, K. (2003). Pelvic floor muscle training during pregnancy to prevent urinary incontinence: A single-blind randomized controlled trial. *Obstetrics and Gynecology*, 101, 313–319.

Mottola, M.F. et al. (2018). 2019 Canadian guideline for physical activity throughout pregnancy. *British Journal of Sports Medicine*, 52, 1339–1346.

Moura, S. et al. (2012). Prevention of preeclampsia. *Journal of Pregnancy*, 2012, Article ID: 435090.

Mustafa, R. et al. (2012). A comprehensive review of hypertension in pregnancy. *Journal of Pregnancy*, 2012, 105918.

Nascimento, S.L. et al. (2013). The effect of physical exercise strategies on weight loss in postpartum women: A systematic review and meta-analysis. *International Journal of Obesity*, DOI: 10.1038/ijo.2013.183. [Epub ahead of print].

Nelson, S.M., Matthews, P., & Poston, L. (2010). Maternal metabolism and obesity: Modifiable determinants of pregnancy outcome. *Human Reproduction Update*, 16, 3, 255–275.

Oken, E. et al. (2006). Associations of physical activity and inactivity before and during pregnancy with glucose tolerance. *Obstetrics & Gynecology*, 108, 5, 1200–1207.

Olson, C.M. (2008). Achieving a healthy weight gain during pregnancy. *Annual Review of Nutrition*, 28, 411–423.

Oteng-Ntim, E. et al. (2012). Lifestyle interventions for overweight and obese pregnant women to improve pregnancy outcome: Systematic review and meta-analysis. *BMC Medicine*, 10, 47.

Padua, L. et al. (2010). Systematic review of pregnancy-related carpal tunnel syndrome. *Muscle & Nerve*, 42, 5, 697–702.

Park, S.H. et al. (2013). Effect of Kegel exercise to prevent urinary and fecal incontinence in antenatal and postnatal women: Systematic review. *Journal of the Korean Academy of Nursing*, 43, 3, 420–430.

Pitkin, R.M. (1999). Energy in pregnancy. *American Journal of Clinical Nutrition,* 69, 4, 583.

Poudevigne, M.S. & O'Connor, P.J. (2005). Physical activity and mood during pregnancy. *Medicine & Science in Sports & Exercise*, 37, 8, 1374–1380.

Procter, S.B. et al. (2014). Position of the Academy of Nutrition and Dietetics: Nutrition and lifestyle for a healthy pregnancy outcome. *Journal of the Academy of Nutrition and Dietetics,* 114, 7, 1099–1103.

Rossi, A. et al. (2011). Quantitative cardiovascular magnetic resonance in pregnant women: Cross-sectional analysis of physiological parameters throughout pregnancy and the impact of the supine position. *Journal of Cardiovascular Magnetic Resonance*, 13, 1, 31.

Sangsawang, B. & Sangsawang, N. (2013). Stress urinary incontinence in pregnant women: A review of prevalence, pathophysiology, and treatment. *International Urogynecology Journal*, 24, 6, 901–912.

Shivakumar, G. et al. (2011). Antenatal depression: A rationale for studying exercise. *Depression & Anxiety*, 28, 3, 234–242.

Society of Obstetricians and Gynaecologists of Canada & Canadian Society for Exercise Physiology (2003). Joint SOGC/CSEP clinical practice guideline: Exercise in pregnancy and the postpartum period. *Journal of Obstetrics and Gynaecology Canada*, 25, 6, 516–522.

Soultanakis, H.N., Artal, R., & Wiswell, R.A. (1996). Prolonged exercise in pregnancy: Glucose homeostasis, ventilatory and cardiovascular responses. *Seminars in Perinatology*, 20, 315–327.

Spinillo, A. et al. (1996). The effect of work activity in pregnancy on the risk of fetal growth retardation. *Acta Obstetricia et Gynecologica Scandinavica*, 75, 531–536.

Sui, Z. & Dodd, J.M. (2013). Exercise in obese pregnant women: Positive impacts and current perceptions. *International Journal of Women's Health*, 5, 389–398.

Szymanski & Satin, A. (2012). Exercise during pregnancy: Fetal responses to current public health guidelines. *Obstetrics & Gynecology*, 119, 3, 603–610.

Tomić, V. et al. (2013). The effect of maternal exercise during pregnancy on abnormal fetal growth. *Croation Medical Journal*, 54, 4, 362–368.

Trogstad, L., Magnus, P., & Stoltenberg, C. (2011). Preeclampsia: Risk factors and causal models. *Best Practice & Research: Clinical Obstetrics & Gynaecology*, 25, 3, 329–342.

Turner, J.A. (2010). Diagnosis and management of preeclampsia: An update. *International Journal of Women's Health*, 2, 327–337.

UK Chief Medical Officers (2019). *Physical Activity Guidelines*. London: Department of Health & Social Care.

U.S. Department of Health & Human Services (2018). *Physical Activity Guidelines for Americans* (2nd ed.). www.health.gov/paguidelines/

Van Zutphen, A.R. et al. (2012). A population-based case-control study of extreme summer temperature and birth defects. *Environmental Health Perspectives*, 120, 10, 1443–1449.

Vleeming, A. et al. (2008). European guidelines for the diagnosis and treatment of pelvic girdle pain. *European Spine Journal*, 17, 6, 794–819.

Wagner, H. et al. (2012). Spinal lordosis optimizes the requirements for a stable erect posture. *Theoretical Biology & Medical Modelling*, 9, 13.

Waller, B., Lambeck, J., & Daly, D. (2009). Therapeutic aquatic exercise in the treatment of low back pain: A systematic review. *Clinical Rehabilitation*, 23, 1, 3–14.

Weissgerber, T.L. et al. (2006). Exercise in the prevention and treatment of maternal-fetal disease: A review of the literature. *Applied Physiology, Nutrition, and Metabolism*, 31, 661–674.

Weissgerber, T.L. et al. (2004). The role of regular physical activity in pre-eclampsia prevention. *Medicine & Science in Sports & Exercise*, 36, 2024–2031.

West, C. et al. (2010). Increased renal α-epithelial sodium channel (ENAC) protein and increased ENAC activity in normal pregnancy. *American Journal of Physiology–Regulatory, Integregrative, & Comparative Physiology*, 299, 5, R1326–R1332.

World Health Organization (2020). *WHO Guidelines on Physical Activity and Sedentary Behavior*. https://www.who.int/publications/i/item/9789240015128

World Health Organization (2013). *Fact Sheet No. 311: Obesity and Overweight*. Retrieved December 20, 2013. www.who.int/mediacentre/factsheets/fs311/en/

Yonkers, K.A., Vigod, S., & Ross, L.E. (2011). Diagnosis, pathophysiology, and management of mood disorders in pregnant and postpartum women. *Obstetrics & Gynecology*, 117, 961–977.

SUGGESTED READING

American College of Obstetricians and Gynecologists (2020). Physical activity and exercise during pregnancy and the postpartum period, ACOG Committee Opinion No. 804. *Obstetrics & Gynecology*, 135, 4, e178–e188.

American Council on Exercise (2016). *ACE Group Fitness Instructor Handbook*. San Diego, Calif.: American Council on Exercise.

Benjamin, D.R., van de Water, A.T., & Peiris, C.L. (2013). Effects of exercise on diastasis of the rectus abdominis muscle in the antenatal and postnatal periods: A systematic review. *Physiotherapy*, S0031-9406(13)00083-7.

Clapp, J.F. & Cramm, C. (2012). *Exercising Through Your Pregnancy* (2nd ed.). Omaha, Nebr.: Addicus Books, Inc.

Currie, S. et al. (2013). Reducing the decline in physical activity during pregnancy: A systematic review of behavior-change interventions. *PLoS One*, 8, 6, e66385.

Lamina, S. & Agbanusi, E.C. (2013). Effect of aerobic exercise training on maternal weight gain in pregnancy: A meta-analysis of randomized controlled trials. *Ethiopian Journal of Health Sciences*, 23, 1, 59–64.

Nascimento, S.L. et al. (2013). The effect of physical exercise strategies on weight loss in postpartum women: A systematic review and meta-analysis. *International Journal of Obesity*, DOI: 10.1038/ijo.2013.183. [Epub ahead of print].

Procter, S.B. et al. (2014). Position of the Academy of Nutrition and Dietetics: Nutrition and lifestyle for a healthy pregnancy outcome. *Journal of the Academy of Nutrition and Dietetics*, 114, 7, 1099–11

Society of Obstetricians and Gynaecologists of Canada & Canadian Society for Exercise Physiology (2003). Joint SOGC/CSEP clinical practice guideline: Exercise in pregnancy and the postpartum period. *Journal of Obstetrics and Gynaecology Canada*, 25, 6, 516–522.

APPENDICES

APPENDIX A
ACE® CODE OF ETHICS

APPENDIX B
EXAM CONTENT OUTLINE

APPENDIX C
NUTRITION FOR
HEALTH AND FITNESS

GLOSSARY

INDEX

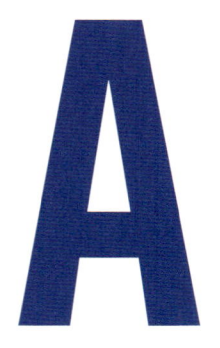

ACE® CODE OF ETHICS

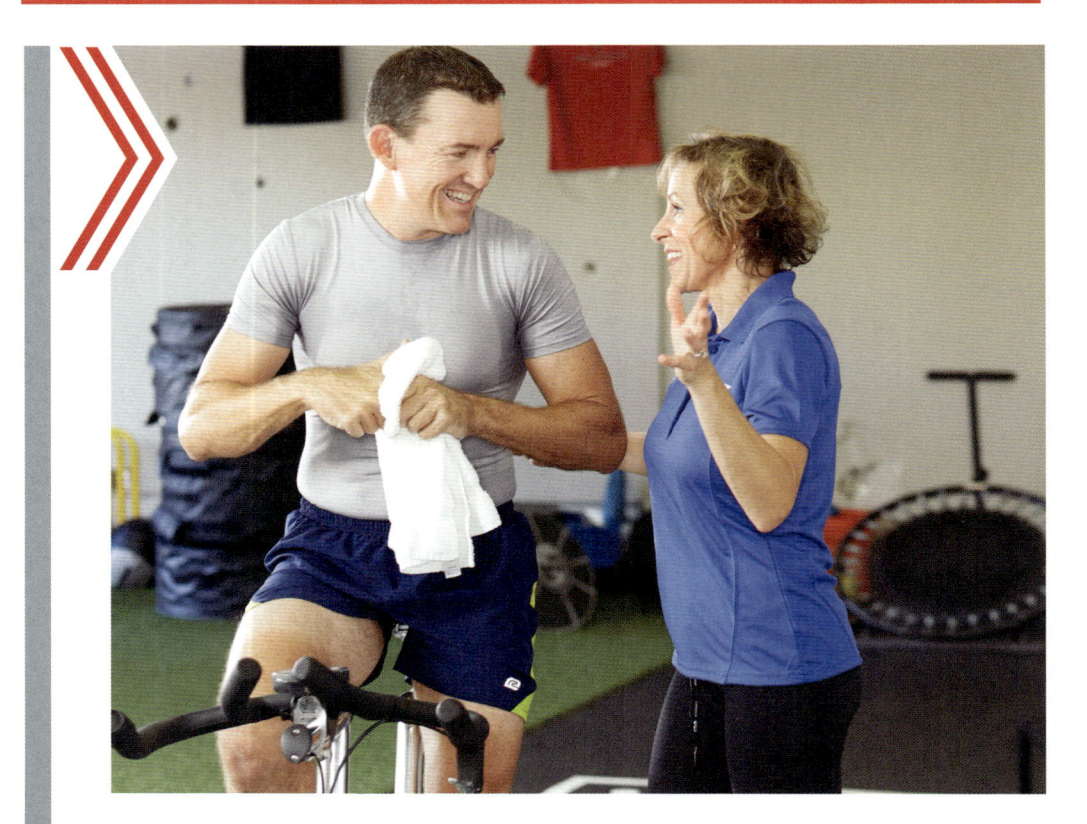

ACE CERTIFIED PROFESSIONALS ARE GUIDED BY THE FOLLOWING principles of conduct as they interact with clients/participants, the public, and other health and exercise professionals.

ACE certified Professionals will endeavor to:

- Provide safe and effective instruction
- Provide equal and fair treatment to all clients/participants
- Stay up-to-date on the latest health and fitness research and understand its practical application
- Maintain current cardiopulmonary resuscitation (CPR) certification and knowledge of first-aid services
- Comply with all applicable business, employment, and intellectual property laws
- Maintain the confidentiality of all client information
- Refer clients to more qualified health or medical professionals when appropriate
- Uphold and enhance public appreciation and trust for the health and fitness industry
- Establish and maintain clear professional boundaries

PROVIDE SAFE AND EFFECTIVE INSTRUCTION

Providing safe and effective instruction involves a variety of responsibilities for ACE Certified Professionals. Safe means that the instruction will not result in physical, mental, or financial harm to the client/participant. Effective means that the instruction has a purposeful, intended, and desired effect toward the client's/participant's goal. Great effort and care must be taken in carrying out the responsibilities that are essential in creating a positive exercise experience for all clients/participants.

Screening

ACE Certified Professionals should have all potential clients/participants complete an industry-recognized health-screening tool to ensure safe exercise participation. If significant risk factors or signs and symptoms suggestive of chronic disease are identified, refer the client/participant to a physician or primary healthcare practitioner for medical clearance and guidance regarding which types of assessments, activities, or exercises are indicated, contraindicated, or deemed high risk. If an individual does not want to obtain medical clearance, have that individual sign a legally prepared document that releases you and the facility in which you work from any liability related to any injury that may result from exercise participation or assessment. Once the client has been cleared for exercise and you have a full understanding of the client's/participant's health status and medical history, including their current use of medications, a formal risk-management plan for potential emergencies must be prepared and reviewed periodically.

Assessment

The main objective of a health assessment is to establish the client's/participant's baseline fitness level in order to design an appropriate exercise program. Explain the risks and benefits of each assessment and provide the client/participant with any pertinent instructions. Prior to conducting any type of assessment, the client/participant must be given an opportunity to ask questions and read and sign an informed consent. The types and order of assessments are dictated by the client's/participant's health status, fitness level, symptoms, and/or use of medications. Remember that each assessment has specific protocols and only those within your scope of practice should be administered. Once the assessments are completed, evaluate and discuss the results objectively as they relate to the client's/participant's health condition and goals. Educate the client/participant and emphasize how an exercise program will benefit the client/participant.

Program Design

You must not prescribe exercise, diet, or treatment, as doing so is outside your scope of practice and implies ordering or advising a medicine or treatment. Instead, it is appropriate for you to design exercise programs that improve components of physical fitness and wellness while adhering to the limitations of a previous injury or condition as determined by a certified, registered, or licensed allied health professional. Because nutritional laws and the practice of dietetics vary in each state, province, and country, understand what type of basic nutritional information is appropriate and legal for you to disseminate to your client/participant. The client's/participant's preferences, and short- and long-term goals as well as current industry standards and guidelines must be taken into consideration as you develop a formal yet realistic exercise and weight-management program. Provide as much detail for all exercise parameters such as mode, intensity, type of exercise, duration, progression, and termination points.

Program Implementation

Do not underestimate your ability to influence the client/participant to become active for a lifetime. Be sure that each class or session is well-planned, sequential, and documented. Instruct the client/participant how to safely and properly perform the appropriate exercises and communicate this in a manner that the client/participant will understand and retain. Each client/participant has a different learning curve that will require different levels of attention, learning aids, and repetition. Supervise the client/participant closely, especially when spotting or cueing is needed. If supervising a group of two or more, ensure that you can supervise and provide the appropriate amount of attention to each individual at all times. Ideally, the group will have similar goals and will be performing similar exercises or activities. Position yourself so that you do not have to turn your back to any client/participant performing an exercise.

Facilities

Although the condition of a facility may not always be within your control, you are still obligated to ensure a hazard-free environment to maximize safety. If you notice potential hazards in the health club, communicate these hazards to the client and the facility management. For example, if you notice that the clamps that keep the weights on the barbells are getting rusty and loose, it would be prudent of you to remove them from the training area and alert the facility that immediate repair is required.

Equipment

Obtain equipment that meets or exceeds industry standards and utilize the equipment only for its intended use. Arrange exercise equipment and stations so that adequate space exists between equipment, participants, and foot traffic. Schedule regular maintenance and inspect equipment prior to use to ensure it is in proper working condition. Avoid the use of homemade equipment, as your liability is greater if it causes injury to a person exercising under your supervision.

PROVIDE EQUAL AND FAIR TREATMENT TO ALL CLIENTS/PARTICIPANTS

ACE Certified Professionals are obligated to provide fair and equal treatment for each client/participant without bias, preference, or discrimination against gender, ethnic background, age, national origin, basis of religion, or physical disability.

The Americans with Disabilities Act protects individuals with disabilities against any type of unlawful discrimination. A disability can be either physical or mental, such as epilepsy, paralysis, HIV infection, AIDS, a significant hearing or visual impairment, mental retardation, or a specific learning disability. ACE Certified Professionals should, at a minimum, provide reasonable accommodations to each individual with a disability. Reasonable simply means that you are able to provide accommodations that do not cause you any undue hardship that requires additional or significant expense or difficulty. Making an existing facility accessible by modifying equipment or devices, assessments, or training materials are a few examples of providing reasonable accommodations. However, providing the use of personal items or providing items at your own expense may not be considered reasonable.

This ethical consideration of providing fair and equal treatment is not limited to behavioral interactions with clients, but also extends to exercise programming and other business-related services such as communication, scheduling, billing, cancellation policies, and dispute resolution.

STAY UP-TO-DATE ON THE LATEST HEALTH AND FITNESS RESEARCH AND UNDERSTAND ITS PRACTICAL APPLICATION

Obtaining an ACE certification required you to have broad-based knowledge of many disciplines; however, this credential should not be viewed as the end of your professional development and education. Instead, it should be viewed as the beginning or foundation. The dynamic nature of the health and fitness industry requires you to maintain an understanding of the latest research and professional standards and guidelines and their impact on the design and implementation of exercise programming. To stay informed, make time to review a variety of industry resources such as professional journals, position statements, trade and lay periodicals, and correspondence courses, as well as to attend professional meetings, conferences, and educational workshops.

An additional benefit of staying up-to-date is that it also fulfills your certification renewal requirements for continuing education credit (CEC). To maintain your ACE Certified status, you must obtain an established amount of CECs every two years. CECs are granted for structured learning that takes place within the educational portion of a course related to the profession and presented by a qualified health and exercise professional.

MAINTAIN CURRENT CPR CERTIFICATION AND KNOWLEDGE OF FIRST-AID SERVICES

ACE Certified Professionals must be prepared to recognize and respond to heart attacks and other life-threatening emergencies. Emergency response is enhanced by training and maintaining skills in CPR, first aid, and using automated external defibrillators (AEDs), which have become more widely available. An AED is a portable electronic device used to restore normal heart rhythm in a person experiencing a cardiac arrest and can reduce the time to defibrillation before EMS personnel arrive. For each minute that defibrillation is delayed, the victim's chance of survival is reduced by 7 to 10%. Thus, survival from cardiac arrest is improved dramatically when CPR and defibrillation are started early.

COMPLY WITH ALL APPLICABLE BUSINESS, EMPLOYMENT, AND INTELLECTUAL PROPERTY LAWS

As an ACE Certified Professional, you are expected to maintain a high level of integrity by complying with all applicable business, employment, and copyright laws. Be truthful and forthcoming with communication to clients/participants, coworkers, and other health and exercise professionals in advertising, marketing, and business practices. Do not create false or misleading impressions of credentials, claims, or sponsorships, or perform services outside of your scope of practice that are illegal, deceptive, or fraudulent.

All information regarding your business must be clear, accurate, and easy to understand for all potential clients/participants. Provide disclosure about the name of your business, physical address, and contact information, and maintain a working phone number and email address. So that clients/participants can make an informed choice about paying for your services, provide detailed information regarding schedules, prices, payment terms, time limits, and conditions. Cancellation, refund, and rescheduling information must also be clearly stated and easy to understand. Allow the client/participant an opportunity to ask questions and review this information before formally agreeing to your services and terms.

Because employment laws vary in each city, state, province, and country, familiarize yourself with the applicable employment regulations and standards to which your business must conform. Examples of this may include conforming to specific building codes and zoning ordinances or making sure that your place of business is accessible to individuals with a disability.

The understanding of intellectual property law and the proper use of copyrighted materials is an important legal issue for all ACE Certified Professionals. Intellectual property laws protect the creations of authors, artists, software programmers, and others with copyrighted materials. The most common infringement of intellectual property law in the fitness industry is the use of music in an exercise class. When commercial music is played in a for-profit exercise class, without a performance or blanket license, it is considered a public performance and a violation of intellectual property law. Therefore, make sure that any music, handouts, or educational materials are either exempt from intellectual property law or permissible under laws by reason of fair use, or obtain express written consent from the copyright holder for distribution, adaptation, or use. When in doubt, obtain permission first or consult with a qualified legal professional who has intellectual property law expertise.

MAINTAIN THE CONFIDENTIALITY OF ALL CLIENT/PARTICIPANT INFORMATION

Every client/participant has the right to expect that all personal data and discussions with an ACE Certified Professional will be safeguarded and not disclosed without the client's/participant's express written consent or acknowledgement. Therefore, protect the confidentiality of all client/participant information such as contact data, medical records, health history, progress notes, and meeting details. Even when confidentiality is not required by law, continue to preserve the confidentiality of such information.

Any breach of confidentiality, intentional or unintentional, potentially harms the productivity and trust of your client/participant and undermines your effectiveness as an exercise professional. This also puts you at risk for potential litigation and puts your client/participant at risk for public embarrassment and fraudulent activity such as identity theft.

Most breaches of confidentiality are unintentional and occur because of carelessness and lack of awareness. The most common breach of confidentiality is exposing or storing a client's personal data in a location that is not secure. This occurs when a client's/participant's file or information is left on a desk, or filed in a cabinet that has no lock or is accessible to others. Breaches of confidentiality may also occur when you have conversations regarding a client's/participant's performance or medical/health history with staff or others and the client's/participant's first name or other identifying details are used.

Post and adhere to a privacy policy that communicates how client/participant information will be used and secured and how a client's/participant's preference regarding unsolicited mail and email will be respected. When a client/participant provides you with any personal data, new or updated, make it a habit to immediately secure this information and ensure that only you and/or the appropriate individuals have access to it. Also, the client's/participant's files must only be accessed and used for purposes related to health and fitness services. If client/participant information is stored on a personal computer, restrict access by using a protected password. Should you receive any inquiries from family members or other individuals regarding the progress of a client/participant or other personal information, state that you cannot provide any information without the client's/participant's permission. If and when a client/participant permits you to release confidential information to an authorized individual or party, utilize secure methods of communication such as certified mail, sending and receiving information on a dedicated private fax line, or email with encryption.

REFER CLIENTS/PARTICIPANTS TO MORE QUALIFIED HEALTH OR MEDICAL PROFESSIONALS WHEN APPROPRIATE

A fitness certification is not a professional license. Therefore, it is vitally important that ACE Certified Professionals who do not also have a professional license (e.g., physician, physical therapist, registered dietitian, psychologist, or attorney) refer their clients/participants to a more qualified professional when warranted. Doing so not only benefits your clients/participants by making sure that they receive the appropriate attention and care, but also enhances your credibility and reduces liability by defining your scope of practice and clarifying what services you can and cannot reasonably provide.

Knowing when to refer a client/participant is, however, as important as choosing to which professional to refer. For instance, when a client/participant complains of symptoms of muscle soreness or discomfort or exhibits signs of fatigue or lack of energy, it is not an absolute indication to refer your client/participant to a physician. Because continual referrals such as this are not practical, familiarize and educate yourself on expected signs and symptoms, taking into consideration the client's/participant's fitness level, health status, chronic disease, disability, and/or background as they are screened and as they begin and progress with an exercise program. This helps you better discern between emergent and non-emergent situations and know when to refuse to offer your services, continue to monitor, and/or make an immediate referral.

It is important that you know the scope of practice for various health professionals and which types of referrals are appropriate. For example, some states require that a referring physician first approve visits to a physical therapist, while other states allow individuals to see a physical therapist directly. Only registered or licensed dietitians or physicians may provide specific dietary recommendations or diet plans; however, a client/participant who is suspected of an eating disorder should be referred to an eating disorders specialist. Refer clients/participants to a clinical psychologist if they wish to discuss family or marital problems or exhibit addictive behaviors such as substance abuse.

Network and develop rapport with potential allied health professionals in your area before you refer clients/participants to them. This demonstrates good will and respect for their expertise and will most likely result in reciprocal referrals for your services and fitness expertise.

UPHOLD AND ENHANCE PUBLIC APPRECIATION AND TRUST FOR THE HEALTH AND FITNESS INDUSTRY

The best way for ACE Certified Professionals to uphold and enhance public appreciation and trust for the health and fitness industry is to represent themselves in a dignified and professional manner. As the public is inundated with misinformation and false claims about fitness products and services, your expertise must be utilized to dispel myths and half-truths about current trends and fads that are potentially harmful to the public.

When appropriate, mentor and dispense knowledge and training to less-experienced exercise professionals. Novice exercise professionals can benefit from your experience and skill as you assist them in establishing a foundation based on exercise science, from both theoretical and practical standpoints. Therefore, it is a disservice if you fail to provide helpful or corrective information—especially when an individual, the public, or other exercise professionals are at risk for injury or increased liability. For example, if you observe an individual using momentum to perform a strength-training exercise, the prudent course of action would be to suggest a modification. Likewise, if you observe an exercise professional in your workplace consistently failing to obtain informed consents before clients/participants undergo fitness testing or begin an exercise program, recommend that they consider implementing these forms to minimize liability.

Finally, do not represent yourself in an overly commercial or misleading manner. Consider the exercise professional who places an advertisement in a local newspaper stating: "Lose 10 pounds in 10 days or your money back!" It is inappropriate to lend credibility to or endorse a product, service, or program founded upon unsubstantiated or misleading claims; thus a solicitation such as this must be avoided, as it undermines the public's trust of health and exercise professionals.

ESTABLISH AND MAINTAIN CLEAR PROFESSIONAL BOUNDARIES

Working in the fitness profession requires you to come in contact with many different people. It is imperative that a professional distance be maintained in relationships with all clients/participants. Exercise professionals are responsible for setting and monitoring the boundaries between a working relationship and friendship with their clients/participants. To that end, ACE Certified Professionals should:

- Never initiate or encourage discussion of a sexual nature
- Avoid touching clients/participants unless it is essential to instruction
- Inform clients/participants about the purpose of touching and find an alternative if the client/participant objects
- Discontinue all touching if it appears to make the client/participant uncomfortable

Take all reasonable steps to ensure that any personal and social contacts between themselves and their clients/participant do not have an adverse impact on the trainer–client, coach–client, or instructor–participant relationship.

If you are unable to maintain appropriate professional boundaries with a client/participant (whether due to your attitudes and actions or those of the client/participant), the prudent course of action is to terminate the relationship and, perhaps, refer the client/participant to another professional. Keep in mind that charges of sexual harassment or assault, even if groundless, can have disastrous effects on your career.

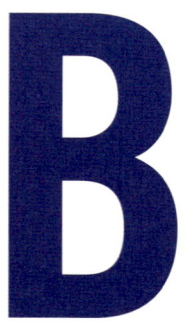

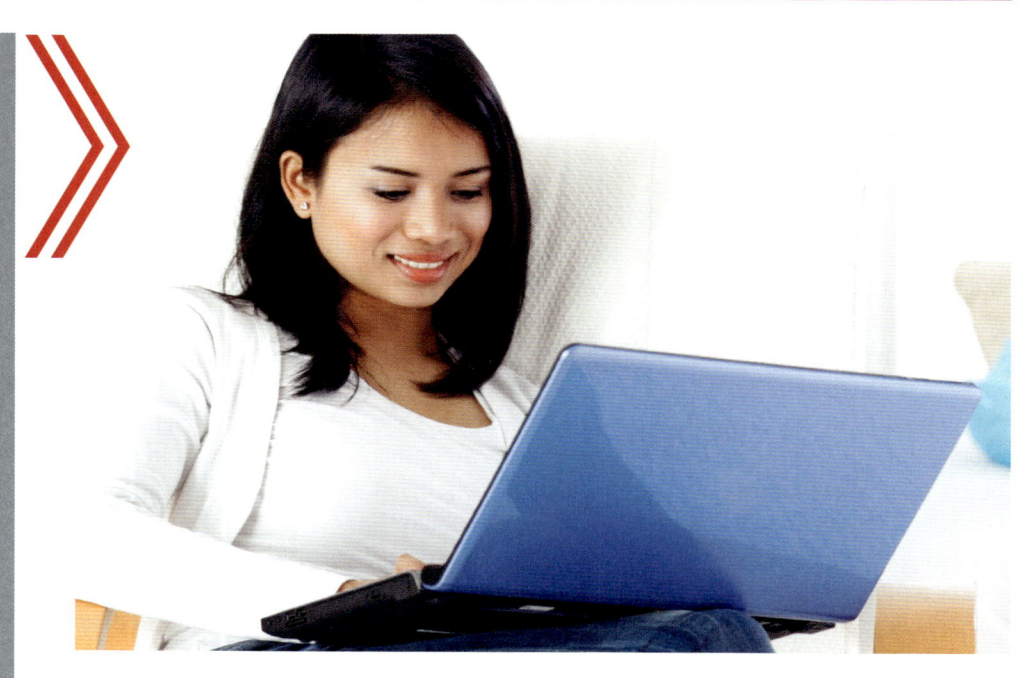

B EXAM CONTENT OUTLINE

For the most up-to-date version of the Exam Content Outline, please go to www.ACEfitness.org/fitness-certifications/certification-exam-content.aspx and download a free PDF.

ATTENTION EXAM CANDIDATES!

When preparing for an ACE® certification exam, be aware that the material presented in this manual, or any other text or educational materials, may become outdated due to the evolving nature of the fitness and healthcare industries, as well as new developments in current and ongoing research. ACE certifications and the exams one must pass to earn these certifications are based on in-depth job analyses and industry-wide validation surveys.

By design, ACE certification exams assess a candidate's ability to analyze multiple case studies that are representative of the work that a certified professional would encounter on a daily, weekly, or monthly basis, and then to apply knowledge of the most current scientifically based professional standards and guidelines to determine the best solution for the scenario presented. *The dynamic nature of this field requires that ACE certification exams be regularly updated to ensure that they reflect the latest industry findings and research. Therefore, the knowledge, skills, and abilities required to pass these exams are not solely represented in this or any other industry text or educational materials.* In addition to learning the material presented on our website, this manual, and associated educational resources, ACE strongly encourages all exam candidates and fitness professionals to keep abreast of new developments, guidelines, and standards from a variety of valid industry sources.

EXAM CONTENT OUTLINE

The Exam Content Outline is essentially a blueprint for the exam. As you prepare for the ACE Certified Medical Exercise Specialist (CMES) exam, it is important to remember that all questions map directly to one of the task statements in this outline.

Target Audience Statement

The ACE Certified Medical Exercise Specialist (CMES) is an integral member of the healthcare team, developing and delivering specific and complementary programming in collaboration with other healthcare providers. The CMES has expertise in conducting assessments and designing comprehensive health and fitness programs to help clients prevent and manage disease, avoid injuries, improve overall wellness and function throughout all phases of medical interventions, and return to desired activities following rehabilitation. The CMES applies the principles of exercise science, health coaching, nutrition, psychology, corrective exercise, therapeutic exercise, and pathophysiology to develop individualized health and fitness programs for special-population clients with clinical issues (e.g., cardiovascular, pulmonary, metabolic, and musculoskeletal) in order to facilitate lasting behavior change and improve client health, function, and well-being.

The following eligibility requirements have been established for individuals to sit for the ACE Certified Medical Exercise Specialist examination:
- Must be at least 18 years of age
- Must hold a current adult cardiopulmonary resuscitation (CPR) certificate, and if living in the U.S.A. or Canada, a current automated external defibrillator (AED) certificate
- Must hold a four-year (bachelor's) degree in exercise science or related field
- Must have 500 hours of work experience designing and implementing exercise programs for apparently healthy and/or at-risk individuals, as documented by a qualified professional

DOMAINS, TASKS, AND KNOWLEDGE AND SKILL STATEMENTS

A Role Delineation Study, or job analysis, was conducted by the American Council on Exercise and Castle Worldwide, Inc., for the ACE Certified Medical Exercise Specialist program. The first step in this process was completed by a panel of subject matter experts in the various disciplines within the field of medical exercise as an advanced specialization within fitness. The primary goal of the panel was to identify the primary tasks performed by Certified Medical Exercise Specialists in helping individuals with a wide variety of special needs (e.g., disease, post-rehabilitation) independently and in cooperation with other qualified healthcare professionals to manage health risks and improve health, fitness, mobility, and quality of life through medical exercise programs.

The panel first identified the major responsibilities performed by a professional Certified Medical Exercise Specialist. These responsibilities are defined as "Tasks," and it was determined that the responsibilities of the professional CMES could be described in 16 task statements. These tasks were then grouped into four Performance Domains, or major areas of responsibility.

The Performance Domains are listed below, with the percentage indicating the portion of the exam devoted to each Domain:
- Domain I: Interviews and Assessments – 27%
- Domain II: Program Design, Implementation, and Modification – 35%
- Domain III: Communication and Behavior Change – 21%
- Domain IV: Professional Conduct and Risk Management – 17%

Each Performance Domain is composed of Tasks, which detail the job-related functions under that particular Domain. Each Task is further divided into Knowledge and Skill Statements that detail the scope of information and understanding required to perform each Task and explain how the skills required to apply that understanding in a practical setting.

The Domains, Task Statements, and Knowledge and Skill Statements identified by the panel of subject matter experts were presented to a large, nationally representative group of current ACE Certified Medical Exercise Specialists through an online survey, and the survey results were used to validate the work of the panel and establish test specifications for the CMES exam. This completed the Role Delineation Study, with the outcome of this study being the ACE Certified Medical Exercise Specialist Exam Content Outline detailed here. Please note that while each question on the CMES exam maps to one of the Tasks in the Exam Content Outline, not all Knowledge and Skill Statements will be addressed on each exam administration, as there are not enough questions on a certification exam to cover every Knowledge and Skill Statement.

DOMAIN I: INTERVIEWS AND ASSESSMENTS   27%

Task 1

Gather health, fitness, and lifestyle information from client interviews and journals, electronic medical records, questionnaires, and communication with other healthcare providers to ensure accurate screening and assessment of the client.

Knowledge of:
  a. Industry standard screening and assessment tools
  b. Key elements of health-risk appraisal (e.g., risk factors, nutrition, lifestyle behaviors, medical history, physical activity)
  c. Additional elements of health-risk appraisal (e.g., social support, psychological well-being)
  d. Legal forms (e.g., informed consent, waivers, physician's release, release of information)
  e. Applicable healthcare regulatory standards (e.g., HIPAA)
  f. Interviewing methods
  g. Healthcare networking and communication practices

Skill in:
  a. Selecting appropriate forms for specific client situations
  b. Requesting and receiving information from healthcare providers in a timely manner
  c. Effective listening
  d. Effective interviewing
  e. Processing information received from various sources

Task 2

Evaluate health, fitness, and lifestyle information using industry guidelines and recommendations to assess an individual's readiness for physical activity, facilitate program design, optimize adherence, identify at-risk clients, and make appropriate referrals.

Knowledge of:
  a. Standard guidelines for determining risk factors, signs and symptoms, and risk stratifications
  b. Health and lifestyle conditions/situations requiring medical release, referral, or further investigation
  c. Program readiness factors (physical, mental, emotional, situational, preferential)
  d. Contraindications for program participation

Skill in:
  a. Using information collected to facilitate program design
  b. Recognizing the need to gather further information
  c. Identifying disease risk factors, signs, and symptoms
  d. Discerning the need for medical clearance or referral
  e. Identifying client readiness, expectations, and personal preferences

Exam Content Outline   APPENDIX B

Task 3

Perform baseline and periodic follow-up screens and assessments using recommended guidelines and protocols in order to optimize program design, ensure safety, and enhance effectiveness.

Knowledge of:
 a. Screening and assessment methods (e.g., blood pressure, blood glucose, posture, gait, cardiorespiratory, strength, flexibility, functional movement)
 b. Population-specific screenings and assessments
 c. Appropriate timing for screenings, assessments, and reassessments
 d. Exercise protocols, guidelines, and techniques
 e. Established norms/benchmarks for various screenings and assessments
 f. Safe and effective programs
 g. Risk stratification (e.g., ACSM, AACVPR)

Skill in:
 a. Selecting appropriate screens and assessments
 b. Performing appropriate screens and assessments
 c. Interpreting screening and assessment results
 d. Applying screening and assessment results to optimize program design
 e. Identifying risk
 f. Referring to appropriate healthcare professionals

DOMAIN II: PROGRAM DESIGN, IMPLEMENTATION, AND MODIFICATION   35%

Task 1

Set realistic and appropriate goals based on client expectations and limitations, assessment data, and recommendations from healthcare professionals.

Knowledge of:
 a. Goal-setting methods (e.g., SMART)
 b. Goal-setting types (e.g., outcome, process, performance)
 c. Effective communication and collaboration styles
 d. Relationships between goal setting and client expectations/limitations

Skill in:
 a. Selecting the appropriate goal-setting method
 b. Helping clients prioritize their wants and needs
 c. Collaborating with clients and healthcare providers
 d. Interpreting and clarifying healthcare provider exercise recommendations/prescriptions
 e. Applying healthcare provider exercise prescriptions appropriately
 f. Creating realistic goals
 g. Helping clients manage expectations

Task 2

Design preventive programs for at-risk clients in order to help them improve health, fitness, and function while mitigating the risk of diseases, disorders, ailments, and injuries.

Knowledge of:
 a. Principles of program design (e.g., specificity, overload, rest and recovery, progression, volume, periodization)

b. Exercise theories and guidelines (e.g., FITT-VP)
   c. Principles of exercise science and nutrition
   d. Risk factors and their application to program design
   e. Pathophysiology (management, treatment, and prevention)
   f. Medications that affect exercise response
   g. Contraindications for exercise (acute and chronic)
   h. Exercise protocols, guidelines, and modalities for specific conditions (e.g., cardiovascular, pulmonary, metabolic, orthopedic, pregnancy, cancer)
   i. Corrective exercise techniques and methods
   j. Dietary recommendations for specific conditions (e.g., cardiovascular, pulmonary, metabolic, pregnancy)
   k. Appropriate regression/progression for special populations

Skill in:
   a. Prioritizing program elements
   b. Interpreting medical information to determine appropriate exercise programming and/or contraindications
   c. Designing appropriate client-specific preventive programs
   d. Integrating healthy behaviors into client's activities of daily living

Task 3

Design programs for clients in all stages of medical intervention in order to complement treatment and improve health, fitness, and function.

Knowledge of:
   a. Principles of program design (e.g., specificity, overload, rest and recovery, progression, volume, periodization)
   b. Exercise theories and guidelines (e.g., FITT-VP)
   c. Principles of exercise science and nutrition
   d. Pathophysiology (management, treatment, and prevention)
   e. Psychological impact of acute and chronic illnesses/injuries
   f. Medications that affect exercise response
   g. Contraindications for exercise (acute and chronic)
   h. Exercise protocols, guidelines, and modalities for specific conditions (e.g., cardiovascular, pulmonary, metabolic, orthopedic, pregnancy, cancer)
   i. Exercise protocols, guidelines, and modalities prior to medical intervention (e.g., bariatric surgery, orthopedic surgery, joint replacements, organ transplants)
   j. Post-treatment exercise protocols, guidelines, and modalities
   k. Corrective exercise techniques and methods
   l. Dietary recommendations for specific conditions (e.g., cardiovascular, pulmonary, metabolic, pregnancy)

Skill in:
   a. Prioritizing program elements
   b. Interpreting medical information to determine appropriate exercise programming and/or contraindications
   c. Designing appropriate client-specific programs
   d. Integrating healthy behaviors into clients' activities of daily living

Exam Content Outline   APPENDIX 3

Task 4

Modify a client's program and goals based on reassessment data; exercise, nutrition, and lifestyle logs; client- and healthcare provider–reported information in order to ensure program safety and success.

Knowledge of:
a. Program modifications for exercise, nutrition, and lifestyle
b. Environmental factors requiring program modification
c. Health and lifestyle conditions/situations requiring program modification
d. Exercise progressions and regressions
e. Exercise guidelines, techniques, and protocols
f. Nutrition guidelines and recommendations
g. Behavioral change strategies
h. Healthy lifestyle practices
i. Relative and absolute criteria for terminating exercise

Skill in:
a. Interpreting client reassessment data
b. Communicating reassessment results to client and healthcare providers
c. Reestablishing goals
d. Determining appropriate program modifications
e. Assessing client health-related lifestyle behaviors
f. Assessing client food intake
g. Identifying signs and symptoms for terminating exercise
h. Modifying programs based on self-monitoring data

Task 5

Collaborate with other members of the healthcare team in order to deliver complementary programs that promote improved health, fitness, and function.

Knowledge of:
a. Roles and responsibilities of various healthcare providers
b. Effective communication styles
c. Tools used in communication with healthcare providers (e.g., assessment summaries, periodic updates, transfer forms, SOAP notes, medical records)
d. Cross-referral procedures
e. Treatment protocols for various diseases/dysfunctions (e.g., hypoglycemia, chest pain, ACL reconstruction, low-back pain)
f. Standard healthcare terminology
g. Factors affecting client health and well-being
h. Relationships between exercise, nutrition, supplements, and medications (prescription and over-the-counter)

Skill in:
a. Providing clarity regarding the role of the exercise specialist in the continuum of care
b. Maintaining detailed documents for all referrals
c. Communicating with healthcare team members

APPENDIX B

DOMAIN III: COMMUNICATION AND BEHAVIOR CHANGE — 21%

Task 1

Develop rapport with clients using purposeful questioning and attentive listening to facilitate communication, compliance, and a positive working relationship.

Knowledge of:
a. Communication styles
b. Personality types
c. Psychological factors related to illness and injury
d. Learning styles
e. Principles of rapport building
f. Interviewing styles

Skill in:
a. Identifying a client's personality type and learning style
b. Interpersonal communication (verbal and nonverbal)
c. Effective listening
d. Effective interviewing
e. Assessing individual differences and responding accordingly

Task 2

Educate the client on specific health behaviors and self-monitoring tools in order to enhance program adherence, safety, and success.

Knowledge of:
a. Self-monitoring tools (e.g., blood glucose monitoring, dyspnea, hydration, rest/recovery, heart rate, RPE, talk test) and their appropriate application
b. Guidelines for exercise participation based on self-monitoring results
c. Signs and symptoms for modifying and/or terminating exercise
d. Healthy behaviors
e. Personality styles
f. Learning styles
g. Behavior-change theories and strategies (e.g., barriers and enhancers, stages of change)
h. Coaching techniques that enhance program adherence and self-efficacy
i. Evidence-based educational resources

Skill in:
a. Selecting teaching techniques to align with client learning styles
b. Interpreting self-monitoring data
c. Identifying stages of change and personality styles
d. Determining behavior-modification needs based on stage of change and/or personality
e. Coaching clients through health-related behavioral change
f. Teaching clients to modify programs based on self-monitoring data

Task 3

Instruct clients on safe and effective exercise techniques using appropriate communication, coaching, and cueing strategies in order to optimize program outcomes and build self-efficacy.

Knowledge of:
  a. Coaching techniques
  b. Cueing and spotting techniques
  c. Exercise theories and guidelines (e.g., FITT-VP)
  d. Proper movement patterns including progressions and regressions
  e. Contraindicated exercises for specific diseases/dysfunctions
  f. Exercise modalities, tools, and safety considerations
  g. Proper exercise techniques and body alignment
  h. Positive reinforcement for correcting exercise technique

Skill in:
  a. Recognizing postural deviations, poor technique, inefficient movements, and signs of fatigue
  b. Teaching focus and concentration skills to help the client develop kinesthetic awareness
  c. Teaching the rationale behind specific exercises/movement patterns
  d. Helping a client implement a safe and effective home exercise program
  e. Constructive cueing

Task 4

Apply coaching strategies in order to facilitate lasting healthy behavioral change.

Knowledge of:
  a. Behavior-change theories and strategies (e.g., barriers and enhancers, stages of change)
  b. Factors affecting program adherence and effectiveness
  c. Goal-setting methods (e.g., SMART)
  d. Goal-setting types (e.g., outcome, process, performance)
  e. Support systems and resources
  f. Signs and symptoms of psychological distress
  g. Personality types
  h. Learning styles
  i. Appropriate referral networks

Skill in:
  a. Identifying personality types and learning styles
  b. Identifying factors affecting program adherence and effectiveness
  c. Coaching clients through lapses
  d. Educating clients in personal change strategies
  e. Cultivating self-efficacy
  f. Identifying barriers to change
  g. Strategic planning to overcome barriers
  h. Identifying stress triggers
  i. Goal creation and compliance
  j. Creating a positive exercise experience

DOMAIN IV: PROFESSIONAL CONDUCT AND RISK MANAGEMENT   17%

Task 1

Maintain detailed records using policies and procedures that adhere to professional guidelines in order to track progress, make appropriate adjustments, and communicate (as necessary) with other healthcare professionals.

Knowledge of:
  a. Industry standards, methods, and regulations for record keeping
  b. Methods for protecting client confidentiality
  c. SOAP notes
  d. Policies and procedures for revising records
  e. Standard healthcare terminology

Skill in:
  a. Recording and revising information in the appropriate format

Task 2

Comply with applicable laws, regulations, ACE Code of Ethics, and industry guidelines in order to protect the interests of all stakeholders and minimize risk.

Knowledge of:
  a. Professional insurance recommendations
  b. ACE Code of Ethics
  c. ACE Professional Practices and Disciplinary Procedures
  d. Facility safety guidelines
  e. Importance of laws and regulations (federal and local)
  f. CMES scope of practice

Skill in:
  a. Providing safe and effective exercise instruction/education
  b. Safeguarding confidential information
  c. Referring clients to more qualified fitness, medical, or health professionals when appropriate
  d. Administering CPR, and AED if accessible
  e. Administering basic injury-management procedures
  f. Enhancing healthcare professionals' confidence in the fitness industry
  g. Establishing and maintaining clear professional boundaries

Task 3

Recognize and respond to acute medical conditions and injuries by following an emergency action plan in order to provide appropriate care and comply with risk-management practices.

Knowledge of:
  a. Components of an emergency action plan
  b. First aid: Prevention, care, and treatment
  c. CPR/AED: Prevention, care, and treatment
  d. Emergency supplies (e.g., personal protective equipment, first aid kit, AED, oxygen)
  e. Signs, symptoms, and risks associated with diseases, dysfunctions, and injuries

Skill in:
  a. Developing an emergency action plan
  b. Recognizing signs and symptoms of an impending health threat
  c. Administering first aid
  d. Administering CPR
  e. Using an AED
  f. Responding to emergencies and injuries

Task 4

Pursue information from professional resources in order to provide services consistent with accepted standards of care.

Knowledge of:
   a. Evidence-based educational resources regarding the following topics (not an exhaustive list):
      o Relationships among exercise, nutrition, supplements, and medications (prescription and over-the-counter)
      o Relationships between nutrition/hydration and disease prevention and treatment
      o Relationships between alternative health practices and disease prevention and treatment
      o Health parameters for certain diseases/dysfunctions
   b. Health and fitness trends
   c. Governing bodies and professional associations that produce guidelines and recommendations for health and fitness (e.g., American Heart Association, American College of Sports Medicine, Centers for Disease Control and Prevention, U.S. Department of Health and Human Services)
   d. Guidelines and recommendations for health and fitness provided by governing bodies and professional associations

Skill in:
   a. Evaluating the credibility of educational resources
   b. Interpreting and applying research findings
   c. Locating appropriate educational resources

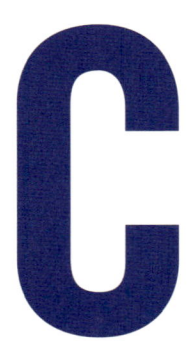

C

NUTRITION FOR HEALTH AND FITNESS

IN THIS APPENDIX

ACE POSITION STATEMENT ON NUTRITION SCOPE OF PRACTICE FOR MEDICAL EXERCISE SPECIALISTS

DIETARY REFERENCE INTAKES AND ACCEPTABLE MACRONUTRIENT DISTRIBUTION RANGES

DIETARY GUIDELINES

KEY GUIDELINE 1: FOLLOW A HEALTHY DIETARY PATTERN AT EVERY LIFE STAGE

KEY GUIDELINE 2: CUSTOMIZE AND ENJOY FOOD AND BEVERAGE CHOICES TO REFLECT PERSONAL PREFERENCES, CULTURAL TRADITIONS, AND BUDGETARY CONSIDERATIONS

KEY GUIDELINE 3: FOCUS ON MEETING FOOD GROUP NEEDS WITH NUTRIENT-DENSE FOODS AND BEVERAGES, AND STAY WITHIN CALORIE LIMITS

KEY GUIDELINE 4: LIMIT FOODS AND BEVERAGES HIGHER IN ADDED SUGARS, SATURATED FAT, AND SODIUM, AND LIMIT ALCOHOLIC BEVERAGES

SUPPORT HEALTHY DIETARY PATTERNS FOR ALL

FOOD LABELS

HISTORY AND PRESENT STATE OF FOOD LABELING

READING THE NUTRITION LABEL

FOOD SAFETY AND SELECTION

PRACTICAL CONSIDERATIONS FOR MEDICAL EXERCISE SPECIALISTS

PROVIDING GROCERY STORE TOURS

COLLABORATING WITH REGISTERED DIETITIANS

FUELING BEFORE, DURING, AND AFTER EXERCISE

PRE-EXERCISE FUELING

FUELING DURING EXERCISE

POST-EXERCISE REPLENISHMENT

FLUID AND HYDRATION BEFORE, DURING, AND AFTER EXERCISE

HYDRATION BEFORE EXERCISE

HYDRATION DURING EXERCISE

POST-EXERCISE HYDRATION

NUTRITIONAL SUPPLEMENTS

NUTRITIONAL SUPPLEMENTS WITH STRONG EVIDENCE TO SUPPORT EFFICACY AND APPARENT SAFETY

NUTRITIONAL SUPPLEMENTS WITH LITTLE TO NO EVIDENCE TO SUPPORT EFFICACY AND/OR APPARENT SAFETY

SUMMARY

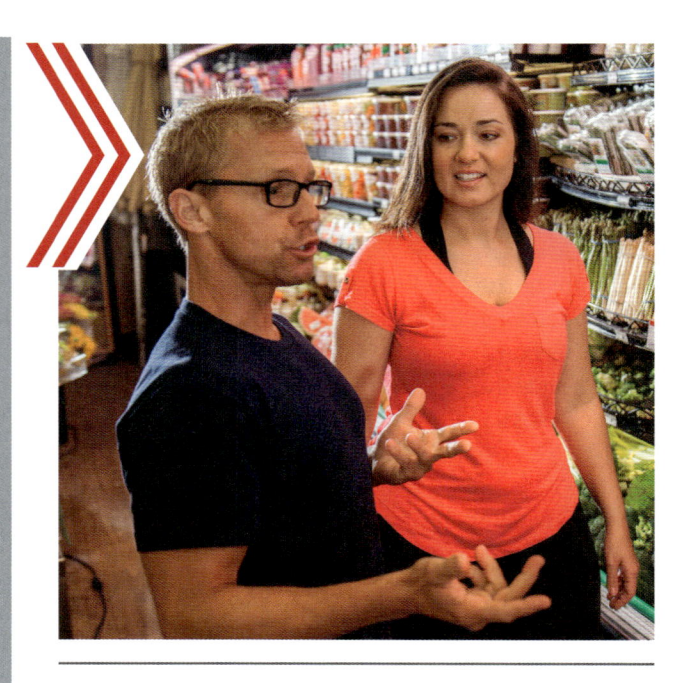

ABOUT THE AUTHOR

Natalie Digate Muth, MD, MPH, RDN, FAAP, FACSM, is a board-certified pediatrician, obesity medicine specialist, and registered dietitian. She directs a healthy weight clinic in Carlsbad, California, and is an Adjunct Assistant Professor at UCLA Fielding School of Public Health. She is a member of the Motivational Interviewing Network of Trainers. Dr. Muth has published over 100 articles, books, and book chapters, including *Coaching Behavior Change* (ACE, 2014), *ACE Fitness Nutrition Manual* (ACE, 2013), *Family Fit Plan: A 30-Day Wellness Transformation* (American Academy of Pediatrics, 2019), *The Picky Eater Project: 6 Weeks to Healthier, Happier Family Mealtimes* (American Academy of Pediatrics, 2016), *"Eat Your Vegetables!" and Other Mistakes Parents Make: Redefining How to Raise Healthy Eaters* (Healthy Learning, 2012), the textbook *Sports Nutrition for Allied Health Professionals* (F.A. Davis, 2014), and several chapters in the *ACE Diabetes Prevention Lifestyle Coaching Handbook* (ACE, 2019). She holds a Bachelor of Science degree in psychology and physiological science from UCLA, and a Master of Public Health and Medical Doctor degree from the University of North Carolina-Chapel Hill.

Natalie Digate Muth

THE ACE® CERTIFIED MEDICAL EXERCISE SPECIALIST (CMES) enjoys the rewarding opportunity to help clients not only improve their fitness but also adopt healthful nutrition habits. The federal government's *Dietary Guidelines for Americans* and MyPlate provide a foundation upon which a CMES can help clients optimize their nutrition and overall health. In addition, use of these resources and tools provides an opportunity to incorporate nutrition into sessions with clients while staying within **scope of practice.**

ACE POSITION STATEMENT ON NUTRITION SCOPE OF PRACTICE FOR MEDICAL EXERCISE SPECIALISTS

It is the position of the American Council on Exercise (ACE) that a CMES not only can but should share general nonmedical nutrition information with their clients.

In the current climate of an epidemic of **obesity,** poor nutrition, and physical inactivity, paired with a multibillion-dollar diet industry and a strong interest among the general public in improving eating habits and increasing physical activity, the CMES is well positioned to partner with clients in the journey to live healthier lifestyles. A CMES provides an essential service to their clients, the industry, and the community at large when they are able to offer credible, practical, and relevant nutrition information to clients while staying within their professional scope of practice.

Ultimately, an individual CMES's scope of practice as it relates to nutrition is determined by state policies and regulations, education and experience, and competencies and skills. While this implies that the nutrition-related scope of practice may vary among professionals, there are certain actions that are within the scope of practice for every CMES.

For example, it is within the scope of practice for the CMES to share evidence-based dietary guidelines and resources, such as those endorsed or developed by the federal government, especially the *Dietary Guidelines for Americans* (www.dietaryguidelines.gov) and the MyPlate recommendations (www.myplate.gov). A CMES who has earned a certification accredited by the National Commission for Certifying Agencies (NCCA) that provides basic nutrition information, such as those provided by ACE, and those who have undertaken nutrition continuing education, should also be prepared to discuss:
- Principles of healthy nutrition and food preparation
- Food to be included in the balanced daily diet
- Essential **nutrients** needed by the body
- Actions of nutrients on the body
- Effects of deficiencies or excesses of nutrients
- How nutrient requirements vary through the lifecycle
- Principles of pre- and post-workout nutrition and hydration
- Information about nutrients contained in foods or supplements

A CMES who does not feel comfortable sharing this information is strongly encouraged to complete continuing education to further develop nutrition competency and skills and to develop relationships with **registered dietitians**

LEARNING OBJECTIVES:

Upon completion of this chapter, the reader will be able to:

» Explain what is within a medical exercise specialist's scope of practice as it relates to nutrition

» Discuss the current *Dietary Guidelines for Americans* and other evidence-based eating patterns

» Dissect a nutrition label to determine the total number of calories; calories from fat, protein, and carbohydrate; and overall nutritional value of a product

» Outline practical strategies within a medical exercise specialist's scope of practice to improve client food literacy

» Explain proper fueling and hydration principles for before, during, and after exercise

» Discuss nutritional supplements with clients while staying within scope of practice

(RDs) or other qualified health professionals who can provide this information as requested by clients. Working with health coaches—or even becoming an ACE Certified Health Coach—may be particularly fruitful, as health coaches can provide much-needed support and guidance around the behavioral aspects of making and sustaining dietary changes. It is within the CMES's scope of practice to distribute and disseminate information or programs that have been developed by an RD or medical doctor. Note that some RDs may elect to use the newer title of registered dietitian nutritionist (RDN) and that there is no difference between the two credentials.

The actions that are outside the scope of practice for the CMES include, but may not be limited to, the following:

- Personalized nutrition recommendations or meal planning other than that which is available through government guidelines and recommendations, or has been developed and endorsed by an RD or physician
- Nutritional assessment to determine nutritional needs and nutritional status, and to recommend nutritional intake
- Specific recommendations or programming for nutrient or nutritional intake, caloric intake, or specialty diets
- Nutritional counseling, education, or advice aimed to prevent, treat, or cure a disease or condition, or other acts that may be perceived as **medical nutrition therapy**
- Development, administration, evaluation, and consultation regarding nutritional care standards or the nutrition care process
- Recommending, prescribing, selling, or supplying nutritional supplements to clients
- Promotion or identification of oneself as a "nutritionist" or "dietitian"

Engaging in these activities can place a client's health and safety at risk and possibly expose the CMES to disciplinary action and litigation. To ensure maximal client safety and compliance with state policies and laws, it is essential that the CMES recognize when it is appropriate to refer to an RD or physician. ACE recognizes that some fitness and health clubs encourage or require their employees to sell nutritional supplements. If this is a condition of employment, ACE suggests that a CMES:

- Obtains complete scientific understanding regarding the safety and efficacy of the supplement from qualified healthcare professionals and/or credible resources. *Note:* Generally, the Office of Dietary Supplements (www.ods.od.nih.gov), the National Center for Complementary and Alternative Medicine (www.nccam.nih.gov), and the Food and Drug

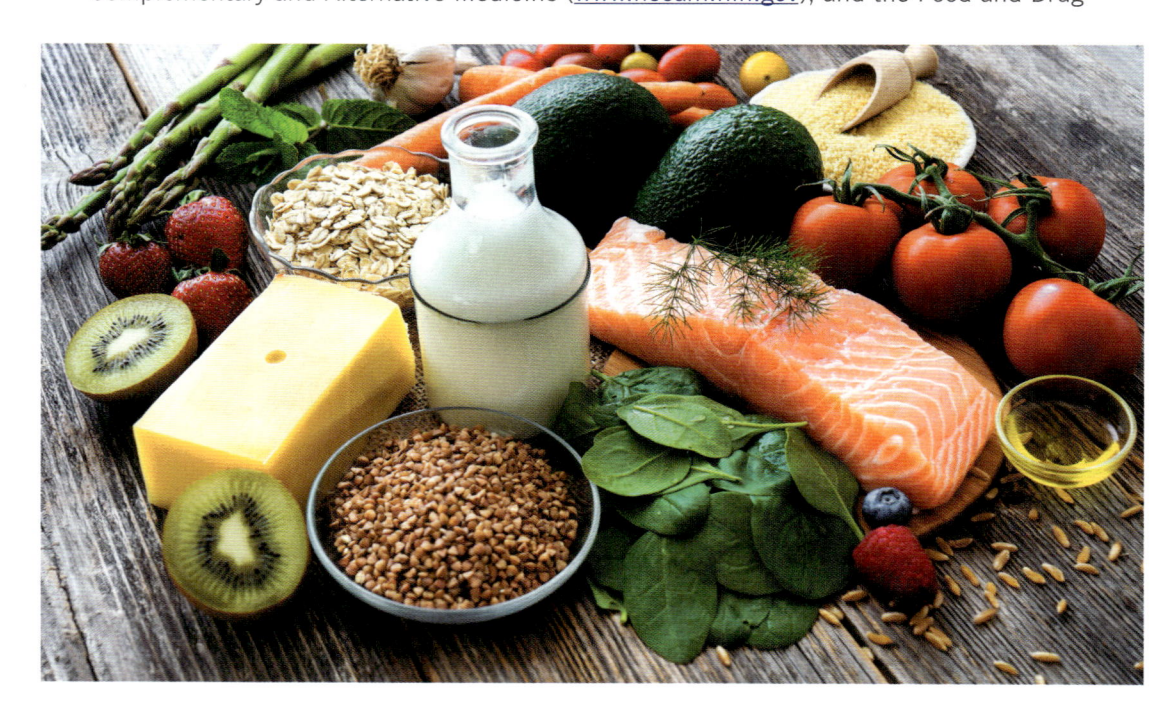

Administration (www.FDA.gov) are reliable places to go to examine the validity of the claims as well as risks and benefits associated with taking a particular supplement. Since the sites are from trusted resources and in the public domain, the CMES can freely distribute and share the information contained on these sites.
- Stays up-to-date on the legal and/or regulatory issues related to the use of the supplement and its individual ingredients
- Obtains adequate insurance coverage should a problem arise

DIETARY REFERENCE INTAKES AND ACCEPTABLE MACRONUTRIENT DISTRIBUTION RANGES

In determining the types and amounts of foods to recommend, the *Dietary Guidelines* rely heavily on the latest scientific evidence as well as established reference intakes for specific nutrients for individuals across age and sex. In fact, much of the information contained within the *2020-2025 Dietary Guidelines for Americans* (9th ed.) [U.S. Department of Agriculture (USDA), 2020] is based upon **Dietary Reference Intakes (DRIs)** published by the National Academy of Medicine, formerly the Institute of Medicine (IOM, 2006). DRI is a generic term used to refer to four types of reference values:

- **Recommended Dietary Allowance (RDA):** The RDA represents the level of intake of a nutrient that is adequate to meet the known needs of practically all healthy persons. If the level is at or above the RDA, then the client almost certainly consumes a sufficient amount (since the RDA covers 97 to 98% of the population).
- **Estimated Average Requirement (EAR):** The EAR is the adequate intake in 50% of an age- and sex-specific group. If a person's intake falls well below the EAR, it is likely that person does not consume enough of the nutrient. If the level is between the EAR and the RDA, then it is likely the client consumes enough of the nutrient (50%+ likelihood).
- **Tolerable Upper Intake Level (UL):** This is the maximal intake that is unlikely to pose a risk of adverse health effects to almost all individuals in an age- and sex-specific group. Comparing a person's usual intake of a nutrient to the UL helps to determine whether they are at risk of nutrient **toxicity.** The UL is set so that even the most sensitive people should not have an adverse response to a nutrient at intake levels near the UL. Thus, many people who have intakes above the UL may never experience a nutrient toxicity, though it is difficult to assess which clients may be most and least at risk for a nutrient overdose.
- **Adequate Intake (AI):** The AI is a recommended nutrient intake level that, based on research, appears to be sufficient for good health. If the nutrient in question has not been adequately studied and too little information is available to determine an EAR (a level good enough for 50% of the population), then it is also not possible to determine an RDA (a level good enough for 97 to 98% of the population). In these cases, the AI is published. If a client's intake is at or exceeds the AI, then it is very likely that they consume enough of the nutrient to prevent deficiency. If intake is below the AI, then it is possible (but not certain) that the client is deficient in that nutrient.

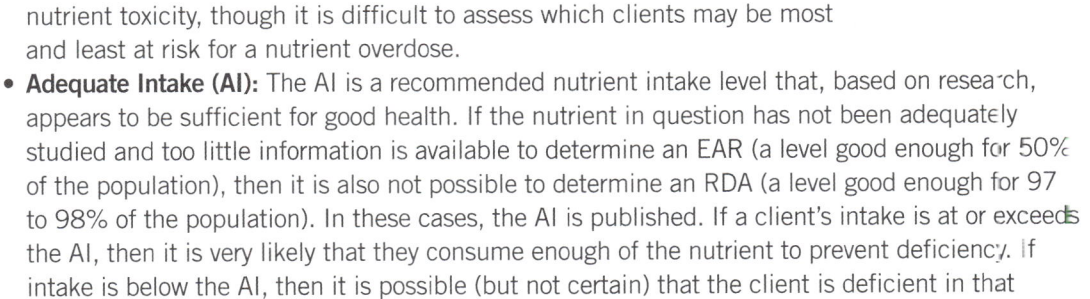

DRIs for specific nutrients are available at www.nationalacademies.org. In addition, the CMES may access the DRI interactive calculator available at www.nal.usda.gov/fnic/dri-calculator/ to determine recommended nutrient needs based on sex, age, height, weight, and activity level.

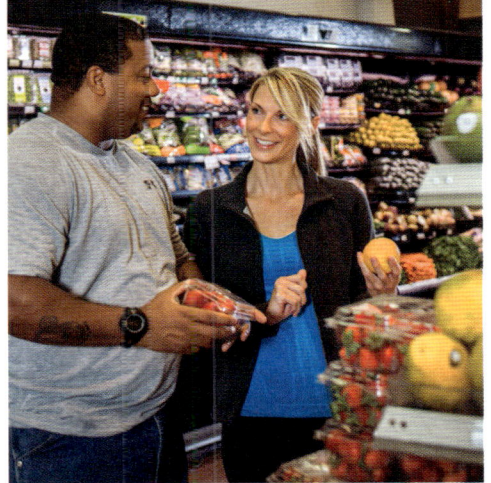

In addition to the DRIs, the IOM has established a range, known as the **Acceptable Macronutrient Distribution Range (AMDR),** for the percentage of **calories** that should come from **carbohydrate, protein,** and **fat** for both optimal health and reduction of chronic disease risk. While many weight-loss diets purport success based on variations from these recommendations, strong evidence supports that it is not the relative proportion of **macronutrients** that determines long-term weight-loss success, but rather calorie content and whether a person can maintain the intake over time.

Select daily nutritional goals by sex and age for the macronutrients are shown in Table 1.

TABLE 1
DAILY NUTRITIONAL GOALS FOR AGE-SEX GROUPS BASED ON DIETARY REFERENCE INTAKES AND DIETARY GUIDELINES RECOMMENDATIONS*

	Source of Goal[A]	Female 14–18	Male 14–18	Female 19–30	Male 19–30	Female 31–50	Male 31–50	Female 51+	Male 51+
Calorie level(s) assessed		1,800	2,200	2,000	2,400	1,800	2,200	1,600	2,000
Macronutrients									
Protein, g	RDA	46	52	46	56	46	56	46	56
Protein, % kcal	AMDR	10–30	10–30	10–35	10–35	10–35	10–35	10–35	10–35
Carbohydrate, g	RDA	130	130	130	130	130	130	130	130
Carbohydrate, % kcal	AMDR	45–65	45–65	45–65	45–65	45–65	45–65	45–65	45–65
Fiber, g	14g/1,000 kcal	25	31	28	34	25	31	22	28
Added sugars, % kcal	DGA	<10%	<10%	<10%	<10%	<10%	<10%	<10%	<10%
Total lipid, % kcal	AMDR	25–35	25–35	20–35	20–35	20–35	20–35	20–35	20–35
Saturated fatty acid, % kcal	DGA	<10%	<10%	<10%	<10%	<10%	<10%	<10%	<10%
Linoleic acid, g	AI	11	16	12	17	12	17	11	14
Linolenic acid, g	AI	1.1	1.6	1.1	1.6	1.1	1.6	1.1	1.6

* Refer to www.dietaryguidelines.gov, Appendix 1, for information about the needs for children and adolescents.

[A] RDA = Recommended Dietary Allowance; AMDR = Acceptable Macronutrient Distribution Range; DGA = *2020-2025 Dietary Guidelines* recommended limit; 14 g fiber per 1,000 kcal = basis for AI for fiber; AI = Adequate Intake

Reprinted from U.S. Department of Agriculture (2020). *2020-2025 Dietary Guidelines for Americans* (9th ed.). www.dietaryguidelines.gov

The *Dietary Guidelines* and The National Academies of Sciences, Engineering, and Medicine offer a number of tables that are excellent resources for the CMES. Be sure to visit www.dietaryguidelines.gov and www.nationalacademies.org and familiarize yourself with the many valuable tools you can share with clients. While it is not necessary to commit each table to memory, it is beneficial to make general observations and consider how you would apply the content in real-world settings.

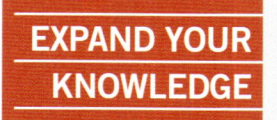

EXPAND YOUR KNOWLEDGE

FINDING CREDIBLE SOURCES OF NUTRITION INFORMATION

While the *Dietary Guidelines for Americans* and MyPlate form the foundation of both this chapter and the ACE Certified Medical Exercise Specialist's scope of practice as it relates to nutrition, these are not the only credible resources. As noted in the following section, the *Dietary Guidelines* are sometimes influenced by political pressure and are therefore criticized for being potentially biased. To broaden their understanding of dietary recommendations, the CMES may want to familiarize themself with other credible resources, including the following:

- Academy of Nutrition and Dietetics (www.eatright.org)
- Canada's Dietary Guidelines for Health Professionals and Policy Makers (https://foodguide.canada.ca/en/guidelines/)
- Harvard University's Healthy Eating Plate (www.hsph.harvard.edu/nutritionsource/healthyeating-plate/)

DIETARY GUIDELINES

Every five years, a panel of nutrition experts from a variety of fields, such as dietetics, medicine, and public health, update the *Dietary Guidelines* through a rigorous process, including a review of the nutrition-related scientific literature and a series of meetings over several years. This committee of experts develops a report that is made available to the public and federal agencies for comment (the scientific report of the 2020 Dietary Guidelines Advisory Committee is available at www.dietaryguidelines.gov/2020-advisory-committee-report). Ultimately, the report is reviewed and edited before it is approved by Congress and becomes the federal government's official nutrition advice for Americans. Once published, the document is intended to be used by health professionals and government officials to develop educational materials and design and implement nutrition-related programs. It is within the scope of practice for the CMES to use and disseminate the information contained within the *Dietary Guidelines*, as well as its associated tools and resources.

Though the development of the *Dietary Guidelines* is influenced by political pressures, efforts are made to ultimately publish scientifically supported evidence for optimal nutrition for the generally healthy population. As such, the *Dietary Guidelines* generally reflect the best evidence on how to eat for optimal health for Americans at every stage of life, from infancy to older adulthood.

The *2020-2025 Dietary Guidelines for Americans* offer four big-picture recommendations that are key to good nutrition and making every bite count. An overview of these four key recommendations, how they pertain to the CMES, and how this information can best be used to support clients in achieving their nutrition goals are provided here. In addition, readers are referred to www.dietaryguidelines.gov for a full review of the report.

Key Guideline 1: Follow a Healthy Dietary Pattern at Every Life Stage

At every life stage, it is important to eat healthfully and almost everyone can benefit from making food and beverage choices that better support healthy dietary patterns. It is never too early or too late to follow a healthy dietary pattern.

The *2020-2025 Dietary Guidelines for Americans* make a point to emphasize overall dietary patterns more so than individual nutrients, recognizing that the overall nutritional value of a person's diet is more than "the sum of its parts." A healthy dietary pattern should not be viewed as a rigid prescription, but rather as a customizable framework featuring core elements that individuals can personalize to make affordable choices that meet traditional and cultural preferences. The main components of a healthy eating pattern include:

- Vegetables of all types—dark green; red and orange; beans, peas, and lentils; starchy; and other
- Fruits, especially whole fruit
- Grains, at least half of which are whole grains
- Dairy, including fat-free or low-fat dairy, including milk, yogurt, cheese, and/or fortified soy products
- Protein foods, including seafood; lean meats and poultry; eggs; beans, peas, and lentils; nuts; seeds; and soy products
- Oils, including vegetable oils and oils in foods, such as seafood and nuts

The three types of healthy dietary patterns discussed at most length in the *Dietary Guidelines* are the **Healthy U.S.-Style Dietary Pattern,** the **Healthy Mediterranean-Style Dietary Pattern,** and the **Healthy Vegetarian Dietary Pattern.**

The Healthy U.S.-Style Dietary Pattern is based on the types and proportions of foods Americans typically consume, but in nutrient-dense forms and appropriate amounts. It is a framework for healthy eating that all Americans can follow.

The Healthy Mediterranean-Style Dietary Pattern is adapted from the Healthy U.S.-Style Dietary Pattern, modifying amounts recommended from some food groups to more closely reflect eating patterns that have been associated with positive health outcomes in studies of Mediterranean-style diets. The Healthy Mediterranean-Style Dietary Pattern contains more fruits and seafood and less dairy, meats, and poultry than does the Healthy U.S.-Style Dietary Pattern. The pattern is similar to the Healthy U.S.-Style Dietary Pattern in nutrient content, with the exception of providing less calcium and vitamin D.

The Healthy Vegetarian Dietary Pattern is adapted from the Healthy U.S.-Style Pattern, modifying amounts recommended from some food groups to more closely reflect eating patterns reported by self-identified **vegetarians** in the National Health and Nutrition Examination Survey (NHANES). Based on a comparison of the food choices of these vegetarians to nonvegetarians in NHANES, amounts of soy products (particularly tofu and other processed soy products), legumes, nuts and seeds, and whole grains were increased, and meat, poultry, and seafood were eliminated (USDA, 2020). Dairy and eggs were included because they were consumed by the majority of these vegetarians. This pattern can be **vegan** if all dairy choices are comprised of fortified soy beverages (soy milk) or other plant-based dairy substitutes. This pattern is similar in meeting nutrient standards to the Healthy U.S.-Style Dietary Pattern, but somewhat higher in calcium and **fiber** and lower in vitamin D.

Each of these patterns provides notable health benefits and can be consumed at varying calorie levels based on individual needs. They can also be adapted to meet cultural and personal preferences. In fact, moderate to strong evidence shows that these healthy dietary patterns are associated with reduced risk of chronic diseases such as **cardiovascular disease, type 2 diabetes,** obesity, and some cancers (USDA, 2020). In all, the most important components of a healthy dietary pattern include high intakes of vegetables and fruits and low intakes of processed meats and poultry, sugar-sweetened beverages (e.g., soda), and refined grains (e.g., processed "junk food" like chips).

MyPlate and MyPlate Daily Food Plan Checklists

While the *Dietary Guidelines* describe these three types of dietary patterns, many of the most robust tools available from the federal government to help translate recommendations into action are based on the Healthy U.S.-Style Dietary Pattern. For example, the MyPlate recommendations aim to translate the *Dietary Guidelines* into a simple image that people can use to guide nutrition choices. MyPlate simplifies the government's nutrition messages into an easily understood and implemented graphic—a dinner plate divided into four sections: fruits, vegetables, protein, and grains, accompanied by a glass of nonfat milk (to represent calcium-rich foods) (Figure 1). The goal is to influence Americans to eat a more balanced diet by encouraging people to make half their plate vegetables and fruits. Free downloadable educational materials to share with clients are available on the MyPlate website (www.myplate.gov).

Figure 1
MyPlate graphic

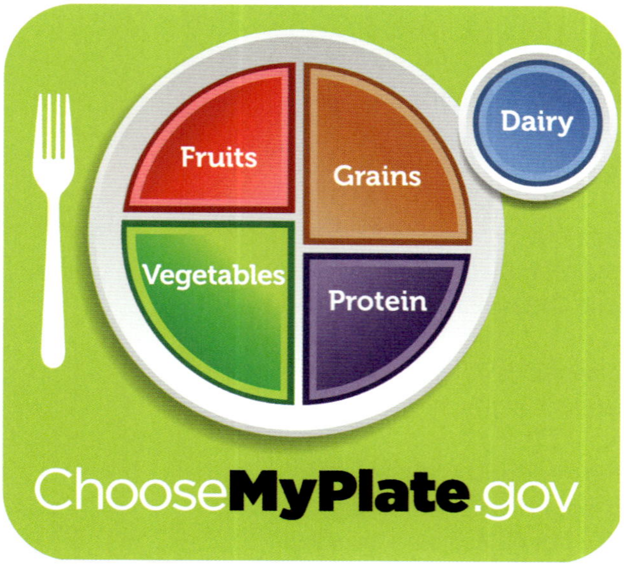

The MyPlate Daily Food Plan Checklists offer a good place to start when working with clients to identify daily calorie and nutrient needs. At www.myplate.gov/myplate-plan, clients can input their age, sex, height, weight, and physical-activity level to get a personalized eating plan to meet calorie needs. Users are categorized into one of 12 different energy levels (from 1,000 to 3,200 calories per day) and are given the recommended number of **servings** to eat from each of the five food groups.

NIH Body Weight Planner

The goal of a dietary intervention to decrease weight is to create a caloric deficit so that fewer calories are consumed than are expended. With about 3,500 calories in a pound of fat, a 500- to 1,000-calorie deficit each day through decreased food intake and increased physical activity leads to about a 1- to 2-pound (0.45 to 0.9 kg) weight loss per week, at least at first. While predicting weight loss based on the equation of 3,500 calories per pound is useful early on in weight loss, as an individual loses weight, metabolism (and thus energy expenditure) changes and the equation becomes less accurate and overpredicts weight loss. While these calculations can help empower clients to take action, it is important to remember that weight management involves a complex interplay among environmental, behavioral, genetic, and hormonal factors.

The NIH Body Weight Planner (https://www.niddk.nih.gov/bwp), a tool initially developed and validated by researchers at the Massachusetts Institute of Technology in partnership with the National Institutes of Health, more accurately accounts for these metabolic changes. It approximates that for every 10-calorie decrease in daily caloric intake, the average adult with **overweight** will lose about 1 pound (0.45 kg). Half of the weight will be lost by one year and 95% of the weight change will occur by three years (Hall et al., 2011). For example, a woman who decreases her daily caloric consumption from 2,200 calories to 2,000 calories would lose about 20 pounds (9.1 kg), with the first 10 pounds (4.5 kg) lost within one year of the lowered caloric intake, and about 10 more pounds (4.5 kg) lost by the end of three years, assuming she maintains the reduction in caloric intake. If she had created a 500-kcal deficit each day, she would lose 25 pounds (11.4 kg) in the first year and about 25 more pounds (11.4 kg) by the end of three years.

Simply enter a client's age, sex, weight, height, current physical-activity level, goal weight, planned activity level, and goal time frame and the NIH Body Weight Planner determines the caloric needs to maintain the current weight, reach a goal weight in a specified amount of time, and sustain the new body weight based on planned physical-activity levels.

EXPAND YOUR KNOWLEDGE

WHAT IS MORE IMPORTANT FOR WEIGHT LOSS: EXERCISE OR NUTRITION?

Many people wonder which is more effective for achieving weight-loss goals, increasing caloric expenditure through exercise or decreasing caloric intake through diet modification. Ultimately, both approaches can lead to weight loss and the most effective method is the one to which clients will adhere. Often, clients begin a weight-loss journey by decreasing caloric intake because the required behavior changes are perceived to be more doable than increasing physical activity. Others find increasing caloric expenditure to be the best starting point. When looking at the various components of a weight-loss program, both calorie reduction and physical activity play vital roles and the combination of these factors can lead to energy expenditure exceeding energy intake. Also, the combined effects of exercise and decreased caloric intake can lead to achieving weight-loss goals in a shorter period of time (Fayh et al., 2013). A randomized clinical trial compared the effects of achieving a 5% reduction in weight through diet or diet plus exercise on cardiovascular parameters of individuals with obesity. Interestingly, during this study, both groups reached the weight-loss goal, showing that making only dietary changes may lead to weight loss. However, the diet plus exercise group achieved a 5% reduction of weight in an average of 66 days compared to 80 days for the dietary intervention–only group, suggesting that that the combination of diet and exercise is more efficient for reaching weight-loss goals (Fayh et al., 2013).

Also, the *Physical Activity Guidelines for Americans* suggest that exercise is essential when making a lifestyle change because it increases the caloric deficit to speed weight loss and is crucial for maintaining weight loss (U.S. Department of Health & Human Services, 2018). Importantly, regular physical activity provides health benefits regardless of how body weight changes over time and helps to reduce **abdominal fat** (or **visceral fat**) and preserve muscle mass during weight-loss efforts.

Key Guideline 2: Customize and Enjoy Food and Beverage Choices to Reflect Personal Preferences, Cultural Traditions, and Budgetary Considerations

Following a healthy dietary pattern should be enjoyable at all life stages and across all ages, racial and ethnic backgrounds, and socioeconomic statuses.

The *Dietary Guidelines* provide a framework intended to be personalized to meet individual, household, and federal program participants' preferences, in addition to the foodways of the diverse cultures in the United States. Recommendations are made at the food-group level to avoid

APPENDIX C

being prescriptive and to allow people to "make it their own" by selecting the meals, beverages, snacks, and healthy foods they prefer and that are specific to their needs.

- *Begin with personal preferences:* From a young age, it is important to expose children to different types of food to develop an interest in, and willingness to eat, a variety of foods. Progressing through each life stage, it is important to ensure that individual and family preferences—in nutrient-dense forms—are built into everyday choices to establish and maintain a healthy dietary pattern.
- *Include cultural traditions:* To help communities across the country to eat and enjoy a healthy dietary pattern, it is important to customize the dietary guidelines framework to respect specific traditions and cultures.
- *Be mindful of budget considerations*: Eating healthfully does not have to be expensive, as a healthy dietary pattern can be affordable and fit within individual or family budgetary constraints. Employing a wide range of strategies, including using a variety of fresh, frozen, dried, and canned options; considering seasonal and regional food availability; and planning ahead, can make it possible to follow a healthy dietary pattern that fits within any budget.

Vegetables

Vegetables are an important contributor to a healthy dietary pattern. Vegetables are classified into five subgroups—dark green; red and orange; beans, peas, and lentils; starchy; and other. While all subgroups are high in nutrients overall, some groups contain higher amounts of certain nutrients. For example, dark green vegetables are highest in vitamin K, while red and orange vegetables are high in vitamin A, beans, peas, and lentils contain the most fiber, and starchy vegetables are highest in potassium. The *Dietary Guidelines* advise Americans to eat vegetables from all of the subgroups. Current vegetable intake compared to recommended intake is shown in Figure 2.

Figure 2
Dietary intakes compared to recommendations: Percent of the U.S. population ages 1 and older who are below and at or above each dietary goal

Reprinted from United States Department of Agriculture *(2020). 2020-2025 Dietary Guidelines for Americans* (9th ed.). www.dietaryguidelines.gov

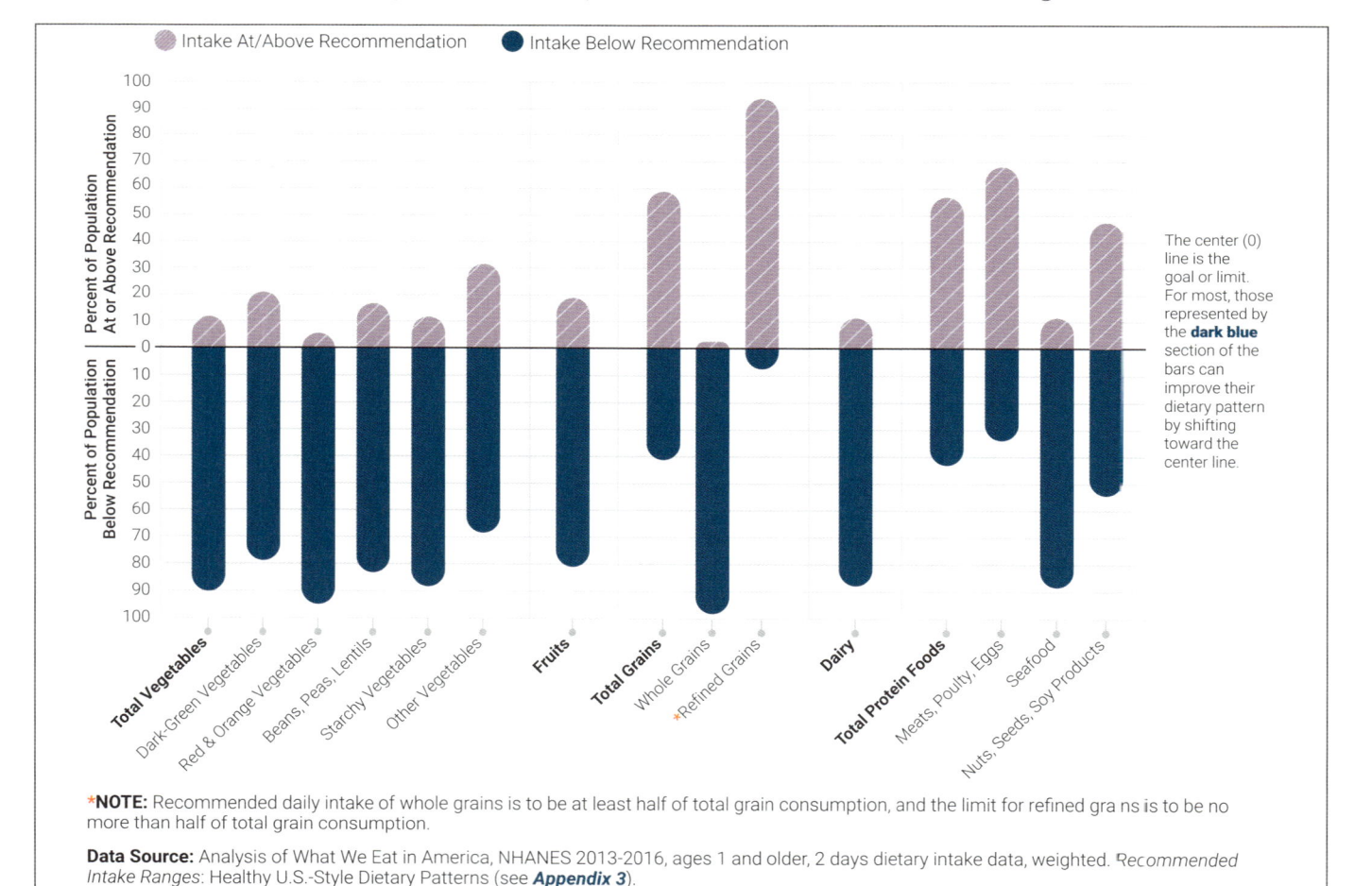

***NOTE:** Recommended daily intake of whole grains is to be at least half of total grain consumption, and the limit for refined grains is to be no more than half of total grain consumption.

Data Source: Analysis of What We Eat in America, NHANES 2013-2016, ages 1 and older, 2 days dietary intake data, weighted. Recommended Intake Ranges: Healthy U.S.-Style Dietary Patterns (see **Appendix 3**).

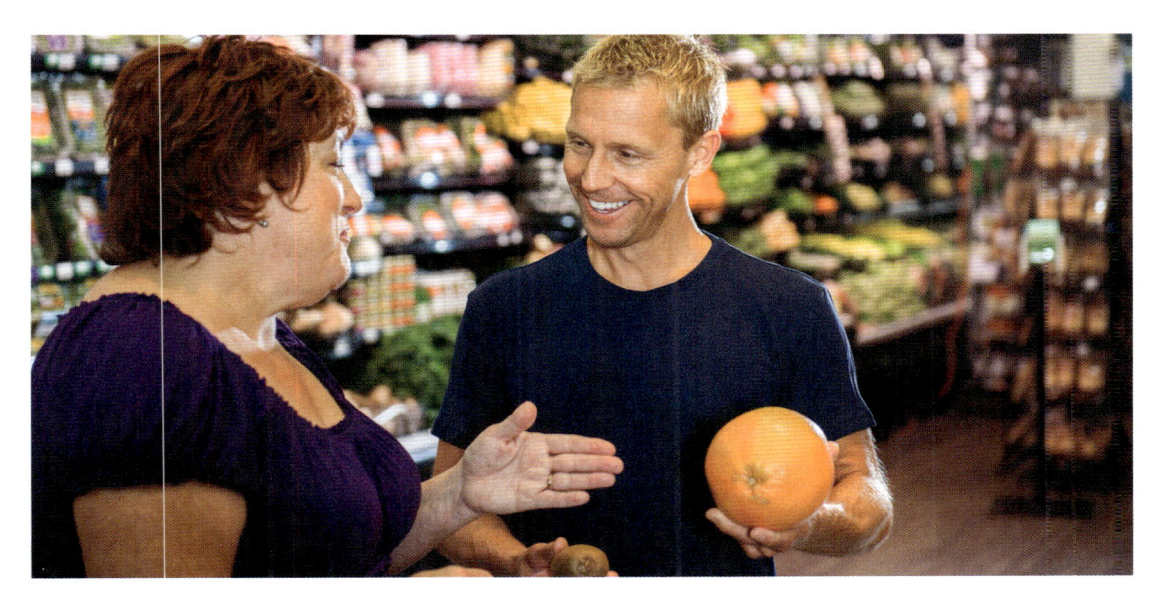

Fruits

Whole fruits, including fresh, frozen, canned, 100% juice, and dried forms, provide key nutrients, including dietary fiber, potassium, and vitamin C. Note that dried and canned fruits and fruit juices "count" as fruits, but are more calorie-dense than fresh and frozen fruits and thus should be consumed with attention to **portion** sizes. The *Dietary Guidelines* advise that no more than half of fruit should come from pasteurized fruit juice that is diluted with water (without added sugars), and that juice that is less than 100% fruit is considered to be a "sugary drink" (and should be avoided, although the *Guidelines* come short of saying that directly, and instead note that added sugars can be accommodated as long as they are less than 10% of total calorie intake per day, while staying within calorie recommendations). Current fruit intake compared to recommended intake is shown in Figure 2.

Grains

Grains include foods such as rice, oatmeal, and popcorn, as well as products that contain grains like bread, cereals, crackers, and pasta. Grains can either be refined or whole. Refined grains are heavily processed and provide limited nutritional value (essentially, through processing, all of the nutrients are removed and then four B vitamins and **iron** are added back thus creating "enriched grains"). Whole grains contain the entire grain kernel and provide health and nutritional value, including fiber, iron, zinc, manganese, folate, magnesium, copper, **thiamin, niacin,** vitamin B6, phosphorus, selenium, **riboflavin,** and vitamin A. Whole grains include foods such as brown rice, quinoa, and oats. The majority of grain consumption should come from whole grains. When choosing foods, it is easiest to identify whole-grain products by looking at the ingredient list on the nutrition label. "Whole grain" should be the first ingredient, or the second after water. Whole grains contain 16 grams of whole grain per 1 ounce-equivalent. Foods that are partly whole grain also can contribute to grain needs and should contain at least 8 grams of whole grain per 1 ounce-equivalent. Examples of "1 ounce-equivalent" include a slice of bread, half a cup of pasta or rice, 1 cup of cereal, or one tortilla. Current grain intake compared to recommended intake is shown in Figure 2.

Dairy and Fortified Soy Alternatives

The dairy and fortified soy group includes milk, yogurt, cheese, and fortified soy beverages. Dairy products are high in calcium, phosphorus, vitamin A, vitamin D (usually through fortification), riboflavin, vitamin B12, protein, potassium, zinc, choline, magnesium, and selenium. The *Dietary Guidelines* do not consider plant "milk," such as coconut, almond, rice, oat, and hemp, as dairy because their overall nutritional value is not similar to dairy milk and fortified soy beverages, though they may contain calcium.

The *Dietary Guidelines* suggest that adults should aim for 3 cups per day of dairy or fortified soy products, while children aged two to eight should consume 2 to 2.5 cups per day depending on the specific calorie level of their dietary pattern. However, the *Dietary Guidelines* also acknowledge that the Healthy Mediterranean-Style Eating Plan, which is lower in dairy products, is comparable in nutritional value to the Healthy U.S.-Style Dietary Pattern. The current dairy intake compared to recommended intake in the Healthy U.S.-Style Dietary Pattern is shown in Figure 2.

Protein Foods

Protein foods include a diversity of foods from plant and animal sources, including the following subgroups: seafood; meats, poultry, and eggs; and nuts, seeds, and soy products. Beans, peas, and lentils also are considered protein foods in addition to being included in the vegetables group. Additionally, many dairy and soy products are high in protein. Protein foods are high in nutrients, such as niacin, vitamin B12, vitamin B6, riboflavin, selenium, choline, phosphorus, zinc, copper, vitamin D, and vitamin E. Some subgroups contain higher levels of specific nutrients than others. For example, meat provides the most zinc; poultry the most niacin; seafood the most vitamin B12, vitamin D, and **omega-3 fatty acids**; eggs the most choline; seeds the most vitamin E; and meat, poultry, and seafood the most heme iron, which is better absorbed than plant sources of iron. Current protein intake compared to recommended intake is shown in Figure 2.

Due to the increasing evidence supporting the health benefits of seafood, the *Dietary Guidelines* recommend that adults consume 8 to 17 ounces of seafood per week, depending on the preferred healthy dietary pattern framework being used and the total calorie level of the pattern. The U.S. Food and Drug Administration (FDA) and the U.S. Environmental Protection agency (EPA) have created joint guidance and advice to help people choose fish and shellfish wisely (FDA.gov/fishadvice). The benefits also hold true for pregnant and breastfeeding women, and a weekly consumption of at least 8 and up to 12 ounces of a variety of lower methylmercury seafood choices is recommended. During pregnancy, however, women should be especially cautious to choose seafood that is low in methylmercury and avoid shark, swordfish, and king mackerel.

Oils

Oils are fats that contain a high percentage of **monounsaturated fats** and **polyunsaturated fats** and are liquid at room temperature. Oils are not a food group; however, the *Dietary Guidelines* recognize them as an important part of a healthy dietary pattern because they contain **essential fatty acids** and vitamin E. Commonly consumed plant oils include canola, corn, olive, peanut, safflower, soybean, and sunflower oils. Oils are naturally present in olives, nuts, seeds, avocados, and seafood. Tropical plant oils such as coconut, palm kernel, and palm oil are not included in the oils category due to their high **saturated fat** content. Americans are advised to consume about 5 teaspoons of oil per day for a 2,000-calorie diet.

Limits on Calories that Remain

The recommended food patterns are intended to meet nutritional needs while staying within calorie limits. For most people who follow the *Dietary Guidelines,* few calories will remain for "other purposes." Approximately 85% of total daily calories are needed to eat healthfully and meet food group recommendations from nutrient-dense forms, leaving 15% of daily calories available for other uses, including saturated fats, added sugars, and alcoholic beverages. If alcohol is consumed, it should be consumed in moderation, defined as up to one drink per day for women and two drinks per day for men. One drink is equivalent to 12 ounces of beer, 5 ounces of wine, or 1.5 ounces of hard liquor.

Nutrition for Health and Fitness

APPENDIX C

FOOD MODELS AND PORTION ESTIMATES

Recommendations are often provided in terms of the number of servings needed to meet a client's needs, so it is important that the CMES is able to effectively estimate intake and teach clients how to do it.

A portion is the amount of food a person chooses to eat, while a serving is a standardized amount of a food used to estimate and/or evaluate one's intake. Increases in portion sizes have been frequently cited as an important contributing factor to the growing rates in obesity seen over the past several decades (Figure 3). Portions are very difficult for some to estimate, and correct estimates could mean the difference between a 1,400-calorie diet and a 2,200-calorie diet.

A CMES can assist clients in a number of ways when estimating their portions. Comparing food portions to common items is a helpful way for clients to visualize the foods they eat, adopt better habits, and eat more appropriate food amounts. For example, in Table 2, servings are compared to common household items for reference.

EXPAND YOUR KNOWLEDGE

TWENTY YEARS AGO

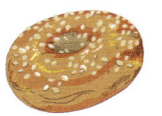

BAGEL
3-inch diameter:
140 calories

CHEESEBURGER
1 portion:
333 calories

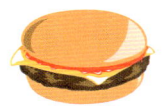

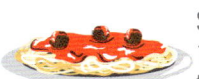

SPAGHETTI AND MEATBALLS
1 cup of spaghetti, sauce, and three small meatballs:
500 calories

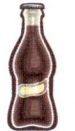

SODA
6.5 oz:
85 calories

FRIES
2.4 oz:
210 calories

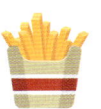

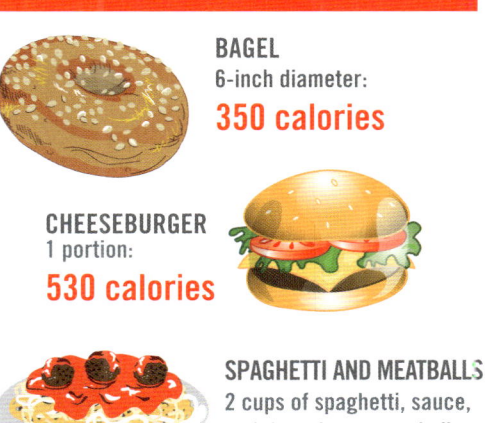

TODAY

BAGEL
6-inch diameter:
350 calories

CHEESEBURGER
1 portion:
530 calories

SPAGHETTI AND MEATBALLS
2 cups of spaghetti, sauce, and three large meatballs:
1,025 calories

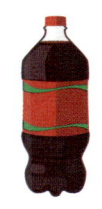

SODA
20 oz:
300 calories

FRIES
6.9 oz:
610 calories

Figure 3
Increases in portion sizes

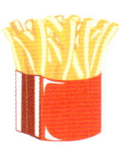

TABLE 2
ESTIMATING PORTION SIZE

Food Group	Key Message	What Counts?	Looks Like …
Grains	Make half your grains whole.	1 oz equivalent = 1 slice of bread 1 cup of ready-to-eat cereal ½ cup cooked rice, pasta, or cooked cereal 5 whole-wheat crackers	CD cover A baseball ½ a baseball

TABLE 2 *(continued)*

Vegetables	Vary your veggies. Make half your plate fruits and vegetables.	1 cup = 1 cup of raw or cooked vegetable 2 cups of raw leafy salad greens 1 cup of vegetable juice	Baseball Softball
Fruits	Make half your plate fruits and vegetables.	1 cup = 1 cup raw fruit ½ cup dried fruit 1 cup 100% fruit juice	Tennis ball 2 golf balls
Milk	Switch to fat-free or low-fat (1%) milk.	1 cup = 1 cup of milk, yogurt, or soy milk 1.5 ounces of natural cheese or 2 ounces of processed cheese	Baseball 1½ 9-volt batteries
Protein Foods	Choose lean proteins.	1 ounce = 1 oz of meat, poultry, or fish ¼ cup cooked dry beans 1 egg 1 Tbsp peanut butter ½ oz nuts or seeds 2 Tbsp hummus	Deck of cards for lean meats (3 oz); checkbook = 3 oz fish ½ golf ball ½ of a Post-it note Golf ball
Oils	Choose liquid oils and avoid solid fats.	3 tsp = 1 Tbsp vegetable oils ½ medium avocado 1 oz peanuts, mixed nuts, cashews, almonds, or sunflower seeds	Tip of thumb

For more specific amounts, please visit www.myplate.gov.

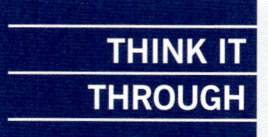

THINK IT THROUGH

ASSESSING NUTRITIONAL INTAKE
- Record your nutritional intake for two weekdays and one weekend day.
- Assess how your intake compares to the recommendations. Which food group recommendations are you meeting? Which are you exceeding? Where are you falling short?
- What changes might you make to improve your nutrition? What are you already doing well?

Key Guideline 3: Focus on Meeting Food Group Needs with Nutrient-dense Foods and Beverages, and Stay within Calorie Limits

Adhere to a dietary pattern that meets the recommendations for vegetables, fruits, grains, dairy, and protein foods consumed at an appropriate calorie level with limited amounts of added sugars, saturated fats, and sodium. Cut back on foods and beverages higher in these components to amounts that fit within healthy dietary patterns.

The *Dietary Guidelines* urge Americans to meet nutritional needs by consuming nutrient-dense foods and beverages, which provide **minerals, vitamins,** and health-promoting elements with no or little added sugars, sodium, or saturated fat, while also staying within daily calorie limits.

Added Sugars

Natural sugars include fruit sugar (**fructose**) and milk sugar (**lactose**). However, most sugars in the typical American diet are added sugars, which can come in many different forms (Table 3). While the body metabolizes natural and added sugars in the same way, most foods high in added sugars have very little nutritional value. These added sugars contribute about 270 calories per day, or more than 13% of the total calories in the American diet. The most commonly consumed food products containing these added sugars are sugar-sweetened beverages, desserts and sweet snacks, sweetened tea and coffee, and candy. The *Dietary Guidelines* recommend that Americans consume less than 10% of calories from added sugars, while staying within calorie limits. Noncaloric sweeteners may be used to reduce caloric intake in the short term, but their long-term value for helping to lose weight and maintain weight loss is still unclear. The primary sources of these added sugars for Americans ages 1 and older are shown in Figure 4.

Added Sugars
Average Intake: 266 kcal/day

- Breakfast Cereals & Bars 7%
- Candy & Sugars 9%
- Higher Fat Milk & Yogurt 4%
- Sugar-Sweetened Beverages 24%
- Desserts & Sweet Snacks 19%
- Sandwiches 7%
- Coffee & Tea 11%
- Other Sources 19%

Within Sugar-Sweetened Beverages:
- Other Sources 1%
- Soft Drinks 16%
- Fruit Drinks 5%
- Sport & Energy Drinks 2%

Within Desserts & Sweet Snacks:
- Other Sources 1%
- Doughnuts, Sweet Rolls, & Pastries 3%
- Cookies & Brownies 6%
- Ice Cream & Frozen Dairy Desserts 5%
- Cakes & Pies 4%

Data Source: Analysis of What We Eat in America, NHANES, 2013-2016, ages 1 and older, 2 days dietary intake data, weighted.

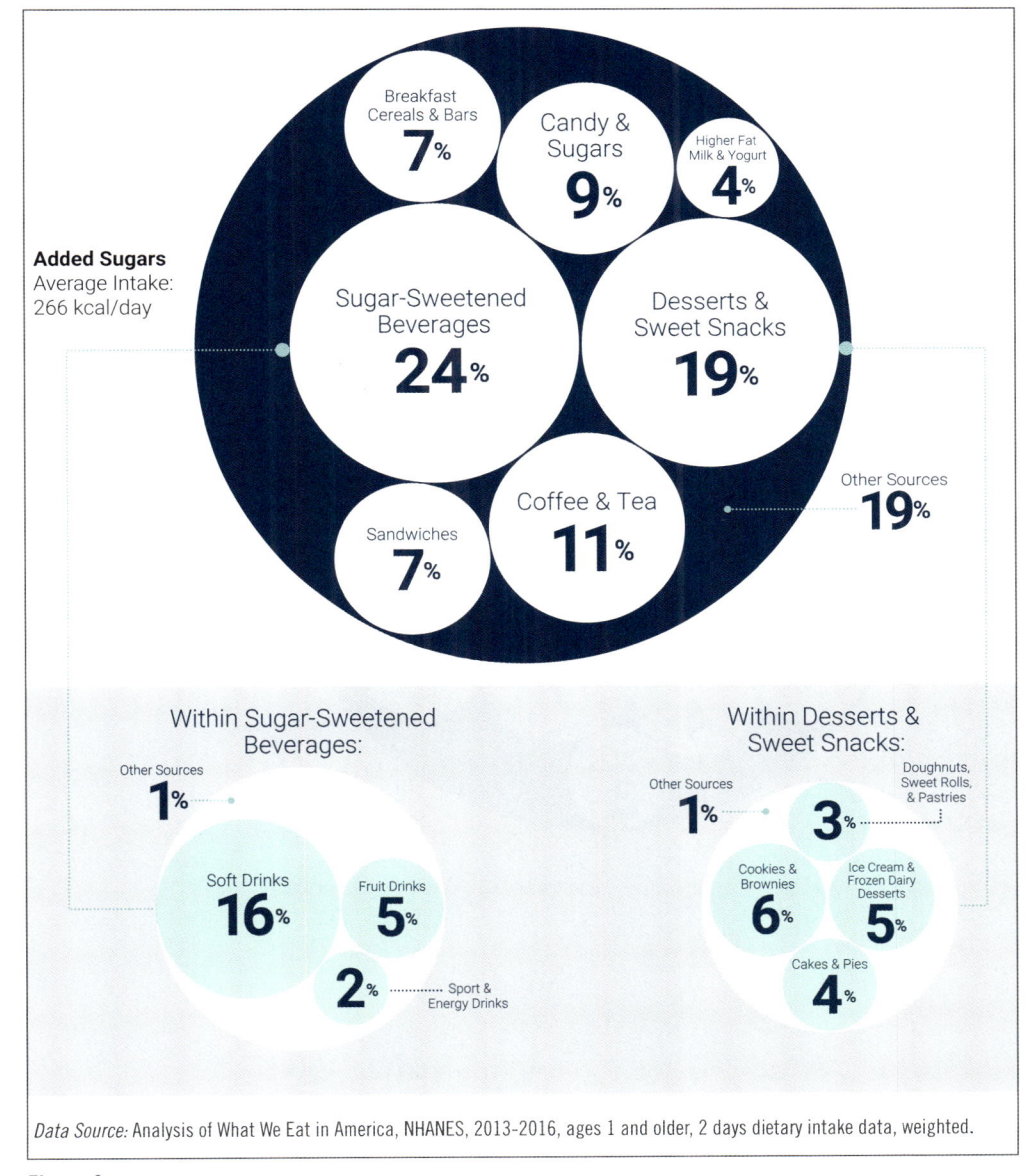

Figure 3
Top sources and average intakes of added sugars: U.S. Population ages 1 and older

Reprinted from United States Department of Agriculture (2020). *2020-2025 Dietary Guidelines for Americans* (9th ed.). www.dietaryguidelines.gov

TABLE 3
THE MANY WAYS TO SAY SUGAR
Agave syrup
Anhydrous dextrose
Brown sugar
Cane juice
Confectioner's powdered sugar
Corn sweetener
Corn syrup
Corn syrup solids
Crystal dextrose
Dextrin
Dextrose
Evaporated corn sweetener
Fructose
Fruit juice concentrate
Fruit nectar
Glucose
High-fructose corn syrup
Honey
Invert sugar
Lactose
Liquid fructose
Malt syrup
Maltose
Maple syrup
Molasses
Nectar
Pancake syrup
Raw sugar
Sucrose
Sugar
Sugar cane juice
Trehalose
Turbinado sugar
White granulated sugar

Saturated Fats

The types of **fatty acids** consumed play a more significant role in health than the amount of fat consumed. "Solid fats" include saturated fats and **trans fats.** A high intake of saturated fat is associated with increased total and **low-density lipoprotein (LDL)** cholesterol—both of which increase the risk of cardiovascular disease. The *Dietary Guidelines* recommend a diet containing <10% of total calories from saturated fat. Major sources of saturated fat for Americans include sandwiches, including burgers, tacos and burritos; desserts and sweet snacks; and rice, pasta, and other grain-based mixed dishes. Evidence suggests that the health benefits are best when saturated fat is replaced with foods higher in polyunsaturated and monounsaturated fats, such as most types of vegetable oils. Salmon, tuna, and other fatty fish and many types of nuts and seeds, such as flaxseeds, are high in polyunsaturated fat. The scientific understanding of saturated fats continues to emerge, and there is debate about whether saturated fats are as harmful to health as was previously believed. That said, the *Dietary Guidelines* emphasize the importance of limiting saturated fats, staying within saturated fat limits, and replacing saturated fat with unsaturated fat to support healthy dietary patterns. This is most important during adulthood because the prevalence of coronary heart disease increases with age and high LDL cholesterol peaks between the ages of 50 and 59 in men and 60 and 69 in women (USDA, 2020). The primary sources of saturated fat for Americans ages 1 and older are shown in Figure 5.

Figure 5
Top sources and average intakes of saturated fat: U.S. population ages 1 and older

Reprinted from United States Department of Agriculture (2020). *2020-2025 Dietary Guidelines for Americans* (9th ed.). www.dietaryguidelines.gov

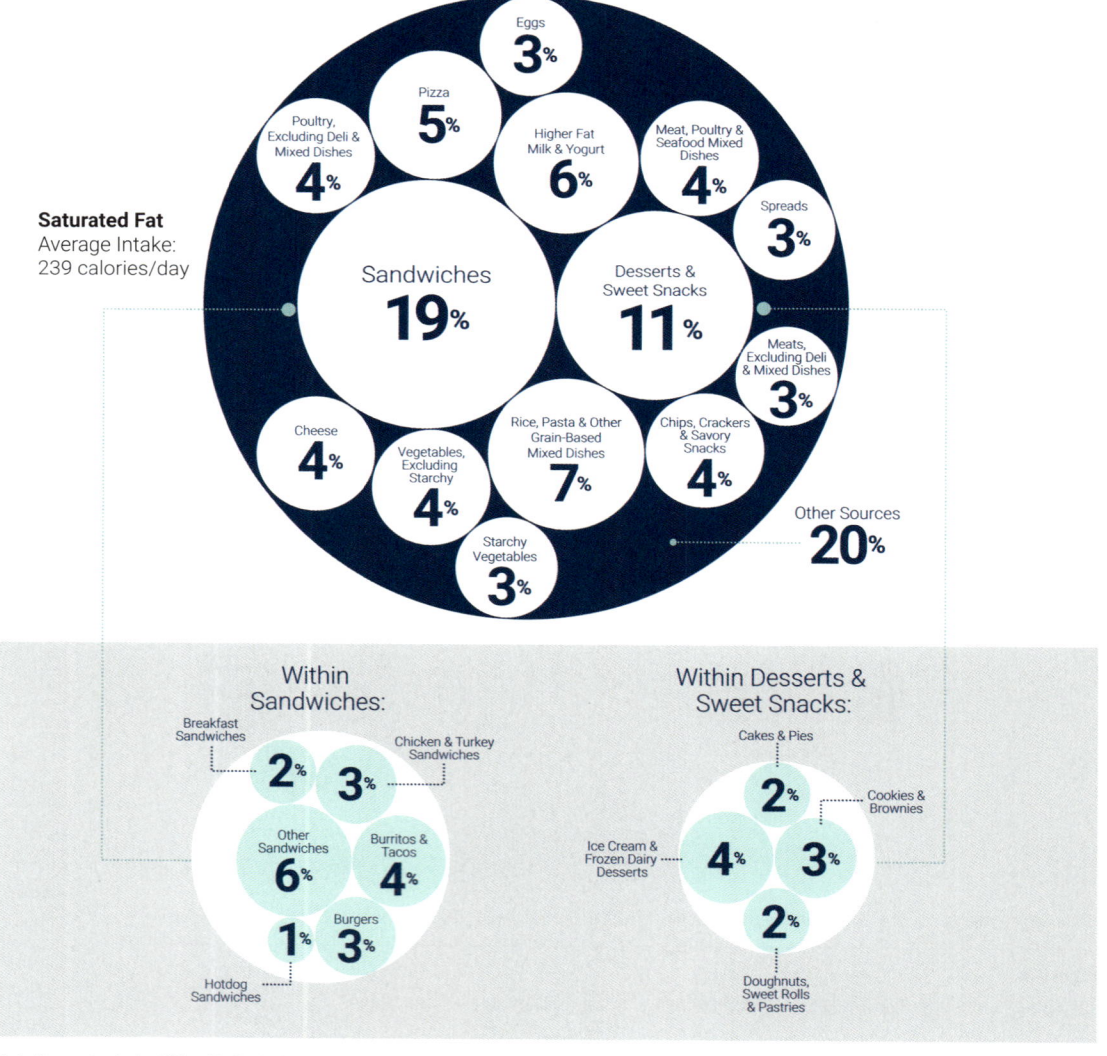

Saturated Fat
Average Intake: 239 calories/day

- Eggs 3%
- Pizza 5%
- Poultry, Excluding Deli & Mixed Dishes 4%
- Higher Fat Milk & Yogurt 6%
- Meat, Poultry & Seafood Mixed Dishes 4%
- Spreads 3%
- Sandwiches 19%
- Desserts & Sweet Snacks 11%
- Meats, Excluding Deli & Mixed Dishes 3%
- Cheese 4%
- Vegetables, Excluding Starchy 4%
- Rice, Pasta & Other Grain-Based Mixed Dishes 7%
- Chips, Crackers & Savory Snacks 4%
- Starchy Vegetables 3%
- Other Sources 20%

Within Sandwiches:
- Breakfast Sandwiches 2%
- Chicken & Turkey Sandwiches 3%
- Other Sandwiches 6%
- Burritos & Tacos 4%
- Hotdog Sandwiches 1%
- Burgers 3%

Within Desserts & Sweet Snacks:
- Cakes & Pies 2%
- Cookies & Brownies 3%
- Ice Cream & Frozen Dairy Desserts 4%
- Doughnuts, Sweet Rolls & Pastries 2%

Data Source: Analysis of What We Eat in America, NHANES, 2013-2016, ages 1 and older, 2 days dietary intake data, weighted.

Trans Fats

Trans fats are found naturally in dairy and meat products ("ruminant trans fats"), but the majority of intake comes from processed foods ("artificial trans fats"). Artificial trans fats increase LDL cholesterol and contribute to increased cardiovascular disease risk. Trans fats are required by law to be listed on the food label, although foods that contain <0.5 grams of trans fat per serving are allowed to claim "0 grams" of trans fat. Consumers can identify these foods by looking on the ingredient list for the words "partially hydrogenated." Americans should consume as little trans fats as possible without compromising the nutritional adequacy of the diet.

Sodium and the Dietary Approaches to Stop Hypertension Eating Plan

Sodium intake is associated with high levels of blood pressure for some people. Maintaining a normal blood pressure decreases the risk of cardiovascular disease, **congestive heart failure,** and kidney disease. The estimated intake of sodium per day for the average American is 3,393 mg, far more than the recommended amount of <2,300 mg. In fact, only 3% of males and 23% of females in America meet sodium goals. This is at least in part due to the fact that sodium is ubiquitous in the food supply, especially in canned, processed, and restaurant-prepared dishes. Added table salt also contributes significantly to daily intake. The primary sources of sodium for Americans ages 1 and older are shown in Figure 6.

Sodium
Average Intake: 3,393 mg/day

Top sources (percent of total sodium intake):
- Sandwiches 21%
- Other Sources 19%
- Rice, Pasta & Other Grain-Based Mixed Dishes 8%
- Vegetables, Excluding Starchy 7%
- Poultry, Excluding Deli & Mixed Dishes 5%
- Pizza 5%
- Meat, Poultry & Seafood Mixed Dishes 5%
- Starchy Vegetables 4%
- Chips, Crackers & Savory Snacks 4%
- Soups 4%
- Desserts & Sweet Snacks 4%
- Yeast Breads & Tortillas 3%
- Deli & Cured Products 3%
- Eggs 3%
- Breakfast Cereals & Bars 3%
- Condiments & Gravies 3%

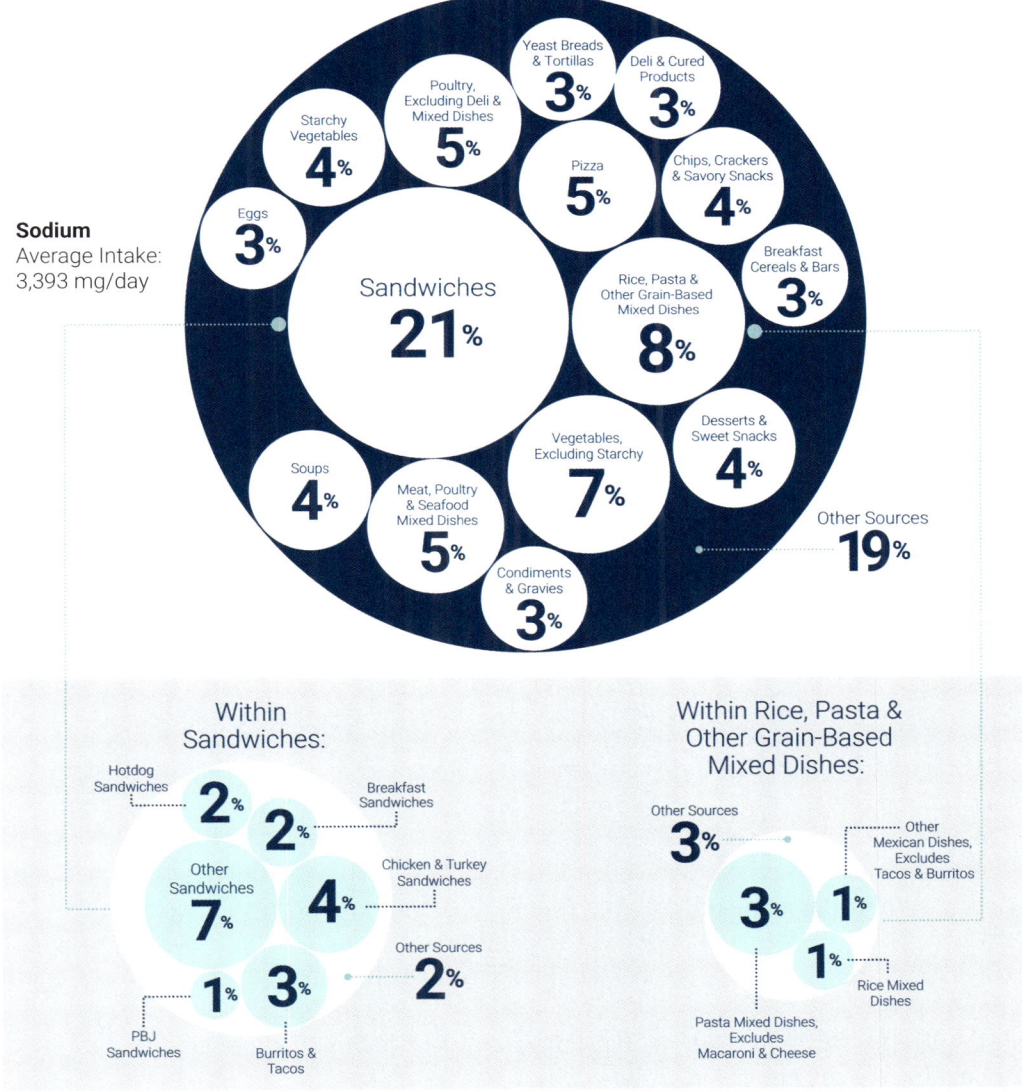

Within Sandwiches:
- Other Sandwiches 7%
- Chicken & Turkey Sandwiches 4%
- Burritos & Tacos 3%
- Hotdog Sandwiches 2%
- Breakfast Sandwiches 2%
- Other Sources 2%
- PBJ Sandwiches 1%

Within Rice, Pasta & Other Grain-Based Mixed Dishes:
- Other Sources 3%
- Pasta Mixed Dishes, Excludes Macaroni & Cheese 3%
- Other Mexican Dishes, Excludes Tacos & Burritos 1%
- Rice Mixed Dishes 1%

Figure 6
Top sources and average intakes of sodium: U.S. Population ages 1 and older

Reprinted from United States Department of Agriculture (2020). *2020-2025 Dietary Guidelines for Americans* (9th ed.). www.dietaryguidelines.gov

Data Source: Analysis of What We Eat in America, NHANES, 2013-2016, ages 1 and older, 2 days dietary intake data, weighted.

The CMES can help clients decrease sodium intake by collaborating to set goals to:
- Read nutrition labels and pay attention to sodium content
- Consume more fresh foods and fewer processed foods
- Eat more home-prepared meals and add little table salt or sodium-containing seasonings
- When eating out, ask that salt not be added
- Reduce calorie intake (since most foods also contain sodium)

In addition, individuals with **hypertension** are advised to follow the low-sodium **Dietary Approaches to Stop Hypertension (DASH) eating plan** to optimize health and decrease blood pressure. The DASH eating plan is low in saturated fat, **cholesterol,** and total fat. The staples are whole grains, fruits, vegetables, and legumes. Fish, poultry, lean meats, nuts, and other unsaturated fats as well as low-fat dairy products are also encouraged. Consequently, it is rich in potassium, magnesium, calcium, protein, and fiber. Red meat, sweets, and sugar-containing beverages are very limited. Thus, it is low in saturated and total fat and cholesterol. The DASH eating plan recommends that men drink two or fewer and women drink one or fewer alcoholic beverages per day. While developed to reduce blood pressure, the DASH eating plan can be adopted by anyone regardless of whether the person has elevated blood pressure. In fact, some studies suggest that the eating plan may also reduce cardiovascular disease risk by lowering total cholesterol and LDL cholesterol in addition to lowering blood pressure (reviewed in Eckel et al., 2014).

The DASH eating plan lowers **systolic blood pressure (SBP)** by about 5 to 6 mmHg and **diastolic blood pressure (DBP)** by 3 mmHg when compared to a typical American diet of the 1990s. This effect on blood pressure holds true across ages, sex, and ethnicity for individuals with blood pressures 120–159/80–95 mmHg (Eckel et al., 2014). Several variations of the DASH eating plan have been studied with even more pronounced results. For example, when 10% of calories from carbohydrates were replaced with an equal number of calories from protein or unsaturated fat, SBP decreased by an additional 1 mmHg compared to the standard DASH eating plan in both hypertensive and nonhypertensive individuals. When looking at only hypertensive individuals, SBP decreased by 3 mmHg compared to the standard DASH eating plan (Eckel et al., 2014).

Note that certain populations, such as individuals participating in intensive physical activity in hot and humid environments, need sufficient sodium intake to replace sodium lost in fluid. The AI for sodium in people nine to 50 years old is 1,500 mg per day and the UL is 2,200 to 2,300 mg per day. Most athletes will meet sodium needs with a sodium intake within this range, although making recommendations regarding the timing and amount of sodium replacement is outside the scope of the *Dietary Guidelines*.

Key Guideline 4: Limit Foods and Beverages Higher in Added Sugars, Saturated Fat, and Sodium, and Limit Alcoholic Beverages

Choose nutrient-dense foods and beverages across and within all food groups in place of less healthy choices. Consider cultural and personal preferences to make these shifts easier to accomplish and maintain.

While the *Dietary Guidelines* advocate an overall healthy and balanced dietary pattern that is low in added sugars, saturated fat, and sodium, the reality is that most Americans eat nothing like the eating patterns recommended by the *Dietary Guidelines,* as shown in Figure 2. By making shifts in dietary patterns, Americans can achieve and maintain a healthy body weight, meet nutrient needs, and decrease the risk of chronic disease by making healthy choices one day at a time.

Overall, the *Dietary Guidelines* advise that Americans shift their eating patterns to:
- Make healthy choices one day at a time
- Make nutrient-dense choices one meal at a time

Nutrition for Health and Fitness

- Consume more vegetables
- Consume more fruits
- Consume more whole grains and fewer refined grains
- Consume more dairy products
- Increase variety in protein food choices and choose more nutrient-dense foods. That is, eat more seafood in place of meat, poultry, or eggs and use beans, peas, and lentils or nuts and seeds in mixed dishes instead of some meat or poultry. Men and teenage boys should consume less protein, especially meat, poultry, and eggs.
- Exchange solid fats for oils
- Reduce added sugar consumption to less than 10% of calories per day
- Reduce saturated fat intake to less than 10% of calories per day
- Reduce sodium intake to less than 2,300 milligrams per day
- When alcohol is consumed, drinking less is better for health than drinking more, and adults of legal drinking age can choose not to drink at all or to drink in moderation by limiting intake to 2 drinks or less for men per day and 1 drink per day for women.

Examples of how these shifts might play out in a daily eating plan include:
- Shift from high-calorie snacks (such as tortilla chips with cheese dip) to nutrient-dense snacks (carrots with hummus dip)
- Shift from fruit products with added sugars (fruit-filled cereal bar) to whole fruit (apple)
- Shift from refined grains (white bread) to whole grains (whole-wheat bread)
- Shift from snacks high in sodium (meat and cheese sticks) to unsalted snacks (unsalted cashews)
- Shift from solid fats (butter in a frying pan) to oils
- Shift from beverages with added sugars (soda) to no-sugar-added beverages (seltzer water)

The *Dietary Guidelines* also acknowledge the importance of regular physical activity for improving health, feeling better, and reducing the risk for developing many chronic diseases (USDA, 2020). Most people would benefit from moving more and sitting less, even if for only a few minutes at a time, because some physical activity is better than none.

Support Healthy Dietary Patterns for All

Everyone has a role in helping to create and support healthy dietary patterns in multiple settings nationwide, where people learn, work, live, gather, and play.

The *Guidelines* charge all sectors of society to play an active role in the movement to make the United States healthier by supporting individuals and families in adopting healthier behaviors that align with the *Dietary Guidelines* and to ensure families have access to safe, healthy, and affordable foods. Food and activity behaviors are best viewed in the context of a **socio-ecological model.** This model can be described as an approach that emphasizes the development of coordinated partnerships, programs, and policies to support healthy eating and active living. In this framework, interventions should extend well beyond providing traditional education to individuals and families about healthy choices, and should help build skills, reshape the environment, and reestablish social norms to facilitate individuals' healthy choices (Figure 7).

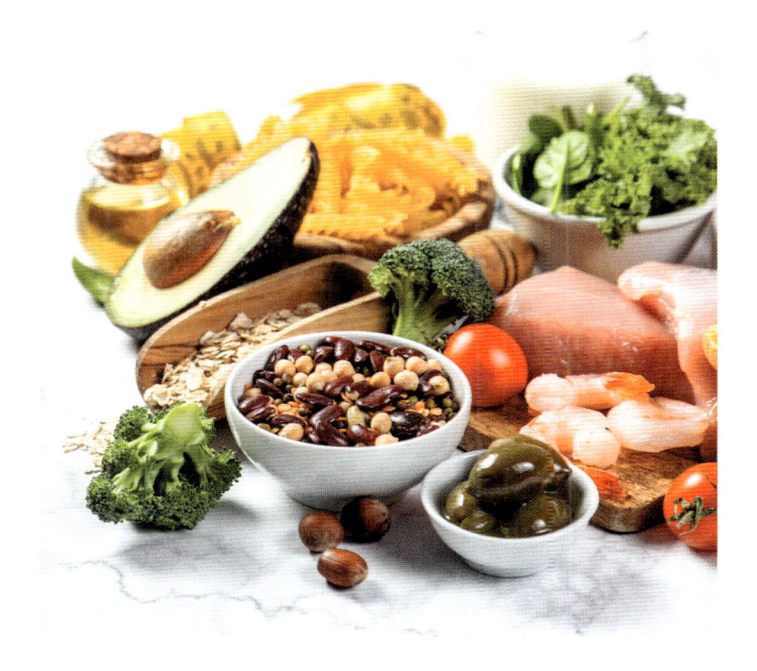

Figure 7
The ecological perspective, with examples of how each level influences food choices

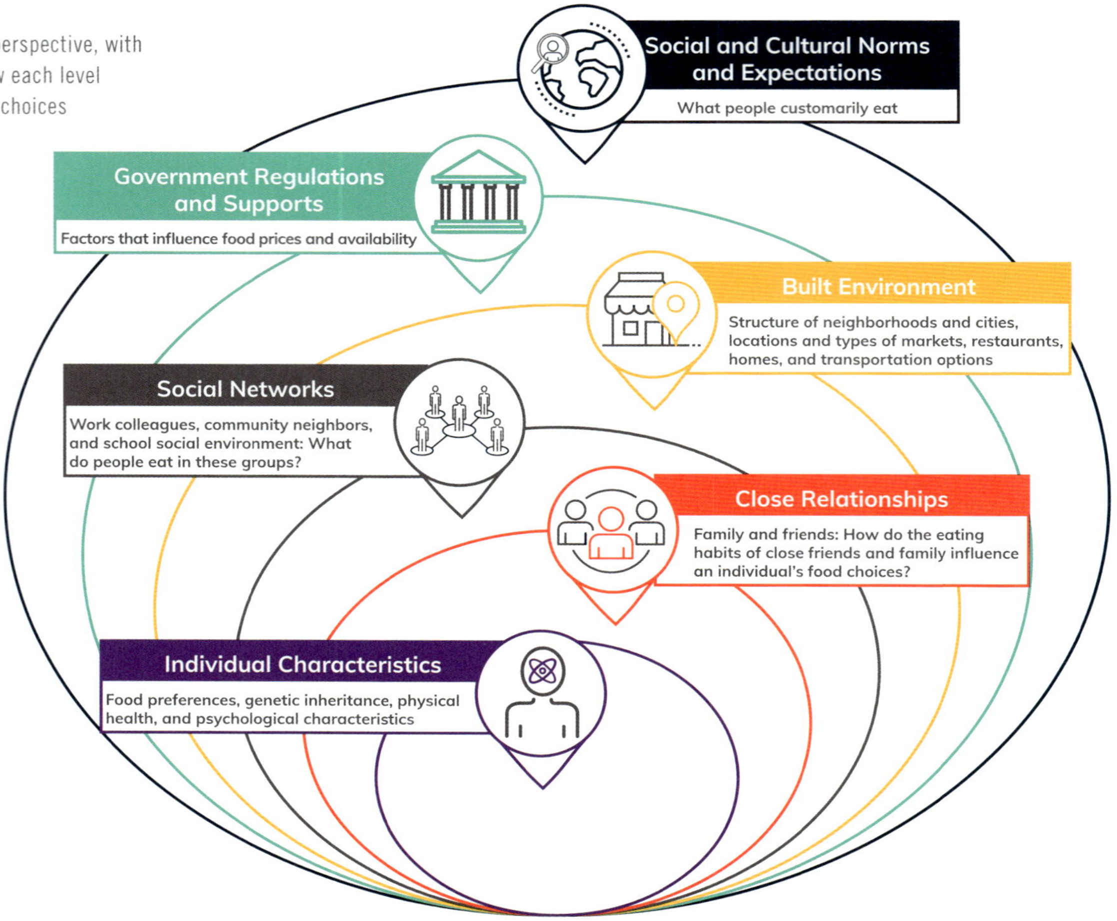

Social and Cultural Norms and Expectations
What people customarily eat

Government Regulations and Supports
Factors that influence food prices and availability

Built Environment
Structure of neighborhoods and cities, locations and types of markets, restaurants, homes, and transportation options

Social Networks
Work colleagues, community neighbors, and school social environment: What do people eat in these groups?

Close Relationships
Family and friends: How do the eating habits of close friends and family influence an individual's food choices?

Individual Characteristics
Food preferences, genetic inheritance, physical health, and psychological characteristics

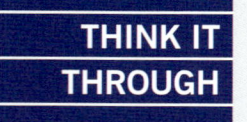

THINK IT THROUGH

THE ECOLOGICAL PERSPECTIVE

Taking an ecological perspective facilitates the understanding of many types of health behaviors, including eating behaviors (Sallis & Owen, 2015).

Consider your own eating behaviors. Using an ecological perspective, list supports and barriers at each level that influence your behavior. How might taking into consideration high-level factors like community design and public policies influence your work as a CMES?

The CMES can best "meet people where they are" to understand individual choices and motivators by paying particular attention to:
- **Food access:** Access to healthy, safe, and affordable food choices is influenced by several factors, including proximity to grocery stores, financial resources, transportation, and neighborhood resources such as average income and availability of public transportation.
- **Household food insecurity:** This occurs when access to nutritious and safe food is limited or uncertain. Food insecurity affects a family's ability to obtain food and make healthy choices and can worsen stress and chronic disease risk.
- **Acculturation:** Acculturation involves moving toward a typical American dietary pattern from what is often a more nutritious pattern of the home country. The recommended dietary pattern is flexible to accommodate personal preferences, cultural traditions, and budgetary considerations.

The most effective interventions are multifaceted, using a combination of strategies to impact behavior change, and also multilevel in that they function across the various aspects of the

socio-ecological model. An impactful intervention might include a combination of changes across one or more of the following domains:
- **Home:** Develop skills in meal planning and cooking. Limit screen time at home and build in time for family physical activity.
- **School:** Commit to offering only healthy meals and snacks; provide nutrition labels and calorie and nutrient information in cafeterias; reach out to parents about making healthy changes at home; increase the amount and quality of nutrition education and school gardens; commit to support physical-activity programs, high-quality physical education, and active play.
- **Worksite:** Offer health and wellness programs, including nutritional counseling, active breaks, and flexible schedules that allow for physical activity and walking meetings. Provide stand-up desks to decrease sitting time.
- **Community:** Support shelters, food banks, farmers markets, community gardens, and walkable communities.
- **Food retail:** Reach out to consumers about making healthy changes; increase access to healthy and affordable food options.

Several specific strategies that the CMES can employ to support clients in shifting eating patterns to improve health and more closely resemble the recommended intakes include the following:
- Partner with individuals to increase awareness of the foods and beverages that make up their own or their family's eating patterns and identify areas where they can make small changes that align with the *Dietary Guidelines,* such as modifying recipes or food selections.
- Enhance self-efficacy with skills like gardening, cooking, meal planning, and label reading.
- Explore ways that individuals can model healthy eating behaviors for friends and family.
- Co-create plans to help clients limit screen time and time spent being sedentary and increase physical activity.

FOOD LABELS

For people to make healthy nutrition decisions, they first have to be able to understand which nutrients contribute to a healthy diet, and second, know which foods contain those nutrients. While the bulk of a healthy diet is made up of whole, unprocessed foods that do not carry food labels, there are processed or prepared foods (e.g., low-fat milk and milk products) that can be part of a healthy diet and do have food labels. The food label, a required component of nearly all packaged foods, can help people turn knowledge into action. It can also be a source of confusion and misunderstanding.

History and Present State of Food Labeling

It was not until the early 1970s, when consumers faced a boom in production of processed foods, that nutrition labels were included on packaged foods. As an increasing number of foods arrived on grocery store shelves, many of which made nutrition claims, the Food and Drug Administration (FDA) proposed regulations in 1972 to require food labels on packaged foods that added nutrients or made nutrition claims. The labels would be voluntary for foods without claims. The first nutrition labels contained basic nutrition information, including calories, protein, carbohydrate, and fat, as well as the RDA for protein and several vitamins and minerals. Inclusion of sodium, saturated fat, and polyunsaturated fat was optional (Food and Nutrition Board, 2010).

As more products arrived on shelves and consumers became increasingly interested in reviewing food labels, food manufacturers responded with a plethora of ambiguous claims touting nutritional value and health benefits, even though FDA regulations had long prohibited mention of disease prevention or health promotion on food labels. Though companies could not explicitly state or imply that a food's nutrient properties could help to prevent, cure, or treat any disease or symptom, ambiguous nutrition claims designed to catch consumers' attention (such as "extremely low in saturated fat") became commonplace. The FDA policy helped to protect consumers against potentially harmful claims. However, it also limited manufacturers' ability to advertise the benefits of foods that provided legitimate health benefits, such as foods that were high in fiber. In 1984, the National Cancer Institute and Kellogg's launched a food-labeling campaign on a high-fiber cereal box linking the high-fiber intake to a possible reduction in some cancers. In the absence of regulatory action, other food manufacturers followed suit, leading to a frenzy of nutrition and health claims on food labels (Food and Nutrition Board, 2010).

In 1990, congress passed the Nutrition Labeling and Education Act (NLEA), which gave the FDA the authority to require nutrition labeling on most food packages and specified the information and nutrients that must be included on the label. It also required specific criteria for approved health claims. The FDA's stated goal in developing the label criteria was to (1) minimize confusion, (2) help consumers choose healthier diets, and (3) provide an incentive to companies to improve the nutritional value of their products. The Nutrition Facts panel with which most of today's consumers are familiar was mandated in 1993. Though trans fats were not initially included on the nutrition label, their inclusion was required by 2003 if the product contained more than 0.5 grams of trans fat per serving. This regulation drastically decreased the amount of trans fats used in food production (Food and Nutrition Board, 2010).

In 2016, the FDA introduced a new Nutrition Facts label. The new label includes a few design changes, including increased font size and bold type for "calories" and "serving size" and the actual amount, in addition to **percent daily value (PDV)** of vitamin D, calcium, iron, and potassium. Content changes to the label include the addition of "added sugars" in grams and a PDV for added sugars. Vitamin D and potassium are required additions to the label, while vitamins A and C no longer must be included. Calcium and iron are still required. "Calories from fat" is no longer required, as the type of fat is more important than the amount. Daily values for some nutrients, such as sodium, dietary fiber, and vitamin D, are updated based on new DRIs from the National Academy of Medicine. Finally, the new label includes updates to serving sizes. Law requires that serving sizes be based on amounts of food and beverages that people commonly consume, not what they should consume. Because people are eating larger portions, the new label includes a serving size as a larger amount. For instance, a serving of ice cream used to be 1/2 cup but is now 2/3 cup. It is important for the CMES to recognize this change and that the serving size is not a recommendation of how much to eat. (In many cases, people should eat less than one serving of a food.) The number of servings per container has long been a source of confusion. Now, packages that are between one and two servings will be required to be labeled as one serving since people commonly consume the whole package in one sitting. For larger package sizes, manufacturers must include two column labels to include the amounts per serving and amounts per package.

Health Claims

The issue of whether or not to allow health claims was addressed by the NLEA. Claims that can be used on food and **dietary supplement** labels include **health claims, nutrient content claims,** and **structure/function claims.**

Health claims describe a relationship between a food or food component and the prevention or treatment of a disease or health-related condition. To be included on a nutrition label, health claims must be authorized by the FDA or be based on an authoritative statement of a scientific body of the federal government or the National Academies of Science, after notification to the FDA. A listing of currently allowed health claims is available at https://www.fda.gov/Food/LabelingNutrition/ucm2006876.htm.

Qualified health claims are allowed on product labels if there is emerging evidence for a relationship between a food or food component and decreased risk of a disease or health condition, but the scientific evidence is not conclusive. The statement must include a qualifying statement saying that the evidence supporting the claim is limited.

Nutrient content claims imply health benefits by describing the level of a nutrient in a product using terms like "free," "high," or "low," or compared to another product using terms like "more," "reduced," and "lite." A product can be labeled as "healthy" if it has "healthy" levels of total fat, saturated fat, cholesterol, and sodium. A listing of nutrient content claims is available at https://www.fda.gov/food/food-labeling-nutrition/nutrient-content-claims.

Structure/function claims are regulated by the **Dietary Supplement Health and Education Act (DSHEA)**. They typically apply to supplements and do not need to be preapproved by the FDA. These types of claims relate a nutrient or dietary ingredient to normal human structure or function, such as "calcium builds strong bones," or describe a benefit related to addressing a nutrient deficiency. It must state a disclaimer that the FDA has not evaluated the claim and that the supplement is not intended to treat, cure, or prevent any disease.

Front-of-Package Labeling

Since 1987, when the American Heart Association first developed the "Heart Guide Initiative" to tag foods that were the most heart healthy, organizations from PepsiCo and General Mills to grocery stores, nonprofits, and academic groups have implemented front-of-package (FOP) labeling to communicate with consumers. While intended to help consumers make healthier choices, the multiple and varied labels have been confusing and, in many cases, misleading. This issue came to public attention in 2009 when a popular sugar-sweetened cereal, along with macaroni and cheese, ice cream, and fruit roll-ups, were given a SmartChoice FOP label. In anticipation of potential regulation on FOP labeling systems, Congress mandated the IOM to develop a two-part report on FOP labeling (Food and Nutrition Board, 2012; Food and Nutrition Board, 2010). The IOM committee concluded that "It is time for a fundamental shift in strategy, a move away from systems that mostly provide nutrition information without clear guidance about its healthfulness, and toward one that encourages healthier food choices through simplicity, visual clarity, and the ability to convey meaning without written information. An FOP system should be standardized and it also should motivate food and beverage companies to reformulate their products to be healthier and encourage food retailers to prominently display products that meet this standard" (Food and Nutrition Board, 2012). The report advised a labeling system that is based on calories, saturated and trans fat, sugar, and salt. As of the time of this writing, no action has been taken.

Reading the Nutrition Label

While the nutrition label provides a large amount of useful nutrition information, it can also be a source of confusion for many consumers. A CMES can play an important role in helping consumers effectively use the nutrition label to guide them in making healthy choices.

A Stepwise Approach

A CMES can assist clients in dissecting the food label (Figure 8) by taking a stepwise approach. Start from the top with the serving size and the number of servings per container. In general, serving sizes are standardized so that consumers can compare similar products. All of the nutrient amounts listed on the food label are for one serving, so it is important to determine how many servings are actually being consumed to accurately assess nutrient intake.

Next, attention should be given to the total calories, which indicate how much energy a person gets from a particular food. Fat contains 9 calories per gram, while carbohydrate and protein contain 4 calories per gram. Americans tend to consume too many calories, without meeting daily nutrient requirements. This part of the nutrition label is the most important factor for weight control. In general, 40 calories per serving is considered low, 100 calories is moderate, and 400 or more calories is considered high [U.S. Food & Drug Administration (FDA), 2004].

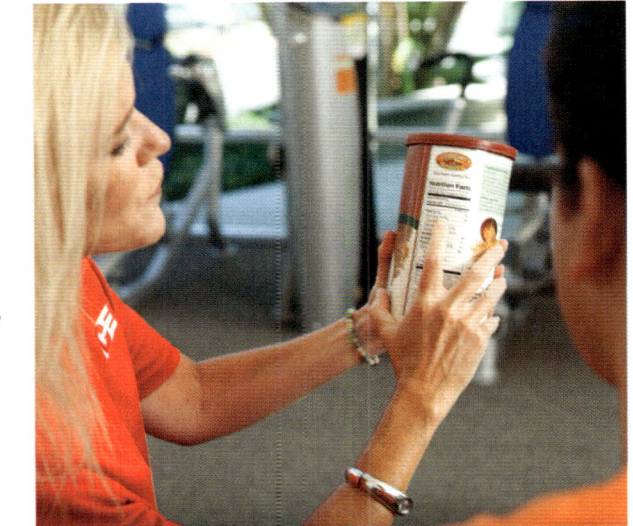

APPENDIX C

Figure 8
Nutrition facts label

① Serving Size
The label presents serving sizes as the amount that most people actually consume in a sitting. This is not necessarily the same as how much one should eat per serving. All of the nutrition information on the label is based on one serving. If you eat twice the serving size shown here, multiply the nutrient and calorie values by two.

② Calories
The number of calories listed represents the total calories from fat, carbohydrate, and protein (manufacturers are allowed to round this value to the nearest 5- or 10-calorie increment). 100 calories per serving is considered moderate, while 400 calories or more per serving is considered high. A 5'4", 138-lb active woman needs about 2,200 calories each day. A 5'10", 174-lb active man needs about 2,900 calories.

③ Total Fat
Fat is calorie-dense and, if consumed in large portions, can increase the risk of weight problems. While once vilified, most fat, in and of itself, is not bad. Adults should consume 20 to 35% of total calories from fat.

④ Saturated Fat
Saturated fat is part of the total fat in food. It is listed separately because it plays an important role in raising blood cholesterol and your risk of heart disease. Eat less than 10% of total calories from saturated fat.

⑤ Trans Fat
Trans fat works a lot like saturated fat, except it is worse. This fat starts out as a liquid unsaturated fat, but then food manufacturers add some hydrogen to it, turning it into a solid saturated fat (that is what "partially hydrogenated" means when you see it in the food ingredients). They do this to increase the shelf-life of the product, but in the body the trans fat damages the blood vessels and contributes to increasing blood cholesterol and the risk of heart disease. Individuals should consume as little trans fat as possible.

⑥ Cholesterol
Many foods that are high in cholesterol are also high in saturated fat, which can contribute to heart disease. Dietary cholesterol itself likely does not cause health problems.

Nutrition Facts

8 Servings Per Container	
Serving Size	2/3 cup (55g)

Amount Per Serving
Calories 230

	% Daily Value*
Total Fat 8g	10%
Saturated Fat 1g	5%
Trans Fat 0g	0%
Cholesterol 0mg	0%
Sodium 160mg	7%
Total Carbohydrate 37g	13%
Dietary Fiber 4g	14%
Total Sugars 12g	
Includes 10g Added Sugars	20%
Protein 3g	
Vitamin D 2mcg	10%
Calcium 260mg	20%
Iron 8mg	45%
Potassium 235mg	6%

* The % Daily Value (DV) tells you how much a nutrient in a serving of food contributes to a daily diet. 2,000 calories a day is used for general nutrition advice.

Daily Value
Daily Values are listed based on a 2,000-calorie daily eating plan. Your calorie and nutrient needs may be a little bit more or less based on your age, sex, and activity level (see https://fnic.nal.usda.gov/fnic/interactiveDRI/). For saturated fat, trans fat, sodium, and added sugars, choose foods with a low % (5% or less) Daily Value. For dietary fiber, vitamins, and minerals, your Daily Value goal is to reach 100% of each.

Ingredients: *This portion of the label lists all of the foods and additives contained in a product, in descending order by weight.*

Allergens: *This portion of the label identifies which of the most common allergens may be present in the product.*

(More nutrients may be listed on some labels)

  mcg = micrograms (1,000 mcg = 1 mg)
  mg = milligrams (1,000 mg = 1 g)
  g = grams (about 28 g = 1 ounce)

⑦ Sodium
You call it "salt," the label calls it "sodium." Either way, it may add up to high blood pressure in some people. So, keep your sodium intake low—less than 2,300 mg each day.

⑧ Total Carbohydrate
Carbohydrates are in foods like bread, potatoes, fruits, and vegetables, as well as processed foods. Carbohydrate is further broken down into dietary fiber and sugars. Consume foods high in fiber often and those high in sugars, especially added sugars, less often. Adults should consume 45 to 65% of total calories from carbohydrates.

⑨ Dietary Fiber
There are two kinds of dietary fiber: soluble and insoluble. Fruits, vegetables, whole-grain foods, and beans, peas, and lentils are all good sources and can help reduce the risk of heart disease and cancer. Individuals should try to eat 14 grams of dietary fiber for every 1,000 calories consumed.

⑩ Sugars
Too much sugar contributes to weight gain and increased risk of diseases like diabetes and fatty liver disease. Foods like fruits and dairy products contain natural sugars (fructose and lactose), but also may contain added sugars. It is recommended to consume less than 10% of total calories from added sugar, or less than 50 g per day based on a 2,000-calorie dietary pattern.

⑪ Protein
To limit saturated fat, eat small servings of lean meat, fish, and poultry. Use skim or low-fat milk, yogurt, and cheese. Try vegetable proteins like beans, grains, and cereals. Adults should consume 10 to 35% of total calories from protein.

⑫ Vitamins and Minerals
Your goal here is 100% of each for the day. Don't count on one food to do it all. Let a combination of foods add up to a winning score.

The next two sections of the label note the nutrient content of the food product. Ideally, intake of saturated and trans fat and sodium should be minimized, and adequate amounts of fiber should be consumed, along with vitamins and minerals, especially vitamin D, potassium, calcium, and iron. The food label includes the total amount of sugars (natural and added), as well as the amount of added sugars.

The PDVs are listed for key nutrients to make it easier to compare products (just make sure that the serving sizes are similar), evaluate nutrient content claims (does 1/3 reduced-sugar cereal really contain less carbohydrate than a similar cereal of a different brand?), and make informed dietary tradeoffs (e.g., balance consumption of a high-fat product for lunch with lower-fat products throughout the rest of the day). In general, 5% daily value or less is considered low, while 20% daily value or more is considered high (USDA, 2020).

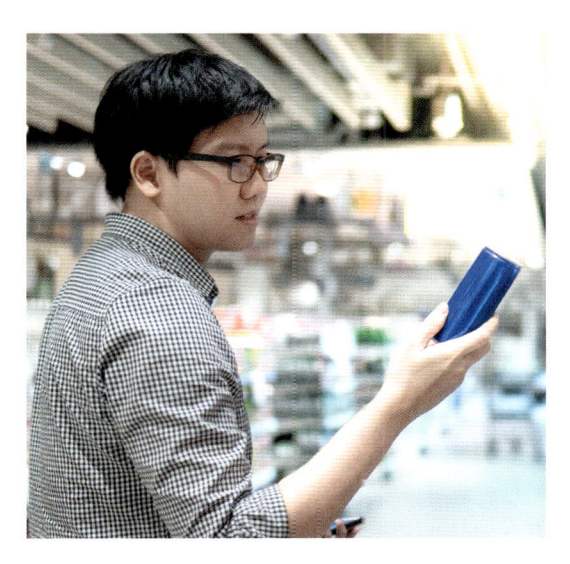

The footnote at the bottom of the label reminds consumers that all PDVs are based on a 2,000-calorie diet. Individuals who need more or fewer calories should adjust recommendations accordingly. For example, 3 grams of fat provides 5% of the recommended amount for someone on a 2,000-calorie diet, but 7% for someone on a 1,500-calorie diet.

Legislation also requires food manufacturers to list all potential food **allergens** on food packaging. The most common food allergens are fish, shellfish, soybean, wheat, egg, milk, peanuts, and tree nuts. This information usually is included near the list of ingredients on the package. Clearly, this information is especially important to clients with food allergies. For clients who follow a gluten-free diet, this is also an easy way to identify if wheat is a product ingredient.

Clients should carefully review the ingredients list. Note that the ingredient list is in decreasing order of substance weight in the product. That is, the ingredients that are listed first are the most abundant ingredients in the product. The ingredient list is useful to help identify whether or not the product contains trans fat, solid fats, added sugars, whole grains, and refined grains.

- **Trans fat:** Although trans fat is included in the "fat" section of the nutrition label, if the product contains <0.5 grams per serving, the manufacturer does not need to claim it. However, if a product contains "partially hydrogenated oils," then the product contains trans fat. Partially hydrogenated oils are a major source of artificial trans fat in the food supply and are no longer generally recognized as safe and are no longer added to foods (USDA, 2020).
- **Solid fats:** If the ingredient list contains beef fat, butter, chicken fat, coconut oil, cream, hydrogenated oils, palm kernel oils, pork fat (lard), shortening, or stick margarine, then the product contains solid fats.
- **Added sugars:** Ingredients signifying added sugars are listed in Table 3. In many cases, products contain multiple forms of sugar.
- **Whole grains:** To be considered 100% whole grain, the product must contain all of the essential parts of the original kernel—the bran, germ, and endosperm. When choosing products, the whole grain should be the first or second ingredient. Examples of whole grains include brown rice, buckwheat, bulgur (cracked wheat), millet, steel-cut oats, popcorn, quinoa, rolled oats, whole-grain sorghum, whole-grain triticale, whole-grain barley, whole-grain corn, whole oats/oatmeal, whole rye, whole wheat, and wild rice.
- **Refined grains:** Refined grains are listed as "enriched." If the first ingredient is an enriched grain, then the product is not a whole grain. This is one way to understand whether or not a "wheat bread" is actually whole wheat or a refined product.

DO THE MATH

NUTRITION LABEL SAMPLE PROBLEM

Using the nutrition label from Figure 8, determine (1) the number of calories per container; (2) the calories from carbohydrate, protein, and fat per serving; and (3) the percentage of calories from carbohydrate, protein, and fat.

1. 230 calories per serving x 8 servings per container = 1,840 calories per container

2. *Carbohydrate:* 37 grams carbohydrate per serving x 4 calories per gram = 148 calories per serving from carbohydrate

   Protein: 3 grams protein per serving x 4 calories per gram = 12 calories per serving from protein

   Fat: 8 grams fat per serving x 9 calories per gram = 72 calories per serving from fat

   Note that the label rounds the 232 calories calculated in question 2 to 230 calories.

3. *Carbohydrate:* 148 calories from carbohydrate/230 calories = 64% carbohydrate

   Protein: 12 calories from protein/230 calories = 5% protein

   Fat: 72 calories from fat/230 calories = 31% fat

Figure 9
Food safety recommendations

Reprinted from United States Department of Agriculture (2020). *2020-2025 Dietary Guidelines for Americans* (9th ed.).
www.dietaryguidelines.gov

FOOD SAFETY AND SELECTION

An important but often underestimated key to healthy eating is to avoid foods contaminated with harmful bacteria, viruses, parasites, and other microorganisms. About one in six Americans, or 48 million people, become sick each year from foodborne illness, 128,000 are hospitalized, and approximately 3,000 die (Centers for Disease Control and Prevention, 2011). Special populations most at risk include pregnant women, infants and young children, older adults, and people who are immunocompromised. The majority of foodborne illnesses are preventable with a few simple precautions (Figure 9).

Follow Food Safety Recommendations

An important part of healthy eating is keeping food safe. Individuals in their own homes can help keep food safe by following safe food handling practices. Four basic food safety principles work together to reduce the risk of foodborne illness—Clean, Separate, Cook, and Chill.

1: Clean — Wash hands and surfaces often.

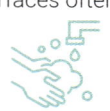

2: Separate — Separate raw meats from other foods.

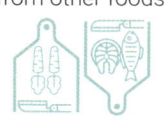

3: Cook — Cook food to safe internal temperatures.

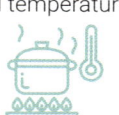

4: Chill — Refrigerate foods promptly.

Some eating behaviors, such as consuming raw, undercooked, or unpasteurized food products, increase the risk of contracting a foodborne illness. Populations at increased risk of foodborne illness, or those preparing food for them, should use extra caution. These include women who are pregnant, young children, and older adults. Specific guidance for these life stages is discussed in subsequent chapters. Individuals with weakened immune systems are also at increased risk for foodborne illness. More information about food safety is available at:

- Your Gateway to Food Safety: **foodsafety.gov**
- USDA Food Safety Education campaigns: **fsis.usda.gov/wps/portal/fsis/topics/food-safety-education/teach-others/fsis-educational-campaigns**
- Fight BAC!®: **fightbac.org** and for Babies and Toddlers: **fightbac.org/kids/**
- CDC 4 Steps to Food Safety: **cdc.gov/foodsafety**
- FDA: Buy, Store & Serve Safe Food at **fda.gov/food/consumers/buy-store-serve-safe-food**

Clients can employ the following tips while grocery shopping to reduce the risk of foodborne illness:
- Check produce for bruises and feel and smell for ripeness.
- Look for a "sell-by" date for breads and baked goods, a "use-by" date on some packaged foods, an "expiration date" on yeast and baking powder, and a "packaged date" on canned and some packaged foods.
- Make sure packaged goods are not torn and cans are not dented, cracked, or bulging.
- Separate fish and poultry from other purchases by wrapping them separately in plastic bags.
- Pick up refrigerated and frozen foods last. Make sure all perishable items are refrigerated within one hour of purchase.

PRACTICAL CONSIDERATIONS FOR MEDICAL EXERCISE SPECIALISTS

While much of the buzz around nutrition often relates to individual ingredients or a proportion of calories from specific macronutrients, there is an increasing movement toward an overall healthy eating pattern based on the consumption of more whole foods. In order to assist clients in translating the most current evidence and recommendations into practical and sustainable nutrition changes while keeping within scope of practice, the CMES can offer further support, guidance, and resources in the following ways.

Providing Grocery Store Tours

The average grocery store in America has about 40,000 products from which to choose. For this reason, grocery shopping can be an overwhelming and confusing experience for many clients. The traditional guidance to stick to the perimeter of the store can help narrow the choices, and as such this advice has been dispensed by health educators and health agencies for quite some time. The outer aisles are usually where most of the whole, fresh foods are located, with the exception of whole grains, beans, and legumes, which are commonly found in the center aisles. Aside from these items, the majority of foods that are located in the center aisles of the store are highly processed and nutrient-deficient. For clients seeking further support and guidance navigating the plethora of options, the CMES may opt to expand their offerings to provide grocery store tours, which have been found to be an effective strategy for helping clients learn healthier shopping and eating practices (Nikolaus et al., 2016).

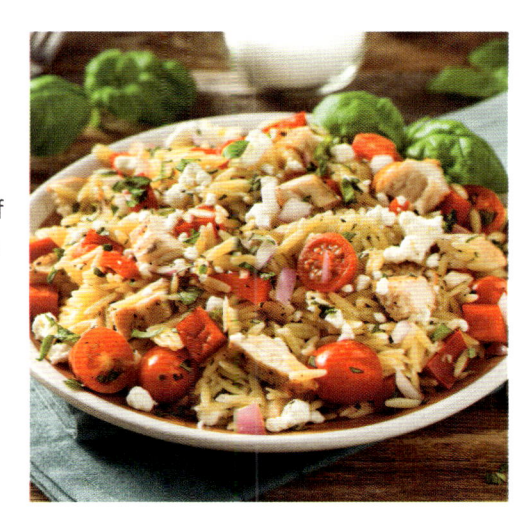

APPLY WHAT YOU KNOW

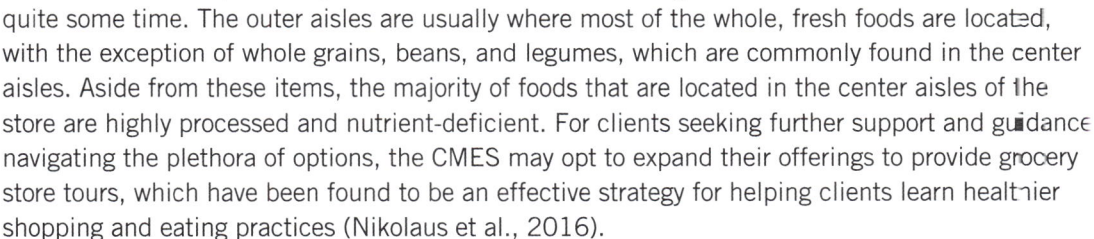

EATING HEALTHY ON A BUDGET

It is estimated that approximately 32% of working families in the U.S. may not have enough money to meet basic needs (Roberts, Povich, & Mather, 2012). Specifically, as of 2019 the USDA reported that 10.5% of Americans were food insecure at least some time during the year, a percentage that rises disproportionately for households with children and people of color (Coleman-Jensen et al., 2018). A CMES will likely work with individuals for which healthy eating is impacted by financial limitations and should therefore be prepared to support individuals in understanding and navigating options. This may include, but is not limited to:
- Supporting clients in accessing additional support as needed through established programs, such as the Supplemental Nutrition Access Program
- Providing resources upon client request, such as a list of local food pantries
- Collaboratively brainstorming money-saving shopping tips, such as buying in bulk, using coupons, purchasing generic or store brands, and considering frozen over fresh produce when most economical

Collaborating with Registered Dietitians

As discussed earlier in this appendix, the issues, questions, and controversies that surround nutrition are numerous and quite nuanced. A CMES should strive to provide clients with the facts and allow for a personalized approach to nutrition, referring them to an RD when needed. Issues that would indicate the need for a referral include, but are not limited to, disordered eating, multiple chronic disease states, client request for meal planning, or a need for detailed nutrition information beyond the scope of practice for a CMES. A CMES can expand their referral networks by visiting http://www.eatright.org/find-an-expert. It is advised that the CMES attend local nutrition-related events and conferences and develop community resources through collaboration with other health and exercise professionals.

FUELING BEFORE, DURING, AND AFTER EXERCISE

Creating and implementing safe and effective exercise programs for clients can be accomplished effectively through the guidelines set forth in the ACE Integrated Fitness Training® Model, which include asking important questions during the initial interview, selecting appropriate assessments, developing programs that are informed by the results of those assessments, and progressing clients as appropriate.

Physically active individuals need the right types and amounts of food before, during, and after exercise to maximize the amount of energy available to fuel optimal performance and minimize the amount of gastrointestinal distress. Sports nutrition strategies should address three exercise stages: pre-exercise, during exercise, and post-exercise (Figure 10).

Figure 10
Sports nutrition strategies

Sports nutrition strategies should address three exercise stages:
1. Pre-exercise: Beginning one week prior to the event, through warm-up
2. During exercise
3. Post-exercise: Up to 36 hours post-exercise

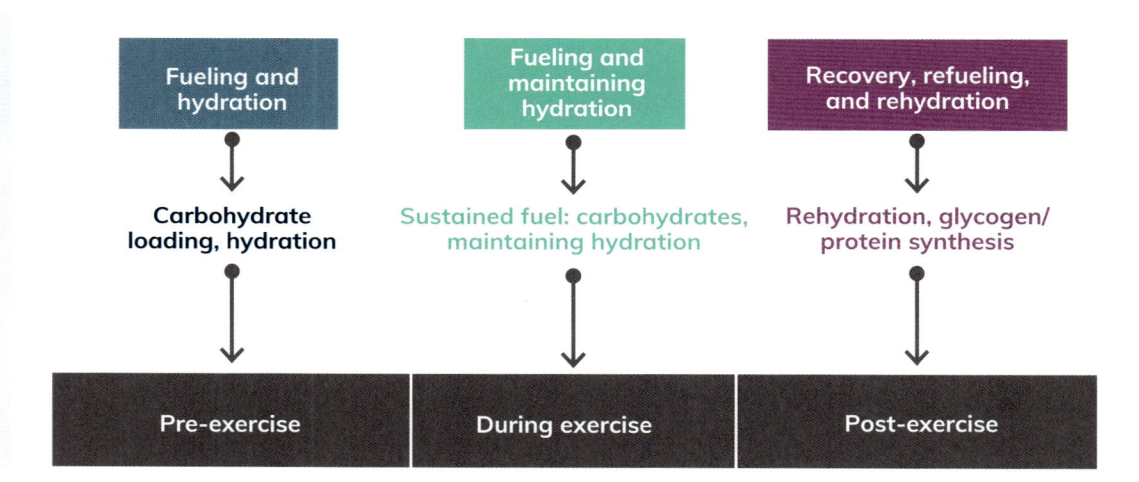

Fueling and hydration	Fueling and maintaining hydration	Recovery, refueling, and rehydration
Carbohydrate loading, hydration	Sustained fuel: carbohydrates, maintaining hydration	Rehydration, glycogen/protein synthesis
Pre-exercise	During exercise	Post-exercise

Pre-exercise Fueling

The two main goals of a pre-exercise snack are to (1) optimize **glucose** availability and **glycogen** stores and (2) provide the fuel needed to support exercise performance. Keeping this in mind, in the days up to a week before a strenuous endurance effort, an athlete should consider what nutritional strategies might set the stage for optimal performance. For example, an individual preparing for a long endurance event might consider the pros and cons of **carbohydrate loading**. On the day of the event or an important training session, the athlete should aim to eat a meal about four to six hours prior to the workout to minimize gastrointestinal distress and optimize performance. Four hours after eating, the food will already have been digested and absorbed; now liver and muscle glycogen levels are increased. To translate this into an everyday, practical recommendation, athletes who plan to work out for an extended duration in the early afternoon should be certain to eat a wholesome, carbohydrate-rich breakfast. Those who exercise in the early morning may benefit from a carbohydrate-rich snack before going to bed.

Some research also suggests that eating a relatively small carbohydrate- and protein-containing snack (e.g., 50 grams of carbohydrate and 5 to 10 grams of protein) 30 to 60 minutes before exercise helps increase glucose availability near the end of long-duration workout and helps to decrease exercise-induced protein **catabolism** (Kreider et al., 2010). The exact timing and size of the snack for peak performance will vary by individual and type of exercise. As a general rule, individuals should try out any snacks or drinks with practice sessions and workouts prior to relying on them to help athletic performance during competition. In general, a pre-exercise or pre-workout meal or snack should be:

- Relatively high in carbohydrate to maximize blood glucose availability (*Note:* Although no DRIs exist for pre-exercise carbohydrate intake, most credible sources recommended 1.0 to 4.5 g of carbohydrate per kg of body weight, depending on the type of food and the time of the exercise or event.)
- Relatively low in fat and fiber to minimize gastrointestinal distress and facilitate **gastric emptying**
- Moderate in protein
- Approximately 400 to 800 calories—an amount that should fuel the exercise without causing noticeable sluggishness or fullness
- Well-tolerated by the individual

Fueling during Exercise

The goal of during-exercise fueling is to provide the body with the essential nutrients needed by muscle cells and to maintain optimal blood glucose levels. During a prolonged endurance effort, such as a marathon, an athlete is at risk of "hitting the wall"—a phenomenon often occurring around mile 20 of a marathon. This is when extreme fatigue sets in due to depleted carbohydrate stores. However, there are gradations on the physical demands of exercise based on the duration of the exercise session. Exercise lasting less than one hour can be adequately fueled with existing glucose and glycogen stores. No additional carbohydrate-containing drinks or foods are necessary. When exercise lasts longer than one hour, blood glucose levels begin to dwindle. After one to three hours of continuous moderate-intensity exercise (65 to 80% $\dot{V}O_2max$), muscle glycogen stores may become depleted. If no glucose is consumed, the blood glucose levels drop, resulting in further depletion of muscle and liver glycogen stores. When this happens, regardless of the athlete's mental toughness or desire to maintain intensity, performance falters. To maintain a ready energy supply during a prolonged, moderate-to-vigorous, continuous exercise session (>60 minutes), athletes should consume glucose-containing beverages and snacks. Athletes should consume 30 to 60 grams of carbohydrate per hour of training (Rodriguez, Di Marco, & Langley, 2009). This is especially important for prolonged exercise and exercise in extreme heat, cold, or high altitude; for athletes who did not consume adequate amounts of food or drink prior to the training session; and for athletes who did not carbohydrate load or who restricted energy intake for weight loss.

Carbohydrate consumption during prolonged exercise should begin shortly after the initiation of the exercise. The carbohydrates will be more effective if the 30 to 60 grams per hour are consumed in small amounts in 15- to 20-minute intervals rather than as a large **bolus** after two hours of exercise (Rodriguez, Di Marco, & Langley, 2009). Some experts believe that adding protein to carbohydrate during exercise will help to improve performance, but the evidence is inconclusive.

Post-exercise Replenishment

The main goal of post-exercise fueling is to replenish glycogen stores and facilitate muscle repair. The average client training at moderate intensities every few days does not need any aggressive post-exercise replenishment. Normal dietary practices following exercise will facilitate recovery within 24 to 48 hours, but athletes following vigorous training regimens, especially those who will participate in multiple training sessions in a single day (e.g., triathletes or athletes participating in training camp for a team sport), will benefit from strategic refueling. Studies show that the best post-workout meals include mostly carbohydrates accompanied by some protein (Kreider et al., 2010). Refueling should begin within 30 minutes after exercise and be followed by a high-carbohydrate meal within two hours (Kreider et al., 2010). The carbohydrates replenish the used-up energy that is normally stored as glycogen in muscle and liver. The protein helps to rebuild the muscles that were fatigued with exercise. A carbohydrate intake of 1.5 g/kg of body weight in the first 30 minutes after exercise and then every two hours for four to six hours is recommended (Rodriguez, Di Marco, & Langley, 2009). After that, the athlete can resume their typical, balanced diet. Of course, the amount of refueling necessary depends on the intensity and duration of the training session. A long-duration, low-intensity workout may not require such vigorous replenishment.

> **APPLY WHAT YOU KNOW**
>
> **POST-WORKOUT SNACK AND MEAL IDEAS**
>
> In the several hours following a prolonged and strenuous workout, consuming snacks and meals high in carbohydrate with some protein can set the stage for optimal glycogen replenishment and subsequent performance. Here are a few snack and meal ideas that fit the bill:
>
> **Snack 1:** In the first several minutes after exercise, consume 16 oz of Gatorade or other sports drink, a power gel such as a Clif Shot or GU, and a medium banana. This quickly begins to replenish muscle carbohydrate stores. *Carbohydrates: 73 g; Protein: 1 g; Calories: 296*
>
> **Snack 2:** After cooling down and showering, grab another quick snack such as 12 oz of orange juice and 1/4 cup of raisins. *Carbohydrates: 70 g; Protein 3 g; Calories: 292*
>
> **Small meal appetizer:** Enjoy a spinach salad with tomatoes, chickpeas, green beans, and tuna and a whole-grain baguette. *Carbohydrates: 70 g; Protein: 37 g; Calories: 428*
>
> **Small meal main course:** Replenish with whole-grain pasta with diced tomatoes. *Carbohydrates: 67 g; Protein: 2 g; Calories: 276*
>
> **Dessert:** After allowing ample time for the day's snacks and meals to digest, finish your refueling program with 1 cup of frozen yogurt and berries. *Carbohydrates: 61 g; Protein: 8 g; Calories: 276*

FLUID AND HYDRATION BEFORE, DURING, AND AFTER EXERCISE

When it comes to fluid balance during exercise, it seems like the proverbial double-edged sword: Drinking too little can lead to **dehydration**—a scary condition exercisers have been cautioned against in every text, handout, and presentation on fluid replacement. However, drinking too much plain water—out of fear of not drinking enough—could lead to **hyponatremia** (i.e., low sodium in the blood), a condition less well known and understood, but equally frightening. Here is the good news: the body is very good at handling and normalizing large variations in fluid intake. For this reason, severe hyponatremia and dehydration are rare and generally affect very specific high-risk populations during specific types of activities [i.e., anyone exercising at a low to moderate intensity for an extended period of time (generally four hours or more) while consuming too much water may be at risk]. Both conditions are highly preventable. To prevent dehydration and hyponatremia, the goal is to drink just the right amount of fluid and/or **electrolytes** before, during, and after exercise to maintain a state of **euhydration,** which is a state of "normal" body water content—the perfect balance between "too much" and "not enough" fluid intake (Table 4).

TABLE 4
FLUID REPLACEMENT RECOMMENDATIONS BEFORE, DURING, AND AFTER EXERCISE

	Fluid	Comments
Before Exercise	• Drink 5–7 mL/kg (0.08–0.11 oz/lb) at least 4 hours before exercise (12–17 ounces for a 154-lb individual)	• If urine is not produced or is very dark, drink another 3–5 mL/kg (0.05–0.08 oz/lb) two hours before exercise. • Sodium-containing beverages or salted snacks will help retain fluid.
During Exercise	• Monitor individual body-weight changes during exercise to estimate sweat loss. • Composition of fluid should include 20–30 mEq/L of sodium, 2–5 mEq/L of potassium, and 5–10% of carbohydrate.	• Prevent a >2% loss in body weight. • Amount and rate of fluid replacement depends on individual sweating rate, environment, and exercise duration.
After Exercise	• Consumption of normal meals and beverages will restore euhydration. • If rapid recovery is needed, drink 1.5 L/kg (23 oz/lb) of body weight lost.	• Goal is to fully replace fluid and electrolyte deficits. • Consuming sodium will help recovery by stimulating thirst and fluid retention.

Reprinted with permission from American College of Sports Medicine (2022). *ACSM's Guidelines for Exercise Testing and Prescription* (11th ed.). Philadelphia: Wolters Kluwer.

Hydration before Exercise

Most people begin exercise euhydrated with little need for a rigorous prehydration regimen. However, if fewer than eight to 12 hours have elapsed since the last intense training session or fluid intake has been inadequate, the individual may benefit from a prehydration program. Some clients may try to hyperhydrate with glycerol-containing solutions that act to expand the extra- and intra-cellular spaces. While glycerol may be advantageous for certain individuals who meet specific criteria, glycerol is unlikely to be advantageous for those who will experience no to mild dehydration during exercise (loss of <2% body weight) and glycerol use may in fact contribute to increased risk of hyponatremia (van Rosendal et al., 2010).

Hydration during Exercise

The goal of fluid intake during exercise is to prevent performance-diminishing or health-altering effects from dehydration or hyponatremia. A CMES can share the following guidelines with clients:

- **Aim for a 1:1 fluid replacement to fluid loss ratio:** Ideally, exercisers should consume the same amount of fluid as they lose in sweat. An easy way to assess post-exercise hydration is to compare pre- and post-exercise body weight. The goal is to avoid weight loss greater than 2%. There is no one-size-fits-all recommendation, though if determining individual needs is not feasible, clients should aim to drink 0.4 to 0.8 L/h (8 to 16 oz/h), with the higher rate for faster, heavier individuals in a hot and humid environment and the lower rate for slower, lighter individuals in a cool environment (Sawka et al., 2007). Because people sweat at varying rates and exercise at different intensities, this range may not be appropriate for everyone. However, when individual assessment is not possible, this recommendation works for most people.
- **Drink fluids with sodium during prolonged exercise sessions:** If an exercise session lasts longer than two hours or a client is participating in an event that stimulates heavy sweat

(and consequently, sodium) losses, then the client should consider consuming a sports drink that contains elevated levels of sodium. In one study, researchers did not find a benefit from sports drinks that contain only the 18 mmol/L (or 100 milligrams per 8 oz) of sodium typical of most sports drinks and thus concluded that higher levels would be needed to prevent hyponatremia during prolonged exercise (Almond et al., 2005). Table 5 presents the sodium content of some popular drinks. The IOM recommends that people exercising for prolonged periods in hot environments consume sports drinks that contain 20 to 30 mEq/L (0.5 to 0.7 g/L) of sodium to stimulate thirst and replace sweat losses and 2 to 5 mEq/L (0.8 to 2.0 g/L) of potassium to replace sweat losses (Rodriguez, Di Marco, & Langley, 2009). Alternatively, exercisers can consume extra sodium with meals and snacks prior to a lengthy exercise session or a day of extensive physical activity. Additional sodium or supplementation with salt tablets seems to be unnecessary based on the limited research on this topic (Hew-Butler et al., 2006; Speedy et al., 2002).

- **Drink carbohydrate-containing sports drinks to reduce fatigue:** Individuals exercising for longer than one hour should also consume carbohydrate with fluids. With prolonged exercise, muscle glycogen stores become depleted and blood glucose becomes a primary fuel source. To maintain performance levels and prevent fatigue, individuals should choose drinks and snacks that provide about 30 to 60 grams of rapidly absorbed carbohydrate for every hour of training. As long as the carbohydrate concentration is about 6 to 8%, it will have little effect on gastric emptying (Rodriguez, Di Marco, & Langley, 2009).

Sports drinks play an important role in replenishing fluids, glucose, and sodium lost during moderate-to-vigorous exercise lasting more than one hour. Although sports drinks may not completely protect against hyponatremia, they serve an important purpose in endurance exercise. Table 5 provides nutritional information for some of the most popular sports drinks.

TABLE 5
EVALUATING SPORTS DRINKS

Beverage	Serving Size (oz)	Calories (kcal)	Sodium (mg)	Carbohydrate (g)	Carbohydrate Concentration (%)	Sugars (g)
Gatorade Thirst Quencher	12	80	160	22	6.2%	21
Gatorade Endurance formula	12	90	300	22	6.2%	13
Pedialyte*	12	35	370	9	2.5%	9
Powerade	12	78	150	21	5.9%	20.4
Propel	12	0	162	0	0%	0
Ultima	12	0	59	0	0%	0
Zico Coconut Water	12	36	50	8	2.2%	6.4

*Although Pedialyte is not marketed as a sports drink, it is sometimes used by athletes as such.

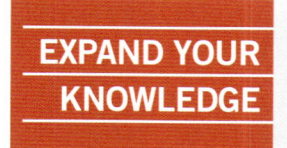

EXPAND YOUR KNOWLEDGE

ENDURANCE TRAINING AND HYDRATION STATUS

Past headlines shared the unlikely but real tragedy of the 28-year-old novice Boston Marathon runner who suffered severe hyponatremia and later died en route to the hospital, as well as the story of the 24-year-old elite runner who collapsed from dehydration while exploring desolate trails in the Grand Canyon's summer heat without sufficient water. In all, a scattering of half marathon and marathon deaths have drawn attention to the safety concerns of these endurance challenges.

Nutrition for Health and Fitness

Underlying heart conditions, dehydration, and hyponatremia most often are the causes of death during races in young athletes. Sadly, it turns out that not many runners are paying serious attention to hydration. In one study, a whopping 65% of the athletes studied were "not at all" concerned about keeping themselves hydrated (Brown et al., 2011). This nonchalance can come at a cost. Drinking too little can lead to dehydration, which results from a sweat rate that exceeds fluid replenishment. Exercising at very high intensities, exercising in humid conditions, and low fluid intake all increase the likelihood of dehydration. Dehydration, along with high exercise intensity, hot and humid environmental conditions, poor fitness level, incomplete heat **acclimatization,** and a variety of other factors can all raise body temperature and together lead to heat stroke.

While dehydration is a serious concern, individuals should also be aware that drinking too much—out of fear of not drinking enough—could lead to hyponatremia, a less well-known and less understood but equally frightening condition characterized by a low blood sodium level. Exertional hyponatremia results from excessive intake of low-sodium fluids during prolonged endurance activities—that is, drinking a greater volume of fluid than the volume lost in sweat—and possibly, to a lesser extent, from inappropriate fluid retention.

A study of 488 Boston Marathon runners published in the *New England Journal of Medicine* found that 13% (22% of women and 8% of men) had hyponatremia, and 0.6% had critical hyponatremia, at the end of the race. Runners with hyponatremia were more likely to be of low **body mass index,** consume fluids at every mile (and more than 3 liters total throughout the race), finish the race in more than four hours, and gain weight during the run. The greatest predictor of hyponatremia was weight gain, which researchers attributed to excessive fluid intake (Almond et al., 2005). Importantly, hyponatremia is not limited to runners. Anyone exercising at a low to moderate intensity for an extended period of time (generally four hours or more) while consuming too much water can be at risk.

MYTH: DRINKING FLUIDS BEFORE AND DURING EXERCISE CAUSES GASTROINTESTINAL DISTRESS

Rationale: Since blood flow is diverted away from the gastrointestinal system during exercise, fluids consumed before or during exercise will just sit around sloshing in the stomach during the workout.

The science: It is true that gastric emptying, or the speed with which the stomach empties its contents into the **small intestine,** slows down during exercise. This is largely because exercise-induced sympathetic stimulation diverts blood flow from the gastrointestinal (GI) system to the heart, lungs, and working muscles. As a result, individuals sometimes experience stomach cramps along with a variety of other uncomfortable GI issues such as reflux, heartburn, bloating, gas, nausea, and vomiting. It turns out, though, that good hydration with the right fluids can help increase gastric emptying and lead to reduced GI problems with exercise. Gastric emptying is maximized when the amount of fluid in the stomach is high. On the other hand, high-intensity exercise (>80% $\dot{V}O_2max$), dehydration, hyperthermia, and consumption of high-energy (>8% carbohydrate), **hypertonic** drinks (like juices and some soft drinks) slow gastric emptying.

A CMES can recommend the following practical tips to prepare the gut for exercise or competition (Brouns & Beckers, 1993):

- Get acclimatized to heat.
- Stay hydrated.
- Practice drinking during training to improve competition-day comfort.
- Avoid eating too much before and during exercise.
- Avoid high-energy, hypertonic food and drinks before (within 30 to 60 minutes) and after exercise. Limit protein and fat intake before exercise.
- Ingest a high-energy, high-carbohydrate diet.
- Avoid high-fiber foods before exercise.
- Limit nonsteroidal anti-inflammatory drugs (NSAIDs) such as ibuprofen and naproxen, alcohol, caffeine antibiotics, and nutritional supplements before and during exercise, as they can cause GI discomfort. The client should experiment during training to identify their triggers.
- Urinate and defecate prior to exercise.
- Consult a physician if GI problems persist, especially abdominal pain, diarrhea, or bloody stool.

EXPAND YOUR KNOWLEDGE

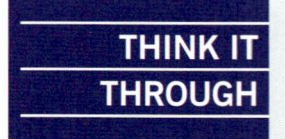

> **THINK IT THROUGH**
>
> **HYDRATION DURING ENDURANCE EXERCISE**
> Individuals who perform extended endurance activities, such as those lasting an hour or longer, can benefit from drinking fluids containing sodium and carbohydrate. What would you say to a client who wants to know the best approach for hydration during a prolonged endurance running event?

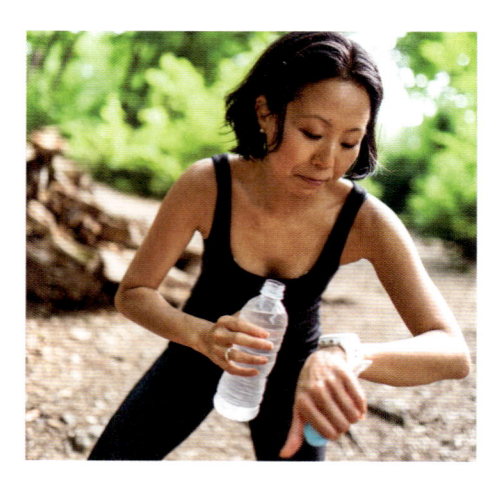

Post-exercise Hydration

Following exercise, the client should aim to correct any fluid imbalances that occurred during the exercise session. This includes consuming water to restore hydration, carbohydrates to replenish glycogen stores, and electrolytes to speed rehydration. If the client will have at least 12 hours to recover before the next strenuous workout, rehydration with the usual meals and snacks and water should be adequate. The sodium in the foods will help retain the fluid and stimulate thirst. If rehydration needs to occur quickly, the clients should drink about 1.5 L of fluid for each kilogram (or 0.70 L of fluid for each pound) of body weight lost (Sawka et al., 2007). This will be enough to restore lost fluid and also compensate for increased urine output that occurs with rapid consumption of large amounts of fluid. A severely dehydrated athlete (>7% body weight loss) with symptoms (nausea, vomiting, or diarrhea) may need intravenous fluid replacement and should seek medical attention immediately. Those at greatest risk of hyponatremia should be careful not to consume too much water following exercise and instead should focus on replenishing sodium.

NUTRITIONAL SUPPLEMENTS

The Dietary Supplement and Health Education Act (DSHEA) dictates supplement production, marketing, and safety guidelines. The following are the highlights of the legislation. A CMES and their clients must be aware that savvy product manufacturers and marketing experts have found ingenious ways to get around some of the rules.

- A dietary supplement is defined as a product (other than tobacco) that functions to supplement the diet and contains one or more of the following ingredients: a vitamin, mineral, herb or other botanical, **amino acid,** a nutritional substance that increases total dietary intake, metabolite, constituent, or extract, or some combination of these ingredients.
- Safety standards provide that the Secretary of the Department of Health & Human Services may declare that a supplement poses imminent risk or hazard to public safety. A supplement is considered **adulterated** if it, or one of its ingredients, presents a "significant or unreasonable risk of illness or injury" when used as directed, or under normal conditions. It may also be considered adulterated if too little information is known about the risk of an unstudied ingredient.
- Supplement labels cannot include claims that the product diagnoses, prevents, mitigates, treats, or cures a specific disease. Instead, they may describe the supplement's effects on the "structure or function" of the body or the "well-being" achieved by consuming the substance. Unlike other health claims, these nutritional support statements are not approved by FDA prior to marketing the supplement.
- Supplements must contain an ingredient label, including the name and quantity of each dietary ingredient. The label must also identify the product as a "dietary supplement" (FDA, 1995).

Many clients experiment with various herbs and supplements. The websites of the FDA (www.fda.gov) and the National Institutes of Health Office of Dietary Supplements (www.ods.od.nih.gov) provide reputable, up-to-date information about numerous supplements and herbs that a CMES can reference. If a client is also on medications, there is risk for drug-supplement interactions, and it is important to recommend that the client disclose and discuss this with a doctor, pharmacist, or highly qualified RD.

The CMES should endeavor to provide clients with evidence-based educational resources on the effectiveness of various nutritional supplements. This will ensure clients are able to make informed decisions and fully understand how consumption of these products will impact their health, performance, and training. The CMES should take a conservative approach to discussing supplements, always being mindful of their scope of practice.

A critical issue that must be initially addressed pertaining to nutritional supplements is safety. In the scientific literature, when no side effects have been reported, this has been interpreted to mean that the nutritional supplement in question is safe for the length of time and dosages evaluated (Kerksick et al., 2018). Nutritional supplements found to have sound theoretical rationale with the majority of available research in relevant populations using appropriate dosing regimens demonstrating their safety are placed into the category of "strong evidence to support efficacy and apparently safe" (Kerksick et al., 2018).

Nutritional Supplements with Strong Evidence to Support Efficacy and Apparent Safety

Creatine

It has been suggested that the most effective supplement available to fitness enthusiasts to increase high-intensity exercise performance and muscle mass is creatine monohydrate (Kerksick et al., 2018). Indeed, there is a mountain of scientific literature demonstrating that creatine supplementation increases skeletal muscle mass during exercise training. Moreover, the long-term safety of creatine monohydrate has been well-established. Creatine is an essential substrate for the **phosphagen energy system** and involved in **adenosine triphosphate (ATP)** regeneration during high-intensity exercise. As such, creatine supplementation has also been shown to result in an enhanced ability to match cellular ATP production and demand during high-intensity and repeated bouts of intense exercise. Creatine supplementation can increase creatine storage in skeletal muscle with a loading phase (20 to 25 grams/day for five to seven days), followed by a maintenance dose of 3 to 5 grams/day.

Caffeine

Caffeine is a natural stimulant found in coffee, tea, and also many nutritional supplements. There is robust scientific evidence demonstrating that caffeine ingestion serves as effective **ergogenic** aid for **aerobic** and **anaerobic** exercise performance. Caffeine ingested orally is quickly absorbed into the bloodstream and peaks within 30 to 60 minutes. Caffeine mechanistically effects the **central nervous system,** primarily by antagonism of adenosine receptors, which results in enhanced mood, reduced perception of pain, and increased attention. At the skeletal muscle level, caffeine ingestion promotes enhanced sodium/potassium pump activity, greater calcium release from the **sarcoplasmic reticulum,** and increased **fat oxidation/glycogen sparing**. Overall, it has been recommended that a dosage of ~3 to 6 mg/kg of body weight of caffeine ingested 30 to 60 minutes prior to exercise will increase work capacity, time to exhaustion, and reduced perceived effort during endurance exercise (Naderi et al., 2016).

Post-exercise Carbohydrate Ingestion

This is a classic nutritional recommendation for recreational enthusiasts and athletes alike. After prolonged and exhaustive endurance-related exercise, the most important factor determining the timeframe to recovery is muscle glycogen replenishment (Ivy, 2004). It has been well established for quite some time that post-exercise carbohydrate ingestion is critical to synthesis of muscle glycogen. More recently, both the precise timing of carbohydrate ingestion and optimal carbohydrate dosage have become better understood (Beelen et al., 2010). Post-exercise muscle glycogen replenishment occurs in two phases—a rapid rate that persists for 30 to 60 minutes after exercise cessation and a considerably reduced rate (60 to 90%) in the time period afterward. There is also evidence for a dose-response relationship between post-exercise dosage of carbohydrate ingestion and the rate of muscle glycogen resynthesis. For example, it has been shown that administration of 1.2 grams/kg/hour of carbohydrate increased muscle glycogen content 150% more than 0.8 grams/kg/hour. However, ingestion of 1.6 grams/kg/hour provided no further increase in muscle glycogen content. Importantly, eating carbohydrates in smaller amounts over time is more effective at restoring muscle glycogen than eating one or two larger amounts less frequently. In summary, to optimize muscle glycogen repletion post-exercise, it has been recommended to ingest 1.2 grams/kg/hour of carbohydrate at 15- to 30-minute intervals immediately upon exercise termination (Beelen et al., 2010).

Protein Supplementation

Many people use protein supplements to boost protein intake and ensure consumption of a particular protein type or amino acid. To aid in efficient **digestion** and **absorption,** most protein supplements are sold as **hydrolysates,** which are short amino-acid chains of partially digested protein. **Whey** and **casein** tend to be the most popular.

Whey, the liquid remaining after milk has been curdled and strained, is a high-quality protein that contains all of the **essential amino acids.** There are three varieties of whey—whey protein powder, whey protein concentrate, and whey protein isolate—all of which provide high levels of the essential and **branched-chain amino acids (BCAAs),** vitamins, and minerals. Whey powder is 11 to 15% protein and is used as an additive in many food products. Whey concentrate is 25 to 89% protein, while whey isolate is 90+% protein; both forms are commonly used in supplements. Notably, while the isolate is nearly pure whey, the proteins can become denatured during the manufacturing process, decreasing the supplements' usefulness. Unlike the other whey forms, the isolate is lactose-free (Hoffman & Falvo, 2004). Studies of whey protein have found that whey offers numerous health benefits, including increased muscle **hypertrophy** and muscular strength (when combined with muscular training) and bone growth (Hayes & Cribb, 2008).

Casein, the source of the white color of milk, accounts for 70 to 80% of milk protein. Casein exists in what is known as a **micelle,** a compound similar to a soap sud that has a water-averse inside and water-loving outside. This property allows the protein to provide a sustained slow release of amino acids into the bloodstream, sometimes lasting for hours. Some studies suggest that combined supplementation with casein and whey offers the greatest muscular strength improvements following a 10-week intensive muscular-training program (Kerksick et al., 2006).

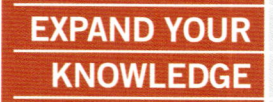

EXPAND YOUR KNOWLEDGE

IS THERE A NEED FOR PROTEIN SUPPLEMENTATION?

Supplemental protein use is a common practice among both recreational exercisers and athletes striving to enhance gains in strength and muscle mass following workouts and is often a controversial topic (Morton et al., 2018). Many Americans consume more protein than the current recommendations for protein intake call for, which includes an AMDR of 10 to 35% for adults 19 and older (USDA, 2020) and an RDA of 0.8 g/kg/day (IOM, 2006). The needs for athletes are 1.2 to 2.0 g/kg/day (Academy of Nutrition and Dietetics, American College of Sports Medicine, and Dietitians of Canada, 2016), with specific needs for optimal adaptation being based on experience level, nutrient needs, athletic goals, and training and competition timing within a periodized program.

So, is supplemental protein needed? According to a systematic review of 49 studies presented by Morton et al. (2018), protein supplementation may augment resistance-training adaptations. The following observations about protein supplementation were made:

- Supplementation augments increases in **one-repetition maximum (1-RM)** strength and **fat-free mass (FFM).**
- Supplementation is more effective in resistance-trained individuals compared to novices but is less effective with increasing chronological age.
- The benefits do not increase with intakes above 1.6 g/kg/day.
- The current RDA may not be enough to maximize strength and FFM with resistance training.
- Resistance training alone is the more important stimulus, and timing of intake plays a minor, if any, role in influencing gains.

Sodium Bicarbonate

It is well known that recovery from **cellular acidosis** is paramount in order to restore the capacity to regenerate ATP from both the phosphagen system and **glycolysis.** Muscle **buffering capacity** can be augmented by nutritional strategies. Indeed, alkalizing agents have been studied extensively for their potential to enhance performance by attenuating the extent to which metabolic acidosis contributes to fatigue during high-intensity exercise performance (Peart et al., 2012). One such alkalizing substance that has been found to improve recovery by increasing the muscle buffering capacity is sodium bicarbonate. The mechanism by which sodium bicarbonate ingestion mediates an ergogenic effect is by promoting removal of protons from the **skeletal muscle milieu.** Given the fact that increased concentrations of proton molecules within the muscle cell are detrimental to skeletal muscle performance, it should be recognized that an increased rate of removal from the skeletal muscle environment will result in a more rapid recovery. This in turn will permit a better performance of subsequent high-intensity exercise bouts.

The main drawback to using sodium bicarbonate is that some individuals experience gastrointestinal distress with its ingestion. Accordingly, it has been recommended to first purposefully experiment with the sodium bicarbonate–loading protocols to maximize the alkalizing effects and minimize the risk of potential symptoms. The recommended dosage and timeframe for sodium bicarbonate ingestion is 0.2 to 0.4 grams/kg with 1 liter of fluids at 60 to 120 minutes pre-exercise (Peart et al., 2012). Sodium bicarbonate can be ingested either in capsule form or in a flavored beverage.

β-alanine

The amino acid -alanineis naturally occurring and found in foods such as fish and meat. β-alanine is also a precursor and rate-limiting molecule for synthesis of carnosine. Carnosine itself is found in skeletal muscle and has numerous important physiological functions, including calcium, **enzyme,** and pH regulation. Therefore, β-alanine supplementation has been heavily studied given its potential mechanistic ergogenic benefits. The case for β-alanine supplementation appears to be quite clear. In a meta-analysis, it was reported that performance of high-intensity exercise lasting between 60 and 240 seconds benefited from β-alanine supplementation (Hobson et al., 2012). In terms of the most efficacious dosage, 3 to 6 grams per day of β-alanine for a duration of four to 10 weeks has been recommended (Naderi et al., 2016). Beyond that timeframe, a maintenance dosage of 1.2 grams per day of β-alanine has been suggested (Naderi et al., 2016).

Nutritional Supplements with Little to No Evidence to Support Efficacy and/or Apparent Safety

A myth can be defined as an untrue explanation for a natural phenomenon. Unfortunately, numerous myths remain pervasive and well-engrained throughout the fitness industry, in particular as it pertains to various nutritional supplements. In this section are a list of nutritional supplements with little to no evidence to support efficacy and/or safety.

Glutamine

Glutamine is an amino acid that is used in the biosynthesis of proteins. It was originally suggested that glutamine supplementation might simulate protein synthesis and thereby promote enhanced muscular performance. However, more recent research has found glutamine supplementation does not benefit muscular performance and, therefore, it has been concluded that there is insufficient scientific evidence to support glutamine supplementation for increases in **lean body mass** and/or muscular performance (Kerksick et al., 2018).

Arginine

Arginine is an amino acid that is used in the biosynthesis of proteins. In the body, arginine changes into the potent **vasodilator** nitric oxide. Given that nitric oxide is known to promote

vasodilation and enhance skeletal muscle blood flow, it has been suggested that arginine supplementation may increase exercise performance (Alvares et al., 2011). However, the majority of the other published scientific literature regarding arginine supplementation have not reported a beneficial ergogenic result (Kerksick et al., 2018).

Carnitine

Carnitine is an ammonium compound produced by the liver and kidneys. It serves as a transporter of long-chain fatty acids into the **mitochondria** to be oxidized for energy production and therefore plays a key role in the regulation of **lipid** metabolism. Accordingly, both scientists and sport nutritionists alike have entertained the notion that supplementation could increase the **bioavailability** of carnitine and enhance overall capacity for lipid metabolism. Nevertheless, to date, the majority of research findings on carnitine supplementation reports it does not significantly alter total muscle carnitine content, enhance lipid metabolism, improve exercise performance, and/or elicit weight loss in individuals with overweight or obesity (Kerksick et al., 2018).

Chronic Use of Antioxidants

It has been conventional wisdom that antioxidant supplementation may benefit exercise performance by countering the increase in **free radicals** associated with exercise because of the long- and well-established link between cell damage and free radicals. Several key studies (Teixeira et al., 2009; Gomez-Cabrera et al., 2008; Close et al., 2006) questioned the effectiveness of the antioxidant supplementation strategy altogether, as it has been demonstrated that antioxidant supplementation hampers favorable exercise training adaptations and interferes with the recovery process.

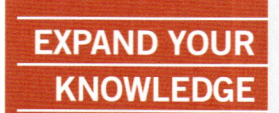

EXPAND YOUR KNOWLEDGE

SUPPLEMENT LABELS

The FDA does not closely regulate dietary supplements and provides no guarantee that the nutrients and ingredients contained in a supplement label are actually what exists in the product. However, the FDA does have some rules for supplement labeling.

When it comes to supplements, the nutrition label is referred to as a Supplement Fact panel. Items that must be listed in the Supplement Fact panel include:
- Names and quantities of dietary ingredients, serving size, and servings per container
- Total calories, total fat, saturated fat, added sugars, cholesterol, sodium, total carbohydrate, dietary fiber, sugars, protein, vitamin D, potassium, calcium, and iron when present in measurable amounts
- Any vitamin, mineral, or other nutrient added to the product for the purpose of supplementation, or if a claim is made about them
- Percent daily values for all ingredients for which the FDA has established daily values (except for protein and when supplements are intended for children less than four years of age)

In addition to the Supplement Fact panel, supplement packaging must include the name of the dietary supplement, the amount of the supplement, the ingredient list, and the name and location of the manufacturer, packer, or distributor.

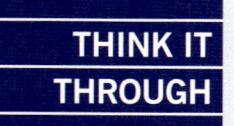

THINK IT THROUGH

DISCUSSING SUPPLEMENTS WITH CLIENTS

Recommending supplements to clients is outside of the CMES's scope of practice. However, a CMES should be prepared to discuss information about the safety and efficacy of supplements, as well as supplement regulation, as can be found within trusted resources and in the public domain. When discussing supplements with clients, it is critical that the information provided does not come across as an endorsement and that a referral is made to a qualified medical professional or RD when considering supplements. How would you respond to a client asking for specific supplement recommendations without advising or endorsing, while making a referral at the same time?

SUMMARY

An individual's health is greatly influenced by the foods they consume. While each nutrient plays a specific role in the body's well-being, it is the balance among these different nutrients that allows for most optimal functioning and prevention of chronic diseases. The *Dietary Guidelines* emphasize a movement away from a focus on specific nutrients toward an overall healthy dietary pattern. The CMES is ideally positioned to not only support and spread this message, but also to use the nutrition tools and tips to empower clients to translate recommendations into real and practical nutrition changes. Ultimately, by having a firm understanding of the *Dietary Guidelines* and its associated tools, a CMES can incorporate nutrition education based upon these resources into their work while simultaneously staying within scope of practice and safely maximizing impact.

REFERENCES

Academy of Nutrition and Dietetics, Dietitians of Canada, and American College of Sports Medicine (2016). Position of the Academy of Nutrition and Dietetics, Dietitians of Canada, and the American College of Sports Medicine: Nutrition and athletic performance. *Journal of the Academy of Nutrition and Dietetics,* 116, 3, 501–528.

Almond, L. et al. (2005). Hyponatremia among runners in the Boston Marathon. *New England Journal of Medicine,* 352, 15, 1550–1556.

Alvares, T.S. et al. (2011). L-arginine as a potential ergogenic aid in healthy subjects. *Sports Medicine,* 41, 233–248.

American College of Sports Medicine (2022). *ACSM's Guidelines for Exercise Testing and Prescription* (11th ed.). Philadelphia: Wolters Kluwer.

Beelen, M. et al. (2010). Nutritional strategies to promote postexercise recovery. *International Journal of Sport Nutrition and Exercise Metabolism,* 20, 515–532.

Brouns, F. & Beckers, E. (1993). Is the gut an athletic organ? Digestion, absorption and exercise. *Sports Medicine,* 15, 242–257.

Brown, S. et al. (2011). Lack of awareness of fluid needs among participants at a midwest marathon. *Sports Health A Multidisciplinary Approach,* 3, 5, 451–454.

Centers for Disease Control and Prevention (2011). *CDC Estimates of Foodborne Illness in the United States.* www.cdc.gov/foodborneburden/PDFs/FACTSHEET_A_FINDINGS_updated4-13.pdf

Close, G.L. et al. (2006). Ascorbic acid supplementation does not attenuate post-exercise muscle soreness following muscle-damaging exercise but may delay the recovery process. *The British Journal of Nutrition,* 95, 976–981.

Coleman-Jensen, A. et al. (2018). *Household Food Security in the United States in 2018.* https://www.ers.usda.gov/webdocs/publications/90023/err256_summary.pdf?v=0

Eckel R.H. et al. (2014). 2013 AHA/ACC guideline on lifestyle management to reduce cardiovascular risk: A report of the American College of Cardiology/American Heart Association Task Force on Practice Guidelines. *Journal of the American College of Cardiology,* 63, 25 Pt B, 2960–2984.

Fayh, A.P.T. et al. (2013). Effects of 5% weight loss through diet or diet plus exercise on cardiovascular parameters of obese: A randomized clinical trial. *European Journal of Nutrition,* 52, 1443–1450.

Food and Nutrition Board (2012). *Front-of-Package Nutrition Rating Systems and Symbols: Promoting Healthier Choices.* Washington, D.C.: National Academies Press.

Food and Nutrition Board (2010). *Examination of Front-of-Package Nutrition Rating Systems and Symbols: Phase 1 Report.* Washington, D.C.: National Academies Press.

Gomez-Cabrera, M.C. et al. (2008). Oral administration of vitamin C decreases muscle mitochondrial biogenesis and hampers training-induced adaptations in endurance performance. *The American Journal of Clinical Nutrition,* 87, 142–149.

Hall, K.D. et al. (2011). Quantification of the effect of energy imbalance on bodyweight. *The Lancet,* 378, 9793, 826–837.

Hayes, A. & Cribb, P.J. (2008). Effect of whey protein isolate on strength, body composition, and muscle hypertrophy during resistance training. *Current Opinions in Clinical Nutrition and Metabolic Care,* 11, 40–44.

Hew-Butler, T.D. et al. (2006). Sodium supplementation is not required to maintain serum sodium concentrations during an Ironman triathlon. *British Journal of Sports Medicine,* 40, 3, 255–259.

Hobson, R.M. et al. (2012). Effects of β-alanine supplementation on exercise performance: A metaanalysis. *Amino Acids,* 43, 25–37.

Hoffman, J.R. & Falvo, M.J. (2004). Protein: Which is best? *Journal of Sports Science and Medicine,* 3, 118–130.

Institute of Medicine (2006). *Dietary Reference Intakes: The Essential Guide to Nutrient Requirements.* Washington, D.C.: National Academies Press.

Ivy, J.L. (2004). Regulation of muscle glycogen repletion, muscle protein synthesis and repair following exercise. *Journal of Sports Science and Medicine,* 3, 131–138.

Kerksick, C.M. et al. (2018). ISSN exercise & sports nutrition review update: Research & recommendations. *Journal of the International Society of Sports Nutrition,* 15, 38.

Kerksick, C.M. et al. (2006). The effects of protein and amino acid supplementation on performance and training adaptations during ten weeks of resistance training. *Journal of Strength and Conditioning Research,* 20, 3, 643–653.

Kreider, R.B. et al. (2010). ISSN exercise & sport nutrition review: Research & recommendations. *Journal of the International Society of Sports Nutrition,* 7, 7.

Morton, R.W. et al. (2018). A systematic review, meta-analysis and meta-regression of the effect of protein supplementation on resistance training-induced gains in muscle mass and strength in healthy adults. *British Journal of Sports Medicine,* 52, 376–384.

Naderi, A. et al. (2016). Timing, optimal dose and intake duration of dietary supplements with evidence-based use in sports nutrition. *Journal of Exercise Nutrition & Biochemistry,* 20, 1–12.

Nikolaus, C.J. et al. (2016). Grocery store (or supermarket) tours as an effective nutrition education medium: A systematic review. *Journal of Nutrition, Education and Behavior,* 48, 8, 544–554.e1.

Peart, D.J. et al. (2012). Practical recommendations for coaches and athletes: A meta-analysis of sodium bicarbonate use for athletic performance. *Journal of Strength and Conditioning Research,* 26, 1975–1983.

Roberts, B., Povich, D., & Mather, M. (2012). *The Working Poor Family Project, Policy Brief: Low-Income Working Families: The Growing Economic Gap.* http://www.workingpoorfamilies.org/wpcontent/uploads/2013/01/Winter-2012_2013-WPFP-Data-Brief.pdf

Rodriguez, N.R., Di Marco, N.M., & Langley, S. (2009). American College of Sports Medicine position stand: Nutrition and athletic performance. *Medicine & Science in Sports & Exercise,* 41, 709–731.

Sallis, J.F. & N. Owen. (2015). Ecological models of health behavior. In: Glanz, K. (Ed.) *Health Behavior: Theory, Research, and Practice* (5th ed.). Hoboken, N.J.: John Wiley & Sons.

Sawka, M.N. et al. (2007). American College of Sports Medicine position stand: Exercise and fluid replacement. *Medicine & Science in Sports & Exercise,* 39, 2, 377–390.

Speedy, D.B. et al. (2002). Oral salt supplementation during ultradistance exercise. *Clinical Journal of Sport Medicine,* 12, 5, 279–284.

Teixeira, V.H. et al. (2009). Antioxidants do not prevent post-exercise peroxidation and may delay muscle recovery. *Medicine & Science in Sports & Exercise,* 41, 1752–1760.

U.S. Department of Agriculture (2020). *2020-2025 Dietary Guidelines for Americans* (9th ed.) www.dietaryguidelines.gov

U.S. Department of Health & Human Services (2018). *Physical Activity Guidelines for Americans* (2nd ed.). www.health.gov/paguidelines/

U.S. Food & Drug Administration (2004). *How to Understand and Use the Nutrition Facts Label.* www.fda.gov/Food/IngredientsPackagingLabeling/LabelingNutrition/ucm274593.htm#calories

U.S. Food and Drug Administration (1995). *Dietary Supplement Health and Education Act of 1994.* https://ods.od.nih.gov/About/DSHEA_Wording.aspx

van Rosendal, S.P. et al. (2010). Guidelines for glycerol use in hyperhydration and rehydration associated with exercise. *Sports Medicine,* 40, 2, 113–129.

SUGGESTED READING

U.S. Department of Agriculture (2020). *2020-2025 Dietary Guidelines for Americans* (9th ed.) www.dietaryguidelines.gov

GLOSSARY

A1GDM Gestational diabetes mellitus that is controlled with only diet and exercise.

A2GDM Gestational diabetes mellitus that requires medication to achieve euglycemia.

Abdominal bracing A mild contraction of the abdominal wall.

Abdominal fat *See* Visceral obesity.

Abdominal hollowing A movement that involves the "sucking in" of the abdomen to activate the transverse abdominis.

Abduction Movement away from the midline of the body.

Absorption The uptake of nutrients across a tissue or membrane by the gastrointestinal tract.

Acceptable Macronutrient Distribution Range (AMDR) The range of intake for a particular energy source that is associated with reduced risk of chronic disease while providing intakes of essential nutrients.

Acclimatization Physiological adaptation to an unfamiliar environment and achievement of a new steady state. For example, the body can adjust to a high altitude or a hot climate and gain an increased capacity to work in those conditions.

Achilles tendinopathy A term used to describe two characteristics of Achilles tendon injury—inflammation and tendinosis (microtears in the tissue and around the tendon caused by overuse).

Actin Thin contractile protein in a myofibril.

Action The stage of the transtheoretical model of behavioral change during which the individual is actively engaging in a behavior that was started less than six months ago.

Activities of daily living (ADL) Activities normally performed for hygiene, bathing, household chores, walking, shopping, and similar activities.

Acute Descriptive of a condition that usually has a rapid onset and a relatively short and severe course; opposite of chronic.

Acute coronary syndrome A sudden, severe coronary event that mimics a heart attack, such as unstable angina.

Adduction Movement toward the midline of the body.

Adenosine trisphosphate (ATP) A high-energy phosphate molecule required to provide energy for cellular function. Produced both aerobically and anaerobically and stored in the body.

Adequate Intake (AI) A recommended nutrient intake level that, based on research, appears to be sufficient for good health.

Adherence The extent to which people follow their plans or treatment recommendations. Exercise adherence is the extent to which people follow an exercise program.

Adipocyte A fat cell.

Adiponectin A hormone related to energy metabolism regulation that facilitates the action of insulin by sending blood glucose into the body's cells for storage or use as fuel, thus increasing the cells' insulin sensitivity or glucose metabolism.

Adipose tissue Fatty tissue; connective tissue made up of fat cells.

Adiposity The state of being fat; fatness; obesity.

Adulterated A supplement is considered adulterated if it, or one of its ingredients, presents a "significant or unreasonable risk of illness or injury" when used as directed, or under normal circumstances.

Aerobic In the presence of oxygen.

Aerobic power *See* $\dot{V}O_2$max.

Afferent nervous system The portion of the somatic nervous system that carries impulses from receptors to the central nervous system.

Affirmation A statement of intended results spoken or written in the first person, present tense; offer of emotional support or encouragement.

Agatston score A test to detect calcification within the coronary arteries. The amount of calcification can give, to some extent, an indication of the overall amount of atherosclerosis.

Agility The ability to rapidly and accurately change the position of the body in space; a skill-related component of physical fitness.

Agonist The muscle directly responsible for observed movement; also called the prime mover.

Aldosterone One of two main hormones released by the adrenal cortex; plays a role in limiting sodium excretion in the urine.

Allergen A substance that can cause an allergic reaction by stimulating type-1 hypersensitivity in genetically susceptible individuals.

Allograft A transplant in which transplanted tissue is sourced from a genetically non-identical member of the same species.

Alzheimer's disease An age-related, progressive disease characterized by death of nerve cells in the brain leading to a loss of cognitive function; the cause of the nerve cell death is unknown.

Amenorrhea The absence of menstruation.

Amino acids Nitrogen-containing compounds that are the building blocks of protein.

Anabolic Muscle-building effects.

Anaerobic Without the presence of oxygen.

Anaerobic glycolysis The metabolic pathway that uses glucose for energy production without requiring oxygen. Sometimes referred to as the lactic acid system or anaerobic glucose system, it produces lactic acid as a by-product.

Android Adipose tissue or body fat distributed in the abdominal area (apple-shaped individuals).

Angina A common symptom of coronary artery disease characterized by chest pain, tightness, or radiating pain resulting from a lack of blood flow to the heart muscle.

Angina pectoris Chest pain caused by an inadequate supply of oxygen and decreased blood flow to the heart muscle; an early sign of coronary artery disease. Symptoms may include pain or discomfort, heaviness, tightness, pressure or burning, numbness, aching, and tingling in the chest, back, neck, throat, jaw, or arms; also called angina.

Anginal threshold The point at which angina symptoms occur.

Annulus fibrosus The outer ring of intervertebral discs.

Anorexia *See* Anorexia nervosa.

Anorexia nervosa (AN) An eating disorder characterized by a restriction of energy intake relative to requirements leading to a significant low body weight in the context of age, sex, developmental trajectory, and physical health; intense fear of gaining weight or becoming fat; and body-image disturbances, including a disproportionate influence of body weight on self-evaluation.

Antagonist The muscle that acts in opposition to the contraction produced by an agonist (prime mover) muscle.

Antecedents Variables or factors that precede and influence a client's exercise participation, including the decision to not exercise as planned.

Anterior Anatomical term meaning toward the front. Same as ventral; opposite of posterior.

Anterior cruciate ligament (ACL) A primary stabilizing ligament of the knee that travels from the medial border of the lateral femoral condyle to its point of insertion anterolaterally to the medial tibial spine.

Anterior shin splints Pain in the anterior compartment muscles of the lower leg, fascia, and periosteal lining. Often induced by exertional or sudden changes in activity.

Anteversion Pelvic position characterized by the ASIS (anterior superior iliac spine) being forward of the pubic symphysis.

Anthropometric Pertaining to the measurement of the human body and its parts, most commonly performed using skinfolds, girth measurements, and body weight.

Antioxidant A substance that prevents or repairs oxidative damage; includes vitamins C and E, some carotenoids, selenium, ubiquinones, and bioflavonoids.

Anxiety A state of uneasiness and apprehension; occurs in some mental disorders.

Aortic aneurysm A general term for any swelling of the aorta, usually representing an underlying weakness in the wall of the aorta at that location.

Apolipoprotein A protein that binds to insoluble lipids to form the soluble lipoproteins, such as high-density lipoprotein (HDL) and low-density lipoprotein (LDL), that transport triglycerides and cholesterol within the body.

Apoptosis The programmed cell death or the deliberate suicide of a cell in a multicellular organism for the greater good of the whole individual.

Arrhythmia A disturbance in the rate or rhythm of the heartbeat. Some can be symptoms of serious heart disease; may not be of medical significance until symptoms appear.

Artery A blood vessel that carries oxygenated blood away from the heart to vital organs and the extremities.

Arthroscopy A minimally invasive surgical procedure in which an examination and sometimes treatment of damage of the interior of a joint is performed using an arthroscope, a type of endoscope that is inserted into the joint through a small incision.

Arthrokinematics The general term for the specific movements of joint surfaces, such as rolling or gliding.

Arthrokinetics The study of joint movement.

Arthroplasty A surgery to repair, reposition, replace, or remove parts in an arthritic joint.

Arthrosis A degenerative disease of a joint.

Articular cartilage Cartilage covering the ends of the bones inside diarthroidial joints; allows the ends of the bones to glide without friction.

Articulation A joint.

Asthma A chronic inflammatory disorder of the airways that affects genetically susceptible individuals in response to various environmental triggers such as allergens, viral infection, exercise, cold, and stress.

Asthma exacerbation An episode of progressively worsening shortness of breath, cough, wheezing, and/or chest tightness that results in decreases in expiratory airflow; also called "asthma attack."

Ataxia Failure of muscular coordination; irregularity of muscular action.

Atherogenesis Formation of atheromatous deposits, especially on the innermost layer of arterial walls.

Atherogenic Tending to promote the formation of fatty plaques in the arteries.

Atherogenic dyslipidemia Formation of atheromatous deposits, especially on the innermost layer of arterial walls due to an abnormal concentration of lipids or lipoproteins in the blood.

Atheroma A deposit or degenerative accumulation of lipid-containing plaques on the innermost layer of the wall of an artery.

Atherosclerosis A specific form of arteriosclerosis characterized by the accumulation of fatty material on the inner walls of the arteries, causing them to harden, thicken, and lose elasticity.

Atherosclerotic cardiovascular disease (ASCVD) A specific form of arteriosclerosis in which an artery wall thickens as a result of invasion and accumulation of white blood cells (WBCs).

Atopy Allergic hypersensitivity.

Atrioventricular node (AV node) The specialized mass of conducting cells in the heart located at the atrioventricular junction.

Atrophy A reduction in muscle size (muscle wasting) due to inactivity or immobilization.

Auscultation Listening to the internal sounds of the body (such as the heartbeat), usually using a stethoscope.

Autogenic inhibition An automatic reflex relaxation caused by stimulation of the Golgi tendon organ (GTO).

Automated external defibrillator (AED) A portable electronic device used to restore normal heart rhythms in victims of sudden cardiac arrest.

Autonomic nervous system The part of the nervous system that regulates involuntary body functions, including the activity of the cardiac muscle, smooth muscles, and glands. It has two divisions: the sympathetic nervous system and the parasympathetic nervous system.

Autonomic neuropathy A disease of the nonvoluntary, non-sensory nervous system (i.e., the autonomic nervous system) affecting mostly the internal organs such as the bladder muscles, the cardiovascular system, the digestive tract, and the genital organs.

Autonomous motivation Engaging in an activity out of free will and the desire to do so.

Avascular necrosis A disease resulting from the temporary or permanent loss of the blood supply to the bones.

Axis of rotation The imaginary line or point about which an object, such as a joint, rotates.

Balance The ability to maintain the body's position over its base of support within stability limits, both statically and dynamically.

Bariatrics The branch of medicine that deals with the causes, prevention, and treatment of obesity.

Baroreceptor A sensory nerve ending that is stimulated by changes in pressure, as those in the walls of blood vessels.

Basal metabolic rate (BMR) The energy required to complete the sum total of life-sustaining processes, including ion transport (40% BMR), protein synthesis (20% BMR), and daily functioning such as breathing, circulation, and nutrient processing (40% BMR).

Base of support (BOS) The areas of contact between the feet and their supporting surface and the area between the feet.

Beta cell Endocrine cells in the islets of Langerhans of the pancreas responsible for synthesizing and secreting the hormone insulin, which lowers the glucose levels in the blood.

Beta receptors Receptors believed to exist on nerve cell membranes of the sympathetic nervous system in order to explain the specificity of certain agents that affect only some sympathetic activities (such as vasodilation and increased heart beat).

Bicipital tendinitis An inflammation of one of the tendons that attach the muscle (biceps) on the front of the upper arm bone (humerus) to the shoulder joint.

Bioavailability The degree to which a substance can be absorbed and efficiently utilized by the body.

GLOSSARY

Bioelectrical impedance analysis (BIA) A body-composition assessment technique that measures the amount of impedance, or resistance, to electric current flow as it passes through the body. Impedance is greatest in fat tissue, while fat-free mass, which contains 70–75% water, allows the electrical current to pass much more easily.

Biotensegrity An area of biological study that looks at the tensional integrity of an anatomical structure.

Blood pressure (BP) The pressure exerted by the blood on the walls of the arteries; measured in millimeters of mercury (mmHg) with a sphygmomanometer.

Body composition The makeup of the body in terms of the relative percentage of fat-free mass and body fat.

Body dysmorphism A type of chronic mental illness in which the afflicted person cannot stop thinking about a flaw in his or her appearance—a flaw that is either minor or imagined.

Body-fat percentage The proportion of body composition representing the relative percentage of body fat. Calculated by dividing the fat mass by the total body mass, then multiplying by 100.

Body mass index (BMI) A relative measure of body height to body weight used to determine levels of weight, from underweight to extreme obesity.

Bolus A food and saliva digestive mix that is swallowed and then moved through the digestive tract.

Bone mineral density (BMD) A measure of the amount of minerals (mainly calcium) contained in a certain volume of bone.

Bone modeling An overall gain in bone mineral that occurs when the rate of bone formation is faster than the rate of bone resorption.

Bone remodeling A locally coordinated activity of osteoclasts and osteoblasts whereby bone can both prevent and repair damage caused by everyday loading. A key feature of remodeling is that it replaces damaged tissue with an equal amount of new bone tissue.

Bradycardia Slowness of the heartbeat, as evidenced by a pulse rate of less than 60 beats per minute.

Branched-chain amino acid (BCAA) An essential amino acid that inhibits muscle protein breakdown and aids in muscle glycogen storage. The BCAAs are valine, leucine, and isoleucine.

Bronchioles The smallest tubes that supply air to the alveoli (air sacs) of the lungs.

Bronchitis Acute or chronic inflammation of the bronchial tubes. *See* Chronic obstructive pulmonary disease (COPD).

Bronchospasm Abnormal contraction of the smooth muscle of the bronchi, resulting in an acute narrowing and obstruction of the respiratory airway.

Buffering capacity The ability of muscles to neutralize proton accumulation during high-intensity exercise, thus delaying the onset of acidosis.

Bursa A sac of fluid that is present in areas of the body that are potential sites of friction.

Bursitis Swelling and inflammation in the bursa that results from overuse.

Calcitonin A hormone that acts to reduce blood calcium (Ca++), opposing the effects of parathyroid hormone (PTH).

Calorie A measurement of the amount of energy in a food available after digestion. The amount of energy needed to increase 1 kilogram of water by 1 degree Celsius. Also called a kilocalorie.

Capsule An anatomical term that refers to a cover or envelope partly or wholly surrounding a structure.

Carbohydrate The body's preferred energy source. Dietary sources include sugars (simple) and grains, rice, potatoes, and beans (complex). Carbohydrate is stored as glycogen in the muscles and liver and is transported in the blood as glucose.

Carbohydrate loading Up to a week-long regimen of manipulating intensity of training and carbohydrate intake to achieve maximal glycogen storage for an endurance event.

Cardiac autonomic neuropathy (CAN) A disease of the non-voluntary, non-sensory cardiovascular system commonly seen in persons with longstanding diabetes mellitus type 1 and 2.

Cardiac output The amount of blood pumped by the heart per minute; usually expressed in liters of blood per minute

Cardiometabolic risk The identification of factors that increase the likelihood of CVD onset. Managing these risk factors can help a person avoid diabetes and heart disease.

Cardiopulmonary resuscitation (CPR) A procedure to support and maintain breathing and circulation for a person who has stopped breathing (respiratory arrest) and/or whose heart has stopped (cardiac arrest).

Cardiovascular disease (CVD) A general term for any disease of the heart, blood vessels, or circulation.

Cardiovascular drift Changes in observed cardiovascular variables that occur during prolonged, submaximal exercise without a change in workload.

Carioca A footwork agility drill in which the participant moves laterally by crossing one foot behind the other; resembles a Brazilian traditional dance.

Carpal tunnel syndrome (CTS) A pathology of the wrist and hand that occurs when the median nerve, which extends from the forearm into the hand, becomes compressed at the wrist.

Catabolism Metabolic pathways that break down molecules into smaller units and release energy.

Catecholamine Hormone (e.g., epinephrine or norepinephrine) released as part of the sympathetic response to exercise.

Cellular acidosis A decrease in muscle pH (below 7) caused by the accumulation of protons in a muscle cell. These protons come from the splitting of adenosine triphosphate (ATP) into adenosine diphosphate (ADP) and inorganic phosphate. Each time this splitting takes place, one hydrogen ion (proton) is released.

Center of gravity (COG) The point around which all weight is evenly distributed; also called center of mass.

Center of mass (COM) *See* Center of gravity (COG).

Central nervous system (CNS) The brain and spinal cord.

Cerebral palsy An umbrella term encompassing a group of non-progressive, noncontagious conditions that cause physical disability in human development.

Cerebral vascular disease A group of brain dysfunctions related to disease of the blood vessels supplying the brain.

Cesarean birth Delivery of a baby through incisions made in the mother's abdomen and uterus.

Chemoprophylaxis The use of drugs, nutritional supplements, or other natural substances to prevent future disease.

Cholesterol A fatlike substance found in the blood and body tissues and in certain foods. Can accumulate in the arteries and lead to a narrowing of the vessels (atherosclerosis).

Chronic Descriptive of a condition that persists over a long period of time; opposite of acute.

Chronic disease Any disease state that persists over an extended period of time.

Chronic obstructive pulmonary disease (COPD) A condition, such as asthma, bronchitis, or emphysema, in which there is chronic obstruction of air flow.

Chronotropic incompetence An inability to appropriately increase heart rate. Can be genetically acquired or pathologic.

Circumduction A biplanar movement involving the sequential combination of flexion, abduction, extension, and adduction.

Cirrhosis A disease of the liver in which normal cells in the liver are replaced by scar tissue. This condition results in the failure of the liver to perform many of its usual functions.

Claudication Cramplike pains in the calves caused by poor circulation of blood to the leg muscles; frequently associated with peripheral vascular disease.

Clinical lipidology A multidisciplinary branch of medicine focusing on lipid and lipoprotein metabolism and their associated disorders.

Closed-ended question A question format that limits respondents with a short list of answer choices such as "yes" or "no."

Co-contraction The mutual coordination of antagonist muscles (such as flexors and extensors) to maintain a position.

Coefficient of friction The ratio of the force that maintains contact between an object and a surface and the frictional force that resists the motion of the object.

Cognitive restructuring Intentionally changing the way one perceives or thinks about something.

Comorbidities Disorders (or diseases) in addition to a primary disease or disorder.

Complex carbohydrate A long chain of sugar that takes more time to digest than a simple carbohydrate.

Compression fracture A collapse of a vertebra due to trauma or due to a weakened vertebra in a person with osteoporosis.

Compressive force A force squashing, squeezing, or pressing down on an object.

Computed tomography (CT) A development of x-ray technology to examine the soft tissues of the body. Involves recording "slices" of the body with a CT scanner. A cross-sectional image is then formed by computer integration.

Concentric A type of isotonic muscle contraction in which the muscle develops tension and shortens when stimulated.

Congestive heart failure (CHF) Inability of the heart to pump blood at a sufficient rate to meet the metabolic demand or the ability to do so only when the cardiac filling pressures are abnormally high, frequently resulting in lung congestion.

Connective tissue The tissue that binds together and supports various structures of the body. Ligaments and tendons are connective tissues.

Contemplation The stage of the transtheoretical model of behavioral change during which the individual is weighing the pros and cons of behavioral change.

Contractile proteins The protein myofilaments that are essential for muscle contraction.

Contractility The ability of muscle tissue (cardiac or skeletal) to contract when stimulated.

Contralateral The opposite side of the body; the other limb.

Controlled motivation Doing a task with a sense of pressure, demand, or coercion.

Coordination The ability to process and execute appropriate actions or motor responses with proper sequence (timing) and magnitude to produce smooth, flowing movement; a skill-related component of physical fitness.

Coronary angiography A medical imaging technique in which an x-ray picture is taken to visualize the inner opening of the coronary arteries.

Coronary artery bypass grafting (CABG) A procedure in which veins are harvested from a patient's leg and sewn from the aorta to the coronary artery past the blockage.

Coronary artery disease (CAD) *See* Coronary heart disease (CHD).

Coronary heart disease (CHD) The major form of cardiovascular disease; results when the coronary arteries are narrowed or occluded, most commonly by atherosclerotic deposits of fibrous and fatty tissue; also called coronary artery disease (CAD).

Corporation A legal entity, independent of its owners and regulated by state laws; any number of people may own a corporation through shares issued by the business.

Cortical bone Compact, dense bone that is found in the shafts of long bones and the vertebral endplates.

Corticosteroid One of two main hormones released by the adrenal cortex; plays a major role in maintaining blood glucose during prolonged exercise by promoting protein and triglyceride breakdown.

Cortisol A hormone that is often referred to as the "stress hormone," as it is involved in the response to stress. It increases blood pressure and blood glucose levels and has an immunosuppressive action.

Cosmesis The preservation or restoration of physical beauty, particularly of the human body.

Crepitus A crackling sound produced by air moving in the joint space; also called crepitation.

Cross-training A method of physical training in which a variety of exercises and changes in body positions or modes of exercise are utilized to positively affect compliance and motivation, and also stimulate additional strength gains or reduce injury risk.

Cryotherapy Treatment of a disorder with ice or by freezing.

Cyanosis A bluish discoloration, especially of the skin and mucous membranes, due to reduced hemoglobin in the blood.

Cytokines Hormone-like low molecular weight proteins, secreted by many different cell types, which regulate the intensity and duration of immune responses and are involved in cell-to-cell communication.

DASH eating plan *See* Dietary Approaches to Stop Hypertension eating plan.

De Quervain's syndrome A pathology of the hand that affects the two tendons that move the thumb away from the hand.

Decisional balance One of the four components of the transtheoretical model of behavioral change; refers to the numbers of pros and cons an individual perceives regarding adopting and/or maintaining an activity program.

Deep vein thrombosis A blood clot in a major vein, usually in the legs and/or pelvis.

Degenerative joint disease A non-infectious, progressive disorder of the weight-bearing joints. The majority of degenerative joint disease is the result of mechanical instabilities or aging-related changes within the joint.

Dehydration The process of losing body water; when severe can cause serious, life-threatening consequences.

Delayed-onset muscle soreness (DOMS) Soreness that occurs 24 to 48 hours after strenuous exercise, the exact cause of which is unknown.

Depression 1. The action of lowering a muscle or bone or movement in an inferior or downward direction. 2. A condition of general emotional dejection and withdrawal; sadness greater and more prolonged than that warranted by any objective reason.

GLOSSARY

Diabetes See Diabetes mellitus.

Diabetes mellitus A disease of carbohydrate metabolism in which an absolute or relative deficiency of insulin results in an inability to metabolize carbohydrates normally.

Diabetic ketoacidosis (DKA) A feature of uncontrolled diabetes mellitus characterized by a combination of ketosis (the accumulation of substances called ketone bodies in the blood) and acidosis (increased acidity of the blood). Symptoms include slow, deep breathing with a fruity odor to the breath; confusion; frequent urination; poor appetite; and eventually loss of consciousness.

Diaphoresis Profuse sweating.

Diastasis recti A separation of the recti abdominal muscles along the midline of the body.

Diastolic blood pressure (DBP) The pressure in the arteries during the relaxation phase (diastole) of the cardiac cycle; indicative of total peripheral resistance.

Dietary Approaches to Stop Hypertension (DASH) eating plan An eating plan designed to reduce blood pressure; also serves as an overall healthy way of eating that can be adopted by nearly anyone; may also lower risk of coronary heart disease.

Dietary Reference Intake (DRI) A generic term used to refer to three types of nutrient reference values: Recommended Dietary Allowance (RDA), Estimated Average Requirement (EAR), and Tolerable Upper Intake Level (UL).

Dietary supplement A product (other than tobacco) that functions to supplement the diet and contains one or more of the following ingredients: a vitamin, mineral, herb or other botanical, amino acid, dietary substance that increases total daily intake, metabolite, constituent, extract, or some combination of these ingredients.

Dietary Supplement and Health Education Act (DSHEA) A bill passed by Congress in 1994 that sets forth regulations and guidelines for dietary supplements.

Digestion The process of breaking down food into small enough units for absorption.

Discogenic back pain Dysfunction or degeneration of lumbar intervertebral discs.

Distal Farthest from the midline of the body, or from the point of origin of a muscle.

Diuretic Medication that produces an increase in urine volume and sodium excretion.

Dorsiflexion Movement of the foot up toward the shin.

Dose-response relationship Direct association between the amount of a stimulus and the magnitude of the desired outcome (e.g., amount of physical activity and good health).

Double product Expressed as a product of heart rate in beats per minute times systolic blood pressure. Bears a close relationship with myocardial work or myocardial $\dot{V}O_2$.

Dual-energy x-ray absorptiometry (DXA) An imaging technique that uses a very low dose of radiation to measure bone density. Also can be used to measure overall body fat and regional differences in body fat. Formerly abbreviated as DEXA.

Dynamic balance The act of maintaining postural control while moving.

Dyslipidemia A condition characterized by abnormal blood lipid profiles; may include elevated cholesterol, triglyceride, or low-density lipoprotein (LDL) levels and/or low high-density lipoprotein (HDL) levels.

Dyslipoproteinemia Blood lipid disorders.

Dyspnea Shortness of breath; a subjective difficulty or distress in breathing.

Dysrhythmia A term for a group of conditions in which there is abnormal electrical activity in the heart.

Eccentric A type of isotonic muscle contraction in which the muscle lengthens against a resistance when it is stimulated; sometimes called "negative work" or "negative reps."

Ecchymosis The escape of blood into the tissues from ruptured blood vessels marked by a black-and-blue or purple discolored area.

Edema Swelling resulting from an excessive accumulation of fluid in the tissues of the body.

Electrical muscle stimulation (EMS) A technique to elicit muscle contraction by delivering electric impulses to the muscles.

Electrocardiogram (ECG) A recording of the electrical activity of the heart.

Electrolyte A mineral that exists as a charged ion in the body and that is extremely important for normal cellular function.

Elevation The action of raising a muscle or bone, or a movement in a superior or upward direction.

Empathy Understanding what another person is experiencing from his or her perspective.

Emphysema An obstructive pulmonary disease characterized by the gradual destruction of lung alveoli and the surrounding connective tissue, in addition to airway inflammation, leading to reduced ability to effectively inhale and exhale.

Employee A person who works for another person in exchange for financial compensation. An employee complies with the instructions and directions of his or her employer and reports to them on a regular basis.

Endocrine Refers to either the gland that secretes directly into the systemic circulation or the substance secreted.

Endorphin Natural opiates produced in the brain that function to reduce pain and improve mood.

Endothelium Thin, single-celled layer of epithelial cells that line the circulatory system.

Energy balance The balance between energy taken in, generally as food and drink, and energy expended through normal living and physical activity; when caloric intake equals caloric expenditure resulting in no change in body weight. A positive or negative energy balance will cause weight gain or weight loss, respectively.

Enzyme A protein that speeds up a specific chemical reaction.

Epimysium A layer of connective tissue that encloses the entire muscle and is continuous with fascia and other connective-tissue wrappings of muscle, including the endomysium and perimysium.

Epinephrine A hormone released as part of the sympathetic response to exercise; also called adrenaline.

Ergogenic Intended to enhance physical performance, stamina, or recovery.

Essential amino acids Eight to 10 of the 23 different amino acids needed to make proteins. Called essential because the body cannot manufacture them; they must be obtained from the diet.

Essential fatty acids Fatty acids that the body needs but cannot synthesize; includes linolenic (omega-3) and linoleic (omega-6) fatty acids.

Essential hypertension Hypertension without an identifiable cause; also called primary hypertension.

Estimated Average Requirement (EAR) An adequate intake in 50% of an age- and gender-specific group.

Estradiol An estrogenic hormone, $C_{18}H_{24}O_2$, produced by the ovaries and used in treating estrogen deficiency.

Estrogen Generic term for estrus-producing steroid compounds produced primarily in the ovaries; the female sex hormones.

Etiology The cause of a medical condition.

Euglycemia A normal glucose response.

Euhydration A state of "normal" body water content.

Eversion Rotation of the foot to direct the plantar surface outward; occurs in the frontal plane.

Exercise physiology The study of how the body functions during physical activity and exercise.

Exercise-induced asthma (EIA) *See* Exercise-induced bronchospasm (EIB).

Exercise-induced bronchoconstriction Transient and reversible airway narrowing triggered by vigorous exercise; also called exercise-induced asthma (EIA).

Extension The act of straightening or extending a joint, usually applied to the muscular movement of a limb.

External rotation Outward turning about the vertical axis of bone.

Extinction The removal of a positive stimulus that has in the past followed a behavior.

Extrinsic feedback Information received from an external source (such as another person) about a completed task (such as an exercise).

Extrinsic motivation Motivation that comes from external (outside of the self) rewards, such as material or social rewards.

Familial hypercholesterolemia A disorder passed down through families, which causes low-density lipoprotein (LDL) ("bad") cholesterol levels to be very high.

Familial hypertriglyceridemia A disorder passed down through families, which causes a higher-than-normal level of triglycerides in a person's blood.

Fascia Strong connective tissue that performs a number of functions, including developing and isolating the muscles of the body and providing structural support and protection.

Fascicle A bundle of skeletal muscle fibers surrounded by perimysium.

Fast-twitch muscle fiber One of several types of muscle fibers found in skeletal muscle tissue; also called type II fibers and characterized as having a low oxidative capacity but a high gylcolytic capacity; recruited for rapid, powerful movements such as jumping, throwing, and sprinting.

Fat An essential nutrient that provides energy, energy storage, insulation, and contour to the body. 1 gram of fat equals 9 kcal.

Fat-free mass (FFM) That part of the body composition that represents everything but fat—blood, bones, connective tissue, organs, and muscle; also called lean body mass.

Fat oxidation The metabolic pathway that, in the presence of oxygen, breaks down fatty acids to produce energy in the form of adenosine triphosphate (ATP).

Fatty acid A long hydrocarbon chain with an even number of carbons and varying degrees of saturation with hydrogen.

Fatty liver The collection of excessive amounts of triglycerides and other fats inside liver cells.

Feedback An internal response within a learner; during information processing, it is the correctness or incorrectness of a response that is stored in memory to be used for future reference. Also, verbal or nonverbal information about current behavior that can be used to improve future performance.

Female athlete triad A condition consisting of a combination of disordered eating, menstrual irregularities, and decreased bone mass in athletic women.

Fiber Carbohydrate chains the body cannot break down for use and which pass through the body undigested.

Fibrinolysis The breakdown of fibrin, usually by the enzymatic action of plasmin.

Fibrosis Excessive formation of fibrous connective tissue.

First ventilatory threshold (VT1) Intensity of aerobic exercise at which ventilation starts to increase in a nonlinear fashion in response to an accumulation of metabolic by-products in the blood.

Flexibility The ability to move joints through their normal full ranges of motion.

Flexion The act of moving a joint so that the two bones forming it are brought closer together.

Fluoroscopy X-ray guidance used to ensure that a medication reaches its intended destination.

Folate A B vitamin that is essential for cell growth and reproduction.

Folic acid A water-soluble, B vitamin required for breaking down complex carbohydrates into simple sugars to be used for energy; pregnant women have an increased need for folic acid, both for themselves and their child, as it is necessary for the proper growth and development of the fetus.

Forced expiratory volume in one second (FEV1) The amount of air exhaled in the first one second of maximal exhalation.

Forced vital capacity (FVC) The total amount of air that can be forcibly exhaled after a maximal inhalation.

Free fatty acid (FFA) A fatty acid that is only loosely bound to plasma proteins in the blood. Fatty acids are used by the body as a metabolic fuel. Antioxidants, such as vitamin C and vitamin E, neutralize free radicals.

Free radical A chemical group that has unshared electrons available for a reaction. Free radicals can damage the integrity of DNA and have been implicated as a cause of cancers.

Frontal plane A longitudinal section that runs at a right angle to the sagittal plane, dividing the body into anterior and posterior portions.

Fructose Fruit sugar; the sweetest of the monosaccharides; found in varying levels in different types of fruits.

Functional capacity The maximal physical performance represented by maximal oxygen uptake.

Gait The manner or style of walking.

Gastric bypass A surgical procedure that creates a very small stomach; the rest of the stomach is removed. The small intestine is attached to the new stomach, allowing the lower part of the stomach to be bypassed.

Gastric emptying The process by which food is emptied from the stomach into the small intestines.

Gastroesophageal reflux disease (GERD) A chronic condition in which the lower esophageal sphincter allows gastric acids to reflux into the esophagus, causing heartburn, acid indigestion, and possible injury to the esophageal lining.

General partnership A type of business arrangement in which each partner assumes management responsibility and unlimited liability and must have at least a 1% interest in profit and loss.

Gestational diabetes mellitus (GDM) An inability to maintain normal glucose, or any degree of glucose intolerance, during pregnancy, despite being treated with either diet or insulin.

Ghrelin A hormone produced in the stomach that is responsible for stimulating appetite.

Glucagon A hormone released from the alpha cells of the pancreas when blood glucose levels are low; stimulates glucose release from the liver to increase blood glucose. Also releases free fatty acids from adipose tissue to be used as fuel.

Glucose A simple sugar; the form in which all carbohydrates are used as the body's principal energy source.

Glycemic index (GI) A ranking of carbohydrates on a scale from 0 to 100 according to the extent to which they raise blood sugar levels.

Glycemic load (GL) A measure of glycemic response to a food that takes into serving size consideration; GL = Glycemic index x Grams of carbohydrate/100.

Glycerol A precursor for synthesis of triacylglycerols and of phospholipids in the liver and adipose tissue.

Glycogen The chief carbohydrate storage material; formed by the liver and stored in the liver and muscle.

Glycogen sparing The use of non-carbohydrates as a source of energy during exercise so that the depletion of muscle glycogen stores is delayed. If fat, for example, makes a greater contribution to an athlete's efforts during the initial stages of a race, more glycogen will be available for the later stages and muscle fatigue will be delayed.

Glycolysis The breakdown of glucose or of its storage form glycogen.

Glycosuria An excretion of glucose in the urine.

Glycosylated hemoglobin (A1c) A form of hemoglobin used primarily to identify the plasma glucose concentration over prolonged periods of time.

Golgi tendon organ (GTO) A sensory organ within a tendon that, when stimulated, causes an inhibition of the entire muscle group to protect against too much force.

Gout A disorder of purine metabolism, occurring especially in men, characterized by a raised but variable blood uric acid level and severe recurrent acute arthritis of sudden onset, resulting from deposition of crystals of sodium urate in connective tissues and articular cartilage.

Ground reaction force The force exerted by the ground on a body in contact with it.

Growth hormone A hormone secreted by the pituitary gland that facilitates protein synthesis in the body.

Gynoid Adipose tissue or body fat distributed on the hips and in the lower body (pear-shaped individuals).

Hatha yoga A yoga system of physical exercises and breathing control.

Health belief model A model to explain health-related behaviors that suggests that an individual's decision to adopt healthy behaviors is based largely upon his or her perception of susceptibility to an illness and the probable severity of the illness. The person's view of the benefits and costs of the change also are considered.

Health claim A statement that describes a relationship between a food or food component and the prevention or treatment of a disease or health-related condition.

Health Insurance Portability and Accountability Act (HIPAA) Enacted by the U.S. Congress in 1996, HIPAA requires the U.S. Department of Health and Human Services (HHS) to establish national standards for electronic health care information to facilitate efficient and secure exchange of private health data. The Standards for Privacy of Individually Identifiable Health Information ("Privacy Rule"), issued by the HHS, addresses the use and disclosure of individuals' health information—called "protected health information"—by providing federal protections and giving patients an array of rights with respect to personal health information while permitting the disclosure of information needed for patient care and other important purposes.

Healthy Mediterranean-Style Dietary Pattern One of three USDA Food Patterns featured in the *Dietary Guidelines for Americans*; modified from the Healthy U.S.-Style Dietary Pattern to more closely reflect dietary patterns that have been associated with positive health outcomes in studies of Mediterranean-style diets.

Healthy U.S.-Style Dietary Pattern One of three USDA Food Patterns featured in the *Dietary Guidelines for Americans;* based on the types and proportions of foods Americans typically consume, but in nutrient-dense forms and appropriate amounts.

Healthy Vegetarian Dietary Pattern One of three USDA Food Patterns featured in the *Dietary*

Guidelines for Americans; modified from the Healthy U.S.-Style Dietary Pattern to more closely reflect dietary patterns reported by self-identified vegetarians.

Heart attack A sudden and sometimes fatal occurrence of coronary thrombosis, typically resulting in the death of part of a heart muscle due to a blockage of blood flow to the area.

Heart failure (HF) A condition in which the heart cannot adequately pump enough blood to the rest of the body.

Heart rate (HR) The number of heart beats per minute.

Heart-rate reserve (HRR) The reserve capacity of the heart; the difference between maximal heart rate and resting heart rate. It reflects the heart's ability to increase the rate of beating and cardiac output above resting level to maximal intensity.

Hemiarthroplasty Partial hip replacement.

Hemodynamic Pertaining to the forces involved in the circulation of blood (e.g., heart rate, stroke volume, cardiac output).

Herniated disc Rupture of the outer layers of fibers that surround the gelatinous portion of the disc.

High-density lipoprotein (HDL) A lipoprotein that carries excess cholesterol from the arteries to the liver.

High-intensity interval training (HIIT) An exercise strategy alternating periods of short, intense anaerobic exercise with less-intense recovery periods.

Homeostasis An internal state of physiological balance.

Homocysteine A normal by-product of metabolism that can promote development of heart disease.

Hormone A chemical substance produced and released by an endocrine gland and transported through the blood to a target organ.

Hydrolysates A product of hydrolysis, in which water reacts with a compound to produce other compounds.

Hydrostatic weighing Weighing a person fully submerged in water. The difference between the person's mass in air and in water is used to calculate body density, which can be used to estimate the proportion of fat in the body.

Hydrotherapy The use of exercises in a pool as part of treatment for physical ailments.

Hypercalcemia An abnormally high level of calcium in the blood, usually more than 10.5 milligrams per deciliter of blood.

Hypercapnia A condition marked by an unusually high concentration of carbon dioxide in the blood as a result of hypoventilation.

Hypercholesterolemia An excess of cholesterol in the blood.

Hyperglycemia An abnormally high content of glucose (sugar) in the blood (above 100 mg/dL).

Hyperinsulinemia High blood insulin levels.

Hyperkalemia An increase in serum potassium levels.

Hyperlipidemia An excess of lipids in the blood that could be primary, as in disorders of lipid metabolism, or secondary, as in uncontrolled diabetes.

Hyperosmolar hyperglycemic nonketotic syndrome (HHNS) An emergency condition in which elevated glucose levels are accompanied by dehydration without ketones in the blood or urine.

Hyperpnea Abnormally deep or rapid breathing.

Hypertension (HTN) High blood pressure, or the elevation of resting blood pressure at or above 130/80 mmHg.

Hyperthermia Abnormally high body temperature.

Hyperthyroidism A condition characterized by hyperactivity of the thyroid gland; the metabolic processes of the body are accelerated.

Hypertonic Having extreme muscular tension.

Hypertriglyceridemia An elevated triglyceride concentration in the blood.

Hypertrophic cardiomyopathy A disease in which the heart muscle becomes abnormally thick, which makes it harder for the heart to pump blood.

Hypertrophy An increase in the cross-sectional size of a muscle in response to progressive resistance training.

Hyperuricemia An unusually high concentration of uric acid in the blood.

Hypoalphalipoproteinemia A deficiency of high-density (alpha) lipoproteins in the blood.

Hypochondriasis A mental disorder characterized by excessive fear of, or preoccupation with, a serious illness, despite medical testing and reassurance to the contrary.

Hypoglycemia A deficiency of glucose in the blood commonly caused by too much insulin, too little glucose, or too much exercise. Most commonly found in the insulin-dependent diabetic and characterized by symptoms such as fatigue, dizziness, confusion, headache, nausea, or anxiety.

Hypoinsulinemia Waning of the insulin dose.

Hyponatremia Abnormally low levels of sodium ions circulating in the blood; severe hyponatremia can lead to brain swelling and death.

Hypotension Low blood pressure.

Hypothyroidism Underactivity of the thyroid gland, leading to reduced secretion of thyroid hormones and a reduction in resting metabolic rate.

Hypoxia A condition in which there is an inadequate supply of oxygen to tissues.

Ideal body weight A term used to describe the weight that people are expected to weigh for good health, based on age, sex, and height. Also called ideal weight or desirable body weight.

IgE antibodies Often high in people with allergies, they cause the immune system to react to foreign substances such as pollen, fungus, and animal dander; found in the lungs, skin, and mucous membranes.

Iliotibial band friction syndrome (ITBFS) A repetitive overuse condition that occurs when the distal portion of the iliotibial band rubs against the lateral femoral epicondyle.

Impingement syndrome Reduction of space for the supraspinatus muscle and/or the long head of the biceps tendon to pass under the anterior edge of the acromion and coracoacromial ligament; attributed to muscle hypertrophy and inflammation caused by microtraumas.

Independent contractor A person who conducts business on his or her own on a contract basis and is not an employee of an organization.

Inferior Located below.

Inflammation A protective tissue response to injury or destruction of tissues, which serves to destroy, dilute, or wall off both the injurious agent and the injured tissues; classic signs include pain, heat, redness, swelling, and loss of function.

Informed consent A written statement signed by a client prior to testing that informs him or her of testing purposes, processes, and all potential risks and discomforts.

Infrared interactance Body-composition assessment method that involves the use of light absorption and reflection to estimate percent fat and fat-free mass; also called near-infrared interactance (NIR).

Insertion The point of attachment of a muscle to a relatively more movable or distal bone.

Instant An event in the gait cycle that designates a component of locomotion such as the heel strike of the right foot.

Insulin A hormone released from the pancreas that allows cells to take up glucose.

Insulin resistance An inability of muscle tissue to effectively use insulin, where the action of insulin is "resisted" by insulin-sensitive tissues.

Insulin-like growth factor Polypeptide structurally similar to insulin that is secreted either during fetal development or during childhood and that mediates growth hormone activity.

Insulin-like growth factor I (IGF-I) *See* Insulin-like growth factor.

Intermediate-density lipoprotein (IDL) Formed from the degradation of very low-density lipoproteins; enables fats and cholesterol to move within the bloodstream.

Intermediate-twitch muscle fiber A muscle fiber that has properties somewhere in between fast-twitch and slow-twitch muscle fibers (i.e., it shares characteristics of both).

Internal rotation A rotation of a limb in a joint toward the midline of the body.

Intrinsic feedback Feedback provided by the clients themselves; the most important type of feedback for long-term program adherence.

Intrinsic motivation Motivation that comes from internal states, such as enjoyment or personal satisfaction.

Inversion Rotation of the foot to direct the plantar surface inward; occurs in the frontal plane.

Ipsilateral On the same side of the body or limb.

Iron An essential dietary mineral necessary for the transport of oxygen (via hemoglobin in red blood cells) and for oxidation by cells; deficiency causes of anemia; found in meat, poultry, eggs, vegetables, and cereals (especially those fortified with iron).

Ischemia A decrease in the blood supply to a bodily organ, tissue, or part caused by constriction or obstruction of the blood vessels.

Ischemic heart disease A disease characterized by reduced blood supply to the heart. Also known as heart disease.

Ischemic stroke A sudden disruption of cerebral circulation in which blood supply to the brain is either interrupted or diminished.

Isokinetic A type of muscular contraction where tension developed within the muscle changes throughout the range of motion; performed with the use of special equipment; also referred to as "variable resistance" exercise.

Isometric A type of muscular contraction in which the muscle is stimulated to generate tension but little or no joint movement occurs.

Isotonic A type of muscular contraction where the muscle is stimulated to develop tension and joint movement occurs.

Joint capsule A ligamentous sac that surrounds the articular cavity of a freely movable joint.

Joint mobility The range of uninhibited movement around a joint or body segment.

Joint stability The ability to maintain or control joint movement or position.

Juvenile arthritis (JA) The most common type of arthritis in children under the age of 17. Juvenile rheumatoid arthritis causes persistent joint pain, swelling, and stiffness. Also known as juvenile idiopathic arthritis (JIA).

Kegel exercise Controlled isometric contraction and relaxation of the muscles surrounding the vagina to strengthen and gain control of the pelvic floor muscles.

GLOSSARY

Ketoacidosis Occurs when a high level of ketones (beta hydroxybutyrate, acetoacetate) are produced as a by-product of fatty-acid metabolism.

Ketone An organic compound (e.g., acetone) with a carbonyl group attached to two carbon atoms.

Ketosis An abnormal increase of ketone bodies in the body; usually the result of a low-carbohydrate diet, fasting, or starvation.

Kinematics The study of the form, pattern, or sequence of movement without regard for the forces that may produce that motion.

Kinesthesia Awareness of movement.

Kinetic chain The concept that compares the body and its extremities being linked together by a series of joints to a chain. Movement at each segment affects all links in the chain.

Kinetics The branch of mechanics that describes the effects of forces on the body.

Korotkoff sounds Five different sounds created by the pulsing of the blood through the brachial artery; proper distinction of the sounds is necessary to determine blood pressure.

Kyphosis Excessive posterior curvature of the spine, typically seen in the thoracic region.

Labrum Fibrocartilage that helps to increase the stability of the shoulder joint.

Lactate threshold (LT) The point during exercise of increasing intensity at which blood lactate begins to accumulate above resting levels, where lactate clearance is no longer able to keep up with lactate production.

Lactic acid A metabolic by-product of anaerobic glycolysis; when it accumulates it decreases blood pH, which slows down enzyme activity and ultimately causes fatigue.

Lactose A disaccharide; the principal sugar found in milk.

Laminectomy Surgical removal of the posterior arch of a vertebra.

Lapses The expected slips or mistakes that are usually discreet events and are a normal part of the behavior-change process.

Latent Weak and inactive (e.g., muscles).

Lateral epicondylitis An injury resulting from the repetitive overloading of the wrist and finger extensors that originate at the lateral epicondyle; often referred to as "tennis elbow."

Laxity Lacking in strength, firmness, or resilience; joints that have been injured or overstretched may exhibit laxity.

Lean body mass (LBM) The components of the body (apart from fat), including muscles, bones, nervous tissue, skin, blood, and organs.

Learned helplessness A psychological state in which people have come to believe that they are helpless in, or have no power or control over, certain situations.

Leptin A hormone released from fat cells that acts on the hypothalamus to regulate energy intake. Low leptin levels stimulate hunger and subsequent fat consumption.

Leukocytes White blood cells.

Liability insurance Insurance for bodily injury or property damage resulting from general negligence.

Ligament A strong, fibrous tissue that connects one bone to another.

Ligand A molecule that binds to another chemical entity to form a larger complex.

Limited liability company (LLC) A company that limits investors' personal financial and legal liabilities but provides flow-through taxation for investors. It is not limited to a certain number of shareholders and owners do not have to be U.S. citizens.

Limited partnership A hybrid organizational form, with both limited and general partners. A limited partner has no voice in management and is legally liable only for the amount of his or her capital contributions, plus any other debt obligations specifically accepted.

Limits of stability (LOS) The degree of allowable sway from the line of gravity without a need to change the base of support.

Line of gravity (LOG) A theoretical vertical line passing through the center of gravity, dissecting the body into two hemispheres.

Lipid The name for fats used in the body and bloodstream.

Lipoprotein An assembly of a lipid and protein that serves as a transport vehicle for fatty acids and cholesterol in the blood and lymph.

Locus of control The degree to which people attribute outcomes to internal factors, such as effort and ability, as opposed to external factors, such as luck or the actions of others. People who tend to attribute events and outcomes to internal factors are said to have an internal locus of control, while those who generally attribute outcomes to external factors are said to have an external locus of control.

Lordosis Excessive anterior curvature of the spine that typically occurs at the low back (may also occur at the neck).

Low-back pain (LBP) A general term to describe a multitude of back conditions, including muscular and ligament strains, sprains, and injuries. The cause of LBP is often elusive; most LBP is probably caused by muscle weakness and imbalance.

Low-density lipoprotein (LDL) A lipoprotein that transports cholesterol and triglycerides from the liver and small intestine to cells and tissues; high levels may cause atherosclerosis.

Lumen The cavity of a tubular organ or part.

Macronutrient A nutrient that is needed in large quantities for normal growth and development.

Macrosomia A condition in which a baby is abnormally large before birth.

Macrovascular disease Atherosclerotic processes affecting the large vessels of the body, including coronary, cerebral, and peripheral arteries.

Magnetic resonance imaging (MRI) A diagnostic modality in which the patient is placed within a strong magnetic field and the effect of high-frequency radio waves on water molecules within the tissues is recorded. High-speed computers are used to analyze the absorption of radio waves and create a cross-sectional image based upon the variation in tissue signal.

Maintenance The stage of the transtheoretical model of behavioral change during which the individual is incorporating the new behavior into his or her lifestyle.

Maximal heart rate (MHR) The highest heart rate a person can attain. Sometimes abbreviated as HRmax.

Medial Toward the midline of the body, or the inside.

Medial epicondylitis An injury that results from an overload of the wrist flexors and forearm pronators; often referred to as "golfers elbow."

Medial tibial stress syndrome (MTSS) Inflammation of the periosteum (connective tissue covering of the bone). Often induced by a sudden change in activity and has been associated with pes planus.

Medical nutrition therapy (MNT) Nutrition counseling provided by a registered dietitian.

Melatonin A hormone that plays a role in regulating biological rhythms, including sleep and reproductive cycles.

Meniscectomy The surgical removal of all or part of a torn meniscus.

Menisci The plural form of meniscus; cartilage disks that act as a cushion between the ends of bones

GLOSSARY

that meet in the knee joint.

Metabolic equivalent (MET) A simplified system for classifying physical activities where one MET is equal to the resting oxygen uptake, which is approximately 3.5 milliliters of oxygen per kilogram of body weight per minute (3.5 mL/kg/min).

Metabolic syndrome (MetS) A cluster of factors associated with increased risk for coronary heart disease and diabetes—abdominal obesity indicated by a waist circumference ≥40 inches (102 cm) in men and ≥35 inches (88 cm) in women; levels of triglyceride ≥150 mg/dL (1.7 mmol/L); high-density lipoprotein levels <40 and 50 mg/dL (1.0 and 1.3 mmol/L) in men and women, respectively; blood-pressure levels ≥130/85 mmHg; and fasting blood glucose levels ≥100 mg/dL (6.1 mmol/L).

Micelle An aggregate of lipid- and water-soluble compounds in which the hydrophobic portions are oriented toward the center and the hydrophilic portions are oriented outwardly.

Microalbuminemia A moderate increase in the level of urine albumin; an early sign of diabetic kidney disease.

Microdiscectomy The surgical removal of herniated disc material that presses on a nerve root or the spinal cord using a special microscope or magnifying instrument to view the disc and nerves.

Micronutrient A nutrient that is needed in small quantities for normal growth and development.

Microvascular disease Atherosclerotic processes affecting small vessels of the body, including retina and renal vessels.

Mineral An inorganic substance needed in the diet in small amounts to help regulate bodily functions.

Minute ventilation ($\dot{V}_E$) A measure of the amount of air that passes through the lungs in one minute; calculated as the tidal volume multiplied by the ventilatory rate.

Mitochondria The "power plant" of the cells where aerobic metabolism occurs.

Mobility The degree to which an articulation is allowed to move before being restricted by surrounding tissues.

Monounsaturated fat *See* Monounsaturated fatty acid.

Monounsaturated fatty acid A type of unsaturated fat (liquid at room temperature) that has one open spot on the fatty acid for the addition of a hydrogen atom (e.g., oleic acid in olive oil).

Morbidity The disease rate; the ratio of sick to well persons in a community.

Mortality The death rate; the ratio of deaths that take place to expected deaths.

Motivation The psychological drive that gives purpose and direction to behavior.

Motivational interviewing (MI) A method of questioning clients in a way that encourages them to honestly examine their beliefs and behaviors, and that motivates clients to make a decision to change a particular behavior.

Motor learning The process of acquiring and improving motor skills.

Multiple sclerosis (MS) A common neuromuscular disorder involving the progressive degeneration of muscle function, including increased muscle spasticity.

Muscular endurance The ability of a muscle or muscle group to exert force against a resistance over a sustained period of time; a health-related component of physical fitness.

Muscular fitness Having appropriate levels of both muscular strength and muscular endurance.

Muscular strength The maximal force a muscle or muscle group can exert during contraction; a health-related component of physical fitness.

Myalgia Diffuse muscular pain, often accompanied by malaise.

Myocardial infarction (MI) An episode in which some of the heart's blood supply is severely cut off or restricted, causing the heart muscle to suffer and die from lack of oxygen. Commonly known as a heart attack.

Myocardial ischemia The result of an imbalance between myocardial oxygen supply and demand, most often caused by atherosclerotic plaques that narrow and sometimes completely block the blood supply to the heart.

Myocardium Muscle of the heart.

Myofascial release A manual massage technique used to eliminate general fascial restrictions; typically performed with a device such as a foam roller.

Myofascial sling A continuous line of action formed by muscles, tendons, ligaments, fascia, joint capsules, and bones that lie in series or in parallel to actively moving joints or muscles.

Myofibril The portion of the muscle containing the thick (myosin) and thin (actin) contractile filaments; a series of sarcomeres where the repeating pattern of the contractile proteins gives the striated appearance to skeletal muscle.

Myopathy A neuromuscular disease in which the muscle fibers do not function for any one of many reasons, resulting in muscular weakness.

Myosin Thick contractile protein in a myofibril.

Myotatic stretch reflex Muscular reflex created by excessive muscle spindle stimulation to prevent potential tissue damage.

Negative energy balance A state in which the number of calories expended is greater than what is taken in, thereby contributing to weight loss.

Negative feedback loop A bodily reaction that causes a decrease in function because of some kind of stimulus.

Negative reinforcement The removal or absence of aversive stimuli following a desired behavior. This increases the likelihood that the behavior will occur again.

Nephropathy Disease of the kidneys.

Nephrotic syndrome A collection of symptoms that occur because the tiny blood vessels in the kidney become leaky, which allows protein to leave the body in large amounts.

Neuropathy Any disease affecting a peripheral nerve. It may manifest as loss of nerve function, burning pain, or numbness and tingling.

Neurotransmitter A chemical substance such as acetylcholine or dopamine that transmits nerve impulses across synapses.

Niacin A B vitamin found in meat, wheat germ, dairy products, and yeast; used to treat and prevent pellagra.

Non-exercise activity thermogenesis (NEAT) Physiological processes that produce heat; a relative newly discovered component of energy expenditure.

Non-HDL cholesterol The level of cholesterol other than high-density lipoprotein (HDL) circulating in the blood.

Nonshivering thermogenesis The cold-induced increase in heat production not associated with the muscle activity of shivering.

Nonsteroidal anti-inflammatory drug (NSAID) A drug with analgesic, antipyretic and anti-inflammatory effects. The term "nonsteroidal" is used to distinguish these drugs from steroids, which have similar actions.

Norepinephrine A hormone released as part of the sympathetic response to exercise.

Normoglycemia *See* Euglycemia.

Nuclear magnetic resonance (NMR) A spectroscopy technique that exploits the magnetic properties of certain nuclei that can provide detailed information on the topology, dynamics, and three-dimensional structure of molecules.

Nucleus pulposus The inner gel of intervertebral discs.

Nutrient A component of food needed by the body. There are six classes of nutrients: water, minerals, vitamins, fats, carbohydrates, and protein.

Nutrient content claim A statement of the implied health benefits of a product that describes the level of a nutrient in a product using terms like "free," "high," or "low," or compared to another product using terms like "more," "reduced," and "lite."

OARS model A tool used to explore a client's values; stands for Open-ended questions, Affirmations, Reflections, and Summarizing.

Obesity An excessive accumulation of body fat. Usually defined as more than 20% above ideal weight, or over 25% body fat for men and over 32% body fat for women; also can be defined as a body mass index of ≥30 kg/m^2 or a waist girth of >40 inches (102 cm) in men and >35 inches (89 cm) in women.

Omega-3 fatty acid An essential fatty acid that promotes a healthy immune system and helps protect against heart disease and other diseases; found in egg yolk and cold water fish like tuna, salmon, mackerel, cod, crab, shrimp, and oyster. Also known as linolenic acid.

Omega-6 fatty acid An essential fatty acid found in flaxseed, canola, and soybean oils and green leaves. Also known as linoleic acid.

One-repetition maximum (1-RM) The amount of resistance that can be moved through the range of motion one time before the muscle is temporarily fatigued.

Onset of blood lactate accumulation (OBLA) The point in time during high-intensity exercise at which the production of lactic acid exceeds the body's capacity to eliminate it; after this point, oxygen is insufficient at meeting the body's demands for energy.

Open-ended question A question that does not allow for a simple one-word answer (yes/no); designed to encourage a full, meaningful answer using the subject's own knowledge and/or feelings.

Operant conditioning A learning approach that considers the manner in which behaviors are influenced by their consequences.

Origin The attachment site of a tendon of a muscle attached to the relatively more fixed or proximal bone.

Orthopnea Form of dyspnea in which the person can breathe comfortably only when standing or sitting erect; associated with asthma, emphysema, and angina.

Orthostatic hypotension A drop in blood pressure associated with rising to an upright position.

Osteoarthritis (OA) A degenerative disease involving a wearing away of joint cartilage. This degenerative joint disease occurs chiefly in older persons.

Osteoblast A bone-forming cell.

Osteoclast A cell that reabsorbs or erodes bone mineral.

Osteonecrosis The destruction and death of bone tissue, which may stem from ischemia, infection, malignant neoplastic disease, or trauma.

Osteopenia Bone density that is below average, classified as 1.5 to 2.5 standard deviations below peak bone density.

Osteoporosis A disorder, primarily affecting postmenopausal women, in which bone density decreases and susceptibility to fractures increases.

Overload The principle that a physiological system subjected to above-normal stress will respond by increasing in strength or function accordingly.

Overtraining Constant intense training that does not provide adequate time for recovery; symptoms include increased resting heart rate, impaired physical performance, reduced enthusiasm and desire for training, increased incidence of injuries and illness, altered appetite, disturbed sleep patterns, and irritability.

Overtraining syndrome The result of constant intense training that does not provide adequate time for recovery; symptoms include increased resting heart rate, impaired physical performance, reduced enthusiasm and desire for training, increased incidence of injuries and illness, altered appetite, disturbed sleep patterns, and irritability.

Overweight A term to describe an excessive amount of weight for a given height, using height-to-weight ratios.

Oxidant A chemical compound that readily transfers oxygen atoms or a substance that gains electrons in an oxidation-reduction (redox) reaction.

Palpation The use of hands and/or fingers to detect anatomical structures or an arterial pulse (e.g., carotid pulse).

Palpitation A rapid and irregular heartbeat.

Pancreatitis An inflammation of the pancreas.

Parasympathetic nervous system A subdivision of the autonomic nervous system that is involved in regulating the routine functions of the body, such as heartbeat, digestion, and sleeping. Opposes the physiological effects of the sympathetic nervous system (e.g., stimulates digestive secretions, slows the heart, constricts the pupils, and dilates blood vessels).

Parathryoid hormone (PTH) A chemical substance produced by the parathyroid glands that is a major element in regulating calcium in the body.

Parasthesia An abnormal sensation such as numbness, prickling, or tingling.

Parkinson's disease (PD) A degenerative disorder of the central nervous system that often impairs the sufferer's motor skills and speech; characterized by muscle rigidity, tremor, a slowing of physical movement and, in extreme cases, a loss of physical movement.

Paroxysmal nocturnal dyspnea Attacks of severe shortness of breath and coughing that generally occur at night.

PAR-Q+ *See* Physical Activity Readiness Questionnaire for Everyone.

Pars intrarticularis The posterior aspect of the spine, where the vertebral body and posterior elements join together.

Partnership A business entity in which two or more people agree to operate a business and share profits and losses.

Patellofemoral pain syndrome (PFPS) A degenerative condition of the posterior surface of the patella, which may result from acute injury to the patella or from chronic friction between the patella and the groove in the femur through which it passes during motion of the knee.

Pathogenesis The pathologic, physiologic, or biochemical mechanism resulting in the development of a disease.

Pathomechanics Mechanical forces that are applied to a living organism and adversely change the body's structure and function.

Pathophysiology The functional changes associated with, or resulting from, disease or injury.

Peak expiratory flow (PEF) A test used to monitor asthma in which the maximal flow of exhaled air following a complete inspiration is recorded.

Peptide YY A satiety hormone that is released from the intestines.

Percent daily value (PDV) A replacement for the percent Recommended Dietary Allowance (RDA) on the newer food labels. Gives information on whether a food item has a significant amount of a particular nutrient based on a 2,000-calorie diet.

Percutaneous transluminal coronary angioplasty (PTCA) A procedure that uses a small balloon at the tip of a heart catheter to push open plaques; usually followed by the insertion of a stent.

Perfusion The passage of fluid through a tissue, such as the transport of blood through vessels from the heart to internal organs and other tissues.

Perimenopausal Related to the transitional period of time before menstruation actually stops; the time nearing menopause.

Periostitis Inflammation of the membrane of connective tissue that closely surrounds a bone.

Peripheral arterial disease All diseases caused by the obstruction of large peripheral arteries, which can result from atherosclerosis, inflammatory processes leading to stenosis, an embolism, or thrombus formation.

Peripheral nervous system (PNS) The parts of the nervous system that are outside the brain and spinal cord (central nervous system).

Peripheral neuropathy Damage to nerves of the peripheral nervous system, which may be caused either by diseases of the nerve or from the side effects of systemic illness.

Peripheral vascular disease A painful and often debilitating condition, characterized by muscular pain caused by ischemia to the working muscles. The ischemic pain is usually due to atherosclerotic blockages or arterial spasms, referred to as claudication. Also called peripheral vascular occlusive disease (PVOD).

Pes cavus High arches of the feet.

Pes planus Flat feet.

Pheochromocytoma An epinephrine-secreting tumor on the adrenal gland.

Phosphagen energy system A system of transfer of chemical energy from the breakdown of creatine phosphate to regenerate adenosine triphosphate (ATP).

Physical Activity Readiness Questionnaire for Everyone (PAR-Q+) A brief, self-administered medical questionnaire recognized as a safe pre-exercise screening measure for low-to-moderate (but not vigorous) exercise training.

Pilates A method of mind-body conditioning that combines stretching and strengthening exercises; developed by Joseph Pilates in the 1920s.

Plantar flexion Distal movement of the plantar surface of the foot; opposite of dorsiflexion.

Plaque An atherosclerotic lesion.

Plasma The liquid portion of the blood.

Plyometrics High-intensity movements, such as jumping, involving high-force loading of body weight during the landing phase of the movement that take advantage of the stretch-shortening cycle.

Polydipsia Excessive thirst.

Polyphagia Excessive appetite or eating.

Polyunsaturated fat A type of unsaturated fat (liquid at room temperature) that has two or more spots on the fatty acid available for hydrogen (e.g., corn, safflower, and soybean oils).

Polyuria Frequent urination

Posterior Toward the back or dorsal side.

Positive energy balance A situation when the storage of energy exceeds the amount expended. This state may be achieved by either consuming too many calories or by not expending enough through physical activity.

Positive feedback loop A process in which a change from the normal range of function elicits a response that amplifies or enhances that change.

Positive reinforcement The presentation of a positive stimulus following a desired behavior. This increases the likelihood that the behavior will occur again.

Posterior Toward the back or dorsal side.

Post-exercise hypotension (PEH) Acute post-exercise reduction in both systolic and diastolic blood pressure.

Postprandial dyspnea Respiratory distress and shortness of breath after a meal.

Postprandial glycemia The concentration of glucose in the blood after eating.

Postprandial lipemia The transient excess of lipids in the blood occurring after the ingestion of foods with a large content of fat; hyperlipemia.

Power The capacity to move with a combination of speed and force; a skill-related component of physical fitness.

Precontemplation The stage of the transtheoretical model of behavioral change during which the individual is not yet thinking about changing.

Prediabetes The state in which some but not all of the diagnostic criteria for diabetes are met (e.g., blood glucose levels are higher than normal but are not high enough for a diagnosis of diabetes).

Preeclampsia A pregnancy complication characterized by high blood pressure and signs of damage to another organ system, most often the liver and kidneys. Usually begins after 20 weeks of pregnancy in women whose blood pressure had been normal.

Premature atrial contraction (PAC) An abnormal heartbeat that originates in the atria and precedes a typical atrial contraction.

Premature ventricular contraction (PVC) A form of irregular heartbeat in which the ventricle contracts prematurely, resulting in a "skipped beat" followed by a stronger beat; also called heart palpitations.

Preparation The stage of the transtheoretical model of behavioral change during which the individual is getting ready to make a change.

Pressor response A disproportionate rise in heart rate during resistance training resulting from autonomic nervous system reflex activity.

Primary hypertension Hypertension without an identifiable cause; also called essential hypertension.

Prime mover A muscle responsible for a specific movement. Also called an agonist.

Progesterone Female sex hormone secreted by the ovaries that affects many aspects of female physiology, including menstrual cycles and pregnancy.

Progressive resistive exercise (PRE) A resistance-training exercise program that employs a systematic increase in repetitions and weight to gradually stress the muscles involved, leading to increased strength.

Pronation Internal rotation of the forearm causing the radius to cross diagonally over the ulna and the palm to face posteriorly.

Prone Lying flat, with the anterior aspect of the body facing downward.

Proprioception Sensation and awareness of body position and movements.

Proprioceptive neuromuscular facilitation (PNF) A method of promoting the response of neuromuscular mechanisms through the stimulation of proprioceptors in an attempt to gain more stretch in a muscle; often referred to as a contract/relax method of stretching.

Prostatitis An inflammation of the prostate.

Protein A compound composed of a combination 20 amino acids that is the major structural component of all body tissue.

Proteinuria The presence of an excess of serum proteins in the urine.

Protraction Scapular abduction.

Proximal Nearest to the midline of the body or point of origin of a muscle.

Pseudoclaudication Pain in the buttock, thigh, or leg that occurs with standing or walking and is relieved by rest in a lying or sitting position, or by flexing forward at the waist.

Pulmonary function tests (PFTs) A group of tests that measure how well the lungs take in and release air and how well they move oxygen into the blood; includes spirometry, lung volume measures, and diffusion capacity.

Punishment The presentation of aversive stimuli following an undesired behavior. Decreases the likelihood that the behavior will occur again.

Q-angle The angle formed by lines drawn from the anterior superior iliac spine (ASIS) to the central patella and from the central patella to the tibial tubercle; an estimate of the effective angle at which the quadriceps group pulls on the patella.

Quantitative computed tomography (QCT) A computerized x-ray technique that uses electronic systems to measure volumetric bone mineral density, plus other measures such as the stress-strain index (SSI) and the geometry of the bone.

Quantitative ultrasound (QUS) A bone density test using sound waves.

Quickness The quality of moving fast.

Radiculopathy Dysfunction of a nerve root that can cause numbness or tingling, muscle weakness, or loss of reflex associated with that nerve.

Radionuclide stress testing A diagnostic test for coronary artery disease that involves injecting a radioactive isotope (typically thallium or cardiolyte) into the person's vein, after which an image of the heart becomes visible with a special camera.

Range of motion (ROM) The number of degrees that an articulation will allow one of its segments to move.

Rapport A relationship marked by mutual understanding and trust.

Rate-pressure product Expressed as a product of heart rate in beats per minute times systolic blood pressure. Bears a close relationship with myocardial work or myocardial $\dot{V}O_2$.

Rating of perceived exertion (RPE) A scale, originally developed by noted Swedish psychologist Gunnar Borg, that provides a standard means for evaluating a participant's perception of exercise effort. The original scale ranged from 6 to 20; a revised category ratio scale ranges from 0 to 10.

Reciprocal inhibition The reflex inhibition of the motor neurons of antagonists when the agonists are contracted.

Recommended Dietary Allowance (RDA) The levels of intake of essential nutrients that, on the basis of scientific knowledge, are judged by the Food and Nutrition Board to be adequate to meet the known needs of practically all healthy persons.

Reduce To restore to the normal place or relation of parts, as to reduce a fracture.

Reflective listening A feature of active listening in which the listener makes a best guess at the underlying meaning of what a client has said.

Registered dietitian (RD) A food and nutrition expert who has met the following criteria: completed a minimum of a bachelor's degree at a U.S. accredited university, or other college coursework approved by the Commission on Accreditation for Dietetics Education (CADE); completed a CADE-accredited supervised practice program; passed a national examination; and completed continuing education requirements to maintain registration.

Relapse In behavioral change, the return of an original problem after many lapses (i.e., slips or mistakes) have occurred.

Relaxin A hormone of pregnancy that relaxes the pelvic ligaments and other connective tissue in the body.

Renal failure The inability of the kidneys to excrete wastes and to help maintain the electrolyte balance; loss of kidney function.

Renin An enzyme of high specificity that is released by the kidneys and acts to raise blood pressure by activating angiotensin.

Renin-angiotensin-aldosterone system (RAAS) A hormone system that helps regulate long-term blood pressure and extracellular volume in the body.

Respiratory synctial virus (RSV) A virus that causes cold-like symptoms but can cause breathing difficulties if the lower respiratory tract (i.e., the lungs) becomes involved.

Resorption The removal stage of the bone remodeling cycle.

Resting heart rate (RHR) The number of heartbeats per minute when the body is at complete rest; usually counted first thing in the morning before any physical activity.

Restenosis Recurrent stenosis, or narrowing, of a blood vessel or tubular organ after a surgical correction such as angioplasty.

Retinopathy Any non-inflammatory disease of the retina.

Retraction Scapular adduction.

Return on investment (ROI) The ratio of the net income (profit minus depreciation) to the average money spent by the company overall or on a specific project. Usually expressed as a percentage, a measure of profitability that indicates whether or not a company is using its resources in an efficient manner.

Reversibility The principle of exercise training that suggests that any improvement in physical fitness due to physical activity is entirely reversible with the discontinuation of the training program.

Rhabdomyolysis The breakdown of muscle fibers resulting in the release of muscle fiber contents into the circulation. Some of these are toxic to the kidney and frequently result in kidney damage.

Rheumatoid arthritis (RA) An autoimmune disease that causes inflammation of connective tissues and joints.

Riboflavin A yellow, water-soluble, B vitamin that occurs in green vegetables, germinating seeds, and in milk, fish, egg yolk, liver, and kidney; essential for the carbohydrate metabolism of cells.

Risk management Minimizing the risks of potential legal liability.

Rotation Movement in the transverse plane about a longitudinal axis; can be "internal" or "external."

Sagittal plane The longitudinal plane that divides the body into right and left portions.

Sarcomere The basic functional unit of the myofibril containing the contractile proteins that generate skeletal muscle movements.

Sarcopenia Decreased muscle mass; often used to refer specifically to an age-related decline in muscle mass or lean-body tissue.

GLOSSARY

Sarcoplasmic reticulum The form of endoplasmic reticulum where calcium is stored to be used for muscle activation; located in striated muscle fibers.

Satiety A feeling of fullness.

Saturated fat *See* Saturated fatty acid.

Saturated fatty acid A fatty acid that contains no double bonds between carbon atoms; typically solid at room temperature and very stable.

Scaling Rating a variable on a numerical scale.

Sciatica Pain radiating down the leg caused by compression of the sciatic nerve; frequently the result of lumbar disc herniation.

Scoliosis Excessive lateral curvature of the spine.

Scope of practice The range and limit of responsibilities normally associated with a specific job or profession.

S-Corp A form of business ownership taxed as though it were a partnership. It provides limited liability and is restricted to 75 shareholders and one class of stock. All shareholders must be U.S. citizens and cannot be corporations or partnerships.

Second ventilatory threshold (VT2) A metabolic marker that represents the point at which high-intensity exercise can no longer be sustained due to an accumulation of lactate.

Secondary hypertension Hypertension with an identifiable cause.

Sedentary Doing or requiring much sitting; minimal activity.

Self–blood glucose monitoring (SBGM) The process of collecting detailed information about blood glucose levels at many time points to enable maintenance of a more constant glucose level.

Self-determination theory (SDT) A psychological theory suggesting that people need to feel competent, autonomous, and connected to others in the many domains of life.

Self-efficacy One's perception of his or her ability to change or to perform specific behaviors (e.g., exercise).

Serape effect A myofascial sling that facilitates rotational movements of the torso.

Serum cholesterol The level of total cholesterol in the bloodstream.

Serving The amount of food used as a reference on the nutrition label of that food; the recommended portion of food to be eaten.

Shaping Designing a new behavior chain, including antecedents and rewards, to encourage a certain behavior, such as regular physical activity.

Shear force Any force that causes slippage between a pair of contiguous joints or tissues in a direction that parallels the plane in which they contact.

Simple carbohydrate A short chain of sugar that is rapidly digested.

Skeletal muscle milieu The biochemical substances that make up the setting in which skeletal muscles are located.

Sleep apnea The general condition in which breathing stops for more than 10 seconds during sleep.

Sliding filament theory The explanation for how muscles produce force involving the thick and thin filaments within the sarcomere.

Slow-twitch muscle fiber A muscle fiber type designed for use of aerobic glycolysis and fatty acid oxidation, recruited for low-intensity, longer-duration activities such as walking and swimming.

Small intestine The part of the gastrointestinal system that is the site of the majority of food digestion and absorption.

SMART goal A properly designed goal; SMART stands for specific, measurable, attainable, relevant, and time-bound.

SOAP note A communication tool used among healthcare professionals; SOAP stands for subjective, objective, assessment, and plan.

Social support The perceived comfort, caring, esteem, or help an individual receives from other people.

Socio-ecological model (SEM) A tool that can be used to help the health coach better understand the health behaviors of their clients and more effectively structure behavior-change programs; examines interrelationships between individuals and the environments in which they live and work, as well as the many levels at which individuals are influenced, both in terms of support for healthy behaviors and barriers to improving health behavior.

Sole proprietorship A business owned and operated by one person.

Somatosensory system The physiological system relating to the perception of sensory stimuli from the skin and internal organs.

Specificity Exercise training principle explaining that specific exercise demands made on the body produce specific responses by the body; also called exercise specificity.

Spirometry Pulmonary function testing that measures lung function by assessing the amount (volume) and/or speed (flow) of air that can be maximally inhaled and exhaled; used in the diagnosis and management of asthma.

Spondylolisthesis Forward displacement of one vertebra over another; usually occurs at the L5-S1 level.

Spondylolysis A stress fracture in the posterior aspect of the spine.

Sprain A traumatic joint twist that results in stretching or tearing of the stabilizing connective tissues; mainly involves ligaments or joint capsules, and causes discoloration, swelling, and pain.

Stability Characteristic of the body's joints or posture that represents resistance to change of position.

Stable angina Typical set of symptoms (discomfort in chest, a heavy, viselike, and/or squeezing pain that often radiates to the shoulders, jaw or neck) that usually occurs at predictable times, such as during stress or exercise; once activity ceases, the pain usually goes away.

Stages-of-change model A lifestyle-modification model that suggests that people go through distinct, predictable stages when making lifestyle changes: precontemplation, contemplation, preparation, action, and maintenance. The process is not always linear.

Stanol A naturally occurring chemical compound in plants known to reduce the level of low-density lipoprotein (LDL) cholesterol in blood when ingested.

Static balance The ability to maintain the body's center of mass (COM) within its base of support (BOS).

Static stretching Holding a nonmoving (static) position to immobilize a joint in a position that places the desired muscles and connective tissues passively at their greatest possible length.

Statute of limitations A formal regulation limiting the period within which a specific legal action may be taken.

Steady-state heart rate (HRss) A state of exercise training where the demands of the active tissues can be adequately met by the cardiovascular system.

Steatosis Accumulation of fat in the liver.

Stenosis The narrowing of any tube-like structure within the body (e.g., coronary artery stenosis, spinal stenosis).

GLOSSARY

Sterol Naturally occurring unsaturated steroid alcohols, typically waxy solids.

Stimulus control A means to break the connection between events or other stimuli and a behavior; in behavioral science, sometimes called "cue extinction."

Strain A stretch, tear, or rip in the muscle or adjacent tissue such as the fascia or tendon.

Stress echocardiography Cardiac ultrasound; the sound waves of an ultrasound are used to produce images of the heart at rest and at the peak of exercise.

Stress urinary incontinence (SUI) The involuntary loss of urine that occurs with physical exertion and a rise in abdominal pressure.

Stretch-shortening cycle (SSC) An active stretch (eccentric action) of a muscle followed by an immediate shortening (concentric action) of that same muscle. A component of plyometrics.

Stroke A sudden and often severe attack due to blockage of an artery into the brain.

Stroke volume (SV) The amount of blood pumped from the left ventricle of the heart with each beat.

Structure/function claim A statement that relates a nutrient or dietary ingredient to normal human structure or function such as "calcium builds strong bones," or describes a benefit related to a nutrient deficiency. It must state a disclaimer that the U.S. Food and Drug Administration has not evaluated the claim and that the supplement is not intended to treat, cure, or prevent any disease.

Subacute The characteristic of a condition intermediate between chronic and acute inflammation, exhibiting some of the characteristics of each.

Subluxation An incomplete dislocation; though the relationship is altered, contact between joint surfaces remains.

Summarizing A feature of active listening in which the coach states back to a client what the coach perceives to be the main points of what the client has said.

Superior Located above.

Supination External rotation of the forearm (radioulnar joint) that causes the palm to face anteriorly.

Supine Lying face up (on the back).

SWOT analysis Situation analysis in which internal strengths and weaknesses of an organization (such as a business) or individual, and external opportunities and threats are closely examined to chart a strategy.

Sympathetic nervous system A branch of the autonomic nervous system responsible for mobilizing the body's energy and resources during times of stress and arousal (i.e., the fight or flight response). Opposes the physiological effects of the parasympathetic nervous system (e.g., reduces digestive secretions, speeds the heart, contracts blood vessels).

Sympathomimetic A characteristic of medications that mimic the effects of the sympathetic nervous system.

Symphysitis Irritation of the pubic symphysis caused by increased motion at the joint.

Synapse The region of communication between neurons.

Syncope A transient state of unconsciousness during which a person collapses to the floor as a result of lack of oxygen to the brain; commonly known as fainting.

Synergist A muscle that assists another muscle in function.

Synergistic dominance A condition in which the synergists carry out the primary function of a weakened or inhibited prime mover.

Synovial cell Fibroblasts lying between the cartilaginous fibers in the synovial membrane of a joint.

Synovial fluid Transparent, viscous lubricating fluid found in joint cavities, bursae, and tendon sheaths.

Synovial joint A freely movable articulation, in which the contiguous bony surfaces are covered with articular cartilage and connected by ligaments lined by synovial membrane. Also called a diarthrodial joint.

Synovial membrane The connective-tissue membrane that lines the cavity of a synovial joint and produces the synovial fluid; also called synovium.

Synovium *See* Synovial membrane.

Systolic blood pressure (SBP) The pressure exerted by the blood on the vessel walls during ventricular contraction.

Tachycardia Elevated heart rate over 100 beats per minute.

Tai chi A Chinese system of slow meditative physical exercise designed for relaxation, balance, and health.

Talk test A method for measuring exercise intensity using observation of respiration effort and the ability to talk while exercising.

Target heart rate (THR) Number of heartbeats per minute that indicate appropriate exercise intensity levels for each individual; also called training heart rate.

Telemetry The process by which measured quantities from a remote site are transmitted to a data collection point for recording and processing, such as what occurs during an electrocardiogram.

Tendinitis Inflammation of a tendon.

Tensegrity The characteristic property of a stable three-dimensional structure consisting of members under tension that are contiguous and members under compression that are not.

Teratogenic Nongenetic factors that can cause birth defects in the fetus.

Testosterone In males, the steroid hormone produced in the testes; involved in growth and development of reproductive tissues, sperm, and secondary male sex characteristics.

Therapeutic Lifestyle Change (TLC) eating plan An eating plan from the National Heart, Lung, and Blood Institute (NHLBI) developed specifically to improve cholesterol levels.

Thermoregulation Regulation of the body's temperature.

Thiamin A water-soluble B vitamin found in meat, yeast, and the bran coat of grains; necessary for carbohydrate metabolism and normal neural activity.

Thromboembolism An obstruction of a blood vessel by a blood clot that has become dislodged from another site in the circulation.

Thyroid hormone Hormones secreted by the thyroid gland and responsible for controlling the metabolic rate.

Tidal volume The volume of air inspired per breath.

Tolerable Upper Intake Level (UL) The maximal intake of a nutrient that is unlikely to pose risk of adverse health effects to almost all individuals in an age- and gender-specific group.

Tonicity The elastic tension of living tissues, such as muscles and arteries.

Torsion The rotation or twisting of a joint by the exertion of a lateral force tending to turn it about a longitudinal axis.

Total peripheral resistance (TPR) The resistance to the passage of blood through the small blood vessels, especially arterioles.

Toxicity The degree to which a substance can be harmful to the body.

Trabecular bone Spongy or cancellous bone composed of thin plates that form a honeycomb pattern; predominantly found in the ends of long bones and the vertebral bodies.

Traction The act of pulling or being pulled.

Trans fat *See* Trans fatty acid.

Trans fatty acid An unsaturated fatty acid that is converted into a saturated fat to increase the shelf life of some products.

Transcutaneous electrical nerve stimulation (TENS) A technique used for pain relief in which nerves are electronically stimulated to block the transmission of pain information to the brain.

Transient ischemia Momentary dizziness, loss of consciousness, or forgetfulness caused by a short-lived lack of oxygen (blood) to the brain; usually due to a partial blockage of an artery, it is a warning sign for stroke.

Transient ischemic attack (TIA) Momentary dizziness, loss of consciousness, or forgetfulness caused by a short-lived lack of oxygen (blood) to the brain; usually due to a partial blockage of an artery, it is a warning sign for a stroke.

Translate The act of moving a rigid body in which all parts move in the same direction at the same speed.

Transverse plane Anatomical term for the imaginary line that divides the body, or any of its parts, into upper (superior) and lower (inferior) parts. Also called the horizontal plane.

Transtheoretical model of behavioral change (TTM) A theory of behavior that examines one's readiness to change and identifies five stages: precontemplation, contemplation, preparation, action, and maintenance. Also called the stages-of-change model.

Trendelenburg gait A drop of the pelvis on the side opposite of the stance leg, indicating weakness of the hip abductors and gluteus medius and minimus on the side of the stance leg.

Trigger *See* Antecedent.

Triglyceride Three fatty acids joined to a glycerol (carbon and hydrogen structure) backbone; how fat is stored in the body.

Trochanteric bursitis The painful inflammation of the bursa surrounding the greater trochanter of the femur.

Type 1 diabetes mellitus (T1DM) Form of diabetes caused by the destruction of the insulin-producing beta cells in the pancreas, which leads to little or no insulin secretion; generally develops in childhood and requires regular insulin injections; formerly known as insulin-dependent diabetes mellitus (IDDM) and childhood-onset diabetes.

Type 2 diabetes mellitus (T2DM) Most common form of diabetes; typically develops in adulthood and is characterized by a reduced sensitivity of the insulin target cells to available insulin; usually associated with obesity; formerly known as non-insulin-dependent diabetes mellitus (NIDDM) and adult-onset diabetes.

Type I muscle fibers *See* Slow-twitch muscle fibers.

Type II muscle fibers *See* Fast-twitch muscle fibers.

Unsaturated fat Fatty acids that contain one or more double bonds between carbon atoms; typically liquid at room temperature and fairly unstable, making them susceptible to oxidative damage and a shortened shelf life.

Unstable angina In contrast to stable angina, unstable angina occurs in individuals at unpredictable times, or even at rest; unstable angina may progress to a myocardial infarction.

Valgus Characterized by an abnormal outward turning of a bone, especially of the hip, knee, or foot.

Valsalva maneuver A strong exhaling effort against a closed glottis, which builds pressure in the chest cavity that interferes with the return of the blood to the heart; may deprive the brain of blood and cause lightheadedness or fainting.

Varus Characterized by an abnormal inward turning of a bone, especially of the hip, knee, or foot.

Vascular inflammation The buildup of plaque within the arterial walls. Commonly referred to as atherosclerosis.

Vasoconstriction Narrowing of the opening of blood vessels (notably the smaller arterioles) caused by contraction of the smooth muscle lining the vessels.

Vasodilation Increase in diameter of the blood vessels, especially dilation of arterioles leading to increased blood flow to a part of the body.

Vasodilator Any drug that causes dilation of blood vessels; typically prescribed for the treatment of hypertension.

Vasopressin Hormone released by the posterior pituitary gland during exercise; reduces urinary excretion of water and prevents dehydration.

Vegan A person who does not consume any animal products, including dairy products such as milk and cheese, eggs, and may exclude honey.

Vegetarian A person who does not eat meat, fish, poultry, or products containing these foods.

Ventilatory rate The number of breaths per minute.

Ventricular function Function of heart muscle's (myocardium) contraction mechanics. For example, ventricular ejection fraction is a measure of ventricular contractility (rate and force with which the myocardium contracts).

Very-low-density lipoprotein (VLDL) A lipoprotein containing a very large proportion of lipids to protein and carrying most cholesterol from the liver to the tissues.

Vestibular system Part of the central nervous system that coordinates reflexes of the eyes, neck, and body to maintain equilibrium in accordance with posture and movement of the head.

Visceral adiposity *See* Visceral obesity.

Visceral fat *See* Visceral obesity.

Visceral obesity Excess fat located deep in the abdomen that surrounds the vital organs; closely related to abdominal girth. Its accumulation is associated with insulin resistance, glucose intolerance, dyslipidemia, hypertension, and coronary artery disease. Abdominal girth measured at the level of the umbilicus with values >40 inches (102 cm) in men and >35 inches (89 cm) in women are strong indicators of visceral obesity.

Visual system The series of structures by which visual sensations are received from the environment and conveyed as signals to the central nervous system.

Vitamin An organic micronutrient that is essential for normal physiologic function.

$\dot{V}O_2$max Considered the best indicator of cardiovascular endurance, it is the maximal amount of oxygen (mL) that a person can use in one minute per kilogram of body weight. Also called maximal oxygen uptake and maximal aerobic power.

$\dot{V}O_2$reserve ($\dot{V}O_2$R) The difference between $\dot{V}O_2$max and $\dot{V}O_2$ at rest; used for programming aerobic exercise intensity.

Vulnerable plaque A collection of white blood cells and lipids in the wall of an artery that is particularly unstable and prone to produce sudden major problems such as a heart attack or stroke.

Waist circumference Abdominal girth measured at narrowest part of the torso (above the umbilicus and below the xiphoid process); values >40 inches (102 cm) in men and >35 inches (89 cm) in women are strong indicators of abdominal obesity and associated with an increased health risk.

Waist-to-hip ratio (WHR) A useful measure for determining health risk due to the site of fat storage. Calculated by dividing the ratio of abdominal girth (waist measurement) by the hip measurement.

Yoga Indian word for "union." A combination of breathing exercises, physical postures, and meditation that has been practiced for more than 5,000 years.

INDEX

A

Abdominal bracing, 672

Abdominal fat, 751b

Abdominal hollowing, 483

Abdominal obliques, 482, 483f

Abduction, standing, 592, 592f

ACC/AHA Pooled Cohort 10-year ASCVD Risk Assessment, 218, 219f

Acceptable Macronutrient Distribution Range (AMDR), 747–748

Access to exercise, communicating with distressed clients on, 123

Accreditation Council for Clinical Lipidology, 237b

Acculturation, 762

ACE Certified Medical Exercise Specialist. *See* Certified Medical Exercise Specialist (CMES)

ACE Code of Ethics, 156b, 728–733

ACEfitness.org, 162b, 163b

ACE Integrated Fitness Training Model, 20–53. *See also specific components and topics*
    activities of daily living in, 23
    behavioral change in, 28b
    Cardiorespiratory Training in, 20–40
    client-centered approach in, 26–28
    components of, 24, 24f (*See also specific components*)
    effectiveness of, 50b–52b, 51f, 52t
    fitness assessments in, 27–28
    function-health-fitness-performance continuum in, 23, 23f
    human development in, restoring function, 25b–26b
    Muscular Training in, 40–49
    origins and purpose of, 22
    overview of, 24, 24f
    Physical Activity Guidelines for Americans and, 21–22, 28, 61
    training parameters in, traditional *vs.* contemporary, 21, 22t

ACE Position Statement on Nutrition Scope of Practice for Medical Exercise Specialists, 745–747

Achilles tendinopathy, 593t, 620–622

Acidosis, cellular, 779

Acromioclavicular joint
    after shoulder injury, pathomechanics of, 635b
    anatomy of, 633
    articulations of, 633f, 634
    pathology of, 633–636

Acromioclavicular joint injuries, 633–636
    acromioclavicular joint sprain in, 633–636, 633f
    case study of, 656
    classification of, 633, 634f

Acromioclavicular joint sprain, 633–636
    early intervention for, 635–636
    mechanism of injury in, 633, 633f
    precautions in, 635
    restorative exercise program for, 636
    signs and symptoms of, 633, 634f

Actin, 491

Action stage, 102t, 103
    movement to, 134

Active agonist contraction, with reciprocal inhibition, 450

Activities of daily living (ADL), 23, 430. *See also specific disorders*

Adaptive postural control, in balance, 480

Adduction
    hip, 421, 421f, 421t
    standing, 592, 592f

Adenosine triphosphate (ATP), 777

Adequate Intake (AI), 747

Adherence, 21, 111–114
    for behavioral modification, 111–112
        shaping in, 112, 112b
        stimulus control in, 112, 112b
        written agreements in, 111
    cognitive behavioral techniques in, 112–114
        feedback in, 114
        goal setting in, 113–114, 113b

Adhesions, collagen, 494

Adiponectin, 319

Adipose tissue, 317, 318
    brown, 318

Aerobic exercise. *See also specific disorders; specific types*
    recommendations, 29, 29t

Aerobic power, age on, 62

Affirmations, 130

Affordable Care Act (ACA), 3

Agatston score, 177b

Age (aging)
    in low-back pain, 662
    on physiological capacity, 62
    on physiological function, 508, 508f

Agenda setting, 121

Agility drills, 510

Agility ladder drills, 510–511, 511f

Agonist contraction, active, with reciprocal inhibition, 450

Agreements, written, for behavioral modification, 111

Alcohol
    for coronary heart disease, 184
    excessive consumption of, on bone, 560
    on physiological capacity, 66

Aldosterone, in blood pressure control, 246–248, 247f
Aldosterone-receptor antagonists, 257
Allergens, in asthma, 277
Allergic hypersensitivity, asthma and, 284
Allergy testing, in asthma, 284
Allograft, anterior cruciate ligament, 610
Alpha blockers, 257
Alpha-glucosidase inhibitors, for diabetes mellitus, 373
American College of Cardiology Foundation (ACCF) recommendations
    cardiorespiratory and muscular-training exercise, 22
    physical activity, for coronary heart disease, 169, 200b
Amphetamines, on physiological capacity, 67
Anaerobic glycolysis, 36
Anaerobic threshold, 31b
Anatomical position, 488f, 621f
Android fat, 317
Angina pectoris, 173, 173t
    in CHD patients during exercise, 194, 194t
    stable, 173, 197b
    unstable, 173
Angiography, coronary, 177
    CT, 178b
Angiotensin, 246–248, 247f
Angiotensin-converting enzyme (ACE), 247, 247f
Angiotensin-converting enzyme (ACE) inhibitors, 257
Angiotensin receptor blockers, 257
Ankle
    in balance, 480, 480f
    eversion of, 407
        resistive, 619f
    in gait, 498
    inversion of, 407
        resistive, 619f
    pronation of, 407–421b, 421f
    pronation/supination assessment of, 418f, 420, 420b–421b, 421f
    resistive dorsiflexion of, 619f
    resistive plantar flexion of, 619f
Ankle hops (hop progressions), 574f
Ankle injury, on kinetic chain, 408b, 408f
Ankle joint movements, 407, 407f
Ankle sprains, 616–620, 617t, 619f–621f
    classification of, 617, 617t
    early intervention for, 617–618
    mechanism of injury in, 616–617
    precautions in, 617
    prevalence of, 616
    restorative exercise program for, 618–620
        Functional Training, 618–620, 619f, 620f
        Movement Training, 593t, 620, 621f
    signs and symptoms of, 617

Annulus fibrosus, 665, 665f
Antecedents, 96
Anterior apprehension test, 637, 637f
Anterior capsule stretch, 463, 464f
Anterior compartment
    sitting stretch for, 615, 616f
    standing "toe drag" stretch for, 615, 616f
Anterior cruciate ligament (ACL), in gait, 498, 498f
Anterior cruciate ligament (ACL) injuries, 608–612
    anatomy and pathophysiology of, 604f, 608
    case study of, 624–625
    early intervention for, 610–611
    mechanism of injury in, 608, 609f
    prevalence of, 608
    restorative exercise program for, 611–614
        Functional Training, 611
        Movement Training, 593t, 612
    signs and symptoms of, 608
    treatment options for
        non-operative management, 608
        non-operative precautions, 609
        post-operative precautions, 610
        surgical, allograft, 610
        surgical, hamstring tendon graft, 610
        surgical, patellar tendon graft, 609–610
Anterior lunge, with medicine ball lift, 518f
Anterior oblique myofascial sling, 501, 502f, 514, 515f–516f
    exercises for, 514, 515f–516f
Anterior shin splints, 614–616, 614f–616f
Anterior shoulder instability, 636–641. See also Shoulder instability, anterior
Anterior superior iliac spine (ASIS) assessment, 422, 422f
Anticipatory postural control, in balance, 479
Antihypertensive medications, 255–258
    actions of, 255, 255f
    aldosterone-receptor antagonists, 257
    alpha blockers, 257
    angiotensin-converting enzyme inhibitors, 257
    angiotensin receptor blockers, 257
    beta blockers, 256–257
    calcium-channel blockers, 258
    centrally acting alpha 2 agonists, 258
    diuretics, 256
    peripheral vasodilators, 258
Antioxidants
    in arthritis, 541t
    chronic use, 780
    for coronary heart disease, 184
Antisense ApoB inhibitors, 222
Anxiety
    in diabetes type 2, exercise on, 376
    from health challenges, 58
Apley's scratch test, 446–447, 447f, 447t
Apolipoprotein B (apo B), 213–214, 214f

INDEX

Apolipoproteins, 214–215, 214f
Apoprotein A1 (apo A1), 213
Apprehension test, anterior, 637, 637f
Arginine, 779–780
Arm lifts, prone, 468f–469f
Arm raise, diagonal, 545, 546, 546f
    in scapula plane, 637, 637f
Arrhythmias, ventricular, 173–174
Arthritis, 526–552
    case study of, 551–552
    CMES focus in, 551b
    diagnostic criteria for, 533–535
        in juvenile arthritis, 534
        in osteoarthritis, 533–534
        in rheumatoid arthritis, 534, 535t
    epidemiology of, 528–530
        in juvenile arthritis, 530
        in osteoarthritis, 528
        in rheumatoid arthritis, 530
    etiology of, 527b
    exercise recommendations for, 540–545
        cardiorespiratory endurance exercise in, 544
        contraindications and precautions in, 544
        flexibility exercise in, 545
        guidelines in, lack of, 538, 540
        guidelines in, summary of, 550b
        with osteoarthritis of the knee or hip, 545b
        resistance exercise in, 544–545
    exercises for, sample, 545–550
        body-weight squat, 548, 548f
        calf raises, 545, 546f
        diagonal arm raise, 545, 546, 546f
        glute bridge, 548, 549f
        heel and toe walking, 545, 546f
        hip ROM complex, 548, 550f
        muscle-recruitment difficulty assessment in, 545, 546f
        programming for, 545
        prone hip extension, 548, 549f
        prone plank, 548, 549f
        for quadriceps strength, 547, 547f
        side bridge, 548, 549f
        single-leg squat, 548, 548f
        standing single-leg balance, 545–546, 546f
        terminal 30-degrees knee extension, 547, 547f
        terminal extensions (closed chain), 547, 547f
        wall slide/squat, 547, 547f
    forms of, 527
    history of osteoarthritis in, 529b
    inactivity on, 536b
    nutrition in, 538–540
        elimination diets for, 540
        fatty acids in, 538–540, 539t
        Mediterranean dietary pattern, 540
        nutrients in, 540, 541t
        supplements in, 540, 542t–543t
    overview of, 530–533
        in juvenile arthritis, 533
        in osteoarthritis, 530–532
        in rheumatoid arthritis, 532
    pathophysiology of, 527
    signs and symptoms of, 527
    treatment options for, 536–538
        exercise treatment, 537–538, 537b–538b
        non-pharmacological, 536
        pharmacological, 536
        surgical, 536–537
Arthritis-attributable activity limitations (AAAL), 528, 530
Arthrokinematics, 406, 406f
Arthrokinetics, 405
Arthroplastic total hip replacement, 595–600. *See also* Hip replacement, total
Arthroplasty, for osteoporosis, 566
Articular cartilage
    in gait, 494–495
    of knee, 531
    in osteoarthritis, 531
    properties of, 531
Articulation, 531. *See also* Joint
Assessments. *See also specific types*
    cardiorespiratory
        in Fitness Training, 35–36, 35f
        ventilatory threshold in, 35–36, 35f
    fitness, 27–28
Assumptions, avoiding, for behavioral change, 108–109
Asthma, 277–298
    atopy and, 284
    case studies of, 296–298
    cause of, 279
    diagnostic testing and criteria in, 282–284
        allergy testing in, 284
        peak expiratory flow in, 284, 284f
        physical findings in, 282
        spirometry in, 282–283, 282f, 283f
    epidemiology of, 277
    exacerbation of, 279
    exercise recommendations for, 292–296
        fitness testing in, 294, 295b, 295f
        guidelines in, general activity, 292b
        guidelines in, summary of, 296b
        maximal heart rate in, 292
        programming and progression in, 293–294
        pulmonary responses to exercise training in, 293
    nutrition in, 289–291
        caffeine in, 289
        for comorbidity management, 291
        fatty acids in, 290
        food allergies in, 291
        fruits and vegetables in, 289–290, 290t
        gastroesophageal reflux disease in, 291
        in management and treatment, 289–290, 290t
        nutrients in etiology of, 290t
        obesity and weight loss in, 291
    pathogenesis of, 277, 278f
    severity of, classification of, 279, 279t

treatment options for, 284–289
    action plan in, 287, 288f
    Borg dyspnea scale in, 287, 287t
    education in, 287
    exacerbation management during exercise in, 289, 289t
    exacerbation management in, 287–289, 288f
    medications in, long-term control, 285, 285t
    medications in, quick-relief, 285, 285t
    stepwise approach to, 286f
    trigger avoidance and comorbid condition control in, 280b–281b, 285
triggers for, 277, 280, 280t
    controlling, 280b–281b
Atherogenesis, 171, 172f
    in diabetes mellitus, 369
Atherogenic dyslipidemia, in metabolic syndrome, 346
Atherosclerosis, 171, 172f
    dyslipidemia in, 209
Atherosclerotic cardiovascular disease, 209
Atopy, asthma and, 284
Atrioventricular node (AV node), 173
Autogenic inhibition, in restorative exercise, 449
Automated external defibrillator (AED), 5, 85, 191
Autonomic nervous system, in blood pressure control, 246
Autonomous motivation, 119
Autonomy
    in self-determination theory, 120b
    on self-motivation, 99
Avocado-soybean unsaponifiable fractions, on arthritis, 542t
Axis of rotation, 489b
    in gait, constantly changing, 495

B

Back pain, low, 660–679. *See also* Low-back pain
Backward lunge, with weighted vest, 573f
Balance, 479–484
    ankle, hip, and knee strategies in, 480, 480f
    assessment of, 507–508, 508f
    case study on, 522–523
    components of, 479
    core in, 481–484
        core anatomy in, 481–483, 482f, 493f
        fundamentals of, 481
        intra-abdominal pressure in, 483–484
        stability model for, 481, 481f
        thoracolumbar fascia gain in, 484
    dynamic, 41, 479
    importance of, 479
    postural control in
        adaptive, 480
        anticipatory, 479
        reactive, 479
    somatosensory system in, 480

vs. stability, 474b
static, 41
vestibular system in, 481
visual system in, 480
Balance training. *See also* Gait exercises
    program for, 513t
Ball, medicine
    anterior lunge and lift of, 518f
    toss of, 677, 677f
Ball, stability, shoulder stabilization on, 639, 639f
Banded lateral step, 575f
Banded monster walk, 576f
Barbell row, bent-over, 518f
Barbell squat, 674
Bariatric surgery, 325–326
    diet before and after, 332
Baroreceptors, 246
Baseline fitness screening and testing plan, 88
Base of support (BOS), 479
    central nervous system in, 499
Base Training, 34
Behavior, health, determinants of, 95–100. *See also* Health behavior, determinants of
Behavioral change, 28b, 94–115. *See also specific topics*
    adherence in, 111–114
        for behavioral modification, 111–112
        cognitive behavioral techniques in, 112–114
    communicating recommendations for, 121
    determinants of health behavior in, 95–100
    health belief model in, 106–107
    strategies for, 28b, 108–111
        avoiding assumptions in, 108–109
        client empowerment in, 110
        communication in, 108
        high-risk situations in, 111
        relapse prevention in, 109
    success in, defining, 109b
    transtheoretical model of behavioral change in, 100–106
Bench press exercises, with shoulder instability, 641b
Bend-and-lift assessment, 430–432, 431f, 431t
Bend-and-lift movements, 46, 46f
Benefits, exercise
    on health, 61–62, 84
    identifying, 84
    volume and, dose-response relationship, 29
Bent-knee marches
    reverse, modified dead bug with, 456f
    supine, 455f
Bent-over barbell row, 518f
Beta blockers, 256–257
Beta-cell stimulants, for diabetes mellitus, 373
Beta receptors, in blood pressure control, 246

INDEX

β-alanine, 779
Biceps curl, in pregnancy, 707f
Bicipital tendinitis, 641b, 641f
Biguanides, for diabetes mellitus, 373
Bilateral cable press, standing, 516f
Bilateral row, standing, in pregnancy, 708f
Bile acid sequestrants, 221
Billing, 155–156
Biotensegrity, 489, 489b
Bird dog, 676, 676f
    in pregnancy, 710f
    quadruped, 517f
Bisphosphonates, for osteoporosis, 564–565, 565t
Blackberry thumb, 654–655, 654f
Blood glucose self-monitoring, 370
Blood lipid disorders, 208–239. *See also* Lipid disorders, blood
    overweight/obesity and, 21
Blood pressure
    cardiovascular disease prevention recommendations for, 181t
    cardiovascular events and, 245
    classification of, 250, 250t
    control of
        long-term neurohormonal, 246–247, 247f
        short-term reflex, 246
    DASH eating plan, 760
    formula for, 246
    in metabolic syndrome, 348
    nutrients on, 261–262, 261t
    sodium on, 261–262
    stress on, 60
Blood-pressure measurement, 250–251
    cuff placement in, 250
    cuff sizes in, 250t
    Korotkoff sounds and phases in, 250–251, 251f
Blood vessels, peripheral, aerobic exercise training on, 264–265
B-mode ultrasound assessment, 179b
Body dysmorphism, 57
Body image, 337b
Body mass index (BMI), 321, 322t
    in diabetes mellitus, 369
    formula for, 321
    for hypertension treatment, 261
    knee osteoarthritis, 43
    in metabolic syndrome, 345
Body-weight squat, 548, 548f
Bone(s)
    factors affecting
        age and sex, 559
        bone mineral, 558–559
        genetics and race, 559
        hormones, 559–560

        lactation, 560
        oral contraceptives, 560
        smoking and alcohol, 560
    in gait, 494
    loading, hormonal and dietary interventions on, 571b
    normal *vs.* osteoporotic trabecular, 558, 558f
    remodeling of, 558
    structure and physiology of, 558
    trabecular and cortical, 558, 558f
Bone mineral density (BMD) diagnostic criteria, 561–563, 561t
    dual-energy x-ray absorptiometry (DXA) in, 561, 562–563
    FRAX tool in, 562, 563b, 563f
    quantitative computed tomography in, 563
    quantitative ultrasound in, 563
Bone response, to physical activity, 569–571
    in children and adolescents, 569
    in men, 570
    in women
        postmenopausal, 570
        premenopausal, 569–570
Bones, in gait, 494
Borg dyspnea scale, 287, 287t
Botanicals, on arthritis, 543t
Branched-chain amino acids (BCAAs), 778
Breathing
    pursed-lip, for COPD, 306b
    yogic, in CHD patients, 199b
Breathlessness, in pregnancy, 696–697
Bridge
    glute, 459f, 520f
        with osteoporosis, 577f
        single-leg supine, 520f
    rolling, 674, 675f
    shoulder, 459f
Bronchitis, chronic, COPD from, 298, 299, 299f. *See also* Chronic obstructive pulmonary disease (COPD)
Bronchoconstriction, exercise-induced
    lifestyle choices for, 63
    pulmonary response to exercise training in, 293
Brown adipose tissue, 318
Buffering capacity, muscle, 779
Bursa, 643, 643f
Bursitis, 643
    trochanteric, 590–593 (*See also* Trochanteric bursitis)
Business description, 159–160
Business-management tools, virtual, 162b–163b
Business strategies, 153–164
    billing and payment policies in, 155–156
    business planning in, 159–162
        business description in, 159–160
        decision-making criteria in, 162
        executive summary in, 159
        marketing plan in, 160

operational plan in, 160
risk (SWOT) analysis in, 161–162, 161f
employment options in
employees, 157
independent contractors, 158
self-employed, 158
legal issues and liabilities in, 156–157
legal risks in, avoiding, 157
marketing for medical referrals in, 153–155
virtual tools in, 162b–164b
business-management, 162b–163b
connected health, 163b–164b

B vitamins, for coronary heart disease, 184

C

Cable chop, high-to-low, 409, 516f, 672
Cable press
standing bilateral, 516f
standing single-arm, 515f
Cable pull, lunge to single-arm, 518f
Cadence, 486
Caffeine
for asthma, 289
on physiological capacity, 67
supplemental, 777
Calcitonin, for osteoporosis, 564, 565t
Calcium, in arthritis, 541t
Calcium-channel blockers, 258
Calcium scoring, coronary, 177, 177b–178b, 178t
Calf raises, 545, 546f
with knee bent, 619f
with knee straight, 619f
Calf stretch
in pregnancy, 711f
wall, 615, 615f
Calories, limiting non-nutritional, 754
Capsule, joint, 531. See also Joint(s)
Capsule stretches
anterior (pectoralis), 463, 464f
inferior, 463, 463f
posterior, 463, 464f
superior, 463, 464f
Carbohydrates
counting, 380t
in obesity, 64–65
post-exercise, 777–778
Carbonated beverages, on physiological capacity, 67
Cardiac dysrhythmias, 173–174
Cardiac event risk stratification, during exercise, 191, 191t
Cardiac output, 246
Cardiac workload, in CHD patients during exercise, 195
Cardiometabolic risk, 220b, 368, 368f
Cardiopulmonary resuscitation (CPR) certification, 5, 15, 85, 191

Cardiorespiratory assessments
Fitness Training, 35–36, 35f
ventilatory threshold, 35–36, 35f
Cardiorespiratory fitness. *See also specific disorders and training*
human development, 25b
Cardiorespiratory Training, 28–40. *See also specific phases*
ACSM and American Heart Association, 29
aerobic exercise recommendations in, 29, 29t
Base Training in, 34
behavioral change in, 28b
Fitness Training in, 34–38
assessments in, cardiorespiratory fitness, 35–36, 35f
goals of, 34–35
human development and, 25b
submaximal talk test in, for VT1, 37–38
talk test in, 36–37
frequency, intensity, and duration in, 28–29
maximal heart rate in, calculation of, 29–30, 30f
overview of, 28–31
Performance Training in, 39–40
VT2 threshold assessment in, 39–40
phases of, 31, 31f, 39, 39t
Physical Activity Guidelines for Americans, 28
three-zone intensity model in, 31, 32f, 32t–33t
volume and health/fitness benefits, dose-response relationships, 29
Cardiovascular disease (CVD), 209. *See also* Atherosclerotic cardiovascular disease
hypertension on risk of, 245
nutrition in prevention of, 180–181, 181t, 182f
overweight and obesity in, 21, 323
physiological capacity in, 63
rheumatoid arthritis and, 533b
risk factors for, 21, 259t
physical activity on, 66b
Cardiovascular endurance exercise. *See* Aerobic exercise; *specific types*
Carnitine, 780
Carpal tunnel syndrome, 651–654
in pregnancy, 702
Cartilage, articular, 531
in gait, 494–495
of knee, 531
in osteoarthritis, 531
properties of, 531
Casein, 778
Catabolism, exercise-induced protein, 771
Cat-cow, 454f
Catheterization, coronary, 177
Cellular acidosis, 779
Centering, abdominal, 483
Center of gravity (COG), 479, 479f
central nervous system in, 499

in Functional Training, 41
in pregnancy, 695

Center of mass (COM), 479

Centrally acting alpha 2 agonists, 258

Central nervous system, in gait, 498–499

Cerebral vascular disease, in diabetes mellitus, 369

Certification
CMES, 3, 11–12
CPR, 5, 15, 85, 191

Certified Medical Exercise Specialist (CMES)
certification of, 3
exam content outline for, 734–743
focus of, 271
in healthcare continuum, 3, 4–5, 5f
in healthcare team, 21
for health conditions, multiple, 21
populations served by, 4
role of, 6–8, 21–22 (See also Role, CMES)
scope of practice of, 4–5, 5f, 8–10, 9b, 10t

Change
optimism for, in communication, 120
readiness to, assessing, 133–134
stages of, 101–103, 102t

Change, processes of, 104–106
decisional balance in, 101, 105, 106b
right assessments in, 105b
self-efficacy in, 101, 104–105, 107

Change talk
for motivation, 134–136
OARS model in, 134–136

Chemoprophylaxis, 12b–13b

Chest pain, in CHD patients during exercise, 194, 194t

Chest press
with osteoporosis, 576f
standing, in pregnancy, 707f

Chest/shoulder stretch, in pregnancy, 712f

Children
lifestyle choices on physiological capacity in, 63
lipid and lipoprotein goals in, 216, 217t
osteoporosis prevention exercises for
physical activity and bone response in, 569
programming and progression in, 571

Child's pose, with osteoporosis, 577f

Cholesterol, 171. *See also* Lipoproteins; *specific types*
in atherosclerosis, 209
guidelines for
ACC/ACH, 216
consensus, 215
nutrition for improving profile of, 229–230, 231t
U.S. trends in levels of, 210t

Cholesterol transport inhibitors, 221

Chondroitin, on arthritis, 542t

Chop
diagonal, in pregnancy, 709f
high-to-low cable, 409, 516f, 672

Chronic bronchitis, COPD from, 298, 299, 299f. *See also* Chronic obstructive pulmonary disease (COPD)

Chronic diseases, 58. *See also specific types*
on physiological capacity, 65

Chronic obstructive pulmonary disease (COPD), 64, 298–308
case study on, 307–308
diagnostic testing and criteria for, 299–300, 300t
epidemiology of, 298
exercise recommendations in, 303–307
cardiovascular and pulmonary responses in, 303, 303f
CMES focus in, 307b
continuum of care in, 305
continuum of care in, CMES role in, 305
exercise testing in, 306
guidelines summary in, 306b
programming and progression in, 305–306
pulmonary rehabilitation in, 304b–305b, 304t
pursed-lip breathing in, 306b
nutrition in, 302–303, 302t
overview of, 299, 299f
risk factors for, 298
spirometry classification of, 300, 300t
treatment of
medications in, 301
oxygen therapy and surgery in, 301
physical activity and rehabilitation in, 300
risk reduction in, for comorbidities, 301
risk reduction in, for exacerbations, 301
smoking cessation in, 300

Chronotropic incompetence, 194

Chylomicrons, 210, 210f

Cissus quadrangularis, on arthritis, 543t

Clamshell exercise, 674, 675f

"Clams," side-lying, for hip external rotators, 592, 593f

Claudication, intermittent, 70

Clavicle rotation, 633

Clearance, physician, 84, 85f

Client-centered approach, 26–28

Clinical lipidology, 209

Closed-ended questions, 130

Closed-kinetic-chain movements, 464b, 465f

Closed-kinetic-chain progressions. *See also specific disorders and types*
for hip osteoarthritis, 593b, 595
for lower-extremity musculoskeletal injuries, 593, 593t

Closed-kinetic-chain strengthening exercises, 588

Closed-kinetic-chain weight shifts, 469f–470f

Cocaine, on physiological capacity, 67

Code of Ethics, ACE, 156b, 728–733

Coefficient of friction, 531
in osteoarthritis, 531–532

Cognitive behavioral techniques, for adherence, 112–114

INDEX

feedback in, 114
goal setting in, 113–114, 113b
Cognitive learning, effective education for, 138–139
Cognitive variables, in health behavior, 100
Collagen adhesions, 494
Collagen preparations, on arthritis, 543t
Communication barriers, 132–133, 152
Communication strategies, 118–139
    for behavioral change, 108
    client in, understanding, 121–124
        client's personal resources in, 122
        illness/injury severity and impact in, 121
        outcome in, expected, 121
    difficult communication in, planning for, 68b
    for distressed clients, 122–124
        access to exercise in, 123
        depression in, 123
        education in, 122
        fear of harm in, 124
        goal setting and positive outlook in, 122–123
        medication side effects in, 123
        multiple health problems in, 123
        pain in, 123
        social support in, 123
    effective, basics of, 127–133
        barriers to, 132–133
        directive and guiding communication styles in, 127–129
        motivational interviewing in, 127–128, 127b–128b
        OARS model in, 129–132, 129f (See also OARS model)
        sample client conversations in, 128b–129b
        work for professional in, 132
    for effective education, 136–139
        cognitive learning in, 138–139
        motor learning in, 136–138
    goals in, 120–121
    importance of, 119
    motivation in, 133–136
        change talk in, 134–136
        intrinsic, 119
        readiness to change in, assessing, 133–134
    for relationship building, 124–126
        first impressions in, 124–125, 125b
        nonverbal communication in, 126
        verbal communication in, 125–126
    self-determination theory in, 119b–120b
Competence
    in self-determination theory, 120b
    on self-motivation, 99
Compression fractures, in low-back pain, 666
Computed tomography (CT)
    coronary angiography, 178b
    coronary calcium scan, 177, 177b–178b, 178t
    quantitative, for bone mineral density, 563
    vascular imaging with, 177

Conditioning, operant, 96–98
Confidentiality issues, 152–153
Congestive heart failure, nutrition in, 185
Connected health tools, 163b–164b
Connection
    in communication, 120–121
    in self-determination theory, 120b
Connective tissue, 45b
Conscientiousness, 99
Consultation, 16, 16t
    mastering initial, 148b–149b
Consultation notes, 147–148, 149b
Contemplation stage, 101, 102t
    change talk for, 134–136
    resistance to change in, 133
Contraceptives, oral, on bone, 560
Contracts, personal-training, 155
Contraindications to exercise
    with arthritis, 544
    with coronary heart disease, 190, 191t
    with low-back pain, 669
    with pregnancy, 690, 691f–692f, 693f–694f
Contralateral shoulder press, single-leg balance with, 519f
Control, locus of, 100
Controlled motivation, 119
Conversations. See Communication
Coordination training, 512
Copper
    daily intake of, by age-sex group, 748t
    function and food sources of, 753t
Core
    anatomy of, 481–483, 482f, 493f
    in balance, 481–484
        fundamentals of, 481
        intra-abdominal pressure in, 483–484
        thoracolumbar fascia gain in, 484
    definition of, 481
    muscles in (See also specific muscles)
        function of, 482
        with low-back pain, 482
        spine and, 482, 483f
    stability model for, 481, 481f
Core exercises
    activation, 451–452, 451f, 451t
    function, 451–453
        quadruped drawing-in with extremity movement 452, 452f, 453t
        supine drawing-in, 451–452, 451f, 451t
Core function assessments, 502–507
    McGill's torso muscular endurance battery in 502–507 (See also McGill's torso muscular endurance battery)
    other assessments in, 507
Coronary angiography (catheterization), 177

INDEX

Coronary artery bypass grafting, 179–180
Coronary artery disease, osteoarthritis and, 537
Coronary calcium CT scan, 177, 177b–178b, 178t
Coronary calcium scoring, 177, 177b–178b, 178t
Coronary CT angiography, 178b
Coronary heart disease (CHD), 168–204
    angina pectoris in, 173, 173t
    case study on, 201–203
    CMES role with, 169–170
    diabetes mellitus and, 369
    diagnostic testing and criteria in, 175–179
        B-mode ultrasound assessment in, 179b
        coronary angiography (catheterization) in, 177
        coronary calcium CT scan in, 177b–178b, 178t
        coronary calcium scoring and CT scan in, 177
        coronary CT angiography in, 178b
        ECG exercise testing in, 176
        electrocardiogram in, 175–176
        intravascular ultrasound in, 179b
        MRI in, high-resolution, 179b
        radionuclide stress test in, 176
        stress echocardiography in, 176
        vascular imaging techniques in, 177, 177b–179b
    dysrhythmias in, cardiac, 173–174
    epidemiology of, 170–171
    exercise training recommendations in, stable CHD, 187–203
        2012 ACCF physical-activity recommendations in, 200b
        benefits of, 187, 188t
        candidates, 188
        contraindications to, 190, 191t
        fitness testing in, 189, 189t
        frequency and duration in, 195
        guidelines summary in, 200b–201b
        intensity in, 194–195, 194t
        interval/intermittent aerobic exercise training in, 196
        mindful exercise in, 198–199, 199t
        mode of exercise in, 195–196
        pedometry in, clinical, 193b
        resistance training in, 197–198, 198t
        stable angina and nitroglycerin administration in, 197b
        stationary exercise machines in, 196
        supervision recommendations in, 190–191, 193t
        weekly exercise energy-expenditure goals in, 189t, 192
        yogic breathing in, 199b
    heart failure in, 175, 175t
    high-risk primary prevention and stable CHD in, 170
    importance of, 169
    myocardial infarction in, 174
    nutrition in, 180–187, 181t
        for cardiovascular disease prevention, 180–181, 181t, 182f
        for congestive heart failure, 185
        for coronary heart disease, 183–185
        eating behaviors in, 182t
        eating plans in, 185–187, 186f
        food choice in, 182f
        registered dietitians and medical nutrition therapy in, 180, 183b
    overview of, 171, 172f
    primary prevention of, LDL treatment in, 222–223
    treatment options in, 179–180
Cortical bone, 558, 558f
Cortisol, stress on, 60
Counter-rotation, of thoracic spine and pelvis, 488, 488f, 490
Cover sheet, fax, 144–145, 145f
C-reactive protein, in metabolic syndrome, 346–347
Creatine, 777
Crepitus, 534
Crossed-pelvis syndrome, 673–674
Crossover crunch, in pregnancy, 709f
Crossover point, 36
CT angiography, coronary, 178b
CT scan. *See* Computed tomography (CT)
Curl, biceps, in pregnancy, 707f
Curl-up, 674, 675f
Curvilinear joint motion, in gait, 495, 495t
Curving movements, in gait exercises, 510, 511f
Cutting movements, in gait exercises, 510, 511f
Cytokines, in overweight and obesity, 319

D

D2 flexion pattern, 646, 646f
Dairy, 753–754
DASH eating plan. *See* Dietary Approaches to Stop Hypertension (DASH) eating plan
Deadlift
    Romanian, 520f
    single-leg Romanian, 517f
Decisional balance, 101, 105, 106b
Decision-making criteria, 162
Deep longitudinal myofascial sling, 500, 500f, 520, 520f–522f
    exercises for, 520, 520f–522f
Degenerative joint disease. *See* Osteoarthritis
Delayed-onset muscle soreness (DOMS)
    after hip replacement, 597
    after shoulder impingement syndrome therapy, 646
Depression
    in diabetes type 1, exercise on, 376
    in distressed clients, communication with, 123
    exercise on, 337b
    in health-challenged, 57
    obesity and, 336b–337b
    postpartum, 715
    in pregnancy, 714

INDEX

de Quervain's tenosynovitis, 654–655, 654f

Description, business, 159–160

Development, human, 25b–26f

Diabetes mellitus, 362–398
  body mass index in, 369
  cardiometabolic risk in, 368, 368f
  case studies on, 395–398
    T1DM, 395–396
    T2DM, 396–398
  CMES focus in, 395b
  complications of, 365t
  diagnostic criteria for, 367–369
    body mass index in, 369
    cardiometabolic risk in, 368, 368f
    general, 367, 368t
    metabolic syndrome in, 369
  epidemiology of, 363–364
  exercise recommendations for, 381–394
    aerobic training in, 381–382
    exercise programming in, T1DM, 386
    exercise programming in, T2DM, 387
    flexibility training in, 382, 382t
    guidelines in, leadership, 387b
    guidelines in, summary of, 394b–395b
    on nephropathy, 393
    on neuropathy, 393–394
    practical tips in, 388t
    progression in, 392–393
    rating of perceived exertion and heart rate in, 381
    resistance training in, 382
    on retinopathy, 393
    risks in, management of, 391–392
    risks in, T1DM and T2DM requiring insulin, 389b–391b, 389f
    screening and client assessment in, preparticipation, 383b–386b
  gestational, 367, 686–687
  nutrition in, 377–381
    carbohydrate counting in, 380b, 380t
    in gestational diabetes, 381
    goal of, 377–378
    medical nutrition therapy in, 381b
    in prediabetes, 378
    in T1DM and T2DM, 378–380
  overweight/obesity and, 21
  pathological consequences of, 369–370
    macrovascular disease in, 369–370
    microvascular disease in, 370
    neural complications in, 370
  treatment options for, 370–377
    emergency, 374b
    exercise, 374–377
    exercise, long-term benefits of, in T1DM, 374–376, 375t
    exercise, long-term benefits of, in T2DM, 375t, 376–377
    fundamentals of, 370
    non-pharmacological, 371–372
    pharmacological, 372–373
    surgical, 374
    team approach to, 370, 371f
    type 1, 363, 364–365, 364t
    type 2, 363, 364t, 365–367, 366f
      sleep deprivation in, 62

Diagnosis of disease, psychological impact of, 58–59

Diagonal arm raise, 545, 546, 546f
  in scapular plane, 637, 637f

Diagonal chop, in pregnancy, 709f

Diagonals, 467f

Diaphoresis, 174

Diastasis recti, 702, 702b–703b, 703f

Diastolic blood pressure (DBP), DASH eating plan, 760

Dietary Approaches to Stop Hypertension (DASH) eating plan, 760
  for diabetes mellitus, 378
  for hypertension, 252t, 260, 262–263, 262t–263t

Dietary Guidelines, 2020-2025, 745, 748b, 749–763
  1: healthy dietary pattern at every life stage, 749–751
  2: customize and enjoy, 751–756
  3: nutrient-dense foods and beverages, calorie limits, 756–760
  4: added sugars, saturated fat, sodium, and alcohol, limiting, 760–761
  calories, limiting remaining, 754
  dairy and fortified soy alternatives, 753–754
  development, 749
  Dietary Approaches to Stop Hypertension eating plan 760
  fats
    saturated, 758, 758f
    trans, 759
  fruits, 753
  grains, 753
  healthy dietary patterns for all, supporting, 751–763, 762f
  Healthy Mediterranean-Style Dietary Pattern, 749–750
  Healthy U.S.-Style Dietary Pattern, 749
  Healthy Vegetarian Dietary Pattern, 750
  MyPlate and MyPlate Daily Food Plan Checklists, 750, 750f
  NIH Body Weight Planner, 750–751
  oils, 754
  protein foods, 754
  sodium, 759–760, 759f
  sugars, added, 757, 757f, 757t
  vegetables, 752, 752f
  weight loss, exercise *vs.* nutrition for, 751b

Dietary intakes, actual *vs.* recommended, 752f

Dietary Reference Intakes (DRIs), 747

Dietary Supplement Health and Education Act, 765

Dietitians, registered. *See also specific conditions*

Diets. *See also* Nutrition; *specific types*
  low-carbohydrate, 65
  recommended intakes *vs.* American diet in, 185, 186f
  for weight loss

low-glycemic index, 330
popular, 330–332
recommended, 329–330
Dipeptidyl peptidase-4 (DDP-4) inhibitors, for diabetes mellitus, 373
Directive communication style, 127–129
overview of, 127
sample client conversation in, 128b–129b
Disc, herniated, 665, 670
Discogenic back pain, 665, 665f
Discounts, 155
Disease. *See also specific types*
psychological impact of, 58–59
Distressed clients
communication strategies for, 122–124 (*See also under* Communication strategies)
in overweight and obese, 337b
Diuretics, 256
Doctors. *See* Physicians
Dominance, synergistic, 412, 412f
Dose-response relationship, volume and health/fitness benefits, 29
Double-leg support, 486f, 487
Double product, 195
Downward-facing dog, modified, in pregnancy, 711f
Drugs, 12b
on physiological capacity
illicit, 67
performance-enhancing, 67
Dual-energy x-ray absorptiometry (DXA), 561, 562–563
Dumbbell wrist extension, 647, 649f
Dynamic balance, 41, 479
Dyslipidemia. *See* Blood lipid disorders
Dysmorphism, body, 57
Dyspnea, 70
assessment of, 287, 287t
in CHD patients during exercise, 194t
with heart failure, 175, 175t
in metabolic syndrome, 351b
Dysrhythmias, cardiac, 173–174

E

Eating behaviors, targeting of, 182t
Ecchymosis, 589b
ECG exercise testing, 176
Echocardiography, stress, 176
Edema, ankle, 70
Education. *See also* Communication strategies
of distressed clients, communication in, 122
effective, communication strategies for
cognitive learning in, 138–139
motor learning in, 136–138

Elbow pathologies, 646–651
lateral epicondylitis, 646–649 (*See also* Epicondylitis, lateral)
medial epicondylitis, 650–651, 650f, 651f
Elderly
low-back pain in, 662
physiological capacity in, 62
physiological function in, 508, 508f
Electrocardiogram (ECG), 175–176
Elongation, passive, 447
Emergencies, medical, preparing for, 85
Emotions. *See also specific types*
reflecting, in listening, 131
Emphysema, 299, 299f. *See also* Chronic obstructive pulmonary disease (COPD)
Employees, 157
Employment options
employees, 157
independent contractors, 158
self-employed, 158
Empowerment, client, 110
"Empty can" position, 644, 645, 645f
Encouraging, in reflective listening, 131
Endothelium, vascular, in atherogenesis, 171, 172f
Endurance training, hydration status and, 774b–776b
Energy balance
mechanisms of, 317
negative, 317
positive, 317
Energy-expenditure goals, in CHD patients for weekly exercise, 189t, 192
Engagement, of learners, 138–139
Entertainment, audience, in teaching, 139
Enzymes, proteolytic, on arthritis, 543t
Epicondylitis, lateral, 646–649
case study on, 655
causes of, 646
early intervention in, 647
forearm muscles in, 646, 646f
mechanism of injury in, 646–647
restorative exercise program for, 647–649
Functional Training, 647, 648f, 649f
Movement Training, 649
passive wrist flexion, 647, 647f
signs and symptoms of, 647, 647f
Epicondylitis, medial, 650–651, 650f, 651f
Epimysium, 493b
Epinephrine, stress on, 60
Equations, power, 677b
Equilibrium, 499
Equilibrium reactions, 499
Erector spinae muscles, 423, 423f

INDEX

Estimated Average Requirement (EAR), 747
Estrogen
    on bone, 559
    for osteoporosis, 564, 565t
Etiology, 527b
Eversion, ankle, 407
    resistive, 619f
Exam content outline
    Medical Exercise Specialist, 734–743
    as study tool, 6b
Executive summary, 159
Exercise. *See also specific types and disorders*
    with asthma, pulmonary responses to, 293
    goals of (*See also specific types of exercise*)
        identifying, 84
    health benefits of, 61–62, 84
    on low-back pain, 663
    volume and, dose-response relationship, 29
    for weight loss, 751b
Exercise-induced asthma (bronchospasm)
    exercise recommendations in, 292
    lifestyle choices in, 63
    pulmonary response to exercise training in, 293
Exercise-induced hyperglycemia, with diabetes mellitus, 390b
Exercise prescription, by physician, 8b
Exercise program
    designing, 88
    planning implementation of, 88–89
Exercise risks. *See also* Contraindications to exercise
    determining acute, 84
    in pregnancy, 690, 695t
Exercise testing
    in coronary heart disease, 188
    ECG, 176
    vs. fitness testing, 188
    with hypertension, before exercise participation, 266
    stopping, indications for, 266, 266t
Expenditures, health care, 3
External hip rotation, seated, 594, 595f
External humeral rotation
    prone extension with, 647, 648f
    prone horizontal abduction with, 647, 648f
External rotators
    myofascial release for, 598, 599f
    side-lying "clams" for, 592, 593f
External shoulder rotation, 645, 645f
    with scapular retraction, 647, 649f
        prone, 647, 648f
        side-lying, 647, 648f
Extinction, 97
Extrinsic feedback, 114

F

Facebook, 162b–163b
Familial hypercholesterolemia, 211
Fascia, 45b, 493b
    in gait, 492–494
    subsystems of, 494, 494t
Fat, body
    abdominal, 751b
    android (visceral), 317
    brown adipose tissue in, 318
    fat tissue in, 318
    visceral, 751b
Fats, dietary
    nutrition label, 766f, 767
    saturated, 758, 758f
    solid, 758
        nutrition label, 766f, 767
    trans, 759
        nutrition label, 766f, 767
Fatty acids
    for arthritis, 538–540, 539t
    for asthma, 290
Fatty liver, 66
Fax cover sheet, 144–145, 145f
Fear
    of harm, communication with, 124
    vs. hope as motivator, 107b
Feedback
    for adherence, 114
    intrinsic and extrinsic, 114
    for motor learning, helpful, 138
Female athlete triad, 560b–561b
Females. *See* Women
Fetal macrosomia, 367, 687
FEV1/FVC, in asthma severity, 279t
Fiber, dietary, 185
Fibrates, 221
Finkelstein's test, 654, 654f
First impressions, in relationship building, 124–125, 125b
F.I.R.S.T. program guidelines, 450t
First ventilatory threshold (VT1). *See* VT1
Fish oil, on arthritis, 542t
Fitness assessments, 27–28
Fitness testing. *See also specific types*
    baseline, 88
    with coronary heart disease, 189, 189t
    informed consent for, 85, 86f–87f
Fitness Training, 34–38, 35f
    assessments in, cardiorespiratory fitness, 35–35, 35f
    goals of, 34–35
    human development and, 25b
    submaximal talk test in, for VT1, 37–38
    talk test in, 36–37
FITT principle, 13–14

INDEX

Flat back, 416f

Flat-back posture, muscle imbalances in, 415, 416f, 416t

Flexibility, 589

Flexibility and muscle-length testing, 439–447
    passive straight-leg raise in, 444, 444f, 444t
    range of motion and movements in
        average, 439, 441t
        lower-extremity, 439, 439f
        lumbar spine, 439, 441f
        shoulder joint, 439, 440f
    for shoulder mobility, 445–447
        Apley's scratch test in, 446–447, 447f, 447t
        for flexion and extension, 445–446, 445f, 446t
        Thomas test for hip flexion/quadriceps length in, 443, 443f, 443t
    worksheets for, 439, 442f

Flexible muscles, lengthened, 449b

Flexion:extension ratio, 507b

Flexor digitorum superficialis, 650, 650f

Floor-roll and scramble-up exercise, 672–673, 673f

Fluid and hydration, exercise, 772–776
    endurance training and hydration status, 774b–776b
    before exercise, 773, 773t
    during exercise, 773–776, 773t
    gastrointestinal distress myth, 775b
    post-exercise, 773t, 776
    principles and recommendations, 772, 773t
    sodium, fluids with, 773–774, 774t
    sports drinks, 774, 774t

Focused practice, for motor learning, 137–138

Folate (vitamin B9), in arthritis, 541t

Folder, client, 147

Food access, 762

Food allergies, on asthma, 291

Food choices. *See also* Nutrition
    influencing, multilevel framework for, 182f
    on physiological capacity, 64–65
    socio-ecological model, 761–762, 762f

Food insecurity, 762

Food labels, 763–768, *See also* Labels, food

Food models, 755f, 755t

Food safety and selection, 768–769, 768b

Foot
    in gait, 498
    on kinetic chain
        pronation of, 420b, 420f
        supination of, 420b, 420f

Foot/ankle complex, in gait, 496, 496t

Foraminal stenosis, 665

Force, formula for, 677b

Force-couple relationships, 411–412
    pelvic, 411, 411f
    shoulder joint, 411–412, 411f, 462

Forced expiratory volume in one second (FEV1), in asthma, 283f

Forced vital capacity (FVC), in asthma, 283f

Force of habit, 324b–325b

Forearm muscles, 646, 646f
    pronator, 650, 650f

Forearm supination, resistive, 641b, 641f

Fortified soy alternatives, 753–754

Fractures. *See also specific types*
    osteoporotic, 557

Framingham 10-year risk algorithm, 218

FRAX tool, 562, 563b, 563f

Free radicals, 780

Frequency, intensity, time, and type (FITT), 22
    aerobic exercise, 29, 29t
    coronary heart disease, 195
    metabolic syndrome, 354
    resistance training exercise, 47, 47t

Friction, coefficient of, 531

Front-of-package labeling, 765

Front plank, 515f
    with hip extension, 515f
    single-arm, 515f

Fruits, 753
    portion size estimates, 756t

Fueling, exercise, 770–772, *See also* Nutrition principles
    before, 770–771, 770f
    during, 770f, 771
    post, replenishment, 770f, 771–772, 772b
    principles and stages, 770, 770f

Functional Training, 41–44, 41f, 49t, *See also specific applications*
    center of gravity in, 41
    joint mobility and stability in, 41–42, 42f
    kinetic chain in, mobility and stability of, 40, 41–43, 41f, 406–407, 407f
    muscle balance in, 42–44, 43f
    pain-compensation cycle in, 42, 42f
    postural assessment in, static, 42
    programming components of, 44, 44f
    restorative exercise, 588

Function-health-fitness-performance continuum, 23, 23f

G

Gait, 484–502
    bones in, 494
    case study on, 522–523
    central nervous system in, 498–499
    control of, 484–485
    definition of, 484
    fascia role in, 492–494, 493b, 494t
    fascia subsystems in, 494, 494t
    foot/ankle complex in, 496, 496t

fundamentals of, 485
gait cycle in, 486–487, 486f, 487t
hip in, 496, 497t
lateral subsystem in, 501b
learning to walk in, 485
lower limbs in, 498
muscle role in, 491–492, 491f
obesity on mechanics of, 335b–336b
single- and double-leg support in, 486–487, 486f
skeletal system in, 494–498
 axis of rotation in, constantly changing, 495
 bones in, 494
 curvilinear joint motion in, 495, 495t
 joint mobility in, 498
 pelvis in, 495
 synovial joints and articular cartilage in, 494–495
thoracic spine in, 496, 497t

Gait analysis, 509, 509f

Gait assessment, 507–508, 507f

Gait cycle, 486–487, 486f, 487t
counter-rotating in, 514
foot stability in, 407
mobility in, 488–490, 488f, 490f

Gait exercises, 510–513
agility ladder drills in, 510–511, 511f
coordination training in, 512
curving movements in, 510, 511f
cutting movements in, 510, 511f
obstacle walking in, 512, 512f
program for, 513t
progression of, 510, 510f
walking drills in, 510, 511f
walking with altered bases of support in, 512

Gait frequency, 486

Gait speed, 486

γ-linolenic acid (GLA), on arthritis, 542t

Gastric emptying, 771

Gastrocnemius, 590, 590f
in gait, 489, 490f

Gastrocnemius/soleus stretch, 615, 615f

Gastroesophageal reflux disease (GERD), in asthma, 291

Gastrointestinal distress, fluid myth, 775b

General partnership, 158

Gestational diabetes mellitus, 367, 381, 686–687

Gestational weight gain, on long-term obesity, 688b–689b, 688t

Get Active Questionnaire for Pregnancy, 691f–692f

Ghrelin, 319–320

Glenohumeral joint, 462
arm movements on, 423, 423f
exercises for proximal mobility of, 462–470 (*See also under* Stability and mobility training exercise examples)
muscles and force-couple relationships in, 411–412, 462

Glucosamine, on arthritis, 542t

Glucose
fasting, in metabolic syndrome, 348
self-monitoring of, 370

Glutamine, 779

Gluteals
myofascial release for, 45, 45f, 598, 599f
retraining of
 barbell *vs.* single-leg squat for, 674
 clamshell exercise for, 674, 675f
 for low-back pain, 673–674

Glute bridge, 459f, 520f, 548, 549f
with osteoporosis, 577f
single-leg supine, 520f

Glute dominance, in squat, 432

Gluteus maximus, 590, 590f
in gait, 489, 490f

Gluteus medius, 590, 590f

Glycemic control, 367

Glycolysis, 779
anaerobic, 36

Glycosuria, in gestational diabetes mellitus, 367

Glycosylated hemoglobin (A1c), 367

Goals. *See also specific topics*
for communication, 120–121
exercise (*See also specific types of exercise*)
 identifying, 84
instructional, clarifying, 138

Goal setting
for adherence, 113–114, 113b
for distressed clients, communication on, 122–123

Golfer's elbow, 650–651, 650f, 651f

Golgi tendon organ (GTO), 449

Grains, 753
portion size estimates, 755t
refined, nutrition label, 766f, 767
whole, nutrition label, 766f, 767

Gravity
center of, 479, 479f
 central nervous system in, 499
 in pregnancy, 695
line of, 418, 418f
in stability, 479

Grocery store tours, 769

Ground reaction forces, 406

Guest speakers, motivational, 139

Guiding communication style, 127–129
overview of, 127
sample client conversation in, 129b

H

INDEX

Habit(s), 98
    changing, step-by-step approach to, 98b
    force of, 324b–325b
Half-kneeling triplanar stretch, 457f–458f
Half roll back, with osteoporosis, 577f
Hamstrings, 423, 423f, 590, 590f
    in gait, 489, 490f
    myofascial release for, 598, 599f
    synergistic dominance in, 412, 412f
Hamstrings exercises
    lying stretch, 458f
    mobility, lying hamstrings stretch, 458f
Hamstring tendon graft, 610
Hand and wrist pathologies, 651–655
    carpal tunnel syndrome, 651–654
    de Quervain's tenosynovitis, 654–655, 654f
Hand tendons, 654, 654f
Harm, communicating with clients fearing, 124
Hatha yoga, for hypertension, 269b–270b
Hawkins-Kennedy test, 644
Head position assessment, 426, 426f, 426t
Healing, tissue, 587–588, 588t
Health behavior, determinants of, 95–100
    habits in, 98, 98b
    operant conditioning in, 96–98
        antecedents in, 96
        implementation of, 97b–98b
        response consequences in, 97
    overview of, 95
    social and individual factors in
        cognitive variables in, 100
        personality traits in, 99
        social support in, 98–99
Health belief model, 106–107
    create hope, not fear in, 107b
    force of habit and, 324b–325b
    self-efficacy in, 107
Healthcare community, working within, 7–8
Healthcare continuum, 3, 4–5, 5f
Healthcare expenditures, 3
Health Care Provider Consultation Form for Prenatal Physical Activity, 693f–694f
Health challenges, 56–89
    chronic diseases in, 58
    client discussion of, 68b
    depression with, 57
    lifestyle choices and impact on physiological capacity in, 62–68
    multiple, monetary impact of, 58
    polypharmacy with, 57
    psychological impact of, 58–62
        disease in, 58–59
        exercise on, 61–62
        stress in, 59–61
    social isolation and body dysmorphism with, 57
    10-step decision-making approach to exercise programming in, 69–89 (See also 10-step decision-making approach, for health-challenged)
Health claims, food labels, 764–765
Health Insurance Portability and Accountability Act (HIPAA) privacy rules, 144, 144b
Health-risk assessment, pre-exercise, 69–84. See also Pre-exercise health-risk assessment
Healthy Mediterranean-Style Dietary Pattern, 185, 187, 749–750
    for arthritis, 540
    for diabetes mellitus, 378
    for metabolic syndrome, modified, 351, 352t
Healthy U.S.-Style Dietary Pattern, 749
Healthy Vegetarian Dietary Pattern, 750
Heart disease, coronary. See Coronary heart disease (CHD)
Heart failure, 175, 175t
Heart rate
    diabetes mellitus, exercise recommendations for, 381
    maximal
        with asthma, 292
        calculation of, 29–30, 30f
    resting, 30
    steady-state, 37
    stress on, 60
    target, 30
    telemetry, 37, 40
Heart-rate reserve, 196b
Heart-rate response, in CHD patients during exercise, 194, 194t
Heel and toe walking, 545, 546f
Heel-off, 487t
Heel strike, 487t, 498, 498f
Helplessness, learned, 100
Hemiarthroplasty, hip, 596
Herbal supplements, 12b–13b
Herniated discs, 665, 670
High-density lipoprotein (HDL), 210f, 211–213, 213t
    in metabolic syndrome, 348
    treatment goals for, 215–216
    U.S. trends in levels of, 210t
High-intensity interval training (HIIT), in CHD patients, 196b
High-risk situations, managing, 111
High-to-low cable chop, 409, 516f, 672
Hip
    anatomy of, 590, 590f, 596f
    anterior musculature of, 422, 422f
    in balance, 480, 480f
    in gait, 496, 497t
    range of motion and movements of, 439, 439f

HIPAA privacy rules, 144, 144b
Hip abduction, single-leg with banded support, 706f
Hip adduction assessment, 421, 421f, 421t
Hip circumference, 321, 322f
Hip extension
  front plank with, 515f
  prone, 548, 549f, 594, 595f
  quadruped, 517f
Hip external rotators
  myofascial release for, 598, 599f
  side-lying "clams" for, 592, 593f
Hip flexion, Thomas test for, 443, 443f, 443t
Hip-flexor mobility exercises
  half-kneeling triplanar stretch, 457f–458f
  lying hip-flexor stretch, 457f
Hip-flexor stretch, lying, 457f
Hip fractures
  epidemiology of, 557–558
  surgery for, 566
Hip hinge, 432, 432f
Hip mobilization exercises
  with glute activation, 459f
  supine 90-90 hip rotator stretch, 460f
Hip musculature, in gait, 489, 490f
Hip musculoskeletal injuries, 590–600. *See also specific types*
  anatomy of, 590, 590f
  case study of, 625–626
  hip replacement
    partial, 596
    total, 595–600 (*See also* Hip replacement, total)
  iliotibial band friction syndrome, 590–593
  osteoarthritis, 594
    exercise recommendations for, 545b
    restorative exercise program for, 594–595, 595f
  trochanteric bursitis, 590–593
Hip replacement, partial, 596
Hip replacement, total, 595–600
  anterior approach to, 597
  case study of, 625–626
  early intervention for, 597
  indications for, 596
  minimally invasive approach to, 599b–600b
  movement restrictions after, 598t
  posterior lateral approach to, 590f, 596–597, 596f
  precautions in, 597
  prevalence of, 595
  procedure in, 595–596
  questions for physician after, 598b
  restorative exercise program for, 597–600
    delayed-onset muscle soreness and pain monitoring in, 597
    Functional Training, 598, 598f
    Movement Training, 599
    purpose and programming of, 597–598
Hip ROM complex, 548, 550f

Hip rotation
  seated
    external, 594, 595f
    internal, 594, 595f
  single-leg lateral, with band, 706f
Hip rotator stretch, supine 90-90, 460f
Hips and thoracic spine proximal mobility exercises, 453–462. *See also under* Stability and mobility training exercise examples
Hmg-CoA reductase inhibitors, 221
Hollowing, abdominal, 483
  on spine, 672
Home-exercise program, 14
Horizontal abduction, prone, with external humeral rotation, 647, 648f
Hormones
  on bone, 559–560
  postmenopausal, for osteoporosis, 564
Hover squat, 576f
Human development, 25b–26b
Humeral rotation
  external
    prone extension with, 647, 648f
    prone horizontal abduction with, 647, 648f
  external and internal, 466f
Hyaluronan, on arthritis, 542t
Hydration, 772–776. *See also* Fluid and hydration, exercise
Hypercalcemia, from inactivity, 65
Hyperglycemia, exercise-induced, with diabetes, 390b
Hyperinsulinemia
  with diabetes mellitus, 390b
  in metabolic syndrome, 348
Hyperlipidemia. *See* Lipid disorders, blood
Hyperosmolar hyperglycemic nonketotic syndrome (HHNS), 366
Hyperpnea, in metabolic syndrome, 351b
Hypertension, 244–272. *See also* Blood pressure
  ACC/AHA guidelines on prevention and management of, 252b–254b, 252t–253t, 254f
  on cardiovascular disease risk, 245
  case studies on, 271–272
  diagnostic criteria for, 250–251
    blood pressure classification in, 250, 250t
    blood pressure measurement in, 250–251, 251f
  epidemiology of, 245
  exercise recommendations for, 263–270
    cardiorespiratory training in, 267–268
    cardiovascular responses to aerobic exercise training in, 264–265
    exercise-related issues in, 266b
    exercise testing before participation in, 266
    guidelines summary in, 270
    mind-body exercise in, 269b–270b
    programming and progression in, 266

resistance training in, 268–269, 269b
stopping exercise test in, 266, 266t
value of, 263–264
medications for, 255–258, 255f (*See also* Antihypertensive medications)
in metabolic syndrome, 346, 348
nutrition in, 260–263
DASH eating plan in, 252t, 260, 262–263, 262t–263t
guidelines for, 260–261
nutrients affecting blood pressure in, 261–262, 261t
overview of, 246–249
blood pressure control in, long-term neurohormonal, 246–247, 247f
blood pressure control in, short-term reflex, 246
cardiac output in, 246
genetics in, 249b
physiology and causes in, 247–249, 248t
overweight/obesity and, 21
primary (essential), 247
secondary, 247
target organ damage from, 249t
on thermoregulation, 265b
treatment options for, 254–260
exercise, 258–260, 259t
non-pharmacological, 254–255
pharmacological, 255–258, 255f (*See also* Antihypertensive medications)
surgical, 258
Hyperthermia, in pregnancy, 697
Hypertonicity, 412
Hypoalphalipoproteinemia, 225
Hypoglycemia, with diabetes mellitus post-exercise, 390b–391b
Hypoinsulinemia, with diabetes mellitus, 390b
Hypotension
orthostatic, 258, 260b
post-exercise, 259

I

IgE antibodies, in asthma, 284
Iliacus, in gait, 489, 490f
Iliotibial band (ITB) complex, 590, 590f
self–myofascial release for, 45, 45f
Iliotibial band friction syndrome (ITBFS), 590–593
etiology and pathology of, 591
precautions in, 591
restorative exercise program for, 592–593
Functional Training, 592, 592f, 593f
Movement Training, 593, 593t
signs and symptoms of, 591
structural abnormalities in, 624b
Impingement syndrome, shoulder, 643–646. *See also* Shoulder impingement syndrome
Implementation

of operant conditioning, 97b–98b
planning exercise program in, 88–89
of restorative exercise programs, 470–474 (*See also* Restorative exercise programs)
safety concerns in, 14
standards of care in, 14
Inactivity. *See* Sedentary clients
Independent contractor, 155, 158
Inferior capsule stretch, 463, 463f
Inflammation
in asthma, 277, 278f
in overweight and obesity, 319
in tissue healing, 588t
vascular, in atherogenesis, 171, 172f
Information gathering, for communication, 121
Informed consent, 85, 86f–87f
for circulatory and respiratory fitness test, 85, 86f–87f
Ingredient list, 767
Inhibition, reciprocal, 412
Insomnia
exercise on, 61–62
health effects of, 62
Instructional media, 139
Insulin, for diabetes mellitus, 372–373
Insulin resistance
from inactivity, 65
maternal, during pregnancy, 686
in obesity, 223–224, 345
Intermediate-density lipoprotein (IDL) cholesterol, 210f, 211
Intermittent claudication, 70
Interval/intermittent aerobic exercise training, for CHD patients, 196
Interviewing, motivational. *See* Motivational interviewing (MI)
Intra-abdominal pressure, 483–484
Intravascular ultrasound, coronary, 179b
Intrinsic feedback, 114
Intrinsic motivation, 119
Introductory letter, 144–145, 145f
Inversion, ankle, 407
resistive, 619f
Iron, in arthritis, 541t
Ischemia, 174
Isothiocyanates, on arthritis, 543t

J

Joint(s). *See also specific joints*
in gait
curvilinear motion of, 495, 495t
mobility of, 498
mobility and stability of, 41–42, 41f, 42f, 406, 434,

498
  pathologies of, causes of, 527b–528b
  protection of, exercise for, 532b
  role of, 531
  synovial, 494–495
Joint injuries. See also specific types
  acute vs. insidious, 528b
  osteoarthritis from, 528b
Joint replacement. See also specific types
  questions for physician after, 598b
Juvenile arthritis. See also Arthritis
  diagnostic criteria for, 534
  epidemiology of, 530
  overview of, 533

K

Karvonen formula, 30
Kegel exercises, 704, 718, 718b, 718f
Kettlebell swing, 521f
Kettlebell Turkish get-up, 522f
Kettlebell windmill, 521f
Kinesthesia, 589
Kinetic chain
  ankle injury on, 408b, 408f
  foot pronation and supination on, 420b, 420f
  mobility and stability of, 40, 41–43, 41f, 406–407, 407f
  open and closed movements of, 464b, 465f (See also Closed-kinetic-chain movements; Open-kinetic-chain movements)
  in static postural assessment, 420b–421b, 420f, 421t
  subtalar joint pronation and supination on, 421b, 421f, 421t
Knee (joint)
  anatomy of, 600, 604, 604f
  articular cartilage of, 531
  in balance, 480, 480f
  in gait, 498, 498f
    musculature of, 489, 490f
  musculature of, anterior, 422, 422f
  osteoarthritis of, 43
  pain in, anterior, 600–604
  pes cavus and, 601
  pes planus and, 600–601
  Q-angle in, 601, 601f
  valgus of, 601
Knee extension, terminal 30-degrees, 547, 547f
Knee musculoskeletal injuries, 600–614. See also specific types
  anterior cruciate ligament, 608–612, 624–625
  case study of, 624–625
  knee anatomy and action in, 600
  meniscal, 604–608
  patellofemoral pain syndrome, 600–604
  total knee replacement for, 593t, 612–614
Knee osteoarthritis

  diagnostic criteria for, 534
  exercise recommendations for, 545b
  exercise treatment for, 537
Knee replacement, total, 593t, 612–614
Knowledge, for special populations, 4–5, 4f
Korotkoff sounds, 250–251, 251f
Krill oil, on arthritis, 542t
Kyphosis, 416f, 489
  muscle imbalances in, 415, 416f, 416t
  thoracic, in pregnancy, 699–700
Kyphosis, muscle imbalances in, 43, 415, 416f, 416t

L

Labels, food, 763–768. See also Food labels
  Dietary Supplement Health and Education Act, 765
  front-of-package labeling, 765
  health claims, 764–765
  history and present state, 763–764
  ingredient list, 767
  Nutrition Facts label, 764, 766f
  nutrition label, reading, 765–768, 766f
  percent daily value (PDV), 764, 766f, 767
  sample problem, 768b
Lactate threshold, 31b
Lactation
  bone loss in, 560
  exercise for mother in, 719
  nutrition in, 714
Lateral epicondylitis, 646–649, 655. See also Epicondylitis, lateral
Lateral lunge, 519f
  in pregnancy, 705f
Lateral myofascial sling, 500, 500f, 519, 519f
  exercises for, 519, 519f
Lateral plank, 519f
Lateral step, banded, 575f
Lateral step-up, 519f
Lateral subsystem, in gait, 501b
Latissimus dorsi, in shoulder stability, 640b
Lat pull-down, 640b, 641f
LDL particle number analysis, 215
Leaning side-bend, in pregnancy, 712f
Leap, side, 575f
Learned helplessness, 100
Learning, lifelong, 15–16
Learning style, client, adapting teaching to, 137
Legal issues, 156–157
Legal risks, avoiding, 157
Leg raise, straight-leg, 603
  passive, 444, 444f, 444t
Lengthened muscles
  flexible, 449b

INDEX

weak, 448b–449b

Length-tension relationship, 409–411, 410f

Leptin, 318–319
  negative feedback loop for, 318

Letter, introductory, 144–145, 145f

Leukocytes, in atherogenesis, 171, 172f

Liabilities, 156–157

Lifelong learning, 15–16

Lifestyle choices, on physiological capacity, 62–68
  alcohol in, 66
  with asthma, 63
  caffeine in, 67
  carbonated beverages in, 67
  with cardiovascular disease, 63
  in children, 63
  food choices in, 64–65
  illicit drugs in, 67
  inactivity in, 65, 66b
  mechanisms of, 62
  performance-enhancing supplements/drugs in, 67
  sun exposure in, 68
  tobacco use in, 64

Limbs, lower. See Lower extremities

Limited liability company (LLC), 158

Limited partnership, 158

Limits of stability, 479

Line of gravity, 418, 418f
  in stability, 479

LinkedIn, 163b

Lipid(s), 209. See also specific types
  therapeutic goals for, 215–216
    in children, 216, 217t

Lipid disorders, blood, 208–239
  case study on, 238–239
  diagnostic criteria for, 217–219
    ACC/AHA Pooled Cohort 10-year ASCVD Risk Assessment tool in, 218, 219f
    assessment tools overview in, 217–218
    Framingham 10-year risk algorithm in, 218
    long-term and lifetime risk assessment in, 218–219
    National Lipid Association ASCVD risk assessment and treatment goals in, 218, 218t
  dyslipidemia in, 209
    atherogenic, in metabolic syndrome, 346
  epidemiology of, 209
  exercise recommendations for, 233–238
    of Accreditation Council for Clinical Lipidology, 237b
    ACSM guidelines in, 234, 234b
    AHA/ACC 2013 guidelines in, 234b
    essential programming steps in, 234b–237b
    guidelines summary in, 238b
    weekly energy expenditures in, 233, 233t
  metabolic syndrome and cardiometabolic risk in, 220b
  nutrition in, 229–233
    cholesterol profile improvement in, 229–230, 231t
    eating plans in, 230–233, 232f, 232t
    triglyceride improvement in, 230
  overview of, 210–217
    cholesterol guidelines in, 216
    cholesterol guidelines in, consensus, 215
    chylomicrons in, 210, 210f
    HDL cholesterol in, 210f, 211–213, 213t
    IDL cholesterol in, 210f, 211
    LDL cholesterol in, 210f, 211, 212f, 212t
    LDL particle number, analysis of, 215
    lipid and lipoprotein therapeutic goals in, 215–216
    lipid and lipoprotein therapeutic goals in, in children, 216, 217t
    non-HDL cholesterol and apolipoprotein B in, 213–214, 214f
    other lipoproteins and associate CVD risk biomarkers in, 214–215
    triglycerides in, 210, 210f
    VLDL cholesterol in, 210f, 211
  treatment options for, exercise, 223–229
    exercise + statin combination therapy in, 227
    HDL response to, 225–226
    inactivity vs., 227
    LDL response to, 224–225
    non-HDL response to, 226
    pathogenesis of, 223–224
    pedometer step counts and, 228b
    for postprandial lipidemia, 227b–228b
    resistance training in, 228–229
    statins and myalgia in, 229b
    triglyceride response to, 226–227
  treatment options for, non-pharmacological, 220
  treatment options for, pharmacological, 221–223
    LDL and CHD prevention in, 222–223
    statins in, 222–223, 223t

Lipidology, clinical, 209

Lipoproteins. See also specific types
  in atherogenesis, 171, 172f
  in atherosclerosis, 209
  non-HDL, subclasses of, 213–214, 214f
  therapeutic goals for, 215–216
  therapeutic goals for, in children, 216, 217t
  U.S. trends in levels of, 210t

Listening, reflective, 130–131, 132b

Load/Speed Training, 47–49, 47t, 48f, 49t

Locomotion, 484. See also Gait

Locus of control, 100

Lombard's paradox, 451b, 489

Lordosis
  lumbar, in pregnancy, 699–700
  muscle imbalances in, 43, 415, 416f, 416t

Low-back pain, 660–679
  activity-related factors in
    exercise, 663

occupation, 663
balance and core training for, 482
biopsychosocial model applied to, 661b–662b
case study on, 522–523, 678
chronic vs. acute, 661
conditions in, 664–666
    discogenic back pain, 665, 665f
    herniated discs, 665, 670
    lumbar canal or foraminal stenosis, 665
    lumbar strain or sprain, 664–665
    microtrauma, 665
    osteoporotic compression fractures, 666
    pseudoclaudication, 665
    sciatica, 665
    spinal stenosis, 665
    spondylolisthesis, 666
    spondylosis, 666
    stress fractures, 664
    visceral disease fractures, 664
core in, 482
diagnostic criteria for, 666
epidemiology of, 661
exercise recommendations for, 669–677
    bird dog in, 676, 676f
    caveats in design of, 671
    clamshell exercise, 674, 675f
    client desire in, 669
    curl-up in, 674, 675f
    floor-roll and scramble-up in, 672, 673f
    lumbar torsion control test in, 672, 673f
    medicine ball toss in, 677, 677f
    muscle-activation patterns in, 670
    program progressions in, 671–677
    program progressions in, stage 1: groove motion/motor patterns and corrective exercise, 672–674, 673f, 675f
    program progressions in, stage 2: build whole-body and joint stability, 674–676, 675f, 676f
    program progressions in, stage 3: increase muscle endurance, 676
    program progressions in, stage 4: build strength, 677
    program progressions in, stage 5: power, 677, 677b, 677t
    push-up with BOSU in, 676, 676f
    push-up with staggered hand placement in, 676, 676f
    rolling bridge in, 674, 675f
    scientific foundation for, 670
    side bridge in, modified, 674, 675f
    single-leg squat matrix in, 674, 675f
    spine health emphasis in, 671
    training for performance vs. health in, 670
    training for stability in, 670
    training for strength and/or endurance in, 670
    training goals in, 670
    wall roll in, 672, 673f
individual factors in
    age in, 662

    smoking in, 662–663
    obesity and, 43
    in pregnancy, 700–701
    psychological factors in, 663–664
    from sedentary lifestyle, 43
    talking to client about, 664b
    treatment options for, 666–669
        contraindications in, 669
        evolution of, 667
        exercise treatment in, 668–669
        goals of, 666
        non-pharmacological, 667
        pharmacological, 667–668
        surgical, 668
    vertebral disc anatomy in, 665, 665f
Low-carbohydrate diets, 65
Low-density lipoprotein (LDL), 211
    cardiovascular disease prevention recommendations for, 181t
    on coronary artery inflammation, 211, 212f
    pharmacologic treatment of and primary prevention of coronary heart disease in, 222–223
    reduction strategies, compared, 211, 212t
    saturated fats, 758
    statin drugs on, 171
    therapeutic goals for, 215–216
        in children, 216, 217t
    trends, U.S., 209, 210f
    U.S. trends in levels of, 210t
Lower-cross syndrome, 423
Lower extremities. See also specific parts; specific types
    in gait, 498
    movements of, 439, 439f
    range of motion of, 439, 439f
Lower extremities, musculoskeletal injuries, 586–626. See also specific types
    case studies of, 624–626
    client screening in, 587
    hip pathologies in, 590–600
    knee pathologies in, 600–614
    lower leg, ankle, and foot pathologies, 614–624
        Achilles tendinopathy, 593t, 620–622
        anatomy and physiology of, 614
        ankle sprains, 616–620, 617t, 619f–621t
        plantar fasciitis, 620f, 622–624, 623f
        shin splints, 614–616, 614f–616f
    restorative exercise principles in, 587–590 (See also Restorative exercise principles)
        balance chain progressions, 593, 593t
        closed-kinetic-chain progressions, 593, 593t
        Functional Training, 588
        Movement Training, 588–599
        tissue healing, 588–589, 589t
    strains in, 589b
    structural abnormalities in, 624b
Low-force, longer-duration static stretches, 449
Lumbar canal stenosis, 665
Lumbar dominance, in squat, 432, 432f

INDEX

Lumbar lordosis, in pregnancy, 699–700

Lumbar pain, in pregnancy, 700–701

Lumbar radiculopathy, 665

Lumbar strain or sprain, 664–665

Lumbar torsion control test, 672, 673f

Lung disease, 276–308. *See also specific types*
    asthma, 277–298
    chronic obstructive pulmonary disease, 64, 298–308

Lunge(s), 514
    anterior, with medicine ball lift, 518f
    backward, with weighted vest, 573f
    lateral, 519f
        in pregnancy, 705f
    "never let the knees go past the toes" in, 433
    sideways, with weighted vest, 574f

Lunge to single-arm cable pull, 518f

Lying hamstrings stretch, 458f

Lying hip-flexor stretch, 457f

M

Macronutrients. *See specific types*

Macrosomia, fetal, 367, 687

Macrovascular disease, in diabetes mellitus, 369–370

Magnetic resonance imaging (MRI), cardiac, high-resolution, 179b

Maintenance stage, 102t, 103

Major depressive disorder. *See also* Depression
    obesity and, 336b–337b

Males. *See* Men

Marble pick-up, for foot intrinsic muscles, 623f

Marijuana, on physiological capacity, 67

Marketing
    for medical referrals, 153–155
    word of mouth, 153–154

Marketing plan, 160

Mass, center of, 479

Maximal heart rate (MHR)
    with asthma, 292
    calculation of, 29–30, 30f

McGill, Stuart M., 669–677. *See also* Low-back pain, exercise recommendations for

McGill's torso muscular endurance battery
    evaluation and application of, 507b
    principles of, 502
    record sheet for, 506, 506f
    trunk extensor endurance test in, 504–505, 505f
    trunk flexor endurance test in, 502–503, 503f
    trunk lateral endurance test in, 503–504, 504f

Medial collateral ligament (MCL), in gait, 498, 498f

Medial epicondylitis, 650–651, 650f, 651f

Medial rotation stretch, with towel, 644, 644f

Medial tibial stress syndrome (MTSS), 614–616, 614f–616f

Medical emergencies, preparing for, 85

Medical Exercise Specialist. *See* Certified Medical Exercise Specialist (CMES)

Medical nutrition therapy (MNT), 180, 183b
    for diabetes mellitus, 381b

Medical referrals, marketing for, 153–155

Medical release form, 84, 85f, 143

Medicine ball lift, anterior lunge with, 518f

Medicine ball toss, 677, 677f

Mediterranean-Style Dietary Pattern, Healthy, 185, 187, 749–750
    for arthritis, 540
    for diabetes mellitus, 378
    for metabolic syndrome, modified, 351, 352t

Men
    bone response to physical activity in, 570
    exercise recommendations for osteoporosis prevention in
        in middle-aged men, 572, 572b
        in older men, 572–573

Meniscal injuries, 604–608
    knee joint anatomy in, 604, 604f
    mechanism of injury in, 604
    postoperative rehabilitation in, 606b–607b
    precautions in, 605
    restorative exercise program for
        Functional Training, 607
        Movement Training, 593f, 593t, 603f, 607–608
    signs and symptoms of, 604–605
    treatment options for
        early intervention, 605–606
        non-operative, 605
        surgical, 605

Meniscectomy, 605
    rehabilitation after, 606b–607b

Menisci, 531

Menopause, in osteoporosis, 561b

Metabolic equivalents (Mets)
    in metabolic syndrome, 351b
    with myocardial infarction, 174

Metabolic syndrome (MetS), 21, 65, 220b, 344–357
    body mass index in, 345
    case study on, 355–357
    clinical implications and disorders with, 347b
    definition of, 345, 345f
    in diabetes mellitus, 369
    diagnostic criteria for, 347–348, 348t
    epidemiology of, 345–346, 346f
    exercise recommendations for, 352–355
        anaerobic exercise in, 353
        frequency in, 354
        guidelines summary in, 355b
        intensity and duration in, 354

resistance exercise in, 353–354
risk factors in, 352
$\dot{V}O_2$ reserve in, 352
walking in, 353, 353b
nutrition in, 351–352, 352t
overweight and obesity in, 345–346, 346f
pathogenesis of, 345, 345f
pathophysiology of, 346–347
physical activity on, 66b
treatment options for, 348–351
exercise treatment, 349–351, 349t, 350f
non-pharmacological, 348, 348t
pharmacological, 349
physiologic responses to exercise in, 351b
surgical, 349

Methylsulfonylmethane (MSM), on arthritis, 542t

Micelle, 778

Micronutrients. *See specific types*

Microsomal triglyceride transfer protein inhibitor, 222

Microtrauma, in low-back pain, 665

Microvascular disease, in diabetes mellitus, 370

Mid-stance, 487t

Military press, with shoulder instability, 641b

Milks
plant, 753–754
portion size estimates, 756t

Mind-body exercise, with hypertension, 269b–270b

Mindful exercise, in CHD patient, 198–199, 199t

Minimally invasive surgery, for total hip replacement, 599b–600b

Minute ventilation ($\dot{V}_E$), 293
in ventilatory threshold assessment, 35, 35f

Mobility
joint, 406, 484
lack of, factors in, 409, 409f
sedentary lifestyle on, 485
shoulder, flexibility and muscle-length testing for, 445–447
thoracic-spine, screen for, 437–438, 438f, 438t

Mobility and stability
joint-by-joint approach to, 408b, 408f
of kinetic chain, 407, 407f

Mobility training. *See* Stability and mobility training exercise examples; *specific applications*

Modified dead bug with reverse bent-knee marches, 456f

Modified disability model, 508, 508f

Modified downward-facing dog, in pregnancy, 711f

Modified side-bridge, 674, 675f

Monetary impact, of multiple health challenges, 58

Monounsaturated fatty acids, for arthritis, 540

Monster walk, banded, 576f

Motion, planes of, 488, 488f, 621f

Motivation, 133–136

autonomous, 119
change talk in, 134–136
controlled, 119
intrinsic, 119
readiness to change in, assessing, 133–134

Motivational guest speakers, 139

Motivational interviewing (MI), 127–128, 127b–128b
for nutritional advice for cardiovascular disease prevention, 181
sample client conversations in, 128b–129b

Motivator, fear *vs.* hope as, 107b

Motor learning
effective education for, 136–138
focused practice for, 137–138

Motor units, muscle, 498–499

Movement(s), 406–412, 484–502. *See also specific types and disorders*
in activities of daily living, 430
body mechanics in gym setting and, 474–475
case study on, 475–476
dysfunctional, factors in, 409, 409f
efficiency of, 406, 406f
five primary types of, 430
force-couple relationships in, 411–412, 411f, 412
gait in, 484–502 (*See also* Gait)
joint-by-joint approach to, 408b, 408f
joint differences in, 406–407, 407f
joint mobility and stability in, 484
kinetic chain mobility and stability in, 40, 41, 41f, 406–407, 407f
length-tension relationship in, 409–411, 410f
of lower extremities, 439, 439f
movement efficiency model in, 484, 484f
neural control in, 412, 412f
pain-compensation cycle in, 412, 413f
physiologic considerations in, 475
posture on, 407
of shoulder joint, 439, 440f
of specific joints, 406–407, 407f (*See also specific joints*)

Movement efficiency model, 484, 484f

Movement efficiency pattern, muscle imbalances on, 417

Movement patterns
five fundamental, 514
during squat, 432, 432f

Movement screens, 430–438
bend-and-lift, 430–432, 431f, 431t
pull assessment, 436–437, 437f, 437t
purpose of, 430
push assessment, 435–436, 436f, 436t
rotation assessment, 437–438, 438f, 438t
single-leg assessment, 433–435, 434t, 435f

Movement Training, *See also specific applications*
human development and, 25b
in restorative exercise, 588–599

MSM, on arthritis, 542t

Multifidi, 482, 482f

Muscle. *See also specific muscles and disorders*
    buffering capacity, 779
    core, 481–482, 482f, 493f (*See also* Core)
    in gait, 491–492, 491f
    pains in, from statins, 229b
    sliding filament theory of, 491, 491f

Muscle balance, 42–44
    movement efficiency pattern and, 43, 43f

Muscle fibers
    type I, in posture, 499
    type II, in bone movement, 499

Muscle imbalance, 405
    in dysfunctional movement, 409, 409f
    in flat-back posture, 415, 416f, 416t
    in kyphosis, 43, 415, 416f, 416t
    in lordosis, 415, 416f, 416t
    on movement efficiency pattern, 417
    in sway-back posture, 415, 416f, 416t

Muscle-length testing, 439–447. *See also* Flexibility and muscle-length testing

Muscle motor units, 498–499

Muscle recruitment, in arthritis, assessing difficulties in, 545, 546f

Muscle shortening
    overactive, 449b
    strong, 448b
    tight, 448b

Muscle strength, differences in, on each side of body, 475

Muscular endurance, 25b

Muscular strength, 25b

Muscular Training, 40–49
    Functional Training in, 41–44, 41f, 49t
        center of gravity in, 41
        joint mobility and stability in, 41–42, 42f
        kinetic chain in, mobility and stability of, 40, 41–43, 41f, 406–407, 407f
        muscle balance in, 42–44, 43f
        pain-compensation cycle in, 42, 42f
        postural assessment in, static, 42
        programming components of, 44, 44f
    human development and, 25b
    Load/Speed Training in, 47–49, 47t, 48f, 49t
    Movement Training in, 46–47, 46f, 49t
    phases of, 41, 42f, 49t
    self–myofascial release in, 45b, 45f

Muscular Training Movement Training, 46–47, 46f, 49t

Musculoskeletal injuries
    of lower extremities, 586–626 (*See also* Lower extremities, musculoskeletal injuries; *specific injuries*)
    of upper extremities, 632–656 (*See also* Upper extremities, musculoskeletal injuries)

Myalgia, from statins, 229b

Myocardial infarction (MI), 174

Myocardial ischemia, 70

Myocardium, 171

Myofascial release
    for gluteals/external rotators, 598, 599f
    for hamstrings, 598, 599f
    for quadriceps, 598, 599f
    self–, 45b, 45f
        of ITB complex, with foam roller, 592, 592f
        for scapulothoracic region and glenohumeral joint, 463

Myofascial sling(s), 494, 494t, 499–502
    anterior oblique, 501, 502f
    deep longitudinal, 500, 500f
    lateral, 500, 500f
    in movement, 499–500
    posterior oblique, 501, 502f

Myofascial sling exercises, 514–522
    for anterior oblique sling, 514, 515f–516f
    for deep longitudinal sling, 520, 520f–522f
    for lateral sling, 519, 519f
    for posterior oblique sling, 517, 517f–518f
    principles of, 514

Myopathy, from statins, 229b

Myosin, 491

Myostatic stretch reflex, 573

MyPlate, 745, 748b, 750, 750f

MyPlate Daily Food Plan Checklists, 750

N

National Lipid Association ASCVD risk assessment and treatment goals, 218, 218t

Neer test, 644

Negative energy balance, 317

Negative reinforcement, 97

Nephropathy, in diabetes mellitus, 370
    exercise on, 393

Network, of licensed professionals, 16, 16t

Networking, 146, 146b–147b

Neural control, faulty, 42

Neuropathy, in diabetes mellitus, 370
    exercise on, 393–394

New skills, slow and clear introduction of, 137

Nicotinic acid, 221
    with statin, 221

NIH Body Weight Planner, 750–751

90-90 hip rotator stretch, supine, 460f

Nitric oxide, from arginine, 779–780

Nitroglycerin administration, exercise guidelines for, 197b

Non-exercise activity thermogenesis (NEAT), 327b

Non-HDL cholesterol, 213–214, 214f
    treatment goals for, 215–216

Non-HDL lipoproteins, subclasses of, 213–214, 214f

Nonverbal communication, in relationship building, 126

Normoglycemia, 366

Notes
- consultation, 147–148, 149b
- progress, 145–146
- SOAP, 8, 149–151, 151b

Nucleus pulposus, 665, 665f

Nut milk, 753–754

Nutrient needs, 47t. *See also* Nutrition

Nutrition, 744–781. *See also specific topics*
- Acceptable Macronutrient Distribution Range, 747–748
- ACE Position Statement on Nutrition Scope of Practice for Medical Exercise Specialists, 745–747
- in arthritis, 538–540
- in asthma, 289–291
- budget, healthy eating on a, 769b
- calories, limiting non-nutritional, 754
- in cardiovascular disease prevention, 180–181, 181t, 182f
- for cholesterol profile improvement, 229–230, 231t
- in chronic obstructive pulmonary disease, 302–303, 302t
- in congestive heart failure, 185
- in coronary heart disease, 180–187, 181t
- daily nutritional goals in, by age-sex groups, 748t
- in diabetes mellitus, 377–381
- dairy and fortified soy alternatives, 753–754
- for diabetes mellitus, 381b
- Dietary Approaches to Stop Hypertension eating plan, 760
- *Dietary Guidelines, 2020-2025,* 745, 748b (*see also Dietary Guidelines, 2020-2025*)
- dietary intakes, actual *vs.* recommended, 752f
- Dietary Reference Intakes, 747
- fats
  - saturated, 758, 758f
  - trans, 759
- fluid and hydration, exercise, 772–776
  - endurance training and hydration status, 774b–776b
  - before exercise, 773, 773t
  - during exercise, 773–776, 773t
  - gastrointestinal distress myth, 775b
  - post-exercise, 773t, 776
  - principles and recommendations, 772, 773t
  - sodium, fluids with, 773–774, 774t
  - sports drinks, 774, 774t
- food labels, 763–768
  - Dietary Supplement Health and Education Act, 765
  - front-of-package labeling, 765
  - health claims, 764–765
  - history and present state, 763–764
  - ingredient list, 767
  - Nutrition Facts label, 764, 766f
  - nutrition label, reading, 765–768, 766f
  - percent daily value, 764, 766f, 767
  - sample problem, 768b
- food models and portion estimates, 755f, 755t
- food safety and selection, 768–769, 768b
- fruits, 753
- fueling, exercise, 770–772
  - during exercise, 770f, 771
  - post-exercise replenishment, 770f, 771–772, 772b
  - pre-exercise, 770–771, 770f
  - principles and stages, 770, 770f
- grains, 753
- grocery store tours, 769
- in hypertension, 260–263
- in lactation, 714
- in lipid disorders, blood, 229–233
- medical nutrition therapy in, 180, 183b
- in metabolic syndrome, 351–352, 352t
- MyPlate, 745, 748b, 750, 750f
- MyPlate Daily Food Plan Checklists, 750
- NIH Body Weight Planner, 750–751
- nutritional supplements, 776–780
  - client discussions, 780b
  - with efficacy and safety, no/little evidence, 779–780
    - antioxidants, chronic use, 780
    - arginine, 779–780
    - carnitine, 780
    - glutamine, 779
  - with efficacy and safety, strong evidence, 777–779
    - β-alanine, 779
    - caffeine, 777
    - carbohydrate ingestion, post-exercise, 777–778
    - creatine, 777
    - protein supplementation, 778, 778b
    - sodium bicarbonate, 779
  - labels, 780b
  - principles, 776–777
- oils, 754
- in osteoarthritis, 528–540, 541t
- in osteopenia, 566–568, 568t
- in osteoporosis, 566–568, 568t
- in overweight and obesity, 328–332
- portion size estimates, 755f, 755t–756t
- practical considerations, 769–770
- in pregnancy, 712–714
- protein foods, 754
- Registered Dietitians, collaborating with, 770
- in rheumatoid arthritis, 528–540, 541t
- scope of practice on, 746
- sodium, 759–760, 759f
- for triglyceride profile improvement, 230
- vegetables, 752, 752f
- for weight loss, 751b

Nutritional supplements, 776–780
- client discussions, 780b
- with efficacy and safety, no/little evidence, 779–780
  - antioxidants, chronic use, 780
  - arginine, 779–780

INDEX

carnitine, 780
glutamine, 779
with efficacy and safety, strong evidence, 777–779
β-alanine, 779
caffeine, 777
carbohydrate ingestion, post-exercise, 777–778
creatine, 777
protein supplementation, 778, 778b
sodium bicarbonate, 779
labels, 780b
principles, 776–777
Nutrition Facts label, 764, 766f
Nutrition Labeling and Education Act (NLEA), 764
Nutrition labels. *See* Labels, food
Nuts, for coronary heart disease, 184

O

OARS model, 129–132, 129f
affirmations in, 130
for change talk, 134–136
open-ended questions in, 129–130
reflective listening in, 130–131, 132b
summarizing in, 132
Obesity
on asthma, 291
insulin resistance in, 223–224, 345
long-term, gestational weight gain on, 688b–689b, 688t
low-back pain and, 43
maternal, in pregnancy, 687–688
Obliques, abdominal, 482, 483f
O'Brien active compression test, 633, 634f
Obstacle walking, 512, 512f
Office visits, 146
Oils, 754
portion size estimates, 756t
Omega-3 fatty acids
for arthritis, 538, 539t
for asthma, 290
for coronary heart disease, 184
Omega-6 fatty acids
for arthritis, 538
for asthma, 290
One-arm row, standing (weight-bearing), 574f
Onset of blood lactate accumulation (OBLA), 31b, 39–40. *See also* VT2
Open-ended questions, 129–130
Open-kinetic-chain movements, 464b, 465f
Open-kinetic-chain strengthening exercises, 588
Operant conditioning
antecedents in, 96
implementation of, 97b–98b
response consequences in, 97

Operational plan, 160
Optimism for change, in communication. *See* Communication
Oral contraceptives, on bone, 560
Oral hypoglycemic agents, for diabetes mellitus, 373
Ornish Diet and Lifestyle Spectrum Plan, 186–187
Orthopnea, 70
Orthostatic hypotension, 258, 260b
Osteoarthritis. *See also* Arthritis
on articular cartilage, 531
brief history of, 529b
coronary artery disease and, 537
course of symptoms in, normal, 532
diagnostic criteria for, 533–534
epidemiology of, 528, 594
exercise recommendations for, 540–545
cardiorespiratory endurance exercise in, 544
contraindications and precautions in, 544
flexibility exercise in, 545
guidelines in, lack of, 538, 540
with knee or hip OA, 545b
resistance exercise in, 544–545
exercises for, sample, 545–550 (*See also under* Arthritis)
of hip, 594–595, 595f
from joint injuries, 528b
of knee, 43
nutrition in, 528–540, 541t
overview of, 530–532
prevalence of, increasing, 529b
treatment options for
exercise treatment, 537–538
exercise treatment, on symptoms, 537b–538b
pharmacological, 536
surgical, 536–537
Osteoblasts, 558
Osteoclasts, 558
Osteonecrosis, 565
Osteopenia. *See also* Osteoporosis
case studies on, 578–580
definition of, 557
diagnostic criteria for, 561–563, 561t
epidemiology of, 557
exercise recommendations for, 569–578
from inactivity, 65
nutrition in, 566–568, 568t
treatment options for, 564–566, 565t
loading, hormonal and dietary interventions, 571b
Osteoporosis, 556–581
bone in
factors affecting, 558–560
structure and physiology of, 558, 558f
case studies on, 578–580
CMES focus in, 578b
definition of, 557
diagnostic criteria for, 561–563, 561t

dual-energy x-ray absorptiometry in, 561, 562–563
FRAX tool in, 562, 563b, 563f
quantitative computed tomography in, 563
quantitative ultrasound in, 563
epidemiology of, 557–558
exercise recommendations for, 569–578
guidelines summary in, with osteoporosis, 578b
guidelines summary in, with osteoporosis risk, 577b
for osteoporotic client, 575–576, 575f–577f
physical activity and bone response in, children and adolescents, 569
physical activity and bone response in, men, 570
physical activity and bone response in, postmenopausal women, 570
physical activity and bone response in, premenopausal women, 569–570
plyometrics in, 573b, 573f (See also Plyometrics)
programming and progression in, children and young adults, 571
programming and progression in, postmenopausal women and older men, 572–573
programming and progression in, premenopausal women and middle-aged adult men, 572, 572b
female athlete triad and, 560b–561b
menopause in, 561b
nutrition in, 566–568, 568t
beneficial, 567, 568t
calcium and vitamin D in, 566–567, 568t
harmful, 567–568
treatment options for, 564–566
exercise treatment, 566
loading, hormonal and dietary interventions, 571b
non-pharmacological, 564
pharmacological, 564–566, 565t
surgical, 566
in women, 560b–561b
Overactive muscles, shortened, 448b
Overhead press, in pregnancy, 708f
Overweight and obesity, 314–340. See also Weight loss
biology of, 318–320
adiponectin in, 319
brown adipose tissue in, 318
fat tissue in, 318
ghrelin in, 319–320
immune hormones in, 319
inflammation in, 319
leptin in, 318–319
peptide YY in, 320
case studies of, 339–340
diagnostic testing and criteria in
assessment methods in, 321, 322t
body mass index in, 321, 322t
hip circumference in, 321, 322f
waist circumference in, 321, 322f
waist-to-hip ratio in, 321, 323t
disorders and diseases related to, 332–333

epidemiology of, 315
exercise recommendations for, 333–336
aerobic program variations in, 335b
after bariatric surgery, 326b
cardiorespiratory exercise in, 335
gait mechanics in, 335b–336b
guidelines summary in, 338b
overview of, 333
physiological effects of, 333, 333t
programming and progressive exercise in, 334
resistance training in, 336
weight loss and weight-gain prevention in, 334
familial connections to, 317b
low-back pain and, 663
maternal, in pregnancy, 687–688
in metabolic syndrome, 345–346, 346f, 347–348
misconceptions and facts about, 315b–316b
nutrition in, 328–332
with bariatric surgery, before and after, 332
caloric intake reduction in, 328–330
dietary approaches to weight loss in, 329–330
popular diets in, 330–332
weight-loss simulator in, 329
overview of, 317
psychological issues in, 336b–337b
sleep-obesity connection in, 320b–321b
treatment options for, 323–328
behavioral therapy, 324
exercise treatment, 326–328, 327b, 327t, 328t
force of habit in, 324b–325b
non-pharmacological, 323–325
pharmacological, 325
small continual changes in, 328t
surgical, 325–326

P

Package plans, 155

Pain. See also specific disorders
distressed clients with, communication with, 123
muscle, from statins, 229b
in restorative exercise, avoiding, 590b
working with clients with, 413b–414b

Pain-compensation cycle, 42, 42f, 412, 413f

Palpitations, 70, 174
in CHD patients during exercise, 194t

Paraphrasing, 131

Parasympathetic nervous system, in blood pressure control, 246

Parathyroid hormone, for osteoporosis, 566

Paroxysmal nocturnal dyspnea, 70

PAR-Q+, 70, 74f–77f

Partial hip replacement, 596

Partnership, 158

Passive elongation, 447

Passive straight-leg raise, 444, 444f, 444t

INDEX

Passive wrist extension, 651, 651f
Passive wrist flexion, 647, 647f
Patellar tendon graft, 609–610
Patellofemoral pain syndrome (PFPS), 600–604
    early interventions for, 602
    mechanism of injury in, 600–601, 601f
    precautions in, 602
    prevalence of, 600
    restorative exercise program for, 602–604
        CKC *vs.* OKC activity, 602–603, 603f
        Functional Training, 603
        Movement Training, 593t, 604
    signs and symptoms of, 601
Payment policies, 155–156
Peak expiratory flow (PEF), in asthma, 282, 284, 284f
Peak flow meter, 284, 284f
Pectoralis major, 482, 483f
Pectoralis stretch, 463, 464f
Pedometer step counts
    for coronary heart disease patient, 193b
    for hyperlipidemia, 228b
Pelvic floor exercises, 718, 718b, 718f
Pelvic floor musculature, 482, 482f
Pelvic force-couples, 411, 411f
Pelvic girdle pain, posterior, in pregnancy, 700–701
Pelvic tilt, 455f
Pelvic tilting assessment, 422–423, 422f, 423b, 423t
Pelvic-tilt progressions
    modified dead bug with reverse bent-knee marches, 456f
    supine bent-knee marches, 455f
Pelvis
    counter-rotation of, 488, 488f
    in gait, 495
Peptide YY, 320
Percent daily value (PDV), 764, 766f, 767
Percutaneous transluminal coronary angioplasty (PTCA), 177, 179–180
Performance-enhancing supplements/drugs, on physiological capacity, 67
Performance Training, 39–40
    in Cardiorespiratory Training phases, 39, 39t
    VT2 threshold assessment in, 39–40
Periostitis, in medial tibial stress syndrome, 614
Peripheral blood vessels, aerobic exercise training on, 264–265
Peripheral vasodilators, 258
Persistence, 107
Personality traits, in health behavior, 99
Personal-training contract, 155
Pes cavus, 601
Pes planus, 600–601

Phosphagen energy system, 777, 779
Physical Activity Readiness Questionnaire for Everyone, 70, 74f–77f
Physician clearance, 84, 85f
Physician-critical pathway in, 6–7, 7f
Physicians
    contact information for, 146
    exercise prescription by, 8b
    referrals from, 153–155
Physiological capacity
    asthma on, 63
    cardiovascular disease on, 63
    chronic diseases on, 63
    lifestyle choices on, 62–68 (*See also* Lifestyle choices, on physiological capacity)
Phytoflavinoids, on arthritis, 543t
Planes of motion, 488, 488f, 621f
Plank
    front, 515f
        with hip extension, 515f
    lateral, 519f
    prone, 548, 549f
    side, 548, 549f
        in pregnancy, 710f
Plantar fascia stretching, 623f
Plantar fasciitis, 620f, 622–624, 623f
    early intervention for, 623
    mechanism of injury in, 622
    precautions in, 623
    prevalence of, 622
    restorative exercise program for
        Functional Training, 623, 623f
        Movement Training, 624
    signs and symptoms of, 622–623
Plant "milk," 753–754
Plant stanols, 184
Plant sterols, 184
Plaques, vulnerable, 171, 172f
Plyometrics, 573b–575b, 573f–575f
    ankle hops or hop progressions, 574f
    backward lunge with weighted vest, 573f
    side leap, 575f
    sideways lunge with weighted vest, 574f
    squat with weighted vest, 573f
    standing (weight-bearing)
        one-arm row, 574f
        shoulder press, 574f
Polypharmacy, 12b–13b, 57
Portion, 755f
Portion size estimates, 755f, 755t–756t
Position
    anatomical, 488f, 621f
    "empty can," 644, 645, 645f
    head, assessment of, 426, 426f, 426t
    scapula, normal, 424, 424f

INDEX

shoulder, assessment of, 423–424, 423f, 424f
Positive emotions, 120
Positive energy balance, 317
Positive outlook, for distressed clients, 122–123
Positive reinforcement, 97
Posterior capsule stretches, 463, 464f, 644, 644f
Posterior mobilization exercises, 462f
Posterior oblique myofascial sling, 501, 502f
　exercises for, 517, 517f–518f
Posterior pelvic girdle pain, in pregnancy, 700–701
Posterior shoulder instability, 641–643, 642f
Post-exercise hypoglycemia, with diabetes mellitus, 390b–391b
Post-exercise hypotension, 259
Postmenopausal hormone therapy, for osteoporosis, 564
Postpartum depression, 715
Postpartum exercise, 716–719
　benefits of, 716
　method of delivery on, 716
　physiological changes in, 717
　programming guidelines and considerations in, 717–719
　　core strengthening in, 719
　　general, 717–718
　　Kegel (pelvic floor) exercises in, 718b, 718f
　　for lactating mother, 719
　research on, 716
Postpartum weight loss, 716b
Postprandial exercise responses, in diabetes mellitus, 391b
Postprandial glycemia, in diabetes mellitus, 373
Postprandial lipidemia, exercise for, 227b–228b
Postural assessment, 412–429
　initial, purpose of, 13f, 412–413
Postural assessment, of static posture, 42, 415–429, 415b
　checklist and worksheets for, 427, 427f–429f
　chronological plan for, 419, 420f
　deviation 1 in: foot pronation/supination, and tibial and femoral rotation, 418f, 420, 420b–421b, 421f
　deviation 2 in: hip adduction, 421, 421f, 421t
　deviation 3 in: pelvic tilting, 411f, 422–423, 422f, 423b, 423t
　deviation 4 in: shoulder position and thoracic spine, 423–424, 423f, 424f
　deviation 5 in: head position, 426, 426f, 426t
　insights from, 415–416
　kinetic chain in, 420b–421b, 420f, 421t
　limitations of, 415b
　muscle imbalances in, 415–417
　　factors in, 417
　　in flat-back posture, 415, 416f, 416t
　　in kyphosis, 43, 415, 416f, 416t
　　in lordosis, 415, 416f, 416t
　　on movement efficiency pattern, 417

　　in sway-back posture, 415, 416f, 416t
　neutral spine alignment in, 415, 415f
　plumb line instructions for, 418–419
　plumb line positions in, 415f, 418f, 419
　postural deviations in, 415–417, 416f
　right-angle rule in, 417–418, 418f
　scapular winging and scapular protraction in, 425, 425f, 425t
Postural compensation, restorative exercises for, 447–450, 450t
　active agonist contraction and reciprocal inhibition in, 450
　goal of, 447
　low-force, longer duration static stretches in, 449
　passive elongation in, 447
　programming steps for, 447, 448t
　stretch-then-strengthen approach in, 449
　terminology in, 448b–449b
Posture
　body mechanics in gym setting and, 474–475
　case study on, 475–476
　interventions for correction of, evidence on, 405b
　on kinetic chain stability and mobility, 407
　occupational and lifestyle, 405
　physiologic considerations in, 475
　poor, 404
Posture, static, 415
　deviations in, 415–417, 416f
　neutral spine alignment in, 415, 415f
Posture correction, seated, 576f
Power equations, 677b
Power training, for performance. See Performance Training
Practice, focused, for motor learning, 137–138
Prebiotics, on arthritis, 543t
Precontemplation stage, 101, 102t
　change talk for, 134–136
　resistance to change in, 133
Preeclampsia, 687
Pre-exercise health-risk assessment, 69–84
　exercise history and attitude questionnaire in, 78, 83f–84f
　health-history questionnaire in, 78, 79f–81f
　health screening algorithm, 70, 71f–72f
　musculoskeletal health questionnaire in, 78, 82f
　PAR-Q+ in, 70, 74f–77f
　preparticipation checklist, 73f
　purpose of, 69
Pregnancy and prenatal period, 684–716
　biomechanical considerations in, 699–704
　　carpal tunnel syndrome in, 702
　　diastasis recti in, 702, 702b–703b, 703f
　　low-back and posterior pelvic girdle pain in, 700–701
　　lumbar lordosis and thoracic kyphosis in, 699–700
　　postural adaptations in, 699–700

INDEX

pubic pain in, 701–702
stress urinary incontinence in, 703–704
case study on, 721
CMES focus in, 720b
exercise during pregnancy in, 685–686
maternal fitness in, 686
physical activity participation rates in, 685–686
exercise techniques in, 704–712
core exercises, 709, 709f–710f
lower-extremity exercises, 704, 704f–706f
stretches, 711, 711f–712f
upper-extremity exercises, 707, 707f–708f
gestational diabetes mellitus in, 367, 381, 686–687
gestational weight gain and long-term obesity in, 688b–689b, 688t
maternal exercise and fetal response in, 689–695
concerns in, 689
contraindications and risk factors in, 690, 691f–692f, 693f–694f
high-risk exercises in, 690, 695t
signs to terminate exercise in, 690
maternal fitness in, 686
maternal obesity in, 687–688
nutrition in, 712–714
alcohol, tobacco, and energy drink avoidance, 713–714
caffeine, 714
fish and seafood intake, 714
fluid intake, 714
foods and caloric intake, 713
lactation, 714
safe food handling, 714
vitamin and mineral intake/supplementation, 713, 713t
physiological changes in, 695–697
cardiovascular system, 695–696
musculoskeletal system, 695
respiratory system, 696–697
thermoregulatory system, 697
preeclampsia in, 687
programming guidelines and considerations in, 697–699
aerobic exercise in, 697–698
musculoskeletal conditioning in, 698
rating of perceived exertion in, 699
recommendations and guidelines in, 697–699, 699t
special considerations in, 698t
psychological considerations in, 714–715
summary guidelines in, 719b–720b
Prenatal period. See Pregnancy and prenatal period
Preparation stage, 102t, 103
Press exercises. See specific types and indications
Press-ups, seated, 639, 639f
Prevention. See also specific diseases
chemoprophylaxis in, 12b–13b
disease, 11–12
of exercise relapse, 109

primary, 11
secondary, 11
tertiary, 11–12
Prevention and Public Health Fund, 3
Pricing, 155
Primary condition, 527b
Primary prevention, 11. See also specific diseases
Privacy issues, 16
Probiotics, on arthritis, 543t
Processes of change, 104–106
decisional balance in, 101, 105, 106b
self-efficacy in, 101, 104–105, 107
right assessments in, 105b
Professional networks, 16, 16t
Professional relationships, 143–153. See also Relationships, professional
Progesterone
on ligaments in pregnancy, 695
for osteoporosis, 564
Program participation, client knowledge of, 111b
Progress note, 145–146
Proliferation, in tissue haling, 588t
Promotional campaigns, in health facility, 146
Pronation
of ankle, 407
assessment of, 418f, 420, 420b–421b, 421f
of foot, on kinetic chain, 420b, 420f
of subtalar joint on feet, tibia, and femur, 421b, 421f, 421t
Prone arm lifts, 468f–469f
Prone extension, with external humeral rotation, 647, 648f
Prone external shoulder rotation, with scapular retraction, 647, 648f
Prone hip extension, 548, 549f, 594, 595f
Prone horizontal abduction, with external humeral rotation, 647, 648f
Prone plank, 548, 549f
Prone trunk lift, 576f
Proprioceptive neuromuscular facilitation patterns, for shoulder impingement syndrome, 646
Protein
foods, 754
portion size estimates, 756t
supplementation, 778, 778b
Proteolytic enzymes, on arthritis, 543t
Pseudoclaudication, 665
Psoas major, in gait, 489, 490f
Psoas minor, in gait, 489, 490f
Psychological impact, of health challenges, 58–62
disease in, 58–59
exercise on, 61–62

stress in, 59–61
Pubic bone assessment, 422, 422f
Pubic pain, in pregnancy, 701–702
Pull-down, lat, 640b, 641f
Pulling movement, 46f, 47, 514
Pulmonary disease, 276–308. *See also specific types*
    asthma, 277–298
    chronic obstructive pulmonary disease, 64, 298–308
Pulmonary function tests, for asthma, 279, 279t
Pulmonary rehabilitation, for COPD, 304b–305b, 304t
Pulmonary responses to exercise training
    with asthma, 293
    with COPD, 303, 303f
Punishment, 97
Pursed-lip breathing, for COPD, 306b
Push assessment, 435–436, 436f, 436t
Pushing movement, 46, 46f, 514
Push-up
    with BOSU, 676, 676f
    with staggered hand placement, 676, 676f
    wall, 639, 639f

Q

Q-angle, 601, 601f
Quadratus lumborum, 482, 482f
Quadriceps
    myofascial release for, 45, 45f, 598, 599f
    strengthening exercises for, in arthritis, 547, 547f
    Thomas test for length of, 443, 443f, 443t
Quadriceps dominance, in squat, 432
Quadruped bird dog, 517f
Quadruped drawing-in with extremity movement, 452–453, 452f, 453t
Quadruped hip extension, 517f
Quadruped shoulder stabilization, 639, 639f
Quantitative computed tomography, for bone mineral density, 563
Quantitative ultrasound, for bone mineral density, 563
Questioning, in reflective listening, 131
Questions
    closed-ended, 130
    open-ended, 129–130

R

Radiculopathy, lumbar, 665
Radionuclide stress test, 176
Range of motion (ROM)
    of ankle, 439f
    assessment of, 44
    average adult, 439, 441t
    of knee, 438f
    of lumbar spine, 441f
    of shoulder joint, 439, 440f
RANKL inhibitors, for osteoporosis, 564, 565t
Rapport, 27
Rate-pressure product, 194–195, 269
    in metabolic syndrome, 353–354
Rating of perceived exertion (RPE), 30
    in coronary heart disease patients, during exercise, 194
    in Fitness Training, 34
    for overweight and obese, 327, 327t
    in pregnancy, 696, 699
Reaction forces, ground, 406
Reactive postural control, in balance, 479
Readiness to change, assessing, 133–134
Reality check, for clients, 14
Reciprocal inhibition, 412
    with active agonist contraction, 450
    Lombard's paradox and, 451b, 489
Recommended Dietary Allowance (RDA), 747
Rectus abdominis, 482, 483f
Referrals, medical, marketing for, 153–155
Refined grains, nutrition label, 766f, 767
Reflective listening, 130–131, 132b
Registered Dietitian Nutritionist, 746
Registered Dietitians, 745–746
    collaborating with, 770
Reinforcement, negative and positive, 97
Relapse, 101, 104b
    dealing with, 109b
    prevention of, 109
Relationship building, client, communication strategies for, 124–126
    first impressions in, 124–125, 125b
    nonverbal communication in, 126
    verbal communication in, 125–126
Relationships, professional, 143–153
    confidentiality issues in, 152–153
    healthcare professionals communication in, 143–152
        barriers to, 152
        client folder in, 147
        consultation notes in, 147–148, 149b
        on deviations from guidelines, 143
        HIPAA privacy rules on, 144, 144b
        initial consultation in, 148b–149b
        introductory letter or fax cover sheet in, 144–145, 145f
        medical release form in, 85f, 143
        networking in, 146, 146b–147b
        office visits in, 146
        options for, 144
        physician contact information in, 146
        progress note in, 145–146
        promotional campaigns in, health facility, 146

SOAP notes in, 8, 149–151, 151b
importance of, 143
Relaxin, on ligaments in pregnancy, 695
Release form, medical, 84, 85f, 143
Remodeling
bone, 558
in tissue healing, 588t
Renin-angiotensin-aldosterone system (RAAS)
aerobic exercise training on, 264
in blood pressure control, 246–248, 247f
Repetitive movement, on mobility, 473b
Research
on ACE IFT Model effectiveness, 50b–52b, 51f, 52t
on postpartum exercise, 716
Resistance training. *See also* Load/Speed Training; *specific disorders*
in coronary heart disease patient, 197–198, 198t
Resistive ankle dorsiflexion, 619f
Resistive ankle eversion, 619f
Resistive ankle inversion, 619f
Resistive ankle plantar flexion, 619f
Resistive forearm supination, 641b, 641f
Resistive wrist extension, 647, 647f
Respiratory syncytial virus (RSV), asthma and, 280
Response consequences, 97
Resting heart rate (RHR), 30
Restorative exercise principles, 587–590
Functional Training in, 588
Movement Training in, 588–599
pain in, avoiding provoking, 590b
tissue healing in, 587–588, 588t
Restorative exercise programs
design and implementation of, 470–474
fundamentals of, 470
implementing restorative exercise in, 472–473
movement screens and flexibility tests in, 472–473
posture assessment in, 472
prioritizing in, 471
process in, 471–474
re-screening in, 473–474
source *vs.* symptom in, 471
using assessment and screening information in, 470–471
for postural compensation, 447–450 (*See also* Postural compensation, restorative exercises for)
repetitive movement on mobility in, 473b
stability *vs.* balance in, 474b
Retinopathy, in diabetes mellitus, 370, 393
Reverse bent-knee marches, modified dead bug with, 456f
Reverse flys with supine 90-90, 468f
Rheumatoid arthritis. *See also* Arthritis
cardiovascular disease and, 533b

classification criteria for, 534, 535t
diagnostic criteria for, 534
epidemiology of, 530
learned helplessness on, 100
nutrition in, 528–540, 541t
elimination diets for, 540
nutrients in, 540, 541t
supplements in, 540, 542t–543t
overview of, 533
stages of, 530b
treatment options for
exercise treatment, 538
pharmacological, 536
surgical, 537
Right-angle rule, 417–418, 418f
Righting reactions, 499
Right-side bridge:left-side bridge, 507b
Risk analysis, 161–162, 161f
Risk management, 15
Risks, exercise. *See also* Contraindications to exercise
determining acute, 84
in pregnancy, 690, 695t
Rocking quadrupeds, 462f
Role, CMES, 6–8, 21–22
disease prevention focus in, 11–12
physician-critical pathway in, 6–7
working within healthcare community in, 7–8
Roll back, half, with osteoporosis, 577f
Rolling bridge, 674, 675f
Romanian deadlift, 520f
single-leg, 517f
Rotation, *See also specific types and exercises*
assessment, 437–438, 438f, 438t
axis of, 489b
Rotational movement, 46f, 47, 514
Rotator cuff, 643
movements of, 463, 463f
muscles of, 638, 638f
tendinitis of, 643
Rotator cuff injury, shoulder impingement syndrome in, 643–646. *See also* Shoulder impingement syndrome
Rotator cuff muscle exercises, 466–470
closed-kinetic-chain weight shifts, 469f–470f
diagonals, 467f
humeral rotation, external and internal, 466f
prone arm lifts, 468f–469f
reverse flys with supine 90-90, 468f
Row
bent-over barbell, 518f
standing, 640, 640f
standing bilateral, in pregnancy, 708f
standing (weight-bearing) one-arm, 574f
Runner's knee, 600–604. *See also* Patellofemoral pain syndrome (PFPS)

S

Sacroiliac (SI) joint dysfunction, pregnancy, 700–701

S-adenosyl-methionine (SAMe), on arthritis, 543t

Safety
    food, 768–769, 768b
    in program implementation, 14

SAMe, on arthritis, 543t

Sarcomere, length-tension relationship in, 409–411, 410f

Sarcopenia, in COPD, 302

Satiety, ghrelin in, 319

Saturated fats, 758, 758f

Scaling, 134

Scaption, 647, 648f

Scapula
    actions of, 462
    arm movements on, 423, 423f
    force-couple relationships in, 411, 411f, 462
    movements of, 423–424, 424f
    normal position of, 424, 424f
    winging and protraction of, 425, 425f, 425t

Scapular plane elevation, with thumb-up position, 647, 648f

Scapular retraction
    external rotation with, 647, 649f
    external rotation with, prone, 647, 648f

Scapulothoracic articulation, muscles acting at, 638, 638f

Scapulothoracic joint
    movements of, 423–424, 424f, 462–463, 463f
    muscle balance and force-coupling in, 462

Scapulothoracic region proximal stability exercises, 462–470. See also under Stability and mobility training exercise examples

Sciatica, 665

Scoliosis, 416f

Scope of practice, CMES, 8–10, 9b, 10t
    coronary heart disease in, stable, 170
    in healthcare continuum, 4–5, 5f
    legal issues and liabilities in, 156
    nutrition, 746
    standards of care in, 13–17 (See also Standards of care)

S-Corp, 158

Screening and testing plan. See also specific types
    for baseline fitness, 88

Seated hip rotation
    external, 594, 595f
    internal, 594, 595f

Seated posture correction, 576f

Seated press-ups, 639, 639f

Seated single-arm overhead press, scapular plane, 48, 48f

Secondary condition, 527b–528b

Secondary prevention, 11

Second ventilatory threshold (VT2). See VT2

Sedentary clients, 485, 716
    anxiety in, exercise on, 337b
    blood pressure in, cardiorespiratory training on, 266
    diabetes mellitus in, 377 (See also Diabetes mellitus)
    elasticity loss in, 494
    energy stores in, 61
    leisure activity time of, 317
    lipid levels in, 227
    metabolic syndrome in [See Metabolic syndrome (MetS)]
    mobility and gait in, 485
    pelvic tilting in, 422
    physiological capacity in, 65, 66b
    plantar fasciitis in, 622
    postpartum, 716
    pregnant, 685, 689b, 690
        physician's clearance for exercise in, 719t–720b
        start of exercise program in, 699
    resistance exercise in, initial, 198
    sensory integration dysfunction in, 63
    stages of change in, 101, 102t
    triglycerides and HDL in, 227
    unstructured exercise in, 327b
    walking in, 268

Selective estrogen-receptor modulators (SERMS), for osteoporosis, 565–566, 565t

Self-blood glucose monitoring (SBGM), 370

Self-determination theory, 119b–120b

Self-efficacy, 21
    in health belief model, 107
    in processes of change, 101, 104–105
    right assessments for, 105b

Self-employed, 158

Self-esteem, exercise on, 337b

Self-monitoring, in behavior modification, 110

Self-motivation, 99

Self-myofascial release, 45b, 45f
    of ITB complex, with foam roller, 592, 592f
    for scapulothoracic region and glenohumeral joint, 463

Sensory integration dysfunction, 62

Serape effect, 500

Serratus punches, 640, 640f

Shaping, for behavioral modification, 112, 112b

Shear forces, 531

Shin splints, 614–616, 614f–616f

Shoulder bridge, 459f

Shoulder extension, 640b, 641f

Shoulder flexion, in scapular plane, 645, 645f

Shoulder-girdle muscles, anterior, 638, 638f

Shoulder impingement syndrome, 643–646
    anatomical structures in, 643, 643f
    early intervention for, 644
    "empty can" position in, 644, 645, 645f

INDEX

mechanism of injury in, 643, 643f
precautions in, 644
restorative exercise program for, 644–646
    Functional Training, 645, 645f
    initial stages of, 644, 644f
    Movement Training, 645–646, 645f, 646f
signs and symptoms of, 644
Shoulder instability, 636
    weight-lifting exercises and, 640–641, 641f
Shoulder instability, anterior, 636–641
    early intervention for, 637, 637f
    mechanism of injury in, 636–637
    precautions in, 637
    restorative exercises for, 638–640, 638f
        Functional Training in, 639, 639f
        Movement Training in, 640, 640f
    signs and symptoms of, 637, 637f
Shoulder instability, posterior, 641–643, 642f
Shoulder joint
    acromioclavicular joint after injury to, 635b
    articulations of, 633f
    muscles and force-couple relationships in, 411, 411f, 462
    range of motion and movements of, 439, 440f
Shoulder mobility assessment, 445–447
    Apley's scratch test in, 446–447, 447f, 447t
    for flexion and extension, 445–446, 445f, 446t
Shoulder packing, 465f
Shoulder pathologies, 636–646
    anterior shoulder instability, 636–641
    posterior shoulder instability, 641–643, 642f
    shoulder impingement syndrome, 643–646
Shoulder position assessment, 423–424, 423f, 424f
Shoulder press
    contralateral, single-leg balance with, 519f
    with shoulder instability, 641b
    standing (weight-bearing), 574f
Shoulder rotation, external, 645, 645f
    prone, 647, 648f
    with scapular retraction, 647, 649f
    side-lying, 647, 648f
Shoulder shrugs, 640, 640f
Shoulder stabilization
    quadruped, 639, 639f
    on stability ball, 639, 639f
Shoulder stretch, in pregnancy, 712f
Shrugs, shoulder, 640, 640f
Side-bend, leaning, in pregnancy, 712f
Side bridge, 548, 549f
    modified, 674, 675f
    in pregnancy, 710f
    rolling, 674, 675f
Side bridge:extension ratio, 507b
Side effects, medication, 123
Side leap, 575f

Side-lying "clams," for hip external rotators, 592, 593f
Side-lying external rotation, 647, 648f
Sideways lunge, with weighted vest, 574f
Signs and symptoms. *See also specific disorders*
    of excessive effort in CHD patients, 194, 194t
Single-arm cable press, standing, 515f
Single-arm front plank, 515f
Single-arm overhead press, seated, scapular plane, 48, 48f
Single-leg assessment, 433–435, 434t, 435f
Single-leg balance
    with contralateral shoulder press, 519f
    standing, 545–546, 546f
Single-leg hip abduction, with banded support, 706f
Single-leg lateral hip rotation, with band, 706f
Single-leg movement, 46, 46f
Single-leg Romanian deadlift, 517f
Single-leg squat, 548, 548f, 674
    in pregnancy, 705f
Single-leg squat matrix, 674, 675f
Single-leg supine hip bridge, 520f
Single-leg support, 486–487, 486f
Sitting stretch, for anterior compartment, 615, 616f
Sit-to-stand squat, 704f
6-minute walk test (6MWT), 294, 295b, 295f
Skeletal system, in gait, 494–498
    axis of rotation in, constantly changing, 495
    bones in, 494
    curvilinear joint motion in, 495, 495t
    joint mobility in, 498
    pelvis in, 495
    synovial joints and articular cartilage in, 494–495
SLAP lesion, 641b
Sleep, exercise on, 61–62
Sleep-obesity connection, 320b–321b
Sleep problems
    exercise on, 61–62
    health effects of, 62
Sliding filament theory, 491, 491f
SMART goals
    for behavioral change, 113
    in stages of change, 103
Smoking
    cessation of, for COPD, 300
    excessive, on bone, 560
    in low-back pain, 662–663
    on physiological capacity, 64
SOAP notes, 8, 149–151, 151b
Social isolation, in health-challenged, 57
Social support
    for client empowerment, 110
    communication with distressed clients on, 123

in health behavior, 98–99
Socio-ecological model, 761–762, 762f
Sodium
    on blood pressure, 261–262
    dietary, 759–760, 759f
    exercise intake, 773–774, 774t
    for hypertension treatment, 261–262
Sodium bicarbonate, supplemental, 779
Soft drinks, on physiological capacity, 67
Sole proprietorship, 158
Soleus stretch, 615, 615f
Solid fats, 758
    nutrition label, 766f, 767
Somatosensory system, in balance, 480
Soy alternatives, fortified, 753–754
Special populations. *See also specific types*
    specific knowledge for, 4–5, 4f
Spinal extensions, 460f–461f
Spinal stenosis, 665
Spinal twists, 461f
Spine
    core and, 482, 483f
    frontal and sagittal views of, 413, 413f
Spirometry
    for asthma, 282–283, 282f, 283f
    of COPD, 300, 300t
Spondylolisthesis, in low-back pain, 666
Spondylosis, in low-back pain, 666
Sports drinks, 774, 774t
Squat (squatting), 514
    barbell, 674
    body-weight, 548, 548f
    dumbbells, 48, 48f
    hover, 576f
    movement patterns in, 432, 432f
    "never let the knees go past the toes" in, 433
    single-leg, 548, 548f, 674
        in pregnancy, 705f
    sit-to-stand, 704f
    with weighted vest, 573f
Squat matrix, single-leg, 674, 675f
Stability
    vs. balance, 474b
    joint, 406, 484
    limits of, 479
Stability and mobility training exercise examples, 451–470
    proximal mobility: hips and thoracic spine, 453–462
        cat-cow, 454f
        goal and principles of, 453–454
        hamstrings mobility (lying hamstrings stretch), 458f
        hip-flexor mobility (lying hip-flexor stretch), 457f
        hip-flexor mobility progression (half-kneeling triplanar stretch), 457f–458f
        hip mobilization (supine 90-90 hip rotator stretch), 460f
        hip mobilization with glute activation (shoulder bridge), 459f
        pelvic-tilt progressions (modified dead bug with reverse bent-knee marches), 456f
        pelvic-tilt progressions (supine bent-knee marches), 455f
        pelvic tilts, 455f
        posterior mobilization (rocking quadrupeds), 462f
        thoracic-spine mobilization exercises: spinal extensions, 460f–461f
        thoracic-spine mobilization exercises: spinal twists, 461f
    proximal stability: core function, 451–453
        quadruped drawing-in with extremity movement, 452–453, 452f, 453t
        supine drawing-in, 451–452, 451f, 451t
    proximal stability of scapulothoracic region and proximal mobility of glenohumeral joint, 462–470
        anterior capsule stretch, 463, 464f
        closed-kinetic-chain weight shifts, 469f–470f
        diagonals, 467f
        goals of, 462
        humeral rotation, external and internal, 465f
        inferior capsule stretch, 463, 463f
        key factors in, 463
        movements in, 462–463, 463f
        muscle balance and force-coupling in, 462
        open- and closed-kinetic-chain movements in 464b, 465f
        posterior capsule stretches, 463, 464f
        prone arm lifts, 468f–469f
        reverse flys with supine 90-90, 468f
        self-myofascial release, 463
        shoulder packing, 465f
        superior capsule stretch, 463, 464f
Stability ball, shoulder stabilization on, 639, 639f
Stable angina, 173
    exercise recommendations for, 197b
Stages of change, 101–103, 102t. *See also specific stages*
    moving forward and backward in, 134
    resistance to change in, 133–134
Stance
    mid-stance, 487t
    phase of, 486–487, 486f
    terminal, 487t
Standards of care, 13–17. *See also specific topics*
    10-step decision-making approach for special populations in, 15
    consultations in, 16, 16t
    knowing one's limits in, 16–17
    lifelong learning in, 15–16
    privacy issues in, 16
    program design components in, 13–14
    risk management in, 15
    safety concerns in program implementation in, 14

INDEX

Standing abduction, 592, 592f
Standing adduction, 592, 592f
Standing bilateral cable press, 516f
Standing bilateral row, in pregnancy, 708f
Standing chest press, 707f
Standing one-arm row, 574f
Standing rows, 640, 640f
Standing shoulder press, 574f
Standing single-arm cable press, 515f
Standing single-leg balance, 545–546, 546f
Standing "toe drag" stretch, for anterior compartment, 615, 616f
Stanols, plant, 184
Static balance, 41
Static posture. *See also* Posture, static
    assessment of, 42, 415–429 (*See also* Postural assessment, of static posture)
Static stretching, low-force, longer duration, 449
Statins, 221, 222–223
    intensive *vs.* moderate therapy with, 223, 223t
    myalgia and, 229b
    with nicotinic acid, 221
Stationary exercise machines, for CHD patients, 196
Step, banded lateral, 575f
Step counts, pedometer
    for CHD patients, 193b
    for hyperlipidemia, 228b
Step frequency, 486
Step length, 486, 486f
Step-up, 520f
    lateral, 519f
Step width, 486, 486f
Sterols, plant, 184
Stimulus control, 96
    for behavioral modification, 112, 112b
Straight-leg raise, 603
    passive, 444, 444f, 444t
Strengthening exercises. *See also specific types and disorders*
    closed-kinetic-chain, 588
    open-kinetic-chain, 588
Stress
    definition of, 59
    on health, 59–61
    psychological, in pregnancy, 715b
Stress echocardiography, 176
Stress fractures, in low-back pain, 664
Stressors
    external, 59
    internal, 59–60
Stress reaction, 60

Stress test, radionuclide, 176
Stress urinary incontinence, in pregnancy, 703–704
Stretches (stretching). *See also specific types and indications*
    in pregnancy, 711, 711f
Stretch-shortening cycle, 493
Stretch-then-strengthen approach, 449
Stride length, 486, 486f
Stroke, in diabetes mellitus, 369
Strong muscles, shortened, 448b
Strontium ranelate, for osteoporosis, 566
Study tools, exam content outline as, 6b
Submaximal talk test, 37–38
Subtalar joint, on feet, tibia, and femur
    pronation of, 421b, 421f, 421t
    supination of, 421b, 421f, 421t
Success, 109b
Sugars, added, 757, 757f, 757t
    nutrition label, 766f, 767
Summarizing, 132
Sun exposure, 68
Superior capsule stretch, 463, 464f
Supination
    of ankle, 407
    of ankle, tests for, 418f, 420, 420b–421b, 421f
    of foot, on kinetic chain, 420b, 420f
    of subtalar joint, on feet, tibia, and femur, 421b, 421f, 421t
Supine 90-90 hip rotator stretch, 460f
Supine bent-knee marches, 455f
Supine drawing-in, 451–452, 451f, 451t
Supplements, 12b–13b
    for arthritis, 540, 542t–543t
    herbal, 12b–13b
    performance-enhancing, 67
    for pregnancy, 713, 713t
Supplements, nutritional, 776–780. *See also* Nutritional supplements
Support, base of, 479
    central nervous system in, 499
Sway-back posture, 416f
    muscle imbalances in, 415, 416f, 416t
Swing phase, 486, 486f, 487t
SWOT analysis, 161–162, 161f
Sympathetic nervous system
    aerobic exercise training on, 264
    in blood pressure control, 246
Symphysitis, in pregnancy, 701–702
Syncope, 70
    with cardiac arrhythmias, 174
Syndrome, 345. *See also specific types*

Synergistic dominance, 412, 412f
Synovial cells, 531
Synovial fluid, in arthritis, 527
Synovial joints, 494–495
  in gait, 494–495
Synovial membrane, 531
Systolic blood pressure (SBP)
  DASH eating plan, 760
  in metabolic syndrome, 351b

T

Tachycardia, 70
Tai chi, for hypertension, 269b
Talk test, 30, 36–37
Target heart rate (THR), 30
Task choice, 107
Telemetry, heart rate, 37, 40
10-step decision-making approach, for health-challenged, 69–89
  overview and value of, 69
  step 1: perform pre-exercise health-risk assessment, 69–84 (*See also* Pre-exercise health-risk assessment)
  step 2: obtain physician clearance, 84, 85f
  step 3: identify exercise benefits and goals, 84
  step 4: determine acute exercise risks, 84
  step 5: prepare for medical emergencies, 85
  step 6: obtain informed consent, 85, 86f–87f
  step 7: plan baseline fitness screening and testing, 88
  step 8: design exercise program, 88
  step 9: plan exercise program implementation, 88–89
  step 10: double-check established guidelines, 89
10-step decision-making approach, for special populations, 15
Tendinitis
  bicipital, 641b, 641f
  rotator cuff, 643
Tendon grafts, for ACL injuries
  hamstring, 610
  patellar, 609–610
Tennis elbow, 646–649, 655. *See also* Epicondylitis, lateral
Tenosynovitis, de Quervain's, 654–655, 654f
Tensegrity, 489b
Tensor fasciae latae (TFL), 590, 590f
Terminal 30-degrees knee extension, 547, 547f
Terminal extensions (closed chain), 547, 547f
Terminal stance, 487t
Tertiary prevention, 11–12
Texting tenosynovitis, 654–655, 654f
Therapeutic Lifestyle Change (TLC) eating plan, 230–233, 232f, 232t
  for metabolic syndrome, 351–352, 352t
Thermogenesis, non-exercise activity, 327b
Thermoregulation
  hypertension on, 265b
  in pregnancy, 697
Thiazolidinediones, for diabetes mellitus, 373
Thomas test for hip flexion/quadriceps length, 443, 443f, 443t
Thoracic kyphosis, in pregnancy, 699–700
Thoracic mobility exercise, with osteoporosis, 575f
Thoracic spine
  assessment of, 423–424, 423f, 424f
  counter-rotation of, in gait, 488, 488f, 490
  in gait, 496, 497t
Thoracic-spine mobility screen, 437–438, 438f, 433t
Thoracic-spine mobilization exercises
  spinal extensions, 460f–461f
  spinal twists, 461f
Thoracolumbar fascia gain, 484
Three-zone intensity model, 31, 32f, 32t–33t
Tidal volume
  in metabolic syndrome, 351b
  in ventilatory threshold assessment, 35
Tight muscles, shortened, 448b
Tissue healing, 587–588, 588t
Tobacco use. *See* Smoking
"Toe drag" stretch, standing, for anterior compartment, 615, 616f
Tolerable Upper Intake Level (UL), 747
Total hip replacement, total, 595–600, 625–626. *See also* Hip replacement, total
Total knee replacement, 593t, 612–614
Total peripheral resistance (TPR), 246
Towel, medial rotation stretch with, 644, 644f
Towel crunches, 618, 620f
Trabecular bone, 558, 558f
Training parameters. *See also specific types*
  traditional *vs.* contemporary, 21, 22t
Trans fats, 759
  nutrition label, 766f, 767
Transtheoretical model of behavioral change, 100–106
  overview of, 100–101
  processes of change in, 104
  relapse in, 101, 104b
  stages of change in, 101–103, 102t
Transverse abdominis, 481, 482, 482f, 483f
  with low-back pain, 482
Trendelenburg gait, in trochanteric bursitis, 591
Triceps surae, 421b, 421f
Triggers, 59–60
  for asthma, 277, 280, 280t
  of COPD exacerbation, 301

Triglycerides, 171, 210, 210f
    in metabolic syndrome, 348
    nutrition for improving profile of, 230
    treatment goals for, 215–216
    U.S. trends in levels of, 210t

Triplanar stretch, half-kneeling, 457f–458f

Trochanteric bursitis, 590–593
    etiology and pathology of, 590
    Functional Training, 592, 592f, 593f
    Movement Training, 593, 593t
    precautions in, 591
    restorative exercise program for, 592–593
    signs and symptoms of, 591

Trunk extensor endurance test, 504–505, 505f

Trunk flexor endurance test, 502–503, 503f

Trunk lateral endurance test, 503–504, 504f

Trunk lift, prone, 576f

Trust, in communication, 120–121

T-spine. *See* Thoracic spine

Turkish get-up, kettlebell, 522f

Twitter, 163b

Type II muscle fibers, in bone movement, 499

Type I muscle fibers, in posture, 499

U

Ultrasound
    B-mode, 179b
    intravascular, coronary, 179b
    quantitative, for bone mineral density, 563

Ultraviolet rays, on physiological capacity, 68

Unstable angina, 173

Unstructured exercise, 327b

Upper extremities, musculoskeletal injuries, 632–656. *See also specific types*
    acromioclavicular joint injuries
        acromioclavicular joint sprain in, 633–636, 633f
        classification of, 633, 634f
    case studies on
        acromioclavicular joint separation, 656
        lateral epicondylitis, 655
    classification of, 634f
    elbow pathologies, 646–651
        lateral epicondylitis, 646–649
        medial epicondylitis, 650–651, 650f, 651f
    shoulder pathologies, 636–646
        anterior shoulder instability, 636–641
        posterior shoulder instability, 641–643
        shoulder impingement syndrome, 643–646
        shoulder joint articulations in, 633f
    wrist and hand pathologies, 651–655
        carpal tunnel syndrome, 651–654
        de Quervain's tenosynovitis, 654–655, 654f

Urinary incontinence, stress, in pregnancy, 703–704

U.S.-Style Dietary Pattern, Healthy, 749

V

Valgus, 538b
    knee, 601

Valsalva maneuver
    with cardiac arrhythmias, 174
    with hypertension, avoiding, 269

Varus, 538b

Vascular imaging techniques, 177, 177b–179b

Vascular inflammation, in atherogenesis, 171, 172f

Vasodilators, peripheral, 258

Vasopressin, in blood pressure control, 246

Vastus medialis oblique (VMO) muscle, in patellofemoral pain syndrome, 601

Vegan, 750

Vegetables, 752, 752f
    portion size estimates, 756t

Vegetarian Dietary Pattern, Healthy, 750

Vegetarians, 750

Velocity, formula for, 677b

Ventilation, minute, 293

Ventilatory threshold
    assessment of, 35–36, 35f
    second, in asthma exercise programming, 298

Ventricular arrhythmias, 173–174

Vertebral disc anatomy, 665, 665f

Vertebral fractures
    epidemiology of, 557
    surgery for, 566

Very-low-density lipoprotein (VLDL) cholesterol, 210f, 211

Vestibular system, in balance, 481

Virtual tools, 162b–164b
    business-management, 162b–163b
    connected health, 163b–164b

Visceral fat, 317, 751b

Visual system, in balance, 480

Vitamin B9 (folate), in arthritis, 541t

Vitamin D, in arthritis, 541t

$\dot{V}O_2$max, 196b
    with asthma, 293
    with coronary heart disease, 175, 175t
    maximal heart rate calculation for, 30

$\dot{V}O_2$peak, 196b

$\dot{V}O_2$reserve ($\dot{V}O_2$R), 196b
    heart rate calculation for, 30
    with metabolic syndrome, exercise for, 352

VT1, 30, 31b
    crossover point and ventilation in, 36
    in Fitness Training, 34
    submaximal talk test for, 37–38
    talk test for, 37
    in three-zone intensity model, 32b, 32f

ventilatory threshold assessment and, 35, 35f

VT2, 30, 31b
- in asthma exercise programming, 298
- onset of blood lactate accumulation and, 31b, 39–40
- talk test and, 37
- in three-zone intensity model, 32b, 32f
- ventilation in, 36
- ventilatory threshold assessment and, 35, 35f

VT2 threshold assessment, 39–40

W

Waist circumference, 321, 322f
- in metabolic syndrome, 347

Waist-to-hip ratio, 321, 323t

Walk. *See also* Gait
- banded monster, 576f

Walking
- energy cost of, 353b
- heel and toe, 545, 546f
- learning, 485
- for metabolic syndrome patients, 353

Walking drills, 510, 511f
- with altered bases of support, 512
- obstacle, 512, 512f

Walk test, 6-minute, 294, 295b, 295f

Wall push-ups, 639, 639f

Wall roll, 672, 673f

Wall slide/squat, 547, 547f

Wall stretch, calf, 615, 615f

Weak muscles, lengthened, 448b–449b

Weighted vest
- backward lunge with, 573f
- sideways lunge with, 574f
- squat with, 573f

Weight loss. *See also* Overweight and obesity
- on asthma, 291
- diets for, 329–332 (*See also* Diets, for weight loss)
- exercise *vs.* nutrition for, 751b

NIH Body Weight Planner, 750–751
- nutrition for, 751b
- for overweight and obesity, 329–330, 334
- postpartum, 716b

Weight-loss simulator, 329b

Whey, 778

Whole grains, nutrition label, 766f, 767

Women
- bone response to physical activity in
  - postmenopausal, 570
  - premenopausal, 569–570
- exercise for osteoporosis prevention in
  - postmenopausal, 572–573
  - premenopausal, 572, 572b

Word-of-mouth marketing, 153–154

Work, formula for, 677b

Wrist and hand pathologies, 651–655
- carpal tunnel syndrome, 651–654
- de Quervain's tenosynovitis, 654–655, 654f

Wrist extension
- dumbbell, 647, 649f
- passive, 651, 651f
- resistive, 647, 647f

Wrist flexion, passive, 647, 647f

Wrist tendons, 654, 654f
- in de Quervain's tenosynovitis, 654, 654f

Written agreements, for behavioral modification, 111

Y

Yoga, for hypertension, 269b–270b

Yogic breathing, in coronary heart disease patients, 199b

Z

Zinc, in arthritis, 541t